Evidence-Based Physical Examination

BEST PRACTICES FOR HEALTH AND WELL-BEING ASSESSMENT

Kate Sustersic Gawlik, DNP, APRN-CNP, FAANP, is an assistant professor of clinical nursing at The Ohio State University. She is certified by the American Nurses Credentialing Center as an adult and family nurse practitioner. She has extensive background in primary care, with experience in family practice, college health, urgent care, and reproductive care. Her clinical interests are evidence-based practice, population health, preventive medicine, clinician well-being, health professionals' education, wellness, and cardiovascular disease prevention. She has served as the project manager for the Million Hearts® initiatives at Ohio State's College of Nursing since 2013. She leads and serves on multiple state and national workgroups targeted at improving cardiovascular population health.

Dr. Gawlik started her nursing career in 2006 and completed her MSc in nursing with a specialization as an adult/geriatric nurse practitioner in 2009 from The Ohio State University. In 2015, she graduated with her DNP and a post-master's certificate as a family nurse practitioner from The Ohio State University. Dr. Gawlik was awarded the Outstanding Faculty Award in 2013 and the Outstanding Leadership Award in 2017 at The Ohio State University. She received an Abstract of Distinction at the Council for the Advancement of Nursing Science Conference in 2016 and the Editor's Pick for 2017 Paper of the Year by the *American Journal of Health Promotion* for "An Epidemiological Study of Population Health Reveals Social Smoking as a Major Cardiovascular Risk Factor." She was awarded the 2018 American Association of Nurse Practitioner State Award for Excellence for Ohio. She was inducted as a fellow into the American Association of Nurse Practitioners in June 2018.

Dr. Gawlik has been teaching nursing students since 2007. She has taught a variety of undergraduate, RN–BSN, and graduate nursing courses and serves as a clinical preceptor for advanced practice nursing students. Her passion lies in teaching in the online platform, both in synchronous and asynchronous classrooms. She has been teaching solely online since 2012. Dr. Gawlik developed an online educational module on cardiovascular population health that is used nationally and internationally. The educational module has led to the cardiovascular screening of over 75,000 people. Her educational interests include the development of new and innovative teaching modalities and pedagogies for online teaching with a focus on advanced assessment, evidence-based practice, and health promotion courses.

This is Dr. Gawlik's first book. She is hopeful that by integrating her three passions—advanced assessment, evidence-based practice, and health promotion—into one book, students will have the opportunity to apply and assimilate these three foundational skills in their journey to become expert clinicians.

Bernadette Mazurek Melnyk, PhD, APRN-CNP, FAANP, FNAP, FAAN, is the vice president for health promotion, university chief wellness officer, and professor and dean of the College of Nursing at The Ohio State University. She is also a professor of pediatrics and psychiatry at Ohio State's College of Medicine. In addition, she is the executive director of the Helene Fuld Health Trust National Institute for Evidence-Based Practice in Nursing and Healthcare. Dr. Melnyk earned her BSc in nursing from West Virginia University, her MSc with a specialization in nursing care of children and as a pediatric nurse practitioner from the University of Pittsburgh, and her PhD in clinical research from the University of Rochester where she also completed her post-master's certificate as a psychiatric mental health nurse practitioner.

She is a nationally/internationally recognized expert in evidence-based practice, intervention research, child and adolescent mental health, and health and wellness and is a frequent keynote speaker at national and international conferences on these topics. Dr. Melnyk has consulted with hundreds of healthcare systems and colleges throughout the nation and globe on how to improve quality of care and patient outcomes through implementing and sustaining evidence-based practice. Her record includes over $33 million of sponsored funding from federal agencies and foundations as principal investigator and over 400 publications.

Dr. Melnyk is coeditor of six other books: *Implementing the Evidence-Based Practice (EBP) Competencies in Healthcare: A Practical Guide for Improving Quality, Safety, and Outcomes*; *Evidence-Based Practice in Nursing & Healthcare: A Guide to Best Practice* (4th Edition), an *American Journal of Nursing Research* Book of the Year Award winner; *Implementing EBP: Real World Success Stories*; *A Practical Guide to Child and Adolescent Mental Health Screening, Early Intervention and Health Promotion* (2nd Edition); *Intervention Research and Evidence-Based Quality Improvement: Designing, Conducting, Analyzing and Funding* (2nd Edition), also an *American Journal of Nursing Research* Book of the Year Award winner; and *Evidence-Based Leadership, Innovation and Entrepreneurship in Nursing and Healthcare*.

Dr. Melnyk is an elected fellow of the National Academy of Medicine, the American Academy of Nursing, the National Academies of Practice, and the American Association of Nurse Practitioners. She served a 4-year term on the 16-member U.S. Preventive Services Task Force and the National Institutes of Health's National Advisory Council for Nursing Research and was a board member of the National Guideline Clearinghouse and the National Quality Measures Clearinghouse (NGC/NQMC). She currently serves as a member of the National Quality Forum's

(NQF) Behavioral Health Standing Committee. Dr. Melnyk also serves as editor of the journal *Worldviews on Evidence-Based Nursing* and is a member of the National Academy of Medicine's Action Collaborative on Clinician Well-Being and Resilience as well as an elected board member of the National Forum for Heart Disease & Stroke Prevention.

Dr. Melnyk has received numerous national and international awards, including the Audrey Hepburn Award, Mary Tolle Wright Excellence in Leadership Award, and the International Nursing Research Hall of Fame Award from Sigma Theta Tau International, the Jessie Scott Award from the American Nurses Association for the improvement of healthcare quality through the integration of research, education, and practice, the 2012 Midwest Nursing Research Society Senior Scientist Award, the NIH/National Institute of Nursing Research's inaugural Director's Lectureship Award, the AANP Sharp Cutting Edge Award, and the National Organization of Nurse Practitioner Faculties Lifetime Achievement Award. She has been recognized as an Edge Runner three times by the American Academy of Nursing for founding and directing the National Association of Pediatric Nurse Practitioners' KySS child and adolescent mental health program, her COPE Program for parents of critically ill children and preterm infants, and her Creating Opportunities for Personal Empowerment (COPE) cognitive-behavioral skills building program for depressed and anxious children, teens, and college students, which is being implemented in 45 states throughout the United States and five countries. She is also the founder of two companies that disseminate her evidence-based intervention programs.

Dr. Melnyk founded the National Interprofessional Education and Practice Consortium to Advance Million Hearts, which is a collaboration of over 170 organizations and academic institutions across the United States. She also created and chaired the first three National Summits on Building Healthy Academic Communities and is the founder of the National Consortium for Building Healthy Academic Communities, a collaborative organization to improve population health in the nation's institutions of higher learning, and served as its first president.

Alice M. Teall, DNP, APRN-CNP, FAANP, is director of graduate health and wellness programming, director of innovative telehealth services, and an assistant professor of clinical nursing at The Ohio State University College of Nursing. An expert in nursing education, Dr. Teall was honored with The Ohio State University Provost Award for Distinguished Teaching by a Lecturer and with the Wright State University Presidential Award for Faculty Excellence. While serving as director of the online Family Nurse Practitioner program, she was chosen as The Ohio State College of Nursing Graduate Educator of the Year for 4 consecutive years.

Alice M. Teall began her nursing career as a diploma graduate of Miami Valley Hospital School of Nursing in 1983. She earned her BSc in nursing from Capital University, her MSc with a specialization as a Family Nurse Practitioner from Wright State University, and her DNP from The Ohio State University. She has certifications as a Family and Pediatric Nurse Practitioner and as an Integrative Nurse Coach. Her clinical expertise and areas of interest include adolescent health, primary care of at-risk youth and families, college health, and recovery from substance use disorder. Dr. Teall has an extensive background in primary care, which includes addressing population health using telehealth technologies and improving access to care through statewide quality improvement initiatives. She has received leadership, alumni, and practice awards and is a Fellow of the American Academy of Nurse Practitioners.

An experienced educator, Alice M. Teall has taught assessment online and on campus for students across nursing programs, including LPN, traditional undergraduate, RN–BSN completion, accelerated graduate entry, traditional master's, BS-to-DNP, post-master's, and doctoral programs. Dr. Teall has published and presented nationally about the effective use of classrooms as engaged and collaborative communities of inquiry, where active learning, timely feedback, diversity of thought, and support for self-care and wellness are norms. Her contributions to advanced practice education include innovative use of synchronous web-conferencing, incorporation of health and wellness coaching techniques in clinical practice, and use of telehealth as an evaluation strategy for distance students. Her doctoral work included an evidence-based quality improvement initiative to improve clinician confidence in addressing health, wellness, and self-management of chronic disease using coaching strategies.

Dr. Teall has taught students nationally and internationally to provide evidence-based, patient-centered, collaborative care for individuals and families. This textbook includes best practice guidance gained from her experience in course and clinical teaching, program administration, and curriculum development. Her hope is that health science students will create authentic connection and partnerships with patients, peers, and faculty as they learn to implement the knowledge, skills, and attitudes required of evidence-based assessment.

Evidence-Based Physical Examination

BEST PRACTICES FOR HEALTH AND WELL-BEING ASSESSMENT

Kate Sustersic Gawlik, DNP, APRN-CNP, FAANP

Bernadette Mazurek Melnyk, PhD, APRN-CNP, FAANP, FNAP, FAAN

Alice M. Teall, DNP, APRN-CNP, FAANP

Editors

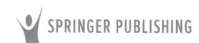
SPRINGER PUBLISHING

Springer Publishing Company, LLC
11 West 42nd Street
New York, NY 10036
www.springerpub.com
http://connect.springerpub.com/home

Acquisitions Editor: Adrianne Brigido
Compositor: S4Carlisle Publishing Services

ISBN: 978-0-8261-6453-7
ebook ISBN: 978-0-8261-6454-4
Instructor's Manual ISBN: 978-0-8261-6462-9
Instructor's PowerPoint Slides ISBN: 978-0-8261-6459-9
Instructor's Test Bank ISBN: 978-0-8261-6458-2 (Also available on Respondus®.)
Instructor's Image Bank ISBN: 978-0-8261-6455-1
Chapter 22 Supplementary Material ISBN: 978-0-8261-6452-0
DOI: 10.1891/9780826164544

Qualified instructors may request supplements by emailing textbook@springerpub.com
Supplementary material for Chapter 22 is available from www.springerpub.com/ebpe.

Visit https://connect.springerpub.com/content/book/978-0-8261-6454-4/chapter/ch00 to access accompanying videos.

20 21 22 23 24 / 5 4 3 2

The author and the publisher of this Work have made every effort to use sources believed to be reliable to provide information that is accurate and compatible with the standards generally accepted at the time of publication. Because medical science is continually advancing, our knowledge base continues to expand. Therefore, as new information becomes available, changes in procedures become necessary. We recommend that the reader always consult current research and specific institutional policies before performing any clinical procedure or delivering any medication. The author and publisher shall not be liable for any special, consequential, or exemplary damages resulting, in whole or in part, from the readers' use of, or reliance on, the information contained in this book. The publisher has no responsibility for the persistence or accuracy of URLs for external or third-party Internet websites referred to in this publication and does not guarantee that any content on such websites is, or will remain, accurate or appropriate.

Library of Congress Cataloging-in-Publication Data

Names: Gawlik, Kate, editor. | Melnyk, Bernadette Mazurek, editor. | Teall, Alice M., editor.
Title: Evidence-based physical examination : best practices for health and well-being assessment / [edited by] Kate Gawlik, DNP, RN, ANP-BC, FNP-BC, Bernadette Mazurek Melnyk, PhD, APRN-CNP, FAANP, FNAP, FAAN, Alice M. Teall, DNP, APRN-CNP, FAANP.
Description: New York : Springer Publishing Company, [2021] | Includes bibliographical references and index.
Identifiers: LCCN 2019046757 (print) | LCCN 2019046758 (ebook) | ISBN 9780826164537 (paperback) | ISBN 9780826164544 (ebook)
Subjects: LCSH: Physical diagnosis. | Evidence-based medicine.
Classification: LCC RC76 .E95 2021 (print) | LCC RC76 (ebook) | DDC 616.07/54—dc23
LC record available at https://lccn.loc.gov/2019046757
LC ebook record available at https://lccn.loc.gov/2019046758

Publisher's Note: New and used products purchased from third-party sellers are not guaranteed for quality, authenticity, or access to any included digital components.

Printed in the United States of America.

This book is dedicated to my husband, Jason, who always believes in me and supports my dreams, no matter how wild and crazy they may be. There is no one else who I would want to be with on this journey. To my parents, Edward and Karen, who made me the person I am today and who never fail to amaze me with their selflessness, patience, and unconditional love. To Hadley, Tyler, Hunter, and Austin—may you continue to see the world the way you see it now. You are going to do great things.

—KATE SUSTERSIC GAWLIK

I dedicate this book to my loving husband, John, who has supported me throughout the past three decades to pursue my dreams; my three wonderful daughters, Kaylin, Angela, and Megan, who have provided understanding and support to me to fuel my passions; and my two awesome grandsons, Alexander and Bradley, who I will continue to encourage to dream, discover, and deliver throughout their life's journeys. In addition, I would like to devote this book to all of my past and current students who have kept my "spirit of inquiry" thriving through their quest to become the best evidence-based providers to ultimately transform health and improve lives throughout the nation and world.

—BERNADETTE (BERN) MAZUREK MELNYK

The value of having someone who believes in you is impossible to measure. To my husband, Tom, this book is dedicated to you. Thank you for believing in me, keeping your sense of humor, and running our household while I spent the time and energy needed to do this work. To Amy, Mallory, Kevin, and Dominique, you are amazing adults, and I love sharing life with you. To my grandchildren, Noah, Aiden, Evan, Emma, Sebastian, and the little one still on the way, you are loved.

—ALICE M. TEALL

Contents

PART III: EVIDENCE-BASED PHYSICAL EXAMINATION AND ASSESSMENT OF SEXUAL AND REPRODUCTIVE HEALTH

PART IV: EVIDENCE-BASED PHYSICAL EXAMINATION AND ASSESSMENT OF MENTAL HEALTH

**PART V: SPECIAL TOPICS IN
EVIDENCE-BASED ASSESSMENT**

Contributors

Melissa Baker, DNP, RN
Director for Prelicensure Programs
College of Nursing
The Ohio State University
Columbus, Ohio
Chapter 5: Approach to the Physical Examination:
General Survey and Assessment of Vital Signs

Angela Blankenship, MS, RN, CPNP-AC/PC
APRN Clinical Leader
The Heart Center, Nationwide Children's Hospital
College of Nursing
The Ohio State University
Columbus, Ohio
Chapter 6: Evidence-Based Assessment of the Heart
and Circulatory System

Sherry Bumpus, PhD, FNP-BC, CME
Associate Professor
College of Nursing
Michigan State University
East Lansing, Michigan
Chapter 20: Evidence-Based Assessment of the
Female Genitourinary System

Amber Carriveau, DNP, FNP-BC
Assistant Professor, Family Nurse Practitioner
Program Director
Michigan State University
East Lansing, Michigan
Chapter 20: Evidence-Based Assessment of the
Female Genitourinary System

Kelly Casler, DNP, APRN, FNP-BC, EBP-C
Assistant Professor of Clinical Practice
College of Nursing
The Ohio State University
Columbus, Ohio
Chapter 6: Evidence-Based Assessment of the Heart
and Circulatory System

Maria Colandrea, DNP, NP-C, CORLN, CCRN, FAANP
Clinical Consulting Associate
Department of Otolaryngology
Duke School of Nursing, Durham VA Medical Center
Durham, North Carolina
Chapter 13: Evidence-Based Assessment of the Ears,
Nose, and Throat

Catherine Davis, LPCC
Forensic Interviewer/Mental Health Advocate
Center for Family Safety and Healing
Nationwide Children's Hospital
Columbus, Ohio
Chapter 24: Evidence-Based Assessment and
Screening for Traumatic Experiences: Abuse, Neglect,
and Intimate Partner Violence

Katharine Doughty, MS, CPNP
Pediatric Nurse Practitioner
Center for Family Safety and Healing
Nationwide Children's Hospital
Columbus, Ohio
Chapter 24: Evidence-Based Assessment and
Screening for Traumatic Experiences: Abuse, Neglect,
and Intimate Partner Violence

Sandy Dudley, MS, BBA, PA-C
Instructor
Digestive Health Institute and Section of Pediatric
Gastroenterology, Hepatology and Nutrition
School of Medicine
University of Colorado
Aurora, Colorado
Chapter 16: Evidence-Based Assessment of the
Abdominal, Gastrointestinal, and Urological Systems

Kristie L. Flamm, DNP, FNP-BC, ACNP-BC, FAANP
Clinical Assistant Professor
College of Nursing
University of Arizona
Tucson, Arizona
*Chapter 6: Evidence-Based Assessment of the Heart
and Circulatory System*

Kate Sustersic Gawlik, DNP, APRN-CNP, FAANP
Assistant Professor of Clinical Nursing
College of Nursing
The Ohio State University
Columbus, Ohio
*Chapter 1: Approach to Evidence-Based Assessment
of Health and Well-Being*
*Chapter 2: Evidence-Based History-Taking Approach
for Wellness Exams, Episodic Visits, and Chronic
Care Management*
*Chapter 3: Approach to Implementing and
Documenting Patient-Centered, Culturally Sensitive
Evidence-Based Assessment*
*Chapter 6: Evidence-Based Assessment of the Heart
and Circulatory System*
*Chapter 8: Approach to Evidence-Based Assessment
of Body Habitus (Height, Weight, Body Mass Index,
Nutrition)*
*Chapter 10: Evidence-Based Assessment of the
Lymphatic System*
*Chapter 11: Evidence-Based Assessment of the Head
and Neck*
*Chapter 15: Evidence-Based Assessment of the
Musculoskeletal System*
*Chapter 16: Evidence-Based Assessment of the
Abdominal, Gastrointestinal, and Urological Systems*
*Chapter 23: Evidence-Based Assessment of Substance
Use Disorder*
*Chapter 28: Evidence-Based Assessment of Personal
Health and Well-Being for Clinicians: Key Strategies
to Achieve Optimal Wellness*
*Chapter 29: Evidence-Based Health and Well-Being
Assessment: Putting It All Together*

Retha D. Gentry, DNP, FNP-C
Assistant Professor, Graduate Programs
College of Nursing
East Tennessee State University
Johnson City, Tennessee
*Chapter 9: Evidence-Based Assessment of Skin, Hair,
and Nails*

Brenda M. Gilmore, DNP, CNM, FNP-BC, CNE, NCMP
Assistant Professor
College of Nursing
University of South Florida
Tampa, Florida
*Chapter 17: Evidence-Based Assessment of the
Breasts and Axillae*

Matt Granger, APRN-CNP
Wexner Medical Center
Ross Heart Hospital
The Ohio State University
Columbus, Ohio
*Chapter 6: Evidence-Based Assessment of the Heart
and Circulatory System*

Martha Gulati, MD, MS, FACC, FAHA, FASPC
Professor of Medicine and Chief of Cardiology
University of Arizona
Phoenix, Arizona
*Chapter 6: Evidence-Based Assessment of the Heart
and Circulatory System*

Emily Hill Guseman, PhD, ACSM-CEP
Assistant Professor
Diabetes Institute
Department of Family Medicine
Heritage College of Osteopathic Medicine
Ohio University
Athens, Ohio
*Chapter 8: Approach to Evidence-Based Assessment
of Body Habitus (Height, Weight, Body Mass Index,
Nutrition)*

Audra Hanners, DNP(c), RN, APRN-CNP, EBP-C
Instructor of Clinical Practice
College of Nursing
The Ohio State University
Columbus, Ohio
*Chapter 6: Evidence-Based Assessment of the Heart
and Circulatory System*

Brittany B. Hay, DNP, APRN, ANP-BC, FNP-BC
Assistant Professor
College of Nursing
University of South Florida
Tampa, Florida
*Chapter 17: Evidence-Based Assessment of the
Breasts and Axillae*

Gail Hornor, DNP, CPNP, AFN-BC
Pediatric Nurse Practitioner
Center for Family Safety and Healing
Nationwide Children's Hospital
Columbus, Ohio
Chapter 24: Evidence-Based Assessment and Screening for Traumatic Experiences: Abuse, Neglect, and Intimate Partner Violence

Catherine Huber, MD
Child Abuse Pediatrician, Center for Family Safety and Healing
Nationwide Children's Hospital
Assistant Professor of Clinical Pediatrics, College of Medicine
The Ohio State University
Columbus, Ohio
Chapter 24: Evidence-Based Assessment and Screening for Traumatic Experiences: Abuse, Neglect, and Intimate Partner Violence

Joyce Karl, DNP, RN, APRN-CNP
Assistant Professor of Clinical Nursing
College of Nursing
The Ohio State University
Columbus, Ohio
Chapter 6: Evidence-Based Assessment of the Heart and Circulatory System

Jennifer Kosla, DNP, APRN-CNP, CPNP-PC, CNE
Assistant Professor of Clinical Practice
College of Nursing
The Ohio State University
Columbus, Ohio
Chapter 4: Evidence-Based Assessment of Children and Adolescents

Pamela Lusk, DNP, RN, FAANP, FNAP
Associate Professor of Clinical Practice
College of Nursing
The Ohio State University
Columbus, Ohio
Chapter 22: Evidence-Based Assessment of Mental Health

Kady Martini, DNP, RN, NEA-BC
Assistant Professor of Clinical Practice
College of Nursing
The Ohio State University
Columbus, Ohio
Chapter 5: Approach to the Physical Examination: General Survey and Assessment of Vital Signs

Bernadette Mazurek Melnyk, PhD, APRN-CNP, FAANP, FNAP, FAAN
Dean and Professor
College of Nursing
The Ohio State University
Columbus, Ohio
Chapter 1: Approach to Evidence-Based Assessment of Health and Well-Being
Chapter 4: Evidence-Based Assessment of Children and Adolescents
Chapter 22: Evidence-Based Assessment of Mental Health
Chapter 28: Evidence-Based Assessment of Personal Health and Well-Being for Clinicians: Key Strategies to Achieve Optimal Wellness

Molly McAuley, DNP, CNL, RN
Assistant Professor of Clinical Practice
College of Nursing
The Ohio State University
Columbus, Ohio
Chapter 5: Approach to the Physical Examination: General Survey and Assessment of Vital Signs

Rosario Medina, PhD, FNP-BC, ACNP, CNS
Assistant Dean of Graduate Programs
College of Nursing
University of Colorado
Aurora, Colorado
Chapter 16: Evidence-Based Assessment of the Abdominal, Gastrointestinal, and Urological Systems

John Melnyk, PhD, OD
Clinical Assistant Professor
Department of Ophthalmology
Wexner Medical Center
Dublin, Ohio
Chapter 12: Evidence-Based Assessment of the Eye

Lisa K. Militello, PhD, MPH, RN, CPNP
Assistant Professor
College of Nursing
The Ohio State University
Columbus, Ohio
Chapter 27: Using Health Technology in Evidence-Based Assessment

Mary Alice Momeyer, DNP, APRN, CNP, AGPCNP-BC
Assistant Professor of Clinical Nursing
College of Nursing
The Ohio State University
Columbus, Ohio
Chapter 6: Evidence-Based Assessment of the Heart and Circulatory System

Hollie Moots, DNP, RN, CNE
Assistant Professor of Clinical Practice
College of Nursing
The Ohio State University
Columbus, Ohio
Chapter 5: Approach to the Physical Examination: General Survey and Assessment of Vital Signs

Emily Neiman, MS, ARPN-CNM, C-EFM
Certified Nurse Midwife
Wexner Medical Center
The Ohio State University
Columbus, Ohio
Chapter 21: Evidence-Based Obstetric Assessment

Lisa E. Ousley, DNP, FNP-C
Assistant Professor, Graduate Programs
College of Nursing
East Tennessee State University
Johnson City, Tennessee
Chapter 9: Evidence-Based Assessment of Skin, Hair, and Nails

Vinciya Pandian, PhD, MBA, MSN, RN, ACNP-BC, FAAN, FAANP
Associate Professor
School of Nursing
Johns Hopkins University
Baltimore, Maryland
Chapter 7: Evidence-Based Assessment of Lungs and Respiratory System

Oralea A. Pittman, DNP, APRN-CNP, FAANP
Assistant Professor of Clinical Nursing
College of Nursing
The Ohio State University
Columbus, Ohio
Chapter 7: Evidence-Based Assessment of Lungs and Respiratory System

Linda Quinlin, DNP, RN, APRN-CNS, APRN-CNP, ACHPN
Assistant Professor of Clinical Nursing
College of Nursing
The Ohio State University
Columbus, Ohio
Chapter 2: Evidence-Based History-Taking Approach for Wellness Exams, Episodic Visits, and Chronic Care Management
Chapter 24: Evidence-Based Assessment and Screening for Traumatic Experiences: Abuse, Neglect, and Intimate Partner Violence

Eileen M. Raynor, MD, FACS, FAAP
Associate Professor, Pediatric Otolaryngology
Duke Head and Neck Surgery & Communication Sciences
Duke University School of Medicine
Durham, North Carolina
Chapter 13: Evidence-Based Assessment of the Ears, Nose, and Throat

Samreen Raza, MD, FACC
Clinical Cardiologist
Baylor Scott & White The Heart Hospital
Plano, Texas
Chapter 6: Evidence-Based Assessment of the Heart and Circulatory System

Kerry Z. Reed, MS, RN, CPNP-PC
Senior Instructor
Digestive Health Institute and Section of Pediatric Gastroenterology, Hepatology and Nutrition
School of Medicine, University of Colorado
Children's Hospital Colorado Anschutz Medical Campus
Aurora, Colorado
Chapter 16: Evidence-Based Assessment of the Abdominal, Gastrointestinal, and Urological Systems

Haley Roberts, BS
Project and Administrative Coordinator
College of Nursing
The Ohio State University
Columbus, Ohio
Chapter 25: Evidence-Based Therapeutic Communication and Motivational Interviewing in Health Assessment

Allison Rusgo, MHS, MPH, PA-C
Assistant Clinical Professor
Physician Assistant Department
College of Nursing and Health Professions, Drexel University
Philadelphia, Pennsylvania
Chapter 6: Evidence-Based Assessment of the Heart and Circulatory System

Debbie Sheikholeslami, BSN, RN
Registered Nurse
University of Iowa Hospitals and Clinics
Iowa City, Iowa
Chapter 25: Evidence-Based Therapeutic Communication and Motivational Interviewing in Health Assessment

Britta Shute, MSN, APRN, FNP-BC
Family Nurse Practitioner
UCONN Health
Farmington, Connecticut
Chapter 18: Evidence-Based Assessment of Sexual Orientation, Gender Identity, and Health

Leslie E. Simons, DNP, ANP-BC
Certified Pain Management Nurse
Assistant Professor, Health Programs
College of Nursing
Michigan State University
East Lansing, Michigan
Chapter 14: Evidence-Based Assessment of the Nervous System

Leigh Small, PhD, RN, CPNP-PC, FNAP, FAANP, FAAN
Associate Dean of Academic Programs
College of Nursing
University of Colorado
Aurora, Colorado
Chapter 16: Evidence-Based Assessment of the Abdominal, Gastrointestinal, and Urological Systems

Tammy Spencer, DNP, RN, CNE, ACNS-BC, CCNS
Assistant Dean of Academic Programs
College of Nursing
University of Colorado
Aurora, Colorado
Chapter 16: Evidence-Based Assessment of the Abdominal, Gastrointestinal, and Urological Systems

Janna D. Stephens, PhD, RN
Assistant Professor
College of Nursing
The Ohio State University
Columbus, Ohio
Chapter 27: Using Health Technology in Evidence-Based Assessment

Zach Stutzman, MS, PA-C, ATC
Physician Assistant, Total Joint Replacement
Sports & Orthopaedic Specialists
Minneapolis, Minnesota
Chapter 15: Evidence-Based Assessment of the Musculoskeletal System

Alice M. Teall, DNP, APRN-CNP, FAANP
Assistant Professor of Clinical Nursing
College of Nursing
The Ohio State University
Columbus, Ohio
Chapter 1: Approach to Evidence-Based Assessment of Health and Well-Being
Chapter 3: Approach to Implementing and Documenting Patient-Centered, Culturally Sensitive Evidence-Based Assessment
Chapter 6: Evidence-Based Assessment of the Heart and Circulatory System
Chapter 7: Evidence-Based Assessment of Lungs and Respiratory System
Chapter 8: Approach to Evidence-Based Assessment of Body Habitus (Height, Weight, Body Mass Index, Nutrition)
Chapter 10: Evidence-Based Assessment of the Lymphatic System
Chapter 11: Evidence-Based Assessment of the Head and Neck
Chapter 12: Evidence-Based Assessment of the Eye
Chapter 19: Evidence-Based Assessment of Male Genitalia, Prostate, Rectum, and Anus
Chapter 23: Evidence-Based Assessment of Substance Use Disorder
Chapter 28: Evidence-Based Assessment of Personal Health and Well-Being for Clinicians: Key Strategies to Achieve Optimal Wellness
Chapter 29: Evidence-Based Health and Well-Being Assessment: Putting It All Together

Kathryn Tierney, MSN, APRN, FNP-BC
Family Nurse Practitioner
Middlesex Health
Middletown, Connecticut
*Chapter 18: Evidence-Based Assessment of Sexual
Orientation, Gender Identity, and Health*

Sharon Tucker, PhD, APRN-CNS, F-NAP, FAAN
Endowed Professor and Implementation Residency
Director
College of Nursing
The Ohio State University
Columbus, Ohio
*Chapter 25: Evidence-Based Therapeutic
Communication and Motivational Interviewing in
Health Assessment*

Marjorie A. Vogt, PhD, DNP, CPNP, CFNP, FAANP
Clinical Professor and DNP Associate Director
College of Health Sciences and Professions
Ohio University
Dublin, Ohio
*Chapter 26: Evidence-Based History and Physical
Examinations for Sports Participation Evaluation*

Sinead Yarberry, MSN, RN, CNS
Instructor of Clinical Practice
College of Nursing
The Ohio State University
Columbus, Ohio
*Chapter 5: Approach to the Physical Examination:
General Survey and Assessment of Vital Signs*

Rosie Zeno, DNP, APRN-CNP, CPNP-PC
Assistant Professor of Clinical Practice
College of Nursing
The Ohio State University
Columbus, Ohio
*Chapter 4: Evidence-Based Assessment of Children
and Adolescents*
Chapter 12: Evidence-Based Assessment of the Eye
*Chapter 19: Evidence-Based Assessment of Male
Genitalia, Prostate, Rectum, and Anus*
*Chapter 24: Evidence-Based Assessment and
Screening for Traumatic Experiences: Abuse, Neglect,
and Intimate Partner Violence*

Preface

"The only way to predict the future is to create it."
—Peter Drucker

We begin this preface by emphasizing that the only way to ensure an accurate diagnosis for an individual's health and well-being is through a thorough history and evidence-based health and well-being assessment. Learning to effectively assess the health and well-being of an individual involves integrating skills of history taking, physical examination, and diagnostic decision-making within the context of patient-centered, culturally sensitive, evidence-based clinical practice. The process of teaching and learning assessment is complex. As experienced faculty who have taught assessment and advanced assessment across educational programs, we recognize that health science students who learn evidence-based, valid, reliable assessment techniques and approaches are better prepared to deliver evidence-based, safe, quality clinical care. Student engagement in learning also requires that they understand and appreciate the importance of wellness for their own health and well-being.

Evidence-Based Physical Examination: Best Practices for Health and Well-Being Assessment was developed to reflect a practical, scientific, and holistic approach to the learning of advanced, as well as basic, assessment. The textbook includes a review of how to approach individuals across the life span, prioritizes a broad understanding of wellness, presents evidence-based recommendations for assessments, and systematically reviews the physical examination components required to inform clinical decision-making.

GOALS OF THIS TEXTBOOK

The overall goal of this textbook is to provide the strategies and best practices needed by clinicians to assess an individual's health and well-being. The rationale for our evidence-based approach is that it creates the foundation for building a comprehensive differential diagnosis or problem list, provides the strategies for triaging the acuity of the patient, and creates the groundwork for the integration of wellness, health promotion, disease prevention, and support for self-efficacy into an individualized, patient-centered plan of care based on the best and latest evidence. Only with comprehensive, accurate, and evidence-based assessment can a clinician ensure patient safety and high-quality cost-effective care. Additional goals of this text include:

1. To promote evidence-based practice at the assessment and diagnostic levels to ensure that clinicians are using valid and reliable examination methods in which to base future decision-making
2. To incorporate an interprofessional, multidisciplinary approach that encompasses cultural competency, social determinants of health, and trauma-informed care while keeping mental health and a wellness perspective at the center of all patient interactions
3. To understand the utilization and integration of modern technology and its role in the assessment process
4. To provide information on specific assessment skills that are often overlooked or misunderstood
5. To summarize abnormal findings for common disease states across the life span
6. To ensure that clinicians are able to conduct a thorough self-assessment of their own personal health and take good self-care, because burnout and poor clinician well-being adversely affect healthcare quality and safety.

DISTINGUISHING FEATURES TO SUPPORT STUDENT LEARNING

Evidence-Based Physical Examination: Best Practices for Health and Well-Being Assessment strives to incorporate the latest and best clinical evidence for physical examination assessment skills that are valuable in everyday clinical practice. It includes assessment of the dimensions of wellness and health behaviors as a routine component of history taking and involves when and how to incorporate specific physical examination techniques. Evidence-based national guidelines are integrated into the recommendations for the history and physical examination for individuals across the life span.

The textbook incorporates several unique features. Each chapter begins with a motivational quote to inspire individuals as they learn evidence-based health and well-being assessments, followed by specific learning objectives. An extensive review of anatomy, physiology, and pathophysiology provides the foundation for the history and physical examination. Life-span considerations are included in every chapter, with an entire chapter dedicated to pediatric and adolescent differences and considerations. Due to their vital contributions to the assessment process, laboratory and imaging sections are included in chapters, when appropriate. These sections provide an overview of commonly ordered labs and imaging studies with an explanation of how they are useful to the assessment and diagnostic processes.

In addition, this textbook offers discrete chapters dedicated to specific populations or disease states that are often overlooked and/or misunderstood. There are entire chapters dedicated to current, priority topics, including the following unique chapters:

- Chapter 8: Approach to Evidence-Based Assessment of Body Habitus (Height, Weight, Body Mass Index, Nutrition)
- Chapter 18: Evidence-Based Assessment of Sexual Orientation, Gender Identity, and Health
- Chapter 23: Evidence-Based Assessment of Substance Use Disorder
- Chapter 24: Evidence-Based Assessment and Screening for Traumatic Experiences: Abuse, Neglect, and Intimate Partner Violence
- Chapter 28: Evidence-Based Assessment of Personal Health and Well-Being for Clinicians: Key Strategies to Achieve Optimal Wellness

INSTRUCTOR RESOURCES

Evidence-Based Physical Examination: Best Practices for Health and Well-Being Assessment is accompanied by an Instructor's Manual and comprehensive instructor resources, which include learning objectives, chapter summaries, case studies, essay questions, multiple-choice questions with rationales, and PowerPoint slides. Instructor resources also include a test bank and an image bank. In addition, all systems chapters have corresponding case study videos for common chief concerns, wellness and chronic disease visits, and mental

health examinations. These videos demonstrate an everyday, clinical practice approach. These videos can be used as a teaching tool for students. Students can view the videos on their own to enhance their history-taking and assessment skills, and the videos can be used as part of classroom teaching and discussion.

Some individual chapter exemplars of teaching tools are noted in the following list:

- Chapter 6: Evidence-Based Assessment of the Heart and Circulatory System
  - Video Case Studies: Hypertension Follow-Up Visit; Chest Pain; Dizziness
  - 10 Multiple-Choice Questions With Rationales
  - Two Essay Questions With Suggested Answers
  - Text Case Studies: Hypertension Follow-Up; Chest Pain
- Chapter 23: Evidence-Based Assessment of Substance Use Disorder
  - Video Case Study: Smoking/Smoking Cessation Visit
  - 10 Multiple-Choice Questions With Rationales
  - Two Essay Questions With Suggested Answers
  - Text Case Study: Illicit Prescription Use

INTENDED AUDIENCE

This textbook is intended for a broad audience of health science students and clinicians who strive to exemplify excellence in evidence-based assessment and practice. Educators who provide instruction to students enrolled in graduate, baccalaureate, and associate degree health science programs who aspire to provide an evidence-based advanced assessment approach to individuals across the life span will appreciate the scientific foundation, holistic perspective, and practical approach to history taking and physical examination. The courses/programs for which this text would be appropriate include:

- Graduate nursing assessment courses
- Undergraduate nursing assessment courses
- Medical student assessment courses
- Family/adult/pediatric/psychiatric nurse practitioner graduate programs
- Programs focused on acute care, primary care, or specialty care management
- Midwifery graduate programs
- School nursing specialty programs
- Child mental health graduate specialty programs
- Maternal–child health graduate programs
- Physician assistant graduate programs
- Pharmacy graduate programs
- Occupational therapy graduate programs

- Physical therapy graduate programs
- Respiratory therapy graduate programs
- Social work programs

Other intended audiences are practicing clinicians, including APRNs (clinical nurse specialists, clinical nurse leaders, nurse practitioners, nurse anesthetists, school nurses, and educators based in clinical settings), nurses, physicians, physician assistants, physical therapists, respiratory therapists, social workers, pharmacists, and occupational therapists who work in clinical and community healthcare settings caring for children, adolescents, adults, older adults, and families.

ORGANIZATION OF THE CONTENT

PART I: FOUNDATIONS OF CLINICAL PRACTICE

The first five chapters of this text identify approaches to assessment. These chapters include how to understand evidence-based guidelines; deliver and document care; include family, social, cultural, and developmental assessments; and adapt assessment strategies based on why the individual is seeking care, whether the individual is experiencing urgent or emergent health needs, and the age and understanding of the individual.

PART II: EVIDENCE-BASED PHYSICAL EXAMINATION AND ASSESSMENT OF BODY SYSTEMS

Chapters 6 through 16 focus on body systems. Each of these chapters includes a thorough review of anatomy, physiology, and pathophysiology as a foundation for interpreting examination findings. Each chapter includes a listing of pertinent components of history and review of systems, examination techniques, life-span considerations, abnormal findings, and clinical pearls.

PART III: EVIDENCE-BASED PHYSICAL EXAMINATION AND ASSESSMENT OF SEXUAL AND REPRODUCTIVE HEALTH

Chapters 17 through 21 continue to use a systems approach, while more thoroughly presenting assessments related to sexual health. Assessment of gender identity and sexual orientation is included as a separate chapter to allow students an opportunity to learn and practice therapeutic communication when discussing sensitive topic areas. Breast assessment, male/female genitalia, and pregnancy assessment are also included as individual chapters.

PART IV: EVIDENCE-BASED PHYSICAL EXAMINATION AND ASSESSMENT OF MENTAL HEALTH

Chapters 22 through 25 focus on advanced assessment of mental health. While mental health assessments are incorporated throughout the text, these chapters provide a thorough review of pertinent anatomy, physiology, and pathophysiology and approaches to history and physical examination. Evidence-based screening tools are included, as are examples of how to apply these tools in clinical practice.

PART V: SPECIAL TOPICS IN EVIDENCE-BASED ASSESSMENT

Chapters 26 through 29 are unique additions to this textbook. Chapter 26 reviews special considerations for pre-participation physical examinations for adolescent athletes. Chapter 27 introduces the concept of how health technology can be incorporated into evidence-based assessments and clinical decision support. Chapter 28 invites the clinician to evaluate his or her own personal health and well-being, a priority in light of the prevalence of clinician burnout and its adverse consequences. The last chapter of the text provides a summary listing of the components of a comprehensive health history and physical examination.

We hope you enjoy using the book as much as we enjoyed creating it.

Kate Sustersic Gawlik, Bernadette Mazurek Melnyk,
and Alice M. Teall

Acknowledgments

Thank you to the authors from across disciplines and across the country who contributed to writing the chapters in this text. Your expertise in health and wellness assessments and insight into the evidence-based foundation of clinical practice will guide future health science students.

Thank you to colleagues who have truly been the "wind beneath our wings." Thank you, Kathy York, for your support, which spans a decade. Thank you to Rosie Zeno, whose pediatric expertise and dedication to this project involved significant contributions to four chapters and whose support in helping us to meet deadlines will be long remembered.

Thanks to all of you who were willing to be a part of the photos and videos associated with this effort, including family, friends, and colleagues who either collaborated to create patient cases or contributed normal and abnormal findings so that others may learn. Special thanks to Mallory Caldwell; your willingness to be a part of this effort is greatly appreciated. Thank you to Jason, Amy, Nathan, Matt, Andrew, Maya, and Portia; your contributions are seen within the pages of this text.

Without the support from our team at Springer Publishing Company, this book would not exist. Thank you for this rewarding opportunity. Adrianne Brigido, your feedback has been invaluable. We are grateful for your work in bringing this text to publication. We are also grateful for the efforts of Robert Pancotti, Senior Content Development Specialist.

To all of the health science students whom we have had the opportunity to teach, thank you for demonstrating a willingness to learn and for your dedication to providing the best, evidence-based, patient-centered care for individuals, families, communities, and populations. You make us proud. We see you as clinicians who focus your clinical practice on partnering with individuals in a way that improves their health and wellness. You are changing the culture of the healthcare delivery system.

List of Videos

Visit https://connect.springerpub.com/content/book/978-0-8261-6454-4/chapter/ch00 to access the videos.

Instructor Resources

Evidence-Based Physical Examination: Best Practices for Health and Well-Being Assessment includes a robust ancillary package. Qualified instructors may obtain access to ancillary materials by emailing textbook@springerpub.com. Available resources:

- Instructor's Manual:
  - Learning Objectives
  - Chapter Summaries
  - Case Studies with Questions and Answers/Rationales
  - Video Links

- Test Bank:
  - Multiple-Choice Questions with Answers/Rationales
  - Essay Questions with Answers/Rationales

- Image Bank

- Chapter-Based PowerPoint Presentations

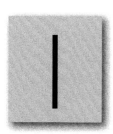

FOUNDATIONS OF CLINICAL PRACTICE

1

Approach to Evidence-Based Assessment of Health and Well-Being

Kate Gawlik, Bernadette Mazurek Melnyk, and Alice M. Teall

"Health is a state of complete physical, mental and social well-being and not merely the absence of disease or infirmity."

—World Health Organization

LEARNING OBJECTIVES

- Describe the rationale for an evidence-based approach to the assessment of health and well-being.
- Apply the principles and steps of evidence-based practice that guide assessment of the dimensions of wellness.
- Identify evidence-based resources to guide health assessment strategies, approaches, and techniques.

SYSTEMATIC APPROACH TO ADVANCED HEALTH AND WELL-BEING ASSESSMENT

Assessment is the action of making an appraisal, judgment, or evaluation. Advanced skills of assessment include an interpretation of findings within the complexity of a situation. To effectively implement advanced assessment skills in clinical practice involves a complex series of steps; a foundation of knowledge; an ability to appreciate the information shared by an individual, patient, or family; and clinical interpretation of the assessments of **health** and **well-being**.

Advanced assessment is the cornerstone of clinical practice. Clinicians use advanced assessment skills as the foundation for delivering quality care. To deliver the highest quality of healthcare and ensure the best

patient outcomes, there has been a dramatic shift in clinical practice to incorporating the latest research or best evidence and to questioning the processes and systems that have been in place for years to determine whether they are the most effective and efficient methods. **Evidence-based practice** (EBP) is a lifelong problem-solving approach to the delivery of care that incorporates the current best evidence with a clinician's expertise and patient or family preferences and values (Melnyk & Fineout-Overholt, 2019). When implemented consistently, EBP results in the highest quality of care, improved population health outcomes, decreased costs, and clinician empowerment, otherwise known as the quadruple aim in healthcare (Bodenheimer & Sinsky, 2014; Melnyk & Fineout-Overholt, 2019). However, even with all of its positive benefits, EBP is not the standard of care in many healthcare systems owing to multiple barriers, including inadequate EBP skills in clinicians and cultures, which promote a philosophy of "that is the way we do it here."

If assessments are not thorough or findings are not interpreted within the context of the best clinical evidence, errors are more likely. Findings from research indicate that approximately 400,000 people die every year from preventable medical errors, and this is now a public health epidemic and the third leading cause of death in the United States (Makary & Daniel, 2016). Although numerous factors influence the occurrence of errors, using the best evidence in clinical assessment and management has been identified as a priority in reducing the number of preventable medical errors and improving population health outcomes. While there has been steady progress in the evidence-based management of clinical problems or diseases over the past 2 decades, incorporating the best evidence in health and well-being assessment has been much slower. Specifically, a number of commonly taught physical assessment techniques have demonstrated a low sensitivity, a low specificity, and negative predictive value (e.g., scoliosis screening), and yet these techniques continue to be incorporated when teaching clinicians assessment skills. Unfortunately, many well-meaning clinicians across the United States are steeped in a practice rooted in the way they were taught years before or are following outdated practices and policies not based on the best evidence. As a result, the quality, safety, and health outcomes of their patients are not as optimal as they could be if these clinicians were consistently steeped in EBP.

This book takes a new approach to the process of advanced health and well-being assessment through rigorous critical appraisal of the evidence underlying history and physical exam techniques, assessment strategies, the use of imaging tests or lab studies, and/or approaches to health and well-being. **Evidence-based assessment** lays the foundation for building comprehensive differential diagnoses or a problem list, provides the strategies for triaging the acuity of the patient, and creates the groundwork for integration of **wellness**, health promotion, and disease prevention into the plan of care based on the best and latest evidence. Thorough history-taking and assessment provide the clinician with key subjective information and tangible, objective information on which to base current and future decision-making. Only with comprehensive, accurate, and evidence-based assessment can a clinician ensure patient safety, quality, and cost-effective care.

THE IMPORTANCE OF EVIDENCE-BASED ASSESSMENT

Kaylin's Story

Kaylin was 8 years old when she went to New Zealand and Australia with her parents for a dream trip. The trip's first layover was at the Los Angeles airport, where Kaylin enjoyed dinner and an ice-cream sundae. She was the picture of health when leaving Los Angeles and was very excited to be going to the land of koala bears. However, approximately 3 hours from New Zealand, Kaylin awakened her mom, who is a pediatric nurse practitioner, from a deep sleep to let her know that she was feeling sick, specifically saying that her "belly hurt." Her mom felt her forehead, which revealed she had a fever. Then, within an hour, Kaylin started vomiting, and her mom suspected early appendicitis. The pattern of fever and abdominal pain that preceded vomiting was the classic picture of appendicitis. Kaylin's mom woke her dad to let him know that Kaylin was

sick and that she suspected early appendicitis. Kaylin's dad was convinced that this was the "gastrointestinal (GI) bug" that he had experienced 4 days earlier.

Kaylin continued to vomit intermittently for the rest of the flight to New Zealand. After landing, Kaylin's parents took her immediately to a 24-hour medical facility, where they conveyed concerns about early appendicitis to the physician who evaluated her. After examining her and running a few lab tests, it was decided that she just had a GI virus and that she could be taken to her hotel. The physician kept emphasizing that Kaylin did not have abdominal rebound, which is a common physical assessment sign of appendicitis.

After 48 hours, Kaylin's temperature dropped, and she stopped vomiting, so the family traveled to their next destination, Sydney, Australia, where they spent 4 days touring the most common attractions. Kaylin did not seem her normal self. She was even complacent about seeing and holding koala bears at the animal preserve, which was unusual since that was all that she talked about before the trip. In Sydney, Kaylin was without fever and did not complain any further about abdominal pain. However, she was pale, lacked an appetite, walked a little humped over, and was not her energetic self.

After 4 days in Sydney, the family flew to a place called Ayers Rock in the Australian outback. The second day there, they went to a dinner called the Sounds of Silence. Kaylin still lacked her appetite and literally fell asleep on the table at dinner. The family was to fly from Ayers Rock to Cairns, Australia, the next morning. During the night, Kaylin began to moan in her sleep with a fever of 104°F. Her mom was now convinced that Kaylin's appendix had ruptured, leading to a serious medical situation with an abdominal abscess. The family took the next flight out of Ayers Rock and, as soon as they landed, took Kaylin to another medical facility. The physician there ordered blood work that showed a 33,000 white blood cell count, 92% neutrophils, and 36 bands/stabs. Immediately after these lab results were known, Kaylin's mom and dad rushed her to the emergency department of the public hospital in Cairns, knowing Kaylin had a very serious medical situation.

In the emergency department, Kaylin was examined by multiple physicians and a surgeon, who had her jumping up and down on her right foot, assuring everyone that this was not an abdominal problem since she was able to do that task. More blood tests and cultures were performed, and, after hours, Kaylin's parents were told that they could take her back to the hotel as it was just a virus, even though her mom was insistent that she had a ruptured appendix. She kept telling the physicians that the severe shift to the left in Kaylin's lab work indicated a severe bacterial, not viral, infection. She begged the physicians for an MRI or ultrasound of her abdomen, but they would not perform the test. Finally, after some time of pleading with the physicians to admit her to the hospital, Kaylin was admitted to the pediatric unit. The head nurse later told Kaylin's parents that she was labeled a "soft admission," but that she was being admitted to the hospital because she was the daughter of a stressed-out nurse mom from the United States who was insistent on her admission.

Throughout the night and during the entire next day, Kaylin was evaluated by at least six physicians. Kaylin's parents told the same story to each physician, insisting that she had a ruptured appendix and was now experiencing an abdominal abscess. Kaylin was looking worse—her fever remained at 104°F, she had tachycardia out of proportion to her fever, and she was starting to look septic. After Kaylin's mom pleaded with multiple physicians, asking them for an ultrasound of her abdomen, the last physician finally agreed to the test. An ultrasound was performed, which revealed a huge abscess from a ruptured appendix in Kaylin's abdomen.

One of the public surgeons came in to communicate the results of the ultrasound to Kaylin's parents. He said that the best treatment was to place Kaylin on IV triple high-dose antibiotics *for 6 weeks* in hopes that her body would wall the abscess off, and, then, an elective surgery could be performed to remove it and what was left of the appendix. Kaylin's mom asked the surgeon for the evidence behind his recommended treatment, but he could not give her a solid answer. As Kaylin's mom was sobbing and wishing they were at home in the United States at a hospital with physicians with whom they were familiar and who would have believed and listened to them, Kaylin's nurse said that, as Americans, they could call for a consult from a private surgeon. They asked her to get them the best surgeon in town, which she did. Without that nurse, Kaylin may have never made it home.

A couple of hours later, the private surgeon walked into the room and evaluated Kaylin. He told Kaylin's parents that he needed to get Kaylin to the theater (operating room) immediately as she was full of infection and on the verge of sepsis. After more than a day of pleading with multiple physicians and asking for the evidence behind decisions that were being made, the family finally had a healthcare clinician who was engaged in evidence-based decision-making.

Kaylin was in surgery for several hours. By the time of surgery, she had full-blown peritonitis and pelvic sepsis, but never had she had classic guarding, which is typically seen with peritonitis. She was not the typical case of appendicitis as she had a retroverted appendix, so she did not have the classic "rebound" that is commonly seen in children with appendicitis. Because of her extensive infection, Kaylin's peritoneal cavity had to be flushed with saline for 2 solid hours. Her parents were never so relieved as to see the surgeon emerge from the operating room and tell them that he believed

Kaylin would have an extensive recovery but that she would be all right.

Kaylin's recovery was very slow. She lost 10 pounds, developed an ileus after surgery, and had extensive infection that was challenging to resolve. After 2 weeks in the hospital, Kaylin finally recovered enough to be taken back to the family's hotel room. With her abdomen still distended, the family could not fly home for another week. During her hospital stay, the surgeon who examined Kaylin in the emergency department came to see them and apologized profusely for missing the diagnosis in the emergency department. Later that week, he conducted grand rounds and reviewed Kaylin's case with numerous physicians so that her atypical case of a ruptured appendix would not be missed again.

Parents know their children best but do not always have clinicians who listen well to the information they have to offer. Kaylin's case is a prime example of how various elements of EBP were not taken into consideration. If Kaylin's mom had not had the knowledge that she did in evidence-based assessment to be a strong advocate for her daughter during this experience, Kaylin might have died. Sadly, hundreds of thousands of people die every year from preventable medical errors, many from clinicians who do not take the family's history and input into thoughtful consideration and who do not consistently deliver evidence-based care.

One out of 10 patients admitted to the hospital will experience a medical error. We also know that EBP results in the highest quality, low-cost healthcare with the best patient outcomes. However, what is often not taught or emphasized enough in EBP is how to factor in a patient or family member's preferences or a clinician's expertise into the evidence-based decision-making process. It is our hope that Kaylin's story will help all clinicians to remember to listen to and heed the wisdom/preferences of patients and their family members and to always listen to their own clinical expertise when making the best evidence-based assessments and decisions about patient care. Through EBP and advocating for what we know is soundly based on the EBP process, medical errors and complications will be avoided and more patient lives will be saved.

Note: Kaylin is the daughter of Bernadette Mazurek Melnyk, coeditor of this book. The full story of Kaylin is included in a book with many other stories on how EBP makes a difference in the lives and health outcomes of patients and families by Melnyk and Fineout-Overholt (2011).

Jennifer's Story

Jennifer was a healthy 38-year-old woman who was 8 weeks pregnant. She had no chronic illnesses and was not taking any medications. She visited a local urgent care center with upper respiratory symptoms. She reported a productive cough, low-grade fever of 99.0°F, fatigue, and some nasal congestion. She reported no leg symptoms. During her visit, a d-dimer blood test was ordered to rule out a pulmonary embolism. The d-dimer test was mildly elevated. It was then recommended that she needed further evaluation owing to concern for a pulmonary embolism (PE). Based on her d-dimer level, Jennifer was advised to go to the local emergency department where she was told she needed to have a pulmonary computed tomography (CT) scan to rule out a PE. She was warned repeatedly of the risks to her fetus of having the CT scan but was still advised by multiple clinicians to complete the imaging study despite these risks. Despite feeling very conflicted about the scan, she completed it. The result of the CT scan was negative, and she was sent home with the diagnosis of an upper respiratory infection.

There were multiple opportunities where clinicians failed to utilize EBP during their assessment of Jennifer. The d-dimer test should never have been ordered. This is a nonspecific test that is often elevated in multiple conditions and always elevated in pregnancy (Goodacre, Nelson-Piercy, Hunt, & Chan, 2015). In fact, the American Thoracic Society/Society of Thoracic Radiology (ATS/STR) Clinical Practice Guideline for the Evaluation of Suspected Pulmonary Embolism in Pregnancy (Leung et al., 2012) recommends specifically against the use of d-dimer to exclude PE in pregnancy. Next, the pulmonary artery CT scan should never have been ordered. The ATS/STR guidelines recommend a chest x-ray as the first radiation-associated procedure. In addition, the Wells Criteria for Pulmonary Embolism is a risk stratification tool used to estimate the probability of an acute PE. If the clinicians in the hospital had utilized the Wells criteria, they would have discovered that Jennifer's risk of having a PE was 3%. The evidence was clear that she did not need the CT scan and that the risks of the CT scan far outweighed the benefits, yet she was still advised by multiple clinicians to proceed with having it done. If the clinicians had utilized EBP during their assessment, Jennifer never would have had the CT scan and put herself and her fetus at risk.

MOVING TO A MODEL OF PREVENTION

Evidence-based assessment requires critical thinking beyond completion of the techniques of physical assessment and includes an understanding of the context of the health and well-being of populations. With the aging baby boomer population and the increasing rates of chronic diseases, patient care is getting more and more complex. Patients are presenting with multiple diagnoses, problems, and needs. Acuity is higher, and the healthcare system is becoming more difficult to navigate. Clinicians practicing today need to holistically approach patients and help them meet their optimal wellness goals by addressing the multiple aspects affecting their health and well-being.

Fully integrating an assessment of wellness into practice involves understanding that being healthy involves more than physical health. Well-being assessment should include the **nine dimensions of wellness**, namely, physical, emotional, financial, intellectual, career, social, creative, environmental, and spiritual (**Figure 1.1**; Melnyk & Neale, 2018a, 2018b). Clinicians need to take each of these dimensions into consideration when assessing individuals and families. Each dimension can impact the other dimensions. Failing to take into account all nine dimensions results in an incomplete well-being assessment, which could lead to inaccurate conclusions and noneffective management. For example, when a patient is struggling financially and has an unstable career (threatened financial and career wellness) to the extent of not being able to feed their family, the patient will forego buying blood pressure medication so as to be able to buy food. In making this decision, the patient is jeopardizing their short-term and long-term physical wellness. The patient's stress level is high owing to constant worry about supporting the family, thereby threatening the patient's emotional wellness. When the patient's basic needs, such as not having a steady food source, are not being met, creative and environmental wellness are not a consideration or a priority. Failing to ask about a patient's ability to pay for their medications and just labeling the patient as

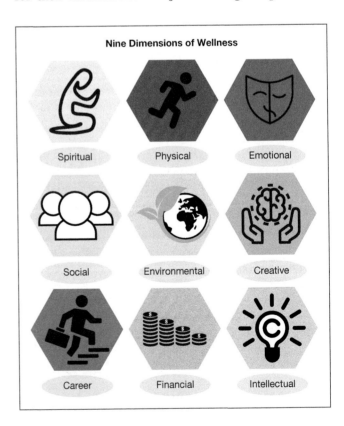

FIGURE 1.1 Nine dimensions of wellness: physical, emotional, financial, intellectual, career, social, creative, environmental, and spiritual.

"noncompliant" can happen in this type of situation if a full well-being assessment is not conducted.

Approaching the steps of assessment in a manner that embodies patient-centered, evidence-based care and taking into account a patient's individual needs and preferences will help to improve patient outcomes and overall population health. The patient's individual well-being needs can be understood and addressed by asking the right questions and taking all dimensions of their wellness into consideration. Using this approach to assessment is imperative for promoting optimal health and preventing disease. Using advanced assessment strategies that are grounded in evidence and focusing on health promotion will help to move patients to a higher level of health and well-being. For all of these reasons, this text begins with a description of EBP and includes best evidence to guide assessment in each chapter.

THE SEVEN STEPS OF EVIDENCE-BASED PRACTICE

Without current best evidence, clinical practice becomes out-of-date, resulting in adverse outcomes to patients. Therefore, clinicians should be skilled in the seven steps of EBP, as described here, in order to provide the highest quality of care (**Box 1.1**; Melnyk & Fineout-Overholt, 2019).

BOX 1.1
THE SEVEN STEPS OF THE EBP PROCESS

0. Cultivate a spirit of inquiry within an EBP culture and environment.
1. Ask the burning clinical question in PICOT format.
2. Search for and collect the most relevant, best evidence.
3. Critically appraise the evidence (i.e., rapid critical appraisal, evaluation, and synthesis).
4. Integrate the best evidence with one's clinical expertise and patient/family preferences and values in making a practice decision or change.
5. Evaluate outcomes of the practice decision or change based on evidence.
6. Disseminate the outcomes of the EBP decision or change.

EBP, evidence-based practice; PICOT, patient population, intervention of interest, comparison intervention, outcome, time.

Source: Used with permission from Melnyk, B. M., & Fineout-Overholt, E. (2019). *Evidence-based practice in nursing and healthcare. A guide to best practice* (4th ed.). Philadelphia, PA: Wolters Kluwer.

STEP #0: CULTIVATE A SPIRIT OF INQUIRY WITHIN AN EBP CULTURE AND ENVIRONMENT

All clinicians need to develop a spirit of inquiry that prompts them to constantly ask questions regarding their practices (e.g., What is the best valid and reliable screening tool for depression in pregnant women? What is the most effective treatment for pneumonia in small children?). Working within an EBP culture and environment will help to support this spirit of inquiry instead of being part of a practice that is steeped in tradition or has the philosophy of "that is the way it is done here."

STEP #1: FORMULATE THE BURNING CLINICAL PICOT QUESTION

In this step of EBP, it is important for clinicians to place their clinical questions in PICOT format (i.e., *P*atient population, *I*ntervention or *Issue* of interest, *C*omparison intervention or group, *O*utcome, and *T*ime frame) to yield the most relevant, efficient, and best evidence search of the literature. For example, a well-designed PICOT question would be: In overweight adults seen for a primary care well visit (the patient population), how does counseling on healthy lifestyle behaviors (the experimental intervention) compared with providing a pamphlet on healthy lifestyles (the comparison intervention) affect physical activity and healthy eating (the outcomes) 2 months after the well visit (the time frame it takes for the interventions to achieve the outcome)? When questions are asked in a PICOT format, searches are conducted in a more targeted and efficient way that saves time and yields an effective search to answer the PICOT question (Melnyk & Fineout-Overholt, 2019). For clinical questions that are not intervention focused, the meaning of the letter *I* can be "issue of interest" instead of "intervention." An example of a nonintervention PICOT question would be: In teenagers (Patient population), how does screening for bullying (the Issue of interest) predict depression (the Outcome) 6 months later (Time)? In this question, there is no appropriate comparison group, so the PIOT is appropriate, yet it is still referred to as a PICOT question.

STEP #2: SEARCH FOR THE BEST EVIDENCE

The search for the best evidence should begin with each of the keywords from the PICOT question, which are entered one at a time, ending with the command to combine all keywords from the PICOT question. The strongest level of evidence (i.e., Level 1 evidence that is comprised of systematic reviews or meta-analyses) should be searched for first. See **Figure 1.2** for an example of an evidence hierarchy that captures the levels of evidence. If there are no systematic reviews or meta-analyses available, then the search proceeds with the next strongest level of evidence to answer the

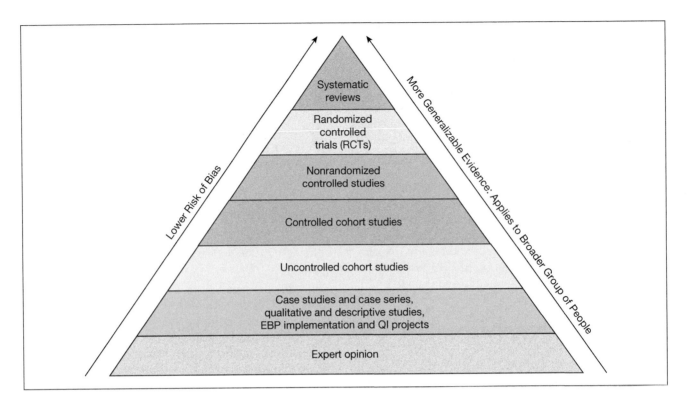

FIGURE 1.2 Hierarchy of evidence pyramid. The hierarchy of evidence pyramid demonstrates the levels of evidence. The strongest level of evidence is at the top of the pyramid (systematic reviews and/or meta-analyses), and the weakest is at the bottom of the pyramid (expert opinion).

EBP, evidence-based practice; QI, quality improvement.

Source: Used with permission from Melnyk, B. M., & Fineout-Overholt, E. (2019). *Evidence-based practice in nursing and healthcare. A guide to best practice* (4th ed.). Philadelphia, PA: Wolters Kluwer.

PICOT question (i.e., Level 2 evidence, which is that generated from at least one well-designed randomized controlled trial [RCT], etc.).

STEP #3: CRITICAL APPRAISAL OF EVIDENCE

This step in the EBP process involves critical appraisal of evidence found from the systematic search. Evaluating and critically appraising evidence involves recognition of when study findings are valid (i.e., as close to the truth as possible), reliable, and applicable to a clinician's patients. Rapid critical appraisal of studies can be conducted in a time-efficient way by answering the following questions (Melnyk & Fineout-Overholt, 2019):

1. **Are the results of the study valid? (Validity)** Validity assesses whether the results of the study are as close to the truth as possible. Did the researchers conduct the study using the best research methods possible? For example, in intervention trials, it would be important to determine whether the subjects were randomly assigned to treatment or control groups, which is the best strategy for controlling confounding variables.

2. **What are the results? (Reliability)** In an intervention trial, this would include (a) whether the intervention worked, (b) how large a treatment effect was obtained, and (c) whether clinicians could expect similar results if they implemented the intervention in their own clinical practice setting (i.e., the preciseness of the intervention effect).

3. **Will the results help the clinician in caring for their patients? (Applicability)** This third rapid critical appraisal question includes asking whether: (a) the subjects in the study are similar to the patients for whom care is being delivered, (b) the benefits are greater than the risks of treatment (i.e., potential for harm), (c) the treatment is feasible to implement in the practice setting, and (d) the patient desires the treatment.

Special Considerations for Health and Well-Being Assessment

Evidence-based assessment involves an appreciation for the evidence that supports implementation of specific techniques and strategies.

Validity

Determining **validity** requires asking the question, is the clinician assessing the right thing in the right way to deliver accurate and useful assessment results? In the context of health assessment, this would refer to the extent to which a screening instrument or assessment technique is measuring what it is intending to measure (Sullivan, 2011). For example, if a clinician is screening a patient for depression and administers the Generalized Anxiety Disorder-7 (GAD-7) questionnaire, this would not be a valid way to determine whether the patient has depression. The clinician would be screening for anxiety, but not depression. In order to screen for depression, the clinician would need to administer a valid and reliable screening tool like the Patient Health Questionnaire-9 (PHQ-9). This screening tool has been validated and would accurately determine whether a patient is at risk for depression (Mitchell, Yadegarfar, Gill, & Stubbs, 2016; Moriarty, Gilbody, McMillan, & Manea, 2015).

Four major types of validity are discussed here: content validity, construct validity, criterion validity, and external validity. Each type estimates validity in a slightly different way.

Content Validity

Content validity is the degree to which the screening tool adequately covers the entire domain or all facets of the content it is seeking to evaluate (Sullivan, 2011). Depression can have a variety of symptoms, including sadness, anhedonia, anger, changes in appetite or sleep patterns, and guilt. Having high content validity would mean the PHQ-9 asks about all of these symptoms to ensure the tool is all encompassing of the range of symptoms that can present when a patient is depressed.

Construct Validity

Construct validity refers to the concept of testing the screening tool or assessment technique against similar measures to determine whether an association exists between measures (Sullivan, 2011). To measure the construct validity of the PHQ-9, for example, researchers have established that there is a strong association between PHQ-9 scores and functional status, disability days, and symptom-related difficulty, all of which assess for depression in different ways (Mitchell et al., 2016; Moriarty et al., 2015).

Criterion Validity

Criterion validity refers to the correlation between how well a screening tool or assessment technique predicts the outcome of another measure. In the case of the PHQ-9, criterion validity was established by having patients also interview with a mental health clinician. When the clinician's interview and the PHQ-9 independently reach the same conclusion, namely, that the patient has a diagnosis of depression, criterion validity is high (Mitchell et al., 2016; Moriarty et al., 2015).

External Validity

External validity, also called **generalizability**, is the ability of the screening tool or assessment technique to be used with similar outcomes in a variety of settings and with a variety of populations. The PHQ-9 tool has been used in hospitals, outpatient clinics, specialty clinics, and with all genders and races, all with the same results. Because the PHQ-9 screening tool has been validated using large, randomized populations across clinical settings and across time, the tool has well-established generalizability, or high external validity (Mitchell et al., 2016; Moriarty et al., 2015).

Reliability

Reliability is focused on the concept of consistency and the degree to which the screening tool or assessment technique produces consistent results (Sullivan, 2011). An important consideration when discussing reliability is the difference between precision and accuracy. Precision is the ability to obtain the same results or outcomes every time the tool or assessment technique is used. Accuracy is the ability to obtain the correct result from a tool or technique. A tool or test can be precise but not accurate, or it can be accurate but not precise. For example, think about a scale used to measure weight. If multiple clinicians weigh a patient using the same scale and they all get the same weight, the scale would be a precise measurement. However, if the scale were improperly calibrated by 5 pounds, despite its being a precise form of measurement, it would not be an accurate measurement. Ideally, a reliable measure is both precise and accurate. There are three main ways to test reliability: test-retest reliability, internal consistency, and inter-rater reliability. Similar to validity, each type estimates reliability in a different way.

Test-Retest Reliability

Test-retest reliability is the ability of a test or technique to be consistent over time. In other words, if a patient completes the PHQ-9 and the same patient completes this test again in 24 hours, the results are considered reliable if the test results continue to be the same. This is measured by a test-retest reliability coefficient test. Results vary between 0 and 1, with 1 indicating perfect reliability and 0 indicating no reliability. Any score of 0.70 or higher is considered acceptable, with an ideal score being a 0.80 or higher (Sullivan, 2011).

Internal Consistency

Internal consistency is the degree of agreement between multiple items within a tool (Sullivan, 2011). In the PHQ-9 example, this screening tool is designed to measure depression. Internal consistency means all nine questions measure depression, both separately and collectively. This is measured with a statistical test called Cronbach's alpha. Cronbach's alpha (α) increases when correlations between test items increase and values range from 0 to 1, with a good reliability being at least 0.70 or higher (Melnyk & Morrison-Beedy, 2019).

Inter-Rater Reliability

Inter-rater reliability, also called interobserver reliability, is the ability of two or more independent raters or observers to draw the same conclusions or results. Using the example of depression, inter-rater reliability would be high if two clinicians make a diagnosis of major depressive disorder after each of them has clinically assessed the same patient. Inter-rater reliability is reported as a kappa statistic (κ), which can range from 1 to −1. One indicates perfect agreement between raters, zero indicates a chance occurrence, and negative one indicates agreement is less than chance (Sullivan, 2011).

Accuracy
Sensitivity and Specificity

Appropriate interpretation of the results of screening tests involves understanding how likely the test is to be accurate. Measures of accuracy include **sensitivity**, or how likely the test will correctly identify individuals who have the condition for which the tool or test was designed (Ranganathan & Aggarwal, 2018a). A highly sensitive test is one in which there are few false negative results or few cases of a disease or condition being missed. The sensitivity of a screening test is related to the probability of detection, so this measure is also known as the true positive rate.

The **specificity** of a test refers to the likelihood that the test will correctly identify those without the condition for which the tool was designed. A highly specific test is one in which there are few false positive results (Ranganathan & Aggarwal, 2018a). Measures of specificity determine the true negative rate.

Predictive Value

One of the noteworthy measures of accuracy of a screening test is the test's predictive value. *Positive predictive value* refers to the proportion of positive tests that are true positives and represents the presence of the disease in the population. *Negative predictive value* refers to the proportion of negative tests that are true negatives and represents the absence of the disease or condition in the population (Ranganathan & Aggarwal, 2018a). The measures of sensitivity, specificity, and negative and positive predictive values are depicted in **Figure 1.3**.

Using the diagram in **Figure 1.3**, sensitivity refers to the number of true positives (A) divided by the total number of those who actually have the condition (A + C). Specificity refers to the number of true negatives (D) divided by the number of those who actually do not have the condition (B + D). Positive predictive value refers to the number of true positives (A) divided by the number of positive results (A + B). Negative predictive value refers to the number of true negatives (D) divided by the number of negative results (C + D). Predictive values are influenced by the prevalence of disease in a population (i.e., when a disease or condition is highly prevalent, the positive predictive value of a screening test will be significantly higher).

Likelihood Ratio

While screening tests or diagnostic tools rarely have the sensitivity and/or specificity to provide 100% certainty in diagnosing a disease or condition, highly sensitive

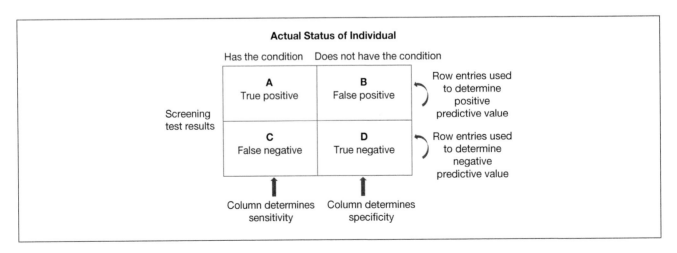

FIGURE 1.3 Sensitivity, specificity, positive predictive value, and negative predictive value. This figure depicts how they are determined and how they are interrelated.

and specific screening tools provide key assessments. The **likelihood ratio**, or LR, is the comparison of how likely the screening test is to detect the condition (true positive) compared with how likely the test is to be accurate when an individual does not have the condition (true negative; Ranganathan & Aggarwal, 2018b). In EBP, the LR is used for determining the value of using a screening or diagnostic test based on accuracy. The LR value depicts how much more likely the individual is to have a positive screening for an existing, undiagnosed condition compared with an individual without the condition (Ranganathan & Aggarwal, 2018b). Unlike predictive values, the LR does not depend on the prevalence of a condition in a population and is more a reflection of the characteristics of the screening test.

The PHQ-9 tool, which has been shown to have content validity and reliability, has also been critically appraised for sensitivity, specificity, and LR characteristics related to screening for mild, moderate, and severe depression. PHQ-9 scores of 10 or greater have an 81.3% sensitivity *and* an 85.3% specificity for major depression (Mitchell et al., 2016). The LRs confirm the association between increasing PHQ-9 scores and the likelihood of depression, as the LR is positive for PHQ-9 scores from 9 to 15 (Mitchell et al., 2016; Moriarty et al., 2015). Evaluating sensitivity, specificity, and LRs confirms that the test is able to identify individuals with and without depression.

When critically appraising study findings and conclusions, the clinician must note study limitations before widely implementing findings in clinical practice. Rigorous research findings provide the evidence needed for clinicians to implement valid, reliable, predictive, sensitive, specific, and generalizable screening tools that can provide important clinical assessments.

STEP #4: INTEGRATE THE EVIDENCE WITH CLINICAL EXPERTISE AND PATIENT/FAMILY PREFERENCES TO MAKE THE BEST CLINICAL DECISION

This step in EBP is integrating the best evidence found from the evidence search with the clinician's expertise and patient/family preferences and values to implement a decision (i.e., putting the evidence found into action). To fully and effectively implement EBP within the context of assessing health and well-being, the clinician must have a broad understanding of health and wellness, screen for episodic and/or chronic problems related to all dimensions of wellness, ask clinical questions, critically appraise evidence, and interpret clinical evidence. Interpreting clinical evidence implies assimilating the steps of EBP within the context of the clinician's expertise, and the patient's history, presentation, and preferences. The interpretation of clinical evidence requires careful reasoning.

Expert clinicians often share the adage that "the patient's diagnosis is found within their history." Listening to the patient is key to diagnosing episodic, chronic, urgent, and/or emergent problems. The patient history is often the predominant determinant of a diagnosis; it typically comprises 80% of the diagnosis being made by a clinician. If a comprehensive thorough history is taken, the likelihood of making a correct diagnosis is extremely high. The physical assessment most often just confirms what a clinician is thinking as a result of a thorough history. The keys to correctly interpreting the clinical evidence that the patient provides are asking the appropriate history questions, deeply listening to the patient's history, and considering appropriate differential diagnoses.

Differential diagnoses are those diagnoses that the clinician is considering based on their interpretation of clinical evidence during the patient encounter. Differential diagnoses are those conditions, problems, diseases, or alterations in health that present with similar signs and symptoms. Clinicians can use the process of establishing differential diagnoses to allow for a systematic and thorough interpretation of assessments obtained during the patient's history and physical exam. Using an evidence-based approach to interpret patient history findings provides the clinician with an opportunity to recognize, interpret, and analyze clinical findings.

Components of the physical exam are determined by interpreting the findings from the patient's history within the context of EBP. Clinicians employ various methods of physical exam (as described within this text) to verify the patient's level of health and well-being across wellness dimensions, including diagnosis of an illness, risk factors for illness, or chronic conditions.

The interpretation of clinical evidence includes the patient's perspective. The key to knowing the patient's perspective is asking about the individual or family concerns, interpretation of findings, and expectations regarding what might be done to support the patient's health and well-being. Remember that the patient is central to the interpretation of clinical evidence. The clinical significance of evidence is best understood within the context of the patient encounter; in other words, best practice for advanced assessment includes patient considerations and clinician expertise. Completing a thorough patient history leads to determination and analysis of clinically important assessments that allow the clinician to make diagnostic and management decisions in partnership with patients and/or families.

The complexity of diagnostic decision-making is on a continuum from straightforward and brief to complex, ongoing, and risk laden. One of the goals of this text is to provide the foundation for assessments across the continuum and to present the evidence to support diagnostic decision-making. The interpretation of clinical findings through an evidence-based framework is intended to lead to clinical interactions that are patient centered, high quality, timely, and accurate.

STEP #5: EVALUATE THE OUTCOMES OF THE PRACTICE CHANGE BASED ON EVIDENCE

This step in EBP is evaluating the evidence-based practice change in terms of how the change affected patient outcomes or how effective the clinical decision was with a particular patient or practice setting. This type of evaluation is necessary to determine whether the change based on evidence resulted in the expected outcomes when implemented in the real-world clinical practice setting. Measurement of outcomes, especially "so-what" outcomes that are important to today's healthcare system (e.g., length of stay, readmission rates, patient complications, turnover of staff, costs) is important to determine and document the impact of the EBP change on healthcare quality and/or patient outcomes (Melnyk & Morrison-Beedy, 2019). If a change in practice, based on evidence, did not produce the same findings as demonstrated in rigorous research, clinicians should ask themselves a variety of questions (e.g., Was the practice delivered in exactly the same way that it was implemented in the study? Were the patients in the clinical setting similar to those in the studies?).

STEP #6: DISSEMINATE THE OUTCOMES OF THE EVIDENCE-BASED PRACTICE CHANGE

The last step in the EBP seven-step process is disseminating the outcomes of the EBP change. Clinicians achieve many positive outcomes by making changes in their care based on evidence, but those outcomes are often not shared with others, even colleagues within their same practice. As a result, others do not learn about the outcomes or the process that led to the change, and clinicians as well as other patients do not benefit from that knowledge. It is important for clinicians to disseminate outcomes of their practice changes based on evidence through such venues as oral and poster presentations at local, regional, and national conferences; EBP rounds within their own practices or institutions; journal and newsletter publications; and lay publications.

EVIDENCE-BASED PRACTICE RESOURCES

There are a variety of excellent EBP resources that are available to assist clinicians in implementing best evidence in their practices. It is important to be familiar with these resources as they are high quality and save clinicians time in searching for best evidence to guide clinical care.

THE UNITED STATES PREVENTIVE SERVICES TASK FORCE EVIDENCE-BASED PREVENTION RECOMMENDATIONS

The United States Preventive Services Task Force (USPSTF) has been a major source of evidence-based prevention recommendations for both children and adults for the past three decades. These recommendations have been widely available to clinicians through the USPSTF website (www.uspreventiveservicestaskforce .org), which provides updated evidence-based recommendations for over 100 primary care screening and behavioral counseling topics.

The USPSTF is an independent panel of 16 national experts in disease prevention and EBP. The Task Force works to improve the health of all Americans by making evidence-based recommendations about clinical preventive services. Task Force members come from the fields of preventive medicine and primary care, including internal medicine, family medicine, pediatrics, behavioral health, obstetrics and gynecology, and nursing. Their recommendations are based on a rigorous review of existing peer-reviewed evidence and are intended to help primary care clinicians and patients decide together whether a preventive service is right for a patient's needs. The Agency for Healthcare Research and Quality (AHRQ) has been authorized by the U.S. Congress to convene the Task Force and to provide ongoing scientific, administrative, and dissemination support to the Task Force. Each year, the Task Force makes a report to Congress that identifies critical evidence gaps in research related to clinical preventive services and recommends priority areas that deserve further examination.

Each topic that is addressed by the USPSTF (e.g., Cervical Cancer Screening; Colorectal Screening; Depression Screening in Children and Adolescents; Depression Screening in Adults; High Blood Pressure Screening in Adults; Obesity Screening in Children and Adolescents; Sexually Transmitted Infections: Behavioral Counseling) undergoes a rigorous systematic review of evidence that is conducted by EBP centers (EPCs) that are contracted by the AHRQ. After the literature review is completed and the evidence is appraised and summarized by the EPC, it is brought to the USPSTF for review and critical appraisal. Reviews are sent to outside experts for peer review, who are asked to provide critical feedback regarding the methods and conclusions of the evidence review. The USPSTF also assesses the "net benefit" of a preventive service by comparing the magnitude of benefits relative to harms associated with the service. Benefits are assessed by reviewing the magnitude of both the relative and the absolute improvements in health outcomes associated with the delivery of the service. The Task Force documents its methods in a procedure manual and other resources to ensure that the recommendations and evidence reviews are of consistently high quality, methodologically sound, scientifically defensible, reproducible, and unbiased. See www.uspreventiveservicestaskforce.org/Page/Name/methods-and-processes for more information. Using both the magnitude of net benefit and the certainty of net benefit assessments, the USPSTF relies on a standard matrix to guide the assignment of a letter grade for its recommendations. After the Task Force releases its new or updated recommendations, they are disseminated on the USPSTF website for public feedback/comment.

The USPSTF assigns each of their recommendations a letter grade (an A, B, C, or D grade or an I statement) based on the strength of the evidence and the balance of benefits and harms of a preventive service. The Task Force does not *consider the costs* of a preventive service when determining a recommendation grade. The recommendations apply only to people who have no signs or symptoms of the specific disease or condition under evaluation, and the recommendations address only services offered in the primary care setting or services referred by a primary care clinician.

The USPSTF recommends services with "A" or "B" letter grades, which should be uniformly recommended for all patients who meet criteria for the service. "C"-rated services are appropriate for selected individuals and should be implemented after a discussion with patients and families about the relatively small net benefit and potential harms. "D"-rated services should not be offered because of the lack of benefit or net harm. The USPSTF recognizes that patients may have questions about or request grade D services. In this case, clinicians should make sure that patients and families are fully informed and make a collaborative decision based on the patients' health status and preferences. Services with an "I" statement also should not be implemented on a routine basis without first introducing shared decision-making with patients and families about the insufficiency of evidence and uncertainty about the net benefit of the service (Table 1.1).

The Electronic Preventive Services Selector (ePSS) is an application designed to help primary care clinicians identify clinical preventive services that are appropriate for their patients. This tool can be downloaded to mobile devices and used in clinical practice to determine appropriate recommended services for patients, based on their sex and age.

EVIDENCE-BASED CLINICAL PRACTICE GUIDELINES

Evidence-based clinical practice guidelines are specific practice recommendations grouped together that have been created from a methodologically rigorous review of the best evidence on a specific topic. Guidelines typically do not answer a single specific clinical question, but rather a group of questions about care. As a result, they have tremendous potential as tools for clinicians to improve the quality of care, the process of care, and patient outcomes as well as reduce variation in care and unnecessary healthcare expenditures (Institute of Medicine Committee on Standards for Developing Trustworthy Clinical Practice Guidelines, 2011).

It is important to note the latest publication date of clinical practice guidelines as many guidelines need updating so that the latest evidence is included in making practice recommendations. It is also important to note

TABLE 1.1 USPSTF Recommendation Grades

Grade	Definition
A	The USPSTF recommends the service. There is high certainty that the net benefit is substantial.
B	The USPSTF recommends the service. There is high certainty that the net benefit is moderate or there is moderate certainty that the net benefit is moderate to substantial.
C	The USPSTF recommends selectively offering or providing this service to individual patients based on professional judgment and patient preferences. There is at least moderate certainty that the net benefit is small.
D	The USPSTF recommends against the service. There is moderate or high certainty that the service has no net benefit or that the harms outweigh the benefits.
I	The USPSTF concludes that the current evidence is insufficient to assess the balance of benefits and harms of the service. Evidence is lacking, of poor quality, or conflicting, and the balance of benefits and harms cannot be determined.

Letter grades are assigned to each recommendation statement. These grades are based on the strength of the evidence on the harms and benefits of a specific preventive service.
USPSTF, United States Preventive Services Task Force.
Source: U.S. Preventive Services Task Force. (n.d.). What the grades mean and suggestions for practice. Retrieved from https://epss.ahrq.gov/ePSS/gradedef.jsp#after2012

the process through which the guidelines were created, as there are many guidelines that have been created by professional organizations that have not followed rigorous processes for development (e.g., systematic reviews; Melnyk et al., 2012). Although clinical practice guidelines have tremendous potential to improve the quality of care and outcomes for patients as well as reduce healthcare variation and costs, their success depends on a highly rigorous guideline development process and the incorporation of the latest best evidence. In addition, guideline success depends on implementation by healthcare clinicians as their dissemination does not equate to implementation.

ECRI Guidelines Trust™

Since 1968, the ECRI Institute has been advancing the science of care throughout the world. Its mission is to protect patients from unsafe and ineffective medical technologies and practices. More than 5,000 healthcare institutions and systems worldwide, including four out of every five U.S. hospitals, rely on the ECRI Institute to guide their operational and strategic decisions. In addition, the Institute serves private payers; federal and state agencies; policy makers; ministries of health; associations; and accrediting agencies. The ECRI Guidelines Trust is a publicly available web-based repository of objective evidence-based clinical practice guideline content. Its purpose is to provide physicians, nurses, other clinical specialties, and members of the healthcare community with up-to-date clinical practices to advance safe and effective patient care. This centralized repository includes evidence-based guidance developed by nationally and internationally recognized medical organizations and medical specialty societies. The ECRI Guidelines Trust provides the following guideline-related content:

- *Guideline briefs*: Summarizes content providing the key elements of the clinical practice guideline.
- *TRUST (Transparency and Rigor Using Standards of Trustworthiness) scorecards*: Ratings of how well guidelines fulfill the IOM Standards for Trustworthiness (see https://guidelines.ecri.org).

The Guidelines International Network

The Guidelines International Network (G-I-N), founded in 2002, encompasses a comprehensive database of clinical practice guidelines. The mission of G-I-N is to "lead, strengthen and support collaboration in guideline development, adaptation and implementation . . . . G-I-N facilitates networking, promotes excellence and helps . . . members create high quality clinical practice guidelines that foster safe and effective patient care" and is comprised of 102 organizations representing 30 countries from all continents (G-I-N, n.d.). See www.g-i-n.net/home.

The Registered Nurses' Association of Ontario Clinical Practice Guidelines

A tool kit to enhance the use of clinical practice guidelines is available from the Registered Nurses' Association of Ontario. It can be downloaded from its website at http://ltctoolkit.rnao.ca.

Research-Tested Intervention Programs and Quality Healthcare Innovations Exchange

Other searchable databases that are helpful to clinicians in making decisions on what evidence-based interventions to implement in their practices are the Research-Tested Intervention Programs (RTIPs) by the National Cancer Institute and the AHRQ Health Care Innovations Exchange. RTIPs is a database of over 200 "evidence-based cancer control interventions and program materials . . . designed to provide . . . practitioners [with] easy and immediate access to research-tested materials" (National Cancer Institute, n.d., "Moving from Research" see https://rtips.cancer.gov/rtips/index.do). Programs listed have undergone rigorous reviews before their inclusion on this website. The Innovations Exchange was created to "speed the implementation of new and better ways of delivering health care" by sharing, learning about, and adopting evidence-based innovations and tools appropriate for a range of healthcare settings and populations (AHRQ, n.d., para. 1). See https://innovations.ahrq.gov.

Choosing Wisely®

In 2010, Howard Brody published "Medicine's Ethical Responsibility for Health Care Reform—The Top Five List" in the *New England Journal of Medicine*. In this piece, Dr. Brody called on U.S. medical specialty societies to identify five tests and treatments that were overused in their specialty and did not provide meaningful benefit for patients (Brody, 2010). Shortly after, the National Physicians Alliance (NPA) piloted the "Five Things" concept through an American Board of Internal Medicine (ABIM) Foundation *Putting the Charter Into Practice* grant and created a set of three lists of specific steps physicians in internal medicine, family medicine, and pediatrics could take in their practices to promote the more effective use of healthcare resources. These lists were first published in *Archives of Internal Medicine*. Building on this work, the ABIM Foundation, along with Consumer Reports, formally launched the *Choosing Wisely* campaign in 2012 with the release of "Top Five" lists from nine specialty societies. The widespread media coverage from nearly every top-tier outlet, along with positive reactions from among the healthcare community, inspired 17 additional societies to join the campaign and release lists in February 2013. More than 70 societies, comprising over

1 million clinicians, are now partners of the *Choosing Wisely* campaign.

In 2013, the ABIM Foundation received a grant from the Robert Wood Johnson Foundation (RWJF) to advance the *Choosing Wisely* campaign by funding 21 state medical societies, specialty societies, and regional health collaboratives to help healthcare clinicians and patients engage in conversations aimed at reducing unnecessary tests and procedures. In 2015, the RWJF awarded a second grant to the ABIM Foundation to continue this important work.

The mission of *Choosing Wisely* is to promote conversations between clinicians and patients by helping patients choose care that is:

- Supported by evidence
- Not duplicative of other tests or procedures already received
- Free from harm
- Truly necessary

To help patients engage their clinician in these conversations and empower them to ask questions about what tests and procedures are right for them, patient-friendly materials were created on the basis of specialty societies' lists of recommendations of tests and treatments that may be unnecessary. *Choosing Wisely* recommendations should not be used to establish coverage decisions or exclusions; they are meant to facilitate conversation about what is appropriate and necessary treatment. As each patient situation is unique, clinicians and patients should use the recommendations as guidelines to determine an appropriate treatment plan together (Choosing Wisely, n.d.). See www.choosingwisely.org/our-mission.

 Key Takeaways

- EBP is a lifelong problem-solving approach to the delivery of care that incorporates the current best evidence with a clinician's expertise and patient/family preferences and values.
- Clinicians should be skilled in the seven steps of EBP in order to provide the highest quality of care.
- Clinicians need to incorporate the EBP process into their health and well-being assessments through rigorous critical appraisal of the evidence underlying history and physical exam techniques, assessment strategies, the use of imaging tests or lab studies, and/or approaches to health and well-being.
- Clinicians should incorporate a well-being assessment into each exam, including the nine dimensions of wellness: physical, emotional, financial, intellectual, career, social, creative, environmental, and spiritual.
- Clinicians should understand and apply the concepts of validity, reliability, sensitivity, specificity, predictive values, and likelihood ratios during the assessment process to improve diagnostic accuracy and ensure high-quality patient care.
- Multiple, high-quality resources exist in which to guide clinicians in making evidence-based decisions.

REFERENCES

Agency for Healthcare Research and Quality. (n.d.). About the AHRQ Health Care Innovations Exchange. Retrieved from https://innovations.ahrq.gov/about-us

Bodenheimer, T., & Sinsky, C. (2014). From triple to quadruple aim: Care of the patient requires care of the provider. *Annals of Family Medicine, 12*(6), 573–576. doi:10.1370/afm.1713

Brody, H. (2010). Medicine's ethical responsibility for health care reform—The top five list. *New England Journal of Medicine, 362*(4), 283–285. doi:10.1056/NEJMp0911423

Choosing Wisely. (n.d.). Our mission. Retrieved from https://www.choosingwisely.org/our-mission

Goodacre, S., Nelson-Piercy, C., Hunt, B., & Chan, W. (2015) When should we use diagnostic imaging to investigate for pulmonary embolism in pregnant and postpartum women? *Emergency Medicine Journal, 32*(1), 78–82. doi:10.1136/emermed-2014-203871

Guidelines International Network. (n.d.). Home page. Retrieved from https://g-i-n.net

Institute of Medicine Committee on Standards for Developing Trustworthy Clinical Practice Guidelines. (2011). In R. Graham, M. Mancher, D. Miller Wolman, S. Greenfield, & E. Steinberg (Eds.), *Clinical practice guidelines we can trust.* Washington, DC: National Academies Press.

Leung, A., Bull, T., Jaeschke, R., Lockwood, C., Boiselle, P., Hurwitz, L., … Tuttle, B. (2012). American Thoracic Society documents: An official American Thoracic Society/Society of Thoracic Radiology clinical practice guideline: Evaluation of suspected pulmonary embolism in pregnancy. *Radiology, 262*(2), 635–646. doi:10.1148/radiol.11114045

Makary, M., & Daniel, M. (2016). Medical error—the third leading cause of death in the US. *British Medical Journal, 353*, i2139. doi:10.1136/bmj.i2139

Melnyk, B. M., & Fineout-Overholt, E. (2011). *Implementing evidence-based practice: Real-life success stories.* Indianapolis, IN: Sigma Theta Tau International.

Melnyk, B. M., & Fineout-Overholt, E. (2019). *Evidence-based practice in nursing and healthcare: A guide to best practice* (4th ed.). New York, NY: Wolters Kluwer.

Melnyk, B. M., Grossman, D. C., Chou, R., Mabry-Hernandez, I., Nicholson, W., Dewitt, T. G., … Flores, G. (2012). USPSTF perspective on evidence-based preventive recommendations for children. *Pediatrics, 130*(2), e399–e407. doi:10.1542/peds.2011-2087

Melnyk, B. M., & Morrison-Beedy, D. (Eds.). (2019). *Intervention research and evidence-based quality improvement: Designing, conducting, analyzing, and funding* (2nd ed.). New York, NY: Springer Publishing Company.

Melnyk, B. M., & Neale, S. (2018a). 9 dimensions of wellness. *American Nurse Today, 13*(1), 10–11. Retrieved from https://www.americannursetoday.com/9-dimensions-wellness

Melnyk, B. M., & Neale, S. (2018b). *9 dimensions of wellness: Evidence-based tactics for optimizing your health and well-being.* Columbus: The Ohio State University.

Mitchell, A., Yadegarfar, M., Gill, J., & Stubbs, B. (2016). Case finding and screening clinical utility of the Patient Health Questionnaire (PHQ-9 and PHQ-2) for depression in primary care: A diagnostic meta-analysis of 40 studies. *BJPsych Open, 2*(2), 127–138. doi:10.1192/bjpo.bp.115.001685

Moriarty, A., Gilbody, S., McMillan, D., & Manea, L. (2015). Screening and case finding for major depressive disorder using the Patient Health Questionnaire (PHQ-9): A meta-analysis. *General Hospital Psychiatry, 37*(6), 567–576. doi:10.1016/j.genhosppsych.2015.06.012

National Cancer Institute. (n.d.). *Research-Tested Intervention Programs (RTIPs).* Retrieved from https://rtips.cancer.gov/rtips/index.do

Ranganathan, P., & Aggarwal, R. (2018a). Common pitfalls in statistical analysis: Understanding the properties of diagnostic tests—Part 1. *Perspectives in Clinical Research, 9*(1), 40–43. doi:10.4103/picr.PICR_170_17

Ranganathan, P., & Aggarwal, R. (2018b). Understanding the properties of diagnostic tests—Part 2: Likelihood ratios. *Perspectives in Clinical Research, 9*(2), 99–102. doi:10.4103/picr.PICR_41_18

Sullivan, G. (2011). A primer on the validity of assessment instruments. *Journal of Graduate Medical Education, 3*(2), 119–120. doi:10.4300/JGME-D-11-00075.1

U.S. Preventive Services Task Force. (n.d.). What the grades mean and suggestions for practice. Retrieved from https://epss.ahrq.gov/ePSS/gradedef.jsp#after2012

World Health Organization. (n.d.) Constitution. Retrieved from https://www.who.int/about/who-we-are/constitution

2

Evidence-Based History-Taking Approach for Wellness Exams, Episodic Visits, and Chronic Care Management

Linda Quinlin and Kate Gawlik

> *"Success is no accident. It is hard work, perseverance, learning, studying, sacrifice and most of all, love of what you are doing or learning to do."*
>
> —PELÉ

 VIDEO

- Well Exam: Adult With Diabetes—History and Physical Exam

LEARNING OBJECTIVES

- Discover the importance and the uniqueness of the wellness exam, episodic visit, and chronic care management visit.
- Identify the components of the wellness exam, episodic visit, and chronic care management visit.
- Recognize modifications to and special considerations in the history and physical exams for special populations.

WELLNESS EXAM, EPISODIC VISIT, AND CHRONIC CARE MANAGEMENT

History taking is the primary way a clinician obtains comprehensive information about the patient and is often the most important aspect of the patient visit for diagnostic decision-making. The approach to **history taking** will change on the basis of the reason for the patient visit. There are different types of health histories that are collected during a patient visit. This chapter will discuss the collection of a history for a wellness exam, an **episodic visit**, and a chronic care management visit and the various components of each. The scope and degree of detail in history taking will depend on the patient's purpose for visiting, their chief concern, the complexity of the patient's medical condition, and the clinician's goals for the visit. Regardless of the type of history, the goal during the interview is to be attentive to the patient and receptive to the patient's needs. Tailor communication, decision-making, and treatment to the purpose of the visit and patient preferences.

Visit https://connect.springerpub.com/content/book/978-0-8261
-6454-4/chapter/ch00 to access the videos.

HISTORY TAKING FOR THE WELLNESS EXAM

Wellness exams are important for preventing illnesses, disease, and health problems. In addition, wellness exams help detect problems at an early stage when treatment is most likely to address the problem identified and target organ damage has not yet occurred. Based on the age of the patient, the wellness exam will vary.

Wellness exams include an age- and gender-appropriate history and physical exam. Wellness exams for a 24-year-old female will vary greatly from a wellness exam for a 60-year-old male, and even for a 60-year-old female. All wellness exams have the same general components (Hill, 2004):

- A comprehensive, culturally sensitive history and physical examination
- Anticipatory guidance, addressing risk factors and the interventions, motivational interviewing, or counseling to reduce the identified risk factors
- Ordering appropriate immunizations, as well as laboratory/diagnostic procedures

When collecting the patient history, effective communication is key. Evidence shows a strong correlation between a clinician's ability to effectively communicate and a patient's ability to adhere to medical advice, practice self-management, and adopt healthy behaviors (Bramhall, 2014; Institute for Healthcare Communication, 2011). Clinicians who have communication skills in explaining, listening, and empathizing can have an impact on the patient's physical and functional health outcomes, as well as having increased patient satisfaction. Clinicians who lack skill in communication have been found to have increased malpractice risk, decrease in patient adherence to their treatment plan, and poorer patient outcomes (Institute for Healthcare Communication, 2011). Refer to **Table 2.1** for core communication skills for clinicians.

KEY HISTORY QUESTIONS AND CONSIDERATIONS

HISTORY OF PRESENT ILLNESS

Patient history collections for wellness exams are not problem-oriented and, hence, do not require a chief concern or history of present illness. Rather, a wellness exam should include a comprehensive history and physical examination appropriate to the patient's age and gender, counseling and anticipatory guidance, risk reduction interventions, the ordering or administration of vaccine-appropriate immunizations, and the ordering of appropriate laboratory and/or diagnostic testing (American College of Obstetricians and Gynecologists, 2018; Owolabi & Simpson, 2012; Wilkinson, 2008). The wellness exam differs from the episodic visit and chronic care management visit because the components of the wellness exam are based on age and risk factors, not a presenting problem (Owolabi & Simpson, 2012).

TABLE 2.1 Core Communication Skills for Clinicians

Open-ended communication	The use of open-ended questions allows the patient to express their true concerns. Allow for silence. Example: *You've reported you have shortness of breath; can you tell me more about that?*
Reflective listening and empathy	The use of reflective listening demonstrates active listening and acknowledges the patient's response. Example: *I can see the news has been upsetting to you.* The patient's emotions are central to effective decision-making. Acknowledging the patient's emotions demonstrates that the clinician appreciates how the patient is feeling. Example: *You are experiencing lots of changes in your health; it's understandable that this would be difficult to accept right now.*
Values and preferences	Understanding a patient's values and preferences allows the clinician to have a deeper understanding of the importance the patient places on their health outcomes. Example: *I hear you say that you value your time with your family, and your preference is to receive treatment for your breast cancer.*

Sources: Bramhall, E. (2014). Effective communications skills in nursing practice. *Nursing Standard, 29*(14), 53–59. doi:10.7748/ns.29.14.53.e9355; Fortin, A. H., Dwamena, F. C., Frankel, R. M., Lepisto B. L., & Smith, R. C. (2019). The middle of the interview: Clinician-centered interviewing. In *Smith's patient-centered interviewing, an evidence-based method* (4th ed., pp. 1–11). New York, NY: McGraw-Hill; Institute for Healthcare Communication. (2011). Impact of communication in healthcare. Retrieved from https://healthcarecomm.org/about-us/impact-of-communication-in-healthcare

PAST MEDICAL HISTORY

For a wellness exam, past medical and surgical history should include:

- Past medical conditions, hospitalizations, surgeries, and injuries: Assess the status of chronic or past medical conditions that may or may not be significant and/or require additional workup at the visit (Owolabi & Simpson, 2012).
- Medications and supplements: Review current medications, including over-the-counter medications, vitamins, supplements, and herbs. Include a review of allergies to medication, food, and environment (Centers for Medicare & Medicaid Services [CMS] Medicare Learning Network® [MLN], 2018). Review age-appropriate immunization status.
  - ○ When reviewing medications, be observant of opioid use. Screening for opioid use during wellness exams can possibly identify the diagnosis of opioid use disorder (OUD). Early identification can assist patients in getting the support they need. In addition, assess for and promote effective nonopioid pain treatments, even if the patient does not have OUD but is possibly at risk (CMS, 2019).

Menstrual/Gynecological/Sexual/Obstetric History

A wellness exam for a woman presents an opportunity to counsel about healthy lifestyle and to minimize health risks. A thorough woman's health history includes the following elements: a menstrual history, a gynecological history, a sexual history, and an obstetric history.

- Menstrual history: Include the age of menarche, the length and frequency of the cycle, the type and amount of menstrual flow, and any associated symptoms, including dysmenorrhea, cramping, mood swings, headaches/migraines, bloating, premenstrual syndrome (PMS), premenstrual dysphoric disorder (PMDD), bleeding between periods or after intercourse, or odor. Note the first day of the last menstrual period (FDLMP). A thorough menstrual history also includes a history of perimenopause or menopause if this is applicable to the patient. Review the patient's current bleeding pattern, if any. If she is no longer bleeding, find out when her last menstrual period was. Discuss if she is experiencing any vasomotor symptoms, including night sweats, hot flashes/flushes, vulvovaginal atrophy or dryness, and/or mood changes. Has she ever been on or does she currently use any form of hormone replacement therapy?

- Gynecological history: Discuss past cervical and vaginal cytology, including the date of her last Pap smear and her results, any history of abnormal Pap smears, any additional treatments or procedures such as a colposcopy, and any follow-up measures. Ask about any medical history of fibroids, abnormal bleeding, gynecological surgeries or procedures, and address any concerns such as abnormal vaginal discharge, odor, dyspareunia, vaginal pruritus, vaginal dryness, and any lesions in the vaginal or inguinal area.
- Sexual history: Ask about current and past sexual activity. Discuss the number of lifetime partners, the current number of partners, and whether she is sexually active with men, women, or both. Does she have any history of sexual abuse, or any history of sexual assault, and does she currently feel safe in her current relationship(s)? Review any history of sexually transmitted infections (STIs) and/or pelvic inflammatory disease. Include dates, treatment of infections, and whether partners also received treatment. Has she had the human papillomavirus vaccine? Discuss current practices to prevent pregnancy and STIs. Discuss her current contraception method, any previous contraception method(s), and the reason(s) for discontinuing other methods. Ask about her ability to achieve orgasm, sexual motivation, and sex drive.
- Obstetric history: When discussing the obstetric history, GPA and TPAL are two commonly used mnemonics to ensure all information is obtained (Table 2.2). In addition to this information, ask about any complications during pregnancy, labor, or postpartum. Did labor happen spontaneously, was it induced, or was it a cesarean delivery? If applicable, what was the reason for the cesarean delivery? Ask about ability to conceive and if any infertility methods or procedures were used.

TABLE 2.2 Common Mnemonics for Obstetric History

G (Gravida)	Number of total pregnancies
P (Para)	Number of viable births
A or Ab (Abortus)	Number of abortions
T	Number of full-term births
P	Number of preterm births
A	Number of abortions
L	Number of living children

FAMILY HISTORY

A wellness exam assessment of family history includes the following:

- Medical history of the patient's grandparents, parents, siblings, and children: Include any conditions that could be hereditary or those conditions that place the patient at increased risk. Review any significant family health history; include the health status, pattern of disease(s), and cause of death of grandparents, parents, siblings, and children.

SOCIAL HISTORY

A wellness exam assessment of social history includes the following:

- Age and gender-appropriate review of significant activities: Include information such as marital status, living arrangement and home conditions, social support system, occupational history, use of illicit drugs, alcohol intake, current or former tobacco use, educational level, religious/spirituality ideals, cultural preferences, and sexual history (Moore, 2010). Also include diet and physical activities in the social history (CMS MLN, 2018).

REVIEW OF SYSTEMS

A review of systems collected during a wellness exam provides a guide to help the clinician gather essential information on current or potential disease processes that may otherwise go unnoticed. The review of systems can identify risk factors pertinent to the patient based on their age, gender, and personal risk factors. During a review of systems, the clinician asks the patient a series of questions, typically arranged by organ system. This series of questions gives the patient an opportunity to discuss their health risks with the clinician that they may not have previously considered reporting. Refer to **Table 2.3** for examples of common review of systems questions.

TABLE 2.3 Examples of Review of System Questions

System	Example
Constitution symptoms	Have you been experiencing any unusual fatigue? Have you been experiencing any weight loss or weight gain? Was the weight loss intentional or unintentional? How much weight have you lost and over what amount of time have you lost the weight? Have you been experiencing any fevers? Do you ever have night sweats? What is your sleep pattern? Do you have any difficulty going to sleep or staying asleep? Have you had any recent illnesses? Do you get frequent infections, or does it take you longer to recover than in the past?
Head	Have you been experiencing any headaches? Have you had any recent falls or head trauma? Have you ever had a concussion or loss of consciousness?
Eyes	Have you been experiencing any vision changes? Do you have blurry vision when you look in the distance or when you are reading? Have you ever worn contacts or glasses? When was the last time you visited to the optometrist? Do you experience sensitivity to light, double vision, blurry vision, or complete vision loss? Do you ever have eye floaters? Do you feel like you can see well at night? Are there rings or halos around things? Do you have any eye pain or discharge?
Ears	Have you been experiencing any hearing loss or marked changes to your hearing? When was the last time a clinician removed the earwax from your ears? Have you ever had your hearing checked by a professional? Do you experience ringing in your ears? Do you have any ear pain or discharge from the ears? Is it painful to touch the ear or surrounding area? Do you have any pain behind your ear? Have you recently been swimming? Does your child seem to be pulling at their ears? Have you ever experienced vertigo or felt like the entire room is spinning around you?
Nose	Have you been experiencing any nasal congestion? Does your nose ever bleed? Have you ever broken your nose? Do you have any seasonal or other known allergies? Have you ever snorted cocaine or other prescription drugs? Do you ever feel any sinus pressure or pain? Have you ever had a nasal polyp?
Mouth and throat	Do you have a sore throat? Do you ever find it difficult to swallow due to pain or any another reason? Do you still have your tonsils? Have you noticed any bleeding from your gums? When was the last time you visited a dentist? How often do you brush your teeth? Do you have any dental pain? Do you have any mouth sores or areas of sensitivity in your mouth? Can you chew your food without pain or difficulty? Do you use, or have you used, chewing tobacco in the past?

(continued)

TABLE 2.3 Examples of Review of System Questions (*continued*)	
System	Example
Cardiovascular	Have you been experiencing any chest pain? Do you have any left arm, jaw, or neck pain? Do you have chest pain when you are active, at rest, or at all times? Do you ever use nitroglycerin to relieve chest pain? Do you have heart palpitations or feel like your heart is beating out of your chest? Have you ever passed out? Do you ever have swelling in your legs or ankles? Do you ever feel pain in your legs after walking or exercising? Have you had any hair loss on your lower legs? Have you ever had a stress test or EKG? How many pillows do you sleep with at night, or do you need to sleep sitting upright?
Respiratory	Have you been experiencing any shortness of breath? Do you have a chronic cough? Do you cough up sputum? Have you ever coughed up blood? Do you have any pain when you inhale or exhale? Do you ever wheeze or feel like your chest is tight? Do you, or have you ever, used an inhaler? Do you currently smoke? Are you exposed to secondhand smoke in your home or work environment? Do you smoke around your children? Are you around any toxic fumes? Have you ever had your home tested for radon? Do you snore, or have you been told that you stop breathing while you are sleeping?
Gastrointestinal	Have you been experiencing any abdominal pain? Are you having regular bowel movements? Has there been any change to your bowel movements? Do you have any diarrhea? Do you ever feel constipated? Do you ever take laxatives or stool softeners? Do you ever see blood in your stool, or do your stools appear black? Do you experience heartburn? Have you ever had hemorrhoids? Have you ever had a colonoscopy? Do you have any food intolerances or sensitivities? How has your appetite been?
Genitourinary	Have you been experiencing frequent urination? Are you experiencing any pain with urination? Does your urine have any unusual odor? Does your urine appear cloudy or look like there is blood in it? Do you urinate more at night when you lie down to sleep? Do you experience any urgency or difficulty making it in time to the bathroom? Do you experience any urinary leakage when you sneeze or jump? Do you have any sores in the genital or buttock areas? Are you experiencing any unusual odor or discharge? Do you experience any pain during intercourse? Are you experiencing any difficulty achieving or keeping an erection? Have you noticed any changes or lumps on your testicles? Do you feel like your urine stream is weak?
Musculoskeletal	Have you been experiencing any pain in your joints? Have you noticed any swelling or restricted movement in your joints? Have you had any recent injuries? Do you have any previous sports or overuse injuries, including any broken bones? Have you noticed your child limping or favoring one leg?
Integumentary	Do you have any rashes or sores? Have you noticed any changes to your skin or moles? Does your skin or do your moles itch or bleed? Do you use any lotions or medications on your skin? Is there any swelling or discharge? Is the rash in one location or all over the body? Have you experienced any hair loss? Have you experienced any changes to your hair, skin, or nails? Have you experienced any recent bug bites? Do you ever bite your nails or pull at your hair?
Neurological	Do you feel any tingling or burning in your lower legs? Do you ever experience weakness or dizziness? Have you ever passed out? Have you ever had a seizure? Do you have any difficulty with remembering things? Do you ever shake or have a tremor? Do you ever have loss of balance or coordination?
Psychiatric	Have you been feeling down, blue, or hopeless? Do you still enjoy things that you have always enjoyed? Do you ever feel nervous or anxious? Do you ever hear or see things that other people do not? Do you ever think about harming yourself or someone else? Do you often feel angry or agitated? Do you ever feel like you have excessive energy or confidence? Do you ever participate in activities that may be considered risky or that get you into trouble? Have you ever been in legal trouble? Have you ever had a panic attack? Do you have any reoccurring nightmares about things that have happened in the past?
Endocrine	Do you ever experience any cold or hot intolerance? Have you noticed any thyroid tenderness or enlargement? Have you ever had a high blood sugar reading?
Hematological/lymphatic	Do you experience any abnormal bleeding when you have an injury? Do you bruise or bleed easily? Do you have any enlarged lymph nodes? Have you ever had a blood clot? Do you have a known clotting or bleeding disorder? Have you ever been told that you are anemic?
Allergic/immunological	Do you have any known seasonal, environmental, or food allergies? Have you ever had an anaphylactic reaction? Have you ever had allergy testing? Do you have asthma or eczema?

Unique Population Considerations for History

Pediatric Patients

Pediatric patients are discussed in Chapter 4, Evidence-Based Assessment of Children and Adolescents.

Patients With Disabilities

The International Classification of Functioning, Disability and Health (ICF) defines *disability* as difficulties occurring in all three areas of functioning: impairments, activity limitations, and participation restrictions. *Impairments* can be defined as having problems in body function or cognition such as paralysis or intellectual disability; *activity limitations* occur when an individual has difficulty completing an activity such as walking; and *participation restrictions* occur when an individual has a problem with any area of life such as facing discrimination in employment (World Health Organization, 2018).

When conducting a health history with a patient who has a disability, it is important for the clinician to conduct the interview as they would with any other patient. Make eye contact and sit down to ensure the patient is at eye level. The clinician needs to be at the patient's eye level so the patient does not have to look up to communicate if they are in a wheelchair or on a motorized scooter (Smeltzer, Mariani, & Meakim, 2017). It is especially important in this population that the patient be seen as an active, not passive, participant in their care and decision-making.

At the start of the interview, the clinician will want to address the patient's disability. It is important to remember that the patient will be the expert on their disability. Patients with disabilities are typically very open to discussing their disability and defining their care goals and needs. An example of how to noninvasively address a patient's disability could be to start with a statement such as "Would it be okay if we talked about your disability?" or "Please tell me about why you are using a hearing aid" (Smeltzer et al., 2017). Be aware of the patient's ability to communicate and participate in the collection of the health history. You should assume the patient can communicate during the exam; don't assume otherwise. Don't overlook the patient and talk only to the family member or caregiver but ensure the patient is always an active participant in the conversation. The clinician should be observant for any accommodations and modifications needed by the patient in order to complete the health history. Examples of accommodations and modifications to consider include the ability of the patient to sign their name, the patient's ability to see the print, and the patient's ability to read and understand the information. It is also important to ensure the patient has enough space for any assistive devices and service animals and provide any extra accommodations for hearing and visual aids (Smeltzer et al., 2017).

Collecting the patient's health history will include asking the same questions that other patients would be asked, in addition to questions about their level of functioning and possible secondary conditions or complications of their disability. Can they manage self-care, complete their activities of daily living (ADLs), follow healthcare instructions, obtain preventive health screenings, and receive follow-up care? Include in the health history a discussion regarding the patient's use of assistive devices or other aids required to maintain their level of current functioning. Specific disabilities are often associated with certain secondary conditions. The clinician needs to be vigilant and proactively monitor for these conditions. For example, a patient with quadriplegia is more likely to have conditions like skin breakdown, urinary tract infections, depression, and upper respiratory infections (Resources for Integrated Care, 2017).

Other unique questions to ask during a patient health history include questions related to abuse or risk of abuse. All types of abuse questions should be included: physical, emotional, financial, and sexual. Ask the patient if they feel safe in their environment and if the patient has ever had any concerns about personal safety. Also assess for fall risk and/or injuries from any previous falls (Smeltzer et al., 2017). Ask about any current transportation issues, personal assistance, mobility equipment, home modifications, and needed supplies.

Patients with disability will need an interprofessional, team-based approach. In addition, depending on the type of disability, the patient will also need community-based support services. Other interprofessional team members may need to be consulted while conducting the history and physical examination and formulating the care plan (Resources for Integrated Care, 2017).

Older Adults

Older adults also have unique history considerations. Their medical histories are often much more complex. Multiple comorbidities are often present, and clinicians are often managing multiple medications and attending to multiple needs. Age-appropriate screenings should be conducted to review a patient's functional ability and level of safety. The use of appropriate screening questions or standardized questionnaires to assess medication appropriateness, ADLs (**Table 2.4**), fall risk, hearing impairment, and home safety should be used for age-appropriate populations (CMS MLN, 2018). There are many commonly used screening tools, including the American Geriatrics Society (AGS) Beers Criteria® for Potentially Inappropriate Medication Use in Older Adults (AGS Beers Criteria Update Expert Panel, 2019), Hendrich II Fall Model (Hendrich, 2016), the Home Fall Prevention Checklist for Older Adults (Centers for Disease Control and Prevention [CDC], 2015), and the

TABLE 2.4 Assessment History Considerations: Activities of Daily Living (ADLs)	
ADLs (Self-Care Activities)	**Instrumental ADLs (Living Independently Activities)**
Do you need help with eating?	Can you complete household chores/work?
Do you need help with dressing?	Can you prepare meals?
Do you need help with bathing?	Can you take your medications correctly?
Do you need help transferring from bed to chair?	Can you manage your finances?
Do you need help toileting?	Can you use a telephone?
Do you ever have loss of your bowel or bladder?	

ADLs, activities of daily living.
Source: Tatum, P. E., Talebreza, S., & Ross, J. S. (2018). Geriatric assessment: An office-based approach. *American Family Physician*, *97*(12), 776–784. Retrieved from https://www.aafp.org/afp/2018/0615/p776.html

Katz Index of Independence in Activities of Daily Living (McCabe, 2019).

Changes in a patient functional assessment can be a first indicator of a mental or physical decline. Identifying functional decline early can trigger interventions that will maximize the patient's independence and safety. Completing a functional screening will help the clinician establish a realistic and patient-focused treatment plan.

Age-appropriate screenings to assess a patient's cognitive function should be conducted initially by direct observation, in addition to any information reported by the patient or concerns raised by family members, friends, caregivers, and others. If it is determined that additional screening is warranted, use validated structured cognitive assessment tools (CMS MLN, 2018) to further assess the patient's cognitive function.

A discussion on advance directives should be conducted with age-appropriate patients. Advance directives assist individuals with end-of-life planning. Advance directives should include a discussion with the patient about future care decisions that may need to be made and identifying a healthcare decision-maker. Advance directives allow patients to share with others their healthcare preferences in the event that they are unable to make their own healthcare decisions.

During a wellness exam, review and assess for patient's risk for depression. Include in the assessment the patient's current and past history of depression or any other mood disorders. Incorporate the use of validated depression screening tools such as the Patient Health Questionnaire-9 (PHQ-9).

PHYSICAL EXAMINATION

The physical examination during a **wellness visit** includes the components recommended by the **U.S. Preventive Services Task Force** (USPSTF) for asymptomatic adults. The exact systems exam and extent

of the physical examination are based on the patient's age, gender, and identified risk factors, rather than a presenting problem (Choosing Wisely, 2017; Hill, 2004). The physical exam should include height, weight, body mass index (BMI), and blood pressure reading (CMS MLN, 2018). Comprehensive routine physical examinations are not recommended for asymptomatic adults (Bloomfield & Wilt, 2011; Choosing Wisely, 2017). There is a lack of evidence supporting comprehensive routine physical examinations in asymptomatic adults aged 18 and older. Routine testing of asymptomatic adults has the potential for overtesting and treatment, increased diagnoses, and increased pharmacological treatment (Choosing Wisely, 2017; Krogsbøll, Jørgensen, & Gøtzche, 2013; Krogsbøll, Jørgensen, Grøhøj, & Gøtzche, 2012; Choosing Wisely, 2017). Comprehensive routine physical examinations of asymptomatic adults can take an inordinate amount of time. The clinician's time is better spent assessing and counseling the patient on age- and gender-appropriate screening tests (**Table 2.5**), preventive interventions such as immunizations, and preventive counseling.

Despite the lack of evidence supporting a comprehensive physical examination for asymptomatic

TABLE 2.5 Screening Versus Assessment	
Screening test	A screening test is used to detect early disease or risk factors for disease in large numbers of healthy individuals.
Diagnostic test	A diagnostic test is used to establish the presence or absence of disease.
Assessment	Provides the clinician with a snapshot of the health status and the health risks of the patient. Assessment is a process of systematically collecting and analyzing the patient's health information to identify, support, and promote healthy behaviors.

adults, the physical examination can be a reassuring part of the patient experience. The placebo effect of a well-administered physical exam can be powerful and therapeutic for patients and has even been shown to change neurotransmitter levels in the brain (Finniss, Kaptchuk, Miller, & Benedetti, 2010; Verghese, Brady, Kapur, & Horwitz, 2011). The context, ritual, setting, clinician's tone of voice, duration of interaction, and clinician's sense of empathy/reassurance/bedside manner can significantly improve both patient outcomes and patient satisfaction (Benedetti, Carlino, & Pollo, 2011; Finniss et al., 2010; Kaptchuk et al., 2008). The clinician should take this information into consideration when completing a wellness visit.

For a complete list of evidence-based recommendations, see Evidence-Based Practice Considerations section.

COUNSELING

During the wellness exam, the clinician should include age- and gender-appropriate counseling and a discussion regarding interventions for identified risk factors. In addition, anticipatory guidance should be provided. For example, anticipatory guidance for the geriatric population should include information on fall prevention. It is important to review age-appropriate safety issues with all patients. Counseling should also include a conversation on USPSTF Grade A/B preventive screenings recommendations for the appropriate gender/age group.

UNIQUE POPULATION CONSIDERATIONS FOR EXAMINATION

Pediatric Patients

Pediatric patients will be discussed in Chapter 4, Evidence-Based Assessment of Children and Adolescents.

Patients With Disabilities

When a patient has a disability, the clinician needs to be flexible and alter their approach for the physical examination to accommodate the patient. Each patient will have different needs based on their disability. A patient who is nonambulatory will have different needs from a patient who is blind. The clinician should check with the patient on specific preferences concerning certain aspects of the exam. Some important considerations are as follows (Smeltzer et al., 2017):

- Is there a way to assist the patient with transfers?
- Does the patient need assistance undressing or dressing?
- When on the examination table, what positions are most comfortable?
- Do there need to be modifications to the examination? Is it appropriate to omit or reduce certain parts

of the exam to ensure patient comfort and better accommodate the patient's disability?
- Are other resources or equipment needed to complete the examination (e.g., lift equipment, special scales or exam table)?
- For future visits, would it be more appropriate to conduct the visit in the patient's own living environment?
- Were common secondary conditions/complications related to the disability screened for and assessed?
- Were preventive care and health promotion considerations screened for and addressed?

Older Adult Population

The physical examination for the older adults begins with a measurement of weight, height, and blood pressure. The clinician should screen for nutritional concerns in older adults by asking the patient if they has lost any weight in the last 6 months without purposefully attempting to lose weight. Medicare defines BMI in older adults as 23 to 30; a BMI less than 23 is associated with increased mortality. The clinician should monitor weight in the older adult and address any modifiable causes of weight loss (Tatum, Talebreza, & Ross, 2018; Winter, MacInnis, Wattanapenpaiboon, & Nowson, 2014). Unintentional weight loss of 5% or more in older adults over 6 months or less requires further evaluation for poor nutrition or other etiologies. The AGS (2015) does not recommend the use of appetite stimulants or high-calorie supplements. These nutritional supplements do not affect quality of life, mood, functional status, or survival. The clinician should encourage social support, discontinue any medications or address any dental issues that could possibly be interfering with eating, provide appealing food and feeding assistance, and discuss the patient's goals (AGS, 2015).

The physical examination should also include assessment of the patient's gait. Falls are common and often unreported in the older adults. Begin with direct observation as soon as the patient enters the examination room. Observe gait speed. Patients with reduced gait speed are more likely to fall. Patients at risk for falls should have an assessment of orthostatic vital signs, visual acuity testing, gait and balance testing, and medication review and discuss environmental hazards in the home. The USPSTF recommends (Grade B) fall prevention for community-dwelling adults who are aged 65 or older or are at risk for falls (Tatum et al., 2018).

Older adults should have hearing and vision screening completed. Clinicians should assess for objective hearing impairment if the patient or family member or caregiver discusses concerns about the patient's hearing or if the patient's cognition or reported depression could be influenced by hearing loss. Use of the whisper test at 2 feet is an effective testing method (Tatum et al., 2018; see Chapter 11, Evidence-Based Assessment of the Head and Neck, for more information on the hearing assessment.) Visual acuity testing is important in the older adults because decreased visual acuity can lead to increased fall risk, fracture, social isolation, and depression. Common causes of visual impairment in the older adult include macular degeneration, cataracts, glaucoma, refractive errors, and diabetic retinopathy. Vision testing using the Snellen chart can be completed in office. (Tatum et al., 2018; see Chapter 12, Evidence-Based Assessment of the Eye, for more information on visual acuity testing.) The American Optometric Association recommends annual eye examinations in adults aged 65 and older.

EVIDENCE-BASED PRACTICE CONSIDERATIONS

PREVENTIVE CARE CONSIDERATIONS

The USPSTF and the CDC have developed a set of evidence-based recommendations for preventive services. These recommendations were developed to help clinicians work with patients to determine whether preventive services are right for patients given their goals of care and needs. Each recommendation is assigned a letter grade by the USPSTF. For USPSTF recommendations grading criteria please refer to www.uspreventives ervicestaskforce.org/Page/Name/grade-definitions. These letter grades indicate the strength of the evidence and the risk versus benefit of a particular service. The recommendations developed by the USPSTF apply to individuals with no signs or symptoms of the disease noted in the recommendation (USPSTF, 2019). The Agency for Healthcare Research and Quality has developed an electronic preventive services selector application for primary care clinicians to help identify gender- and age-appropriate clinical preventive services. This can be downloaded by accessing the following website: https://epss.ahrq.gov/PDA/index.jsp.

The following are Grade A and B recommendations. Preventive Services with Grade A recommendations are services with a high certainty that the net benefit is substantial (USPSTF, n.d.-a). The suggestion for practice is to offer or provide this service. Grade A recommendations include the following (USPSTF, n.d.-b):

- **Blood pressure screening** in individuals aged 18 years or older; measurements should be obtained outside the office setting prior to confirming or before starting treatment for hypertension (HTN)
- **Cervical cancer screening:**
  ○ Women aged 21 to 29:
    ▪ Cervical cytology alone every 3 years
  ○ Women aged 30 to 65 years:

  ▪ Cervical cytology alone every 3 years
  ▪ High-risk human papillomavirus testing alone every 5 years *or*
  ▪ High-risk human papillomavirus testing in combination with cervical cytology every 5 years
- **Colorectal cancer screening** using fecal occult blood testing, sigmoidoscopy, or colonoscopy in adults, beginning at age 50 years and continuing until age 75 years
- **HIV infection screening** in adolescents and adults aged 15 to 65; younger adolescents and older adults who are at an increased risk should also be screened
- **Syphilis screening** in pregnant and nonpregnant persons at increased risk for infection
- **Tobacco use counseling and interventions** in all adults; advise them to quit using tobacco, and provide behavioral interventions and FDA-approved pharmacotherapy for smoking cessation to nonpregnant adults

Preventive Services with Grade B recommendations are services with a high certainty that the net benefits are moderate or there is moderate certainty that the net benefit is moderate to substantial (USPSTF, n.d.-a). The suggestions for practice are to offer or provide these services. Grade B services include the following (USPSTF, n.d.-b):

- **Abdominal aortic aneurysm (AAA) screening** should be done for men aged 65 to 75 who have ever smoked. The USPSTF and CDC recommend one-time screening for AAA by ultrasonography. Men over age 65 who have ever smoked are at the highest risk of an AAA. Men and women can have an AAA, but it is more common in men (U.S. Department of Health and Human Services, 2019b).
- **Alcohol misuse screening and counseling** should be done for adults aged 18 years or older. Clinicians should provide persons who are at risk for hazardous drinking brief behavioral counseling interventions to reduce alcohol misuse. If patients choose to drink, they should be advised to do so only in moderate amounts. A moderate amount of alcohol means up to 1 drink a day for women and up to 2 drinks a day in men (U.S. Department of Health and Human Services, 2019a). One drink equals 12 ounces of beer, 5 ounces of wine, and 1.5 ounces of liquor. Women who are pregnant or are trying to get pregnant and individuals who have certain health conditions or who take certain medications should be advised to abstain completely from drinking alcohol.
- **Low-dose aspirin** should be initiated for the primary prevention of cardiovascular disease and colorectal cancer in adults aged 50 to 59 who have a 10% or greater 10-year cardiovascular risk, who are not

at increased risk for bleeding, have a life expectancy of at least 10 years, and are willing to take low-dose aspirin daily for at least 10 years.

- **Depression screenings** are recommended in the general adult population, including pregnant and postpartum women. Depression screenings should be implemented with adequate systems in place to ensure accurate diagnosis, effective treatment, and appropriate follow-up.
- **Diabetes screenings** for abnormal blood glucose as part of cardiovascular risk assessment in adults aged 40 to 70 who are overweight or obese. Individuals with abnormal blood glucose should be offered or referred for intensive behavioral counseling interventions to promote a healthy diet and physical activity.
- **Healthy diet and physical activity counseling** to prevent cardiovascular disease should be offered to patients who are overweight or obese and have additional cardiovascular disease risk factors.
- **Fall prevention** for the community-dwelling adult aged 65 years or older who is at an increased risk for falls. Exercise interventions or physical therapy are recommended for those adults at risk.
- **Hepatitis B screening** for adults at high risk for infections. USPSTF strongly recommends screening for hepatitis B virus infection in pregnant women at their first prenatal visit.
- **Hepatitis C virus screening** for adults at high risk for infection. It is also recommended to offer a one-time screening for hepatitis C virus infection to adults born between 1945 and 1965.
- **Lung cancer screening** annually with low-dose computed tomography for adults aged 55 to 80 who have a 30-pack-year smoking history and currently smoke or have quit within the past 15 years. Screening should be discontinued once the individual has not smoked for 15 years or a health problem develops that will substantially limit their life expectancy or the ability or wish to have curative lung surgery.
- **Mammography** is recommended biennially for women aged 50 to 74.
- **Obesity screening and counseling** should be offered to adults with a BMI of 30 or higher. These individuals should be referred or offered intensive, multicomponent behavioral interventions.
- **Behavioral counseling** should be offered for the prevention of STIs for all sexually active adolescents and adults who are at an increased risk for STIs.
- **Low-to-moderate-dose statin use** in adults aged 40 to 75 with no history of cardiovascular disease, one or more cardiovascular disease risk factors, and a calculated 10-year cardiovascular disease event risk of 10% or greater. Lipid screening in adults aged

40 to 75 is required to identify dyslipidemia and calculate the 10-year cardiovascular disease risk.
- **Tuberculosis screening** should be provided for latent tuberculosis infection in adults at increased risk.

Patients should be given appropriate vaccines during the wellness exam. The Advisory Committee on Immunizations (ACIP) is a group of medical and public health professionals who develop evidence-based recommendations on the use of vaccines. The immunizations schedule for adults aged 19 and older developed by the ACIP is as follows (CDC, 2019):

- Influenza: administer one dose annually
- Tetanus, diphtheria, and pertussis (Tdap): administer one dose Tdap, then tetanus diphtheria (Td) booster every 10 years
- Measles, mumps, and rubella (MMR)
  - If not immune (if born in 1957 or later), administer 1 dose of MMR
  - Contraindicated during pregnancy, HIV infection with CD4 count less than 200 cells/microliter, and severe immunocompromising conditions
- Varicella
  - If not immune (if born in 1980 or later), administer 2-dose series of Varicella 4–8 weeks apart if adult never received Varicella containing vaccines (Varicella or measles-mumps-rubella-varicella vaccine for children)
  - If adult previously received 1 dose of Varicella, then wait at least 4 weeks after first dose prior to administering second dose of Varicella
  - Contraindicated during pregnancy, HIV infection with CD4 count less than 200 cells/microliter, and severe immunocompromising conditions
- Pneumococcal:
  - For adults aged 65 or older who have not previously received any pneumococcal vaccine or those with unknown vaccination history:
    - Administer 1 dose of pneumococcal conjugate vaccine (PCV13)
    - Administer 1 dose of pneumococcal polysaccharide vaccine (PPSV23) at least 1 year after PCV13 and at least 5 years after last dose of PPSV23
  - For those adults who previously received 1 dose of PPSV23 at age 65 or older and have not received any doses of PCV13:
    - Administer 1 dose of PCV13 at least 1 year after the dose of PPSV23
    - When both PCV13 and PPSV23 are indicated, administer PCV13 first (PCV13 and PPSV23 should not be administered during same visit)

- Herpes zoster:
  - ○ Recombinant Zoster Vaccine (RZV; preferred)
    - ▪ Administer 2 doses of RZV 2 to 6 months apart to adults aged 50 years or older regardless of receipt of zoster vaccine live (ZVL)
    - ▪ Administer RZV at least 2 months after ZVL
    - ▪ Consider delaying RZV until after pregnancy
  - ○ ZVL
    - ▪ Administer one dose ZVL at age 60 or older if not previously vaccinated (RZV preferred over ZVL)
    - ▪ Contraindicated during pregnancy, HIV infection with CD4 count less than 200 cells/microliter, and severe immunocompromising conditions

CASE STUDY: Wellness Exam

History of Present Illness

A 47-year-old adult female patient, well known to the office, presents for a wellness exam. She voices no acute concerns.

Past Medical History

- Medical history: Varicella, 1977, age 6; seasonal allergies diagnosed age 32; bronchitis March 2016
- Surgical history: Tonsillectomy, April 1983, age 12, no complications
- Obstetric/gynecological: None. Menstruation age 12, 1983. Periods 28-day cycle. Normal bleeding; no cramps
- Health maintenance: Spinning class 3 days a week. Flu vaccine October 2018. Cervical cancer screening October 2017—negative; HIV screening 2017—negative
- Medications: Loratadine 10 mg 1 po q day prn for allergic rhinitis; tylenol as needed for pain and fever, last dose 2 months ago for menstrual cramps; no herbal medications
- Allergies: No drug allergies, no food allergies; seasonal allergies

Family History

- No children
- Father: Deceased age 47, motor vehicle accident
- Mother: Deceased age 45, motor vehicle accident
- Sister: Age 30, alive and in good health
- Brother: Age 32, alive, in good health, has HTN
- Maternal grandmother: Deceased age 100, cause of death Alzheimer's, no other medical conditions
- Maternal grandfather: Deceased age 75, cause of death pneumonia, chronic conditions include HTN
- Paternal grandmother: Deceased age 90, cause of death chronic obstructive pulmonary disease (COPD), chronic conditions include HTN
- Paternal grandfather: Deceased age 95, cause of death complications of a fall, chronic conditions include COPD

Social History

Patient lives in an apartment by herself. She teaches seventh grade. She participates in spinning class 3 days a week. She maintains a low-carbohydrate diet. She wears a seat belt and wears a bike helmet. She has smoke detectors in her home. There are no guns in her home, neighborhood, or work environment. She denies using tobacco or illicit drugs. Drinks one glass (5 ounces) of red wine 4 nights a week. She is heterosexual. Currently, not in a sexual relationship. She feels safe in her home, neighborhood, and work. She has a master's degree in education.

Review of Systems

- Constitutional: Good appetite, denies weight loss, denies fatigue, denies fevers
- Eyes: Denies drainage, denies redness, denies changes in vision, recent eye exam
- Ears: Denies ear pain, denies hearing difficulty
- Nose: Positive for clear drainage during spring and fall season
- Mouth: Denies mouth pain
- Throat: Denies difficulty swallowing, denies having a sore throat
- Cardiovascular: Denies chest pain, denies palpitations
- Respiratory: Denies shortness of breath, denies cough
- Gastrointestinal: Denies abdominal pain, denies constipation or diarrhea, denies heartburn
- Genitourinary: Denies frequent urination, denies urgency
- Musculoskeletal: Denies joint pain or swelling, denies restricted motion
- Integumentary: Denies rashes, changes in moles
- Neurological: denies numbness or tingling, denies burning
- Psychiatric: Denies nervousness, anxiety, depression
- Endocrine: Denies heat or cold intolerance

(continued)

CASE STUDY: Wellness Exam (*continued*)

- Hematological/lymphatic: Denies abnormal bleeding
- Allergic/immunological: Positive for seasonal allergies during spring and fall

Physical Examination
- Vitals: Temperature 98.6°F, pulse 76 beats/min, O_2 saturation 98% on room air, respiration rate 20 breaths/min, blood pressure 125/70 mmHg, 125 lb, BMI 24 kg/m^2
- Constitutional: In no acute distress, pleasant, African American female, dresses appropriately for weather, answers questions appropriately, alert and oriented
- Eyes: Acuity by Snellen chart OD 20/20, OS 20/20. Extraocular movements smooth, symmetrical, no nystagmus. No ptosis. No redness, discharge. Conjunctiva and sclera moist and smooth. Sclera clear, no erythema. Pupils are equal in size and reactive to light and accommodation. Pupils converge evenly. Visual fields full by confrontation. Snellen chart, PERRLA (pupils equal, round, reactive to light and accommodation)

Counseling/Anticipatory Guidance
- PHQ-2 negative
- No falls
- Independent with ADLs
- Advance directive discussion completed; patient not ready to complete advance directives at this time
- Cervical cancer screen every 3 years, last screening 2017, due 2020
- Declines HIV screen
- Fasting blood sugar 90
- Counseled on healthy diet
- Influenza vaccine given at today's visit
- Varicella immune
- Contraception and safe sex discussed
- Dental exam April 2018
- Eye exam May 2018

Laboratory
- No laboratory due at this time

Diagnostics
- No diagnostics due at this time

Clinical Pearls

- Use active listening when collecting a patient's history. Hear what the patient is telling you *and* interpret the words that are both spoken and unspoken to understand the significance of the information being provided.
- Make eye contact and appear engaged during the **patient interview**. Avoid staring at the computer screen while obtaining the history.
- If using an interpreter or if the patient is nonverbal, make sure to speak directly to the patient and not the interpreter or family member. This will ensure the patient does not feel disconnected or disrespected.
- Be cognizant of your dress and appearance. Professional appearance provides credibility and helps to establish trust in your abilities as the clinician.
- Avoid referring to a patient by their disease/condition (e.g., diabetic). Instead, reference the individual as the patient with the disease/condition (e.g., patient with diabetes).

- When documenting, remember the difference between subjective and objective signs and symptoms (**Table 2.6**). Subjective information is what the patient is telling you. Objective information is what you see or observe.

TABLE 2.6 Examples of Subjective Versus Objective Signs and Symptoms

Subjective	Objective
Reports photophobia	Patient comes into office wearing sunglasses due to reported photophobia.
Reports feeling nauseous	Patient has an episode of emesis during visit.
Reports leg pain	Patient is limping.
Reports sore throat	Patient's posterior pharynx is erythematous.
Reports feeling sad	Patient has an elevated PHQ-9 score.

PHQ-9, Patient Health Questionnaire-9.

THE EPISODIC VISIT

The episodic visit, visit for an acute problem, accounts for the majority of visits to the clinician (Yawn, Goodwin, Zyzanski, & Stange, 2003). Episodic care visits focus on a specific concern voiced by the patient. The patient can be either an established patient or a new patient. An established patient refers to a patient who has received professional services from a clinician or clinicians within the same group practice within the previous 3 years. A new patient refers to a patient who has not received any professional services from any clinician within the same group practice within the previous 3 years (CMS MLN, 2017). For an episodic visit, the extent of the history collection and examination is variable and based on the clinician's judgment and the patient's presenting symptom. For new patients, a comprehensive health history should be conducted. For established patients, a more limited health history is collected, tailored to the chief concern. The following list provides the general framework for the elements of history taking. Each element will be explained further within this section.

- Chief concern (CC)
- History of present illness (HPI)
- Past medical history (PMH)
- Family history (FH)
- Social history (SH)
- Review of systems (ROS)

Collecting the history for a first-time visit with a new patient will include all components of the history noted previously: CC, HPI, past medical history, family history, social history, and ROS. In established patients who have been previously evaluated, collecting the history will usually include CC; HPI; a brief update of past medical history, family history, and social history; and ROS (Fortin, Dwamena, Frankel, Lepisto, & Smith, 2019).

Gathering the patient's history is the key to developing the differential diagnosis list and determining the diagnosis. It is important to develop patient-centered interviewing skills. Patient-centered interviewing allows the patient to state what is important to them; expressing personal ideas, concerns, and expectations. Patient-centered interviewing skills are used in conjunction with clinician-centered interviewing skills. With clinician-centered interviewing, clinicians take charge of the patient encounter, gathering data on the patient's symptoms and other information that will aid in determining a diagnosis (Fortin et al., 2019).

Conducting the patient history begins with patient-centered interviewing skills to obtain the patient's perspective. It is important to ask open-ended questions. Open-ended questions allow a patient to articulate on their symptoms, including both personal and emotional information. Open-ended questions delve deeper and often obtain discriminating features of which the patient may not even be aware. Asking open-ended questions and allowing a patient to elaborate on their symptom(s) ultimately saves the clinician time, in addition to providing critical clues to the diagnosis. Clinician-centered interviewing often uses closed-ended questions to obtain answers based on the clinician's perspective. Closed-ended questions elicit a "yes" or "no" or short-phrase response from the patient. Closed-ended questions often make the patient feel like the subject of an interrogation and limits both the patient and the clinician from developing a relationship (Fortin et al., 2019).

KEY HISTORY QUESTIONS AND CONSIDERATIONS

HISTORY OF PRESENT ILLNESS

The HPI begins with the CC. The CC is the patient's main reason for the episodic visit. The CC describes the symptom, problem, condition, or diagnosis for the visit (CMS MLN, 2017). The CC is in the patient's own words. An example of a CC is: "My left elbow hurts," or the patient complains of a painful left elbow.

The HPI is often the most helpful component in developing the differential diagnosis list and determining the diagnosis. In the HPI, the patient provides detailed reasons for the visit. The history of the present illness contains eight core elements:

- Location (e.g., left elbow)
- Quality (e.g., aching, sharp)
- Severity (e.g., 5 on a 1–10 scale)
- Duration (e.g., started 2 days ago)
- Timing (e.g., constant)
- Context (e.g., plays tennis every day, injury)
- Modifying factors (e.g., pain relief on ice application)
- Associated signs and symptoms (e.g., left hand weakness)

To ensure the eight core elements are met, consider using the mnemonic PQRSTU and OLD CARTS. Refer to **Table 2.7**.

It is important for clinicians to allow the patient tell their own story about the reason for the visit. This is part of providing culturally competent care. How the patient perceives their illness is just as important a factor when eliciting the patient history. Consider asking questions such as "What do you think caused your health problems?" "Why do you think it started when it did?" and "What kind of treatment do you think you should receive?" (Kleinman, Eisenberg, & Good, 1978). These questions can provide insight into how to approach the patient's examination, care, and treatment.

TABLE 2.7 Mnemonics for the History of Present Illness

PQRSTU	OLD CARTS
P: Provocation/Palliation What started the symptom? What makes it better or worse? What triggers the symptom?	**O: Onset** When did it start?
Q: Quality/Quantity Explain how the symptom feels: sharp, dull, stabbing, burning, crushing, throbbing, nauseating, shooting, twisting, or stretching	**L: Location** Where is it located?
R: Region/Radiation Where is the symptom located? Does it radiate? Where?	**D: Duration** How long does it last?
S: Severity Scale How severe is the symptom on a scale of 1–10?	**C: Character** Describe in words the quality of the symptom: sharp, dull, stabbing, burning, crushing, throbbing, nauseating, shooting, twisting, or stretching
T: Timing When did the symptom start? How long does it last? Constant? Intermittent?	**A: Aggravating Factors/Associated Symptoms** What makes it worse? What symptoms are associated with the symptom?
U: You How does the symptom affect you?	**R: Relieving Factors** What makes it better?
	T: Timing When did the symptom start? How long does it last? Constant? Intermittent?
	S: Severity How severe is the symptom on a scale of 1–10?

HPI, history of present illness.

PAST MEDICAL HISTORY

During an episodic visit, the past medical history is the point in history taking where the patient identifies important past medical information. This past medical history should include the patient experiences with illnesses both acute and chronic (include pertinent childhood illnesses), surgeries, obstetric/gynecological issues, and hereditary conditions that could place the patient at risk. Also included in the past medical history is health maintenance, for example immunizations and screening tests (Srivastava, 2014).

Within the past medical history, medications and other treatments are reviewed. Review all medications taken: prescribed, over-the-counter, and/or herbal. Review the dose, duration of use, reason for use, and side effects. Review allergies, including allergies to medications, food, and environment. Ascertain allergic reaction with exposure to the allergen (Fortin et al., 2019).

FAMILY HISTORY

The family history is a review of the immediate family members' history related to medical events, illnesses, and hereditary conditions that place the patient's current and future health at risk. Include a review of psychiatric history, addiction, or allergies. Immediate family includes parents, grandparents, siblings, children, and grandchildren. If possible, obtain family history for at least two generations. When the patient is providing the family history, inquire if the person whose history is being provided is alive or deceased. If the person is deceased, ask about the age at death and the cause of death, especially for first-degree relatives (Srivastava, 2014). It's important to inquire about the cause of death, which may identify risk factors for a patient due to family history.

Family genetics can give clues to the clinician as to medical conditions that run in a family. Completing a family history can indicate when a patient has an increased risk of developing a particular condition. Family genetics can identify family members with a higher than usual chance of having a disorder. Family genetics does not indicate that a patient will definitely develop that condition, but that they are at risk for developing that disorder. Some disorders that affect multiple family members are caused by gene mutations. These gene mutations can be passed down to other family members; for example, from parent to child. Gene mutations do not cause all conditions affected by multiple family members. Some conditions are caused by a combination of gene mutations and environmental factors. A genetics professional may be helpful to determine whether conditions in a family are inherited and have a genetic component (U.S. National Library of Medicine, 2019).

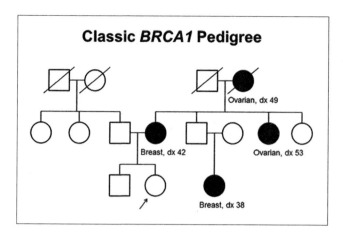

FIGURE 2.1 Classic *BRCA1* pedigree. This pedigree shows some of the classic features of a family with a deleterious *BRCA1* mutation across three generations, including affected family members with breast cancer or ovarian cancer and a young age at onset. *BRCA1* families may exhibit some or all of these features. As an autosomal dominant syndrome, a deleterious *BRCA1* mutation can be transmitted through maternal or paternal lineages, as depicted in the figure.
Source: National Cancer Institute. (2013). Visuals online: Classic BRCA1 pedigree. Retrieved from https://visualsonline.cancer.gov/details.cfm?imageid=10436

Understanding a patient's family genetics and risks helps the clinician to encourage regular checkups or testing for any medical condition that runs in a patient's family. The use of a genogram or pedigree is a graphic representation of a patient's family health history and can be helpful when reviewing a genetic history (**Figure 2.1**). The genogram displays the family's generation and the health disorders that may have moved from one generation to the next. For clinicians, the genogram is an important tool as it can help predict diseases for which the patient may be at risk. Patients can do their own genogram at the CDC website titled *My Family Health Portrait* (https://phgkb.cdc.gov/FHH/html/index.html). Genetic conditions can be inherited in a variety of patterns, depending on the gene involved (e.g., autosomal dominant [**Figure 2.2**], autosomal recessive, X-linked dominant, X-linked recessive [**Figure 2.3**], Y-linked, codominant, mitochondrial, and polygenic). If any red flags are present, as represented in **Box 2.1**, a referral to genetic counseling is necessary.

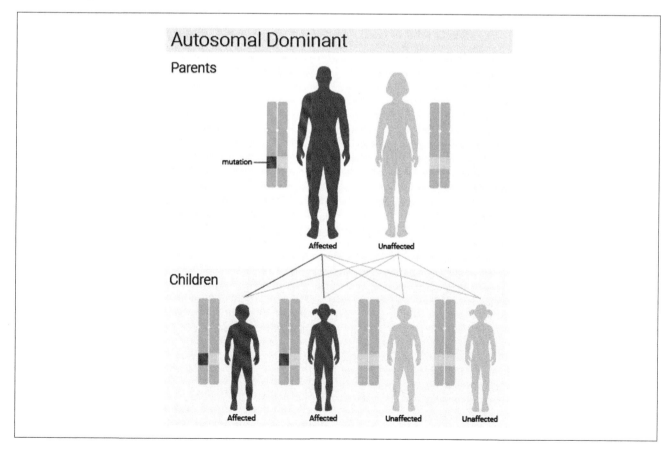

FIGURE 2.2 Autosomal dominant inheritance pattern by one parent.
Source: U.S. National Library of Medicine Genetics Home Reference. (2015a). *Autosomal dominant inheritance.* Bethesda, MD: The Library. Retrieved from https://ghr.nlm.nih.gov/gallery

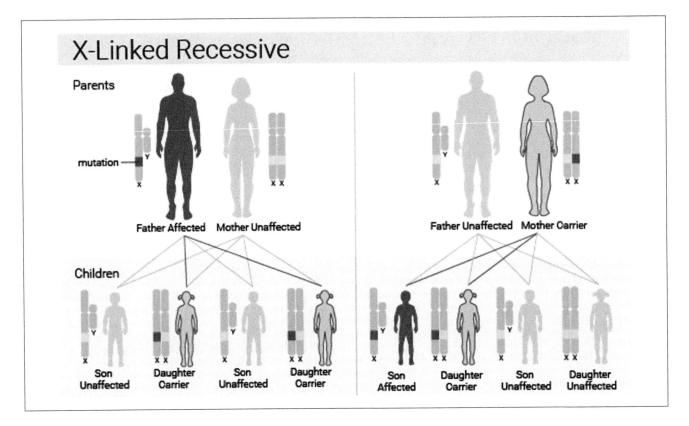

FIGURE 2.3 X-linked recessive inheritance pattern.

Source: U.S. National Library of Medicine Genetics Home Reference. (2015b). *X-linked recessive inheritance.* Bethesda, MD: The Library. Retrieved from https://ghr.nlm.nih.gov/gallery?start=60

BOX 2.1
RED FLAGS THAT REQUIRE GENETIC COUNSELING

- Significant family medical history—breast, ovarian, prostate, colon, melanoma, pancreatic, or other cancers
- Cancer occurs in every generation
- Early age of onset (<50 years)
- Condition in the less-often-affected sex (e.g., male breast cancer)
- Bilateral cancer, or multiple primary cancers in one individual
- Known family genetic mutation
- Ethnicity predisposition to certain genetic disorders (e.g., Ashkenazi Jewish ancestry)
- Consanguinity

Sources: Aiello, L. B., & Chiatti, B. D. (2017). Primer in genetics and genomics, article 4-inheritance patterns. *Biological Research for Nursing, 19*(4), 465–472. doi: 10.1177/1099800417708616 and Crockett-Maillet, G. (2010). Know the red flags of hereditary cancers. *Nurse Practitioner, 35*(7), 39–43. doi:10.1097/01.NPR.0000383660.45156.40

SOCIAL HISTORY

The patient's social history provides information regarding the patient's life, which includes the patient's behaviors and personal choices that may impact disease risk, disease severity, and health outcomes (Fortin et al., 2019). These questions can identify risk factors, which open the door to addressing unhealthy behaviors, and provide insight into potential vulnerabilities of the patient.

The social history addresses (Fortin et al., 2019):

- Occupation: Note exposure to toxic chemicals, injuries, industry-specific job hazards, and stress.
- Health promotion: Assessing diet and screening for bulimia/anorexia is important owing to increasing incidence of obesity and identifying eating disorders. Identify exercise patterns versus sedentary lifestyle.
- Safety: Screen for use of seat belts, bicycle/motorcycle helmets, smoke detectors in home, and guns in home, neighborhood, and at work.
- Substance use:
  - Tobacco: Include all forms of tobacco (pipe, snuff, chewing tobacco, e-cigarettes, hookah, dissolvable products, cigars, and cigarettes). Determine

quantity. For cigarettes, ask about number of pack years for cigarettes (packs smoked per day multiplied by number of years of smoking). Currently using tobacco? Used tobacco in the past? Assess age at which patient started using tobacco; if no longer using tobacco ask about quit date. Assess for type of tobacco.

○ Alcohol: If the patient drinks alcohol, ask about quantity. How often? What type of alcohol?

○ Illicit drugs: Assess type of illicit drug(s) and frequency of use. Assess quantity of use. Consider asking, "Do you currently take, or have you taken in the past, any illicit drugs? If so, which ones?" (Srivastava, 2014).

○ Living arrangement and personal relationships: Does the patient live in an apartment, home, dormitory, prison, assisted living, and so on? Whom does the patient live with: mom, dad, spouse, children, and so on?

○ Sexuality: Assess for patient's sexual orientation or practices. Assess gender identity. Tailor questions to the particular patient encounter (Srivastava, 2014).

○ Intimate partner violence/abuse: Assess for safety in current relationship. Report abuse as required by state law. Provide resources needed for a safe place and for an emergency.

○ Stress: Assess amount of stress, whether it is acute or chronic, and whether it occurs across multiple settings. What are the primary causes of their stress?

○ Mood: Screen for depression using a valid, reliable screening tool such as the PHQ-9 or PHQ-2 to confirm diagnosis and its severity.

○ Health literacy: Health literacy assessment assesses the patient's ability to obtain, process, and understand health information. This, in turn, affects the patient's ability to make healthcare decisions regarding prevention and treatment. Be mindful of a patient's health literacy (Srivastava, 2014).

○ Social determinants: Social determinants of health include the patient's circumstances in which they are born and live and how this affects their health. These circumstances include socioeconomic and cultural factors, accessibility to healthcare and education, safe environmental conditions, safe neighborhoods, utility needs, housing instability, and the availability of healthy food on a reliable basis (NEJM Catalyst, 2017).

REVIEW OF SYSTEMS

The ROS assesses the other systems or problems not already discussed in the history of the present illness (Fortin et al., 2019). It is a review of body systems

obtained by asking open-ended questions to note signs and/or symptoms the patient may be or has been experiencing. There are three different types of ROS: the problem-pertinent ROS, the extended ROS, and the complete ROS. An example of the systems included in the ROS is as follows:

- Constitution systems (include fatigue, weight loss, fever)
- Head, eyes, ears, nose, mouth, throat (HEENT)
- Cardiovascular
- Respiratory
- Gastrointestinal
- Genitourinary
- Musculoskeletal
- Integumentary
- Neurological
- Psychiatric
- Endocrine
- Hematological/lymphatic
- Allergic/immunological

Problem-Pertinent Review of Systems

A problem-pertinent ROS includes a review of the systems directly related to the CC, the problem identified in the history of the present illness. Example:

- Chief concern: "My left elbow hurts."
- System reviewed: Musculoskeletal
- ROS:
  ○ Musculoskeletal: Positive for left elbow joint pain; denies left elbow joint swelling or restricted motion in the left elbow joint

Extended Review of Systems

An extended ROS includes a review of the system directly related to the CC in addition to a limited number of (2–9) additional systems reviewed. Example:

- Chief concern: "My left elbow hurts."
- Systems reviewed: Constitutional, musculoskeletal, neurological
- ROS:
  ○ Constitutional: Denies fatigue, weight loss, or fever
  ○ Musculoskeletal: Positive for left elbow joint pain; denies swelling or restricted motion in the left elbow joint
  ○ Neurological: Denies numbness, sensation loss, or burning in left upper extremity and hand (CMS MLN, 2017)

Complete Review of Systems

With a complete ROS, the system related to the CC, or presenting symptom, is reviewed along with a minimum of 10 other systems. The system reviewed should have positive and negative findings documented. The following is an example of a complete ROS:

- Chief concern: "My left elbow hurts"
- Systems reviewed: Constitutional, HEENT, cardiovascular, respiratory, gastrointestinal, genitourinary, musculoskeletal, integumentary, neurological, and hematologic/lymphatic
- ROS:
  - Constitutional: Denies fatigue, weight loss, or fever
  - HEENT: Denies blurred vision, hearing loss, nasal drainage, or sore throat
  - Cardiovascular: Denies chest pain, denies palpitations
  - Respiratory: Denies shortness of breath on exertion
  - Gastrointestinal: +Good appetite, denies nausea
  - Genitourinary: Denies incontinence, denies burning
  - Musculoskeletal: Positive for left elbow joint pain; denies swelling or restricted motion in the left elbow joint
  - Integumentary: Denies rashes, lesions, or calor to left elbow or arm.
  - Neurological: Denies numbness, sensation loss, or burning in left upper extremity and hand (CMS MLN, 2017)
  - Psychiatric: Denies feeling down, depressed, or hopeless
  - Hematologic/lymphatic: Denies bruising or enlarged lymph nodes (CMS MLN, 2017)

PHYSICAL EXAMINATION

Like history taking, the type and extent of the physical examination is directed by the CC (the presenting problem), the patient's history, and the clinician's judgment. Findings from the patient history will lead the clinician to clues for conducting the physical examination. The physical examination may involve several organ systems, a single organ system, several body areas, or a single body area. There are four types of physical examinations—the problem-focused, expanded problem-focused, detailed exam, and the comprehensive exam.

- *Problem-focused*: Limited exam of the affected body area or organ system
- *Expanded problem-focused*: Limited exam of the affected organ system or body area and other related or symptomatic organ systems or body areas
- *Detailed exam*: Expanded exam of the affected organ system or body area and other related or symptomatic organ systems or body areas

- *Comprehensive*: Multisystem exam or a complete examination of a single organ system

When documenting the physical examination, include a description of objective abnormal and relevant negative findings of the physical examination of a particular organ system or body area. In addition, include a description of any abnormal or unexpected findings from the physical examination of any asymptomatic organ system or body area (CMS MLN, 2017). The body systems of the physical examination are as follows. Refer to the chapter noted for the exam technique for that particular body system:

- Constitutional (Chapters 5 and 8)
- Skin (Chapter 9)
- Lymphatics (Chapter 10)
- HEENT (Chapters 11–13)
- Neck (Chapter 11)
- Respiratory (Chapter 7)
- Heart (Chapter 6)
- Breast (Chapter 17)
- Abdomen (Chapter 16)
- Genitourinary:
  - Male genitalia (Chapter 19)
  - Female genitalia (Chapter 20)
- Musculoskeletal (Chapter 15)
- Vascular (Chapter 6)
- Neurological (Chapter 14)
- Psychiatric (Chapter 22)

The body areas of the physical examination include:

- Head, including the face
- Neck
- Chest, including breast and axillae
- Abdomen
- Genitalia, groin, buttocks
- Back, including spine
- Extremities

EVIDENCE-BASED PRACTICE CONSIDERATIONS

When considering laboratory and imaging considerations, refer to Choosing Wisely® (www.choosingwisely.org). Choosing Wisely promotes conversations between clinicians and patients aimed at reducing unnecessary tests and procedures. Choosing Wisely is supported by evidence to assist in reducing unnecessary tests and treatments in healthcare and works with clinicians to overcome barriers to delivering high-value care (Choosing Wisely, n.d.). Referring to Choosing Wisely will assist the clinician in ordering only necessary testing and diagnostics, which will aid in reducing the healthcare burden for both the patient and the healthcare system.

CASE STUDY: Episodic Visit

Chief Concern

"I have had a cough for about a week that is keeping me up at night."

History of Present Illness

This is a 47-year-old female patient, well known to the office, presenting with a cough for 1 week. Cough has become progressively worse over the past week. Patient states the cough is nonproductive. Patient denies fever but reports increased fatigue and sore throat. Has tried generic cough medicine every 8 hours, without relief. Cough is worse at night. No sick contacts. No recent travel. Had a cough like this last year, diagnosed with seasonal allergies.

Past Medical History

- Surgical history: Benign cyst removal from neck in 2010
- Medical history: HTN, environmental allergies
- Obstetric/gynecological: None
- Health maintenance: Spinning class 3 days a week. Flu vaccine October 2018
- Medications: Losartan 25 mg every day for HTN; dextromethorphan 2 tsp every 8 hours (last dose today at 2 p.m.) for cough, tylenol as needed for pain and fever, last dose 2 months ago; no herbal medications
- Allergies: No drug allergies, seasonal allergies

Family History

- No children
- Father: Deceased age 47, motor vehicle accident
- Mother: Deceased age 45, motor vehicle accident
- Sister: Age 30, alive and in good health
- Brother: Age 32, alive, in good health, has HTN
- Maternal grandmother: Deceased age 100, cause of death Alzheimer's, no other medical conditions
- Maternal grandfather: Deceased age 60, cause of death heart attack, chronic conditions include HTN, coronary artery disease
- Paternal grandmother: Deceased age 90, cause of death COPD, chronic condition HTN
- Paternal grandfather: Deceased age 75, cause of death heart attack, chronic conditions COPD, coronary artery disease

Social History

Patient lives in an apartment by herself. She teaches seventh grade. She participates in spinning class 3 days a week. She maintains a low-carbohydrate diet. She wears seat belts and wears a bike helmet. She has smoke detectors in her home. There are no guns in her home, neighborhood, or work environment. She denies any tobacco use or illicit drugs. Drinks one glass of red wine four nights a week. She is heterosexual and currently not in a sexual relationship. She feels safe in her home, neighborhood, and work. She has a master's degree in education.

Review of Systems

- Constitutional: Good appetite, denies weight loss
- Eyes: Denies drainage, denies redness
- Ears: Denies ear pain
- Nose: Reports some clear drainage, nasal congestion
- Throat and mouth: Denies difficulty swallowing, positive for sore throat; denies mouth pain
- Cardiovascular: Denies chest pain
- Respiratory: Denies shortness of breath
- Gastrointestinal: Denies abdominal pain, denies constipation or diarrhea
- Psychiatric: Denies anxiety, denies depression

Physical Examination

- Vitals: Temperature 97.5°F, pulse 76 beats/min, O_2 saturation 98% on room air, respiration rate 20 breaths/min, blood pressure 125/70 mmHg
- Constitutional: In no acute distress, pleasant, African American female, dresses appropriately for weather
- Head: Atraumatic, normocephalic, no pain with palpation
- Eyes: PERRLA, EOM intact, conjunctiva pink, sclera white
- Ears: External ears no lesions, nontender, tympanic membranes pearly gray, translucent bilateral
- Nose: Septum midline, inferior and middle turbinates boggy
- Throat and mouth: Teeth present in good dentition, tongue no lesions, gums and mucosa no bleeding, pharynx erythematous bilateral, tonsils 1+ without edema or exudate
- Neck: Normal ROM, trachea midline
- Lungs: Respirations regular and unlabored; lung fields resonant to percussion; all lung fields clear to auscultation without adventitious breath sounds
- Heart: Heart rate and rhythm regular, S1 heard best at apex, normal intensity, S2 heard best at base, no clicks, rubs, gallops, or murmurs

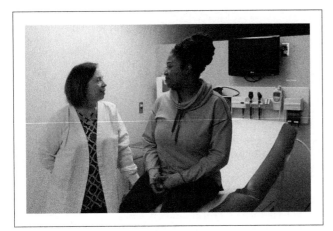

FIGURE 2.4 Clinician demeanor during history taking, remaining cognizant of personal biases, facial expressions, and body language.

 Clinical Pearls

- Use sensitivity and respect when collecting a patient's social history; display nonjudgmental behavior. Social history questions can be personal, and a patient may be reluctant to share social history for fear of embarrassment and being judged.
- Be cognizant of personal biases, facial expressions, and body language (**Figure 2.4**).
- Repeat what the patient has said in your own words to ensure you understand what is being said. This also reassures the patient that you are engaged and listening.
- Use simple words and avoid medical jargon during the clinical interview.

THE CHRONIC CARE MANAGEMENT VISIT

Six in ten adults in the United States have a chronic condition, and four in ten adults in the United States have two or more chronic diseases (CDC, n.d.-d). Chronic conditions are among the leading causes of death and disability. They include the following:

- Heart disease
- Cancer
- Chronic lung disease
- Stroke
- Alzheimer's disease
- Diabetes
- Chronic kidney disease

Quality chronic care management for patients with multiple chronic conditions requires ongoing care by the clinician. Patients receiving chronic care management have at least two or more chronic conditions that are expected to last at least 12 months. These chronic conditions place the patient at risk for adverse health events. Chronic care management includes face-to-face visits along with non–face-to-face visits. Examples of non–face-to-face visits include communicating with the patient via telephone and email, coordinating care with other clinicians, and managing medication refills (Garwood, Korkis, Mohammad, Lepczyk, & Risko, 2016).

The focus of chronic care management is the patient's relationship with the healthcare team (not just the clinician); establishing and achieving individual health goals; coordination of community and social services; medical, functional, and psychosocial assessment; and preventive care (Garwood et al., 2016). The results from the medical, functional, and psychosocial assessment are used to develop the patient's comprehensive treatment plan. The treatment plan should include lifestyle modifications, pharmacological interventions, self-management support, and education. When developing the treatment plan, it is important to take into account the patient's health literacy, functional abilities, cognitive abilities, socioeconomic status, social determinants, and the patient's motivation and willingness to change (Timpel et al., 2017). A comprehensive care plan includes the following (CMS MLN, 2019):

- Problem list
- Expected outcome and prognosis
- Measurable treatment goals
- Symptom management
- Planned interventions and identification of the individuals responsible for interventions
- Medication management
- Community/social services ordered
- A description of how services of agencies and specialists outside the practice will be directed/coordinated
- Schedule for periodic review and, if needed, revision of the care plan

Lifestyle plays an important role in the risk for chronic disease. Tobacco use and exposure to secondhand smoke, poor nutrition, lack of physical activity, and excessive alcohol use have been found to be key contributors to increasing a patient's risk of acquiring a chronic disease (CDC, n.d.-c). Poor lifestyle choices in diet and exercise have lead to 39.8% of United States adults being obese (BMI 30 or greater; CDC, n.d.-a) and 18.5% of children and adolescents being obese (CDC, n.d.-b). Chronic conditions also contribute to an individual's capability of performing one or more ADLs. For example, individuals diagnosed with diabetes between the ages of 20 and 74 are at increased risk for further complicating chronic conditions such as kidney failure, nontraumatic lower extremity amputations, and blindness, which can all contribute to a patient's inability to perform their ADLs (Zamosky, 2013). A patient's inability to perform ADLs can have significant consequences for the patient, often leading to loss of personal independence and possible placement in an assisted living or long-term care facility.

Because of the huge impact that a patient's lifestyle has on the risk of chronic disease, greater emphasis during **chronic care visits** is placed on counseling for lifestyle modifications and risky behaviors. Time must be spent on motivation interviewing and mutual decision-making as to the kind of treatments and behavior modifications that are needed over a longer period of time (Zamosky, 2013). Successful lifestyle modifications include self-monitoring, feedback, and problem-solving, as well as motivation and support. Patients need ongoing support from family and friends and counseling from healthcare professionals (Ylimäki, Kanste, Heikkinen, Bloigu, & Kyngäs, 2015).

To better manage chronic care conditions, innovative strategies have been put into place, including health coaching, team-based care, and group visits. Health coaching improves quality of care and can be cost effective for patients with chronic conditions. Health coaches work with patients to set small achievable goals, develop action plans, overcome barriers, and reinforce the clinician's treatment plan. Health coaches encourage and reinforce patient's self-management strategies (Gastala, Wingrove, Gaglioti, Liaw, & Bazemore, 2018).

Team-based care allows the clinician to delegate services to trained members of the healthcare team. Team-based care improves quality of care, reduces healthcare costs, and provides a more patient-centered type of care. Possible members of a healthcare team include the clinician, nurse, medical assistant, health coach, pharmacist, social worker, dietitians, and exercise specialists. Teams work together with the patient to achieve shared goals, often coordinating care across settings (Szafran, Kennett, Bell, & Green, 2018).

Group visits are another innovative strategy that have been proven to be effective in chronic care management. Group visits allow individuals with the same chronic condition, such as diabetes, to share the same visit. Group visits allow the clinician to spend more time with patients; in addition, patients have an opportunity to interact with other patients who have the same chronic condition. Group visits are an effective way to encourage patients and provide shared strategies to better manage chronic conditions. Group visits

improve patient satisfaction and improve outcomes (Zamosky, 2013).

KEY HISTORY QUESTIONS AND CONSIDERATIONS

HISTORY OF PRESENT ILLNESS

The HPI details the specific reason(s) why the patient is presenting to the clinician. Chronic care visits allow the clinician to monitor the patient's chronic disease process, making it sometimes difficult to document the elements included in the HPI. There are two options for documenting the chronic care visit for a stable condition. One option is to document the elements of the history of the present illness, but another option is to document the status of the chronic or active conditions being addressed in the visit instead of the elements of the history of the present illness (Caux-Harry, 2014). Let's take the example of a patient with poorly controlled diabetes, stable HTN, and stable hyperlipidemia presenting for a chronic care visit to monitor the status of the patient's chronic conditions. For this example, the clinician decides to document the status of the chronic conditions. The documentation would be: "the patient presents today for a follow-up on his type 2 diabetes, which is currently not controlled, medication-controlled HTN, and hyperlipidemia, which is controlled with diet and exercise." The documentation notes the three chronic conditions and the status of each. But what if the clinician decides to document using the elements of the history of the present illness. This documentation would be as follows: "The patient states his blood sugars have been found to be low over the past few days, especially early morning. He has been working evening shift and has not been eating a snack before bed. The patient states he awakens early morning feeling dizzy and sweating. He states after he eats breakfast his blood sugar readings return to normal."

- Severity: Moderate
- Duration: Over the past few days
- Timing: Early morning
- Context: Not eating a snack at night
- Modifying factors: Eating breakfast
- Associated signs and symptoms: Dizziness and sweating

PAST MEDICAL, FAMILY, AND SOCIAL HISTORY

Collecting the past medical, family, and social histories for a chronic care management visit incorporates the same collection techniques as in the wellness exam and episodic visit. For more details on collecting this portion of the history, refer to the wellness and episodic visit sections.

REVIEW OF SYSTEMS

The ROS is the patient's self-report of their experience with the organ systems associated with the chronic condition, along with any new presenting symptom. The ROS includes the pertinent positive and negative findings. The ROS is subjective information provided by the patient, not the clinician's observation (Phillips, 2017). Collecting the ROS during the chronic care management visit focuses on the chronic conditions, a review of any additional organ system related to each chronic condition, and an assessment for comorbidities, which are common in patients with chronic illnesses. The ROS for the chronic care management exam is no different than the collection of the ROS previously discussed. See the wellness exam's ROS and the episodic visit's ROS sections for complete details on collecting a ROS.

REVIEW OF SYSTEMS, PAST MEDICAL HISTORY, FAMILY HISTORY, AND SOCIAL HISTORY

Often, when a patient presents for a follow-up visit for a stable chronic condition, it is difficult to document any changes in the ROS, past medical history, family history, and social history from the previous patient encounter. It is important to note that the entire ROS, past medical history, family history, and social history do not have to be repeated if there is evidence that the clinician reviewed the information and updated any previous information from an earlier patient encounter. An example of updating previous information includes describing any new ROS information, past medical history, family history, and social history information, and also noting if there have been any changes to the information previously collected. The clinician must include in the documentation the date and location of the earlier patient encounter (Moore, 2010).

PREVENTIVE CARE CONSIDERATIONS

Preventive care considerations for a chronic care management visit can be found in the Wellness Exam section under the Evidence-Based Practice Considerations heading, preventive care considerations. Chronic conditions also feature a unique set of preventive considerations aimed at reducing complications of the disease and positively affecting short- and long-term health outcomes. Current evidence-based clinical guidelines for the specific chronic condition(s) should be incorporated into each visit.

PHYSICAL EXAMINATION

The physical exam for a chronic care visit is system based and will be directed by the chronic conditions, the patient's subjective history, and the clinician's judgment. The patient's chronic conditions and findings from the patient history collection will lead the clinician to the organ systems or body areas to be assessed during the physical examination. The physical examination for a patient with multiple chronic conditions should involve several body systems (CMS MLN, 2017). The physical examination completed in the management of chronic conditions is generally not as time intensive as the physical examinations for episodic visits. Chronic care examinations have a greater percentage of time spent in history taking, assessing medication adherence, overcoming patient barriers, and discussing preventive care services. In addition, a large amount of time is also spent providing advice regarding lifestyle modifications and risk reductions such as advice regarding exercise, nutrition, and health promotion strategies (Yawn et al., 2003).

The four types of physical examinations discussed in the episodic visit section are to be used during the chronic care management physical examination. These four visit types are problem-focused, expanded problem-focused, detailed exam, and the comprehensive exam. Refer to the episodic visit's Physical Examination section for complete details regarding the physical examination.

LABORATORY CONSIDERATIONS

Laboratory consideration for chronic care exams are based on the chronic condition, the patient's history, physical exam findings, current evidence-based guidelines recommendations, patient preference, and the clinician's judgment.

EVIDENCE-BASED PRACTICE CONSIDERATIONS

Clinical practice guidelines are evidence-based resources that provide guidance and recommendations on the management of a specific condition. Clinical practice guidelines are based on clinical evidence and expert opinion (Graham, Mancher, Wolman, Greenfield, & Steinberg, 2011). Using clinical practice guidelines for clinical decision-making in the management of a chronic condition is an effective way to improve the quality of healthcare for patients with a chronic condition. But for those adults with multiple chronic conditions (six in ten adults in the United States have a chronic condition, and four in ten adults in the United States have two or more chronic diseases [CDC, n.d.-d]), using clinical practice guidelines for each chronic condition may result in care that is ineffective and impractical and may place an unsustainable treatment burden on the patient. Clinical practice guidelines give detailed recommendations for managing a single condition, but the guidelines often fail to address the needs and priorities unique to patients with multiple chronic conditions (Timpel et al., 2017). Caring for patients with multiple chronic conditions requires a balance between following clinical practice guidelines and adjusting the recommendations for individual patient needs and unique situations (Boyd et al., 2005; Timpel et al., 2017). Clinical practice guidelines are evidence-based recommendations that require the clinician's clinical judgment and patient preferences when used in the management of patients with multiple chronic conditions. Clinical practice guidelines should be used to enhance the clinician and patient's collaboration for developing treatment plans.

CASE STUDY: Chronic Care Management

History of Present Illness

A 47-year-old adult female patient, well known to the primary care clinician, presents today for a follow-up visit on her stable type 2 diabetes, medication-controlled HTN, and hyperlipidemia, which is controlled with diet and exercise. Patient states her blood sugars have been well controlled with diet and exercise; fasting blood sugar ranges from 80 to 110 every morning. HTN controlled with losartan 25 mg daily. Blood pressure readings at home range from a high of 124/70 mmHg to a low of 110/62 mmHg. Hyperlipidemia controlled with diet and exercise. Attends spinning class 3 days a week, lifts weights 2 days a week. Follows an 1,800 calorie azodicarbonamide (ADA) diet. Last visit to this primary care office was 3 months ago, August 2018.

Past Medical History

Past medical (including medications and allergies), family, and social histories have been reviewed from patient's most recent visit 3 months ago, August 13, 2018. There have been no changes to the past medical history, medications or allergies, family history, or social history collected 3 months ago, August 13, 2018, at this primary care office.

Review of Systems

ROS has been reviewed from patient's most recent visit 3 months ago, August 13, 2018. There have been no changes to the ROS collected 3 months ago, August 13, 2018, at this primary care office.

Physical Examination
- Vitals: Temperature 97.5°F, pulse 76 beats/min, O_2 saturation 98% on room air, respiration rate 20 breaths/min, blood pressure 120/70 mmHg, 125 lb, BMI 24 kg/m^2
- Constitutional: In no acute distress, pleasant, African American female, dresses appropriately for weather

- Head: Atraumatic, normocephalic
- Eyes: PERRLA, EOM intact, conjunctiva pink, sclera white, vision grossly intact and fundoscopic examination is unremarkable, positive red reflex bilateral; Snellen 20/20 bilateral
- Ears: External ears no lesions, nontender, TMs gray, translucent bilateral
- Nose: Septum midline, inferior and middle turbinates boggy
- Throat and mouth: Teeth present in good dentition, tongue no lesions, gums and mucosa no bleeding, pharynx pink, tonsils 1+ bilateral
- Neck: Normal ROM, trachea midline, no JVD, thyroid palpable, thyroid and cartilages move with swallowing, no nodules, no tenderness
- Lungs: Respirations regular, unlabored; lung fields resonant to percussion; lungs clear to auscultation in all lung fields, no adventitious breath sounds
- Heart: Heart rate and rhythm regular, S1 heard best at apex, normal intensity; S2 heard best at base, normal splitting, and no clicks, rubs, gallops, or murmurs
- Abdomen: No tenderness with palpation
- Skin: No acanthosis nigricans noted, no rashes
- Neurological: Gait steady, cranial nerves II–XII intact, sensation intact bilateral
- Foot exam: Positive DP and PT pulses, positive monofilament sensation, warm to touch, vibration felt in toes bilaterally; nails trimmed; no callus, no wounds, no deformities bilaterally; +2 Achilles reflexes
- Vascular: No edema bilaterally

Counseling/Anticipatory Guidance
- PHQ-2 negative
- Influenza vaccine given at today's visit
- Dental exam April 2018
- Podiatrist exam July 2018
- Physical activity: At least 150 min/wk of moderate intensity aerobic physical activity

(continued)

CASE STUDY: Chronic Care Management (*continued*)

- Foot care: Avoid going barefoot, test water temperature before stepping into tub, trim toenails to shape of toe, wash and check feet daily, shoes should be not be tight, socks should fit and be changed daily
- Self-management of blood sugar fasting every morning
- Self-management of blood pressure
- Continue losartan 25 mg every day, continue baby aspirin every day

Referrals
- Dilated and comprehensive eye examination by an ophthalmologist annually, last visit November 2017

- Dietitian referral for medical nutrition therapy (has never had referral)

Laboratory
- Hemoglobin A1C (A1C; last lab 3 months ago August 2018, 6.5%)
- Thyroid function tests (last lab 1 year ago)
- Fasting lipid profile (last lab 1 year ago)
- Serum creatinine and glomerular filtration rate (GFR) (last lab 1 year ago)
- Microalbuminuria (last lab 1 year ago)

Diagnostics
No diagnostics

Clinical Pearls

- The use of silence is important to any visit. Silence allows the patient time to reflect on the question and provide a more accurate response (Figure 2.5).

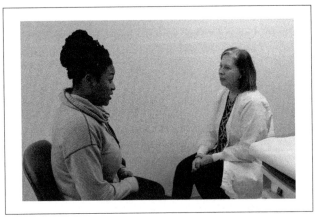

FIGURE 2.5 Clinician remaining silent to allow the patient time to reflect on the question and provide a more accurate response.

Key Takeaways

Wellness, episodic, and chronic care management visits are the three main types of patient visits.

- The approach to history taking and physical examination will change depending on the reason for the patient visit.
- Clinicians should incorporate open-ended communication, reflective listening, empathy, and the patient's values and preferences into every visit.
- A thorough patient history consists of the chief concern, history of present illness, past medical history, medication and allergy history, family history, social history, and review of systems.
- Clinician visits with older adults and patients with disabilities have unique considerations.
- Preventive care considerations should be addressed at every type of visit and should be evidence-based.

REFERENCES

Aiello, L. B., & Chiatti, B. D. (2017). Primer in genetics and genomics, article 4-inheritance patterns. *Biological Research for Nursing, 19*(4), 465–472. doi:10.1177/1099800417708616

American College of Obstetricians and Gynecologists. (2018). *Medicare screening services 2018.* Retrieved from https://www.acog.org/-/media/Departments/Coding/Screening-Services-2018_final.pdf

American Geriatrics Society. (2015). *Ten things clinicians and patients should question.* Retrieved from http://www.choosingwisely.org/societies/american-geriatrics-society

American Geriatrics Society Beers Criteria Expert Panel. (2019). American Geriatrics Society 2019 updated AGS Beers Criteria for potentially inappropriate medication use in older adults. *Journal of the American Geriatric Society, 67*(4), 674–694. doi:10.1111/jgs.15767

Benedetti, F., Carlino, E., & Pollo, A. (2011). How placebos change the patient's brain. *Neuropsychopharmacology*, *36*, 339–354. doi:10.1038/npp.2010.81

Bloomfield, H. E., & Wilt, T. J. (2011, October). Evidence brief: Role of the annual comprehensive physical examination in the asymptomatic adult. In Department of Veterans Affairs (Ed.), *VA evidence-based synthesis program evidence briefs* [Internet]. Washington, DC: Department of Veterans Affairs. Retrieved from https://www.ncbi.nlm.nih.gov/books/NBK82767

Boyd, C. M., Darer, J., Boult, C., Fried, L. P., Boult, L., & Wu, A. W. (2005). Clinical practice guidelines and quality of care for older patients with multiple comorbid diseases: Implications for pay for performance. *The Journal of the American Medical Association*, *294*(6), 716–724. doi:10.1001/jama.294.6.716

Bramhall, E. (2014). Effective communications skills in nursing practice. *Nursing Standard*, *29*(14), 53–59. doi:10.7748/ns.29.14.53.e9355

Caux-Harry, R. (2014). E & M Guidelines: HPI and chronic conditions. Retrieved from https://www.3mhisinsideangle.com/blog-post/em-guidelines-hpi-and-chronic-conditions

Centers for Disease Control and Prevention. (n.d.-a). Adult obesity facts. Retrieved from https://www.cdc.gov/obesity/data/adult.html

Centers for Disease Control and Prevention. (n.d.-b). *Childhood obesity facts*. Retrieved from https://www.cdc.gov/obesity/data/childhood.html

Centers for Disease Control and Prevention. (n.d.-c). *National Center for Chronic Disease Prevention and Health Promotion (NCCDPHP): About chronic diseases*. Retrieved from https://www.cdc.gov/chronicdisease/about/index.htm

Centers for Disease Control and Prevention. (n.d.-d). *National Center for Chronic Disease Prevention and Health Promotion (NCCDPHP): Chronic diseases in America*. Retrieved from https://www.cdc.gov/chronicdisease/resources/infographic/chronic-diseases.htm

Centers for Disease Control and Prevention. (2015). *Check for safety: A home fall prevention checklist for older adults*. Retrieved from https://www.cdc.gov/steadi/pdf/check_for_safety_brochure-a.pdf

Centers for Disease Control and Prevention. (2019). *Recommended adult immunization schedule for ages 19 years or older, United States, 2019*. Retrieved from https://www.cdc.gov/vaccines/schedules/downloads/adult/adult-combined-schedule.pdf

Centers for Medicare & Medicaid Services. (2019). *CMS roadmap: Fighting the opioid crisis*. Retrieved from https://www.cms.gov/About-CMS/Agency-Information/Emergency/Downloads/Opioid-epidemic-roadmap.pdf

Centers for Medicare & Medicaid Services Medicare Learning Network. (2017, August). *Evaluation and management services*. Retrieved from https://www.cms.gov/Outreach-and-Education-Medicare-Learning-Network-MLN/MLNProducts/Downloads/eval-mgmt-serv-guide-ICN006764.pdf

Centers for Medicare & Medicaid Services Medicare Learning Network. (2018, August). *Annual wellness visit*. Retrieved from https://www.cms.gov/Outreach-and-Education/Medicare-Learning-Network-MLN/MLNProducts/downloads/awv_chart_icn905706.pdf

Centers for Medicare & Medicaid Services Medicare Learning Network. (2019, July). *Chronic care management services*. Retrieved from https://www.cms.gov/Outreach-and-Education/Medicare-Learning-Network-MLN/MLNProducts/Downloads/ChronicCareManagement.pdf

Choosing Wisely. (n.d.). *Our mission*. Retrieved from http://www.choosingwisely.org/our-mission

Choosing Wisely. (2017). *Health checkups: When you need them and when you don't*. Retrieved from http://www.choosingwisely.org/patient-resources/health-checkups

Crockett-Maillet, G. (2010). Know the red flags of hereditary cancers. *Nurse Practitioner*, *35*(7), 39–43. doi:10.1097/01.NPR.0000383660.45156.40

Finniss, D. G., Kaptchuk, T. J., Miller, F., & Benedetti, F. (2010). Biological, clinical, and ethical advances of placebo effects. *Lancet*, *375*(9715), 686–695. doi:10.1016/S0140-6736(09)61706-2

Fortin, A. H., Dwamena, F. C., Frankel, R. M., Lepisto, B. L., & Smith, R. C. (2019). *Smith's patient-centered interviewing, an evidence-based method* (4th ed., pp. 1–11). New York, NY: McGraw-Hill Education.

Garwood, C. L., Korkis, B., Mohammad, I., Lepczyk, M., & Risko, K. (2016) Implementation of chronic care management services in primary care practice. *American Journal of Health-System Pharmacy*, *73*(23), 1924–1932. doi:10.2146/ajhp150985

Gastala, N. M., Wingrove, P. M., Gaglioti, A. H., Liaw, W., & Bazemore, A. (2018). The growing trend of health coaches in team-based primary care training: A multicenter pilot study. *Family Medicine*, *50*(7), 526–530. doi:10.22454/FamMed.2018.459897

Graham, R., Mancher, M., Wolman, D. M., Greenfield, S., & Steinberg, E. (Eds.). (2011). *Clinical practice guidelines we can trust*. Washington, DC: National Academies Press. Retrieved from https://www.ncbi.nlm.nih.gov/books/NBK209539/pdf/Bookshelf_NBK209539.pdf

Hendrich, A. (2016). Fall risk assessment for older adults: The Hendrich II Fall Risk Model. Try This: Best Practices in Nursing Care to Older Adults, 8. Retrieved from https://consultgeri.org/try-this/general-assessment/issue-8.pdf

Hill, E. (2004). Making sense of preventive medicine. *Family Practice Management*, *11*(4), 49–54. Retrieved from https://www.aafp.org/fpm/2004/0400/p49.html

Institute for Healthcare Communication. (2011). Impact of communication in healthcare. Retrieved from https://healthcarecomm.org/about-us/impact-of-communication-in-healthcare

Kaptchuk, T. J., Kelley, J. M., Conboy, L. A., Davis, R. B., Kerr, C. E., Jacobson, E. E., … Lembo, A. J. (2008). Components of placebo effect: Randomized controlled trial in patients with irritable bowel syndrome. *BMJ*, *336*, 999–1003. doi:10.1136/bmj.39524.439618.25

Kleinman, A., Eisenberg, L., & Good, B. (1978). Culture, illness, and care: Clinical lessons from anthropological and cross-cultural research. *Annals of Internal Medicine*, *88*(2), 256. doi:10.7326/0003-4819-88-2-251

Krogsbøll, L. T., Jørgensen, K. J., & Gøtzsche, P. C. (2013). General health checks in adults for reducing morbidity and mortality from disease. *The Journal of the American Medical Association*, *309*(23), 2489–2490. doi:10.1001/jama.2013.5039

Krogsbøll, L. T., Jørgensen, K. J., Grøhøj, L. C., & Gøtzsche, P. C. (2012). General health checks in adults for reducing morbidity and mortality from disease. *Cochrane Database of Systematic Reviews, 2012*(10), CD009009. doi:10.1002/14651858.CD009009.pub2

McCabe, D. (2019). Katz Index of Independence in Activities of Daily Living (ADL). *Try This: Best Practices in Nursing Care to Older Adults, 2*. Retrieved from https://consultgeri.org/try-this/general-assessment/issue-2.pdf

Moore, K. (2010). Documenting history in compliance with Medicare's guidelines. *Family Practice Management, 17*(2), 22–27. Retrieved from https://www.aafp.org/fpm/2010/0300/p22.html#

National Cancer Institute. (2013). Visuals online: Classic BRCA1 pedigree. Retrieved from https://visualsonline.cancer.gov/details.cfm?imageid=10436

NEJM Catalyst. (2017, December). Social determinants of health (SDOH). Retrieved from https://catalyst.nejm.org/social-determinants-of-health

Owolabi, T., & Simpson, I. (2012). Documenting and coding preventive visits: A physician's perspective. *Family Practice Management, 19*(4), 12–16. Retrieved from https://www.aafp.org/fpm/2012/0700/p12.html

Phillips, A. (2017, November). A detailed review of systems: An educational feature. *Journal of Nurse Practitioners, 13*(10), 681–686. doi:10.1016/j.nurpra.2017.08.012

Resources for Integrated Care. (2017). *Disability-competent care self-assessment tool*. Retrieved from https://www.resourcesforintegratedcare.com/sites/default/files/DCCAT_Final.pdf

Smeltzer, S., Mariani, B., & Meakim, C. (2017). Assessment of a person with disability. Retrieved from http://www.nln.org/professional-development-programs/teaching-resources/ace-d/additional-resources/assessment-of-a-person-with-disability

Srivastava, S. B. (2014). The patient interview. In C. D. Lauster & S. B. Srivastava (Ed.), *Fundamental skills for patient care in pharmacy practice* (pp. 1–35). Burlington, MA: Jones & Bartlett. Retrieved from http://samples.jbpub.com/9781449652722/9781449645106_ch01_001_036.pdf

Szafran, O., Kennett, S. L., Bell, N. R., & Green, L. (2018). Patients' perceptions of team-based care in family practice: Access, benefits and team roles. *Journal of Primary Health Care, 10*(3), 248–257. doi:10.1071/HC18018

Tatum, P. E., Talebreza, S., & Ross, J. S. (2018). Geriatric assessment: An office-based approach. *American Family Physician, 97*(12), 776–784. Retrieved from https://www.aafp.org/afp/2018/0615/p776.html

Timpel, P., Lang, C., Wens, J., Contel, J. C., Gilis-Januszewska, A., Kemple, K., & Schwarz, P. E. (2017). Individualizing chronic care management by analyzing patients' need: A mixed method approach. *International Journal of Integrated Care, 17*(6), 1–12. doi:10.5334/ijic.3067

U.S. Department of Health and Human Services. (2019a). *Drink alcohol only in moderation*. Retrieved from https://healthfinder.gov/HealthTopics/Category/health-conditions-and-diseases/heart-health/drink-alcohol-only-in-moderation

U.S. Department of Health and Human Services. (2019b). *Talk to your doctor about abdominal aortic aneurysm*. Retrieved from https://healthfinder.gov/HealthTopics/Category/doctor-visits/screening-tests/talk-to-your-doctor-about-abdominal-aortic-aneurysm

U.S. National Library of Medicine Genetics Home Reference. (2015a). Autosomal dominant inheritance [Image file]. Bethesda, MD: The Library. Retrieved from https://ghr.nlm.nih.gov/gallery

U.S. National Library of Medicine Genetics Home Reference. (2015b). X-linked recessive inheritance [Image file]. Bethesda, MD: The Library. Retrieved from https://ghr.nlm.nih.gov/gallery?start=60

U.S. National Library of Medicine. (2019, October). *What does it mean if a disorder seems to run in my family?* Retrieved from https://ghr.nlm.nih.gov/primer/inheritance/runsinfamily

U.S. Preventive Services Task Force. (n.d.-a). Grade definitions. Retrieved from https://www.uspreventiveservicestaskforce.org/Page/Name/grade-definitions

U.S. Preventive Services Task Force. (n.d.-b). USPSTF A and B recommendations. Retrieved from https://www.uspreventiveservicestaskforce.org/Page/Name/uspstf-a-and-b-recommendations

U.S. Preventative Services Task Force. (2019). About the USPSTF. Retrieved from https://www.uspreventiveservicestaskforce.org/Page/Name/about-the-uspstf

Verghese, A., Brady, E., Kapur, C., & Horwitz, R. I. (2011). The bedside evaluation: Ritual and reason. *Annuals of Internal Medicine, 155*(8), 550–553. doi:10.7326/0003-4819-155-8-201110180-00013

Wilkinson, D. (2008). *Coding preventive care services. Journal of AHIMA, 79*(3), 80–82. Retrieved from http://library.ahima.org/doc?oid=78679#.W9tW2dVKiM9

Winter, J. E., MacInnis, R. J., Wattanapenpaiboon, N., & Nowson, C. A. (2014). BMI and all-cause mortality in older adults: A meta-analysis. *American Journal of Clinical Nutrition, 99*(4), 875–890. doi:10.3945/ajcn.113.068122

World Health Organization. (2018). Disability and health. Retrieved from http://www.who.int/news-room/fact-sheets/detail/disability-and-health

Yawn, B., Goodwin, M. A., Zyzanski, S. J., & Stange, K. C. (2003). Time use during acute and chronic illness visits to a family physician. *Family Practice, 20*(4), 474–477. doi:10.1093/fampra/cmg425

Ylimäki, E.-L., Kanste, O., Heikkinen, H., Bloigu, R., & Kyngäs, H. (2015). The effects of a counselling intervention on lifestyle change in people at risk of cardiovascular disease. *European Journal of Cardiovascular Nursing, 14*(2), 153–161. doi:10.1177/1474515114521725

Zamosky, L. (2013). Chronic disease: PCPs called on to meet growing health challenge. *Medical Economics, 90*(15), 30–32, 35–36.

3

Approach to Implementing and Documenting Patient-Centered, Culturally Sensitive Evidence-Based Assessment

Alice M. Teall and Kate Gawlik

"In diversity there is beauty and there is strength."

—Maya Angelou

LEARNING OBJECTIVES

- Examine the concepts of health and well-being within the context of family, community, and culture.
- Recognize the impact of health literacy, age, race, gender, ethnicity, socioeconomic status, and culture on the provision of care.
- Document components of a patient-centered, culturally sensitive assessment of health and well-being.

HEALTH AND WELL-BEING IN THE CONTEXT OF FAMILY, COMMUNITY, AND CULTURE

Implementing the best practices of evidence-based assessment begins with being patient-centered. To be patient-centered regarding health and well-being involves having a broad understanding of the dimensions of wellness. An individual's understanding of health, experience of well-being, ability to implement a healthy lifestyle, and achieve health in all dimensions can change over time and is affected by their **family**, **community**, and culture.

FAMILY AND FAMILY SYSTEMS

The societal definition and understanding of family, and what constitutes a family, has undergone remarkable change. For the purposes of advanced assessment, asking an individual who they consider to be their family is key. According to **family systems** theory (Bowen, 1966), a family functions and interacts emotionally within boundaries and patterns that create interconnectedness and interdependence. The dynamic nature of the family over time can impact an individual's emotional and developmental needs.

The clinician can assess the impact of the family system during the assessment of an individual's family health history and social history. Asking an individual whom they live with and who they consider their support system can provide insight into family relationships, structure, function, developmental stage, and health behaviors.

COMMUNITY, DISPARITIES, AND POPULATION HEALTH

Individuals live and interact with communities, that is, groups of people with common interests, locations, or characteristics (Merriam-Webster, n.d.). Examples of communities include neighborhoods, religious groups, and online groups with shared interests who meet through social media. The health status of communities impacts an individual's health.

For the clinician assessing the health and well-being of an individual, asking about the environments in which an individual resides, works, learns, plays, worships, and connects socially offers insight into the impact of community on their lives. One example is the assessment of safety concerns; recommending to someone to take daily walks outside without assessing the safety of their neighborhood may have a detrimental impact on the person's well-being if the neighborhood is unsafe. If the person in this example has support for wellness in their workplace or school, increasing activity during the time spent at work or school may be a more viable option. Another key assessment related to the economic stability of a community is whether or not an individual is experiencing food insecurity, that is, lacks access to a sufficient quantity of nutritious food; adults who are food insecure are at increased risk of negative health outcomes (Office of Disease Prevention and Health Promotion [ODPHP], n.d.). Socioeconomic conditions, public safety, and the availability of resources in a community are examples of **social determinants of health** that affect the well-being of individuals within communities. **Table 3.1** lists key areas to assess related to social determinants that may impact an individual's health. When there are significant barriers to meeting health and wellness needs within a community, the population of the community experiences **health disparities** or greater burden of illness, injury, disability, and mortality (ODPHP, n.d.).

Clinicians can assess the health of specific groups of patients whom they serve within a community; these types of assessments can lead to interventions to improve **population health**. The term *population health* refers to the health outcomes and concerns of a specific group or population within a community; population health initiatives address ways that resources can be allocated to overcome poorer health conditions and health disparities (Centers for Disease Control and Prevention [CDC], n.d.-b). Clinician support for health and well-being within communities can have significant positive impact on the individuals and families within those communities. Community-based programs and population health initiatives play a key role in preventing disease, improving health, and enhancing quality of life for individuals, families, and communities (ODPHP, n.d.).

CULTURE, CULTURAL IDENTITY, AND HEALTH BELIEFS

An individual's understanding of health, wellness, and illness, and the health literacy skills that they use, reflects their **culture** (CDC, n.d.-a). Culture can be defined by race, ethnicity, geography, or language or seen as a collection of values, beliefs, and behaviors (CDC, n.d.-a). An important role of the clinician is to allow each individual to identify their own culture, ethnicity, race, and language, as cultural identity is not determined by physical characteristics. Culture is a broad term. Healthcare professionals, for example, can be considered as having their own culture, that is, clinicians have a language, belief system, and way of behaving that are unique. Individuals are often influenced by more than one culture, and how they identify with that culture varies uniquely.

TABLE 3.1 Assessments Related to Social Determinants of Health	
Economic Stability	Access to employment and job training Access to resources to meet daily needs, including food
Physical Environment	Access to safe, affordable housing Public safety; exposure to violence, toxic substances, physical hazards
Healthcare System	Availability of evidence-based healthcare services Access to clinicians with linguistic and cultural competency Access to insurance coverage and care meeting health literacy needs
Social Context	Availability of recreational and leisure-time activities Socioeconomic conditions; cohesion and social support Experiences of discrimination, isolation, bias
Education	Access to quality education, including early childhood education Access to Internet, smartphones, and emerging technologies

Source: From Office of Disease Prevention and Health Promotion. (n.d.). *Social determinants of health.* Retrieved from https://www.healthypeople.gov/2020/topics-objectives/topic/social-determinants-of-health

The influence of culture on health beliefs, behaviors, practices, perceptions, and approaches is vast. Symptoms are often interpreted differently on the basis of cultural understanding. Beliefs about health and illness, wellness practices, faith-based influences, approach to food and nutrition, communication styles, and level of involvement of the family and others for support are all aspects of well-being that are influenced by culture. An evidence-based approach to implementing assessment requires sensitivity to cultural norms. Learning to be culturally sensitive goes beyond asking an individual about their "cultural practices," as most individuals are unable to articulate the inherent and significant influence of culture on their health and well-being. Instead, this text incorporates a culturally sensitive and humble approach to history taking and physical examination that allows the individual to have the time and respect required to express concerns and perspectives. Without a respectful approach, insensitivity to cultural perspectives can exacerbate health disparities and have a negative impact on the well-being of individuals, families, and communities.

ROLE OF THE CLINICIAN IN ASSESSING HEALTH AND HEALTH DISPARITIES

CLINICIAN–PATIENT PARTNERSHIP

Implementing evidence-based assessment requires prioritizing the establishment of a partnership with the patient; this partnership begins with therapeutic communication, that is, listening, responding, and interacting with the focus on the patient's health and well-being. In order to implement best practice, clinicians need to consider whether the time and space allowed are conducive to effectively listening to the patient's history, responding to patient concerns, and completing a physical exam, as indicated. Whether an individual is presenting to the clinician as a new or established patient, for a wellness exam, for an acute concern, or for management of a chronic illness, the role of the clinician includes taking the time to listen to patient concerns, respond to questions, and evaluate patient understanding.

RECOGNITION OF BARRIERS

This process of creating a partnership through effective communication and responsiveness can be negatively impacted by barriers. Recognizing that the individual presenting for a visit may have different priorities, perspectives, and concerns regarding health, and that these differences are related to family, social, cultural, or community influences, may not be readily apparent or may be confusing to the clinician, even if the clinician is prioritizing patient wellness. Research studies suggest that all clinicians, regardless of their desire to be equitable, have **implicit bias**, or unconscious perceptions or beliefs related to sexual orientation, gender identity, ethnicity, mental health, religion, and/or socioeconomic status (The Joint Commission, 2016). While implicit bias differs significantly from the conscious attitudes and behaviors of explicit or overt bias, either type of bias can exacerbate health disparities and create barriers to care. Recognizing one's own inherent biases is a reflection of self-awareness. Not all implicit biases are negative; affiliations can inherently be viewed positively. Making an effort to identify situations in which implicit biases impact clinician behavior is key.

CULTURAL SENSITIVITY

Despite the inherent nature of implicit or unconscious bias, a therapeutic patient relationship can be established and maintained if preferences, diversity, and biases are recognized and evaluated (Gonzalez et al., 2018). This requires both sensitivity and humility in the assessment of family, social, and cultural influences on health, as well as an openness to views, perspectives, and strategies related to achieving wellness and implementing healthy lifestyle behaviors. For individuals who have language barriers, having an interpreter available is best practice. Assessing each individual's understanding of symptoms, priorities for wellness, and expectations regarding health interventions is considered evidence-based, culturally sensitive, patient-centered, best practice.

EVIDENCE-BASED PRACTICE CONSIDERATIONS

QUADRUPLE AIM AND THE PROCESS OF CULTURAL HUMILITY

The Institute for Healthcare Improvement (IHI) prioritizes better care for individuals, better health for populations, and lower per capita cost of healthcare through the IHI Triple Aim Initiative (IHI, n.d.). To reach the goals of the Triple Aim, the IHI recommends a systematic, evidence-based approach to healthcare focused on individuals, families, communities, and population health in the provision of culturally sensitive primary care. Numerous organizations and health systems have added a fourth initiative, self-care of the clinician, based on evidence that attaining joy in work allows clinicians to better pursue health equity for all; this **Quadruple Aim** notes that clinician burnout has a detrimental effect on the patient experience (IHI, 2019). Chapter 28 provides further detail about the importance of health, wellness, and self-care for the clinician as a key component of implementing evidence-based, advanced assessment. The clinician who is well is able to effectively work toward the IHI Aims of improving the patient experience and providing care that is culturally sensitive.

To be culturally sensitive requires recognition that cultural beliefs, values, traditions, norms, and institutions do change over time. How culture influences each individual is unique. To assess cultural differences and address social determinants of health effectively requires **cultural humility**. Cultural humility is a lifelong process that involves self-reflection and critique and requires the clinician to be other-centered, self-aware, supportive, and open (Foronda, Baptiste, Reinholdt, & Ousman, 2016). The process of cultural humility results in mutual empowerment, partnership, optimal care, and lifelong learning (Foronda et al., 2016).

In each chapter of this text, history questions specific to each system are listed; many are specific to the patient's chief concern, or reason for seeking care. The questions are intended to be asked in a confidential, sensitive manner and will reveal the patient's perspectives about health, wellness, and illness. As each chapter is reviewed, remember to spend time in self-reflection and consider how to sensitively ask and respond to patient assessments. Implementing evidence-based, patient-centered advanced assessment requires sensitivity and openness to the patient's responses as specific details of their history and perspectives are shared. Remember to consciously avoid stereotyping an individual based on age, gender, sexual orientation, ethnicity, socioeconomic status, religion, or lifestyle behaviors. Recognize that asking patients about their beliefs and behaviors is part of advanced assessment. Respectfully assessing family, social, and cultural beliefs and influences can reveal the impact of health beliefs and practices on an individual's management of illness and dimension of wellness.

QSEN COMPETENCIES AS A FOUNDATION FOR ASSESSMENT

Competencies have been identified to ensure that clinicians are prepared with the knowledge, skills, and attitudes to practice in healthcare with a focus on continuously improving healthcare systems. These competencies, created as a component of the QSEN project, are a result of a collaborative effort of health professionals and have been guided by the Institute of Medicine, National Association for Healthcare Quality, National Patient Safety Foundation, National Committee for Quality Assurance, and the Academy for Healthcare Improvement (QSEN Institute, 2019). These competencies include:

- Patient-centered care
- Teamwork and collaboration
- Evidence-based practice

- Quality improvement
- Safety
- Informatics

The evidence-based foundation of a patient-centered, culturally sensitive, holistic, and empathetic approach to assessment includes the **QSEN competencies** and the Quadruple Aim. As clinicians learn to interact with individuals with respect for family, community, and cultural influences, and to become part of a collaborative team focused on quality, health disparities can be addressed, and a renewed focus on the wellness of communities and populations can occur.

Note that informatics is included as one of the QSEN competencies. As the use of technologies and telecommunications continues to expand exponentially in healthcare, the importance of prioritizing patient-centered, evidence-based, safe, effective, quality care cannot be overstated. Chapter 27 of this text presents a framework for evidence-based review of advancing technologies. Computer-based charting systems, or **electronic medical records (EMRs)**, allow for communication with multiple members of the healthcare team. Thorough documentation of advanced assessment in a clear, concise manner supports quality improvement in the provision of evidence-based care.

DOCUMENTATION OF AN EVIDENCE-BASED ASSESSMENT OF HEALTH AND WELL-BEING

Documentation is an important part of the clinical encounter. Twenty-five to fifty percent of a clinician's time is spent on documentation (Clynch & Kellett, 2015). There are clinical, legal, ethical, and financial aspects that the clinician must take into account when completing relevant documentation about a patient encounter, evaluation, and treatment. The patient record provides an opportunity for the clinician to document the care provided at the visit and track how both the patient's status and subsequent care evolve over time. It also provides the clinician with a place to store an ongoing record of such things as chronic illnesses, surgeries, medications, and treatment responses. Documentation should be thorough yet concise and demonstrate the clinical story of the patient. This is the clinician's opportunity to remember the encounter for future visits and to provide other clinicians with the opportunity to review what the visit entailed. Documentation should be factual, respectful, accurate, and free of bias. The clinician should craft the documentation with consideration for the fact that the patient, their family members, and/or other clinicians may read it in the future.

The clinical record also serves as liability prevention. Failure to document relevant information and data on patient care is considered a significant breach of and deviation from the standard of care and can have significant clinical and legal implications. Quality and safety of patient care are directly dependent on optimal communication among clinicians, which often occurs through documented patient notes. Being proficient at clinical documentation and ensuring documentation integrity are essential parts of the clinician's role.

In the past, documentation was primarily handwritten in patient charts. As of 2017, the majority of office-based clinicians (roughly 86%) were using an electronic system to store patient records for their practice. Hospitals had even higher rates, with 99% of large hospitals, 97% of medium-sized hospitals, 95% of small urban hospitals, and 93% of small rural hospitals having adopted an **electronic health record** (**EHR**; The Office of the National Coordinator for Health Information Technology, 2019a). EHR is often used interchangeably with EMR, although they are different. An EMR is an electronic version of a patient's medical and treatment history for one practice, but the information

remains in that single practice (**Figure 3.1**). An EHR is a "digital version of the patient's chart" (The Office of the National Coordinator for Health Information Technology, 2019b) that can be accessed throughout a patient's healthcare system. EHRs are intended to improve patient care by allowing healthcare clinicians and facilities (i.e., outpatient clinics, hospitals, laboratories, specialists, pharmacies, emergency rooms, etc.) access to a single patient record that contains all information on current and ongoing care. EHRs provide a broader perspective of a patient's care and act as a "hub" for a patient's medical history, diagnoses, medications, treatment plans, immunization dates, allergies, radiology images, and laboratory and test results.

The Health Information Technology for Economic and Clinical Health (HITECH) Act was enacted in 2009 as part of the American Reinvestment & Recovery Act. The HITECH Act (also known as meaningful use) set the goal of modernizing healthcare's infrastructure through the use of interoperable EHRs. Meaningful use is defined as "the use of certified EHR technology in a meaningful manner" (CDC, n.d.-c, para. 2). There are five pillars of health outcomes that meaningful use

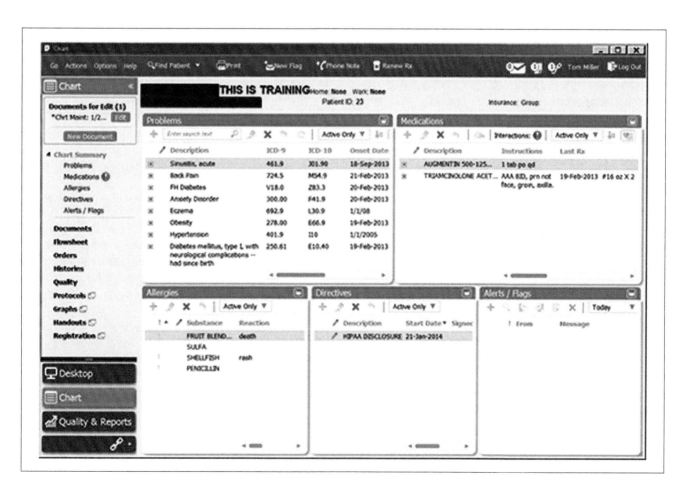

FIGURE 3.1 Sample electronic medical record.

strives to achieve. These pillars (CDC, n.d.-c) are as follows:

1. Improve quality, safety, and efficiency, and reduce health disparities.
2. Engage patients and families in their health.
3. Improve care coordination.
4. Improve population and public health.
5. Ensure adequate privacy and security protection for personal health information.

GENERAL GUIDELINES FOR DOCUMENTATION

Since documentation takes up such a large portion of a clinician's workload, learning to document efficiently is imperative. Clinical documentation does not need to be lengthy to provide an accurate clinical record and serve as liability protection for the clinician. Efficient documentation relies on several guiding principles (Gutheil, 2004).

First, the documentation note needs to convey that a risk–benefit analysis was utilized and should reflect the clinician's decision-making process. Often, clinicians document what the risks of a plan, treatment, or intervention are but fail to adequately recognize and document the benefits. For example, when prescribing a medication, the side effects (risks) are often documented as having been discussed with the patient, but the benefits of taking the medication and, furthermore, the risks of *not taking* the medication are often entirely absent from the charting. By charting both the pros and cons of taking the medication, the clinician's decision-making process is better understood to individuals outside of the patient case.

Second, documentation needs to reflect the use of clinical judgment at all critical decision-making points. This involves documenting what was assessed, both subjectively and objectively, in the clinical encounter and then documenting an appropriate, evidence-based response to the scenario. The patient assessment should be congruent with the response. For example, a charting note that reads: "*Patient actively suicidal. Sent home. Will see back in 1 week*" would be incongruent with the standard of care.

Third, the documentation needs to reflect the patient's capacity to participate in and understand their care. For example, documentation needs to include that the patient understands who to call in an emergency or what symptoms would necessitate an emergency department visit when applicable. And, finally, the documentation needs to support and justify the level of examination that was coded/billed for a particular patient encounter. Reimbursement is tied to documentation, so ensuring that the clinical documentation matches coding and billing details will ensure proper reimbursement. All clinicians should receive and participate in continuing education about coding and billing.

CLINICAL RECORD AS A LEGAL DOCUMENT

It is important to remember that the patient record in any form (written or EMR) serves as a legal document. The medical record is owned by the medical facility where the care was provided, but the information contained within the record is owned by the patient. If the patient or their legal representative requests the medical record, it must be released. The Privacy Rule gives the patient "the right to inspect, review, and receive a copy of [their] medical records and billing records" (U.S. Department of Health and Human Services, 2017).

The healthcare facility has the duty to protect the patient's privacy and maintain confidentiality. The Health Insurance Portability and Accountability Act (HIPAA) Security Rule and the Privacy Rule protect a patient's rights to privacy and control over the disclosure of certain health information. The HITECH Act also gives the patient the right to know who has accessed their medical record.

The collection of records that are kept regarding patient assessments and evaluation that support treatment decisions and justify billing are termed the **designated record set**. Designated record sets are able to be subpoenaed for court and/or may be subject to disclosure under certain circumstances. Patients, as owners of their medical information, have the right to request that inaccurate or incomplete information be amended, a list of disclosures be made, and restrictions be enforced. While a patient can request that the record be changed, the clinician must agree that the request is necessary to correct an incomplete or inaccurate record.

IMPORTANT DOCUMENTATION CONSIDERATIONS

Clinicians employ various methods to complete their documentation. The majority of clinicians type their own clinical notes. However, more clinicians are starting to utilize audio recognition software and the use of scribes. There are pros and cons to each of these methods. Whatever method is determined to be the best for the individual clinician and/or the healthcare facility, care should be taken to minimize error and maximize accuracy and safety. **Table 3.2** reviews the pros and cons of these various documentation methods.

When documenting a clinical encounter, it is important to remember that there are many patient safety issues surrounding how the encounter is written. Abbreviations are frequently misinterpreted, can be dangerous to patient care, and should be discouraged (Hamiel et al., 2018). The Joint Commission has an official "Do Not Use" list of abbreviations (**Table 3.3**). Many healthcare organizations have adopted policies regarding abbreviations and may include more abbreviations than those noted in **Table 3.3**. It is important to check with the policy of the individual healthcare organization(s) before using any abbreviations.

TABLE 3.2 Advantages and Disadvantages of Various Methods of Documentation

Method of Documentation	Advantages	Disadvantages
Typing	• Completed by the clinician so does not need the degree of proofreading as needed with other methods • Lower cost than other methods	• Time consuming • Difficult to maintain eye contact with the patient • Must pay for an EMR/EHR • Must be trained on system software
Audio Transcription/Voice Recognition	• Saves time for the clinician • Allows clinician to focus on the patient	• Must proofread for accuracy • Must be trained on system software
Scribe	• Saves time for clinician • Can be done in real time • Improves accuracy having a second perspective • Allows clinician to focus on patient	• Must pay salary or hourly wage • Must proofread for accuracy • Possible patient discomfort with having another individual present
Written	• Low cost • Time consuming • No training or extra investment	• Concerns for legibility • Cannot be locked • Hard to share with other clinicians • May hinder reimbursement process • Does not track time or provide safety alerts • Phasing out with new legal requirements

EHR, electronic health record; EMR, electronic medical record.

TABLE 3.3 The Joint Commission's Official "Do Not Use" List

Do Not Use	Potential Problem	Use Instead
U, u (unit)	Mistaken for "0" (zero), the number "4" (four), or "cc"	Write "unit"
IU (International Unit)	Mistaken for IV (intravenous) or the number 10 (ten)	Write "International Unit"
Q.D., QD, q.d., qd (daily) Q.O.D., QOD, q.o.d., qod (every other day)	Mistaken for each other Period after the Q mistaken for "I" and the "O" mistaken for "I"	Write "daily" Write "every other day"
Trailing zero (X.0 mg)* Lack of leading zero (.X mg)	Decimal point is missed	Write X mg Write 0.X mg
MS MSO_4 and $MgSO_4$	Can mean morphine sulfate or magnesium sulfate Confused for one another	Write "morphine sulfate" Write "magnesium sulfate"

*Exception: A "trailing zero" may be used only where required to demonstrate the level of precision of the value being reported, such as for laboratory results, imaging studies that report size of lesions, or catheter/tube sizes. It may not be used in medication orders or other medication-related documentation.

Note: Applies to all orders and all medication-related documentation that is handwritten (including free-text computer entry) or on preprinted forms.

Source: The Joint Commission. (2019). Facts about the official "do not use" list of abbreviations. Retrieved from https://www.jointcommission.org/facts_about_do_not_use_list

More than 40% of patients have inaccuracies on their medication lists and even more often have no record about medication allergies and intolerances (Silvestre, Santos, de Oliveira-Filho, & de Lyra, 2017). Medication discrepancies, in particular, often occur during the transfer of care from one facility to another, or from one clinician to another. Asking about current medication with each visit is important to create and ensure an accurate medication list. It may be necessary to contact the patient's pharmacy to verify medications currently prescribed, including doses and frequencies.

Similar to the medication list, it is also important to keep an updated problem list. Problems that are most severe, for example, acute myocardial infarction, and that require the highest levels of involvement, for example, diabetes, should be listed as first or top priorities. All problems should be listed with their date of onset. This is also a good place to list things like *allergy to amoxicillin, which causes anaphylaxis*. The problem list provides a quick reference point for both the primary clinician as well as other clinicians who are providing care. By keeping all problems documented in one area, clinicians gain a better understanding of the patient as a whole and at a glance.

Considerations for safe and accurate documentation include the use of appropriate abbreviations, updated medication and problem lists, and efficient use of a charting system. **Box 3.1** lists additional considerations and includes ways to avoid errors.

The potential for EHR-related patient safety hazards has increased for a number of reasons. The increased scope and complexity of tasks clinicians can perform using EHRs, the pressure to rapidly adopt EHRs (as a result of the incentives created by the HITECH Act), and the diversity of EHR systems available have all increased the potential for errors. EMRs/EHRs have designed internal checks to help safeguard against many documentation pitfalls (e.g., forgetting to code a visit), which can be helpful when appropriately utilized. **Box 3.2** lists ways to avoid common pitfalls associated with electronic clinical documentation.

BOX 3.1
AVOIDING COMMON DOCUMENTATION PITFALLS

1. Be cognizant of the tone in clinical documentation. The tone should remain professional and free from bias. Any sarcasm, joking, demeaning comments/terminology, or negativity should not be included.
2. Avoid being complacent with check-off assessments.
3. Never document an abnormality found during the physical examination without documenting the corresponding intervention.
4. Always document a baseline mental status.
5. Keep the subjective information in the history and the objective information in the physical exam sections of the charting note.
6. Be sure to include pertinent negatives. For example, with a chief concern of chest pain, it would be important to note: *No shortness of breath; no left arm, jaw or neck pain; no nausea; no dizziness; no episodes of syncope*, and so on.
7. Complete the chart at the time of the visit. It is easy to forget certain aspects of the visit after seeing multiple patients or to completely forget to complete the chart. As the saying goes, "If it isn't documented, then it wasn't done."
8. Be specific when describing abnormalities. A *2×2 cm firm, fixed, nontender, slightly pink nodule on the left anterior lower leg approximately five in. Inferior to the patella* is a much more specific description than *a pink nodule on the left lower leg*. Using diagrams can be helpful to show an anatomic location.
9. Describe what is *and* is not seen. The notation *Tympanic membranes visualized* is made more specific by adding: *Tympanic membranes pearly gray without erythema or edema*.
10. Don't forget to sign the chart as this is the official, legal record of care.

BOX 3.2
AVOIDING COMMON EMR AND EHR DOCUMENTATION PITFALLS

1. Clinicians should ensure that they have received adequate training on the EMR/EHR system. Training should include practice time and reinforcement classes when EMR/EHR updates are made. Ask for more training to achieve a level of comfort with the charting system.
2. Don't copy/paste from another visit. Every field needs to be reviewed and modified based on the patient's unique visit that day.
3. Don't rely solely on templates, especially when they are preloaded. Templates can save time when appropriately used, but they can also add in extraneous information to the visit. Templates need to be tailored to what was done, seen, and heard on that day.

(continued)

4. Avoid inconsistencies (e.g., a patient comes in with the concern of headache, then *no headaches* is listed under the review of systems in the template).
5. Be sure to append a patient's medical record and not alter it. Many EMR/EHR systems safeguard against this and do not allow the clinician to alter the original document after it has been locked. Altering a chart without proper documentation is a red flag in a legal case.
6. If the EHR uses drop-down menus, but assessment findings, diagnosis, or other components are not listed, make sure to use the type-in feature to add the specific finding, diagnosis, and/or other components.
7. Don't carry over findings, diagnoses, or medications that are no longer applicable to the patient's care.
8. Don't ignore system alerts. EMR/EHR systems have designed these alerts for a purpose and to improve system processes, patient care, and safety.
9. Don't click every box in hopes of getting a higher reimbursement or safeguarding against liability. For example, if a clinician documented that he or she inspected the skin of a patient's abdomen without actually having done so and the patient is seen several hours later with Cullen's sign noted on the abdomen, this would be seen as negligence since action was not taken at that time of initial assessment.

EHR, electronic health record; EMR, electronic medical record.

CLINICAL DOCUMENTATION: EXAMPLE

Documentation is typically completed in one of two formats: (a) SOAP note of subjective history, objective findings, diagnostic assessment, and plan of care, or (b) a problem-oriented medical record. Both formats are acceptable and should capture the same pertinent clinical information. Documentation format is determined by the individual clinician's preference, the EMR/EHR system being used, and/or the institution or practice. Chapter 2 provides an extensive overview of information to include and other considerations for each of these sections.

SOAP Note
- **S**ubjective data (i.e., the history or what the patient reports)
- **O**bjective data (i.e., the exam including clinician observations)
- **A**ssessment (i.e., the diagnosis or diagnostic assessment with rationale)
- **P**lan (i.e., the plan of care for the patient, including nonpharmacologic interventions, pharmacologic interventions, and/or patient education)

Problem-Oriented Medical Record (POMR)
- Complete physical exam
- Problem list
- Assessment and plan
- Baseline, lab, and imaging findings
- Series of progress notes or SOAP notes

Sample SOAP Note

The documentation example included is for a 30-year-old female patient who is seeking care for fatigue. Note that the plan of care is included to appreciate the format of the SOAP note; clinical decision-making related to treatment is beyond the scope of advanced assessment.

S: Patient is a full-time graduate student who is married with two children under age 5. Nine months ago, she began to experience increased fatigue and difficulty staying focused. Came in to see Dr. R at the clinic and had multiple labs done, all of which were normal. After this, she has continued to have fatigue, even though she sleeps well at night, and also feels "disconnected" from her daily activities. She does not have difficulties meeting her home and school obligations. She feels sad most days (this began about 3 weeks ago), has some anhedonia, denies weight loss or weight gain, has difficulty getting to sleep, feels tired all the time and feels that her thoughts are slower than normal, has impaired concentration, has some feelings of guilt, denies any thoughts of harming herself or harming others, and denies feelings of anxiety or having any anxiety attacks. Past medical history includes preeclampsia with pregnancy and a hernia repair 10 years ago. Denies past history of depression, postpartum depression, anxiety, or other mental health disorders. Denies smoking, alcohol use, or drug use. She has no known drug allergies and does not take any medications or vitamins. Has no family history of depression or anxiety. Is married and states relationship with her husband is supportive, feels safe in her relationship and at home, and denies ever being a victim of violence. Denies any recent illness, fevers, night sweats, weight loss, or weight gain. Denies abdominal pain, nausea, vomiting. Has regular menses and reports mild mood liability before but states this has not been worse than normal. Is not using a contraceptive method; husband has had vasectomy.

O: Vital signs: BP = 114/72, R = 16, Temp 98.3°F, Pulse 74, BMI 23. Pt appears well nourished. Pt is alert and oriented ×3. Patient has a flat affect. Pt is tearful throughout the exam. Thyroid: smooth, soft, nontender bilateral. Heart: regular rate and rhythm. PHQ-9 score: 15 and GAD score: 8.

A: This is a 30-year-old female with a 9-month history of increased fatigue, disconnection from activities, and episodes of tearfulness. Patient meets DSM V criteria for major depression, and PHQ-9 indicates moderately severe depression. Discussed options of trying cognitive behavioral therapy and starting an antidepressant medication. Discussed doing one versus the other versus doing both. She is very responsive to trying both therapy and medication and believes this to be the best option for her.

P: Recommended bupropion XL 150 mg q day. Chose this medication as it can also be energizing and patient reports increased fatigue. Discussed with patient the possible side effects and that she may feel worse for a period of time before feeling better as medication may take up to 6 weeks to be effective. Also discussed potential side effects of bupropion. Referral sent for cognitive behavioral therapy. Reviewed information about healthy lifestyle behaviors related to mood. Has decided to set goal to walk 30 minutes daily. Follow-up appointment made for 2 weeks. Instructed to call if she begins to feel worse, has thoughts of suicidal/homicidal ideation, or has any questions. Instructed to go to an emergency department if she is in need of immediate help.

Clinical Pearls

- Cultural humility is a process of learning to have an approach that is other-oriented.
- Connectedness to family, community, and culture can positively impact health and well-being.
- Active listening requires the clinician to eliminate distractions and focus on an individual's verbal and nonverbal responses.
- Listening and responding empathetically to an individual's history serves to establish a therapeutic partnership, improves patient and clinician satisfaction, and results in improved health outcomes.
- Self-reflection is required to identify implicit bias and is a step of evidence-based assessment.

- Providing interpreter services for individuals with limited English proficiency improves their access to quality healthcare.
- A critical component of effective assessment is documentation.

Key Takeaways

- Responding to individuals in a culturally sensitive, patient-centered, and evidence-based manner allows the clinician to uniquely understand and document an individual's health status and health risks.
- Abbreviations should not be used in patient documentation to ensure quality and safety of patient care.
- Documentation is an essential part of the clinician's role and provides an ongoing, working record on clinical progress of patients in addition to providing liability protection.

REFERENCES

Bowen, M. (1966). The use of family theory in clinical practice. *Comprehensive Psychiatry*, *7*(5), 345–374. doi:10.1016/S0010-440X(66)80065-2

Centers for Disease Control and Prevention. (n.d.-a). *Culture and health literacy*. Retrieved from https://www.cdc.gov/healthliteracy/culture.html

Centers for Disease Control and Prevention. (n.d.-b). *Population health training: What is population health?*. Retrieved from https://www.cdc.gov/pophealthtraining/whatis.html

Centers for Disease Control and Prevention. (n.d.-c). *Public health and promoting interoperability programs: Introduction*. Retrieved from https://www.cdc.gov/ehrmeaningfuluse/introduction.html

Clynch, N., & Kellett, J. (2015). Medical documentation: Part of the solution, or part of the problem? A narrative review of the literature on the time spent on and the value of medical documentation. *International Journal of Medical Informatics*, *84*(4), 221–228. doi:10.1016/j.ijmedinf.2014.12.001

Foronda, C., Baptiste, D.-L., Reinholdt, M. M., & Ousman, K. (2016). Cultural humility: A concept analysis. *Journal of Transcultural Nursing*, *27*, 210–217. doi:10.1177/1043659615592677

Gonzalez, C. M., Deno, M. L., Kintzer, E., Marantz, P. R., Lypson, M. L., & McKee, M. D. (2018). Patient perspectives on racial and ethnic implicit bias in clinical encounters: Implications for curriculum development. *Patient*

Education and Counseling, 101, 1669–1675. doi:10.1016/j.pec.2018.05.016

Gutheil, T. G. (2004). Fundamentals of medical record documentation. *Psychiatry (Edgmont (Pa.: Township)), 1*(3), 26–28. Retrieved from https://www.ncbi.nlm.nih.gov/pmc/articles/PMC3010959/pdf/PE_1_3_26.pdf

Hamiel, U., Hecht, I., Nemet, A., Pe'er, L., Man, V., Hilely, A., & Achiron, A. (2018). Frequency, comprehension, and attitudes of physicians towards abbreviations in the medical record. *Postgraduate Medical Journal, 94*(1111), 254–258. doi:10.1136/postgradmedj-2017-135515

Institute for Healthcare Improvement. (n.d.). *Initiatives: The IHI Triple Aim.*. Retrieved from http://www.ihi.org/Engage/Initiatives/TripleAim/Pages/default.aspx

Institute for Healthcare Improvement. (2019). The Triple Aim: Why we still have a long way to go. Retrieved from http://www.ihi.org/communities/blogs/the-triple-aim-why-we-still-have-a-long-way-to-go

The Joint Commission. (2016). *Implicit bias in health care.* Retrieved from https://www.jointcommission.org/assets/1/23/Quick_Safety_Issue_23_Apr_2016.pdf

The Joint Commission. (2019). *Facts about the official "do not use" list of abbreviations.* Retrieved from https://www.jointcommission.org/facts_about_do_not_use_list

Merriam-Webster. (n.d.). Definition of community. Retrieved from https://www.merriam-webster.com/dictionary/community

Office of Disease Prevention and Health Promotion. (n.d.). *ODPHP* (n.d.). Social determinants of health. Retrieved from https://www.healthypeople.gov/2020/topics-objectives/topic/social-determinants-of-health

The Office of the National Coordinator for Health Information Technology. (2019a). *Quick stats.* Retrieved from https://dashboard.healthit.gov/quickstats/quickstats.php

The Office of the National Coordinator for Health Information Technology. (2019b). What is an electronic health record (EHR)? Retrieved from https://www.healthit.gov/faq/what-electronic-health-record-ehr

QSEN Institute. (2019). QSEN competencies. Retrieved from http://qsen.org/competencies

Silvestre, C., Santos, L., de Oliveira-Filho, A., & de Lyra, J. (2017). 'What is not written does not exist': The importance of proper documentation of medication use history. *International Journal of Clinical Pharmacy, 39*(5), 985–988. doi:10.1007/s11096-017-0519-2

U.S. Department of Health & Human Services. (2017). *Your medical records.* Retrieved from https://www.hhs.gov/hipaa/for-individuals/medical-records/index.html

4

Evidence-Based Assessment of Children and Adolescents

Rosie Zeno, Jennifer Kosla, and Bernadette Mazurek Melnyk

"You are not a drop in the ocean. You are the entire ocean in a drop."

—RUMI

 VIDEOS

- Well Exam: Well-Child—History and Physical Exam
- Well Exam: Infant Exam
- Patient History and Counseling: Adolescent With Depression and Anxiety Symptoms

LEARNING OBJECTIVES

- Discuss the anatomic and physiologic differences of children compared with adults.
- Describe the adaptive approach necessary to obtain a health history from the pediatric patient and family.
- Discuss the challenges and considerations unique to pediatric health history taking.
- Develop age-appropriate questions to use when completing the focused interview.
- Discuss the skills and techniques that are required to facilitate the health history and physical exam of the pediatric patient.
- Understand the special considerations and rationale behind shared decision-making for the pediatric patient.

Visit https://connect.springerpub.com/content/book/978-0-8261-6454-4/chapter/ch00 to access the videos.

ANATOMIC AND PHYSIOLOGIC VARIATIONS IN CHILDREN AND ADOLESCENTS

Human growth and **development** occurs across the life span. Infancy through young adulthood is a period of dynamic structural and functional changes. The clinician should be aware of key anatomic and physiologic differences between adults and children. While pediatric considerations are reviewed in assessment chapters throughout this text, this section is intended to provide broad and detailed pediatric information regarding these variations for careful review.

HEAD, EYES, EARS, NOSE, AND THROAT

Fetal development occurs in a head-to-toe direction known as "cephalocaudal." This pattern of development causes the head to be disproportionately larger than the lower part of the body. This disproportion in body ratio is present at birth and persists through 2 years of age. An additional key anatomic difference in the assessment of the head of children is that the newborn skull is comprised of five bones that may override one another slightly prior to fusion. Therefore, it is normal to palpate bumps and ridges along the suture lines of a newborn's skull.

It can also be normal for **infants** and young **children** to have an asymmetric head shape. Plagiocephaly is a term that describes asymmetry of the skull. Positional plagiocephaly is most common, which is an unintended consequence of safe sleep ("back to sleep") since infants spend a large portion of their time supine, thus placing pressure on the occipital region. Other causes of plagiocephaly include position in the womb, prematurity, muscular torticollis, and craniosynostosis. Craniosynostosis is a more serious condition in which the sutures or bones of the skull close too early, resulting in increased pressure and problems with brain growth. This condition requires prompt referral and management with a neurosurgeon.

The **pediatric** ear canal exam differs from that of the adult as the external auditory canal is short and often curves inward and upward in children under 3 years old; after 3 years of age, the canal is more downward and forward (Chiocca, 2015). Eustachian tube dysfunction is a common problem in children under 2 years old as the tube is shorter and wider and lies in a more horizontal plane, delaying the drainage of secretions. This positioning may result in the presence of middle ear effusions or more frequent ear infections. A common treatment for eustachian tube dysfunction is the placement of myringotomy ear tubes. If the child has had this procedure performed, the clinician may visualize the presence of the tube in the tympanic membrane. The tube should be assessed for placement, patency, and presence of drainage in the ear canal.

The pediatric eye exam has few **physical** differences compared with that of the older adolescent and adult; however, visual development is rapidly taking place in the first few years of life. It is essential for all children to have a regular eye exam and vision **assessment** to ensure early detection and prompt referral for any abnormalities. The pupillary light reflex is underdeveloped until 5 months of age, and transient nystagmus can be a normal finding in infants younger than 6 months. Extraocular muscle function is not well established in the first 6 months of age; therefore, intermittent phorias/strabismus may be observed. Poor muscle coordination and abnormal ocular alignment after 6 months of age may warrant referral and further evaluation. Normal visual acuity in the newborn ranges from 20/100 to 20/400 and gradually develops to 20/20 by 5 to 6 years of age.

Newborns and young infants display a preference for nasal breathing over mouth breathing, which is often referred to as "obligate nose breathing." This does not mean that young infants are unable to breathe through their mouths, since they often do when crying. The preference for nasal breathing is notable because infants must be able to breathe and swallow simultaneously when breast- or bottle-fed. During times of respiratory illness, nasal breathing can become challenging. When young infants are unable to breathe and

feed simultaneously, conditions such as choanal atresia that impair nasal patency should be considered.

The paranasal sinuses virtually reach adult size around age 12 but continue to complete their full development through age 20 in many children. Maxillary and ethmoid sinuses are present at birth. Sphenoid and frontal sinus development is variable, but they are usually distinguishable by age 2 and 8, respectively. Paranasal sinus development should be considered, especially when evaluating young children and **adolescents** for rhinosinusitis, as this condition is grossly overdiagnosed in children.

The presence of "shotty" lymph nodes, especially in the anterior and posterior cervical chains, is a common and normal finding in young children. They generally appear small and often firm. The term is derived from the fact that they have a similar feel to buckshot, or pellets, under the skin. Normal lymph nodes in most regions are ≤ 1 cm but may be up to 1.5 cm in cervical and inguinal nodes for a short period. The lymph system is easily often activated in children by everyday antigens and pathogens. However, *palpable supraclavicular, epitrochlear, or popliteal nodes are never normal.*

Dental eruption usually begins between 6 and 8 months of age with the primary central mandibular incisors. By 30 months of age, all 20 deciduous teeth (baby teeth) should have erupted except for the second molars, which erupt by 3 years of age. Children with delayed tooth eruption (no erupted teeth by age 18 months) should be referred to a pediatric dentist.

Tonsils develop throughout infancy and can usually be visualized by age 6 to 9 months. In comparison with adolescents and adults, children have larger appearing palatine tonsils in proportion to their posterior oropharynx (+2, +3, and even +4 touching or "kissing tonsils"). The enlarged appearance persists throughout childhood and becomes problematic only if children experience frequent pharyngeal infections or if the airway becomes obstructed by hypertrophied tonsils, as evidenced by snoring or symptoms of obstructive sleep apnea.

CHEST

The newborn's chest is more barrel shaped in comparison with that of the older child. The anterior–posterior diameter equals the transverse diameter. Chest circumference is measured at the nipple line and is performed as part of the newborn exam, but not at routine wellness visits. Until 12 to 18 months of age, the chest circumference closely approximates the head circumference, after which chest circumference begins to exceed head circumference.

From birth to 3 years of age, the ribs lie in a horizontal plane, which can restrict the infant's ability to expand the chest fully. Furthermore, the ribs are flexible and provide little structural support to the lungs, which can lead to negative intrathoracic pressure and increased work of breathing (Chiocca, 2015). This explains why children present with accessory muscle use in times of respiratory distress. The clinician is more likely to observe nasal flaring, as well as suprasternal, intercostal, substernal, and subcostal retractions, in small infants and children with respiratory illness than in adults. Nasal flaring and suprasternal retractions are more common in upper airway obstruction, whereas substernal, intercostal, and subcostal retractions are more common in lower airway obstruction. Young infants and children have a higher rate of oxygen consumption as well as increased metabolic rates, which increase the risk of respiratory compromise and collapse. The clinician must identify these conditions and act quickly.

The presence of functional or physiologic murmurs may be detected in children because of their thin chest wall. Murmurs can become even louder when children are scared, ill, or have a fever. Innocent murmurs are often heard in two-thirds of preschool and school-age children and may intensify or change with the child's position (upright versus supine) or respiratory pattern. In innocent heart murmurs, the flow can be heard pumping through the heart normally. Innocent murmurs are usually heard best over one cardiac landmark and do not radiate or move to other landmarks. A systolic murmur is heard when the heart contracts, whereas a diastolic murmur is heard when the heart relaxes. A murmur that occurs throughout contraction and relaxation is known as a continuous murmur. Heart murmurs are graded on a scale of 1 to 6 on the basis of their loudness. The most common types of murmurs in children are Still's murmur, a pulmonary flow murmur, and a venous hum, which is heard in the upright position and dissipates when the child turns their head or lies down. A Still's murmur is a benign flow murmur across the aortic valve from high cardiac output and/or increased contractility; it is typically heard over the left lower sternal border. Pulmonary flow murmurs are high-pitched harsher murmurs heard at the upper left sternal border; they usually disappear with a change in positioning or a Valsalva maneuver. A venous hum is a low-pitched continuous murmur that results from blood returning from the great veins to the heart. Splitting of the second heart sound (i.e., an S2 split) can also be typically heard on inspiration. It is caused when the closure of the aortic valve and the closure of the pulmonary valve are not synchronized during inspiration. A fixed S2 split is abnormal and requires further evaluation as it almost always indicates an atrial septal defect. As children grow, usually by adolescence, innocent murmurs will lessen and eventually disappear. A murmur associated with a palpable thrill (a vibration that can be felt), a murmur heard during diastole, or a murmur with an intensity grading of 4, 5, or 6 should always be considered pathologic and warrants further evaluation. Children with innocent heart murmurs have no associated symptoms, unlike children with pathologic murmurs who often have accompanying symptoms, such as poor feeding, difficulty breathing, fatigue with exercise, cough, chest pain, or dizziness or fainting.

Owing to the normal physiologic increase in the heart and respiratory rates in children, it can be challenging to discern adventitious heart and lung sounds. Heart and respiratory rates vary by age; normal vital signs by age are listed in **Table 4.1**. Therefore, parameters for clinical signs like tachycardia and tachypnea will vary according to age.

ABDOMEN

The abdomen in infants and young children can be more prominent, protruding, and cylindrical. This is a result of a physiologically small pelvis relative to the

TABLE 4.1 Pediatric Vital Signs			
Age	Heart Rate (Beats/Minute)	Blood Pressure (mmHg)	Respiratory Rate (Breaths/Minute)
Premature	110–170	SBP 55–75 DBP 35–45	40–70
0–3 months	110–160	SBP 65–85 DBP 45–55	35–55
3–6 months	110–160	SBP 70–90 DBP 50–65	30–45
6–12 months	90–160	SBP 80–100 DBP 55–65	22–38
1–3 years	80–150	SBP 90–105 DBP 55–70	22–30
3–6 years	70–120	SBP 95–110 DBP 60–75	20–24
6–12 years	60–110	SBP 100–120 DBP 60–75	16–22
>12 years	60–100	SBP 110–135 DBP 65–85	12–20

DBP, diastolic blood pressure; SBP, systolic blood pressure.

volume of abdominal contents. The normal shape of an infant abdomen can be mistaken for distention. Umbilical hernias, small epigastric hernias, and diastasis recti are common normal findings in children, but not in adults. As children grow, the abdomen assumes a more adult-like appearance.

The abdominal wall is thinner in children than in adults and often easier to palpate. The spleen tip may be palpated in a few infants or children. A spleen palpable > 2 cm below the left costal margin is abnormal and should be investigated. However, kidneys are rarely palpable except in a very thin child or newborn infant. Even then, only very skilled clinicians can typically palpate a kidney.

The normal liver span varies in the pediatric patient and is dependent on the child's age. At 2 months of age, the liver span averages 5.5 cm, and by age 5, it averages 8.2 cm. The liver border of infants and young children may be palpable 1 to 2 cm below the right costal margin. A liver border of greater than 3.5 cm in a newborn or greater than 2 cm in children below the right costal margin suggests hepatomegaly and should be investigated.

PUBERTY

Puberty is the physical transition from childhood to adulthood. The normal onset of puberty is between ages 8 to 13 in females and ages 9 to 14 in males. The Sexual Maturity Rating (SMR), also commonly referred to as "Tanner Staging," is the staging of sexual development by inspection. Female sexual development is staged according to breast development, while male sexual development is staged according to genitalia size. Male and female sexual development is also staged according to the distribution of pubic hair. The scale is from 1 (prepubertal) to 5 (adult-like). Chapters 19 and 20 provide additional information regarding assessment of the stages of sexual development. Clinicians should be familiar with the stages of sexual maturity and, if necessary, use standardized pictures demonstrating sexual development for comparison. It can be challenging to estimate SMR when children are between stages or when they groom or shave their pubic hair.

It is most important to note early onset or lack of secondary sexual characteristics outside the expected time frame. Children who exhibit secondary sex characteristics before age 8 (females) or age 9 (males) should be evaluated for precocious puberty. Children with an absence of secondary sex characteristics by age 13 (females) or age 14 (males) should be evaluated for delayed puberty. The cause of these conditions is often idiopathic, but pathology of the hypothalamus–pituitary–gonadal (HPG) axis, adrenal or gonadal conditions, or intracranial pathology must be considered.

MUSCULOSKELETAL

Overall, the skeletal structure is immature and more pliable in children under 8 years of age. Skeletal maturity, or closure of the growth plates, occurs near the end of puberty. Skeletal maturity is typically reached by 14 to 15 years of age in females and 17 to 18 years of age in males. Until then, growth plates are primarily comprised of cartilage and are structurally weaker than calcified bone. Sprains (ligament) and strains (tendons) are less common in younger children than adolescents and adults. Since their growth plates are weaker than the muscles or tendons, young children are more prone to the development of plastic deformities (buckling and bowing) and occult fractures as opposed to more apparent, "clean break" fractures in older adolescents and adults. Clinicians should maintain a high suspicion for growth plate injury for any child presenting with musculoskeletal trauma. Injuries to the growth plate may result in complications such as growth arrest, limb deformity, and shortening of the long bones. Therefore, efficient evidence-based management of bone trauma with close follow-up is crucial to preserving skeletal function and positive outcomes.

Newborns can have a normal physiologic laxity, or instability, of the hip joint in the first month of life. In most cases, this laxity resolves spontaneously. In some cases, the instability of the joint will require intervention. Developmental dysplasia of the hip (DDH) is a term describing a spectrum of abnormalities of the hip joint, from mild dysplasia to complete dislocation. DDH can occur in any infant but is more likely with the following risk factors: female, first-born, Caucasian, family history of DDH, breech position *in utero*. The American Academy of Pediatrics (AAP) clinical practice guideline advises clinical assessment for DDH at birth and every wellness visit until the child is walking normally, as well as selective radiologic imaging for infants with risk factors, especially those with a history of breech positioning *in utero* (Shaw et al., 2016). Long term, DDH can lead to leg-length discrepancies and arthritis in early adulthood.

DEVELOPMENTAL APPROACH TO HISTORY TAKING

There are several key differences in obtaining the health **history** of a child or adolescent compared with an adult. The pediatric population is unique and dynamic in its ongoing and often rapid periods of growth and development. The human brain develops, both structurally and functionally, through adolescence and into the mid-20s (Giedd et al., 1999), with rapid periods of development in infancy and adolescence. Infancy and adolescence are also periods of accelerated physical growth. Moreover, children are continuously developing their motor, language, cognitive, and psychosocial skills. As such, the clinician must employ a developmental approach to the history taking and physical exam of children and adolescents.

HISTORY OF PRESENT ILLNESS

The history of present illness (HPI) provides a chronologic description of the chief concern from the onset of symptoms to the present. There are eight elements to the HPI:

- Location: Where is the site of the problem? Multiple sites?
- Duration: When did the problem start? How long has this been a problem? Is this problem acute or chronic?
- Timing: Does the problem come and go, or is it constant?
- Quality: Is the pain sharp, dull, achy? Is the drainage clear, thick, yellow?
- Severity: Is the problem interrupting sleep, activity, school attendance? Rated on a scale of 1 to 10?
- Context: Is the problem associated with a particular activity, food, or place?
- Modifying factors: What makes the problem better or worse? Any treatments or medications tried?
- Associated signs and symptoms: Pertinent review of systems; for example, fevers, nausea, vomiting, diarrhea, rashes, headache, pain

The main difference between collecting the health history for infants and children compared with the case for adults is that the caregiver becomes the primary historian. As children mature developmentally, they become more able to participate in providing their health history. Therefore, the clinician must be prepared to adjust the approach to history taking accordingly.

Caregivers as Historians

By virtue of their age, infants and young children lack the language development to provide their own health history. Some older children and adolescents may be nonverbal secondary to developmental disabilities. Therefore, clinicians must often depend on caregivers as the historians who give history regarding the child's illness or injury. This requires relying on the caregiver's interpretation of the child's signs and symptoms, which may be inaccurate. For example, a caregiver may report that the child has a "tummy ache" because the child abruptly refuses to eat. However, the child may actually be refusing to eat because of painful lesions in the posterior oropharynx that accompany common viral infections. The clinician may need to adjust wording or rephrase questions to elicit the most accurate

clinical data. For example, instead of "How long has he had leg pain?" the clinician might ask, "When did you first notice him limping?" It is also helpful to begin with open-ended questions—for example, "Can you tell me about his rash?"—and follow up with more specific and objective questions if needed—"Has he been scratching the rash?"

Whereas adults are able to express the severity of their symptoms or rate their pain on a scale from 1 to 10, infants and young children are not reliably able to express the severity of their symptoms. The more severe the symptoms of illness and injury, the more likely there may be interruptions in appetite, sleep, elimination, and activity. To elicit valuable clinical insight into the severity of the child's condition, ask, "How is he eating/sleeping/peeing/pooping?" and "Is he playing like he usually does?" For example, the ill child who is not eating or drinking may be at increased risk for dehydration or suffering pain from their illness. The child who continues to be active and at play indicates normal behaviors despite being ill, whereas the child who refrains from play or is choosing not to participate in activities they usually enjoys may indicate a more serious issue. Likewise, changes in elimination patterns can also alert the clinician to specific disease processes (urinary tract infection, constipation, dehydration, diabetes mellitus), which can further guide the focused history and physical assessment.

If a child is presenting with a mental health or behavioral issue, the use of a screening tool along with the history can be useful with caregivers. For example, the Pediatric Symptom Checklist (PSC) is a valid and reliable 35-item instrument that assesses a variety of mental health/behavioral issues (e.g., internalizing and externalizing disorders) in children and youth between 4 and 18 years of age. There is a 17-item valid and reliable short version of the scale as well. The PSC has been adapted for young children, 18 to 60 months of age, and for children younger than 18 months (Sheldrick et al., 2012; Sheldrick et al., 2013). The scales are freely downloadable and available in multiple languages at www .massgeneral.org/psychiatry/services/treatment programs.aspx?id=2088.

School-Aged Children

A child over age 4 to 5 can usually provide some of their own health history. It is essential to ask questions in an age-appropriate manner according to the developmental age and level of understanding. The clinician should pay close attention to nonverbal cues of comprehension and adjust the questions and terminology as needed. It is more important for the clinician to avoid the use of medical jargon or complex phrasing. For example, the terms "pain" or "discomfort" may be unfamiliar to a child, whereas "ouchies," "boo-boos," or "where it hurts" may be more relatable. Instead of

"Do you have painful bowel movements?" ask, "Does it hurt when you poop?" Instead of "Is the pain persistent or does it come and go?" ask, "Does it hurt all the time or just sometimes?" Instead of "Do you have a history of abdominal pain?" ask, "Has your belly hurt like this before?" Or instead of "Have you had any nausea or vomiting?" ask, "Have you felt like throwing up? Did you puke?"

Adolescents

Adolescence is the transition from childhood to adulthood. As such, it is important to gather history from both the caregiver and the adolescent when possible. While caregivers can offer a valuable perspective regarding the adolescent's health history, clinicians should also prioritize the opportunity for a one-on-one conversation with the adolescent. The clinician can support the adolescent's development of autonomy and responsibility for the latter's own health and wellness.

Adolescents are prone to engage in high-risk behaviors that cause substantial morbidity and mortality, such as substance abuse, reckless driving, and unprotected sex; moreover, many of the health behaviors that contribute to chronic illnesses in adulthood originate in adolescence, such as diet, activity, and tobacco use (Kann et al., 2016). Ensuring an opportunity for a private, confidential conversation with the clinician will improve the accuracy and integrity of the history provided by the adolescent. Studies demonstrate that a guarantee of confidentiality increases not only the number of adolescents willing to divulge private information, but also the number of adolescents willing to seek healthcare (Britto, Tivorsak & Slap, 2010; Lehrer et al., 2007). It is crucial for clinicians to be aware of their federal and state laws regarding adolescent consent and confidentiality, as these laws can vary from state to state.

The clinician should always start the health history with an adolescent by telling them that what they disclose is confidential unless they share information about hurting themselves or hurting someone else, which the clinician must share. Adolescents should also be informed that the same questions that are being asked of them are also asked of other adolescents in order to normalize history taking (Melnyk & Jensen, 2013).

When interviewing adolescents (aged 11–21 years), it is important to be sincere and allow for open-ended dialogue. With adolescents, the clinician can use more adult language; however, extensive medical jargon should still be limited to avoid confusion. If it seems the adolescent does not understand what is being asked, the question should be rephrased. The clinician should ask questions in a respectful, nonjudgmental manner. If a clinician appears to disapprove or make negative assumptions or seems uncomfortable asking sensitive questions, the adolescent may not be comfortable answering the questions. A nonjudgmental attitude is vital in establishing a rapport with adolescents. Teenagers may be distrusting of the intentions and motivations of healthcare clinicians, and they can also detect insincerity and disapproval. This type of rapport can have a damaging effect on the clinical relationship.

A point to note when asking about high-risk behaviors (substance misuse, sexual activity) is that if the teen pauses before answering, it may indicate that they is choosing what information to share or not share. Instead of asking adolescents whether they have ever used drugs or had sex, it is best to ask "When was the first time you ever used drugs, such as marijuana, cocaine, or 'painkillers' that were not prescribed to you?" To establish a more trusting environment, the clinician may wish to rephrase questions and normalize the behavior. For example, "Some teens your age have tried drinking alcohol or vaping; have you or any of your friends tried these things?" The same approach can be used when talking about potential romantic partners and sexual activity. Do not presume to know the adolescent's sexual orientation or gender identity; additional information about the assessment of gender identity and sexual orientation and dialogue to guide this assessment are detailed in Chapter 18. Clinicians should avoid medical jargon and use terminology that is common and direct. "What do you consider sex?" "Do you have sex with males, females, or both?" "What percentage of the time do you use condoms?" "Has anyone made you have sex when you didn't want to?" Establishing a trusting rapport and straightforward dialogue can assist the clinician in obtaining the most accurate health history to care for the adolescent. Motivational interviewing can be an effective method for coaching and counseling the adolescent.

Clinicians should take a thorough psychosocial history at each adolescent health supervision visit. The HEEADSSS (or HE^{2}ADS^3) instrument asks questions in the following psychosocial domains: Home, Education/Employment, Eating, Activities, Drugs, Sexuality, Suicide/Depression, and Safety (Smith & McGuinness, 2017). The tool is an effective method of engaging in an open discussion with the adolescent regarding risk-taking behaviors and risk for depression. The United States Preventive Services Task Force (USPSTF) "recommends screening for major depressive disorder (MDD) in adolescents aged 12 to 18 years. Screening should be implemented with adequate systems in place to ensure accurate diagnosis, effective treatment, and appropriate follow-up" (USPSTF, 2016a, "Recommendation"). The clinician should use a standardized depression-screening tool for depression, like the Patient Health Questionnaire for Adolescents (PHQ-A). The 9-item PHQ-A has the highest positive predictive value for depression in children and adolescents compared with other available depression screens (USPSTF, 2016). If the adolescent is depressed, a suicidal risk assessment should be performed, in which they should be asked about any plan and means to commit suicide. The adolescent should also be assessed for bipolar disorder and other mental health disorders, such as anxiety and substance abuse.

The Guidelines for Adolescent Preventive Services (GAPS) also is a well-established, self-report tool for assessing the special needs of adolescents (Elster & Kuznets, 1994). In addition, the AAP recommends screening all adolescents for tobacco, drugs, and alcohol use with the CRAFFT (Car, Relax, Alone, Forget, Friends, Trouble) tool. This screening tool takes less than 2 minutes to administer, has good sensitivity and specificity, and can help clinicians identify those adolescents that may be experiencing the consequence of substance use or abuse (Moyer, 2014). The CRAFFT is freely available at https://crafft.org/get-the-crafft. Clinicians should be prepared to provide the necessary counseling and referrals when particular concerns are identified.

PAST MEDICAL HISTORY

Collection of past medical history in children and adolescents does not differ significantly from the process used with adults. The clinician should take care to ask about the following aspects:

- Chronic illnesses (physical, mental health/ behavioral)
- Hospitalizations
- Surgeries
- Emergency department or urgent care visits
- Medications
- Allergies to drugs, foods, or the environment

Clinicians should be aware that the ability of children, adolescents, and caregivers to understand common medical terms is widely variable. It is important to phrase questions in a way that most people would understand. For example, instead of asking, "Any past history of hospitalizations?" ask, "Has your child ever had to stay in the hospital overnight?" Instead of asking, "Any past medical history of chronic illnesses?" ask, "Have you ever been told your child has diabetes or asthma?" Two important aspects of past medical history that should not be overlooked in young children are birth history and immunizations.

Birth History

For children aged 0 to 2 years, it is particularly important to inquire about birth history, especially when the child presents with a concern for poor growth, delay in development, respiratory illness, or infectious disease in the newborn.

- Prenatal care; planned or unplanned pregnancy
- Maternal health during pregnancy (infections, hypertension, diabetes, trauma, medications, depression/anxiety, substance use, smoking)
- Gestation at delivery and birth weight
- Labor and delivery complications (premature labor, breech position, fetal distress, birth injuries, hypoxia)
- Type of delivery (vaginal, cesarean, induction, instrumentation)
- Apgar scores
- Newborn infections or respiratory distress; respiratory support required
- Prolonged hospital stay, neonatal intensive care unit (NICU) stay
- Hyperbilirubinemia, hypoglycemia, feeding problems
- Universal hearing screen passed
- Vitamin K administration; hepatitis B vaccination
- Newborn screening results (varies by state)

Immunizations

Children typically receive the majority of their lifetime immunizations in the first year and a half of life. Therefore, infants and young children are particularly vulnerable to vaccine-preventable diseases. When evaluating children for infectious diseases, it is important to ask whether the child's vaccines are up to date, delayed, or behind. It is best to review an up-to-date vaccine record, if available, or access a state-based vaccine registry for accuracy, as some caregivers may be unsure of their child's vaccination status. Childhood vaccines immunize children against the following pathogens:

- Hepatitis B (Hep B)
- Pneumococcal
- Diphtheria/Tetanus/Pertussis (DTaP)
- Polio (IPV)
- Haemophilus influenza type b (Hib)
- Rotavirus
- Measles/Mumps/Rubella (MMR)
- Varicella, hepatitis A (Hep A)
- Meningococcal
- Human papilloma virus (HPV)
- Influenza virus

FAMILY HISTORY

- Chronic illnesses (cardiac disease, hypertension, obesity, diabetes, cancer, epilepsy, asthma, bleeding disorders)
- Intellectual disabilities, learning disorders, chromosomal abnormalities, congenital anomalies, developmental delays
- Mental health disorders (anxiety, depression, bipolar disorder, attention deficit hyperactivity disorder [ADHD], schizophrenia)

SOCIAL HISTORY

Children do not exist independently of their caregivers or their family context. They rely on caregivers to meet their needs and ensure their health and safety. The environment in which children grow and develop is critical to their health and wellness. It is imperative for the clinician to have a proper understanding of a child's psychosocial environment by investigating the following factors:

- Living conditions: single-family home, multigenerational family home, apartment
- Who lives in the home
- Composition of the family
- Occupation of the caregivers
- Day care, attending school, homeschooling
- Extracurricular, intramural activities
- Family violence
- Substance use, smoking
- Relationships, bullying

Social determinants of health (SDH) are the economic, environmental, and psychosocial conditions that affect the growth and development and the health and wellness of children. Early recognition and intervention can positively impact the outcomes of SDH on morbidity and mortality that not only affect at-risk children but also persist into adulthood. Systematic screening of SDH during routine health maintenance visits improves families' receipt of community resources (Garg, Toy, Tripodis, Silverstein & Freeman, 2015). The AAP recommends screening for SDH, such as poverty, adverse childhood experiences (ACEs), food insecurity, and housing (AAP, 2016). Common screening tools can be located at https://screeningtime.org/star-center.

DEVELOPMENTAL HISTORY

The AAP recommends that clinicians perform developmental surveillance at every routine health encounter and a standardized developmental screening at ages 9, 18, and 24 or 30 months (Hagan, Shaw, & Duncan, 2017). **Developmental surveillance** refers to the process of recognizing children who may be at risk for developmental delays. The clinician performs surveillance through physical observation of the child's development and by asking the caregiver whether the child has met age-appropriate developmental milestones. **Developmental screening** refers to the use of standardized tools to identify children at risk for delays in the developmental domains of motor (gross and fine), language, cognitive, emotional, and psychosocial. See **Table 4.2** for commonly used, valid, and reliable developmental screening tools.

All clinicians working with children should be familiar with early childhood developmental milestones as outlined in **Table 4.3**. When a child is not developing skills in one or more domains according to the expected time frame, the child has a *developmental delay*. When a child exhibits mental or physical impairment (or a combination of both) that results in functional limitations of the activities of daily living, the child has a *developmental disorder* or *developmental disability*. Identification of a developmental problem or delay should prompt further diagnostic evaluation and referral for early intervention services if indicated. *Early intervention* (EI) is a collective term describing programs or services that

TABLE 4.2 Developmental Screening Tools		
Screening Tool	**Ages**	**Type of Screening**
Ages & Stages Questionnaires® (ASQ®-3) (Squires & Bricker, 2009)	1–66 months	Developmental screening: communication, gross/fine motor, problem-solving, and personal/social skills
Ages & Stages Questionnaire—Social Emotional (ASQ:SE-2) (Squires, Bricker, & Twombly, 2015)	1–72 months	Social/emotional screening: self-regulation, compliance, social communication, adaptive functioning, autonomy, affect, and interaction with people
Parents' Evaluation of Developmental Status (PEDS©) (Glascoe, 2016)	0–8 years	Surveillance and screening of development, behavior, and mental health
Parents' Evaluation of Developmental Status— Developmental Milestones (PEDS: DM) (Glascoe & Robertshaw, 2016)	0–8 years	Surveillance and screening of development and mental health: expressive/receptive language, fine/gross motor skills, self-help, academics, and social/emotional skills
The Modified Checklist for Autism in Toddlers, Revised, with Follow-Up™ (M-CHAT-R/F) (Robins, Fein, & Barton, 2009)	16–30 months	Risk of autism spectrum disorder (ASD)

TABLE 4.3 Developmental Milestones of Early Childhood

Age	Social/Emotional	Language/Communication	Cognitive	Motor
2 months	Smiles Makes eye contact with caregiver Self-soothes briefly	Coos, makes gurgling sounds Turns head toward sounds	Pays attention to faces and follows with eyes	Develops head control and smoother movement in arms and legs
4 months	Smiles spontaneously at people; copies some facial expressions	Begins to babble Copies sounds Cries in different ways when hungry, tired, or in pain	Responds to affection Reaches for things Follows movement Recognizes familiar people from a distance	Holds head steady Rolls front to back Brings hands to mouth; uses hands and eyes together
6 months	Knows familiar faces Recognizes strangers Responds to others' emotions; likes to look at self in mirror	Responds to sounds by making sounds Responds to own name	Brings things to mouth Shows curiosity about things out of reach Passes things from one hand to another	Rolls back to front Begins to sit without support; when standing, supports weight on legs
9 months	May have stranger anxiety Has favorite toys	Understands "no" Copies sounds and gestures Uses finger to point	Plays peek-a-boo Develops object permanence (looks for things out of sight)	Stands, holding on Sits without support Pulls to standing Crawls
1 year	Cries when caregiver leaves Has favorite things and people Plays games such as pat-a-cake	Responds to simple requests Waves bye-bye Shakes head "no" Says words like "mama," "dada," "uh oh!"	Copies gestures Puts things in a container and takes things out of it Explores things by shaking, banging, throwing	Pulls up to standing Cruises (walks while holding on) May stand alone May take a few steps
18 months	Plays simple pretend, like feeding a doll May have temper tantrums Shows affection to familiar people	Says several single words Points to show someone what they want, points to pictures in a book	Knows what ordinary things are, like brush, spoon, phone Points to one body part; scribbles Follows command like "sit down"	Walks alone Drinks from a cup Eats with a spoon Pulls toys or carries toys while walking; may walk up stairs
2 years	Imitates others Gets excited when with other children and begins to involve them in games and play Shows more independence and defiance	Says sentences of 2–4 words Points to things in a book Follows simple commands Knows names of familiar people and body parts	Begins to sort shapes and colors Plays simple make-believe games Builds a tower of 4 cubes; finds things when hidden	Stands on tiptoe Kicks a ball Begins to run Climbs onto and down from furniture without help Walks up and down stairs while holding on
3 years	Copies adults and friends Shares, cooperates, shows concern and affection without prompting Dresses and undresses self	Follows instructions with 2 or 3 steps Understands prepositions (on, in, under); words are 75% understandable to strangers	Can button, complete puzzles with 3 or 4 pieces, copy a circle Turns book pages one at a time Builds towers of more than 6 blocks	Climbs well Runs easily Jumps forward Pedals a tricycle Walks up and down stairs, one foot on each step

(continued)

TABLE 4.3 Developmental Milestones of Early Childhood (*continued*)

Age	Social/Emotional	Language/ Communication	Cognitive	Motor
4 years	Enjoys doing new things, remembers parts of stories, uses scissors, starts to understand time Brushes teeth	Can say first and last names, uses pronouns correctly; can sing a song or recite a nursery rhyme from memory	Names some colors, numbers; draws a person with 2–4 body parts; plays board games, card games Can print some letters	Hops, stands on one leg for 2 seconds, catches a bounced ball most of the time Climbs stairs, alternating feet
5 years	Likes to sing, dance, act, participate in imaginative play Knows the difference between real and make-believe	Speaks clearly Tells a simple story with complete sentences; uses future tense Says name and address	Prints letters and numbers; copies a triangle and shapes Knows about everyday things (e.g., food, money) Draws a person with at least 6 body parts	Stands on one foot for 10 seconds or longer; may be able to skip, somersault Uses toilet on own Swings, climbs

Source: Adapted from Centers for Disease Control and Prevention. (2019). *Milestone checklist.* Retrieved from https://www.cdc.gov/ncbddd/actearly/pdf/checklists/Checklists-with-Tips_Reader-2019_508.pdf

support development for children aged 0 to 3 years with developmental delays or disabilities. EI might include speech therapy, physical therapy, occupational therapy, or other supports based on child and family need. EI is more likely to be effective in improving the developmental trajectory for the child if provided earlier in life. Children aged 0 to 3 years have greater neuroplasticity and therefore higher capacity for improved outcomes the earlier services are established.

PREVENTIVE CARE CONSIDERATIONS

Review recommended screenings and preventive measures (needed or completed) to maintain the health and well-being of infants, children, and teens. These include:

- The Advisory Council on Immunization Practices (ACIP) of the Centers for Disease Control and Prevention (CDC, n.d.) publishes recommended vaccine schedules annually. Every healthcare encounter is an opportunity to administer the recommended vaccines.
- The Subcommittee on Screening and Management of High Blood Pressure in Children and Adolescents recommends that blood pressure (BP) measurements should be checked annually at each routine health supervision visit for all children beginning at age 3 years (Flynn et al., 2017).
- The AAP recommends that body mass index (BMI) should be evaluated annually beginning at age 2 years at each routine health supervision visit (Barlow & The Expert Committee, 2007). The USPSTF recommends assessing BMI for all children

and adolescents aged 6 years and older and providing or referring for behavioral interventions for weight management (USPSTF, 2017a).
- All children living in communities with increased risk for lead exposure should have blood lead–level testing between 12 and 24 months of age (Council on Environmental Health, 2016). The Centers for Medicare and Medicaid Services (n.d.) require universal lead screening for all Medicaid-eligible children aged 12 and 24 months or any child between 24 and 72 months not previously screened.
- Children should receive hemoglobin screening for anemia routinely at 12 months of age, and at any other health encounter based on nutritional risk (Hagan et al., 2017).
- Children should be screened for dyslipidemia once between ages 9 and 11 and 17 and 21 years (National Heart, Lung, Blood Institute [NHLBI], 2012).
- Application of fluoride varnish is recommended for children aged 6 months to 5 years once teeth are present (USPSTF, 2014).
- The AAP recommends considering fluoride supplementation for those children who live in areas where the primary water source is deficient in fluoride (Clark & Slayton, 2014).
- Adolescents who are 12 to 18 years old should be screened for MDD. Screening should be implemented with adequate systems in place to ensure accurate diagnosis, effective treatment, and appropriate follow-up (USPSTF, 2016).
- The AAP Committee on Adolescence and Society for Adolescent Health and Medicine (2014) recommends annual screening of all sexually active

females and males who have sex with males (MSM) for chlamydia and gonorrhea. Consider screening other sexually active males based on individual- and population-based risk factors.

- Adolescents should be screened for HIV once between the ages of 15 and 18 years; and those at increased risk (sexually active, injection drug use, being tested for other sexually transmitted infections) should be tested annually (USPSTF, 2013).
- The USPSTF (2019) recommends that clinicians provide or refer pregnant and postpartum persons who are at increased risk for perinatal depression to counseling interventions. The AAP recommends that pediatric clinicians perform routine postpartum depression screening at a child's 1-, 2-, 4-, and 6-month health supervision visits (Weitzman & Wegner, 2015). The USPSTF (2019) endorses the Edinburgh Postnatal Depression Scale (EPDS) for pregnant and postpartum women.
- The AAP recommends that sensory screening (vision and hearing) be performed at routine intervals throughout early childhood and adolescence (Hagan et al., 2017). The USPSTF (2017b) recommends vision screening at least once in all children aged 3 to 5 years to detect amblyopia or its risk factors, like strabismus.

DEVELOPMENTAL APPROACH TO PHYSICAL EXAMINATION

Most pediatric clinicians employ the "quiet to active" approach when examining infants and young children (Duderstadt, 2019). It can also be thought of as "least distressing to most distressing." This approach requires that any aspect of the physical exam that necessitates the most cooperation, or that may be potentially uncomfortable, should be performed last. While many clinicians prefer to develop a systematic approach to the physical exam, it is important to modify the order of the exam according to the child's comfort or cooperation level. These aspects may be different from child to child; therefore, clinicians should be prepared to adjust the exam as they go. For example, the clinician may start a child's physical exam by auscultating heart and lung sounds and subsequently notice that the child is apprehensive about the ear exam; thus, the clinician will move on and save it for last. Any exam technique that will potentially make the child cry should be postponed until the end of the exam. Once an infant or child is distressed and crying, it is very difficult to auscultate heart and lung sounds or perform an eye exam.

When performing a focused physical assessment for system-specific complaints, the clinician should aim to perform the assessment in an orderly fashion, if possible: inspection, palpation, percussion, and auscultation.

Except when performing the abdominal exam, it is ideal to reorder the exam approach: inspection, auscultation, percussion, and palpation—especially if the child is presenting with a gastrointestinal or abdominal complaint.

INSPECTION

When performing a head-to-toe physical assessment, the clinician should carefully inspect each system. When evaluating a child for any complaint, it is of particular importance to assess general appearance on entering the exam room:

- Alert, listless, lethargic, or irritable
- Acute distress—mild, moderate, severe
- Well-appearing; ill-appearing; toxic appearance
- Age-appropriate behavior; affect

Furthermore, valuable clinical data can be gathered by simply observing the child closely throughout the encounter. For instance, does the child exhibit age-appropriate motor skills (sitting, crawling, standing, walking, and/or climbing)? Are the child's movements and neuromuscular tone symmetric? Is there evidence of child–caregiver attachment?

Is the clinician able to engage the child in play or interaction? The clinician should capture every opportunity to perform inspection and observation throughout the entirety of the health encounter, especially while performing other aspects of the physical exam.

A challenging aspect of pediatric physical assessment is the otoscopic exam. This is an essential skill for the clinician to master. To examine the auditory canal and tympanic membrane, the clinician should apply traction to the auricle in a downward and backward direction, as opposed to an upward and backward direction (as with adolescents and adults). This will open and align the canal for optimal visualization of the tympanic membrane in the infant or younger child. For maximum visualization, it is also important to use pediatric-sized specula.

PALPATION

Palpation is a key assessment technique, particularly when assessing abnormal skin and soft tissue lesions, organ size, abnormal masses, and injury or deformity. If pain is the presenting complaint, palpate the site of pain last. The clinician should be aware of several considerations regarding the use of palpation when examining the pediatric population compared with adults.

- The head of infants and young toddlers should be palpated to assess fontanel size and closure. Normal fontanels should be soft (open) and flat—not bulging (increased intracranial pressure) or sunken (dehydration). The posterior and anterior fontanels should close by the age of 2 months and 18 months, respectively. Location of the fontanels is depicted in **Figure 4.1**.

- The AAP recommends periodic surveillance for DDH with the following techniques: observing for leg-length discrepancy, asymmetric thigh or gluteal creases, or restricted motion (especially abduction). Ortolani and Barlow tests for hip stability are useful maneuvers to detect dislocation and limited motion in infants under 12 weeks of age. The Ortolani and Barlow maneuvers are shown in **Figure 4.2**. Infants with positive findings, especially those with risk factors, should receive a hip ultrasound. After 4 months of age, the infant should receive hip radiographs if there are limitations or concerns (anteroposterior and frog-leg pelvis views; Shaw et al., 2016). Refer to a pediatric orthopedist as indicated. The AAP recommends DDH surveillance through 1 year of age.

- Young children may exhibit shotty, mobile, nontender lymph nodes, especially in anterior/posterior cervical chains. When palpating lymph nodes in children, it is important to employ a systematic approach while carefully noting whether enlarged nodes are generalized, localized, or unilateral/bilateral.

- When evaluating infants and children for abdominal or gastrointestinal complaints, it is important to perform palpation last following inspection, auscultation, and percussion. Move from light palpation to deep palpation. If a child is complaining of pain in a particular quadrant, palpate that quadrant last to delay any potential discomfort. It is ideal to palpate the abdomen of infants and children when they are relaxed. The abdomen can become very firm when the child is crying, straining, or laughing. The ticklish child may require a gentle but firm touch to avoid sensitivity. It can help for the clinician to place one hand over the top of the child's hand to alleviate the ticklish reflex and facilitate the abdominal exam as depicted in **Figure 4.3**.

- In infants, the femoral pulse should be palpated simultaneously with the brachial or radial pulse. A delayed or diminished femoral pulse in comparison with the brachial or radial pulse is suggestive of the coarctation of the aorta.

- Clinicians should palpate both testicles of the infant male to ensure that they have both descended and can be brought down into the lower third of the scrotal sac. If the testes cannot be palpated, the infant should be referred to a pediatric urologist between the ages of 4 and 6 months.

- The USPSTF (2011; Nelson et al., 2016) does not recommend routine clinical breast or testicular exams as cancer screening in asymptomatic patients of any age because there is insufficient evidence that these exams reduce mortality or improve outcomes.

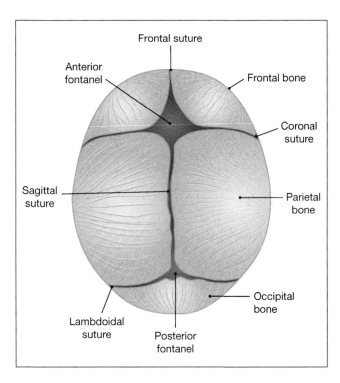

FIGURE 4.1 Anterior and posterior fontanels of an infant's skull.

PERCUSSION

The use of percussion is not routinely employed but can be helpful to the skilled clinician in determining organ size, solid- or air-filled structures, or abnormal masses and lesions. Solid (liver) or fluid-filled (bladder) structures will produce a dull sound, while air-filled structures (bowel, lungs) will produce tympany. One aspect of percussion that is often overlooked is the skill of eliciting costovertebral angle (CVA) tenderness. **Figure 4.4** illustrates this technique. Urinary tract infections are a common and potentially critical issue for infants, children, and adolescents. The maneuver can help distinguish between upper or lower UTIs. CVA tenderness is a finding indicative of kidney inflammation or infection, like pyelonephritis.

AUSCULTATION

The pediatric assessment is very similar to the adult exam in terms of auscultation of heart, lung, and bowel sounds. However, the clinician should avoid using an adult-sized stethoscope or large diaphragm when auscultating heart and lung sounds in infants and young children as this may yield overlapping, confusing findings. The use of a high-quality infant or pediatric stethoscope is encouraged (**Figure 4.5**). During auscultation of the heart sounds, the bell should be used to detect low-frequency sounds, and the diaphragm should be used to detect high-frequency sounds. S1 is generated by the closure of the atrioventricular valves and is best

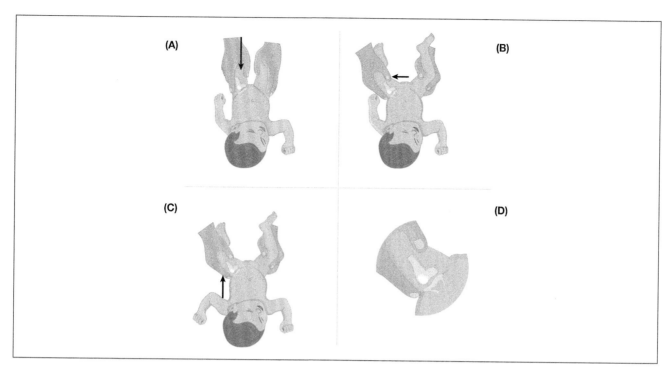

FIGURE 4.2 Barlow and Ortolani maneuvers. A. Barlow testing: From an abducted (thighs outward) position, flex the infant's knees to 90 degrees and apply posterior pressure or force. B, C. Ortolani testing: From the knee-bent position, abduct each of the infant's legs by moving the thigh outward (B) and apply anterior, upward pressure or force (C). D. Testing is positive when maneuvers result in a felt or heard "clunk" or when limited motion in either hip or thigh is noted. Positive testing indicates that the femoral head is partially or completely dislocated from the acetabulum.

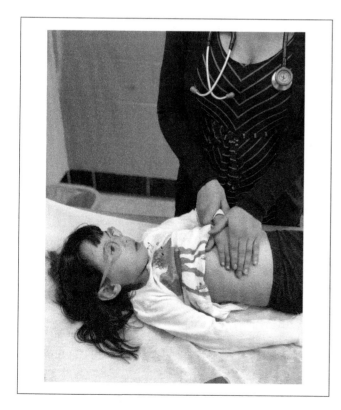

FIGURE 4.3 Abdominal exam technique for ticklish children.

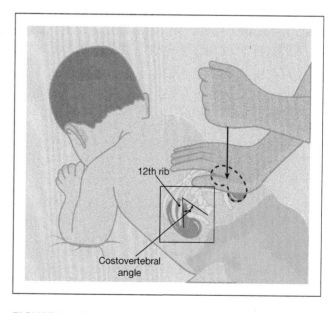

FIGURE 4.4 Percussion for costovertebral angle tenderness.

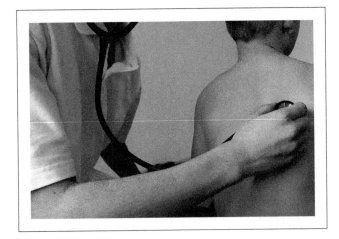

FIGURE 4.5 Clinician using a pediatric stethoscope for auscultation.

heard at the apex or lower left sternal border. The presence of a split S1 is a rare finding and may be benign in children. S2 is produced with the closure of the semilunar valves and marks the beginning of diastole. The physiologic splitting of S2 can occur with respiration and is considered a normal finding in children. A widely split and fixed S2 may be abnormal and may indicate a pathologic condition, such as an atrial septal defect.

Growth Assessment

Accurate and reliable growth measures are essential. Deviations in growth trajectories may be indicative of neglect, chronic illness, malnutrition, hormonal conditions, or congenital syndromes. The CDC (2010) recommends using the World Health Organization (WHO) international growth charts for children aged 0 to 23 months and the 2002 CDC growth charts for children and adolescents aged 2 to 18 years. **Figures 4.6** (p. 69) and **4.7** (p. 70) include the growth charts for ages birth through 24 months for girls and boys. Because children are continuously growing, growth measurements are interpreted differently than in the case of adults. Weight, height/length, BMI, weight for length, and head circumference trends are compared with a reference population of children of the same age and sex and reported as a percentile. These measures should be assessed and documented to allow the clinician to monitor changes over time. **Figures 4.8** (p. 71) and **4.9** (p. 72) include the head circumference for age and weight-for-length percentiles for girls and boys.

Infants and young children under age 2 should be measured lying supine with a recumbent infant length board or examining table, as shown in **Figure 4.10** (p. 73), and should be weighed nude or in a clean, dry disposable diaper on an accurately calibrated scale (**Figure 4.11**, p. 74). Head circumference should be measured for all children up to age 3. This measurement should be obtained with a flexible, but nonelastic measuring tape.

The measuring tape should be placed just above the brow line anteriorly and over the occipital prominence posteriorly, as depicted in **Figure 4.12** (p. 74). It is advisable to measure the head circumference three times in one encounter to ensure the accuracy of the recording.

Length, weight, length-for-weight percentile, and head circumference measurements should be plotted according to age on the WHO growth chart designated for the infant's natal sex. The newborn is expected to lose up to 10% of their birth weight in the first few days of life. Greater than 10% weight loss in the newborn should be urgently investigated. Normal weight gain for the newborn is 15 to 30 g/day (0.5–1 oz/day). It is normal for breastfed newborns to gain weight on the lower end of the normal range. The newborn should recover birth weight by at least 2 weeks of age. The average infant will double their birth weight by 6 months of age and triple it by 12 months. The average newborn length is 20 to 21 inches (51 cm). Linear growth velocity averages 2.5 cm/month from birth to 6 months, 1.3 cm/month from 7 to 12 months, and about 7.6 cm/year between 12 months and 10 years of age on average.

Infants with poor weight gain or growth measurements that trend downward or fall below the third percentile may have a failure to thrive (FTT), and the cause should be investigated. If neglect, organic disease, or severe malnutrition is suspected, the child should be hospitalized for evaluation. An upward-trending head circumference may indicate hydrocephalus or other intracranial pathology. A head circumference that stalls in growth may indicate a premature fusion of sutures/fontanels or a congenital syndrome associated with microcephaly.

For adolescents and children older than age 2, height, weight, and BMI should be plotted on the CDC growth chart relative to the child's natal sex. Young children and adolescents who can stand steadily without assistance should be weighed with a calibrated electronic scale or beam balance scale (**Figure 4.13**, p. 74). Height should be measured with a portable or wall-mount stadiometer, with the child standing erect, looking forward, with heels and occiput against the wall (**Figure 4.14**, p. 74). Height and weight should be obtained without shoes. Prior to the accelerated growth period in adolescence, school-aged children typically grow an average of 2.5 inches and gain an average of 5 to 7 pounds/year.

BMI is calculated by dividing weight in kilograms by the square of height in meters (kg/m^2). While BMI does not measure body fat specifically, it does correlate with direct measures of body fat. A statistical definition of obesity, based on calculation of BMI compared with an age- and sex-specific reference population, is utilized for children and adolescents. Obesity in children is indicated by a BMI greater than or equal to the 95th percentile on the CDC standardized growth chart. A BMI between the 85th and the 95th percentiles is considered overweight. A BMI between the 5th and the

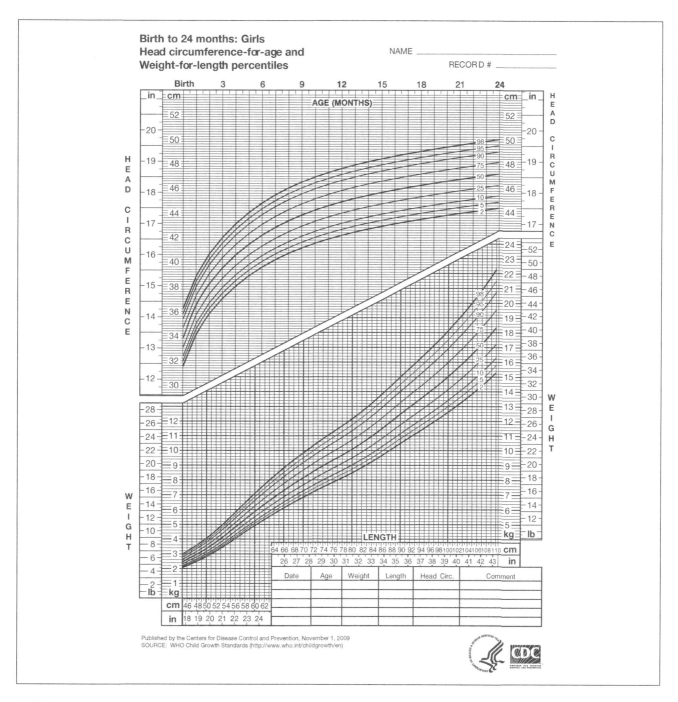

FIGURE 4.6 Growth chart for girls: birth to 24 months.

Source: World Health Organization. (2009b). *Birth to 24 months: Girls head circumference-for-age and weight-for-length percentiles.* Retrieved from https://www.cdc.gov/growthcharts/data/who/GrChrt_Girls_24HdCirc-L4W_9210.pdf

85th percentiles is considered normal weight. BMI calculators can be located on the CDC website: www.cdc .gov/healthyweight/bmi/calculator.html.

Children who fall off their growth curves for height or weight should be evaluated for an underlying condition. A progressive decrease in weight or BMI, or below the third percentile, may warrant further investigation. Older children and adolescents should be asked about intentional weight loss and evaluated for an eating disorder if indicated.

Specialized growth charts provide useful growth references for special populations of children whose growth measures might vary from typically developing children. These charts help to monitor growth among children in comparison with their peers with similar atypical growth and development, such as Down

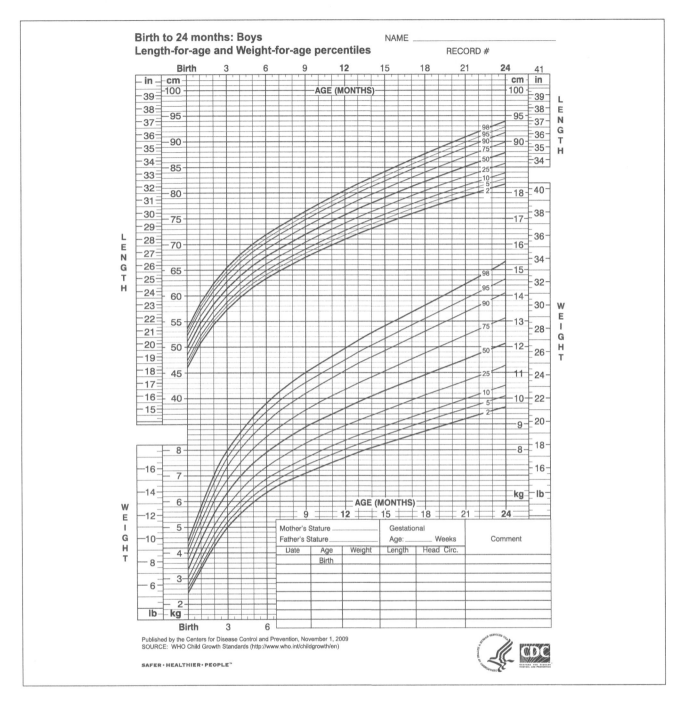

Birth to 24 months: Boys
Length-for-age and Weight-for-age percentiles

FIGURE 4.7 Growth chart for boys: birth to 36 months.

Source: World Health Organization. (2009a). *Birth to 24 months: Boys head circumference-for-age and weight-for-length percentiles.*
Retrieved from https://www.cdc.gov/growthcharts/data/who/GrChrt_Boys_24HdCirc-L4W_rev90910.pdf

Syndrome (Zemel et al., 2015). All growth charts are available for download at no cost from the CDC website: www.cdc.gov/growthcharts/index.htm.

Vital Signs

Vital signs for infants and children can vary greatly in comparison with the normal range for adults (see **Table 4.1**).

- The technique for temperature measurement is age dependent. Rectal temperature is preferred for infants and young children, while the oral temperature can be obtained when the child is developmentally able to hold and maintain the oral thermometer under the tongue (**Figure 4.15**, p. 75). Axillary temperature measurements are adequate, but they usually measure lower than oral

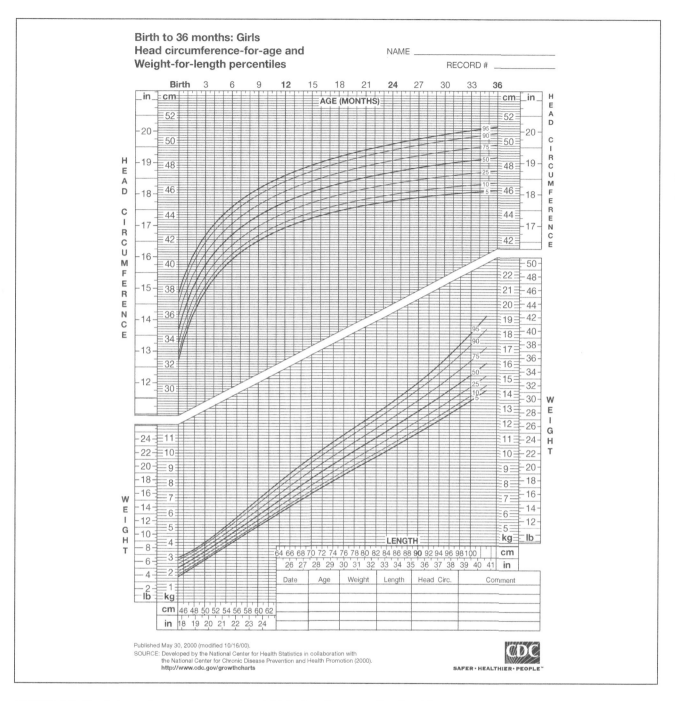

FIGURE 4.8 Head circumference-for-age and weight-for-length percentiles for girls.

Source: National Center for Health Statistics & National Center for Chronic Disease Prevention and Health Promotion. (2000b, October 16). *Birth to 36 months: Girls head circumference-for-age and weight-for-length percentiles.* Retrieved from https://www.cdc.gov/growthcharts/data/set2clinical/cj41c070.pdf

or rectal temperatures, and since axillary temperatures can vary widely, no standard conversion to core temperature exists. In general, fever is defined by a temperature ≥100.4°F. However, it is important to note that newborns and some children with neurologic conditions may not exhibit fever, even in the presence of serious infection. Rather, these children may demonstrate a lower than normal temperature.

- Heart rate can be assessed via auscultation of the apical pulse or palpation of the radial (older children, adolescents), brachial, or femoral pulse (infants). Heart rate also varies with age and may also be increased by activity, illness, or high fever.

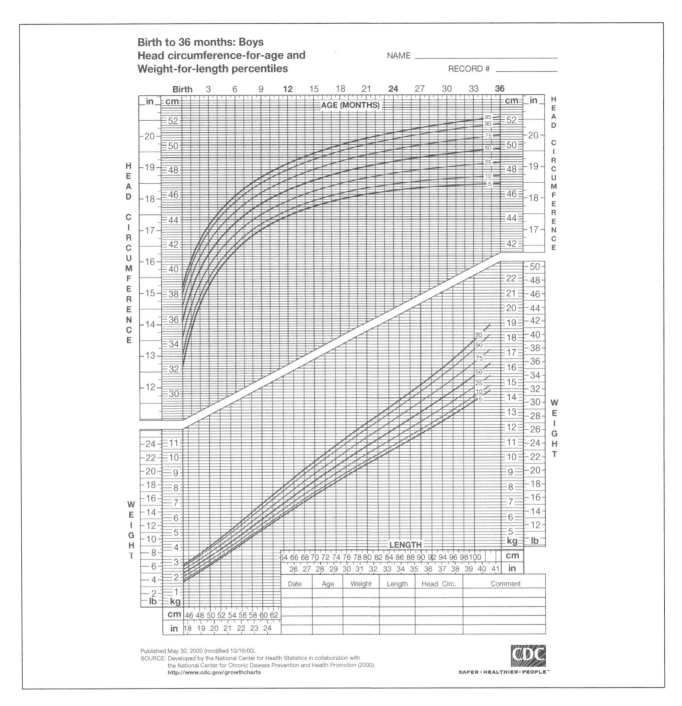

FIGURE 4.9 Head circumference-for-age and weight-for-length percentiles for boys.

Source: National Center for Health Statistics & National Center for Chronic Disease Prevention and Health Promotion. (2000a, October 16). *Birth to 36 months: Boys head circumference-for-age and weight-for-length percentiles.* Retrieved from https://www.cdc.gov/growthcharts/data/set2clinical/cj41c069.pdf

- Respiratory rate varies not only with age but also with activity or distress. Respiratory rate is most accurately assessed for a full minute while the infant or young child is calm or sleeping.
- BP measurement in children not only varies with age, but is also evaluated against standard reference population of sex and height percentile. BP is routinely taken annually, beginning at age 3. Before this

age, BP is taken in response to other findings suspicious of underlying cardiac or renal disease. It is imperative to use an appropriately sized BP cuff to obtain an accurate measurement. The cuff should cover approximately two-thirds of the upper arm. A cuff that is too big will result in a measurement that is too low, while a cuff that is too small will result in a measurement that is too high. Many young children

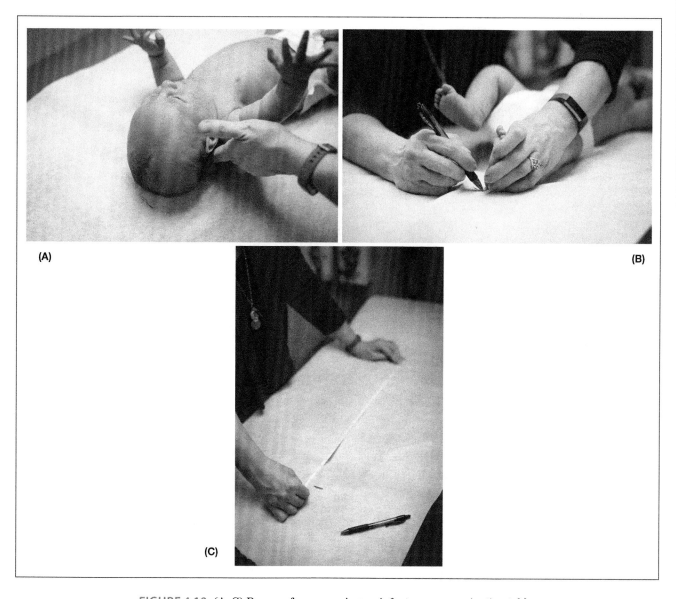

(A)

(B)

(C)

FIGURE 4.10 (A–C) Process for measuring an infant on an examination table.

are fearful of BP measurements. To facilitate the BP measurement and alleviate fear, the clinician can allow the child to examine or play with the equipment first (**Figure 4.16**, p. 75). Clinicians should be mindful of the language they use in preparing children for the procedure, especially for preschool children who engage in magical thinking. Instead of saying, "This will squeeze your arm" or "This is going to get tight," the clinician can say, "This is going to give your arm a hug" or "We are going to check your muscles."

KEY DEVELOPMENTAL CONSIDERATIONS
Infants and Children

Newborns (0–1 month) and young infants (1–6 months) generally prefer to stay warm and secure. The clinician should perform as much of the physical exam as possible prior to removing blankets, clothes, or diapers. By keeping the infant comfortable, the clinician can facilitate an efficient and successful head-to-toe physical exam. In fact, many physical exam elements can be performed while the caregiver is holding the "quiet" infant. In particular, this is an ideal time to auscultate heart and lung sounds. When it is time for the "active" aspects of the exam, the clinician should perform the remainder of the exam with the infant lying supine safely on the exam table. The active aspects of the exam may include the otoscopic ear exam, oropharynx, abdomen, genitalia, and hips. Conversely, the clinician can also seize the opportunity when an infant is already crying to perform an effective exam of the mouth, dentition, and posterior oropharynx.

Chess and Thomas (1987) conducted a longitudinal study to investigate the differences in behavioral traits throughout childhood and adolescence. The study

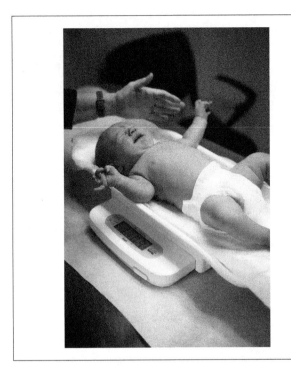

FIGURE 4.11 Infant weighed on calibrated scale.

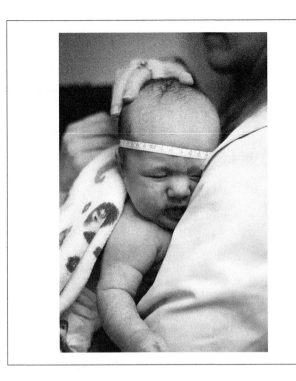

FIGURE 4.12 Measurement of occipito-frontal circumference.

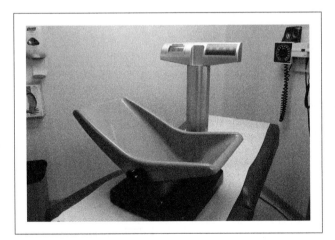

FIGURE 4.13 Calibrated electronic scale.

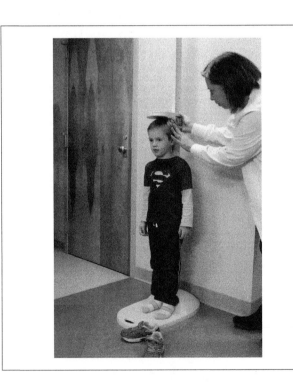

FIGURE 4.14 Stadiometer for standing height measurements.

describes three basic temperament types: easy, diffi-cult, and slow-to-warm-up. Infants and children with a difficult or slow-to-warm-up temperament can be challenging for the clinician. Furthermore, "stranger anxiety" peaks between 6 and 12 months and generally resolves around 2 years of age. However, a child of any age may be wary of strangers and apprehensive when the clinician enters the room. If a child appears fearful or nervous, start the encounter by placing yourself at a physical distance from the child. The clinician should consider beginning the clinical encounter sitting across the room while gathering history from the caregiver, as

demonstrated in **Figure 4.17**. The clinician appears less threatening when sitting than when standing and towering over the child. The child will watch and listen as you build a rapport with the caregiver. Often, once

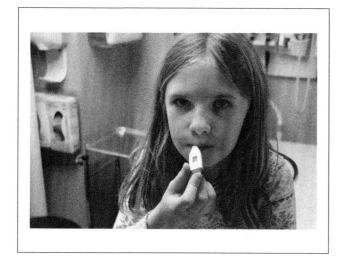

FIGURE 4.15 Measurement of temperature using an oral thermometer.

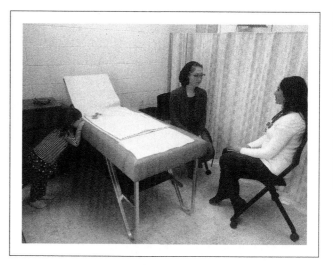

FIGURE 4.17 Clinician with fearful child.

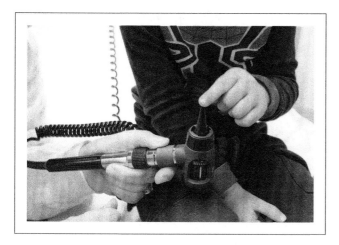

FIGURE 4.16 To alleviate fear, the clinician should allow the child to examine or play with equipment before using it.

the child realizes that the parent is comfortable with you, the child will relax as well. Young children frequently look to their caregivers for social cues. This is called "social referencing."

For older infants (6–12 months) and young children (1–4 years), the aspects of the physical exam that typically feel most worrisome are the otoscopic ear exam; the oral exam with tongue depressor; and/or lying down for abdominal palpation or anogenital exam. Plan to reserve these exam aspects for last. Children develop in all developmental domains (motor, language, cognitive, and psychosocial skills) through play. Play can be an effective tool for the clinician. Learning to transform the physical exam into *play* for the child can help the clinician increase cooperation.

The clinician can use toys, games, or other distractions to facilitate the exam. Ask, "Can you open your mouth big like an alligator?" "Can you show me how you climb up on this table?" Be sure to give positive reinforcement when the child plays along. The clinician should demystify the equipment (otoscope, stethoscope). Even though it is not invasive, some older infants and toddlers are fearful of the stethoscope. The clinician can demonstrate assessment techniques on the child's stuffed animal or a sibling/caregiver before performing them on the child to promote trust and confidence in the clinician. Some children enjoy "having a turn" with the stethoscope to hear their own heart. Furthermore, the clinician might ask, "Do you want to see my flashlight? I use this to look in ears." Let children touch the otoscope speculum to see that it does not hurt. Children are also pleased to see that it can light up their fingers. Then you can say, "Now I am going to use my flashlight to look in your ears."

Do not give the child choices for things that are not optional. For example, if the clinician asks, "Can I look in your ears?" the child may reply no. If the clinician must examine the ears, then it is not optional for the child. Instead, you might ask, "Should I look in your ears or your mouth first?" This approach gives the child some control and can generate cooperation.

The child, whether cooperative or not, must be secured and properly positioned for certain aspects of the physical exam. Safety is paramount. Safe positioning may require caregiver assistance to ensure the child's safety while effectively performing the exam, although it is always preferred to obtain assistance from another healthcare clinician whenever possible so that the caregiver remains in the role of a "comforter" for the child. **Figure 4.18** demonstrates safe positioning to examine the ears of a young infant. The clinician gently immobilizes the infant's head and pulls the auricle downward and backward to align the ear canal. The safest way to hold

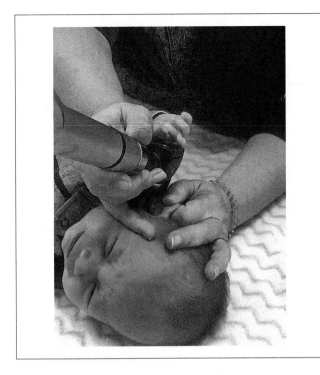

FIGURE 4.18 Infant ear exam technique.

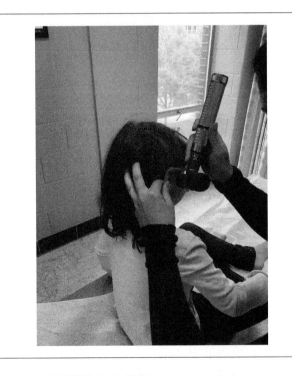

FIGURE 4.19 Child ear exam technique.

the otoscope is upside down, between the thumb and the first finger while using the pinky finger as a fulcrum, especially for infants and young children who might move unexpectedly; this is demonstrated in **Figure 4.19**. For older infants, the caregiver may need to assist the clinician by holding the infant's hands. For older children and adolescents, the auricle should be pulled upward and backward.

Young children can be safely secured on a caregiver's lap with their head and arms secured to assist the clinician in performing a safe exam of the ears or posterior oral pharynx. **Figure 4.20** demonstrates three positioning holds with the assistance of the caregiver. It is helpful to know that children cry and become combative when they are afraid or when they are not happy about being restrained, not necessarily because they are in pain. If the exam is being performed with the child safely secured, it should not cause pain.

ADOLESCENTS

The period of early to late adolescence begins around age 10 and ends around age 21. It is a transition from dependence to independence for the patient and requires facilitation by both the caregiver and the clinician. Although parents are largely responsible for their adolescent's care, the goal is to prepare teens with the tools necessary to self-advocate and manage their healthcare needs as they approach adulthood. The need for privacy during the health history and interview should take priority and be offered during the visit. The clinician can begin the visit with the caregiver present and then conclude the interview with the caregiver outside of the exam room. Adolescents are more likely to divulge private information and ask important questions without their parent or caregiver present. Confidentiality should be maintained and align with the limits of the state law and the clinician's area of practice.

The clinician can implement a typical head-to-toe physical exam sequence and the same techniques used for adults when examining the adolescent. Providing privacy and preserving modesty is paramount. The clinician should keep all parts of the body covered when not being assessed. Adolescents often have concerns regarding their developing bodies, and they feel self-conscious. It is important to reassure the adolescent when everything is normal.

The AAP asserts that if an adolescent patient requires a physical examination of the genitalia or female breasts (for system-specific complaints, or for SMR staging), the use of a chaperone is recommended; however, this should be a shared decision between the clinician and the adolescent (Curry et al., 2011). Some states have mandatory chaperone laws, so it is important for clinicians to be aware of their respective state laws. A chaperone can be a caregiver or another healthcare clinician, but this should be the adolescent's choice.

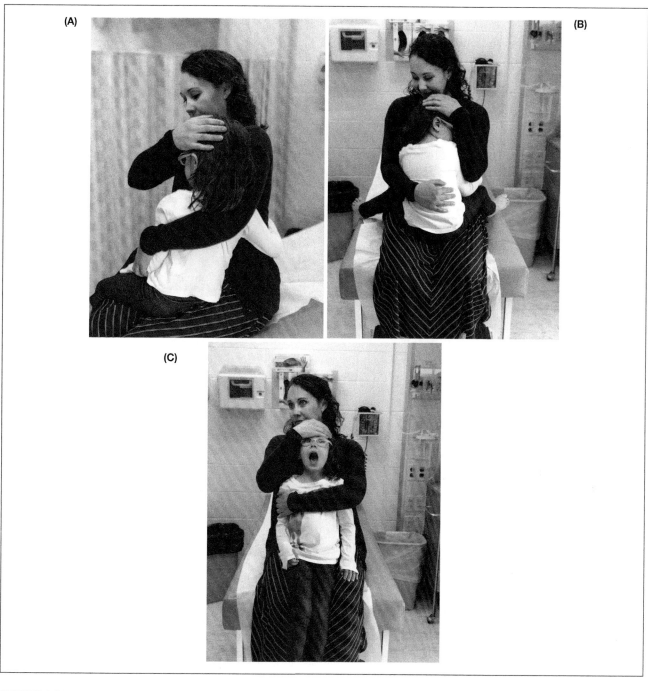

FIGURE 4.20 Positioning holds with caregiver. (A) Sideways. (B) Facing parent. (C) Face-front hold for oral exam/ throat swab.

KEY DIAGNOSTIC AND IMAGING CONSIDERATIONS

Although clinical decision-making surrounding the use of imaging and diagnostics will be discussed in further detail throughout the textbook chapters, there are general practice guidelines that should be considered in pediatric care. Children are different from adults in terms of body surface area and organ development. Children are 10 times more radiosensitive than adults and have a longer lifetime to express any changes, including secondary malignancy or cancer. The use of imaging and exposure to radiation should be used with caution. Owing to the wide use and availability of interventional procedures and imaging, the risk for exposing patients to frequent, sometimes unnecessary, doses of radiation has increased.

Clinicians must consider minimizing exposure to radiation when possible. The Society for Pediatric Radiology developed the ALARA (As Low as Reasonably Achievable) principle, which advocates for radiation dose reduction in the pediatric population (Voss, Reaman, Kaste, & Slovis, 2009). Clinicians must consider how necessary imaging is to the final clinical impression and examine whether alternative options are available to answer the clinical question. For example, the use of ultrasound as opposed to computed tomography (CT) for evaluating a source of abdominal pain can mitigate radiation exposure and achieve the same diagnosis necessary for further management. Additional information and resources on this subject are available through Image Wisely and The Image Gently Alliance. The alliance serves to increase national education and awareness and provides clinical checklists and additional information on its website at www.imagegently.org.

Key Takeaways: Evidence-Based Practice Considerations

- Children are not just small adults.
- Assessment and management of pediatric conditions cannot be scaled down from an adult approach.
- It is imperative that any clinician caring for an infant, child, or adolescent be familiar with current, evidence-based guidelines and resources. Reliable pediatric guidance can be sought at the AAP (www.aap.org), the USPSTF (www.uspreventiveservicestaskforce.org), and the National Association of Pediatric Nurse Practitioners (https://napnap.org).
- *Bright Futures: Guidelines for Health Supervision of Infants, Children, and Adolescents* (Hagan et al., 2017) is a seminal resource for interprofessional healthcare clinicians caring for the pediatric population. The tool kit and resources can be located at https://brightfutures.aap.org.

REFERENCES

American Academy of Pediatrics. (2016). Poverty and child health in the United States. *Pediatrics, 137*(4), e20160339. doi:10.1542/peds.2016-0339

American Academy of Pediatrics, Committee on Adolescence and Society for Adolescent Health and Medicine. (2014). Screening for nonviral sexually transmitted infections in adolescents and young adults. *Pediatrics, 134*, e302–e311. doi:10.1542/peds.2014-1024

Barlow, S., & The Expert Committee. (2007). Expert Committee recommendations regarding the prevention, assessment, and treatment of child and adolescent overweight and obesity: Summary report. *Pediatrics, 120*(Suppl. 4), S164–S192. doi:10.1542/peds.2007-2329C

Britto, M., Tivorsak, T., & Slap, G. (2010). Adolescents' needs for health care privacy. *Pediatrics, 126*(6), e1469–e1476. doi:10.1542/peds.2010-0389

Centers for Disease Control and Prevention. (n.d.). ACIP vaccine recommendations and guidelines. Advisory Committee on Immunization Practices (ACIP). Retrieved from https://www.cdc.gov/vaccines/hcp/acip-recs/index.html

Centers for Disease Control and Prevention. (2010). Use of World Health Organization and CDC growth charts for children aged 0-59 months in the United States. *Morbidity and Mortality Weekly Report, 59*(RR09), 1–15. Retrieved from https://www.cdc.gov/mmwr/pdf/rr/rr5909.pdf

Centers for Disease Control and Prevention. (2019). *Milestone checklist*. Retrieved from https://www.cdc.gov/ncbddd/actearly/pdf/checklists/Checklists-with-Tips_Reader-2019_508.pdf

Centers for Medicare and Medicaid Services. (n.d.). *Lead screening*. Retrieved from https://www.medicaid.gov/medicaid/benefits/epsdt/lead-screening/index.html

Chess, S., & Thomas, A. (1987). Temperamental individuality from childhood to adolescence. *Journal of Child Psychiatry, 16*, 218–226. doi:10.1016/S0002-7138(09)60038-8

Chiocca, E. M. (2015). *Advanced pediatric assessment* (2nd ed.). New York, NY: Springer Publishing Company.

Clark, M. B., & Slayton, R. L. (2014). Fluoride use in caries prevention in the primary care setting. *Pediatrics, 134*(3), 626–633. doi:10.1542/peds.2014-1699

Council on Environmental Health. (2016). Prevention of childhood lead toxicity. *Pediatrics, 138*(1), e20161493. doi:10.1542/peds.2016-1493

Curry, E., Hammer, L. D., Brown, O. W., Laughlin, J. J., Lessin, H. R., Simon, G. R., & Rodgers, C. T. (2011). Policy statement: Use of chaperones during the physical examination of the pediatric patient. *Pediatrics, 127*(5), 991–993. doi:10.1542/peds.2011-0322

Duderstadt, K. G. (2019). *Pediatric physical examination: An illustrated handbook* (3rd ed.). St. Louis, MO: Mosby.

Elster, A. B., & Kuznets, N. J. (1994). *AMA guidelines for adolescent preventive services (GAPS): Recommendations and rationale*. Baltimore, MD: Williams & Wilkins.

Flynn, J. T., Kaelber, D. C., Baker-Smith, C. M., Blowey, D., Carroll, A. E., Daniels, S. R., . . . Thaker, V. (2017). Clinical practice guidelines for screening and management of high blood pressure in children and adolescents. *Pediatrics, 140*(3), e20171904. doi:10.1542/peds.2017-1904

Garg, A., Toy, S., Tripodis, Y., Silverstein, M., & Freeman, E. (2015). Addressing social determinants of health at well-child care visits: A cluster RCT. *Pediatrics, 135*(2), e296–e304. doi:10.1542/peds.2014-2888

Giedd, J. N., Blumenthal, J., Jeffries, N. O., Castellanos, F. X., Hong, L., Zijdenbos, A., & Rapoport, J. L. (1999).

Brain development during childhood and adolescence: A longitudinal MRI study. *Nature Neuroscience, 2*(10), 861–863. doi:10.1038/13158

Glascoe, F. P. (2016). *Parents' Evaluation of Developmental Status (PEDS©)*. Nolensville, TN: PEDStest.com.

Glascoe, F. P., & Robertshaw, N. S. (2016). *Parents' Evaluation of Developmental Status—Developmental Milestones (PEDS©: DM)*. Nolensville, TN: PEDStest.com.

Hagan, J. F., Shaw, J. S., & Duncan, P. (2017). *Bright futures: Guidelines for health supervision of infants, children and adolescents* (4th ed.). Elk Grove Village, IL: American Academy of Pediatrics.

Kann, L., McManus, T., Harris, W., Shanklin, S., Flint, K., Hawkins, J., & Zaza, S. (2016). Youth risk behavior surveillance—United States, 2015. *MMWR Surveillance Summary, 65*(6), 1–174. doi:10.15585/mmwr.ss6506a1

Lehrer, J. A., Pantell, R., Tebb, K., & Shafer, M. A. (2007). Forgone health care among U.S. adolescents: Associations between risk characteristics and confidentiality concern. *Journal of Adolescent Health, 40*(3), 218–226. doi: 10.1016/j.jadohealth.2006.09.015

Melnyk, B. M., & Jensen, P. (Eds.). (2013). *A practical guide to child and adolescent mental health screening, early intervention, and health promotion* (2nd ed.). New York, NY: National Association of Pediatric Nurse Practitioners.

Moyer, V. A. (2014). Primary care behavioral interventions to reduce illicit drug and nonmedical pharmaceutical use in children and adolescents: U.S. Preventive Services Task Force recommendation statement. *Annals of Internal Medicine, 160*, 634–639. doi:10.7326/M14-0334

National Center for Health Statistics & National Center for Chronic Disease Prevention and Health Promotion. (2000a, October 16). Birth to 36 months: Boys head circumference-for-age and weight-for-length percentiles. Retrieved from https://www.cdc.gov/growthcharts/data/set2clinical/cj41c069.pdf

National Center for Health Statistics & National Center for Chronic Disease Prevention and Health Promotion. (2000b, October 16). Birth to 36 months: Girls head circumference-for-age and weight-for-length percentiles. Retrieved from https://www.cdc.gov/growthcharts/data/set2clinical/cj41c070.pdf

National Heart, Lung, Blood Institute. (2012). *Expert panel on integrated guidelines for cardiovascular health and risk reduction in children and adolescents* (Report No. 12-7486). Bethesda, MD: National Institutes of Health. Retrieved from https://www.nhlbi.nih.gov/files/docs/peds_guidelines_sum.pdf

Nelson, H. D., Fu, R., Cantor, A., Pappas, M., Daeges, M., & Humphrey, L. (2016). Effectiveness of breast cancer screening: Systematic review and meta-analysis to update the 2009 U.S. Preventive Services Task Force recommendation. Retrieved from https://www.uspreventiveservicestaskforce.org/Page/Document/evidence-summary-screening-for-breast-cancer/ breast-cancer-screening1

Robins, D. L., Fein, D., & Barton, M. (2009). *The Modified Checklist for Autism in Toddlers, Revised, with Follow-Up (M-CHAT-R/F)*™. Retrieved from https://mchatscreen.com/wp-content/uploads/2015/09/M-CHAT-R_F_Rev_Aug2018.pdf

Shaw, B. A., Segal, L. S., Otsuka, N. Y., Schwend, R. M., Ganley, T. J., Herman, M. J., . . . Smith, B. G. (2016). Evaluation and referral for developmental dysplasia of the hip in infants. *Pediatrics, 138*(6), e1–e11. doi:10.1542/peds.2016-3107

Sheldrick, R. C., Hensen, B. S., Merchant, S., Neger, E. N., Murphy, J. M., & Perrin, E. C. (2012). The preschool pediatric symptom checklist (PPSC): Development and initial validation of a new social/emotional screening instrument. *Academic Pediatrics, 12*(5), 456–467. doi:10.1016/j.acap.2012.06.008

Sheldrick, R. C., Hensen, B. S., Neger, E. N., Merchant, S., Murphy, J. M., & Perrin, E. C. (2013). The baby pediatric symptom checklist: Development and initial validation of a new social/emotional screening instrument for very young children. *Academic Pediatrics, 13*(1), 72–80. doi:10.1016/j.acap.2012.08.003

Smith, G. L., & McGuinness, T. M. (2017). Adolescent psychosocial assessment: The HEEADSS. *Journal of Psychosocial Nursing and Mental Health Services, 55*(5), 24–27 doi:10.3928/02793695-20170420-03.

Squires, J., & Bricker, D. (2009). *Ages & Stages Questionnaires® (ASQ®-3)*. Baltimore, MD: Brookes Publishing.

Squires, J., Bricker, D., & Twombly, E. (2015). *Ages & Stages Questionnaire®—Social Emotional (ASQ®:SE-2)*. Baltimore, MD: Brookes Publishing.

U.S. Preventive Services Task Force. (2011). Testicular cancer: Screening. Retrieved from https://www.uspreventiveservicestaskforce.org/Page/Document/UpdateSummaryFinal/testicular-cancer-screening

U.S. Preventive Services Task Force. (2013). Human immunodeficiency virus (HIV) infection: Screening. Retrieved from https://www.uspreventiveservicestaskforce.org/Page/Document/UpdateSummaryFinal/human-immunodeficiency-virus-hiv-infection-screening

U.S. Preventive Services Task Force. (2014). Final recommendation statement: Dental caries in children from birth through age 5 years: Screening. Retrieved from https://www.uspreventiveservicestaskforce.org/Page/Document/RecommendationStatementFinal/dental-caries-in-children-from-birth-through-age-5-years-screening#Pod12

U.S. Preventive Services Task Force. (2016). Depression in children and adolescents: Screening. Retrieved from https://www.uspreventiveservicestaskforce.org/Page/Document/UpdateSummaryFinal/depression-in-children-and-adolescents-screening1

U.S. Preventive Services Task Force. (2017a). Obesity in children and adolescents: Screening. Retrieved from https://www.uspreventiveservicestaskforce.org/Page/Document/UpdateSummaryFinal/obesity-in-children-and-adolescents-screening1

U.S. Preventive Services Task Force. (2017b). Vision in children ages 6 months to 5 years: Screening. Retrieved from https://www.uspreventiveservicestaskforce.org/Page/Document/UpdateSummaryFinal/vision-in-children-ages-6-months-to-5-years-screening

U.S. Preventive Services Task Force. (2019). Perinatal depression: Preventive interventions. Retrieved from https://www.uspreventiveservicestaskforce.org/Page/Document/UpdateSummaryFinal/perinatal-depression-preventive-interventions

Weitzman, C., Wegner, L., & the Section on Developmental and Behavioral Pediatric, Committee on Psychosocial Aspects of Child and Family Health, Council on Early Childhood, and Society for Developmental and Behavioral Pediatrics. (2015). Promoting optimal development: Screening for behavioral and emotional problems. *Pediatrics, 135*(2), 384–395. doi:10.1542/peds.2014-3716

World Health Organization. (2009a). *Birth to 24 months: Boys head circumference-for-age and weight-for-length percentiles.* Retrieved from https://www.cdc.gov/growthcharts/data/who/GrChrt_Boys_24HdCirc-L4W_rev90910.pdf

World Health Organization. (2009b). *Birth to 24 months: Girls head circumference-for-age and weight-for-length percentiles.* Retrieved from https://www.cdc.gov/growthcharts/data/who/GrChrt_Girls_24HdCirc-L4W_9210.pdf

Voss, S. D., Reaman, G. H., Kaste, S. C., & Slovis, T. L. (2009). The ALARA concept in pediatric oncology. *Pediatric Radiology, 39,* 1142–1146. doi:10.1007/s00247-009-1404-5

Zemel, B. S., Pipan, M., Stallings, V. A., Hall, W., Schadt, K., Freedman, D. S., & Thorpe, P. (2015). Growth charts for children with Down syndrome in the U.S. *Pediatrics, 136*(5), e1204–e1211. doi:10.1542/peds.2015-1652

5

Approach to the Physical Examination: General Survey and Assessment of Vital Signs

Melissa Baker, Hollie Moots, Sinead Yarberry, Molly McAuley, and Kady Martini

"Great things are done by a series of small things brought together."

—Vincent van Gogh

VIDEO

- Well Exam: Complete Physical Exam

LEARNING OBJECTIVES

- Identify components of a general survey used to appraise signs of illness and wellness.
- Describe techniques used to accurately assess vital signs.
- Differentiate the types of pain and associated signs and symptoms.
- Evaluate normal and abnormal findings related to vital signs and the general survey.

GENERAL SURVEY APPROACH TO PHYSICAL EXAMINATION

As a clinician approaches an individual to complete a history and physical exam, the clinician first assesses the situation and the environment to ensure their own

Visit https://connect.springerpub.com/content/book/978-0-8261 -6454-4/chapter/ch00 to access the videos.

personal safety and to note any risks related to completing the assessment. Much of this determination is dependent on where the assessment is taking place, as unfamiliar settings or environments may have unknown risks. Whether an assessment is being done in the community or in a healthcare setting, however, an immediate observation for the clinician's safety is warranted. This immediate observation includes assessment of the environment, which might involve exposures to toxins, chemicals, extreme heat, cold, electric currents, or infectious agents. Clinician considerations include whether gloves, gown, or mask may need to be worn to avoid exposures and/or whether additional help may be needed for an unstable patient.

Once the environment is determined to be safe, and appropriate cautions are taken, an evidence-based advanced assessment begins with a **general survey**, that is, a systematic assessment of the individual's health status.

INITIAL STEPS TO DETERMINE PHYSIOLOGIC STABILITY

The initial assessments of a general survey are completed to determine whether the individual being evaluated is in distress. Observing whether a patient is well or unwell is essential and can be completed quickly. The components of assessment that determine whether an individual has **physiologic stability** can be remembered using the mnemonic *ABCDE*, that is, airway, breathing, circulation, disability, and exposure; note that each of these assessments is vital, with "C" being given the highest priority in adults (American Heart Association [AHA], 2018). **Table 5.1** lists the immediate assessments needed to identify signs and symptoms of emergent or urgent medical problems. For the patient who is physiologically unstable, that is, is unconscious, unresponsive, or not breathing normally, the clinician will need to respond to the situation appropriately, which may require initiating cardiopulmonary resuscitation (CPR) while continuing to assess the emergent situation.

This chapter includes a significant review of vital signs and **pain**, key assessments in determining patient stability. Subsequent chapters will review additional priority assessments, including signs and symptoms of respiratory distress, hypoxia, heart failure, and neurologic disorders. Completing the general survey of an individual allows the clinician to determine an appropriate, subsequent history and physical exam.

COMPONENTS OF A GENERAL SURVEY

Once the clinician has completed the initial steps of the general survey to determine that an individual is or is not experiencing acute distress, the next steps of advanced assessment involve observation of the individual's appearance, behavior, and cognition. These next steps requiring systematic observation can be remembered using the mnemonic *ABC*. **Table 5.2** lists components of each of these broad *ABC* categories, which include observational assessments of mental and physical status.

Assessment of Mental Status

A **mental status** assessment gives the clinician an understanding of the patient's cognitive, emotional, personality, and psychological functioning. Fundamental to the assessment of mental status is identifying the patient's orientation to person, place, time, and situation. Assessment of a patient's affect, mood, attention, judgment, and memory will provide the clinician with additional data regarding the patient's mental and neurologic functioning.

Changes in orientation are noted in a variety of conditions, so the clinician must consider these findings in addition to other pertinent assessment data. Older adults with physical disorders such as urinary tract

---

TABLE 5.1 Initial General Survey Assessments to Determine Physiologic Stability

Mnemonic ABCDE		
A	Airway	Assess for airway obstruction. Signs may include paradoxical chest and abdominal movements with respirations, cyanosis, diminished breath sounds, noisy breath sounds, or wheezing and stridor.
B	Breathing	Assess respiratory rate, depth, rhythm. Signs of respiratory distress include wheezing, stridor, cyanosis, dyspnea, hypoxia, retractions, and inability to speak in full sentences.
C	Circulation*	Palpate pulses to determine rate, rhythm, and adequacy. Assess for bleeding, cyanosis. Measure blood pressure. Signs may include chest pain, dyspnea, decreased perfusion, tachycardia, or bradycardia.
D	Disability	Assess level of consciousness. Examine pupils for size, equality, and reaction to light. Signs of disability or neurologic instability include confusion, irritability, vomiting, or nonresponsiveness.
E	Exposure	Expose the areas of assessment to determine critical conditions and complete the exam, while appropriately ensuring safety, stability, privacy, dignity, and comfort.

*Highest priority for assessment in adults.

TABLE 5.2 Assessments of Appearance, Behavior, and Cognition: Observational Assessments Included as Components of a General Survey

Mnemonic ABC		
A	Appearance	Affect (facial expression), posture, hygiene, and grooming; body habitus (height, weight, waist circumference)
B	Behavior	Verbal or nonverbal expressions of pain, anxiety, or illness; body movements and mobility, coordination
C	Cognition	Orientation to time, person, place; attention and concentration, pattern and pace of speech, judgment, memory, and mood

infections, pneumonia, or the flu may present with confusion or disorientation as their primary symptoms. In children, mental status changes can be the result of a high fever due to acute infections. Multiple medications can also cause a change in orientation or mental status, especially for individuals with multiple chronic illnesses and the elderly. Being careful to note subtle or obvious changes in orientation is essential to completing an accurate general survey.

Measurements of Body Habitus

Height and Weight

Measurements of height and weight are important components of the general survey assessment. These measures provide objective data regarding an individual's risk for chronic illnesses and/or likelihood of underlying genetic disorders, hormonal imbalances, or disease complications. Examples include the association of obesity with type 2 diabetes and changes in weight associated with eating disorders or depression. Weight gain can also be noted in patients with heart failure due to fluid retention. Short stature can be the result of hypothyroidism or nutritional deficiencies in childhood, and tall stature can be found in patients with genetic disorders such as Marfan syndrome.

Body Mass Index (BMI)

BMI is a measure of body size used to determine a weight category; BMI is calculated by the person's weight in kilograms divided by the square of height in meters. **Table 5.3** lists the formulas for calculating BMI.

TABLE 5.3 BMI Calculation

Units of Measurement	Formula to Calculate BMI
Kilograms and meters (or centimeters)	Weight (kg)/(height [m])^2
Pounds and inches	Weight (lb.)/(height [in])^2

BMI, body mass index.

TABLE 5.4 BMI Evaluation

BMI	Weight Status
Below 18.5	Underweight
18.5–24.9	Normal or healthy weight
25.0–29.9	Overweight
30.0 and above	Obese

BMI, body mass index.

Table 5.4 identifies the weight status associated with the BMI.

While BMI does not directly measure body fat, research studies have shown that BMI is more accurate in measuring body fat than other methods such as skinfold thickness (Centers for Disease Control and Prevention [CDC], n.d.). BMI appears to be strongly correlated with various diseases (National Heart, Lung, and Blood Institute [NHLBI], n.d.) and is an inexpensive and easy method for identifying a patient's weight category. While BMI is an effective screening tool, it is not diagnostic to the health of an individual. To determine whether a high BMI is a health risk, further assessments such as evaluation of diet, physical activity, family history, and other appropriate health screenings are warranted. The correlation between BMI and body fat is strong, but even if two people have the same BMI, their level of body fat may differ. In general, the following considerations apply (CDC, 2017):

- At the same BMI, women tend to have more body fat than men.
- At the same BMI, Blacks have less body fat than Whites, and Asians have more body fat than Whites.
- At the same BMI, older adults, on average, tend to have more body fat than younger adults.
- At the same BMI, athletes have less body fat than nonathletes.

When calculated using the same formula, BMI is interpreted differently for children and teens. Interpretation of BMI in children and adolescents requires the consideration of age and gender, as body fat percentages differ as children develop. The CDC BMI-for-age growth charts reflect these differences and visually show BMI as a percentile ranking. See **Figures 5.1** and **5.2** to review CDC BMI Growth Charts. Obesity among 2- to 19-year-olds is defined as a BMI at or above the 95th percentile.

Waist Circumference

Measuring waist circumference helps screen for possible health risks associated with being overweight and/or obese. People who carry excess fat around their waist, rather than their hips, are at a higher risk for heart disease and type 2 diabetes (NHLBI, n.d.). This risk increases significantly for women with a waist circumference greater than 35 inches (80 cm) and men who are greater than 40 inches (94 cm). Waist circumference is a less accurate measure for specific ethnic populations, including individuals from South Asia, China, or Japan, as they display a greater amount of visceral fat; waist circumference is also not a predictor of risk during pregnancy or for individuals with medical conditions causing ascites.

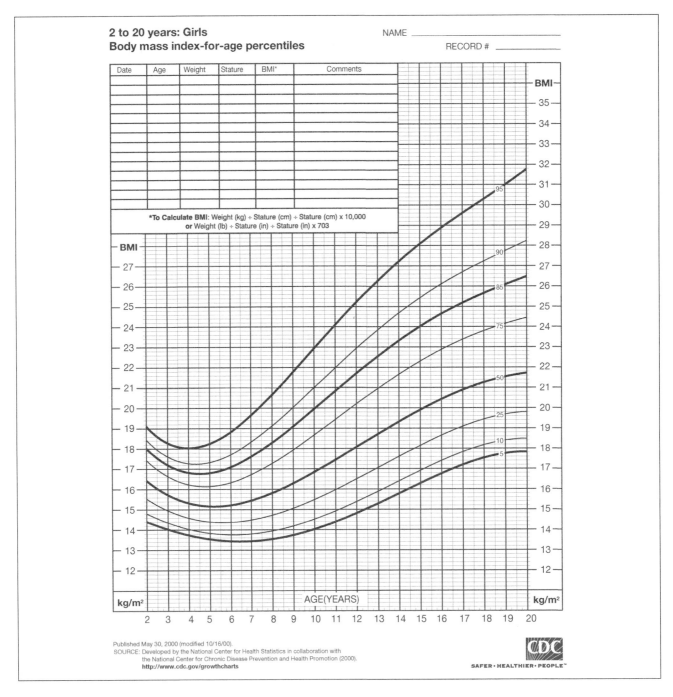

FIGURE 5.1 Body mass index (BMI) growth chart for girls: 2 to 20 years.

Source: National Center for Health Statistics & National Center for Chronic Disease Prevention and Health Promotion. (2000b). *2 to 20 years: Girls body mass index-for-age percentiles.* Retrieved from https://www.cdc.gov/growthcharts/data/set1clinical/cj41c024.pdf

ANATOMY AND PHYSIOLOGY

Assessment of vital signs (e.g., temperature, pulse rate, respiratory rate, and blood pressure [BP]) is essential for detecting acute changes in a patient's condition. Vital signs and pain assessments allow for the identification of signs and symptoms that indicate improvement, instability, and/or deterioration of an individual's physiologic status. Assessment of changes in these clinical parameters plays a fundamental role in the early detection of patient deterioration, but only if the clinician has a foundational understanding of the anatomy and physiology being reflected.

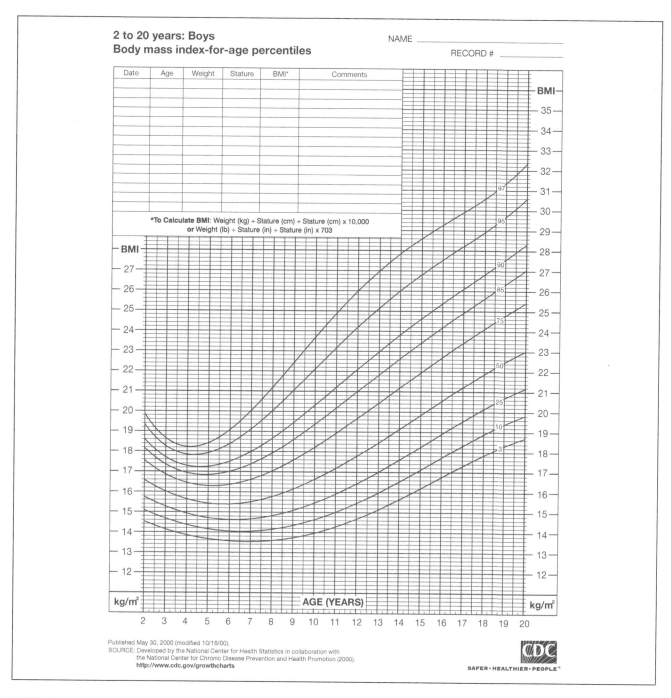

2 to 20 years: Boys
Body mass index-for-age percentiles

NAME _____

RECORD # _____

Date	Age	Weight	Stature	BMI*	Comments

*To Calculate BMI: Weight (kg) ÷ Stature (cm) ÷ Stature (cm) x 10,000
or Weight (lb) ÷ Stature (in) ÷ Stature (in) x 703

Published May 30, 2000 (modified 10/16/00).
SOURCE: Developed by the National Center for Health Statistics in collaboration with
the National Center for Chronic Disease Prevention and Health Promotion (2000).
http://www.cdc.gov/growthcharts

FIGURE 5.2 Body mass index (BMI) growth chart for boys: 2 to 20 years.

Source: National Center for Health Statistics & National Center for Chronic Disease Prevention and Health Promotion. (2000a). *2 to 20 years: Boys body mass index-for-age percentiles.* Retrieved from https://www.cdc.gov/growthcharts/data/set1clinical/cj41c023.pdf

BODY TEMPERATURE

The hypothalamus regulates **body temperature** by maintaining a balance between heat production and loss. Heat can be produced through the chemical reactions of metabolism and through skeletal muscle contractions with exercise. Body heat is lost through evaporation (sweat on the skin), radiation (heat leaving the body into the cooler surrounding air), convection (movement of air/water molecules across the skin), and conduction (physical contact with an item cooler than body temperature). Normal body temperature is 98.6°F (37°C) with a range of 96.4°F to 99.1°F (35.8°C–37.3°C). Body temperature fluctuates 1°F to 1.5°F (0.6°C–0.9°C) over the course of a day, with temperature at its lowest early in the morning and highest in the evening.

PULSE RATE

The arterial pulse results when blood is pumped into an already full aorta during ventricular contraction. This action creates a fluid wave that travels throughout the arterial system from the patient's heart to the peripheral arteries. This recurring wave, called a pulse, is palpable at locations on the body where an artery crosses a bone or firm tissue. The number of beats counted in 1 minute is called the **pulse rate**. Normal pulse rate for an adult is 60 to 100 beats/minute or bpm.

RESPIRATORY RATE

The function of the respiratory system is to carry air into the lungs and to facilitate the diffusion of oxygen into the bloodstream. The respiratory system also receives the waste product, carbon dioxide, from the blood and exhales it. The breathing cycle of inspiration and expiration enables these processes. During inspiration, the diaphragm moves downward, and the intercostal muscles pull the rib cage up and out. This increases lung volume, and air is drawn into the lungs. During expiration, the diaphragm and intercostal muscles relax, and the rib cage moves both downward and inward, reducing the volume of the chest cavity, which forces air out of the lungs. The normal respiratory rate for an adult is 12 to 20 breaths/minute.

BLOOD PRESSURE

A **BP** measurement reflects the force that is exerted by blood on the arterial vessel walls during systole and diastole, which reflects cardiac output and systemic vascular resistance (SVR). An individual's BP is a measure of their hemodynamic stability. The systolic blood pressure (SBP) is the force exerted when the ventricles contract and varies with blood volume, cardiac output, and artery compliance. The diastolic blood pressure (DBP) is the force exerted by the peripheral vascular resistance as the ventricles relax and are filling. The BP reading is noted by the SBP/DBP. The pulse pressure is the difference between the SBP and the DBP. Normal BP is defined as SBP <120 mmHg and DBP <80 mmHg, although the definitions of normal and elevated BP vary, depending on age, individual health factors, and guidelines. BP measurements will fluctuate throughout the day, and many extraneous variables such as smoking, caffeine intake, and room temperature can influence the readings. The key to accurate assessment of BP is the evidence-based guideline(s) for obtaining BP measurements.

PAIN

Pain is an unpleasant sensory experience associated with actual or potential tissue damage. It is a complex experience for patients. The experience of pain is initiated by the receiving of sensory information from a noxious stimulus, but can also be interpreted differently based on individual perspectives. Specialized nerve endings, nociceptors, detect and transmit painful sensations. Noxious or painful stimuli can be mechanical, chemical, or thermal, and are received in the periphery. Nociceptors then carry the signal to the central nervous system (CNS) via sensory fibers. There are two types of sensory fibers—Aδ and C fibers. Aδ fibers have an insulation and are larger in diameter and can transmit a pain signal to the CNS very rapidly. Stimulated Aδ fibers produce localized, sharp sensations that are not long lasting. C fibers are smaller and not insulated, and as a result, they transmit the signal more slowly. Sensations from the C fibers can be described as aching and persist for longer than Aδ pain signals.

Noxious stimuli from injured tissue leads to the release of chemicals (neurotransmitters) that potentiate or inhibit the pain response. Action potential, or the pain message that results from the stimuli, moves along the nerve fiber until it reaches the spinal cord. This initial process is called transduction. The next step in the process is transmission, or the movement of the pain impulse from the spinal cord to the brain. The brain then perceives the pain impulse in the third phase. The final phase of the pain pathway is known as modulation. Modulation allows the pain response to be inhibited. Certain neurotransmitters slow down the pain impulse, blocking some of the effect. When there is injury, disease, or damage to the nerve fibers that transmit painful stimuli, the typical pathway is altered, and abnormal sensations, including continuous and/or episodic pain experiences, can result. The resultant neuropathic pain can be associated with peripheral nerve damage from diseases like diabetes, shingles, or spinal stenosis.

Pain is typically designated or described according to its duration. Acute pain is short term and usually resolves after healing occurs. Some examples of acute pain are surgical and traumatic injury. Chronic or persistent pain is diagnosed when pain has been present for at least 6 months. Patients who have cancer, musculoskeletal disorders, or peripheral neuropathies can experience chronic pain.

LIFE-SPAN CONSIDERATIONS FOR THE PHYSICAL EXAMINATION

Pediatric Vital Signs

Assessment of temperature in newborns is a priority. Infants, especially those with low birth weight, can have difficulty maintaining body temperature. Infants have less subcutaneous fat and hence less insulation. Their small size, increased ratio of body surface to body weight, and inability to shiver impair the infant's ability to conserve heat. Cold stress in a newborn can lead to hypoglycemia, hypoxia, and hypothermia. Fever in an infant under 6 weeks old can be a sign of sepsis and requires immediate further evaluation.

Normal pulse rate for children varies with age. Normal pulse rates are (Van Kuiken & Huth, 2016):

- Neonates, 110 to 160 bpm
- Infants, 100 to 160 bpm
- 1 to 2 years of age, 90 to 150 bpm
- 2 to 5 years of age, 80 to 120 bpm
- 6 to 12 years of age, 70 to 120 bpm
- Older than 12 years of age, 60 to 100 bpm

In children under 2 years old, pulse rate is best assessed by auscultating the apical pulse. The apical pulse is located just left of the midclavicular line at the fifth intercostal space in children younger than 7 years and at the left midclavicular line at the fifth intercostal space in children over 7. In children over the age of 2 years, pulse rate can be determined by palpating the temporal, carotid, femoral, apical, brachial, popliteal, radial, posterior tibial, and dorsalis pedis pulses.

Causes of abnormal pulse rates or rhythms in children should be noted prior to assessing the pulse rate; these include changes in body temperature, hypoxia, anxiety, sepsis, pain, medications, and/or crying. Further investigation is warranted if a child has an irregular heart rhythm, and the child should be assessed for signs of disruption in cardiac output, such as weak, thready pulse; increased rate; cyanosis; tachypnea; fussiness; decreased activity; and poor feeding. Infants and young children commonly have sinus arrhythmia, that is, the heart rate varies with respiration, which is not associated with heart problems.

Infants with suspected cardiovascular or renal abnormalities can be assessed for BP using a neonatal sized cuff. For noncritical infants, it is best practice to use an oscillometer device, at least 1.5 hours after a feeding or medical intervention, taken in the supine or prone position, using the proper size cuff on the right upper arm, and taken while the infant is asleep or in a quiet awake state. Normal BP is determined by postconceptual age in weeks.

Vital Signs During Pregnancy

There is an overall decrease in SVR during pregnancy likely caused by progesterone-mediated smooth muscle relaxation; however, the exact mechanism is unknown (Antony, Racusin, Aagaard, & Dildy, 2017). Decreasing BP is seen around 8 weeks' gestation because of decreased SVR. The decrease in SVR allows the BP to remain stable despite an increase in the cardiac output (CO) that occurs normally in pregnancy. BP monitoring should take place during prenatal visits to identify early signs of hypertension in pregnancy. Hypertension during pregnancy is a major health concern that can have significant complications and consequences for mothers and babies.

Considerations for Older Adults

With advanced age, the body's thermoregulatory measures are less effective. Older adults are less capable of adapting to extreme environmental temperatures, putting them at risk for both hypothermia and heat-related illness. Older adults are also less likely to develop a fever with infection, making body temperature a less reliable indicator of their health status.

Because the older adult's heart takes longer to recover from activity and stress, if an older adult presents with tachycardia, the clinician should review the activities that preceded the assessment to determine whether they are related to the elevated pulse rate. Allow an older adult to rest after a period of activity that may have increased their pulse rate, and reassess.

Geriatric patients have risks for both hypertension and hypotension. The elevated BP associated with hypertension remains a leading risk factor for ischemic heart disease and stroke and has a prevalence rate of 60% to 80% in the geriatric population (Heflin, 2019). Although strict or aggressive BP management does reduce the overall mortality rate, this population may have adverse effects from treatment that led the Eighth Joint National Commission (JNC 8) to change the target BP for those ≥60 years old to a SBP <150 mmHg and DBP <90 mmHg (James, 2014). Orthostatic hypotension is more common in the geriatric population (20%) partly because of diminished baroreceptor sensitivity. Studies have shown that antihypertensive medications may also play a role in postural hypotension, which demonstrates the need to discuss risks, benefits, and patient preference when managing hypertension in this population (James, 2014).

KEY HISTORY QUESTIONS AND CONSIDERATIONS

HISTORY OF PRESENT ILLNESS

Presenting problems that can be noted during the general survey include:

- Syncope, loss of consciousness
- Choking, wheezing, respiratory distress, hypoxia, tachypnea
- Chest pain, dizziness, hypertension, hypotension, bradycardia, tachycardia
- Pulselessness
- Diaphoresis, cyanosis
- Fever (see the text that follows)
- Pain: acute, recurrent, episodic, chronic
- Underweight, overweight, obesity
- Inattention, impulsivity, distraction, anxiety
- Confusion, disorientation, depressed mood

EXAMPLE OF PRESENTING PROBLEM: FEVER

Fever is a temporary increase in body temperature as regulated by the hypothalamus in response to internal or external factors. Fever can help the body respond to infections by creating an inhospitable environment for bacteria and viruses. A patient with a fever may present with chills or shivering, body aches, loss of appetite, weakness/fatigue, and dehydration. The temperature elevation that is considered "abnormal" can depend on the age, the site of measurement, and the clinical condition of the patient. In general, body temperature elevated above 100.4°F (38°C) rectally is commonly considered a fever, while a body temperature above 101°F (38.3°C) is the elevation at which the American Academy of Pediatrics recommends consideration for antipyretics (Ward, 2019). Note that consideration for fever-lowering medications does not indicate a requirement for them. The key to evaluation of fever is critical. The clinical reasoning and assessment of the fever depend on the patient's age, symptoms, and health status, with infants and the elderly being at the highest risk for associated serious illnesses and complications. The elevation of an individual's temperature is not the only indicator of the seriousness of an illness. History of present illness considerations include:

- Chief concern: Fever
- Onset: Recent, chronic; sudden versus insidious, recurrent
- Location: Area of the body assessed for fever; measurement
- Duration: High body temperature increasing, persistent, or intermittent
- Character: Warmth or coolness to touch
- Associated symptoms: Sweating, erythema, shivering, fatigue, body aches
- Aggravating factors: Loss of appetite, vomiting, or diarrhea; identified source of infection
- Relieving factors: Over-the-counter or prescribed medication, cool compresses, fluids
- Temporal factors: Recent or past illness/infection, surgery, or travel

PAST MEDICAL HISTORY

- Recent infection, recent use of antibiotics or antivirals
- Chronic diseases (including cancers, genetic disorders, autoimmune disorders, cardiac disease)
- Recent injury, trauma, or skin infection
- Recent strep throat or mononucleosis
- Birth history (especially for pediatric patients)
- Allergies
- Allergic reactions
- Tuberculosis (recent testing)

FAMILY HISTORY

- Cancer
- Infectious disease
- Immune disorders
- Febrile seizures
- Tuberculosis or positive TB reading

SOCIAL HISTORY

- Smoking history/history of tobacco use/exposure to secondhand smoke
- Medications prescribed/not prescribed; substance use
- Recent travel out of the country
- Sleep history
- Sexual history (including risk factors for HIV exposure)
- Animal or food contact
- Insect bites

REVIEW OF SYSTEMS

- General: Mental status, fatigue, lymphadenopathy, pain, changes in vital signs, weight changes
- HEENT: Headache, ear pain, nasal congestion, sinus pain, sore throat
- Cardiovascular/Respiratory: Shortness of breath at rest or with exertion, cough, chest pain, orthopnea
- Gastrointestinal/Genitourinary: Abdominal pain, nausea, vomiting, difficulty swallowing, black or tarry stools, dysuria, urgency, pelvic pain, vaginal/penile discharge, dyspareunia
- Neurologic: Weakness, numbness, irritability, dizziness, syncope (fainting)
- Endocrine: Changes to skin, hair; temperature intolerance
- Hematologic: Bruising, bleeding, jaundice, paleness, cyanosis
- Integumentary: Rashes, itching
- Psychiatric: Changes in memory, concentration, or mood; confusion

PREVENTIVE CARE CONSIDERATIONS

- Healthy lifestyle behaviors
- Immunization history, including yearly flu vaccination
- Regular handwashing
- Proper food handling and cooking
- Washing of fruits and vegetables
- Consumption of raw or unpasteurized foods/drinks

DIFFERENTIAL DIAGNOSES

- Bacterial or viral infections of the ears, nose, throat, sinuses
- Bacterial or viral infections, including influenza, common cold, infectious mononucleosis, and upper or lower respiratory infections
- Sepsis, meningitis, bronchitis, pneumonia

- Bacterial infections of the bladder or kidneys, gastroenteritis, sexually transmitted infections
- Dehydration, lupus, gout, sarcoidosis, malaria, tuberculosis, endocarditis

PHYSICAL EXAMINATION AND FINDINGS

MEASUREMENT OF TEMPERATURE

Temperature can be measured through multiple routes, including oral, rectal, axillary, temporal artery, tympanic membrane, and skin. Consider the advantages and disadvantages of each route when selecting the best method for measuring temperature in a given patient. **Table 5.5** provides a summary of the sites for temperature measurement, including the advantages, disadvantages, and associated contraindications.

Oral Temperature

The oral route is generally considered the easiest and most reliable means of measuring body temperature. To obtain an oral temperature, the thermometer probe is positioned in either the right or the left posterior sublingual pocket, which has a rich blood supply and offers an indirect reflection of core temperature. **Figure 5.3** depicts how an individual should close their mouth around the probe during measurement. Most electronic thermometers will alert with an audible tone once the body temperature is registered. Disposable sheaths or probe covers offer protection from transmission of infection between patients.

Rectal Temperature

The rectal route of temperature measurement is considered the most reliable as it is the best reflection of core temperature compared with other less invasive routes. However, it is used less frequently in practice owing to patient preference. Do not use oral thermometers rectally as these can cause injury. Rectal thermometers have a security bulb designed specifically for safely taking rectal temperatures. To take a rectal temperature, place the patient in the Sims position. Lubricate the tip of the electronic thermometer's probe cover. While wearing gloves, insert the thermometer probe 1 to 1½ inches into the adult rectum (½ inch for babies), and hold it in place until the temperature is registered. Care should be given to ensure patient privacy throughout the procedure. On average, rectal temperatures are about 1° higher than oral temperature readings.

Axillary Temperature

Measurement of body temperature in the axilla is most commonly conducted using an electronic thermometer. The probe is placed in the middle of the axilla, and the corresponding arm is held against the body to keep the probe in place until the audible tone is heard and the temperature is recorded on the thermometer. The axilla provides greater surface vasculature in newborns and infants than in adults, making it a better reflection of core temperature and a more appropriate site for temperature assessment in these young patients. Axillary temperatures are about 1° lower, on average, than oral temperature readings.

Temporal Artery Temperature

The temperature of the temporal artery in the forehead is measured using an infrared scanning thermometer. To take a temporal artery temperature, place the thermometer probe flat on the center of the patient's forehead. Press and hold the thermometer's scan button. Keeping the sensor flat against the skin, slide the thermometer across the forehead to the hairline. If perspiration is present on the forehead, continue to depress the scan button, lift the probe from the forehead, and touch the probe to the neck behind the earlobe. This will account for the potential cooling effect of perspiration. Release the scan button and remove the thermometer from the skin. The thermometer will display the patient's temperature reading. Accuracy of temperatures taken temporally can vary greatly according to the technique of the user. **Figure 5.4** depicts placement of the sensor on the forehead of a child.

Tympanic Temperature

Tympanic thermometers use infrared scanning to measure the temperature at the tympanic membrane in the ear. To take a tympanic temperature, gently pull the ear back to help straighten the canal (pull up and back for adults; pull down and back for children under 3). Insert the thermometer probe into the ear to seal the canal. Press and hold the thermometer's scan button until an audible tone is noted (1–3 seconds). Remove from the ear canal, and the thermometer will display the patient's temperature. Disposable probe covers should be used to prevent cross-contamination between patients.

ASSESSMENT OF PULSE RATE

Normally in adults, the pulse rate is 60 to 100 beats/minute, or bpm. Numerous factors affect the heart rate, including environmental temperature, body position, body size, medication usage, and the patient's physical activity level. When assessing a pulse, the clinician should note the pulse rate (number of beats/minute), rhythm (pattern or regularity of the beats), and the amplitude (strength of the pulse). To determine the rate, the clinician should count the number of beats for a full 60 seconds, or 30 seconds and multiply times two. Note that counting for any less than 30 seconds could result

TABLE 5.5 Routes for Measurement of Body Temperature		
Advantages	Disadvantages	Contraindications
Oral		
Reflects core temperature Easy, convenient, noninvasive Comfortable for most patients	Patient must be able to hold mouth closed Eating, drinking, and smoking can impact accuracy	Patients who have had oral surgery or are comatose or confused/cannot follow directions Not recommended for patients under age 3 years
Rectal		
Reflects core temperature Appropriate for all ages Useful for patients who cannot follow directions (as necessary with oral method)	Invasive Embarrassing and uncomfortable for patient Requires more time; slower to reflect core temperature changes than oral method	Patients who have heart conditions or have had cardiac surgery owing to potential stimulation of the vagus nerve Patients who are immunosuppressed or at risk for bleeding Patients who have had rectal surgery or who have hemorrhoids
Axillary		
Safe and comfortable for most patients Increased reliability in newborns and infants owing to greater surface vasculature	Less reflective of core temperature Longer measurement time Easy to dislodge—requires positioning and constant monitoring Temperature reading affected by diaphoresis	Not recommended for routine temperature monitoring in adults and children
Temporal Artery		
Fast, easy, convenient, noninvasive Comfortable for most patients Reflects rapid change in core temperature	Temperature readings affected by diaphoresis or anything that prevents heat from dissipating (e.g., hats, hair) Accuracy highly dependent on user technique	Appropriate for screening but not recommended as sole measurement for making treatment decisions
Tympanic Membrane		
Fast, easy, convenient Minimally invasive Shares vasculature with the hypothalamus; reflects rapid change in core temperature Not influenced by factors that affect oral temperature (eating, drinking, smoking)	Careful positioning necessary to ensure accuracy Reading impacted by numerous factors (obstruction by ear hair or wax, patient crying, ambient temperature)	Patients who have had recent ear surgery or a current ear infection Not recommended for patients under age 2
Skin		
Easy and noninvasive Provides continuous monitoring Useful when other methods are contraindicated	Least accurate—skin temperature lags behind other sites with changes to core temperature Reading impacted by environmental temperature	Appropriate for screening but not recommended as sole measurement for making treatment decisions

in an incorrect assessment. Additionally, if the rhythm of the pulse is irregular, default to using the full 60 seconds to calculate a rate.

Peripheral pulses can be assessed at multiple locations, including over the carotid, brachial, radial, femoral, popliteal, dorsalis pedis, and posterior tibial arteries. A general survey of an individual should include assessment of a pulse rate, which can be done by gently compressing the radial artery, or auscultating the apical pulse.

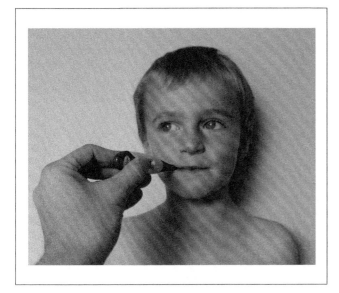

FIGURE 5.3 Oral temperature being assessed for a pediatric patient. Note how the individual should close their mouth around the probe during measurement.

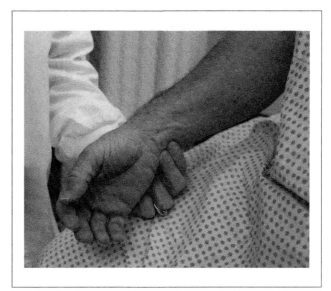

FIGURE 5.5 Palpation of radial pulse.

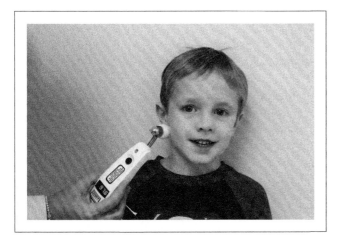

FIGURE 5.4 Use of a scanning thermometer for a pediatric patient.

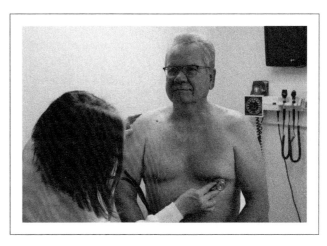

FIGURE 5.6 Auscultation of the apical pulse.

Radial Pulse, Apical Pulse, and the Apical–Radial Pulse

The most common site for assessing the pulse is over the radial artery. **Figure 5.5** shows the location of the pulse site, inside the wrist and superior to the thumb. Gently compressing the radial artery with the fingertips of the middle and index fingers allows for easy assessment of the pulse rate.

The apical pulse is located over the apex of the heart. **Figure 5.6** depicts the location of the apical pulse, at the fifth intercostal space left of the midclavicular line. The landmarks of the chest wall are further explained in Chapter 6, Evidence-Based Assessment of the Heart and Circulatory System. The clinician should place the

bell of the stethoscope over this area and listen, noting the rhythm and amplitude of the heartbeats, as well as the heart rate.

The apical–radial pulse is assessed by counting apical and radial beats simultaneously. To do this, one clinician determines the rate by auscultating at the apex of the heart, and the second clinician counts by palpating the radial pulse. Sometimes heartbeats detected at the apex of the heart cannot be detected at peripheral sites. When the apical pulse rate is higher than the radial pulse rate, the discrepancy is known as the pulse deficit. A pulse deficit may be associated with irregular cardiac rhythms, such as atrial fibrillation. If two clinicians are unavailable for the apical–radial pulse assessment, this can be completed by one clinician. The clinician solely assessing apical–radial pulse would use one hand to hold the stethoscope while auscultating the apical pulse and the other hand to palpate the radial pulse. The clinician would be assessing for discrepancies between the apical impulse heard and the radial pulses felt.

ASSESSMENT OF RESPIRATORY RATE

The National Institute for Clinical Excellence (2007) states that the **respiratory rate** is the most sensitive marker of a deteriorating patient and the first observation to indicate a problem. To assess the respiratory rate, observe the rise and fall of the chest, and count the number of breaths that occur in 1 minute. In practice, clinicians do not always count respirations for a full minute, but instead count for 30 seconds and multiply by two. This practice should be avoided as it decreases the accuracy of the respiratory assessment, especially in the younger populations. It may be useful to calculate respiratory rate at the same time as pulse rate. This will give a more accurate measurement and minimize any subconscious influence, as patients may alter their breathing if they know they are being watched. If the patient is sitting, the feet must be flat on the floor as sitting with legs suspended can reduce venous return, which may increase heart rate and subsequently respiratory rate.

The expected respiratory rate by age can be found in **Table 5.6**. The normal rate of respirations depends on several factors, including age of the individual, recent physical activity, and level of alertness, that is, waking or sleeping states. Additionally, respiration rates may increase with fever, illness, and other medical conditions. Clinicians should assess for tachypnea, an elevated respiratory rate, and bradypnea, an abnormally slow breathing rate. If either condition exists, further assessment is warranted.

TABLE 5.6 Range of Normal Respiratory Rate by Age	
Age	Respiratory Rate (Breaths/Minute)
Premature	40–70
0–3 months	35–55
3–6 months	30–45
6–12 months	22–38
1–3 years	22–30
3–6 years	20–24
6–12 years	16–22
>12 years	12–20

BLOOD PRESSURE MEASUREMENT

There are three evidence-based, effective methods to measure and monitor BP; these are ambulatory blood pressure monitoring (ABPM), home BP monitoring, and office-based BP monitoring (Thomas & Pohl, 2019).

Ambulatory Blood Pressure Monitoring

Using this method, the patient wears a device programmed to obtain BP readings every 15 to 20 minutes during the day and every 30 to 60 minutes during sleep over a 24- to 48-hour period to determine the average day and night BP readings. If a 24- to 48-hour period is not feasible, then 6 hours of ABPM may be acceptable.

The United States Preventive Services Task Force (2015) and the American College of Cardiology (ACC)/AHA (Whelton et al., 2018) recommend out-of-office BP measurements to confirm, treat, and manage hypertension; these authorities note that ABPM is considered the reference standard for a hypertension diagnosis and is a better predictor of cardiovascular events. However, when ABPM is not feasible for want of resources or access, traditional home BP monitoring is an acceptable alternative (Townsend, 2019).

Home Blood Pressure Monitoring

Given the expense and decreased availability of ABPM, more attention has been given to home BP monitoring with inexpensive (USD $40–$60) semiautomatic devices (Thomas & Pohl, 2019). There is a lack of consensus on the optimal schedule for obtaining home BP readings, but evidence suggests that a minimum of 12 to 14 readings taken both during the day and evening over the course of 1 week is best practice (Townsend, 2019). All home monitors should be checked for accuracy at initiation of use and then annually. The patient should also demonstrate competency with correct technique when obtaining BP measurements from their home device and use the proper cuff size.

Office-Based Blood Pressure Monitoring

Currently in the United States, office-based BP monitoring is the standard of care for the screening, diagnosis, and management of hypertension. This is likely to continue for many reasons, including lack of financial resources, reimbursement, and support for ABPM and home BP devices, and the continued use of office-based BP measurements in the randomized trials that provide the evidence for treatment recommendations (Thomas & Pohl, 2019). The correct measurement of an office-based BP requires attention to be paid to all of these factors: time of measurement (including the time of day and potential extraneous variables such as smoking, caffeine intake, and room temperature), type of device, cuff size, cuff placement, technique of measurement, and number of measurements. Studies suggest that many clinicians do not follow one or more of these evidence-based recommendations required to accurately assess, diagnose, and manage hypertension (Thomas & Pohl, 2019).

Selection of the correct cuff size is essential. The length of the BP cuff bladder should be 80% of the circumference of the upper arm and the width at least 40% of the circumference of the upper arm. Using a cuff that is too small will result in artificially high BP readings, and using a cuff that is too large will result in artificially low BP readings. **Figure 5.7** depicts sizes of BP cuffs.

Proper patient positioning is also essential to obtaining an accurate BP reading. The patient should be seated, with the back supported, legs uncrossed, and the arm supported at the level of the heart (**Figure 5.8**). The patient should be allowed to sit quietly for 5 minutes before the BP is measured. Other factors that can influence the measured BP include bladder distention, background noise, and talking. Note that the patient's arm should be free of clothing. Do not roll the sleeve up, as this can create a tourniquet effect and alter the BP reading. Place the midline of the cuff bladder over the palpated brachial artery pulsation. The lower end of the cuff should be 2 to 3 cm above the antecubital fossa to minimize artifact noise from the stethoscope rubbing the cuff. The cuff should fit snugly on the patient's arm. Once the BP cuff is placed, the arm should remain supported at the level of the heart, and neither the patient nor the clinician should talk.

The estimated systolic pressure should be palpated initially to avoid misinterpretation of the BP, which is more likely if the patient has an auscultatory gap (McGrath & Bachmann, 2019). An auscultatory gap is a period of diminished or absent Korotkoff sounds during the measurement of the BP, which can be missed if the cuff is inflated without first palpating the SBP. To palpate the SBP, place the fingers of one hand over the brachial or radial artery, and feel for the pulsation. Rapidly inflate the cuff with the hand bulb 30 mmHg above the point at which the pulse was not palpable. Slowly deflate the cuff at a rate of 2 to 3 mmHg/second until the pulse is palpated again, which is the estimated SBP, then quickly deflate the cuff completely. Once the palpable SBP has been determined, place the bell of the stethoscope lightly over the brachial artery, and inflate the cuff quickly to 30 mmHg above the palpable SBP. Slowly release the cuff, at a rate of 2 to 3 mmHg/second, and listen for the first audible pulse (Korotkoff sound), which is the SBP. Continue to deflate the cuff slowly below the SBP, and listen for the beginning of muffled sounds; approximately 8 to 10 mmHg below the muffled sounds, there is a disappearance of sound, which is the DBP. Once the DBP has been noted, rapidly deflate the cuff completely.

The evidence-based recommendation for accurate BP measurement is to take at least two BP readings,

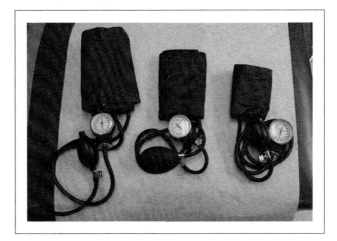

FIGURE 5.7 Various sizes of blood pressure (BP) cuffs. Selection of the correct cuff size is essential. Using a cuff that is too small will result in artificially high BP readings, and using a cuff that is too large will result in artificially low BP readings.

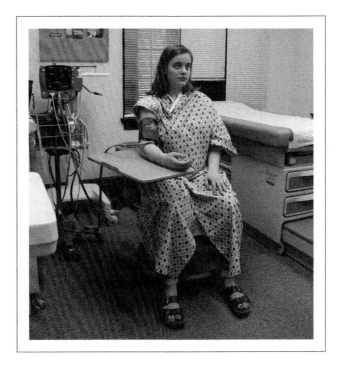

FIGURE 5.8 In-office blood pressure measurement.

spaced 1 to 2 minutes apart, while the individual is seated, one from each arm (Thomas & Pohl, 2019). If there is a substantial (>10 mmHg) and consistent systolic BP difference between the arms, the arm with the higher BP values should be used for future measurements.

For suspected coarctation of the aorta, BP readings should also be obtained from the leg. Principles to obtain a leg BP reading are the same as in the arm. The

SBP in the leg is expected to be 10% to 20% higher than in the brachial artery. The ACC/AHA (Whelton et al., 2018) does not recommend wrist or finger BP monitors owing to unreliable results; however, for obese patients for whom a properly fitted cuff is not available, obtaining a BP reading in the wrist is acceptable. The wrist should be kept at the level of the heart during measurement to avoid a falsely high reading.

Box 5.1 provides a summary of the guidelines and considerations for accurate BP measurement.

ASSESSMENT OF PAIN

There are several assessment findings associated with pain. A patient may exhibit tenderness on palpation or guarding of an area to prevent further injury. Verbalization of pain is the most common way to identify pain, but nonverbal indicators may also exist. A patient may demonstrate an increase in heart rate, BP, and respiratory rate as a response to pain. A patient may also exhibit other physical symptoms, such as nausea, a reduction in appetite, or an inability to sleep.

Self-Reporting Pain Rating Scales

There are several forms of evidence-based self-reporting pain scales. An important factor is the patient's comprehension of the tool. Using the patient's native language and making modifications for sight or hearing impairment(s) are essential to assure accuracy.

Overall pain assessment tools can be effective in obtaining more information about the type of pain being experienced. One example, the Initial Pain Assessment, requires the clinician to ask the patient eight questions regarding the location, duration, quality, intensity, and factors that aggravate or relieve the pain. Numeric rating scales ask a patient to choose a number that best indicates the individual's current level of pain, with 0 being no pain and 10 being the worst pain the patient can imagine. Descriptor scales use key words that describe different levels of pain intensity, such as no pain, moderate pain, and severe pain. A Visual Analog Scale may also be used, which combines a numeric scale and descriptor words, and uses a red–yellow–green color scheme depending on the level of pain. The Wong–Baker FACES Scale (https://wongbakerfaces.org/) can be used for children who can verbalize their pain level but may not be able to correlate it with a number. This evidence-based scale uses a series of faces with different expressions to demonstrate varying levels of pain. Ensuring cognitive level and understanding is crucial before attempting to use any self-reporting scale. Clinical context and the type of pain are also important factors.

Assessing Pain Behaviors

Proper pain assessment includes assessment of pain behaviors, even if a self-report is given. Because pain involves autonomic responses as well as being a protective mechanism, changes to baseline vital signs may be noted. Most commonly, increased respirations, pulse, and BP may be seen.

Newborns and Infant

For neonatal infants, several pain scores consider gestational age in determining their experience of pain. The cutoff age for the use of each of these scales differs but is typically 1 month old. For infants older than 1 month, there are pain scores that use observation of an infant's behavior to determine pain level. For example, the Face, Legs, Activity, Cry, Consolability (FLACC) Score is one reliable tool used in infants that uses the infant's facial expression, leg movement, activity level, crying, and ability to be consoled to determine a standardized score that results in a total number between 0 and 10 (Beltramini, Milojevic, & Pateron, 2017). Utilizing caregivers to help identify pain in nonverbal patients is also a helpful strategy.

Children

Pain behaviors in children are dependent on the cognitive level of the child. For children or adolescents who are nonverbal, a Revised FLACC Score was developed to rate pain based on behavior (Beltramini, Milojevic, & Pateron, 2017). Observing a child's behavior is necessary if they cannot self-report their pain. Changes in vital signs, facial expression, vocalization, increased or decreased movement, and holding or touching the area that is in pain are some of the potential behaviors.

Pregnant Patient

Pain in pregnant patients should be assessed regularly. Traditional pain assessments may be used if they are appropriate for the patient. Frequent pain assessment and intervention during labor is crucial to facilitate healthy delivery. Pain behaviors during pregnancy may include changes in vital signs, especially an increase in respiratory rate and heart rate. Changes to facial expression and vocalization may also occur to indicate pain.

Older Adults

Pain behavior in the older adult may be complicated by chronic conditions or cognitive decline. Identifying changes in behavior may help to recognize pain in the older adult. For example, changes to sleep or appetite could indicate pain.

ADDITIONAL GENERAL SURVEY ASSESSMENTS

In addition to the assessment of vital signs and the assessment of pain, completing the general survey includes objectively noting the appearance, behavior, and cognitive thought processes of the individual. These

BOX 5.1
GUIDELINES FOR THE MEASUREMENT OF BLOOD PRESSURE

Patient Conditions

Posture

Check for postural changes by taking readings after being supine for 5 minutes, then immediately, and 2 minutes after standing. This is particularly important for older adults, diabetics, or patients taking antihypertensive medication.

Sitting is the recommended position for routine BP. The patient should be sitting quietly with back supported for 5 minutes, arm supported at heart level.

Circumstances

No caffeine in the hour preceding the BP reading

No smoking in the 30 minutes preceding the BP reading

No exogenous adrenergic stimulants, such as decongestant medications containing phenylephrine or eye drops for pupillary dilatation

Quiet, warm environment

Home readings should be taken in varying circumstances.

Equipment

Cuff Size

The bladder length should be 80% and bladder width 40% of the upper arm circumference.

Manometer

Aneroid gauges should be calibrated every 6 months.

Technique

Number of Readings

Take at least two readings per visit, separated by as much time as possible. If readings vary by more than 5 mmHg, take additional readings until two consecutive readings are close.

For the diagnosis of hypertension, take three readings at least 1 week apart.

Initially, assess the BP in both arms; if pressures differ, use the arm with the higher pressure.

If the arm pressure is elevated, take the pressure in one leg, particularly in patients under 30 years of age.

Performance

Inflate the cuff quickly to 20 mmHg above the estimated systolic pressure.

Deflate the cuff at a rate of 2–3 mmHg/second.

Record the Korotkoff phase V sound (disappearance) as the diastolic pressure, except in children. In children, the use of phase IV (muffling) may be preferable.

If the Korotkoff sounds are weak, have the patient raise the arm, open and close the hand 5–10 times, then inflate the cuff quickly.

Recordings

Note the pressure, patient position, arm, and cuff size: e.g., 130/80, seated, right arm, standard adult cuff.

BP, blood pressure.

Source: From Thomas, G., & Pohl, M. A. (2019). Blood pressure measurement in the diagnosis and management of hypertension in adults. In G. L. Bakris, L. Kunins, & J. P. Forman (Eds.), UptoDate. Retrieved from https://www.uptodate.com/contents/blood-pressure-measurement-in-the-diagnosis-and-management-of-hypertension-in-adults

assessments are completed while vital signs and the presence of pain are assessed, and include evaluating:

- Level of consciousness
- Responsiveness to voice, light, sound
- Orientation to person, place, time
- Affect and mood, facial expression, speech
- Dress, grooming, and hygiene
- Body habitus (height, weight, waist circumference)
- Body movements, mobility, and coordination

EVIDENCE-BASED PRACTICE CONSIDERATIONS

Wearable technologies and applications for smartphones or at-home devices to monitor vital signs, noting significant changes or abnormalities of pulse, heart rate or rhythm, BP, and even subtle changes in physical activity, is increasingly available and reliable. Chapter 27, Using Health Technology in Evidence-Based Assessment, outlines an evidence-based approach to the use of digital technologies in assessment. New evidence is suggesting that measurement of vital signs and physiologic status by digital technologies may be beneficial for patients to use while at home, especially for older adults (Dias & Paulo Silva Cunha, 2018). More research is needed as the expanded use of digital technologies within assessment is changing the reach of advanced assessment and the information available to the clinician.

NORMAL AND ABNORMAL FINDINGS

HYPERTENSION

Hypertension remains prevalent in the United States and worldwide, is one of the most common reasons for office visits in nonpregnant adults, and is the most significant modifiable risk factor for early cardiovascular disease. The pathophysiology for primary hypertension (formerly called essential hypertension) remains poorly understood; however, a combination of genetic and environmental factors plays a role in the development. Several modifiable risk factors for primary hypertension include smoking; obesity; poor diet, including excessive alcohol and sodium intake; and physical inactivity. There are also nonmodifiable risk factors, including age, family history, race, and reduced number of nephrons.

Secondary hypertension is caused by a specific medication or disease state. Medications that can elevate BP include oral contraceptives, nonsteroidal anti-inflammatories (NSAIDs), decongestants, stimulants, and erythropoietin, to name a few. It is important to obtain a full list of prescription and nonprescription

TABLE 5.7 Definitions of Hypertension for Adults

Blood Pressure	ACC/AHA 2017	JNC8
<120/<80	Normal	Normal
120–129/80	"Prehypertension"	"Elevated"
130–139/80–89		Stage 1 HTN
140–159/90–100	Stage 1 HTN	Stage 2 HTN
≥169/≥100	Stage 2 HTN	

ACC/AHA, The American College of Cardiology/American Heart Association; HTN, hypertension; JNC8, Eighth Joint National Committee.

medications when completing the patient's health history. Medical conditions that cause hypertension include obstructive sleep apnea (OSA), primary renal disease, pheochromocytoma, Cushing's syndrome, hyperthyroidism, and coarctation of the aorta.

When obtaining subjective data from the patient's history, early primary hypertension may be asymptomatic. Severe hypertension may present with headaches, blurred vision, dyspnea, or encephalopathy. Objective data will include multiple readings using proper measurement techniques as described earlier in this chapter. There is controversy regarding the definition of hypertension across two major guidelines: The ACC/AHA and the Eighth Joint National Committee (JNC8; Basile & Bloch, 2019). Each set of evidence-based guidelines is the result of large randomized controlled trials that yielded slightly different conclusions for identification and treatment. The BP measurements, defined as normal, prehypertensive or elevated, stage one hypertension, and stage two hypertension, are listed in **Table 5.7** for both evidence-based guidelines.

Although differences in defining hypertension exist, there are similarities. Both the JNC8 and the ACC/AHA national guidelines recognize the importance of lifestyle modification (weight loss, Dietary Approaches to Stop Hypertension [DASH] diet, smoking cessation, and exercise) as first-line interventions to reduce morbidity and mortality associated with elevated BP. Both also highlight the importance of proper BP measurement and encourage home BP monitoring. The recommendations for medication management are also similar between the two guidelines. In addition, evidence-based recommendations include early recognition of elevated BP in children; **Table 5.8** lists the BP measurements considered hypertensive for the pediatric population.

PAIN

Nociceptive pain results from activation of the normally functioning nervous system. Neuropathic pain,

TABLE 5.8 Definitions of Hypertension for Children

	Children Aged 1–12 Years	Children Aged 13 Years and Older
Normal BP	Systolic and diastolic BP <90th percentile	Systolic BP <120 mmHg and Diastolic BP <80 mmHg
Elevated BP	Systolic and diastolic BP ≥90th percentile to <95th percentile OR 120/80 mmHg to <95th percentile (whichever is lower)	Systolic BP 120–129 mmHg and Diastolic BP <80 mmHg
Stage 1 HTN	Systolic and diastolic BP ≥95th percentile to <95th percentile + 12 mmHg or 130/80 to 139/89 mmHg (whichever is lower)	130/80 to 139/89 mmHg
Stage 2 HTN	Systolic and diastolic BP ≥95th percentile +12 mmHg or ≥140/90 (whichever is lower)	≥140/90 mmHg

BP, blood pressure; HTN, hypertension.

Source: Flynn, J.T., Kaelber, D.C., Baker-Smith, C.M., Blowey, D., Carroll, A.E., Daniels, S.R., de Ferranti, S.D., . . Urbina, E. M. (2017). Clinical practice guideline for screening and management of high blood pressure in children and adolescents. *Pediatrics, 140*(3). doi:10.1542/peds.2017-1904

TABLE 5.9 Comparison of Nociceptive and Neuropathic Pain

Nociceptive Pain	Neuropathic Pain
Usually responsive to nonopioid and opioid pain medication. Examples of nociceptive pain include somatic and visceral pain: • *Somatic pain*: Originates from musculoskeletal tissue. Can be sharp or dull and is usually well localized (patient can point to where it hurts). Example is postoperative pain. • *Visceral pain*: Originates from internal organs. Often poorly localized and accompanied by symptoms of autonomic nervous stimulation, such as nausea, vomiting, or diaphoresis. Example is distention and inflammation of abdominal organs like appendicitis.	Typically poor response to traditional analgesic medications. Adjuvant medications in combination with nonpharmacologic intervention may be necessary for pain control. Results from damage to the brain, spinal cord, or peripheral nerves; it is pathologic, meaning that the disease is within the system. Associated with radiculopathy. Patients will describe pain as "sharp," "shooting," "tingling," or "burning."

however, occurs because of abnormal processing of the pain message from the central or peripheral nervous systems. This type of pain is often difficult for the clinician to assess and treat. A comparison of nociceptive and neuropathic pain is found in **Table 5.9.**

HYPOTHERMIA AND HYPERTHERMIA

Hypothermia occurs when the body loses heat faster than it produces heat and is typically defined by a body temperature <95°F. Hypothermia occurs primarily because of prolonged exposure to cold air or water but can also be induced to treat certain medical conditions. Treatment typically involves warming the body back to normal temperature.

Hyperthermia is an elevation in body temperature. For more information, see assessment of fever as discussed throughout this chapter.

SHOCK

Shock is a life-threatening condition due to lack of blood flow that leads to hypotension and hypoxia. While the effects of shock are initially reversible, shock can rapidly lead to multisystem organ failure and death. Identifying the cause of shock early is essential to saving lives. Types of shock include:

• Septic shock in response to overwhelming infection
• Systemic inflammatory response syndrome (SIRS), which results from noninfectious conditions like burns, amniotic fluid embolism, air embolism, and crush injuries
• Neurogenic shock as a result of severe traumatic brain or spinal cord injury
• Anaphylactic shock, which results from severe allergic reactions to insect stings, foods, or medications
• Cardiogenic shock as a result of myocardial infarction

- Hypovolemic shock, which can occur from hemorrhagic or nonhemorrhagic fluid loss (Hemorrhagic shock is the most common type of shock seen in emergency departments in the United States.)

- Endocrine shock associated with adrenal failure
- Drug- and toxin-induced shock, which can be associated with drug overdoses, snakebites, transfusion reactions, and poisonings

CASE STUDY: Annual Well Exam

Mr. Smith is a 58-year-old who presents to the primary care office for an annual well exam. His BP reads 152/94 mmHg at the beginning of the visit. He states that he has occasionally had a high BP reading.

History

Mr. Smith, an accountant, shares that he has felt fine but also describes his office environment as one of high stress. He states that he feels worried during the day trying to get his work completed and meet business expectations. He notes that he has a short temper and gets frustrated with traffic on the way home. He is married, has a good relationship with his wife, and has two grown children. Mr. Smith denies having headaches, chest pain, blurred vision, or dyspnea. He takes his dog for a walk after work to manage his stress level. He denies feeling down, depressed, or hopeless. He denies a history of depression. He is not a smoker, does not take prescribed medication, and denies use of prescription medications not prescribed to him. Mr. Smith occasionally takes Tylenol or ibuprofen for "aches and pains," and has 1 to 2 drinks of alcohol at night. He denies a past medical history for conditions that may contribute to hypertension, including OSA, kidney disease, and endocrine disorders. He has

never been hospitalized. A family history reveals that both of his parents are alive and have hypertension, hyperlipidemia, and heart disease. He has an older brother who recently completed treatment for melanoma. He feels safe in his home and has never been a victim of violence.

Physical Examination

Mr. Smith has the following vital signs: 98.7°F, pulse 78, respirations 16, BP 152/94 mmHg (right arm), BP 150/94 mmHg (left arm), and a pain rating of 0. He has a BMI of 30. HEENT exam is normal, including retinal exam. Heart rate and rhythm are regular, and lungs are clear to auscultation bilaterally. Carotid arteries are without bruits. The thyroid is smooth, nonenlarged, and without nodules or tenderness. The abdomen is soft, nontender, and nondistended with no organomegaly. Peripheral pulses are 2+ bilateral. Cap refill brisk. No lower extremity edema is noted.

Differential Diagnoses
- Primary Hypertension
- Secondary Hypertension

Final Diagnosis
Primary Hypertension

Clinical Pearls

- Evidence-based assessment begins with observation. Skilled, systematic observation is essential for accurate clinical evaluation.
- For some individuals, especially a younger patient, obtaining vital signs can be anxiety provoking. Be sure to take time to answer questions and alleviate concerns before beginning these assessments as anxiety can increase a patient's pulse rate, respiratory rate, and BP.
- Subtle findings can have a *big* impact on patient outcomes! A thorough and comprehensive assessment can recognize potential problems before they progress to a serious situation. Remember not to overlook the "little things."

Key Takeaways

- Before beginning an assessment, clinicians should assure their safety and the safety of the individual being assessed.
- Initial general survey includes assessing for problems, instability, or alterations in airway, breathing, circulation, and neurologic status, which involves exposing an individual as needed in order to safely and effectively complete the exam.
- Assessments of mental and physical status include the general survey, measurements of vital signs and body habitus, and evaluation of pain.

REFERENCES

American Heart Association. (2018). *Highlights of the 2018 focused updates to the American Heart Association guidelines for CPR and ECC: Advanced cardiovascular life support and pediatric advanced life support.* Retrieved from https://eccguidelines.heart.org/wp-content/uploads/2018/10/2018-Focused-Updates_Highlights.pdf

Antony, K. M., Racusin, D. A., Aagaard, K., & Dildy, G. A. (2017). Maternal physiology. In S. G. Gabbe, J. R. Niebyl, J. L. Simpson, M. B. Landon, H. L. Galan, E. R. Jauniaux, . . . W. A. Grobman (Eds.), *Obstetrics: Normal and problem pregnancies* (7th ed., pp. 38–63). Philadelphia, PA: Elsevier.

Basile, J., & Bloch, M. J. (2019). Overview of hypertension in adults. In G. L. Bakris, W. B. White, L. Kunins, & J. P. Forman (Eds.), *UptoDate.* Retrieved from https://www.uptodate.com/contents/overview-of-hypertension-in-adults/print

Beltramini, A., Milojevic, K., & Pateron, D. (2017). Pain assessment in newborns, infants, and children. *Pediatric Annals, 46*(10), e387–e395. doi:10.3928/19382359-20170921-03

Centers for Disease Control and Prevention. (n.d.). *Healthy weight: About adult BMI.* Retrieved from https://www.cdc.gov/healthyweight/assessing/bmi/adult_bmi/index.html

Dias, D., & Paulo Silva Cunha, J. (2018). Wearable health devices—Vital sign monitoring, systems and technologies. *Sensors, 18*(8), 2414. doi:10.3390/s18082414

Flynn, J.T., Kaelber, D.C., Baker-Smith, C.M., Blowey, D., Carroll, A.E., Daniels, S.R., de Ferranti, S.D., . . Urbina, E. M. (2017). Clinical practice guideline for screening and management of high blood pressure in children and adolescents. *Pediatrics, 140*(3). doi:10.1542/peds.2017-1904

Heflin, M. T. (2019). Geriatric health maintenance. In K. E. Schmader & J. Givens (Eds.), *UptoDate.* Retrieved from https://www.uptodate.com/contents/geriatric-health-maintenance

James, P. A. (2014). 2014 evidence-based guideline for the management of high blood pressure in adults: Report from the panel members appointed to the Eighth Joint National Committee (JNC 8). *The Journal of the American Medical Association, 311*(5), 507–520. doi:10.1001/jama.2013.284427

McGrath, J. L., & Bachmann, D. J. (2019). Vital signs measurement. In J. R. Roberts, C. B. Custalow, & T. W. Thomsen (Eds.), *Roberts and Hedges' clinical procedures in emergency medicine and acute care* (pp. 1–22). Philadelphia, PA: Elsevier.

National Center for Health Statistics & National Center for Chronic Disease Prevention and Health Promotion. (2000a). *2 to 20 years: Boys body mass index-for-age percentiles.* Retrieved from https://www.cdc.gov/growthcharts/data/set1clinical/cj41c023.pdf

National Center for Health Statistics & National Center for Chronic Disease Prevention and Health Promotion. (2000b). *2 to 20 years: Girls body mass index-for-age percentiles.* Retrieved from https://www.cdc.gov/growthcharts/data/set1clinical/cj41c024.pdf

National Heart, Lung, and Blood Institute. (n.d.). *Assessing your weight and health risk.* Retrieved from https://www.nhlbi.nih.gov/health/educational/lose_wt/risk.htm

Thomas, G., & Pohl, M. A. (2019). Blood pressure measurement in the diagnosis and management of hypertension in adults. In G. L. Bakris, L. Kunins, & J. P. Forman (Eds.), *UptoDate.* Retrieved from https://www.uptodate.com/contents/blood-pressure-measurement-in-the-diagnosis-and-management-of-hypertension-in-adults

Townsend, R. (2019). Ambulatory and home blood pressure monitoring and white coat hypertension in adults. In G. L. Bakris & B. J. Gersh (Eds.), *UpToDate.* Retrieved from https://www.uptodate.com/contents/ambulatory-and-home-blood-pressure-monitoring-and-white-coat-hypertension-in-adults

U.S. Preventive Services Task Force. (2015). *Final recommendation statement: High blood pressure in adults: Screening.* Retrieved from https://www.uspreventiveservicestaskforce.org/Page/Document/RecommendationStatementFinal/high-blood-pressure-in-adults-screening#copyright-and-source-information

Van Kuiken, D., & Huth, M. M. (2016). What is 'normal?' evaluating vital signs. *Nephrology Nursing Journal, 43*(1), 49–59. Retrieved from https://library.annanurse.org/anna/articles/1280/view

Ward, M. (2019). Fever in infants and children: Pathophysiology and management. In M. S. Edwards (Ed.), *UpToDate.* Retrieved from https://www.uptodate.com/contents/fever-in-infants-and-children-pathophysiology-and-management

Whelton, P. K., Carey, R. M., Aronow, W. S., Casey, D. E., Jr., Collins, K. J., Dennison Himmelfarb, C., . . . Wright, J. T., Jr. (2018). 2017 ACC/AHA/AAPA/ABC/ACPM/AGS/APhA/ASH/ASPC/NMA/PCNA guideline for the prevention, detection, evaluation, and management of high blood pressure in adults: A report of the American College of Cardiology/American Heart Association Task Force on Clinical Practice Guidelines. *Journal of the American College of Cardiology, 71*(19), e127–e248. doi:10.1016/j.jacc.2017.11.006

EVIDENCE-BASED PHYSICAL EXAMINATION AND ASSESSMENT OF BODY SYSTEMS

6

Evidence-Based Assessment of the Heart and Circulatory System

Kristie L. Flamm, Matt Granger, Kate Gawlik, Allison Rusgo, Angela Blankenship, Audra Hanners, Kelly Casler, Joyce Karl, Mary Alice Momeyer, Samreen Raza, Martha Gulati, and Alice M. Teall

> *"Start each day with a positive thought and a grateful heart."*
>
> —ROY T. BENNET

 VIDEOS

- Follow-Up Exam: Adult With Hypertension
- Patient Case: Woman With Chest Pain

LEARNING OBJECTIVES

- Describe the structure and function of the heart and circulatory system.
- Identify differences and considerations in the anatomy and physiology of the cardiovascular system across the life span.
- Understand the components of a comprehensive, evidence-based history and physical examination of the cardiovascular system.
- Distinguish between normal and abnormal findings in the cardiovascular system.

Visit https://connect.springerpub.com/content/book/978-0-8261 -6454-4/chapter/ch00 to access the videos.

ANATOMY AND PHYSIOLOGY OF THE HEART AND CIRCULATORY SYSTEM

The **cardiovascular system**, comprising the heart and great vessels, is the body's circulatory mechanism. The right side of the heart receives deoxygenated blood from the superior and inferior venae cavae (SVC and IVC) while the left side of the heart pumps oxygenated blood into the aorta for distribution to all organs and tissues (**Figure 6.1**). As this circulatory process is vital for survival, it is imperative that clinicians understand the anatomy and physiology of the cardiovascular system. This knowledge will allow clinicians to evaluate this body system thoroughly and aid in the diagnosis of patients with cardiac-related concerns.

From a surface anatomy perspective, the heart and roots of the great vessels are surrounded by the pericardial sac located in the middle of the thorax. The **heart**, approximately the size of a fist, is bordered laterally and posteriorly by the lungs and anteriorly by the sternum and the third through fifth ribs on the left (**Figure 6.2**). It is located at the body's midline and appears slightly tilted with the base of the heart at the top and the apex of the heart at the bottom.

THE PERICARDIAL AND CARDIAC MEMBRANE

The heart is encased by the pericardium, a double-walled membrane located posterior to the sternum and the costal cartilage between the fifth and eighth thoracic

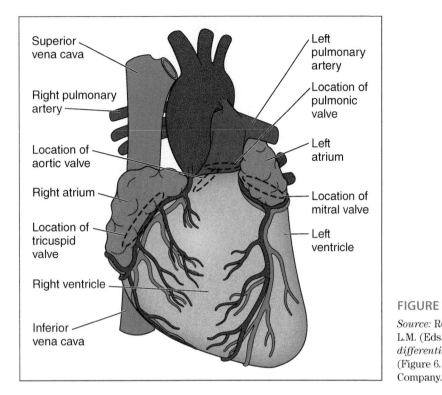

FIGURE 6.1 Anatomy of the heart.

Source: Reproduced from Myrick, K.M., & Karosas, L.M. (Eds.). (2021). *Advanced health assessment and differential diagnosis: Essentials for clinical practice* (Figure 6.1A). New York, NY: Springer Publishing Company.

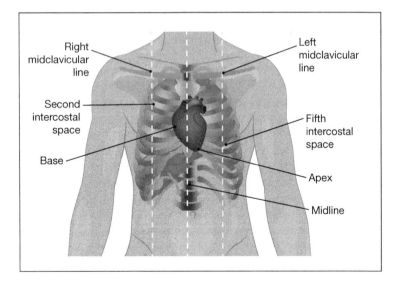

FIGURE 6.2 Cardiac anatomy and surface landmarks.

vertebrae. The pericardium is composed of outer fibrous and inner serous layers. The fibrous pericardium affixes the heart to the mediastinum, which helps maintain its shape and position within the chest. The serous pericardium is further divided into parietal and visceral components. The parietal pericardium is fused to the fibrous pericardium, whereas the visceral pericardium forms the epicardium or outer surface of the heart. In between the visceral and parietal layers is the pericardial space, which contains a small amount of serous fluid to lubricate and protect the heart from injury (**Figure 6.3**).

Similar to the multilayered pericardial sac, the heart is also composed of three layers. The outermost membrane is the epicardium, which functions as the visceral pericardium. The right and left coronary arteries lie upon the epicardial surface and perfuse the heart. The myocardium is the thick middle layer composed of cardiac muscle, and the endocardium is the innermost layer that lines the heart (**Figure 6.4**).

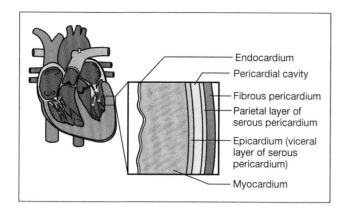

FIGURE 6.3 Pericardial anatomy.

Source: Reproduced from Tkacs, N., Herrmann, L., & Johnson, R. (Eds.). (in press). *Advanced physiology and pathophysiology: Essentials for clinical practice* (Figure 10.2A). New York, NY: Springer Publishing Company.

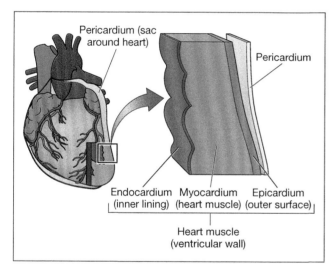

FIGURE 6.4 Anatomical layers of the heart. Depiction of the three layers of the cardiac wall.

Source: Adapted from Betts, J. G., Young, K. A., Wise, J. A., Johnson, E., Poe, B., Kruse, D. H., . . . DeSaix P. (2013). *Anatomy and physiology* (Figure 19.5). Retrieved from https://openstax.org/books/anatomy-and-physiology/pages/19-1-heart-anatomy#fig-ch20_01_04

THE CARDIAC CHAMBERS

The heart contains four chambers—a right and left atria and a right and left ventricle. The right atrium (RA) is located at the right heart border. It receives deoxygenated blood from the SVC, IVC, and coronary sinus, the latter of which connects to the cardiac veins that drain the myocardium. The inferior portion of the RA is a muscular wall with individual openings for the SVC, IVC, and coronary sinus. The outlet of the right atrium is through the tricuspid valve which empties into the right ventricle (RV; **Figure 6.5**).

The RV comprises the majority of the anterior and inferior portions of the heart. The RV meets the pulmonary artery at the sternal angle, which is the *base* of the heart. The RV receives deoxygenated blood from the RA through the aforementioned tricuspid valve. The tricuspid valve apparatus is made up of three valvular cusps, tendinous chords, and three papillary muscles. Once the RV receives deoxygenated blood, it is ejected through the right ventricular outflow tract, through the pulmonary valve and into the pulmonary artery. Blood then enters the lungs through the branch pulmonary arteries where gas is exchanged. Blood becomes saturated with oxygen, and returns to the left atrium via the pulmonary veins. Another important component of the RV is the right bundle branches of the AV bundle. This anatomical feature is an integral part of the heart's electrical conduction system, as it allows for organized cardiac contractions. Last, the interventricular septum is located between the right and left ventricles. This muscular barrier separates the ventricles, and a significant portion of the ventricular septum encroaches into the RV due to the increased pressure from the powerful flow of blood through the left ventricle (LV; see **Figure 6.5**).

The LA encompasses the majority of the heart's base. This chamber has a thicker muscular wall when compared with the RA, and this helps maintain its integrity against forceful blood flow. Within the LA, two superior and two inferior pulmonary veins converge at its posterior wall and allow for the transfer of oxygenated blood from the lungs. The LA also has a left AV aperture where blood is pushed into the LV for distribution to the rest of the body (see **Figure 6.5**). The LV is located slightly posterior and leftward of the RV. It covers the majority of the pulmonary and diaphragmatic aspects of the heart, which equates to the organ's left lateral border.

The tip of the LV also forms the **cardiac apex**, which is an important landmark in the cardiac physical examination. Using palpation during the physical exam, the clinician can appreciate the **point of maximal impulse** or **PMI**, which is located at the apex. Anatomically, this pulsation is helpful when delineating the heart's left lateral border and should be located at the fifth intercostal space in the left midclavicular line. The location of the PMI is also an important factor when evaluating patients with conditions such as hypertension (HTN) and congestive heart failure (CHF), and this will be discussed in future sections of this chapter.

The LV needs to be stronger than the RV because it withstands a powerful contraction as oxygenated blood moves into the aorta. Therefore, its walls are significantly thicker and more muscular than the RV. An important landmark within the LV is the mitral valve, which is used to funnel blood from the LA. This valve is designed to maintain its integrity and prevent the backflow of blood into the LA despite the high-pressure environment generated by strong contractions from the

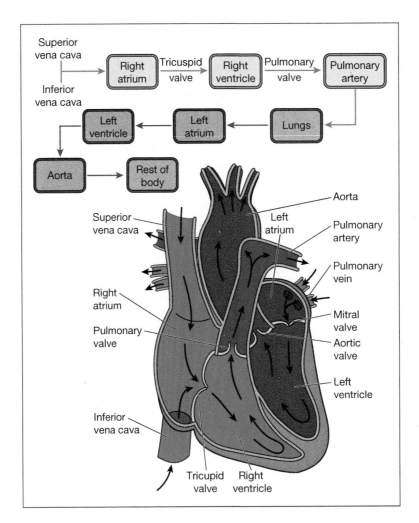

FIGURE 6.5 Cardiac circulatory pathway. Tracing the flow of deoxygenated blood from the venae cavae, through the right side of the heart, and into the lungs where it is oxygenated and returned to the left side of the heart and pumped to the aorta and the rest of the body.

LV. Also located inside the chamber is the aortic orifice, which is encased by a fibrous ring that is connected to the aortic valve. This valve allows for blood flow from the LV to the ascending aorta, which is the final destination of oxygenated blood before it is forced into all other organs and tissues (see **Figure 6.5**).

CARDIAC CIRCULATION

When the atria and ventricles contract, a designated amount of blood is forced into the pulmonary arteries and aorta, and this determines the cardiac output (CO). CO equates to the volume of blood that is discharged from the LV in 60 seconds; the CO is the amount of work done by the heart in response to the body's need for oxygen. It is composed of two components—heart rate and stroke volume, the latter of which is the amount of blood ejected per heartbeat. Both heart rate and stroke volume can vary on the basis of three factors—preload, afterload, and the contractile ability of the heart.

Preload is defined as a given volume of blood that causes cardiac cells to stretch before contraction. This corresponds to the amount of blood that remains in the ventricles at the end of diastole or cardiac relaxation. Afterload is the pressure the heart has to work against in order to eject blood during its contractile phase. It can also be thought of as the amount of pressure that the atria and ventricles have to create in order to successfully eject a sufficient amount of blood into the circulatory system and pulmonary arteries. Contractility is guided by the cardiac muscle cells' ability to work against a given volume of blood—myocardial fibers stretch when under pressure and their recoil allows the atria and ventricles to contract.

The concepts of preload, afterload, and cardiac contractility are especially important when evaluating patients with suspected heart failure (HF). For example, in one type of HF, the ventricles dilate. When this occurs, the chambers require a greater amount of pressure (preload) to overcome the aortic pressure (afterload) needed to eject an adequate amount of blood to maintain adequate cardiac output. Over time, the cardiac cells develop an inability to compensate with these higher pressures and cardiac output is compromised, leading to symptoms of HF. Although there are various types, severity levels, and underlying etiologies for CHF, in many instances preload, afterload, and contractility are affected. Therefore, it is important for clinicians to understand these physiological mechanisms to ensure that patients who present with signs and symptoms of cardiac compromise can receive proper treatment and management.

Cardiac Valves

Cardiac circulation is guided by a series of valves that function on a pressure gradient system. These valves are very important for maintaining proper blood flow through the heart. The mitral and tricuspid valves are located between the LA and LV and the RA and RV, respectively. They are also known as the atrioventricular or AV valves. The pulmonic and the aortic valves are located between the RV and pulmonary artery and between the LV and aorta, respectively. The pulmonary and aortic valves are also known as the semilunar valves due to their half-moon appearance. As each of these valves open and close, the vibrations from the valve leaflets in conjunction with the movement from the blood itself and the individual cardiac structures generate the familiar "lub-dub" sounds heard during cardiac auscultation. Clinically, these normal heart sounds are defined as S1 and S2. There are also two pathological sounds, termed S3 and S4. If a clinician does appreciate one of the abnormal heart sounds, this can signify diseases such as HF or ischemia.

THE CARDIAC CYCLE AND HEART SOUNDS

The **cardiac cycle** is another important physiological concept because it forms the basis for understanding circulatory blood flow as well as valvular and cardiac chamber function. These components are integral portions of the cardiac exam and can help clinicians better evaluate and treat patients with cardiac diseases. By definition, the cardiac cycle describes the period of time between the origination of one heartbeat to the next. Two important terms are systole, the period of ventricular contraction, and diastole, the period of ventricular filling and relaxation. To start the cycle, diastole begins as the aortic and pulmonic valves close. This process prevents the backflow of blood into the LV (from the aorta) and the RV (from the pulmonary artery). Also during diastole, the mitral valve is open to allow blood to move from the LA into the LV. This filling process helps the LV prepare for its contraction of blood into the aorta during systole. The tricuspid valve

is also open during diastole so that blood can flow into the RV from the RA. Atrial contraction occurs at the end of diastole. This creates an increased pressure gradient across the valves and systole begins. During systole, the tricuspid and mitral valve close to prevent regurgitation of blood into the LA and RA, respectively. Additionally, the aortic and pulmonic valves open so that blood can move into the ascending aorta (from the LV) and pulmonary artery (from the RV; **Figure 6.6**).

Focusing on the concept of heart sounds, the S1 and S2 sounds equate to the timing of systole and diastole. The "lub" sound (or S1) occurs when the mitral and tricuspid valves are closed by the pressure generated by ventricular contraction, and the "dub" (or S2) is caused by the closure of the aortic and pulmonic valves following ventricular contraction. During diastole, the pressure in the atria is slightly higher than in the ventricles and the mitral and tricuspid valves are open so that blood can flow from the LA and RA to the LV and RV. During systole, the ventricles contract, which raises their internal pressure. In addition, this accentuates the pressure difference between the LA and LV; thus, the mitral valve is forced closed and the S1 heart sound is generated. As the pressure in the LV continues to rise, it exceeds the pressure in the ascending aorta; thus, the aortic valve opens and blood can move from the LV into the aorta. Once the LV has discharged most of its blood, its pressure decreases below the pressure inside the aorta and the aortic valve subsequently closes. This creates the S2 heart sound. This also prompts another cycle of diastole to begin with the opening of the mitral and tricuspid valves.

There are several heart sounds that can be heard if a patient has a cardiac pathology related to valvular or chamber dysfunction. Typically, when the mitral valve opens during diastole, this is silent. However, if a patient has a stenotic or stiff valve, one might appreciate a snap-like sound as the valve leaflets "pop" open to allow blood to flow between the LA and LV. In adults, a clinician might hear an S3 heart sound, which can indicate ventricular failure or myocardial ischemia. This occurs because of an abrupt deceleration of blood flow across the mitral valve. In children and older adolescents, however, the S3 sound can be a normal variant heard during cardiac auscultation. Last, an S4 sound, also pathological in adults, occurs immediately before S1 and represents ventricular dysfunction, typically stiffness (**Figure 6.7**).

In addition to each of the heart sounds, the clinician may also appreciate a separation, or splitting, of the S1 or S2 heart sounds (**Figure 6.7B**). This finding can be a normal variant or indicative of a cardiac pathology. When auscultating the right side of a patient's heart, one may appreciate two discernable sounds for S2. This is defined as an A2 and P2—the former representing the aortic valve closing and the latter equating to the

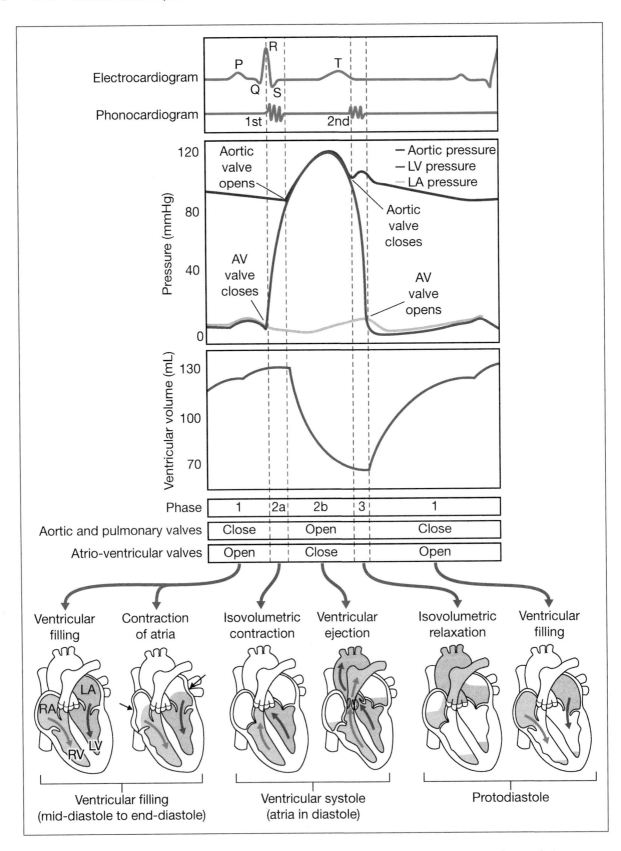

FIGURE 6.6 Elements of the cardiac cycle. The top figure is an EKG representation of the cardiac cycle in conjunction with corresponding pressures, volumes, and valvular activity during each phase. The contraction of each chamber and direction of blood flow during each portion of the cycle are also depicted.

AV, atrioventricular; LA, left atrium; LV, left ventricle; RA, right atrium; RV, right ventricle.

Source: Reproduced with permission from Marieb, E. N. (2005). *Essentials of human anatomy and physiology* (8th ed., Figure 18.20).

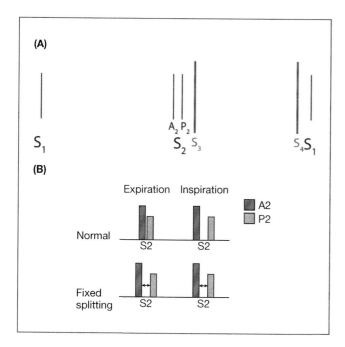

FIGURE 6.7 (A) Physiological and pathological heart sounds. An S3 heart sound in an adult can be pathological and indicate ventricular failure or myocardial ischemia. In a child or adolescent, this is a normal variant. An S4 heart sound, also pathological in adults, occurs immediately before S1 and represents ventricular dysfunction, typically stiffness. (B) Splitting of the S2 heart sound during the cardiac cycle. When performing cardiac auscultation, one may appreciate a split or two discernable sounds for S2 defined as A2 and P2. This finding can be physiological or pathological, thus requiring further investigation. The splitting of S2 into A2 and P2 can be a normal variant during inspiration; however, if it is also appreciated during expiration, it can signify cardiac abnormalities such as valvular disease or septal irregularities.

pulmonic valve closing. During the cardiac cycle, this phenomenon occurs because events that occur on the left side of the heart occur slightly before those on the right side of the heart. To determine the clinical value of this finding, the clinician should coordinate the auscultation with a patient's respiratory cycle. During inspiration, the time required to fill the right side of the heart is slightly increased. This process delays the closing of the pulmonic valve (as compared with the aortic valve); therefore, each valve closure's sound is appreciated separately. When a clinician is investigating heart splitting, it is best heard between the second and third intercostal spaces near the sternum, where A2 is slightly louder than P2 due to the increased pressure within the aorta. An S2 split (into A2 and P2 components) can occur physiologically during inspiration; however, if it persists during exhalation, it is defined as a fixed split. This finding is pathological if the interval between A2 and P2 fails to lengthen during inspiration and requires

further evaluation for underlying valvular diseases or other structural abnormalities, particularly within the septal walls. There are also additional variants such as a wide S2 split or a paradoxical split, which signal the presence of cardiac pathology.

The S1 heart sound is normally a single sound but can also be split when pathology is present, such as a right bundle branch block; however, it does not vary with respiration. S1 is a composite sound made by the near-simultaneous closure of the mitral and tricuspid valves. When splitting occurs, the distinct sounds can be labeled M1 (mitral closure) and T1 (tricuspid closure). The mitral aspect is significantly louder than the tricuspid sound because pressures are higher on the left side of the heart, which causes the mitral valve to close more forcefully and create a louder sound. The clinician can best auscultate the mitral component of S1 at the cardiac apex. The sound of the tricuspid valve closing can be heard best along the left sternal border near the RV.

Cardiac Murmurs

In conjunction with the four heart sounds, heart **murmurs** are also distinct sounds that one might appreciate during a cardiac assessment. In adults, the majority of heart murmurs are indicative of valvular pathology and can affect any of the atrioventricular or semilunar valves; however, benign murmurs can occur in high cardiac output states such as pregnancy, anemia, or fever. Conversely, nearly all murmurs in children are benign or "innocent" and can disappear as the child or adolescent grows into adulthood.

Distinguishing benign murmurs from pathological murmurs can be challenging, even for experienced clinicians. Knowledge of cardiovascular anatomy and physiology, along with experience through clinical practice, will allow clinicians to become more adept at recognizing and characterizing cardiac murmurs. In general, heart murmurs are generated by turbulent blood flow. As blood is forced from one chamber to the next, if a valve is not functioning properly, the smooth flow of blood is disrupted and this creates an abnormal vibratory sound at a given precordial location, which corresponds to the affected valve. The two primary types of valvular disease are stenosis and regurgitation. These findings can occur because of various underlying disease etiologies, or secondary to normal aging. When a valve narrows, blood is forced through a smaller-than-usual aperture and this creates the characteristic murmur of stenosis. Conversely, valves may become incompetent when damaged by trauma or infection. They may also lose function as cardiac chambers enlarge, stretching the valve annulus until the leaflets can no longer coapt properly. As blood flows across this defective valve, some blood flows backward; this backward flowing blood can be forced at high pressure through a relatively small opening, which causes turbulence and creates an audible sound of varying intensity.

Anatomically, it is important to remember where each of the heart valves is located on the precordium. This will increase the likelihood of not only appreciating a heart murmur but also understanding which valve is dysfunctional. Murmurs of the aortic valve are best heard near the cardiac base at the right second intercostal space, and this corresponds to its location between the LV and the ascending aorta. Mitral stenosis (MS) and regurgitation are usually heard near the cardiac apex because this valve is located between the LA and LV. Murmurs that affect the tricuspid valve are usually the loudest near the lower aspect of the left sternal border, which corresponds to its location between the RA and RV. Last, abnormalities associated with the pulmonary valve are best heard near the left second intercostal spaces, which correspond to its location near the RV and the pulmonary artery.

Given this anatomical information, it is apparent that the locations of some murmurs can overlap. To help differentiate, one can note characteristics such as timing during the cardiac cycle, sound radiation, and pitch. **Table 6.1** provides information on the typical characteristics of heart murmurs. This information will increase a clinician's diagnostic accuracy when evaluating a patient with suspected valvular heart disease.

CARDIAC CONDUCTION

To fulfill its role as the circulatory hub for the body, the heart maintains a coordinated electrical system that allows for synchronous cardiac muscle contraction and relaxation. The main components of cardiac conduction are the sinoatrial (SA) node, atrioventricular (AV) node, the bundle of His, the left and right bundle branches, and the Purkinje fibers. These components create a unified pathway for cardiac electrical impulses to travel.

An action potential occurs when there is a change in voltage across a cellular membrane. As charged particles travel between the inside and outside of a cell, the membrane potential changes. When this occurs, a cardiac impulse can be generated as electrical currents travel from cell to cell causing a wave of depolarization to spread across the myocardium. As each cell reaches a critical voltage, muscle contraction is stimulated. This process continues as each cell triggers its neighbor to depolarize and contract. The process is repeated until the impulse has traveled through the entire heart, stimulating each myocardial cell along the way. Action potentials from the heart differ slightly from those created by other cells because they have automaticity. This means that the specialized cells at the SA node can create their

---

TABLE 6.1 Characteristics of Heart Murmurs

Type of Murmur	Precordial Location	Timing in Cardiac Cycle	Radiation	Pitch	Sound Quality	Special Maneuvers
Aortic stenosis	Right second and third intercostal spaces	Mid-systolic	Toward carotid arteries	Crescendo–decrescendo; medium	Harsh	Best heard with patient sitting and leaning forward
Mitral stenosis	Apex	Diastole	None	Decrescendo; low	Rumbling	Use bell of stethoscope at PMI; best heard with patient in left lateral decubitus position
Aortic regurgitation	Left second to fourth intercostal spaces	Diastole	Toward apex	High	Blowing	Best heard with patient sitting and leaning forward with breath held following exhalation
Mitral regurgitation	Apex	Holosystolic	Toward left axilla	Medium/high	Harsh	Murmur should not vary with respiration
Tricuspid regurgitation	Lower left sternal border	Holosystolic	Toward xiphoid process	Medium	Blowing	Murmur will increase with inspiration
Pulmonic stenosis	Left second and third intercostal spaces	Mid-systolic	May radiate to left shoulder	Crescendo–decrescendo; medium	Harsh	None

PMI, point of maximal impulse.

own action potentials without relying on nervous system activity. The main ions that are involved are sodium (Na), potassium (K), and calcium (Ca) in conjunction with various membrane transport proteins that move the charged particles against the electrochemical gradient. As the ions travel between the inside and outside of the cardiac cells, the voltage across the membranes alternates between (+) and (−); this allows the cardiac chambers to depolarize or repolarize on the basis of the given voltage potential. On a macro level, this electrochemical process sets the heart's rate and allows it to rhythmically contract and relax. It also helps to create the cardiac cycle that is depicted graphically via EKGs to show the heart's underlying cardiac activity.

The SA node is a 13.5-mm structure within the RA near the superior vena cava. It is the pacemaker of the heart because it is composed of a group of specialized cardiac cells that can generate impulses that travel to all other cardiac tissues. In a well-functioning heart, the SA node creates approximately 60 to 90 impulses/minute, which match one's normal resting heart rate. This unique electrical property ensures that the SA node is the only designated area for the initiation of cardiac impulses. The SA node is innervated by sympathetic nerves and branches from the vagus nerve and its surrounding tissues function via calcium channel activation. These properties allow impulses from the SA node to travel in a slow and decremental fashion. The node is also directly connected to the cardiac cells of the right atrial wall, and this allows impulses to travel between the SA node and the next point in the cardiac circuit.

Once a impulse is generated by the SA node, it moves slowly to the atrial tissues and then funneled quickly to the AV node, which is approximately 5 mm in size. This small structure is also a group of specialized cardiac cells and is located between the atrial and ventricular septi. It serves as a transition zone where each impulse is temporarily held before moving toward the ventricles. This slight delay at the AV node corresponds to the P-R interval on an EKG and allows for ventricular filling. The next portion of the conduction system is the bundle of His, which is a collection of myocardial cells surrounded by a fibrous outer sheath. Anatomically, this structure is very important because it is the only direct connection for impulses to travel between the atria and the ventricles. The bundle of His then bifurcates into left and right bundle branches, which move through the interventricular septum independently. At this juncture, the left bundle travels toward the apex of the LV while the right bundle branch moves toward the apex of the RV. Last, the two bundle branches further divide into the Purkinje fibers, which disperse into the subendocardium of the myocardium. Once an electrical impulse travels through the bundle branches to the Purkinje fibers, the ventricles contract and one impulse of the cardiac cycle is complete (**Figure 6.8**).

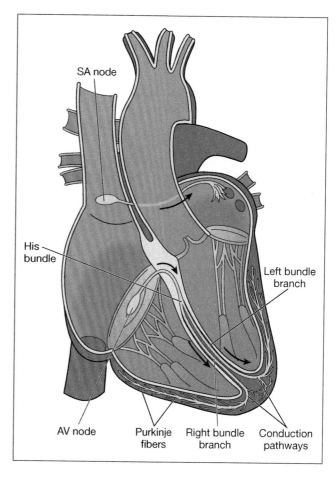

FIGURE 6.8 Electrophysiological pathway of cardiac conduction. Tracing an impulse from the SA node to the AV node through the bundle of His, where it bifurcates into the left and right BBs and terminates at the Purkinje fibers to allow the ventricles to contract and complete one impulse of the cardiac cycle.

AV, atrioventricular; BBs, bundle branches; SA, sinoatrial.

Conceptually, one can understand the heart's **electrical conduction system**; however, it cannot be seen during a physical exam. Therefore, one way to evaluate a patient with a suspected conduction abnormality is an EKG. This diagnostic test is useful because its individual waveforms represent the electrical impulses of the heart, specifically its contraction and relaxation phases. The main components of an EKG are the P-wave, QRS complex, and T-wave (**Figure 6.9**). The EKG begins with the P-wave, which is atrial activation or depolarization (**Figure 6.10**). The QRS complex represents ventricular depolarization and the T-wave equates to ventricular repolarization. Specific heart sounds and timing of the cycle can also be applied to the EKG's waveforms. For example, S1 can be mapped to the QRS complex because it corresponds to ventricular contraction when the mitral valve closes and the aortic valve opens during systole. In addition, S2 represents

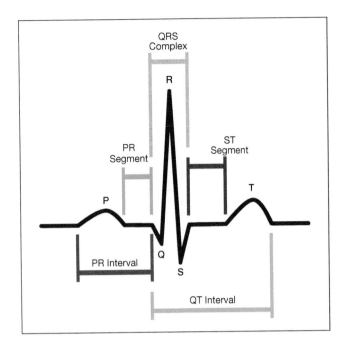

FIGURE 6.9 Electrocardiogram wave.

Source: Adapted from Anthony Atkielski.

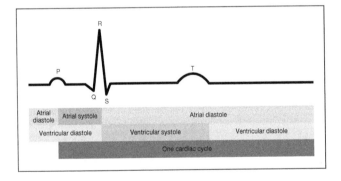

FIGURE 6.10 Cardiac cycle and electrocardiogram.

Source: Betts, J. G., Young, K. A., Wise, J. A., Johnson, E., Poe, B., Kruse, D. H., . . . DeSaix P. (2013). *Anatomy and physiology* (Figure 19.28). Retrieved from https://openstax.org/books/anatomy-and-physiology/pages/19-3-cardiac-cycle

the beginning of diastole with the closing of the aortic valve and the opening of the mitral and tricuspid valves. Finally, the ventricles relax; this is represented by the EKG's T-wave.

THE VASCULAR SYSTEM

Blood is circulated throughout the body by a network of **blood vessels (Figures 6.11** and **6.12**). Arteries carry oxygenated blood away from the heart. Arteries branch into increasingly smaller vessels termed arterioles then even smaller ones called capillaries. At the level of the

capillary, nutrients and wastes are exchanged, causing deoxygenation of the blood and providing the cells with nutrients. The capillaries are connected to venules (smaller vessels) that then form veins. Veins return the deoxygenated blood to the heart. This circulatory process is termed the systemic circuit. Once at the heart, the blood goes through the pulmonary circuit. This is where deoxygenated blood is carried exclusively to the lungs for gas exchange. Gas exchange occurs and the freshly oxygenated blood is pumped back out into systemic circulation.

Blood Pressure

An additional component of the cardiac physical exam is the evaluation of **blood pressure (Figure 6.13)**. While this information is technically documented as a vital sign, it is something to be mindful of during a cardiac exam because blood pressure has a direct correlation with cardiovascular health. As blood circulates during the cardiac cycle and moves into the arterial system, a **pulse** is created. The force that is generated during this process is essentially a measure of one's blood pressure. During cardiac contraction or systole, the pressure reaches its highest level and then falls to its nadir during diastole or relaxation. The pressure at these two extremes are the two numbers that comprise a patient's systolic and diastolic blood pressures that are measured with a sphygmomanometer (blood pressure cuff). The difference between the systolic and diastolic blood pressures is defined as pulse pressure and it can be narrowed or widened in various cardiac conditions. There are also several factors that affect blood pressure such as left ventricular stroke volume, vascular stiffness, volume of blood in the arterial system, and integrity of the aorta.

Although blood pressure is helpful in the evaluation of cardiac abnormalities, it cannot be used to directly assess pressures within the heart. One noninvasive method to assess a patient's overall volume status is to examine the jugular venous system. The jugular veins can help provide an estimation of the pressures within the RA, pericardium, and RV (specifically right ventricular end diastolic pressure).

During a cardiac physical exam, the clinician should evaluate the jugular veins (**Figure 6.14**). As the pressures fluctuate in the RA during contraction and relaxation, the waveform is transmitted to the jugular vein and pulsations can be appreciated via inspection. Jugular venous pressures (JVPs) will increase when there is an excess of fluid in the cardiovascular system. This often occurs in patients who are suffering from exacerbations of HF. The JVP can also fall in settings of hypotension and acute blood loss. The procedure for properly examining and measuring the JVP will be reviewed later in this chapter when reviewing the steps of the cardiac physical examination.

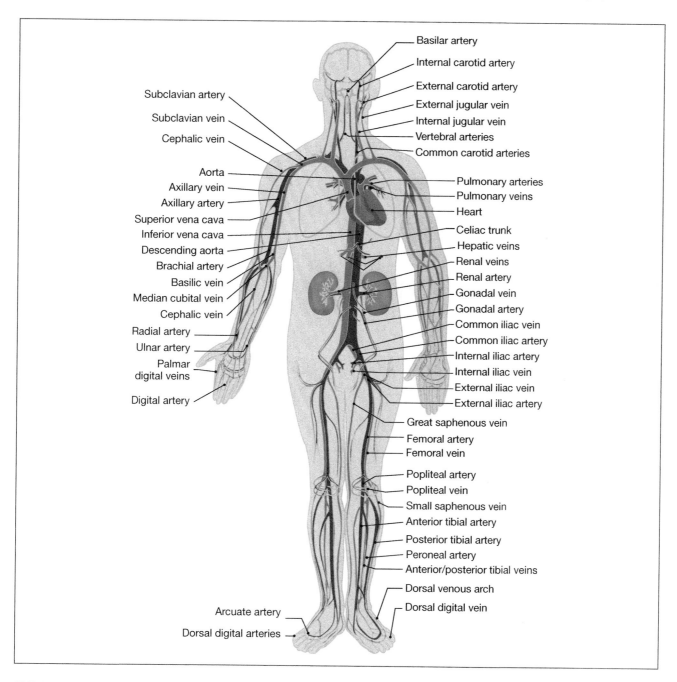

FIGURE 6.11 Circulatory system.

Source: Image courtesy of Mariana Ruiz Villarreal.

PEDIATRIC ANATOMICAL AND PHYSIOLOGICAL CONSIDERATIONS

FETAL HEART DEVELOPMENT

The heart is the first organ to form and supports the development of the rapidly growing embryo. The heart forms from a primary cardiac tube that then splits into two endocardiac tubes (**Figure 6.15**). These tubes fuse together around 21 days and form into a truncus, the bulbus cordis and primitive atrium and ventricles. The tube loops upon itself to form the atrium and ventricles. Further development of the atria and ventricles occurs through the bulging of the tissues forming them. Ingrowth of tissue further forms the atrium and ventricle into separate chambers. This septation of the ventricles occurs around 28 days and the heart is fully

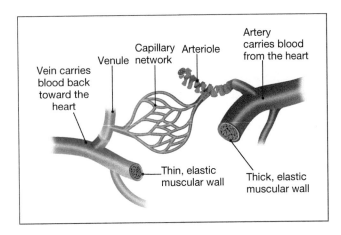

FIGURE 6.12 Blood vessels of cardiovascular system.

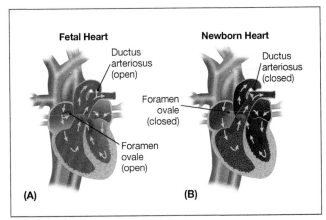

FIGURE 6.15 Fetal heart and newborn heart. (A) Heart development at 35 days. (B) Heart development at 8 weeks.

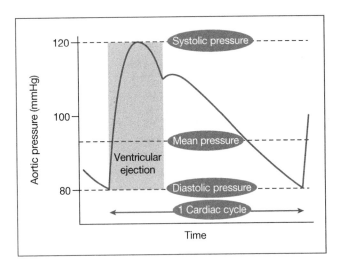

FIGURE 6.13 Blood pressure in the cardiac cycle.

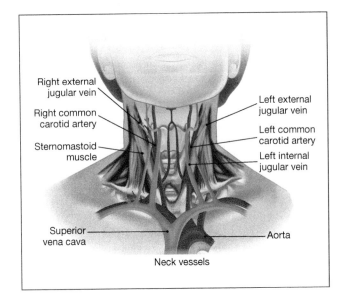

FIGURE 6.14 Blood vessels of the neck.

formed by 35 days. Formation of a congenital heart defect can occur at any of these stages as the heart forms. The stage of the embryonic development where there is a disruption in the fetal development determines the congenital heart defect that occurs. Disruption in the fetal development can occur from unknown reasons as well as known risk factors such as maternal health and/or drug use.

In the development of the fetus, there are two connections that occur and may persist after the birth of the infant. These are the patent ductus arteriosus (PDA) and the patent foramen ovale (PFO). In-utero, the fetal circulation runs in two parallel circuits, and the PDA functions to allow maternal blood flow from the umbilical vein to the IVC. Blood returns to the RA and oxygenated blood flows into the LA through the PFO. This blood flow across the PFO accounts for the majority of blood flow to the LA in fetal circulation. After birth, as the infant begins to breathe, oxygen levels begin to rise, prostaglandin levels fall, and the PDA closes. The PFO closes after birth with increased left atrial filling from the pulmonary veins and decreased return from PDA. A flap valve of the septum primum closes the PFO. In most infants, these connections will close within hours to days after birth; however, in many congenital heart defects, the persistence of these connections may be essential for continued blood flow and oxygenation.

GERIATRIC ANATOMICAL AND PHYSIOLOGICAL CONSIDERATIONS

Age-related changes in the structure and muscular contractility of the heart may or may not produce symptoms depending on disease states, activity level, and stress. In the absence of specific disease, the heart size generally decreases. At rest, there is no significant change in heart rate or CO.

Arterial walls thicken and stiffen due to atherosclerotic changes, predisposing the older adults to isolated systolic HTN and widening pulse pressure. The myocardium loses elasticity and the walls of the atria and ventricles hypertrophy, decreasing cardiac reserve and ability to respond to stress and activity. Heart valves thicken, sclerose, and valve leaflets do not close efficiently. Resulting turbulent blood flow may produce murmurs, many benign. Age-related changes in the electrical system, including a decrease in pacemaker cells in the SA node, predisposing older adults to dysrhythmias. Clinically, cardiovascular disease (CVD) may be difficult to detect and diagnose because it may be asymptomatic or present with vague, atypical symptoms in the older adult population.

KEY HISTORY QUESTIONS AND CONSIDERATIONS

HISTORY OF PRESENT ILLNESS

Common Presenting Symptoms

Chest pain, palpitations, lower-extremity edema

Example: Chest Pain/Pressure/Discomfort

- Onset: Time of onset, manner in which symptoms began, sudden or insidious
- Location: Site of pain (left, right, anterior, posterior), does it radiate
- Duration: Progression and persistence of chest pain since onset
- Character: Intensity, quality, and radiation of pain to the arm, jaw, or neck
- Associated symptoms: Presence or absence of numbness, tingling, weakness, nausea, vomiting, fever, neck pain; heartburn/gastroesophageal reflux disease (GERD), hemoptysis, shortness of breath
- Aggravating factors: Worse with activity, rest, lying flat, food, stress, or movement; painful to touch
- Relieving symptoms: Pharmacological, including nitroglycerin, antacids; nonpharmacological, including rest
- Timing or temporal factors: Worse at night, early morning

DIFFERENTIAL DIAGNOSES

Acute coronary syndrome (ACS), acute myocardial infarction (MI), HF, acute pericarditis, GERD, pneumonia, pulmonary embolus, musculoskeletal strain, panic disorder/attack, acute thoracic aortic dissection

PAST MEDICAL HISTORY

- HTN or history of elevated blood pressures
- Hyperlipidemia
- Diabetes (insulin or non-insulin dependent)
- Obstructive sleep apnea
- Kidney disease
- Stroke
- Blood clots
- ACS
- Acute myocardial infarction (AMI)
- Depression
- Anxiety
- Stress (acute or chronic)
- Adverse childhood experiences (ACES)
- Maternal illnesses, illicit drug use, and medication use when pregnant
- Personal history of congenital heart disease (CHD) and any correctional surgeries
- Previous surgeries, emergency department visits
- Medications or history of medication, dose, and frequency
- Herbal medications/dietary supplements, including fish oil, coenzyme Q10, garlic, niacin
- Allergies (drug, environmental, and food with reaction)

FAMILY HISTORY

- AMI (especially if occurred at a young age)
- CHD
- Coronary artery disease (CAD)
- Depression
- Diabetes
- Down syndrome
- Hyperlipidemia
- HTN
- Inherited hypercoagulable conditions, including factor V Leiden, prothrombin gene mutation, and/or deficiencies of natural proteins that prevent clotting (such as antithrombin, protein C, and protein S)
- Long QT syndrome
- Stroke
- Sudden cardiac death

SOCIAL HISTORY

- Tobacco use (type, pack years)
- Alcohol intake (type, amount, daily intake)
- Recreational drug use (specifically cocaine, heroin use)
- Stress level
- Sleep (patterns, duration)
- Diet (specifically sodium intake, trans fats, red meat consumption)
- Exercise (frequency, duration, type)

REVIEW OF SYSTEMS

- General: Fever, fatigue, dizziness, weight changes, recent travel (long car or plane ride)
- Head, eyes, ears, nose, throat (HEENT): Visual disturbances/visual difficulty, periodontal disease, recent strep infections or history of untreated/undertreated strep infections
- Respiratory: Shortness of breath, orthopnea, snoring with or without witness apneas
- Cardiovascular: Chest pain (with activity, at rest, or both); left arm, jaw, or neck pain; use of nitroglycerin; palpitations; racing heart rate; lower-extremity edema; pain in lower extremities during activity; hair loss on the lower legs; history of stress test or EKG with results
- Gastrointestinal (GI): Abdominal pulsations, abdominal pain, GERD
- Genitourinary (GU): Use of oral contraceptives
- Neurologic: Weakness, numbness and tingling, syncope, headache, falls, dizziness
- Musculoskeletal: Weakness, recent activity or overuse
- Psychiatric: Depression; anxiety; changes in mentation, memory, or mood; current stress level; coping mechanisms

PREVENTIVE CARE CONSIDERATIONS

- Aspirin (taken for primary prevention)
- Low-sodium, high-fiber diet
- Smoking cessation
- Medication to reduce blood pressure and cholesterol
- Exercise

PHYSICAL EXAMINATION OF THE HEART AND CIRCULATORY SYSTEM

INITIAL OBSERVATIONS

The initial cardiovascular and peripheral vascular assessment of an individual, like the assessment of other body systems, begins with the general survey. This survey does not differ from the general survey outlined in Chapter 5, Approach to the Physical Examination: General Survey and Assessment of Vital Signs; however, its focus is primarily related to the cardiac and peripheral vascular systems (PVS). Important general observations include:

- Does the patient appear comfortable? Those presenting with chest pain or shortness of breath should especially be observed for an urgent or emergent situation.

- Observe skin color, respiratory effort (refer to this chapter for specifics), and mental status. Abnormalities in these parameters may indicate cardiovascular (CV) compromise.
- Assess vital signs. All vital signs should be obtained as discussed in Chapter 5, Approach to the Physical Examination. Blood pressure, pulse and respiratory rate, temperature, and pulse oximetry are all indices of the cardiovascular system (CVS). An increase in an individual's weight over a relatively short period of time may be due to vascular congestion and volume retention due to conditions such as CHF. Assessment of height allows for determination of body mass index (BMI). Extreme variations in height may be due to genetic syndromes, which can have associated cardiovascular abnormalities.
- Discoloration or ulceration of the skin of exposed extremities may indicate peripheral vascular disease (PVD).

Refer to **Table 5.1** for a reminder of the assessment to determine physiological stability. If the patient's status is unstable, immediate intervention is warranted.

Blood Pressure Assessment

As noted in Chapter 5, Approach to the Physical Examination, many studies identify that clinicians do not follow evidence-based guidelines when obtaining BP. Proper positioning of the patient is crucial to an accurate reading. Blood pressure is often obtained with the patient sitting on the exam table, which can produce inaccurate readings. It is imperative that the clinician confirm the BP (and indeed all vital signs) was taken properly.

During the initial assessment of a patient with known or suspected CVD or PVD, the BP should be taken in both arms for comparison. Significant differences in the BPs may be due to vascular disease, such as subclavian artery stenosis or other peripheral artery disease (PAD). The proper position for assessing a patient's BP is seated with the arm free of any clothing, the back supported, legs uncrossed, and the arm supported at the level of the heart (**Figure 6.16**). The patient is to be seated quietly for 5 minutes before measurement of the BP. See **Table 5.7** for definitions of blood pressure according to the Eighth Joint National Committee and American College of Cardiology (ACC)/American Heart Association (AHA, 2018) 2017 guidelines.

Abnormal Blood Pressure and Pulse Assessment

Several abnormalities may be observed during BP measurement and are relevant to the cardiovascular exam. As discussed in Chapter 5, Approach to the

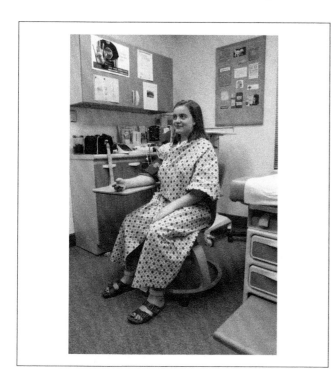

FIGURE 6.16 Proper position to assess blood pressure.

Physical Examination, an auscultatory gap is more common in elderly and hypertensive patients due to poor arterial compliance. Pulsus paradoxus occurs when there is a >10 mmHg drop in systolic pressure during inspiration. When pulsus paradoxus is present, the peripheral pulse may also decrease or disappear, called a paradoxical pulse. This finding can occur with cardiac tamponade, acute airway obstruction, exacerbations of chronic obstructive pulmonary disease (COPD), and asthma. An evidence-based approach suggests that pulsus paradoxus is most reliable for cardiac tamponade when there is a known pericardial effusion (Elder, Japp, & Verghese, 2016). Pulsus alternans occurs when the pulse differs in force between strong and weaker impulses. This occurs with a regular rhythm and may only be noted during BP measurement if there is minimal difference between the strong and weak impulses. Evidence suggests that pulsus alternans is moderately specific for left ventricular (LV) failure; however, its sensitivity is limited for the condition (Elder et al., 2016).

APPROACH TO THE PHYSICAL EXAMINATION

A systematic approach to the CV and PV exams should be taken to ensure that all components of the exam are completed. The cardiovascular exam is completed with the individual in the seated, supine, or left lateral positions, and in some cases the standing/squatting position (Chizner, 2002). Position changes alter the hemodynamics of the heart, causing some sounds to be augmented and others to be dampened. Changes in heart sounds during these position changes provide clues to structural abnormalities and disease. Inform the individual and provide rationale for the position changes they will be asked to make. The exam described here begins with the precordial exam of the seated patient, followed by the precordial exam of the supine patient. Portions of the peripheral vascular exam, such as examination of the extremities, can occur with the patient either seated or supine. Often, the patient is first examined in the seated position as this is the position during which the history is taken. The exam sequence can be modified according to the patient presentation, particular requirements of the patient and/or clinician, and integration of the exam into other regional exams. For example, portions of the PV exam may be completed during the neurologic or musculoskeletal exam.

As with most components of the physical examination, evaluation of the patient is done with the relevant body region exposed. For the cardiac and peripheral vascular exams, this means exposing the chest and extremities, utilizing modest coverage for individuals. Gowns or drapes may be used, asking the patient for permission and/or enlisting their help to expose the area being examined. Ensure that the room temperature is appropriate and that the exam is conducted maintaining the patient's privacy. Patients can be asked to assist with the exam by moving their breast out of the way during palpation and auscultation.

The cardiovascular and peripheral vascular exams follow the typical order of most system exams: (1) inspection, (2) palpation, (3) percussion, and (4) auscultation. Some techniques are not completed in all positions or for all portions of the CV and PV exams. Keep in mind the location of the heart valves and chambers—the second right (aortic valve) and left (pulmonic valve) intercostal spaces (ICS), the left lower sternal border (LSB; mitral valve and right ventricular area), and the fifth ICS mid-clavicular line (MCL; mitral valve and left ventricular area)—as you complete the exam. See **Figure 6.17** for depiction of these sites.

CARDIOVASCULAR EXAMINATION OF THE PATIENT: SEATED POSITION

There is varying opinion and a paucity of evidence regarding the utility of the precordial cardiovascular examination (Silverman & Gertz, 2015). Many

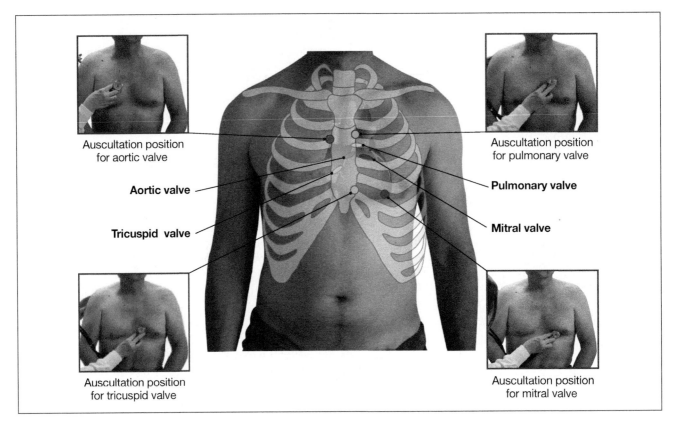

FIGURE 6.17 Auscultatory sites for heart sounds. Positioning for the aortic valve, pulmonary valve, tricuspid valve, and mitral valve.

clinicians fail to perform a complete cardiovascular exam due to perception of its inaccuracy and the ease with which an echocardiogram may be obtained (Gardezi et al., 2018; Heckerling et al., 1991, 1993; Silverman & Gertz, 2015). Quality evidence supports many aspects of the bedside CV exam as an aid in the determination of a variety of cardiac and peripheral vascular abnormalities including valvular disorders, CHD, abdominal aneurysm, PAD, renovascular disease, HF, and cardiomegaly (Elder et al., 2016; Heckerling et al., 1991, 1993; Patel, Tomar, Singh, & Bharani, 2016; Roldan, Shively, & Crawford, 1996). The evidence base for particular portions of the cardiac exam will be discussed within the appropriate sections in the text that follows.

Inspection

Assessment of the chest begins with visual inspection of the chest surface. While inspecting, the clinician should pay special attention to skin color, scars (which may be evidence of prior surgery or an implanted cardiac pacemaker or defibrillator), apparent heaves, lifts, or abnormal pulsations. Heaves and lifts are abnormal outward thrusting or focal movement of the chest wall during the cardiac cycle that may indicate enlarged

chambers, aneurysm, or an underlying valvular disorder. The apical impulse is visualized at the same anatomic location where the PMI is palpated. This normal pulsation is observed, in normal-size hearts, in the left fifth ICS at or just medial to the MCL. Reference any abnormalities to the known cardiac anatomical landmarks so that consideration is given to the area during palpation of the chest wall.

Palpation and Percussion

Palpation and percussion of the chest are typically done during the supine portion of the exam and will be discussed in the text that follows.

Auscultation

Before auscultation, ensure that the room is quiet. Inform the patient that you will be listening in multiple locations throughout the chest in order to perform a thorough exam. Attempt to block out distractions, concentrating solely on the heart sounds. Auscultate the apical pulse, noting the heart rate and rhythm. The rhythm should be regular and the rate should be between 60 and 100 impulses/minute. As noted in Chapter 5, Approach to the Physical Examination, there are multiple factors that affect the heart rate.

For any irregular rhythm, note whether there is a regular or irregular pattern. Assess the radial pulse in conjunction with auscultation of the apical pulse. Any difference between the apical rate and the radial pulse rate is noted as a pulse deficit and may indicate an abnormal cardiac rhythm.

Identify S1 and S2. These heart sounds will allow the clinician to identify systole and diastole, and assist in identifying the timing of abnormal heart sounds. S1 indicates the beginning of systole and is heard as a "lub." S1 also coincides with the carotid artery pulse. Auscultate the apical pulse while gently palpating the carotid artery (refer to carotid pulse palpation later in this chapter for correct carotid palpation technique) to ensure the sound is S1. S1 is heard with each pulsation of the carotid artery. S2 indicates diastole, follows S1, and is heard as "dub." S1, representative of the closure of the mitral and tricuspid valves (atrioventricular [AV] valves), is heard best at the apex and is louder than S2 at this location. S2, indicating the closure of the aortic and pulmonic (semilunar) valves, is heard best at the base and is louder than S1 here.

Listen to the two sounds individually, denoting systole from diastole. A split in the S1 sound (heard best along the LSB) is normal and indicates that the clinician is hearing the sequential closing of the AV valves. Likewise, a physiological S2 split (heard best at the left second and third ICS) is normal and is heard in some individuals during inspiration when the aortic valve closes just before the pulmonic valve. This physiological split resolves with expiration. Persistent S2 splitting may indicate underlying conduction or valvular disorder. A fixed S2 split with no variation with respiration is concerning for an atrial septal defect (ASD) or a ventricular septal defect (VSD). An evidence-based approach to the utility of the S2 split actually lies in the absence of the split heart sound. The absence of a split S2 is useful in excluding ASD (Elder et al., 2016). A paradoxical S2 split in which splitting occurs on expiration and disappears on inspiration is a result of delay of the closure of the aortic valve and may be present with a left bundle branch block (BBB).

Auscultation of the precordium follows an orderly approach guaranteeing a complete auscultatory exam in the four valvular regions during systole and diastole with both the diaphragm and the bell of the stethoscope. Inching the stethoscope along the chest wall is recommended as valves may produce sounds all over the precordium. The diaphragm best picks up relatively high-pitched sounds, such as S1 and S2 and high-pitched murmurs of pulmonic, aortic, and tricuspid regurgitation. The bell is used to auscultate low-pitched sounds, such as S3 and S4 and murmurs

such as mitral and tricuspid stenosis. The bell can function as a diaphragm by pressing it firmly down on the chest. The auscultatory exam may start at the apex or the base of the heart—either is appropriate. Regardless of the approach used, follow a "Z" pattern inching along the path, listening throughout systole and diastole at each site. Starting at the base of the heart, from the second right ICS (**Figure 6.17A**) move the stethoscope in turn to the second left ICS (**Figure 6.17B**), the right sternal border (RSB; **Figure 6.17C**), and the apex in the fifth ICS near the MCL (**Figure 6.17D**). The order is reversed if starting at the apex. Listen with the bell first, then repeat the pattern listening with the diaphragm. Before completing the seated portion of the cardiac exam, the patient is asked to lean forward and hold the breath after full exhalation while the clinician uses the diaphragm to listen along the left LSB. This position brings the left ventricular outflow tract closer to the chest wall and enhances the high-pitched sounds of the semilunar valves. The murmur of aortic regurgitation (AR) can best be heard in this position. Murmurs are discussed more fully in the text that follows.

At each precordial site, listen first for systole and then diastole relative to S1 and S2. Once these are identified, listen carefully for abnormal or extra heart sounds, such as the third (S3) and fourth (S4) heart sounds or murmurs. S3 and S4 may be auscultated in diastole and can be normal or abnormal. S3, occurring right after S2, may be confused with a split S2; however, S3 is heard best at the apex or left LSB, does not vary with respiration, and is lower in pitch than S2. A physiological (normal) S3 may occur in children and young adults in the supine position. It typically resolves with sitting up. A pathological S3 is also referred to as a ventricular gallop and indicates decreased compliance of the ventricle and volume overload, as might occur in HF or high CO states. Although not often detected in the outpatient setting, evidence strongly supports the utility of an S3 in the diagnosis of HF (Elder et al., 2016). S4, occurring immediately before S1, is a soft sound with low pitch. It is heard best with the bell of the stethoscope when the patient is in the left lateral position. A pathological S4, or atrial gallop, may occur as a result of decreased compliance of the ventricle and increased afterload.

A variety of abnormal heart sounds may be auscultated over the precordium. These can include a variety of murmurs and pericardial friction rubs. Murmurs may be heard as a whooshing, clicking, snapping, vibrating, rumbling, or blowing sound. Examples of some murmurs include a high-pitched click, like the mid-systolic click of mitral valve prolapse (MVP), or a high-pitched snap, like the opening snap of MS or the blowing sound of aortic stenosis (AS). The duration of a murmur is longer than a heart sound and results from turbulent blood flow. Murmurs can be benign (physiological) or pathological, related to congenital or acquired abnormalities, such as valvular disease and CHD. Murmurs are described according to eight characteristics: timing, loudness, pitch, pattern, quality, location, radiation, and posture. Interpretation of these characteristics can help to determine the cause of the turbulent blood flow. These characteristics are further outlined in **Table 6.2**.

Innocent or functional murmurs are associated with no valvular or structural heart abnormality but may be due to increased blood flow through the heart (such as with anemia, fever, pregnancy, or hyperthyroidism). These murmurs are typically (a) early systolic with a soft pitch and intensity of 1–2/6; (b) located between the second and fourth left ICS along the LSB; and (c) decrease or disappear with maneuvers that decrease left ventricular end diastolic volume (LVEDV) such as the Valsalva maneuver and standing. Based on evidence, intensity and duration of a murmur are most important in differentiating functional murmurs from pathological murmurs (Elder et al., 2016).

An evidence-based approach to auscultation of the heart recognizes the importance of this facet of the CV exam in identifying heart murmurs (Elder et al., 2016; Patel et al., 2016; Roldan et al., 1996). Comparison of heart auscultation to echocardiography supports the importance of auscultation in the initial diagnosis of valvular disorders, especially when more severe murmurs are present (Elder et al., 2016; Gardezi et al., 2018; Patel et al., 2016). Murmurs and other abnormal heart sounds are further discussed in the Abnormal Findings of the Heart and Circulatory System section.

CARDIOVASCULAR EXAMINATION OF THE PATIENT: SUPINE POSITION

General Approach

The precordial exam is also completed with the patient supine. Lower the head of the bed so that the patient's head and chest are at a 30° to 45° angle. Young patients and healthy patients with no known or suspected cardiopulmonary disease may be examined lying flat.

Inspection

Visual inspection of the chest with the patient in the supine position replicates the inspection completed while in the seated position (see "Inspection" in the Cardiovascular Examination of the Patient: Seated section).

TABLE 6.2 Description of Heart Murmurs

Characteristic	Specifics
Timing in the cardiac cycle	Systolic or diastolic: • Early, mid, or late systole • Early, mid, or late diastole • Throughout systole or diastole: Holosystolic/pansystolic • Holodiastolic
Intensity	Six grades: • Grade 1—barely audible (1/6) • Grade 2—clearly audible but faint (2/6) • Grade 3—moderately loud (3/6) • Grade 4—loud, palpable thrill* (4/6) • Grade 5—very loud, able to be heard with portion of stethoscope off chest, associated thrill (5/6) • Grade 6—loudest, heard with stethoscope just off chest, associated thrill (6/6)
Pitch	• High • Medium • Low
Pattern during the cardiac phase (systole or diastole)	• Crescendo—increasing intensity • Decrescendo—decreasing intensity • Crescendo–decrescendo—increasing then decreasing intensity
Quality	• Click • Snap • Musical • Blowing • Harsh • Rumbling
Location	Valve area or intercostal space of maximum intensity
Radiation	Sound transmitted in direction of the blood flow: • Neck • Back • Axilla
Posture	Murmur disappears or increases in intensity with position change: • Sitting, leaning forward • Left lateral position • Standing • Squatting

*Abnormal pulsation of the precordium, typically palpated over the site of significant murmurs.

Palpation

Precordial palpation begins with palpating the apical impulse. The apical impulse represents the brief contraction of the LV and, as such, is located at the apex of the heart, approximately fifth ICS MCL. The apical impulse is the PMI in patients with normal-sized hearts and surrounding anatomy. PMI locates the left border of the heart and is typically in the fifth ICS, 7 to 9 cm lateral to the mid-sternal line (MSL). Palpation of the apical impulse and PMI provides information about the size of the heart. Displacement of the apical impulse suggests increased LVEDV and left ventricular mass (Elder et al., 2016).

The apical impulse is palpated with the patient in the supine position, but can also be performed in the left lateral position if there is difficulty identifying it while the patient is supine. Patients may be asked to lift their breast up and to the left to aid in identification of the pulse. The apical pulse may not be felt in obese patients or those with thick chest walls. The amplitude and duration of the apical pulse may be more pronounced in pregnant individuals and those with high CO states.

Palpating with the palm of the hand (**Figure 6.18A**) and then the pad(s) of the finger(s), locate the apical pulse. It is less than 2.5 cm in diameter, approximately the size of a quarter. Note the location, size, amplitude (upstroke), intensity (strength/force), and duration of the pulse. Next, palpate over the heart region (**Figure 6.18B**) to determine any thrills, lifts, or heaves. A thrill is a palpable murmur, and any grade 4/6 mumur or louder will have an accompanying palpable thrill. Evidence demonstrates a systolic thrill to be strongly suggestive of significant valvular disease (Elder et al., 2016).

Percussion

Percussion of the heart is thought to be the least useful CV assessment technique. Percussion is a method of tapping on a surface to determine whether the underlying structure is air filled, fluid filled, or solid. In the case of the precordial exam, percussion has been used to delineate cardiac borders. Recent evidence supporting precordial percussion does not exist. Two historical studies, one a replication of the other, support CV percussion to discriminate between those individuals with and without cardiomegaly (Heckerling et al., 1991, 1993). This lack of evidence base for and minimal literature on this technique underscores percussion's place as least valuable during examination of the CV system, and the authors would refer clinicians to inspection, palpation, auscultation, and appropriate imaging and testing if/when there are concerns about cardiac enlargement, or cardiomegaly, as a result of HTN or CAD.

Auscultation

Auscultation of the heart with the patient in the supine position is identical to the exam completed in the seated position, listening over all auscultatory sites with both the bell and the diaphragm (**Figure 6.19**). In addition, the patient is asked to turn to the left lateral position and the clinician auscultates over the apex of the heart, left fifth ICS MCL, with the bell (**Figure 6.20**). In this position, the LV is closer to the chest wall accentuating S3, S4 and mitral murmurs, specifically mitral valve stenosis.

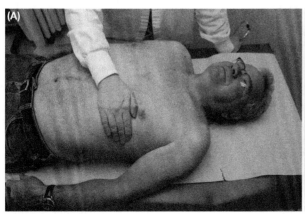
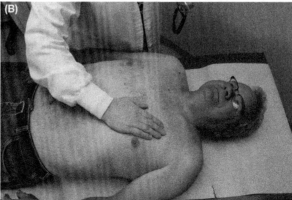

FIGURE 6.18 Palpation of the chest. (A) Palpation with palm of hand to locate the apical pulse. (B) Palpation over the heart region to determine thrills, lifts, or heaves.

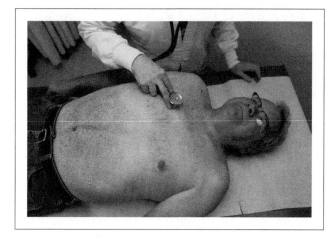

FIGURE 6.19 Auscultation of the precordium while supine.

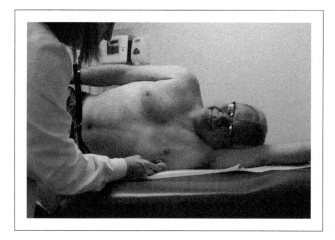

FIGURE 6.20 Auscultation of the apex for heart murmurs.

PERIPHERAL VASCULAR EXAMINATION OF THE PATIENT: SUPINE POSITION

With the patient still in the supine position, the PV exam begins. This portion of the exam includes evaluation of the carotid artery, JVP, and vascular aspects of the abdomen and extremities. As noted previously, the PV exam of the extremities may be performed with the patient seated. For individuals in whom vascular disease is suspected, it is important to examine the legs supine and seated as color changes can indicate certain disorders.

Jugular Venous Pressure

Estimation of JVP is done by inspection and measurement of the highest level of pulsation of the jugular vein. JVP reflects the central venous pressure (CVP), or pressure in the RA. An elevated JVP, and thus elevated right heart pressure, is a sign of HF. Traditionally, the

right internal jugular vein has been used for this measurement; however, it can be difficult to locate. Studies affirm that using either the right or left internal jugular or right or left external jugular vein provides accurate results (Elder et al., 2016). In obese patients, it can be difficult to visualize the jugular veins, making a measurement problematic and likely impossible.

Technique is important in the evaluation of JVP. The following are recognized as important aspects for improved visualization of the jugular veins:

- Raise the head of the bed (HOB) 30° to 45° for visualization of the jugular vein and measurement of JVP. The angle may be more or less depending on at what elevation or height the jugular column (venous meniscus) is visualized. For patients suspected of hypovolemia, the HOB may need to be lowered for visualization of the jugular pulsation. For those suspected of fluid overload, the HOB may need to be raised higher.
- Use a folded pillow or blanket behind the patient's head to elevate the head off the mattress while maintaining the shoulders on the mattress.
- Turn the patient's head away and elevate the jaw slightly.
- Shine a tangential light across the neck to help visualize the venous motion.

Inspection

Identify the jugular vein to be used for measurement of JVP. The internal jugular vein lies deep in the sternomastoid muscle and can be difficult to see. Its pulsation is best visualized in the sternal notch. The top of the external jugular vein is visualized where it overlies the sternomastoid muscle.

To distinguish the jugular veins from the carotid artery, note the following:

- The carotid pulse is palpable wherein venous pulsations are typically not palpable.
- Pulsations of the carotid pulse cannot be eliminated by pressure, as the pulsations of the jugular veins can be.
- The height of the carotid pulsation does not change with the position of the HOB as venous pulsations do.

The angle of Louis, or the sternal angle, is used at the reference point for the JVP measurement. The sternal angle is the bony prominence on the sternum below the sternal notch. Place a ruler vertically on the sternal angle. Use another straight edge as the horizontal reference line. Place the straight edge perpendicular to the ruler across the highest point of the internal jugular pulsation or the point just above where the external jugular appears to collapse (**Figure 6.21**). Round the

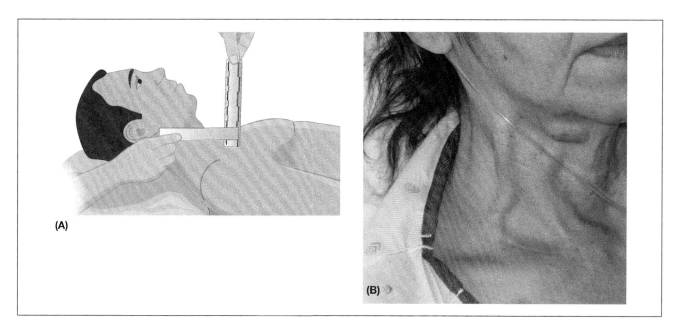

FIGURE 6.21 Assessment for jugular venous distention (JVD) or pressure measurement. (A) Location of internal and external jugular veins. (B) Presence of JVD.

Source: Image courtesy of Ferencga.

identified measurement to the nearest centimeter. If a jugular pulsation is not noted, it may lie below the level of the sternum and, as such, the venous pressure is not elevated. A measurement of 3 cm above the sternal angle indicates an elevated JVP.

There has been concern as to whether measurement of JVP is an accurate reflection of the CVP. Evidence suggests that it is the approximation of the measurement as either high or low, rather than a specific JVP measurement, that is most useful and reliable in determining CVP and HF (Drazner, Rame, Stevenson, & Dries, 2001; Elder et al., 2016; Vinayak et al., 2006). Evidence-based practice for interpretation of the JVP identifies 3 cm above the sternal angle as the cutoff point. A JVP above 3 cm, regardless of the position of the HOB, has a high likelihood (LR+ of 10.4) for an elevated CVP of more than 12 cm H_2O, indicative of increased right heart pressure. Likewise, a JVP of less than 3 cm has a moderately high likelihood (LR+ 8.4) of a CVP below 5 cm H_2O, a normal right heart pressure (Elder et al., 2016).

The presence of prominent jugular venous distention (JVD) may be obvious on visual inspection, precluding the method outlined previously. Other techniques have been identified as acceptable evaluation of JVP to ascertain elevated CVP:

- Visual pulsation of the jugular above the clavicle with the HOB at 45° or the patient in the seated position is consistent with a CVP above 10 cm H_2O, an

elevated right heart pressure (Miranda & Nishimura, 2017; Sinisalo, Rapola, Rossinen, & Kupari, 2007; Weiner, Brown, & Houston, 2017).
- Jugular veins should collapse with deep inspiration or a vigorous nasal sniff. Visualization of jugular veins that do not collapse with one of these two maneuvers is consistent with elevated CVP (Chua Chiaco, Parikh, & Fergusson, 2013; Conn & O'Keefe, 2012).
- If the external jugular vein is initially collapsed, applying light pressure at the base of the neck will cause it to distend. This distention clears rapidly, after release of pressure, if JVP is not elevated. If the external jugular vein remains distended, proceed with evaluation of the JVP by visualization of the internal jugular vein (Chua Chiaco et al., 2013).
- If venous pulsations are not visualized in the neck, JVP is likely normal. Lower the HOB until a pulsation is visualized to ensure that the pressure is not so high that it cannot be visualized (Miranda & Nishimura, 2017).

If JVP is elevated, perform the hepatojugular reflux (HJR), also known as the abdominojugular reflux. This maneuver adds, into the system, venous blood returning to the right side of the heart. If the heart is able to accommodate this increased blood volume, the RV pressure (and thus CVP) is likely not elevated. With the patient supine, the clinician places they right hand over the mid-abdomen below the right costal margin and pushes firmly for 10 to 15 seconds, observing the right jugular. If the jugular rises for a few seconds and then returns to baseline, the CVP is considered normal. Sustained elevation of the jugular is consistent with elevated CVP. In conjunction with an elevated JVP, positive HJR increases the likelihood (LR+ 8.0) of elevated venous pressure (Elder et al., 2016). Some sources cite that abdominal pressure should be applied for 30 seconds during the HJR maneuver; however, evidence suggests that 10 to 15 seconds of sustained firm pressure is appropriate for interpretation of the maneuver (Ewy, 1988; Sochowski, Dubbin, & Naqvi, 1990).

Carotid Arteries

Examination of the carotid arteries is completed with the patient in the supine position and the HOB elevated to 30° to 45°. The assessment begins with palpation.

Palpation

The carotid artery is located just medial to the sternomastoid muscle. Palpate the right and left arteries in turn. Do not apply firm pressure or palpate both carotids at the same time as this can compromise blood flow to the brain, causing syncope. Using several fingers, palpate the artery at the level of the cricoid cartilage. Use the right fingers to palpate the left carotid pulse and the left fingers to palpate the right carotid pulse (**Figure 6.22**). Avoid palpating near the top of the thyroid cartilage, the location of the carotid sinus, as pressure on this may cause slowing of the heart rate. Note the symmetry, rhythm, rate, amplitude (or upstroke), and intensity (or strength, force) of the pulse. The pulse should be smooth with a brisk upstroke. A weak or thready pulse may indicate hypovolemia or shock. A bounding pulse may occur with such things as fever, exercise, hyperthyroidism, or anemia. See **Table 6.3**

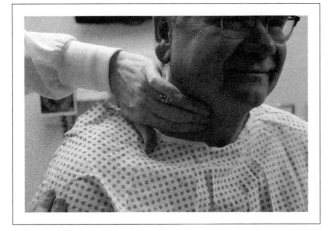

FIGURE 6.22 Palpation of carotid artery.

for other abnormal pulse findings, several of which, as noted earlier in the chapter, may also be noted during BP auscultation. Palpable thrills are abnormal and may indicate a carotid artery murmur or stenosis. The carotid pulses should be symmetric. Palpation of the carotid artery may be done in conjunction with cardiac auscultation during identification of S1 and S2 (refer to the Cardiovascular Examination of the Patient: Seated Position section). Palpation of the carotid and femoral arterial pulses simultaneously is done for suspected coarctation of the aorta. With this condition, there is delayed transmission and amplitude of the femoral pulse as compared with the carotid.

Auscultation

Carotid artery auscultation is completed after palpation, when there is an indication of neurologic signs or symptoms consistent with decreased cerebral blood flow, as occurs with carotid artery stenosis, or when a palpable bruit is identified. The U.S. Preventive Services Task Force (USPSTF; LeFevre, 2014) and Choosing Wisely (American Academy of Family Physicians, 2013) advise against routine screening for carotid artery stenosis, including auscultation of the carotid arteries. However, a 2012 meta-analysis found that auscultation of carotid bruits is of moderate value in detecting clinically significant carotid stenosis, and its authors contend carotid auscultation should be done during routine exams (McColgan, Bentley, McCarron, & Sharma, 2012). Arguably, listening for carotid bruits in the elderly and those with suspected cardiac disease or PVD may be appropriate.

To auscultate the carotid arteries, place the bell of the stethoscope over the identified carotid artery (**Figure 6.23**). Ask the patient to take a breath, exhale, and hold the breath. Holding the breath helps to avoid interpreting tracheal sounds as turbulent blood flow. This technique also avoids contraction of the levator scapulae muscle in the neck from dampening the sound. As when listening for other turbulent blood flow, note a blowing or swishing sound. This is a carotid bruit. Cardiac murmurs may be transmitted from the heart to the carotids. To avoid interpreting a heart murmur for a bruit, perform a complete precordial exam.

Abdomen

The abdominal peripheral vascular exam is classically integrated into the abdominal assessment. Please refer to Chapter 16, Evidence-Based Assessment of the Abdominal, Gastrointestinal, and Urological Systems, for a complete discussion of this exam. Remember to ask the patient to flex their legs in order to relax the abdomen. When completed in conjunction with the rest of the peripheral vascular exam, the standard exam sequence is used, excluding percussion as there is no concern for disrupting peristalsis.

TABLE 6.3 Abnormal Pulse Findings

Type of Pulse	Description	Possible Causes
Anacrotic	Slow notched or interrupted upstroke	AS
Corrigan's or water-hammer	Sharp rise and rapid fall-off	Severe AR or PDA
Bifid or bisferiens	Two systolic peaks	Advanced AR or HCM
Pulsus bigeminus	Every other impulse comes early or a normal impulse is followed by an early impulse	Conduction disorders, premature atrial or premature ventricular contractions
Pulsus alternans	Force varies, alternating impulses of large and small amplitude	Left ventricular failure, valvular heart disease, chronic HTN, or cardiomyopathy
Pulsus paradoxus	Weaker amplitude with inspiration, stronger with expiration	Cardiac tamponade, severe bronchospasm, or acute asthma

AR, aortic regurgitation; AS, aortic stenosis; HCM, hypertrophic cardiomyopathy; HTN, hypertension; PDA, patent ductus arteriosus.

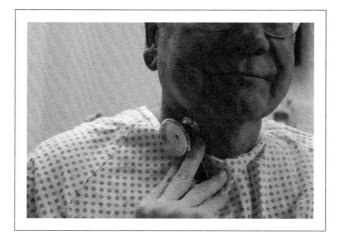

FIGURE 6.23 Auscultation of carotid artery.

Inspection

The abdomen is inspected for skin color, abnormal vascular patterns, and pulsations.

Palpation

Palpate the width of the aorta in the upper abdomen. The clinician may use the thumb and index finger of one hand or the fingers of both hands to palpate each side of the aorta. Press deeply into the abdomen just above the umbilicus and slightly left of midline to identify the aortic pulsation. Normal aortic pulsation is anterior and is visualized most often in thin patients. The normal width of the aorta is approximately 2.5 cm. Aortic width measuring more than 3 cm or the presence of a palpable pulsatile abdominal mass is concerning for abdominal aortic aneurysm. The sensitivity of palpation for an abdominal aneurysm increases with the size of the mass and the decrease in abdominal girth of

the patient (Roldan et al., 1996). The aorta may not be palpable in obese patients. During routine palpation of the remainder of the abdomen, note any other abnormal pulsations.

Auscultation

Auscultation of the abdomen includes the aorta and the renal, iliac, and femoral arteries. Using the bell of the stethoscope, listen in turn over the aorta, right and left renal arteries, right and left iliac arteries, and right and left femoral arteries. Note the location, pitch, and timing of any auscultated vascular sounds. For abnormal vascular sounds, delineate between a venous hum, which is a continuous sound, and the blowing or swooshing sound of a bruit. Refer to Chapter 16, Evidence-Based Assessment of the Abdominal, Gastrointestinal, and Urological Systems, for pictorial representation of the location of the abdominal arterial auscultation sites.

Extremities

Inspection

Inspect the extremities. Note the skin color (keeping in mind the patient's ethnicity) and assess the color of the nails, noting any cyanosis. Check capillary refill. Apply pressure to the nail beds to blanche, then release and note the time, in seconds, until the color returns. Capillary refill of 1 to 2 seconds is considered normal. Note any clubbing of the nails by viewing the nails in profile. The normal angle between the base of the nail bed and the proximal nail fold where it meets the nail is 160° or less. A flattening of the nail base relative to the distal finger or an angle of more than 160° is termed "Schamroth's sign" and is indicative of chronic hypoxia, as can occur in chronic hypoxic lung disease such as COPD, CHD, or other cardiac

TABLE 6.4 Assessments Associated With Cardiovascular Disease

Assessment	Description	Significance
AV nicking	With fundal exam of the eye, indentation or nicking of retinal veins is seen where stiffened retinal arteries cross	Sign of chronic HTN that may indicate additional arterial damage
Clubbing	Painless overgrowth of connective tissues and edema that result in bulbous enlargement of the ends of one or more fingers or toes and excessive sponginess or bogginess of the nail base	Sign of chronic tissue hypoxia
Corneal arcus or arcus senilis	Grey-white-blue ring or arc around the periphery of the cornea formed by lipid deposits; common with aging (in >70% of those over 60)	May be a sign of hyperlipidemia, impaired lipid metabolism
Ear lobe crease	Diagonal crease or deep wrinkle of ear lobe extending from tragus to auricle; may be unilateral or bilateral and signify loss of collagen fibers, elastin	May be associated with CAD; warrants follow-up (Agouridis, Elisaf, Nair, & Mikhailidis, 2015)
Gingivitis and/or periodontitis	Inflammatory diseases of the gums and/or supporting structures of the teeth caused by bacteria; bleeding from the gums after brushing teeth can lead to bacteremia	IE results from bacteremia and is caused by the same bacteria that colonize teeth
Janeway lesions	Irregular, erythematous, flat, painless macules on the palms, soles, thenar, and hypothenar eminences of the hands, tips of the fingers, and plantar surfaces of the toes; rare in clinical practice; from micro-embolisms	Sign of IE
Malar flush	Deep red or purple facial rash of facial cheeks and nasal bridge; can be caused by lupus, rosacea, erysipelas, or vascular stasis associated with pulmonary hypertension	Associated with mitral stenosis (chronic or severe disease)
Musset's sign	Rhythmic nodding or bobbing of the head in synchrony with the heartbeat, a sign of insufficiency—incompetence of the aortic valve	Associated with severe aortic regurgitation
Osler's nodes	Acutely painful purplish nodules on the palms of the hands and the soles of the feet; differ from painless Janeway nodules	Sign of IE
Quincke's pulse	When applying gentle pressure to tip of fingernail, alternate filling and blanching of the capillary bed concomitant with the cardiac cycle is seen; widened pulse pressure results in capillary pulsation	Sign of severe aortic valve insufficiency in aortic regurgitation
Retinopathy	Damage to the small blood vessels of the retina causes visual impairment; uncontrolled HTN and high glucose levels damage retinal vasculature	Sign of hypertensive retinopathy and diabetic retinopathy are the two most common causes
Roth spots	Retinal hemorrhages (red) with white or pale centers; nonspecific finding associated with multiple systemic conditions that cause endothelial damage, including preeclampsia, anemia, leukemia, HIV, retinopathies	Sign of bacterial endocarditis and hypertensive retinopathy
Splinter hemorrhages	Nonblanching red-brown longitudinal hemorrhages appearing under the fingernail plate; can be associated with psoriasis, vasculitis, systemic disease	Sign of subacute endocarditis, especially if associated fever, Osler's nodes, Janeway lesions, Roth spots, or a murmur
Xanthelasma	Yellowish plaques that occur most commonly near the inner canthus of the eyelid, more often on the upper lid than the lower lid; xanthelasma palpebrarum is the most common cutaneous xanthoma	Sign of hyperlipidemia, impaired lipid metabolism
Xanthomas	Deposits of yellowish cholesterol-rich material that can appear anywhere in the body in various disease states; cutaneous manifestations of lipid accumulation within the skin	Sign of hyperlipidemia, impaired lipid metabolism

AV, arteriovenous; CAD, coronary artery disease; HTN, hypertension; IE, infective endocarditis.

disease causing right to left shunting of blood. Fingernails should be smooth. Thick-ridged nails can result from arterial insufficiency and splinter hemorrhages (thin red or brown lines running the length of the nail) can occur with bacterial endocarditis. Clubbing and splinter hemorrhages are assessments that can be associated with CVD. Additional assessments that can be associated with HTN, endocarditis, hyperlipidemia, heart defects, and heart disease are listed in **Table 6.4**. Note that appreciating the abnormal findings would require a comprehensive physical exam, including head, eyes, ears, heart, lungs, and upper and lower extremities.

Arms and legs should be symmetric in size. Examine the lower extremities for skin color, hair distribution, lesions, and edema. Decreased hair distribution, cool skin, skin ulcerations, pale legs on elevation, and dusky red skin in the dependent position may be signs of PAD. Of these signs, cool skin and skin ulceration are more supportive of PAD than the others. However, evidence is lacking for use of a lower extremity exam noting these signs as a screening mechanism for PAD in asymptomatic individuals (Elder et al., 2016). Brown pigmentation or petechiae of the skin, cyanosis with leg dependency, stasis dermatitis (dry, scaling, hyperpigmented skin), and ulcerations may indicate venous insufficiency. Note any varicosities (engorged veins) of the legs. Note edema of the lower extremities as this may indicate poor venous return (as in venous insufficiency) or fluid retention, as occurs in HF.

Palpation
Palpate the arms and legs for skin temperature, texture, turgor, and edema (**Figure 6.24A**). Lower-extremity edema is identified as either pitting or nonpitting, with pitting edema graded 1 to 4. Press firmly and gently with the thumb over the dorsum of the foot and pretibial area of the lower leg (shin). Hold the pressure for 5 seconds. Pitting is present if an indentation remains in the tissue after the thumb is removed (**Figure 6.24B**).

Some degree of pitting edema may be normal in those who stand on their feet all day or are pregnant. Grade the pitting and note the extent to which the edema ascends the extremity. The following scale is used to grade pitting edema:

- 1+ Mild pitting with only slight indentation and no appreciable extremity edema
- 2+ Moderate pitting, thumb indentation resolves rapidly
- 3+ Deep pitting, indentation remains for brief period of time and appreciable extremity edema present
- 4+ Severe pitting, indentation remains for a long time and the extremity is obviously swollen

Nonpitting edema is identified according to severity—mild, moderate, or severe—and the extent to which the edema ascends the extremity (e.g., moderate nonpitting edema of the feet, ankles, and halfway up the calf). If unilateral edema is present, use a tape measure to document the difference between the two extremities. Measure at the smallest and largest difference of the calf and the circumference of the mid-thigh (if edema is present here). While there is a slight difference in the measurement of extremities, right to left, a difference of more than 1 to 2 cm is considered abnormal. Unilateral edema may be due to an injury, a venous thrombosis, lymphatic obstruction, or impaired venous return from a proximal obstruction.

Peripheral pulses are palpated as part of the peripheral vascular exam. Note the symmetry, rate, rhythm, amplitude (or upstroke), and intensity (strength or force) of the pulse. Gently apply pressure over pulse with the index and middle fingers, using the finger pads. Radial pulses are located at the distal flexor surface of the right wrist overlying the radial artery (**Figure 6.25A**). Brachial pulses are palpated medially at the elbow bend, overlying the brachial artery (**Figure 6.25B**). The femoral pulse, supplied by the femoral artery, is palpated in the anterior groin, just below the inguinal ligament. If there is trouble palpating this pulse, ask the patient to flex at the knee and externally rotate the hip (**Figure 6.25C**). The popliteal pulse, also an extension of the femoral artery, is palpated behind the knee. This pulse also can be difficult to locate. Place the fingers of both hands behind the knee and press firmly into the popliteal fossa (**Figure 6.25D**). The posterior tibial (PT) pulse is palpated behind the medial malleolus (**Figure 6.25E**). Dorsalis pedis (DP) pulse is palpable on the dorsum of the foot just lateral to the flexor tendon of the great toe (**Figure 6.25F**). Light pressure on the pulse is important as firm pressure may obliterate the pulsation. In some adults, this pulse may be absent bilaterally. During a routine exam, the ulnar pulse is not typically palpated unless there is concern regarding arterial supply to the hand.

Historically, pulses are graded on a 3-point scale according to the strength or force of the pulse:

- 3+ Bounding
- 2+ Normal
- 1+ Weak
- 0 Absent

A bounding pulse may be due to a high cardiac output state, as occurs with exercise or fever. Bilateral weak pulses are concerning for shock or hypovolemia. A weak unilateral pulse may indicate arterial insufficiency in the affected limb. Refer to **Table 6.3** for more on abnormal pulses.

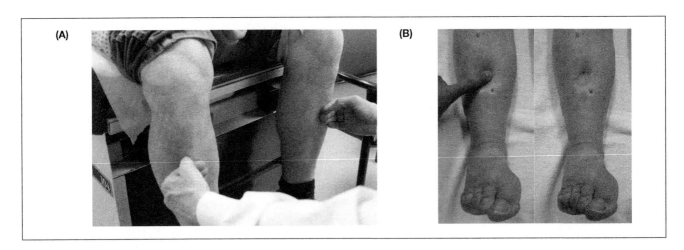

FIGURE 6.24 (A) Palpation of the legs. (B) Pitting edema.
Source: Part B image courtesy of James Heilman, MD.

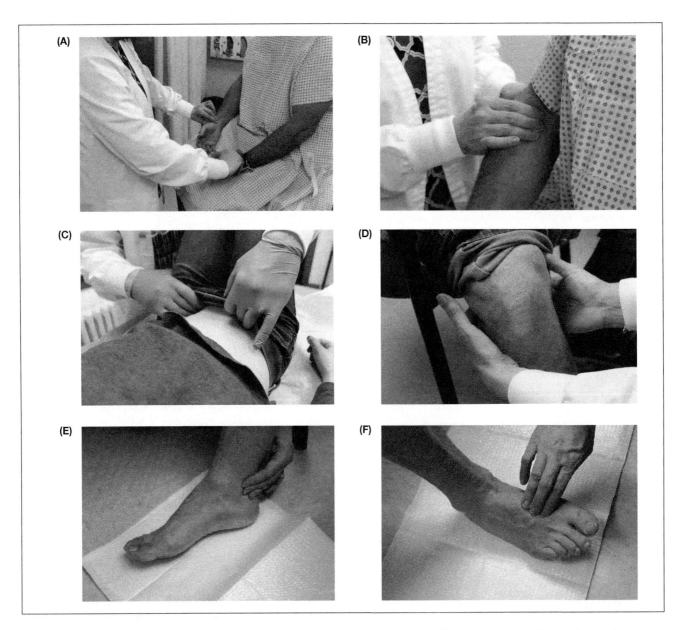

FIGURE 6.25 Palpation of peripheral pulses: (A) radial pulses, (B) brachial pulse, (C) femoral pulse, (D) popliteal pulse, (E) posterior tibial pulse, (F) dorsalis pedis pulse.

CARDIOVASCULAR AND PERIPHERAL VASCULAR EXAMINATION OF THE PATIENT: SPECIAL MANEUVERS

Auscultation

Patients in whom a systolic murmur has been identified should be examined in additional positions in an attempt to further delineate the origin of the murmur. Examining a patient in the squatting and standing positions can help to distinguish between the systolic murmurs of AS and hypertrophic cardiomyopathy (HCM). AS is best heard in the second right ICS while the murmur of HCM is best heard in the third to fourth left ICS. With the patient in the standing position, and preferably using the exam table for balance, the clinician stands next to the patient and places the stethoscope on the chest. The clinician asks the patient to squat and then stand while auscultating the heart. The patient is asked to momentarily pause while in the squatting position, then rise. The murmur of AS intensifies while the murmur of HCM deceases in intensity during the squatting phase as a result of increased arterial blood pressure, stroke volume, and left ventricular volume. The standing phase decreases arterial blood pressure, stroke volume, and left ventricular volume, thus decreasing the intensity of the AS murmur and intensifying the murmur of HCM. Patients may also be asked to perform the Valsalva maneuver (bear down) while supine. The murmur of HCM intensifies during the Valsalva. The squatting and standing positions and the Valsalva maneuver have been demonstrated in a small number of studies to alter venous return, increasing the likelihood of diagnosing such disorders (Cheng, 2010; Elder et al., 2016).

PEDIATRIC CARDIAC EXAMINATION CONSIDERATIONS

Many aspects of the physical exam in infants and children are the same as adults. Auscultation of heart sounds may indicate different disease processes in the pediatric population; however, they occur at the same landmarks and are described and classified in the same fashion (**Figure 6.26**). General appearance of the infant or child (happy or cranky), as well as nutritional and respiratory status are very important in infants and children. Subtle changes in these systems can signal warning signs for CHD. Palpation of pulses is another very important exam technique in infants and children as differentials in pulses between extremities can be indicative of a coarctation of the aorta while bounding pulses may be indicative of a shunt lesion (PDA or AV fistula; Park, 2016). Finally, blood pressure evaluation in children is just as important as it is in adults and can help screen for heart diseases. Clinicians should be familiar with appropriate techniques for obtaining blood pressure as well as normative blood pressure ranges for infants and children by age.

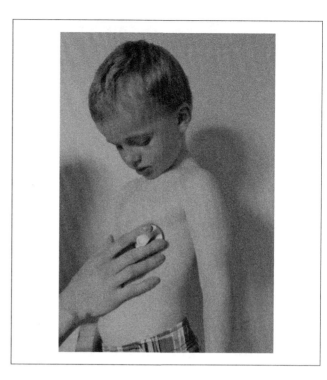

FIGURE 6.26 Assessment of pediatric heart sounds.

See Chapter 4, Evidence-Based Assessment of Children and Adolescents, for normal blood pressures by age for children and adolescents.

LABORATORY CONSIDERATIONS FOR THE HEART AND CIRCULATORY SYSTEM

LABORATORY TESTS TO ASSESS FOR CARDIAC DISORDERS AND CARDIOVASCULAR STATUS

The following lab tests are used to assess cardiac status and function. The list is not intended to be exhaustive, but to provide clinicians with an explanation of the common laboratory tests seen in cardiac conditions and how they can help determine cardiac diagnoses. See **Table 6.5** for labs that should be considered in the initial workup for hypertension per the ACC/AHA (2018) 2017 hypertension guidelines.

- **Atrial natriuretic hormone (ANH)** is a hormone secreted by the cardiac muscle cells (i.e., cardiomyocytes) in the atria in response to volume and pressure changes. ANH levels are elevated in HF, volume overload, and cardiovascular conditions with high atrial filling pressures.
- **Brain natriuretic peptide or B-type natriuretic peptide (BNP)** or **N-terminal pro-B-type natriuretic peptide (NT-proBNP)** are hormones secreted by cardiomyocytes in the ventricles of the

TABLE 6.5 Basic and Optional Laboratory Tests for Primary Hypertension

Basic testing	Fasting blood glucose Complete blood count Lipid profile Serum creatinine with eGFR* Serum sodium, potassium, and calcium* Thyroid-stimulating hormone Urinalysis Electrocardiogram
Optional testing	Echocardiogram Uric acid Urinary albumin to creatinine ratio

* May be included in a comprehensive metabolic panel.
eGFR, estimated glomerular filtration rate.
Source: American College of Cardiology/American Heart Association Task Force on Clinical Practice Guidelines. (2018). 2017 ACC/AHA/AAPA/ABC/ACPM/AGS/APhA/ASH/ASPC/NMA/PCNA guideline for the prevention, detection, evaluation, and management of high blood pressure in adults. *Journal of the American College of Cardiology, 71*(19), e127–e248. doi:10.1016/j.jacc.2017.11.006

heart, usually in response to stretching caused by increased ventricular blood volume. BNP and NT-proBNP levels are elevated in HF and are currently used as biomarkers for the condition. These levels can be helpful in evaluating patients presenting with dyspnea to differentiate cardiac versus pulmonary etiology. BNP and NT-proBNP may also be elevated in asymptomatic left ventricular dysfunction, arterial and pulmonary HTN, valvular heart disease, cardiac arrhythmia, and ACS.

- **Calcium (serum levels)** may be elevated with thiazide diuretic use due to increased renal absorption. Hypercalcemia can cause EKG changes (short QT, Osborn/delta waves) and arrhythmia (ventricular irritability, ventricular fibrillation). Low calcium levels can lead to prolonged QT intervals as noted on EKG.
- **Complete blood count (CBC)** is used to detect anemia, which can mimic symptoms of or contribute to HF. CBCs are also used to identify possible infection, inflammation, dehydration, vitamin deficiencies, leukemia, or effects and/or side effects of medications.
- **Liver function tests** (bilirubin, alanine aminotransferase [ALT], aspartate aminotransferase [AST], alkaline phosphatase [ALP] levels, and albumin levels) are used to detect hepatic congestion, cardiac hepatopathy (liver damage caused by cardiac disorders), or volume overload. Elevated levels of bilirubin, ALT, AST, and ALP and low levels of albumin may be found in HF.
- **Magnesium (serum levels)** may be decreased with diuretic use due to excessive renal loss or

following cardiopulmonary bypass. Hypomagnesemia can cause EKG changes (QT prolongation, atrial and ventricular ectopy) and arrhythmia (torsades de pointes, atrial tachyarrhythmia). Although rare and usually iatrogenic, hypermagnesemia can lead to EKG changes (increased PR and QRS duration, peaked T waves, and flattened P waves) and arrhythmia (complete AV block, asystole).

- **Novel HF biomarkers** (e.g., galectin-3 [Gal-3], soluble suppression of tumorigenicity 2 [sST2], other inflammation, fibrosis and injury markers) are prognostic biomarkers used in the diagnosis and management of HF and other cardiac conditions. Elevated levels of Gal-3 and sST2 proteins in the blood may indicate increased risk of HF complications and the need for more aggressive treatment (Piek, Du, de Boer, & Silljé, 2018).
- **Renal function tests** are often completed to assess renal status, volume status, and to rule out a renal etiology in cardiac disorders such as HTN or HF. Decreased glomerular filtration rate (GFR) or estimated glomerular filtration rate (eGFR) indicate decreased renal blood flow or renal insufficiency. Elevated serum creatinine and blood urea nitrogen (BUN) are often found in HF. Additional renal function tests based on the medication regimen may be appropriate primarily on the basis of expert opinion (Al-Naher, Wright, Devonald, & Pirmohamed, 2018).
- **Serum electrolyte levels** (sodium, potassium, carbon dioxide, chloride) to detect electrolyte imbalances that can worsen HF, cause EKG changes and arrhythmia, or decrease medication effectiveness.
- **Thyroid-stimulating hormone (TSH) level** to detect thyroid disorders. Both hyperthyroidism and hypothyroidism can be potential causes of HF and contribute to other cardiac disorders such as HTN, tachycardia, and atrial fibrillation.
- **Urinalysis** can also help to detect signs of renal disease or diabetes as a potential cause(s) of cardiac conditions.

LABORATORY TESTS TO ASSESS FOR MYOCARDIAL INJURY AND MYOCARDIAL INFARCTION

- **Troponins/cardiac troponins** (cardiac troponin T [cTnT] and cardiac troponin I [cTnI]) are used to evaluate clinical suspicion of acute myocardial ischemia or injury. The timing and level of elevation are diagnostic and predictive of morbidity and mortality risk. Levels are elevated in ACS, but may also be elevated in HF, atrial fibrillation, sepsis, hypovolemia, pulmonary embolism, myocarditis, myocardial contusion, and renal failure.
- **Creatinine kinase-MB Isoenzyme (CK-MB)** is elevated in MI, myocarditis, pericarditis, cardiac defibrillation, cardiac surgery, cardiomyopathy,

hypothermia, muscular dystrophy, extensive rhabdomyolysis, and strenuous exercise such as in marathon runners. The timing and ratio of CK-MB elevation can be diagnostic for MI.

LABORATORY TESTS TO CONSIDER FOR ALTERNATIVE CAUSES

- **Arterial blood gases (ABGs)** to assess for hypoxia, acid–base balance, and pulmonary disease.
- **Blood cultures** to assess for potential infectious processes (endocarditis, blood or systemic infection).
- **Human immunodeficiency virus (HIV) testing**. HIV-associated cardiomyopathy (decreased left ventricular [LV] ejection fraction [EF] or dilated LV by imaging studies, with or without symptoms of HF) is currently recognized as a major long-term complication of HIV-1 infection in both developed and developing countries (Remick et al., 2014).
- **Lyme serology** should be considered as a potential rare cause of bradycardia/AV block and to assess for Lyme carditis, a viral perimyocarditis (Scheffold, Herkommer, Kandolf, & May, 2015).
- **Serum ferritin level and/or transferrin saturation** to assess for iron deficiency, macrocytic anemia, or hemochromatosis.
- **Thiamine level** to detect deficiency, beriberi, or alcoholism.

LABORATORY TESTS TO ASSESS FOR SELECTED COMORBID CONDITIONS

- **Glycated (glycosated) hemoglobin or hemoglobin A1c (HbA1c)** to evaluate for diabetes mellitus. Elevated HbA1c levels and diabetes mellitus are associated with increased risk of coronary heart disease and CVD.
- **Lipid profile** to evaluate for hypercholesterolemia and hypertriglyceridemia. Elevated levels of total cholesterol, low-density lipoprotein, and triglycerides increase cardiovascular risk and contribute to atherosclerosis.
- **Toxicology screening and drug levels** can be considered if illicit substances or nontherapeutic medication levels are suspected.

DIAGNOSTIC CONSIDERATIONS FOR THE HEART AND CIRCULATORY SYSTEM

ANKLE-BRACHIAL INDEX

Ankle-Brachial Index (ABI) is the standard test used to diagnose peripheral artery disease (PAD) and has shown clinical correlation to lower-extremity arterial angiograms identifying 50% or more stenosis (Aboyans et al., 2012). ABIs are reported as the ratio of the ankle systolic pressure to the arm systolic pressure and are abnormal when the ratio is less than or equal to 0.90. This cutoff creates a specificity of 83% to 99% but a low sensitivity (69%–79%; Aboyans et al., 2012). Much of the sensitivity issues are related to gender, genetic, ethnic, and race differences. Therefore, when clinical history and findings are suspicious for PAD, but the ABI is 0.91 to 1.00, it should be considered a borderline result. Performing an ABI immediately post-exercise improves the sensitivity of ABI and is recommended in patients with borderline and even normal ABI results (0.91–1.40) who have symptoms of claudication or for whom there is high clinical suspicion for PAD (Aboyans et al., 2012; Gerhard-Herman et al., 2017). Variability occurs between clinicians in performance of the ABI, which will influence validity and reliability of the findings. Therefore, it is paramount to reference current guidelines to ensure standard techniques are followed during ABI performance, including use of Doppler technique and avoidance of oscillometric blood pressure cuffs (Aboyans et al., 2012).

ELECTROCARDIOGRAM

An EKG is a noninvasive test that measures the electrical activity of the heart. It uses electrodes placed on the skin to measure voltage changes as the heart beats. By measuring the voltage across several vectors, an EKG can evaluate a variety of aspects of cardiac structure and function. It is a very effective way of evaluating the status of the conduction system, detecting arrhythmias, and identifying signs of ischemia. It can be used to detect structural change in the heart, such as chamber hypertrophy and enlargement, valve disease, and pericarditis. EKG can also be helpful in the assessment of patients with syncope, suspected drug toxicities or side effects, electrolyte imbalances, and metabolic disorders. EKG is often ordered for the initial evaluation of patients with cardiovascular complaints.

One example of a common rhythm abnormality identified by EKG is atrial fibrillation (**Figure 6.27**). Atrial fibrillation is a rhythm in which the organized atrial activity is lost. Instead of contracting, the atria fibrillate, or quiver. The ventricular rhythm becomes irregular and can at times become very fast. The loss of atrial contraction leads to a modest reduction in CO, which can be further impaired by the lack of diastolic filling with faster heart rates. Under the right circumstances, in people with underlying heart disease, new onset atrial fibrillation can lead to HF symptoms. Restoration of sinus rhythm is important, especially for those in whom atrial fibrillation is causing symptoms. Atrial fibrillation is an important rhythm to detect because it (as well as atrial flutter) can lead to blood clots forming in the atria where blood flow is stagnant due to the loss of contraction. If these blood clots are ejected

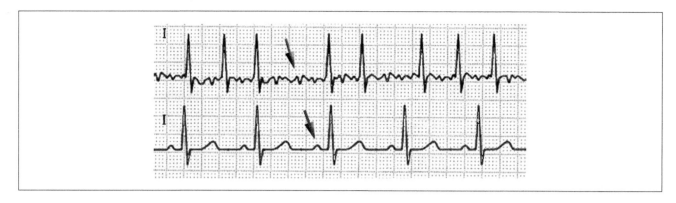

FIGURE 6.27 Atrial fibrillation. Abnormal electrocardiogram of atrial fibrillation (top) and sinus rhythm (bottom). The purple arrow indicates a P-wave, which is lost in atrial fibrillation.

Source: Image courtesy of J. Heuser.

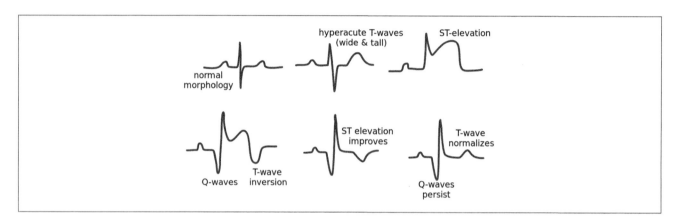

FIGURE 6.28 Electrocardiogram (EKG) changes associated with myocardial infarction. The EKG manifestations of the evolution of a myocardial infarction.

Source: Image courtesy of Oldblueday.

from the heart, they can cause MI, stroke, and other peripheral embolic phenomenon. For this reason, anticoagulation is often recommended for people who develop atrial fibrillation and have preexisting risk factors for CVD.

Myocardial ischemia occurs when there is mismatch between cardiac oxygen supply and oxygen demand. Oxygen supply and demand mismatch happens if there is a sudden reduction in oxygen delivery to the cardiac tissues because of a thrombus or other occlusion. This can also happen when a sudden increase in oxygen demand occurs in the presence of a significant obstruction in a coronary artery from atherosclerotic plaque. If there is a complete occlusion of blood flow to the myocardium, eventually tissue death will occur, also known as infarction. Along with elevation of biomarkers in the blood, EKG is a key component in the diagnosis and management of ACS, which occurs with sudden myocardial ischemia or infarction. EKG changes associated with ischemia include ST-segment depression or

T-wave inversion. EKG changes associated with infarction include ST elevation, ST depression, and the development of Q waves. Chronic changes in the EKG such as ST depression and T-wave inversion can also occur because of obstructive CAD, and Q waves from a prior MI can become permanent features on a person's EKG (**Figure 6.28**).

Heart block is a conduction system abnormality in which the electrical communication between the atria and ventricles is abnormal. In first-degree heart block, conduction through the atrioventricular node is prolonged. This is identified as a prolonged PR interval on EKG. In second-degree heart block, some of the impulses generated by the atria fail to be conducted to the ventricles. This can be noted by absent QRS complexes after P waves and can be associated with a gradually prolonging PR interval (Mobitz I) or a fixed PR interval (Mobitz II; **Figure 6.29**). Mobitz I heart block can be a normal finding in young people and in athletes, whereas Type 2 Mobitz II is always pathological. In third-degree

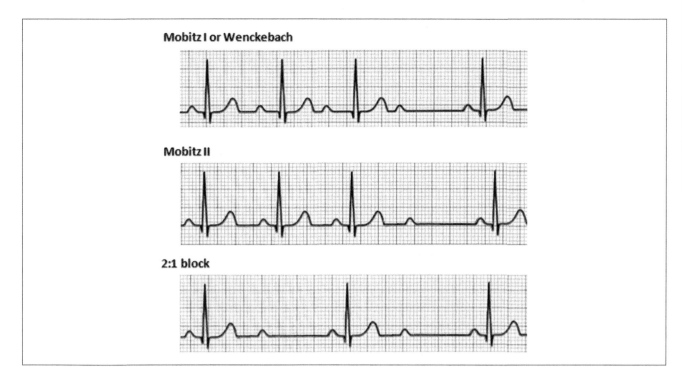

FIGURE 6.29 Heart block. Examples of electrocardiogram depicting second-degree heart block.
Source: Image courtesy of N. Patchett.

heart block, there is complete failure of the atrioventricular node to conduct impulses, and the atria and ventricles are essentially electrically isolated from each other. When this occurs, the ventricles contract independently of the atria. Since the ventricles can no longer respond to impulses originating in the sinoatrial node, pacemaker cells from other cardiac tissue such as the His bundle take over pacing duties and an escape rhythm forms. This rhythm is typically less than 60 impulses/minute, depending on the origin of the escape rhythm, and has the potential for causing hemodynamic instability. If no reversible cause is identified, then a pacemaker is often implanted.

Premature impulses can occur when the normal heart rhythm is interrupted by an electrical impulse from an ectopic origin. Ectopic impulses originating in the atria are called premature atrial contractions (PAC) and have a narrow QRS complex. If an ectopic impulse arises from the ventricles, the QRS complex is wide and this is termed a premature ventricular contraction (PVCs). PACs and PVCs are usually benign and do not cause symptoms. In some instances, they can occur more frequently due to underlying conditions such as HF or ischemia (**Figure 6.30**).

Ventricular fibrillation (VF; **Figure 6.31**) and ventricular tachycardia (VT; **Figure 6.32**) are life-threatening heart rhythms that require immediate attention. Ventricular tachycardia may occur briefly and resolve spontaneously or can be sustained. Sustained VT left

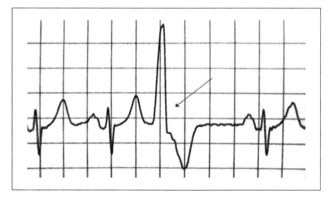

FIGURE 6.30 Premature ventricular contraction.
Source: Image courtesy of James Heilman, MD.

untreated may be stable for a relatively short period of time or can lead to cardiac arrest. VT can also degenerate into ventricular fibrillation and cardiac arrest. Both unstable VT and VF are treated with unsynchronized electrical cardioversion to attempt to restore normal rhythm.

Ambulatory Electrocardiographic Monitors

Ambulatory electrocardiographic monitors are portable battery-powered devices that are worn continuously for varying lengths of time to record and/or transmit EKG information (often via phone) from the patient's

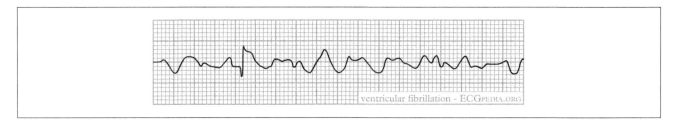

FIGURE 6.31 Ventricular fibrillation.
Source: Image courtesy of CardioNetworks.

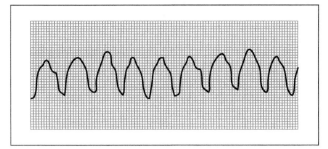

FIGURE 6.32 Ventricular tachycardia.

location to a healthcare setting/clinician where information can be downloaded and analyzed. These monitors are helpful in identifying episodes of concern such as intermittent heart rate or rhythm abnormalities and for evaluating such conditions as atrial fibrillation or syncope.

- Holter monitor is worn continuously for several days.
- Cardiac event recorders (closed loop or looping recorder, symptom event recorder) are activated by patients when they are experiencing symptoms.

CHEST RADIOGRAPH

A chest radiograph or x-ray is a fast, relatively inexpensive test that can provide helpful clues to guide decision-making when faced with a patient with symptoms suspected to involve the heart. The test takes only 10 to 15 minutes with the patient sitting, standing, or lying. A small amount of radiation is passed through the chest from either anterior to posterior or vice versa. Lateral-view images can also be obtained. The x-ray beams that pass through the chest are picked up by a detector, and an image is created. A chest x-ray provides information about cardiac anatomy via the size and shape of its silhouette but, combined with other findings, can be diagnostic for various pathologies. The cardiac silhouette itself may be enlarged if the patient has a condition such as dilated cardiomyopathy, hypertensive heart disease, pericardial effusion, or CHD. The shape of the heart silhouette can also be useful to determine

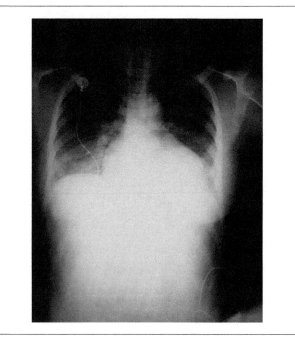

FIGURE 6.33 Chest x-ray to evaluate cardiac size. Anteroposterior x-ray of a 28-year-old who presented with heart failure that was secondary to chronic hypertension. Note the presence of an enlarged cardiac silhouette. Fluid is accumulating in lungs bilaterally.

Source: Image courtesy of Dr. Thomas Hooten/Centers for Disease Control and Prevention. Retrieved from https://phil.cdc.gov/Details .aspx?pid=6241

which of the chambers are enlarged. For instance, if the silhouette extends beyond the right sternal border, this suggests right atrial or ventricular enlargement (**Figure 6.33**).

Other findings that might give clues to underlying cardiac pathology are pleural effusions; diffuse haziness or prominent interstitial lung markings, which suggest pulmonary edema; and enlarged pulmonary arteries, which suggest pulmonary HTN. Chest x-rays can also provide information about a patient's medical and surgical history by revealing implantable devices and objects such as pacemakers or pacemaker wires, prosthetic valves, sternal wires, and surgical clips.

ECHOCARDIOGRAM

Transthoracic Echocardiogram

A transthoracic echocardiogram (TTE) uses ultrasound (US) waves to create 2D and 3D pictures of the heart by detecting the reflection of the sound waves as they encounter tissue and blood. The speed and direction of blood flow can also be determined using Doppler imaging. **Figure 6.34** shows an example of a 2D image depicting a short-axis view of the base of the heart, with a closed aortic valve in the center of the image. A transthoracic echocardiogram is performed by placing a US transducer on various parts of the chest wall while the patient lies in the left lateral semirecumbent position. Images taken by the sonographer are stored and later interpreted by a cardiologist. This test is a useful way of determining the size and strength of the cardiac chambers and obtaining information about the structure and function of heart valves. It can also evaluate portions of the aorta, pulmonary arteries, and central veins. One of the limitations of transthoracic echocardiography is that the image quality depends on adequate acoustic windows. Acoustic windows can be adversely affected if a patient has lung disease, obesity, breast implants, or other conditions that may interfere with sound transmission. IV contrast material can sometimes be used in these instances to gain basic information such as left ventricular function.

Transesophageal Echocardiogram

A transesophageal echocardiogram (TEE) is similar to a TTE in its ability to obtain 2D, 3D, and Doppler images of the heart, but with one important difference: greater image quality. A TEE is performed by inserting a flexible probe that is tipped with a transducer into the esophagus and stomach. This positions the transducer directly behind the heart with very little tissue in between, so the image quality is much higher and allows for identification and measurement of small structures that may not be detected by TTE, such as valvular vegetations, thrombi, congenital defects, and aortic dissections, and can better define valvular function when TTE images are inadequate. Transesophageal echocardiograms require sedation as well as local anesthetic to the posterior pharynx to avoid stimulating the patient's gag reflex while the probe is inserted.

STRESS TESTING

Stress testing refers to the process of evaluating the cardiovascular response to exercise. This can be done to look for evidence of cardiac pathology such as CAD, or to evaluate other parameters such as blood pressure response to exercise or the presence of arrhythmias, which may be induced by exercise. All stress testing involves inducing cardiovascular stress either with exercise or by pharmacological methods. Stress testing is most often performed to unmask cardiac ischemia in response to a reported patient symptom such as chest pain or pressure. A stress test is also frequently performed before surgery to determine whether underlying cardiac disease is present and stratify the risk of major adverse cardiac events. Guidelines recommend against the use of stress testing in all patients before surgery, but advocate for their use in a selected patient population with poor or unknown functional capacity,

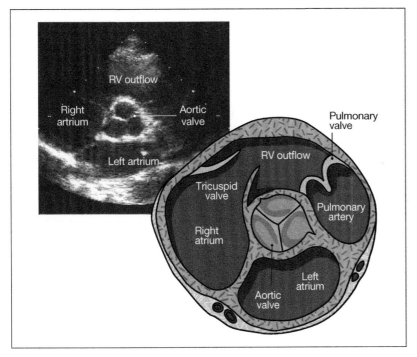

FIGURE 6.34 Short-axis view of aortic valve.

Source: Image courtesy of Patrick J. Lynch and C. Carl Jaffe.

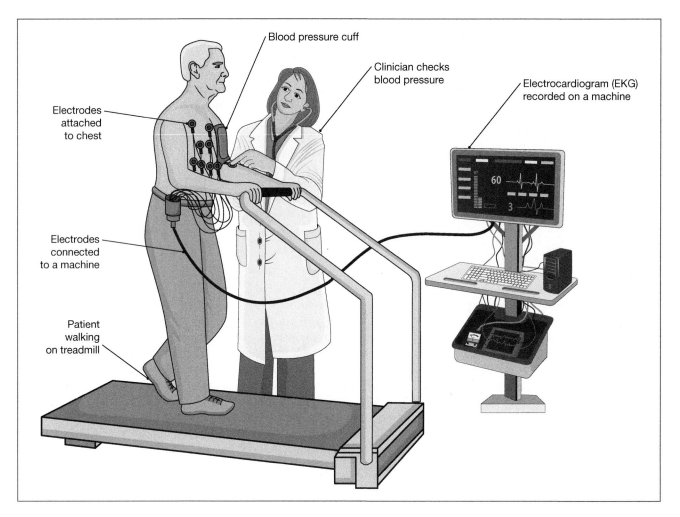

FIGURE 6.35 Treadmill stress testing.

Source: Adapted from the National Heart, Lung, and Blood Institute.

who are at elevated risk for perioperative complications, and for whom the results of stress testing would impact decision-making or perioperative planning (Fleisher et al., 2014).

Interpreting the results of a stress test relies heavily on the patient's individual pretest probability. The pretest probability can be designated as either low, intermediate, or high risk of having disease. In the case of stress testing to detect CAD, the pretest probability is determined by considering the patient's age, gender, and symptoms. In general, patients who have low pretest probability for CAD should not undergo stress testing because the risk of a false-positive test result is higher than their pretest probability of disease. The same is true for high-risk patients, in that the risk of a false-negative test result is greater than the chance that they do not have disease present. For this reason, stress testing should only be performed in individuals with intermediate probability for disease (Fihn et al., 2012).

Treadmill Stress Electrocardiogram

A treadmill stress EKG is a diagnostic test in which an EKG is performed during exercise. Before the test, patients have EKG electrodes placed across their chest in the same fashion as they would have for a resting EKG. During the test, patients walk on a treadmill, and the intensity of exercise is gradually increased by adjusting the speed and incline of the treadmill at specified intervals according to the Bruce protocol or modified Bruce protocol. Heart rhythm, rate, and blood pressure are measured at regular intervals before, during, and after the test. A continuous 12-lead EKG runs throughout the entire test and for a few minutes into recovery (**Figure 6.35**). During exercise, changes in the EKG such as T-wave inversions, ST-segment depression or elevation, or frequent premature ventricular contractions may be provoked, which indicate underlying myocardial ischemia. Typically, a positive treadmill EKG is followed up with another test, such as a stress test with imaging or a coronary angiogram.

Stress Echocardiogram

Stress echocardiography (echo) is another method of evaluating the cardiovascular response to stress. Like a treadmill stress EKG, stress echo is useful for detecting cardiac ischemia by electrocardiogram, and in fact an exercise EKG is performed during a stress echo. But in addition to the stress EKG, a stress echo allows visualization of cardiac wall motion as CO is increased in response to exercise. Stress echocardiograms are useful when a treadmill EKG is not sufficient to evaluate for ischemia because the patient cannot exercise, has a left BBB, or the EKG is indeterminate and there is ongoing suspicion for ischemia. During a stress echocardiogram, patients are connected to an EKG machine in the same fashion as the treadmill EKG described previously. Exercise is then performed on a treadmill, and once peak exertion is achieved, the patient is instructed to move to a table where a limited echocardiogram is performed. Careful attention is paid to the way in which the heart contracts. If a segment of the myocardium shows a reduced or absent ability to contract with exercise, this suggests that blood supply to that area of the heart is limited by an atherosclerotic plaque. If a patient is unable to exercise, external pacing or drugs such as dobutamine, dipyridamole, and adenosine can be infused to simulate stress. Stress echocardiogram sensitivity and specificity for detection of coronary artery stenosis of greater than 50% of the luminal diameter is 88% and 83%, respectively (Pellikka, Nagueh, Elhendy, Kuehl, & Sawada, 2007).

Single-Photon Emission Computed Tomography

Single-photon emission computed tomography (SPECT) imaging is another highly accurate way to detect cardiac ischemia. It involves the use of a radioactive tracer, usually technetium-99m or thallium-201, which is injected into the bloodstream. This tracer is then taken up by the myocardium in areas where there is adequate tissue blood supply. A gamma camera takes resting pictures of the heart to establish baseline perfusion images that will be compared with stress images. After 2 to 3 hours have passed so the radioactive tracer has sufficiently decayed, the patient is exercised or given a drug such as adenosine or regadenoson to simulate the effects of exercise on the heart. Another injection of radioactive tracer is given at peak exercise and absorbed by the myocardium in areas of sufficient blood supply. Then another set of images is taken of the heart with the gamma camera. If cardiac ischemia is present, there will be areas of uptake visible in the resting images, which are absent in the stress images. Some variations of this test exist, such as performing rest and stress images on different days or using different tracers, but the overall concept is the same. According to the 2013 AHA guidelines for exercise testing, SPECT has a sensitivity between 87% and 90% and a specificity of 73% to 89% (Fletcher et al., 2013).

Other Methods of Stress Testing

In addition to the previously described methods, there are other methods for noninvasive detection of CAD. These include stress cardiac magnetic resonance imaging (MRI), cardiopulmonary stress testing (CPET), and positron emission tomography (PET).

CORONARY COMPUTED TOMOGRAPHY ANGIOGRAPHY AND CORONARY CALCIUM SCORING

In contrast to the previously described methods of stress testing, which use physiological data to detect CAD, computed tomography (CT) angiography of the coronary arteries and calcium scoring are methods to detect CAD via an anatomical assessment. Coronary calcium scoring is based on the known relationship between the presence of vascular calcification and CAD as an indicator of vascular disease. For this test, a patient lays flat on a table that is moved into the CT scanner. Images are taken for about 10 minutes, and contrast dye is not used. A calcium score is determined by the amount of calcium within the walls of the coronary arteries. A total coronary artery calcium (CAC) score is then reported. A score of 0 indicates no disease is present, and a score of 400 or greater indicates extensive CAD is present (Nasir, Michos, Blumenthal, & Raggi, 2005). Coronary calcium score is also an independent predictor of coronary heart disease events (Pletcher, Tice, Pignone, & Browner, 2004) and can be used to assist in risk stratification for individuals who are at intermediate risk for developing CVD and to inform decision-making regarding lifestyle changes and medical therapy (Arnett et al., 2019).

CT angiography is performed in a similar way to calcium scoring, with the important exception that contrast dye must be used. With any CT test, CT contrast dye must be used with caution or avoided in persons with severe chronic kidney disease or who have previously demonstrated an allergy to contrast. A CT angiogram of the coronary arteries is able to recreate a detailed picture of the coronary artery anatomy and is able to detect narrowing due to plaques of 50% or greater with a sensitivity of 95% and a specificity of 83% (Budoff et al., 2008). This test can be helpful when there is a need to noninvasively identify the presence of CAD, but a stress test is unable to be performed.

CORONARY ANGIOGRAPHY

Coronary angiography is an invasive procedure in which contrast dye is injected into a coronary artery.

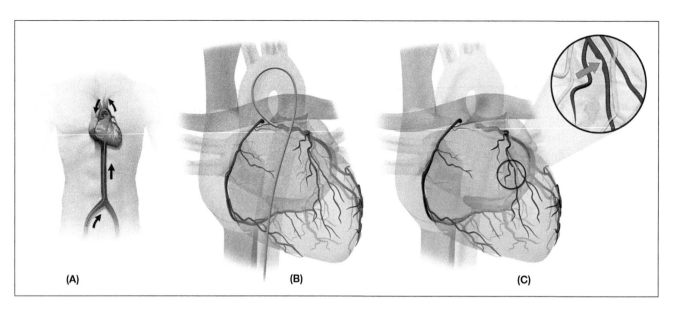

FIGURE 6.36 Coronary angiography to evaluate blood flow. (A) Catheter is inserted in leg and guided up the aorta. (B) Catheter tip stops at left coronary artery. (C) Contrast agent is injected into arteries. X-ray imaging shows stenosis in left coronary artery.

Source: Image courtesy of Bruce Blaus.

The dye is injected through a catheter that has been passed through an artery until it reaches the aortic root. From there, the separate right and left coronary systems can be engaged. When contrast is injected, its passage through the coronary arteries is visualized in real time using fluoroscopy, which is a special x-ray camera (**Figure 6.36**). Visual inspection of the coronary arteries enables their anatomy to be defined, and plaques or thrombi within the vessel can be identified and intervened upon if necessary. Coronary angiography is the gold standard for the detection of CAD by which all other tests are measured. It is useful in cases of ACS or when there is high clinical suspicion for myocardial ischemia and a diagnosis is needed. Coronary angiography can be performed as a stand-alone diagnostic test or may be followed by a percutaneous coronary intervention (PCI) such as balloon angioplasty or coronary stenting. Risks from the procedure are rare but serious and include death, MI, stroke, arterial embolization, perforation, bleeding, and others. Because of these risks, this procedure is only carried out when the benefits from diagnosis or treatment of disease outweigh the risks.

CARDIOVASCULAR MAGNETIC RESONANCE IMAGING

Cardiovascular magnetic resonance imaging (CMR) uses magnetic fields and radiofrequency to create 3D images of the heart and great vessels. The images that are created have very high spatial and temporal resolution and allow for creation of cinematic sequences that can evaluate many aspects of cardiac structure and function with great precision. CMR allows for highly accurate assessment of ventricular function and can perform tissue characterization. It can also detect inflammation and edema within the myocardium, presence of iron overload or fibrosis within the myocardial walls, and provide information about valvular function. One of the main benefits of CMR is that it avoids exposure to radiation. Gadolinium contrast agent is frequently used during CMR, and although gadolinium does not have the same nephrotoxicity as CT contrast, it must nonetheless be used carefully in people with documented reactions. People with moderate-to-severe chronic kidney disease are also at risk of developing nephrogenic systemic fibrosis if given gadolinium, so this is often avoided in this population. Patients with metallic implants such as pacemakers are often unable to have CMR because of the risk of injury. Some implanted devices such as prosthetic heart valves or surgical clips are CMR safe but may cause imaging artifacts. The website www.mrisafety.com contains a comprehensive list of implantable medical devices and information about their CMR safety. When having a CMR, patients must lie flat on a table for up to an hour. Many patients who are claustrophobic require preprocedural treatment with anxiolytics such as benzodiazepines.

CARDIAC COMPUTED TOMOGRAPHY

Cardiac CT is another form of advanced cardiac imaging. Like CMR, it can provide detailed cardiac anatomical and functional data with great precision. The process for this test is like the other CT tests described previously. Contrast media is necessary for this test, so it must be used with caution in those with documented sensitivities to contrast media or people with moderate-to-severe chronic kidney disease. Cardiac CT is an excellent choice for gathering data noninvasively on people who have implanted ferromagnetic material and cannot have CMR. Because of the time required to obtain images, cardiac CT is limited by the fact that the patient's heart rate must be near 60 impulses/minute. Radiation exposure is also a consideration with any CT test.

EVIDENCE-BASED PRACTICE CONSIDERATIONS FOR THE HEART AND CIRCULATORY SYSTEM

AMERICAN COLLEGE OF CARDIOLOGY AND THE AMERICAN HEART ASSOCIATION

- HTN is a leading risk factor for mortality and disability. With its association with heart disease, stroke, HF, and chronic kidney disease, HTN is second only to cigarette smoking as a preventable cause of death in the United States.
- Given demographic trends and the increasing prevalence of HTN with increasing age (79% of men and 85% of women >75 years old have HTN), the consequences of HTN are expected to increase. Individuals should be counseled on their risk for development of atherosclerotic cardiovascular disease (ASCVD; **Box 6.1**).

UNITED STATES PREVENTIVE SERVICES TASK FORCE RECOMMENDATIONS

- For all adults aged 18 years and older, the USPSTF recommends screening for high blood pressure. Measurements should be obtained outside of the clinical setting for diagnostic confirmation before starting treatment (Grade A; USPSTF, 2015). Current evidence is insufficient to recommend screening for primary HTN in asymptomatic children and adolescents to prevent subsequent CVD in childhood or adulthood (Grade I; USPSTF, 2013). Benefits and harms should be individually assessed.
- For adults at low risk for a cardiovascular event, it is not recommended to do an EKG for screening and prevention purposes (Grade D). If adults are deemed to be at an intermediate or high risk, the benefits and harms of screening should be assessed (Grade I; USPSTF, 2018b).
- The USPSTF concludes that the current evidence is insufficient to assess the balance of benefits and harms of adding the ABI, high-sensitivity C-reactive

---

BOX 6.1
RISK CALCULATOR FOR ESTIMATING 10-YEAR RISK FOR ATHEROSCLEROTIC CARDIOVASCULAR DISEASE*

Calculation Information:

- Age, gender, race
- Systolic and diastolic blood pressure
- Total cholesterol, HDL, and LDL
- History of diabetes, smoking (current, former, never)
- Current (yes/no) medications for HTN, statin, or on aspirin therapy

Factors Increasing ASCVD Risk Included in Clinician-Patient Risk Discussion:

- Family history of premature ASCVD
- Primary hypercholesterolemia
- Metabolic syndrome
- Chronic kidney disease
- Chronic inflammatory conditions
- History of premature menopause
- History of pregnancy-associated conditions that increase later ASCVD risk (e.g., preeclampsia)
- High-risk race/ethnicity (e.g., South Asian ancestry)
- Lipids/biomarkers associated with increased ASCVD risk

10-Year Risk for ASCVD:

- Low-risk (<5%)
- Borderline risk (5%–7.4%)
- Intermediate risk (7.5%–19.9%)
- High risk (≥20%)

*Calculations are for those without ASCVD only. Calculator can be found online at http://tools.acc.org/ASCVD-Risk-Estimator-Plus/#!/calculate/estimate

ASCVD, atherosclerotic cardiovascular disease; HDL, high-density lipoprotein; HTN, hypertension; LDL, low-density lipoprotein.

---

protein (hsCRP) level, or CAC score to traditional risk assessment for CVD in asymptomatic adults to prevent CVD events (Grade I; USPSTF, 2018a).
- In men ages 65 to 75 years who have ever smoked, a one-time screening for abdominal aortic aneurysm (AAA) with ultrasonography should be completed (Grade B). In men ages 65 to 75 years who have never smoked, clinicians should selectively offer screening for AAA based on risk (Grade C). In women ages 65 to 75 years who have ever smoked, the current evidence is insufficient to assess the balance of benefits

and harms of screening for AAA (Grade I). Last, in women who have never smoked, screening for AAA is not recommended (Grade D; USPSTF, 2014).

CHOOSING WISELY® RECOMMENDATIONS

Considerations from the Choosing Wisely Initiative set forth by the ACC (2019) and the American Society of Nuclear Cardiology (ASNC; 2012) regarding cardiac imaging and testing for patients are as follows:

- Do not perform stress cardiac imaging or advanced noninvasive imaging in the initial workup of asymptomatic patients unless high-risk markers are present. High-risk markers are as follows: diabetes in patients more than 40 years old, PAD, or more than 2% yearly risk for CAD events.
- Do not perform annual stress cardiac imaging or advanced noninvasive imaging as part of a serial or scheduled pattern in asymptomatic patients. Exceptions to this rule include patients more than 5 years after a bypass operation, more than 2 years after a stenting procedure, or after having a stent placed in the left main coronary artery.
- Do not perform stress cardiac imaging, EKG, or advanced noninvasive imaging as a part of the preoperative assessment for patients undergoing low-risk, non-cardiac surgery.
- Do not perform echocardiography as routine follow-up for mild, asymptomatic native valve disease in adult patients unless there is a change in clinical status.

ABNORMAL FINDINGS OF THE HEART AND CIRCULATORY SYSTEM

Heart disease is the leading cause of death for both men and women in the United States. Coronary heart disease is the most common type of heart disease. Knowing the early and major warning signs are key to saving lives. In this section, definitions, risk factors, and key history and physical findings of these diagnoses are provided. Common and severe forms of CVD and peripheral vascular disorders associated with increased morbidity are reviewed.

ACUTE CORONARY SYNDROME

ACS is a prolonged period of decreased myocardial oxygenation due to decreased blood flow in coronary arteries resulting in sections of necrosis in the heart muscle known as MI. ACS is a constellation of symptoms due to myocardial ischemia. Ischemia occurs due to mismatch of myocardial oxygen demand and delivery, often resulting from partial or total occlusion of a coronary artery. ACS includes both non-ST-segment elevation myocardial infarction (NSTEMI) and ST-segment elevation myocardial infarction (STEMI; Sweis & Jivan, 2018). NSTEMI is not associated with infarction and necrosis. The different classifications involve acute coronary artery ischemia and are differentiated on the basis of symptoms, EKG findings, and cardiac biomarker levels (Sweis & Jivan, 2018). The term *syndrome* is used because although signs and symptoms in patients can be similar, the actual disease process that causes the reduced blood to the heart flow may differ (Norton, 2017). For example, ischemia of the heart could be due to one of the previous classifications; however, the result of tissue injury or death of the myocardium is the same if left untreated.

The most common cause of ACS is atherosclerosis, an inflammatory disease that causes remodeling of the coronary arteries. Specifically, rupture of a thrombus in an atherosclerotic plaque is the main cause of ACS (Norton, 2017). The thrombus creates a blockage in the coronary artery, resulting in partial or full occlusion of the vessel. Risk factors suggesting ACS (LR ≥+2.0 and CI that excluded 1.0) were a history of an abnormal stress test, history of PAD, pain radiation to both arms, pain similar to ischemia, and change in pain pattern over the past 24 hours with no benefit from nitroglycerin (Fanaroff, Rymer, Goldstein, Simel, & Newby, 2015). Other risk factors are similar to all CVDs, including older age, diabetes, smoking, HTN, hyperlipidemia, lack of exercise, unhealthy diet, overweight/obese, and family history of heart disease. Patients with a history of ACS experience a decrease in ability to perform ordinary activities, and experience other comorbidities and mental health issues that affect their quality of life (QoL; Ye et al., 2019). About 10% of patients who present with acute chest pain are diagnosed with ACS (Fanaroff et al., 2015). A comprehensive systematic review found that History, EKG, Age, Risk Factors, and Troponin (HEART) or Thrombolysis in Myocardial Infarction (TIMI) risk scores that incorporate the first cardiac troponin provided more diagnostic information than history, physical exam, and EKG alone (Fanaroff et al., 2015).

Key History and Physical Findings
- Risk factors as previously noted
- Chest pain that is described as aching, pressure, tightness, or burning
- Chest pain occurs either at rest or with activity and does not change with respiration or position, lasting more than 20 minutes
- Nausea/vomiting
- Shortness of breath
- Diaphoresis
- Recent cocaine use
- Pain radiating to both arms, left arm, jaw, or neck

- Change in pain pattern over the past 24 hours with no benefit from nitroglycerin
- Fatigue
- Dizziness, lightheadedness
- Syncope
- EKG abnormalities (ST depression)
- Elevated cardiac serum markers (troponin)
- HEART risk score range 7 to 10
- TIMI risk score 5 or higher

ABDOMINAL AORTIC ANEURYSM

An aortic aneurysm is a ballooning or weakening of the aortic wall that is predisposed to rupturing. A true aneurysm is defined as a segmental, full-thickness dilation of a blood vessel that is 50% greater than the normal aortic diameter. Although aneurysms have a strong genetic predisposition, the most common cause is atherosclerosis (Goolsby & Grubbs, 2019). Aging, HTN, cigarette smoking, and being a male Caucasian have all been described as risk factors. There are usually no associated pain symptoms. The finding of a palpable, pulsatile mass on examination has a significant likelihood of being an AAA +LR = 8.0; McGee, 2018). A strong bounding pulse can be found on palpation, but most often this condition is diagnosed with US. A comprehensive systematic review found that when US is used for a suspected AAA there was a significant reduction in mortality as a result of sequelae from the aneurysm in males age 65 to 79 years; however, there was insufficient evidence to demonstrate a positive benefit from this screening strategy in women suspected of an AAA (Cosford, Leng, & Thomas, 2007).

Key History and Physical Findings

- Asymptomatic in the majority of patients
- Pulsatile abdominal mass
- Bounding pulse
- If symptomatic but not ruptured, pain is typically near the position of the aneurysm (epigastric region of the abdomen, back, flank, or pelvic region) and has an indolent onset
- Pain does not change with position or movement
- Syncope or feeling faint
- Ruptured AAA triad: severe acute pain, a pulsatile abdominal mass, and hypotension occurs in approximately 50% of patients

ATHEROSCLEROSIS AND CORONARY ARTERY DISEASE

Atherosclerosis is the most common type of arteriosclerosis, a general term for a condition causing thickening and loss of elasticity of the arterial wall due to plaques (**Figure 6.37**). The plaques, called atheromas, consist of inflammatory cells, lipids, smooth muscle cells, minerals, and connective tissue. The accumulation of

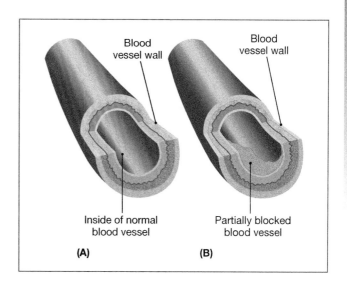

FIGURE 6.37 Atherosclerosis. (A) Normal blood vessel. (B) Partially blocked blood vessel.

these atheromas may result in the narrowing of the arterial lumen (Stary et al., 1995; Thanassoulis & Afshar, 2019). Even if a plaque does not cause narrowing of the arterial lumen, it may be clinically significant because of potential complications that can suddenly develop (Stary et al., 1995). Atherosclerosis is most clinically relevant because it causes CAD and CVD (Thanassoulis & Afshar, 2019). The histological composition of atheromas is used to classify advancement of the disease process. The different stages of atherosclerosis (mild disease to advanced disease and then to complications from the ruptured plaque) are initiated or augmented by inflammatory cytokines that are released when endothelial injury occurs (Thanassoulis & Afshar, 2019).

Mild atherosclerosis and CAD are typically asymptomatic. Signs and symptoms of transient ischemia (e.g., stable angina, transient ischemic attacks [TIAs]) may appear when lesions decrease blood flow by narrowing the arterial lumen by 70% or more and/or by rupturing and acutely occluding a major artery (Thanassoulis & Afshar, 2019). Atherosclerosis and CAD can also lead to aneurysms, arterial dissection, or sudden death without any prior symptoms of angina. Risk factors include abdominal obesity, diabetes, metabolic syndrome, endothelial dysfunction, inflammatory and immunological factors, insulin resistance, and smoking (Catapano et al., 2016; Thanassoulis & Afshar, 2019).

Key History and Physical Findings

- Hyperlipidemia
- History of smoking
- Asymptomatic in mild disease
- Symptoms of moderate-to-severe arteriosclerosis depend on the arteries affected but can include:
  - Angina

- ○ Intermittent claudication (IC)
- ○ TIAs
- ○ Stroke
- ○ HTN
- ○ Weak pulses
- ○ Bruits
- ○ Decreased blood pressure in limbs
- ○ Elevated inflammatory biomarkers (C-reactive protein)
- ○ CAC score >100 (moderate disease), >300 (severe disease)
- ○ Ankle-Brachial Index <0.9 or >1.4

ATRIAL SEPTAL DEFECT

An ASD (**Figure 6.38**) is an opening between the RA and the LA, or the upper two chambers of the heart. ASD is common in combination with other heart defects and is often critical to blood flow and oxygenation in some CHD (Wernovsky et al., 2020). As an isolated heart defect, ASD accounts for approximately 8% to 10% of congenital heart defects in children (Allen, Shaddy, Penny, Feltes, & Cetta, 2016). Young infants and children with ASD are often asymptomatic and may be found only incidentally while undergoing other testing such as an EKG or echocardiogram. Occasionally an infant with isolated ASD may present as symptomatic with signs of CHF. It is unclear in this rare instance how these patients differ from those who are asymptomatic (Allen et al., 2016; Wernovsky et al., 2020). Older children may present with mild fatigue or dyspnea due to long-standing left to right shunting across the atrium. The amount of left to right shunting that occurs is dependent on the size of the ASD as well as pulmonary pressures. Shunting between the atrium can cause both RA and LA dilation over time. Adults with an unrecognized or untreated ASD may develop right-sided HF, pulmonary HTN, or Eisenmenger's syndrome.

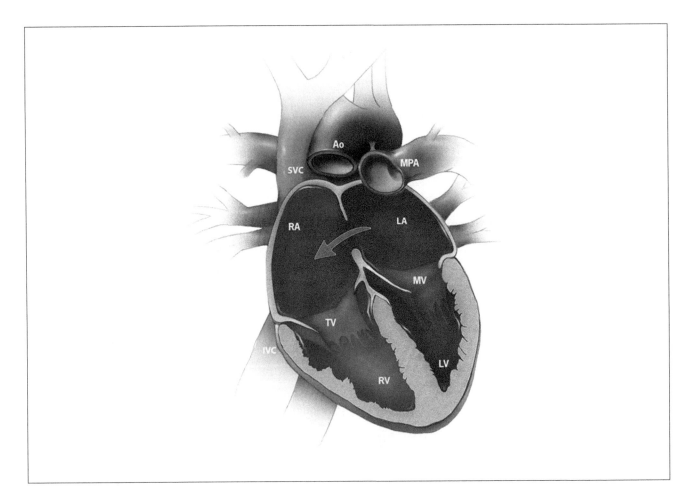

FIGURE 6.38 Atrial septal defect.

Ao, aorta; IVC, inferior vena cava; LA, left atrium; LV, left ventricle; MPA, main pulmonary artery; MV, mitral valve; RA, right atrium; RV, right ventricle; SVC, superior vena cava; TV, tricuspid valve

Source: Courtesy of the Centers for Disease Control and Prevention.

Key History and Physical Findings

- Family history of ASD
- Genetic syndromes: Holt–Oram syndrome, trisomy 21, Noonan's syndrome
- Wide fixed split S2: hallmark finding
- Systolic ejection murmur at the left parasternal area (midway between sternal border and midclavicular line); murmurs may be very soft in early childhood
- Those with long-standing left to right shunting: left precordial bulge, and prominent RV impulse
- Cardiomegaly on chest X-ray
- EKG: Normal sinus rhythm (NSR), may have prolonged QRS
- Transesophageal Echocardiogram: Demonstrate size and location of ASD, gold standard for diagnosis

CHRONIC VENOUS INSUFFICIENCY

Chronic venous insufficiency (CVI) is a condition caused by stasis and reflux of venous blood flow. Important mimics of CVI that should be differentiated during the clinical reasoning process are masses that obstruct the venous system. CVI exists along a continuum that progresses from small telangiectasic "spider" veins to varicose veins, and, in severe cases, venous ulcers. At least 25 million adults in the United States have CVI, and approximately 25% of these affected adults have advanced CVI such as venous ulcer disease (Eberhardt & Rafetto, 2014). CVI can occur at various anatomical levels, including superficial, deep, and perforating veins. Duplex venous scanning is recommended by guidelines for all patients with suspected CVI (Gloviczki et al., 2011). For patients with more advanced disease, CT venography or MR venography are sometimes used (Gloviczki et al., 2011). A cardinal sign/symptom of CVI is pitting edema. When edema is assessed, it is important to assess for presence or absence of pitting by gently pushing into the edema. When present, pitting is graded from 0 to 4 on the basis of how deep of an indentation is made and how fast the pitting recovers. An absence of pitting should clue the clinician to look for causes of nonpitting edema such as lymphedema, lipidemia, and myxedema. Venous eczema, or stasis dermatitis, is an inflammation of the skin overlying venous disease. It is frequently seen in patients with CVI and is sometimes confused with cellulitis since both conditions can be painful, erythematous, and warm to touch (Grey, Harding, & Enoch, 2006). However, cellulitis, in contrast to stasis dermatitis, is usually unilateral and the erythema is more demarcated than that seen in stasis dermatitis. **Table 6.6** reviews the differences in clinical findings between CVI and PAD.

TABLE 6.6 Signs and Symptoms of Chronic Venous Insufficiency Versus Peripheral Artery Disease

Sign/Symptom	CVI	PAD
Edema	Common	Uncommon
Ulcer location	Medial or lateral ankle	Toes or feet
Moisture	Common	Uncommon
Pain	Less common	More common
Other findings	Hyperpigmentation, lipodermatosclerosis	Absent pulses

CVI, chronic venous insufficiency; PAD, peripheral artery disease. *Sources:* Grey, J. E., Harding, K. G., & Enoch, S. (2006). Venous and arterial leg ulcers. *BMJ, 332*(7537), 347–350. doi:10.1136/bmj.332.7537.347; Spentzouris, G., & Labropoulos, N. (2009). The evaluation of lower extremity ulcers. *Seminars in Interventional Radiology, 26*(4), 286–295. doi:10.1055/s-0029-1242204

Key History and Physical Findings

- History of prolonged sitting or standing throughout the day
- Obesity
- Physical inactivity
- Older age
- Female gender
- Prior injury to the extremity
- Pregnancy
- Can be asymptomatic, especially early in disease
- Aching in lower legs is the most commonly reported symptom
- Heaviness and itching in lower legs
- Pitting edema in lower legs
- Varicose veins
- Will often see combined edema and hyperpigmented skin, sometimes called "brawny edema" (**Figure 6.39**)
- Reduced ankle motion
- Hyperpigmentation and lipodermatosclerosis (inflamed and thickened skin) signal more advanced disease
- Lower-extremity ulcerations
- Location of venous ulcers can be a clue to location of disease:
  - Medial ankle ulcers are most often seen with greater saphenous vein disease.
  - Lateral ankle ulcers are seen with small saphenous vein disease (Labropoulos et al., 1994).
- Normal sensory and motor exams (helps exclude diabetic neuropathy)

- Abdominal exam should be normal and helps exclude abdominal mass as cause for venous insufficiency.
- Varicosities in the perineal, vulvar, or groin are a clue to obstruction of the iliac veins from a mass or tumor (Gloviczki et al., 2011).
- Varicosities in the scrotum can occur with gonadal vein incompetence and, of more concern, inferior venal cava lesions, renal carcinoma, or left renal vein occlusion from nutcracker syndrome (Gloviczki et al., 2011).

- Limb-length discrepancies, varicosities in the neonate, and capillary malformations raise concern for congenital venous malformations (such as Klippel–Trenaunay syndrome).

See **Figure 6.40** for varicosities, and **Figure 6.41** for venous ulcerations.

COARCTATION OF THE AORTA

Coarctation of the aorta (**Figure 6.42**) is a defect of the aortic arch involving a narrowing of the arch and represents approximately 7% of CHD (Wernovsky et al., 2020). This narrowing often occurs at the insertion site of the ductus arteriosus. Coarctation is described as an obstructive lesion in which blood flow is diminished or nonexistent past the area of the obstruction. Coarctation can present in varying degrees depending on the amount of narrowing. Many infants will present within the first week of life as the ductus arteriosus closes and hence limiting blood flow past the obstruction. Infants with a critical obstruction to blood flow will present with acute symptoms of shock, metabolic acidosis, renal failure, and necrotizing enterocolitis (Wernovsky et al., 2020). This is defined as a ductal-dependent circulation and these infants require prostaglandin (PGE) to reopen the ductus arteriosus, allowing blood flow past the area of obstruction. These infants may require resuscitation and may have depressed ventricular function until blood flow is restored through resuscitation efforts and PGE infusion. Critical coarctation in the infant is a life-threatening condition if not quickly recognized

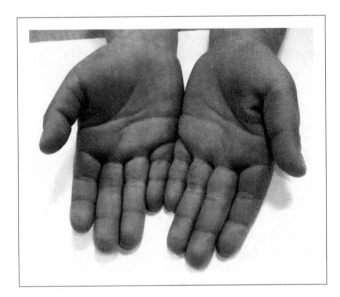

FIGURE 6.39 Brawny edema.

Source: Image courtesy of Dong Soo Kim.

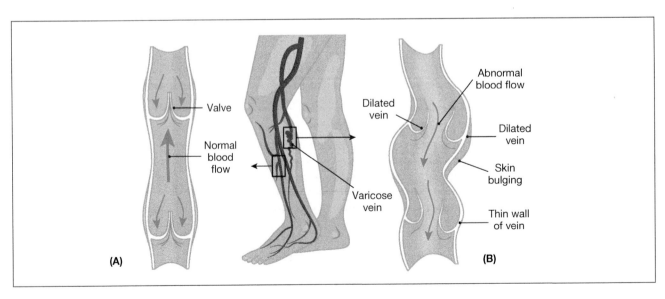

FIGURE 6.40 Varicosities. (A) Vein with normal blood flow. (B) Varicose vein.

Source: Adapted from the National Heart, Lung, and Blood Institute.

and treated. Some infants who do not have a significant obstruction will present later in the first few months of life with symptoms of HF. Older children and adults can also present with coarctation due to

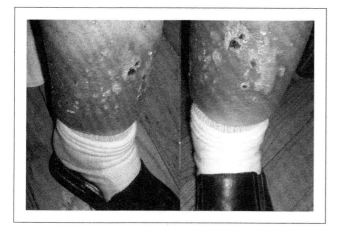

FIGURE 6.41 Venous ulcerations.

a narrowing that was not significant enough in childhood to cause symptoms or development of collateral vessels (Wernovsky et al., 2020). It is possible for coarctation to go undetected in infancy and for older children and adults to present with coarctation. The older child or adult may present with systemic HTN and a murmur. If pulses are palpated, femoral pulses will be weak and a delay between upper extremity and lower-extremity pulses will be appreciated. Coarctation can be repaired with surgery or by stenting the narrowed segment. Children or adults with repaired coarctation require lifelong cardiology follow-up, as they can have re-coarctation or complications arising from the intial surgical repair.

Key History and Physical Findings

- Family history of coarctation
- Genetic syndromes: Turner's syndrome, 22q11.2 (DiGeorge's) syndrome
- Murmur: Systolic ejection murmur along the left sternal border

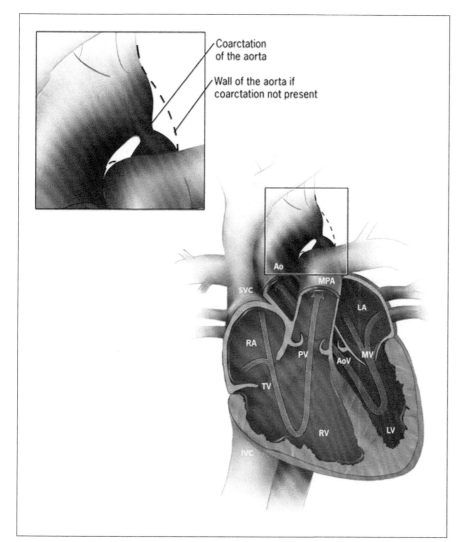

FIGURE 6.42 Coarctation of the aorta.

Ao, aorta; AoV, Aortic valve; IVC, inferior vena cava; LA, left atrium; LV, left ventricle; MPA, main pulmonary artery; MV, mitral valve; PV, pulmonary valve; RA, right atrium; RV, right ventricle; SVC, superior vena cava; TV, tricuspid valve

Source: Courtesy of the Centers for Disease Control and Prevention.

- Gallop rhythm common
- Signs of CHF
- Weak or absent femoral pulses
- Tachypnea and tachycardia
- Skin mottling, delayed capillary refill, and peripheral cyanosis
- Chest x-ray abnormalities:
  - Infants: Cardiomegaly and increased pulmonary vascular markings
  - Older child or adult: Figure-3 sign on the left border of the mediastinum and rib notching. Figure-3 sign is due to an abnormal contour of the aortic arch with indentation at the coarctation site. Rib notching is an erosion of the inferior surface of the rib due to dilated and tortuous intercostal arteries (Allen et al., 2016). In late presentation of coarctation, blood flow to the intercostal arteries is increased in order to bypass the area of coarctation.
- EKG abnormalities:
  - Infants: Normal right ventricular dominance with right axis deviation
  - Older child or adult: Left ventricular hypertrophy (LVH)
- Echocardiogram: Initial diagnostic test of choice. Location and degree of coarctation as well as velocity measurements to determine severity.

DEEP VEIN THROMBOSIS

Deep vein thrombosis (DVT) occurs when clots develop in the deep venous systems of the extremities. DVT most commonly involves the lower extremities, but upper extremity DVT is possible. Although it is a common condition, there is risk for serious sequelae, like pulmonary embolus, especially if the diagnosis is missed. There is a lack of key history and physical exam findings that offer strong predictive value for DVT. Therefore, clinical history and exam should be combined with diagnostic testing when evaluating patients (Bates et al., 2012). The two most commonly used diagnostic tests for DVT are D-dimer and US (Bates et al., 2012). D-dimers are performed in patients with low or moderate pretest probability for DVT, and when negative in this setting, D-dimer effectively rules out DVT (Bates et al., 2012; Mousa, 2018). D-dimers are underutilized in clinical practice even though they are moderate to highly sensitive and are useful to "rule out" DVT. However, D-dimers lack specificity because they can also be elevated in non-DVT disorders/conditions like atrial fibrillation or pregnancy (Bates et al., 2012; Mousa et al., 2018). If there is high pretest probability for DVT, either compression US of the proximal veins or whole leg US should be the first-step diagnostic test and D-dimer is not performed. Establishing pretest probability for lower-extremity DVT is accomplished

with clinical prediction rules, of which the Wells' criteria (**Table 6.7**) is the best studied and recommended for clinical use. The Wells' criteria should not be used for inpatients due to poor accuracy in this setting (Silviera et al., 2015).

Key History and Physical Findings

- Active cancer (positive likelihood ratio of this finding is 2.9)
- History of recent immobilization or surgery
- Recent travel
- Unilateral leg edema
- In the outpatient, a score of one or less on the Wells' criteria combined with a negative D-dimer test reduces the probability of DVT to less than 2% (Geersing et al., 2014)
- Erythema, skin tenderness, cool extremities, palpable cord, and Homan's sign are not useful in confirming or negating the presence of DVT (McGee, 2018; **Figure 6.43**)

HEART FAILURE

HF is a complex syndrome caused by ventricular dysfunction and results in the inability of the heart to

TABLE 6.7 Wells' Clinical Prediction Tool	
Criteria	Point
Active cancer	1
Immobilization or paralysis of lower extremity	1
Recent bed restrictions	1
Tenderness along the deep venous system	1
Leg swelling (ankle to thigh)	1
Symptomatic leg swollen >3 cm compared with asymptomatic leg	1
Pitting edema of symptomatic leg > asymptomatic leg	1
Prior DVT	1
Visible collateral superficial veins other than varicose veins	1
Other diagnosis than DVT more or as likely	−2
Low pretest probability of DVT = score of 1 or less High pretest probability = score of 2 or higher	

DVT, deep vein thrombosis.
Source: Wells, P. S., Anderson, D. R., Bormanis, J., Guy, F., Mitchell, M., Gray, L., . . . Lewandowski, B. (1997). Value of assessment of pretest probability of deep-vein thrombosis in clinical management. *The Lancet, 350*(9094), 1795–1798. doi:10.1016/S0140-6736(97)08140-3

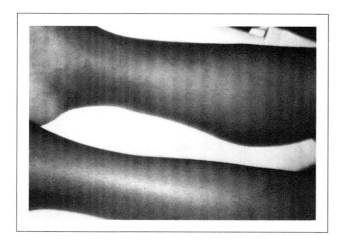

FIGURE 6.43 Deep vein thrombosis.

Source: Image courtesy of Dr. Sellers/Emory University/Centers for Disease Control and Prevention. Retrieved from https://phil.cdc.gov/Details.aspx?pid=1345

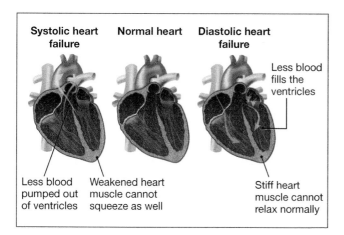

FIGURE 6.44 Heart failure.

sufficiently meet the body's metabolic needs required to sustain life (**Figure 6.44**). It is a result of structural or functional impairment of ventricular filling or ejection of blood (Shah, 2017; Yancy et al., 2013). The term *heart failure* is not the same as *cardiomyopathy* or *LV dysfunction* because the latter two terms describe structural or functional abnormalities that cause HF. There are two main classifications of HF based on EF of LV; HF with preserved ejection fraction (HFpEF) and HF with reduced ejection fraction (HFrEF; Yancy et al., 2013). HFrEF is defined as HF with LVEF ≤40%, and HFpEF is HF with LVEF ≥50% EF. More recently, patients with an LVEF between 40% and 50% have been classified as HF mid-range EF (HFmrEF; Yancy et al., 2013). HF classification is important because it helps describe severity and development of disease progression. It can also guide therapy choices. There are several different

classification systems. The New York Heart Association functional classification system and the ACC/AHA classification are two of the most widely used.

HF has a significant impact on health-related quality of life (HRQoL), including higher rates of depression, higher BMI, low perceived control, and uncertainty about prognosis (Yancy et al., 2013). Risk factors include obesity, smoking, sedentary lifestyle, diet, HTN, diabetes, and history of an AMI. Diagnosis requires a combination of a careful history and examination with evaluation of cardiac structure and function in patients suspected of HF. Because some signs and symptoms (e.g., fatigue, dyspnea, or edema) are nonspecific, it makes obtaining an accurate health history and identifying key physical findings vital (Shah, 2017).

Key History and Physical Findings

- Fatigue
- Anorexia
- Nausea
- Medical history of AMI, LVH
- Weakness
- Arrhythmia or tachycardia
- Dyspnea at rest or with exertion
- Abdominal fluid accumulation (ascites)
- Chest pain, heaviness, or tightness (if caused by an AMI)
- Jugular venous distention
- Cough with white or pink blood-tinged exudate
- Edema, swelling
- Weight gain (can be rapid from fluid retention)
- Nocturia
- Elevated ANH, BNP
- Elevated Gal-3 and sST2 proteins

HYPERTENSION

HTN, or high blood pressure, long known as the silent killer, is a leading risk factor for mortality and disability. In 2018, the ACC and the AHA released updated clinical guidelines advocating for tighter blood pressure control. This is an effort to reduce life-threatening heart attacks and strokes through earlier diagnosis and treatment. Approximately 90% to 95% of individuals with high blood pressure are asymptomatic and have essential (or primary) HTN in which there is no identifiable etiology. HTN can be related to secondary causes, which may include polycystic kidney disease, renovascular disease, Cushing's syndrome, and pheochromocytoma.

Key History and Physical Findings

- Positive family history of cardiac disease and/or HTN
- Diabetes
- Overweight or obese
- Physical inactivity/sedentary lifestyle

- Tobacco use
- Alcohol abuse
- Unhealthy dietary intake, including excessive salt and saturated fats
- Majority are asymptomatic
- History of headaches, nosebleeds
- Elevated blood pressure measurements per guidelines (see Chapter 5, Approach to the Physical Examination, Table 5.7)
- Presence of arteriovenous (AV) nicking, hemorrhages, papilledema, or exudates on fundoscopy
- Distended neck veins, presence of carotid bruits, thyromegaly
- Displacement of PMI, clicks, murmurs, arrhythmias, S3 and S4 heart sounds
- Abdominal bruits, abnormal aortic pulsation, enlarged kidneys
- Lower-extremity edema

INFECTIVE ENDOCARDITIS

Infective endocarditis (IE) is defined as an infection of the endocardial surface of the heart, which may include one or more heart valves, the mural endocardium, or a septal defect (American Heart Association, 2015). It causes severe valvular insufficiency, which may lead to intractable CHF and myocardial abscesses. IE is commonly associated with dental disease and intravenous (IV) drug use. Many organisms have been identified as causative agents; however, *Staphylococcus aureus* has become the primary pathogen of endocarditis. Untreated, it is often fatal. IE presents with a wide range of symptoms from generalized vague malaise to more focal cardiac or neurologic signs.

Key History and Physical Findings

- Fever, chills, malaise
- Dyspnea, cough
- Joint pains
- Petechiae: Common, but nonspecific, finding
- Subungual (splinter) hemorrhages: Dark-red, linear lesions in the nail beds
- Osler's nodes: Tender subcutaneous nodules usually found on the distal pads of the digits
- Janeway lesions: Nontender maculae on the palms and soles
- Focal neurologic deficits, including paralysis, hemiparesis, aphasia
- Delirium
- Gallops
- Rales
- Cardiac arrhythmias
- Pericardial or pleural friction rub

MITRAL VALVE PROLAPSE

MVP is characterized by displacement or prolapse of the mitral valve leaflets into the LA during systole (**Figure 6.45**). The most common cause is due to idiopathic degeneration of the connective tissue of the mitral valve and chordae tendineae (Armstrong, 2018). Development of MVP can lead to the most common complication, mitral regurgitation (MR), that can be further complicated by sudden chordae tendineae rupture (Nishimura et al., 2014). There appears to be a strong hereditary link to the development of MVP. It can be associated with connective tissue diseases or in patients with Graves' disease, sickle cell, or rheumatic heart disease (RHD; Armstrong, 2018). There is evidence that suggests a good prognosis exists with MVP; however, there are instances of serious complications such as sudden cardiac death, endocarditis, or severe MVP (Hayek, Gring, & Griffin, 2005). The degree of leaflet thickness can help ascertain the severity of disease as it is associated with a 14-fold higher risk of complications, including sudden death (Armstrong, 2018; Hayek et al., 2005).

Key History and Physical Findings

- Can be asymptomatic
- Mid-systolic click on auscultation of heart
- Chest pain
- Fatigue
- Dyspnea on exertion
- Anxiety
- Heart palpitations or arrhythmias
- Mitral valve leaflet thickness ≥5 mm by echocardiography

PERICARDITIS

Pericarditis is an inflammation of the pericardium, which is the fibroelastic membrane that surrounds the heart (**Figure 6.46**). The etiology of pericarditis can be an infectious disease process (viral, bacterial, or fungal infections) or a noninfectious disease process

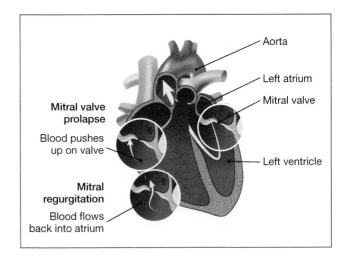

FIGURE 6.45 Mitral valve prolapse and mitral regurgitation.

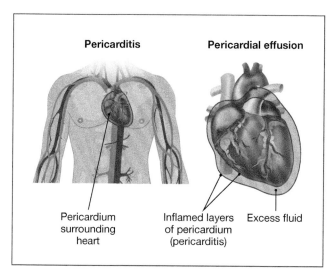

Pericarditis   Pericardial effusion

Pericardium surrounding heart

Inflamed layers of pericardium (pericarditis)

Excess fluid

FIGURE 6.46 Pericarditis.

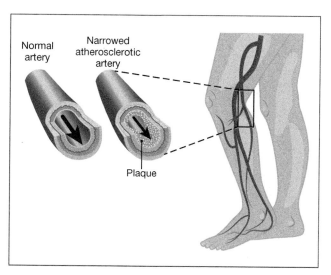

Normal artery

Narrowed atherosclerotic artery

Plaque

FIGURE 6.47 Peripheral artery disease.

(metabolic disorders, trauma, tumors, and autoimmune or autoinflammatory diseases). On rare occasions, it can be drug related, but most causes are labeled idiopathic (Hoit, 2019; Imazio, Gaita, & LeWinter, 2015). Pericarditis may be secondary to a systemic disease process or a primary process unrelated to another systemic disease (Imazio et al., 2015). It can be acute or chronic. The disease can cause cardiac tamponade, which is the presence of fluid in the pericardial sac (Imazio et al., 2015; Shah, 2017).

Key History and Physical Findings

- History of acute trauma
- Chest pain that worsens with breathing and lying down
- Chest pain that improves with sitting upright or leaning forward
- Tachypnea and nonproductive cough
- Fever >100.4°F
- Chills or weakness
- Pericardial friction rub
- If cardiac tamponade (pressure on heart secondary to accumulation of fluid in the pericardial sac) occurs, additional signs (rare) are cool extremities, cyanosis, hypotension, decreased systolic BP >10 mmHg during inspiration

PERIPHERAL ARTERY DISEASE

PAD is an atherosclerotic disease that affects the arteries of the lower extremities (**Figure 6.47**). Disease can occur in the iliac, femoral, popliteal, peroneal, and/or tibial arteries and can be bilateral or unilateral. Patients with PAD may experience IC, an exercise-induced pain in the calves or other parts of the lower extremity. IC occurs because of atherosclerotic obstruction of the

lower-extremity vasculature and is similar to the anginal symptoms in patients with CAD. Traditionally, IC has been considered the hallmark symptom of PAD. However, although it has high specificity for PAD, the absence of IC should not exclude the possibility of PAD because only about a third of patients have typical IC symptoms (Criqui & Aboyans, 2015; McDermott et al., 2001). Other patients have atypical symptoms (like claudication symptoms at rest) and nearly 20% can be asymptomatic (Criqui & Aboyans, 2015; McDermott et al., 2001). The ulcers that are commonly associated with PAD can be difficult to differentiate between PAD and CVI. See **Table 6.6** for common differences in presentation.

Key History and Physical Findings

- Past or present smoking history
- Diabetes
- Chronic kidney disease
- African-American race
- Metabolic syndrome
- Hypertension
- Hyperlipidemia
- Older age (>65)
- Locations of the pain from IC may vary on the basis of the level of the atherosclerosis
- Most commonly causes calf pain
- Aortoiliac disease causes buttock or thigh pain
- Tibial artery disease can cause foot pain
- Femoral and iliac bruits (present in advanced and/or proximal disease)
- Weak or no posterior tibialis and/or dorsalis pedis pulses
- Asymmetric temperature to feet
- Hairless lower extremities and atrophic skin

- Lower-extremity ulcers/wounds usually found on the toes and feet and have a well-demarcated border
- Ulcers are painful and lack edema

RAYNAUD'S PHENOMENON

Raynaud's phenomenon occurs from vasomotor dysfunction that affects the distal arterial circulation of the fingers, toes, earlobes, face, nipples, or nose (**Figure 6.48**). Symptoms occur in response to stress or cold temperatures and the occlusion and spasm of arteries cause distinct episodes of pallor (Wigley & Flavahan, 2016). Traditionally, exacerbations

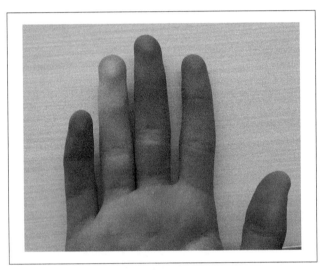

FIGURE 6.48 Raynaud's phenomenon.
Source: Image courtesy of Thomas Galvin.

of Raynaud's phenomenon have been described with a "tricolor" phase of symptoms (from white to blue to red), but it is unusual for patients to experience all three color changes (Dean, 2018). As the recovery of pallor ensues, the affected extremities can become hyperemic and patients may experience pain, numbness, and tingling. Raynaud's phenomenon is divided into two types: primary and secondary. Symptoms are similar between the two types, but there are a few distinctions, which are described in **Table 6.8**. Raynaud's phenomenon is primarily diagnosed through history and physical exam; however, diagnostic tests can be used. Capillaroscopy, thermography, and cold "challenge" or stimulation tests may be used to determine diagnosis, although more research is needed to determine best practice for diagnosis beyond history and presentation (Maverakis et al., 2014).

Key History and Physical Findings

- Female gender
- Family history of Raynaud's
- History of co-occurring vascular diseases like PAD and CVI (Dean, 2018)
- Thinner patients
- Color change of digits, triggered by cold or stress
- Vasospasms last a few minutes to a few hours (Pope, 2013).
- Most commonly, the fingers (index, middle, and ring fingers) are affected, followed by the toes.
- Can affect a single digit or only part of a digit
- Sclerodactyly, or thickening and tightness of the skin of the affected areas, is highly associated with Raynaud's phenomenon (Herrick & Murray, 2018; Maverakis et al., 2014).

TABLE 6.8 Characteristics of Primary and Secondary Raynaud's Phenomenon

Primary Raynaud's Phenomenon	Secondary Raynaud's Phenomenon
- Also called Raynaud's disease - Most common of the two types; usually there is no underlying disease - Does not cause complications like ulcerations (Herrick & Muir, 2014; Pope, 2013) - History of occupational or other upper extremity vibration exposure is common (Pope, 2013; Wigley & Flavahan, 2016) - Capillaroscopy is usually normal.	- Also called Raynaud's syndrome - Due to an underlying disease - Exacerbations are more often asymmetric, more frequent, and more severe. - May cause ulcerations (Herrick & Muir, 2014; Pope, 2013) - History may reveal beta-blocker medications, carpal tunnel syndrome, cancer, hypothyroidism, or kidney disease (Wigley & Flavahan, 2016) - Suspect when presenting symptoms occur after age 40 or in a male (Pope, 2013) - May have underlying history of connective tissue disorders or rheumatoid arthritis (underlying history may not yet be recognized/confirmed at time of evaluation). For example, Raynaud's phenomenon is the most common presenting symptom of systemic sclerosis. - Anti-centromere, anti-RNA polymerase antibody, and antinuclear antibodies used to assess for underlying connective tissue disease (Maverakis et al., 2014) - Capillaroscopy is usually abnormal.

RHEUMATIC HEART DISEASE

RHD is sequelae of rheumatic fever (RF) and is characterized by permanent damage to the heart valves (**Figure 6.49**). RF is an inflammatory response in the body that is a result of strep throat and/or scarlet fever. RHD disproportionately affects those living in poverty with little access to healthcare and untreated

exposure to group A *streptococcus* (Gewitz et al., 2015). Most commonly, the mitral valve is damaged but the aortic valve can also be affected. Usually, the symptoms of RHD show up 10 to 20 years after the original illness. RHD can be prevented by preventing strep infections or treating them with antibiotics when they do occur.

Key History and Physical Findings

- History of suspected rheumatic fever
- History of untreated or undertreated strep throat
- Socioeconomic status
- Pathological heart murmur (mitral or aortic valve stenosis or regurgitation)
- Children may not have any initial symptoms.
- Joint pain and/or arthritis symptoms
- Chest pain or swelling due to myocarditis or pericarditis

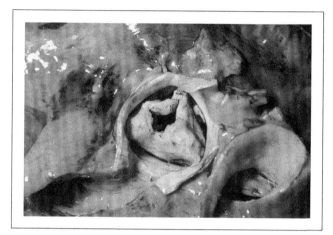

FIGURE 6.49 Rheumatic heart disease with thickened, fused valve leaflets, and severe stenosis, or stricture of the aortic lumen.

Source: Image courtesy of Dr. Edwin P. Ewing, Jr./Centers for Disease Control and Prevention. Retrieved from https://phil.cdc.gov/Details.aspx?pid=848

TETRALOGY OF FALLOT

Tetralogy of Fallot (TOF; **Figure 6.50**) is the most common form of cyanotic congenital heart defects and accounts for approximately 3.5% of CHD (Wernovsky et al., 2020). TOF comprises four different defects: VSD, overriding aorta, pulmonary stenosis (PS), and RV hypertrophy. Because of advances in fetal imaging, there is a high incidence of prenatal diagnosis—up to 70% are diagnosed prenatally and with a 90% accuracy (Allen et al., 2016). TOF has a varied presentation that

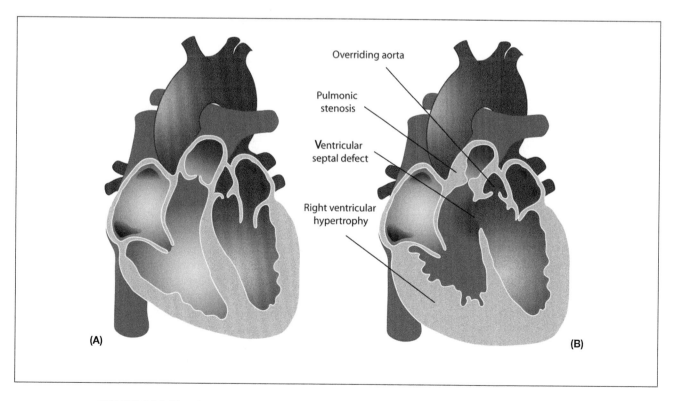

FIGURE 6.50 Tetralogy of Fallot. (A) Normal heart. (B) Heart with Tetralogy of Fallot defects.

is related to the degree of PS or, in some cases, pulmonary atresia (an imperforate pulmonary valve). In TOF, blood flows from the RA to the RV; some blood from the RV may go out the narrowed RV outflow tract (RVOT) depending on the degree of PS, whereas some blood is directed across the VSD to the LV and out the aorta that is situated overriding both ventricles above the VSD. The degree of RVOT obstruction from the PS or pulmonary atresia determines the amount of blue blood that is shunted across the VSD and out the aorta to the systemic circulation. Infants with significant RVOT obstruction from PS may present as very cyanotic in the neonatal period and require earlier surgical intervention. Some infants with pulmonary atresia may have significant major aortopulmonary collateral arteries (MAPCAs) at birth and therefore may not present as cyanotic.

A somewhat unique symptom in TOF from other congenital heart defects is hypercyanotic spells, also known as "Tet spells." In a hypercyanotic spell, the infant experiences an acute decrease in blood across the RVOT, causing the infant to suddenly develop deep blue skin, nails, and lips after crying or feeding. This may be due to hypovolemia or agitation that causes dynamic obstruction from the hypertrophied RV. Infants with hypercyanotic spells may respond well to medical management, but this may also be a consideration for earlier surgery. Infants who have adequate pulmonary blood flow may often go home to feed and grow for several weeks to months before returning for a surgical repair. Infants with TOF who are discharged home before surgery need to be monitored carefully for weight gain as well as symptoms of too little or too much pulmonary blood flow. This presents as hypoxia if there is too much pulmonary blood flow. Either condition can lead to poor liquid intake and failure to thrive in these infants. Most infants with TOF do well with surgical intervention and survive into adulthood.

Key History and Physical Findings

- Family history of CHD
- Genetic syndromes:
  - 22q11.2 deletion (DiGeorge's syndrome)
  - Trisomy 21, 18, 13
  - Holt–Oram syndrome
  - Alagille's syndrome
- Murmur: Systolic ejection murmur at left lower sternal border with a single S2
- Cyanosis: Varying degrees
- Chest x-ray: "Boot-shaped" heart related to RV hypertrophy; may not be as prominent in early diagnosis

- EKG: Shows NSR with rightward axis deviation and RV hypertrophy; may see a right BBB in the postoperative patient
- Echocardiogram: Initial diagnostic test of choice. Degree of PS or atresia with velocity measurements to determine severity, presence of MAPCAs

VENTRICULAR SEPTAL DEFECT

VSD (**Figure 6.51**) is an opening between the RV and the LV. The incidence of VSD is difficult to determine as many spontaneously close. It is estimated to occur in anywhere from 5 to 50 per 1,000 live births. As with an ASD, a VSD often occurs in combination with other heart defects as well as in isolation. VSDs are also classified and described by location along the septum as well as in relation to the atrioventricular valves. The significance of a VSD also depends on the size and location of the defect as well as the pulmonary and systemic vascular resistance. A large defect with left-to-right shunting can result in LV dilation and eventually CHF. Infants with a large VSD may initially be asymptomatic due to elevated pulmonary pressures at birth but may develop symptoms of CHF as lung pressures fall. Small VSDs on the other hand are pressure restrictive, and infants do not develop volume overload or CHF symptoms. Smaller defects may spontaneously close over time. Large VSDs that are left untreated can result in development of CHF, pulmonary vascular disease, and Eisenmenger's syndrome (Wernovsky et al., 2020).

Key History and Physical Findings

- Family history of VSD
- Genetic syndromes:
  - Trisomy 13, 18, and 21
  - Holt–Oram syndrome
- Maternal use of marijuana, cocaine, and paint stripping
- Murmur: Dependent on the size of defect:
  - Large defect: May not have a significant murmur or may have a short systolic ejection murmur
  - Small defect: Loud holosystolic murmur often recognized in early infancy
- Chest x-ray: Small defect may be normal. Large defect may suggest cardiomegaly and increased pulmonary vascular markings.
- EKG: Nonspecific for defect, reflects the hemodynamic state; typically NSR, may demonstrate biventricular hypertrophy in large defects
- Echocardiogram: Demonstrates size and location of VSD as well as volume loading of ventricle; first choice for diagnostic testing

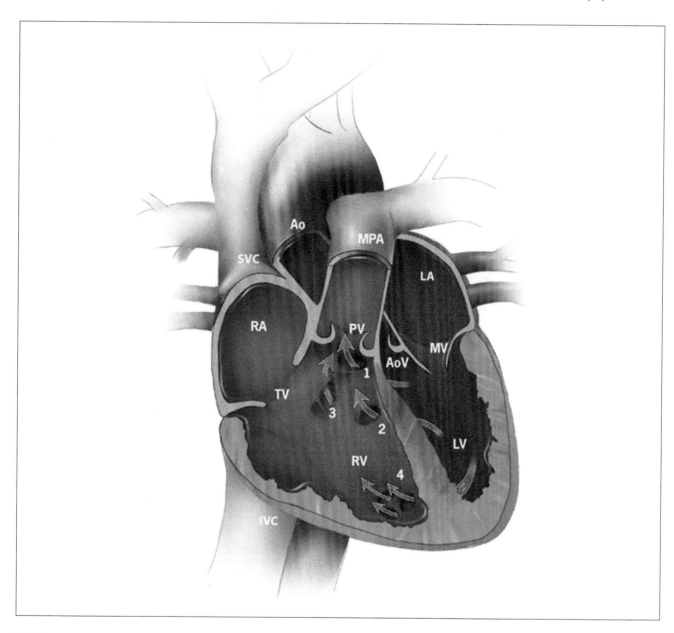

FIGURE 6.51 Ventricular septal defect.

Ao, aorta; AoV, Aortic valve; IVC, inferior vena cava; LA, left atrium; LV, left ventricle; MPA, main pulmonary artery; MV, mitral valve; RA, right atrium; RV, right ventricle; SVC, superior vena cava; TV, tricuspid valve; 1, conoventricular, malaligned; 2, perimembranous; 3, inlet; 4, muscular

Source: Courtesy of the Centers for Disease Control and Prevention.

CASE STUDY: Chest Pain

Presenting Symptoms

AJ is a 52-year-old black woman with chest pain and nausea that started today. Vital signs: Temp 101°F, pulse 88 and irregular, respiratory rate 20/minute, and BP 162/108. BMI 30.

History of Present Illness, Past Medical History, and Review of Symptoms

AJ begins the visit by sharing that she started having suprasternal chest pain early this morning. She first noticed the pain after exercise; the dull, aching, pressure resolved until she was at work. She associates the chest pain that she experienced at work with movement, although it has been sharp, tight, and unremitting. When AJ's coworkers noticed that she was sweating and holding her hands to her chest, they called for an ambulance. She is currently being seen in the emergency department.

AJ shares no personal health history of hypertension, heart disease, or diabetes and has never had this type of pain previously. Family history (father) of "heart problems." AJ is a previous smoker. She quit 2 years ago, after smoking 1/2 pack/day for 30 years. She takes no routine, prescribed medications; takes acetaminophen and ibuprofen as needed; and was given aspirin en route.

Associated symptoms include nausea and lightheadedness; no syncope. She denies shortness of breath. AJ rates her pain as an "8" on a 1 to 10 scale and admits to feeling worried; she has a sense that "something is wrong." She became lightheaded during the assessment. She feels more comfortable supine, but continues to clutch her chest throughout history-taking.

Differential Diagnoses

Unstable angina; AMI; ACS; pericarditis; costochondritis; musculoskeletal strain; GERD; acute gastritis; cholelithiasis; biliary colic; pneumonia; pulmonary embolism

Physical Examination

- General: Diaphoretic; mucosa pink; no rashes; cap refill brisk; no edema; no clubbing
- Head/neck: No carotid bruits; no lymphadenopathy; no obvious JVD
- Cardiovascular: Tachycardia with irregular rhythm; split S2 and soft S1; peripheral pulses equally palpable
- Lungs: No retractions noted; breath sounds full, equal, with scattered wheezes to auscultation; negative tactile fremitus, no egophony noted; O_2 Sat 96%
- Abdomen: Soft, nontender, nondistended; no hepatosplenomegaly, HJR negative
- Neurologic/psychiatric: Speech is clear and distinct; appearance, behavior, and cognition appropriate for the circumstances

Laboratory and Imaging

- 12-lead EKG: Confirmed ST-segment elevation (>1 mm in two anatomically contiguous leads), presence of Q waves
- Cardiac troponin: Significantly elevated
- Comple blood count: Slight elevation in white blood cell count, otherwise normal results; no anemia
- Comprehensive metabolic panel: Normal potassium, magnesium, and creatinine levels; normal blood glucose level
- Color-flow Doppler transthoracic echocardiography: Abnormal wall motion consistent with AMI. *Note that this echo was completed in consultation with cardiology, and the patient was evaluated immediately in the cardiac catheterization lab.*

Final Diagnosis

ST-elevation myocardial infarction (STEMI)

CASE STUDY: Hypertension Follow-Up

Presenting Symptoms

AT is a 40-year-old white female who presents for hypertension and hyperlipidemia follow-up. Vital signs: Temp 98°F, pulse 80, respiratory rate 12/minute, and BP 120/82 in right arm and 122/80 in left arm. BMI 26 (unchanged). Charting note indicates that most recent lipid panel was much improved, with total cholesterol of 198 and LDL of 96. These results were reviewed by phone with AT before this visit.

Review of Wellness and Self-Management of Chronic Disease

- Functional and psychosocial assessment: AT begins the visit by sharing that she is feeling well overall. She monitors her BP twice weekly, and those have been "around 120/80." While she tracks her results, she did not bring the log to the visit today. She is taking lisinopril and atorvastatin daily and denies side effects to medications, is able to afford medications, and remembers to take daily using a pill organizer.
- Assessment of wellness, healthy lifestyle behaviors, and individual health goals: AT is prioritizing exercise and has incorporated 30 minutes of walking into daily routine, minimally 2 or 3 times weekly. She had recent dental and eye exam within the past 6 months.
- Review of collaborative management: AT met with the dietician to discuss sodium intake and verbalized understanding that she should "limit salt" to 1,500 mg daily or less. She states, "I also learned a lot about different hidden salts that are in processed foods."
- Self-management support: AT states she is reading food labels now to identify salt/sodium content. She discussed and reviewed information about sodium content in canned and frozen food.

Review/Update of Family and Social History

- No change in family health history since last visit
- Never a smoker, denies tobacco use, illicit drug use in any form
- Alcohol intake limited to a glass of wine once or twice a year

Focused Review of Systems

- Constitution: Denies recent illnesses, unusual fatigue; no changes in weight
- HEENT: Denies headaches, nosebleeds
- Cardiovascular: Denies chest pain; neck pain; left shoulder, arm, or jaw pain
- Respiratory: Denies cough, shortness of breath
- GI/GU: Denies nausea or vomiting; no changes in menstrual cycle
- Psychiatric: States stress level has been manageable and believes that she has good coping mechanisms for stress; denies feeling low, down, or depressed in the past 2 weeks; has activities that she is able to enjoy

Differential Diagnoses

Hypertension, controlled; hyperlipidemia

Physical Examination

- General: In no distress; comfortably sitting on exam table; alert and oriented
- Eyes: Conjunctiva, sclera clear; red reflex present, fundoscopic exam normal with no AV nicking or retinal hemorrhages noted
- Head/neck: Thyroid palpable, smooth, no palpable nodularity; no lymphadenopathy; no carotid bruits to auscultation, no obvious JVD
- Cardiovascular: S1 and S2 distinct, heart rate/rhythm regular with no murmurs or gallops noted
- Lungs: Breath sounds full, equal, and clear bilaterally; no adventitious sounds
- Peripheral vascular: Peripheral pulses palpable and equal bilaterally; no edema of lower extremities
- Abdomen: No aortic, renal, or iliac bruits; soft, nontender, nondistended
- Neurologic/psychiatric: Speech is clear and distinct; appearance, behavior, and cognition appropriate for the circumstances

Laboratory and Imaging

Consider lipid profile before next follow-up visit

Final Diagnoses

Hypertension, controlled; hyperlipidemia, controlled

Clinical Pearls

- Auscultation is a sensitive, specific, and effective method for detecting how the cardiac system is functioning. The heart sound S1 indicates the beginning of systole and coincides with the apical pulse. S2 indicates diastole, closure of the aortic and pulmonic valves, and thus is heard best at the base.
  - Systolic murmurs occur between S1 and S2, during ventricular contraction. Systolic murmurs include aortic stenosis, mitral regurgitation, and tricuspid regurgitation.
  - Diastolic murmurs occur after S2 and before S1, during heart muscle relaxation between impulses. Diastolic murmurs include MS and AR.
  - Physiological split S2 sounds are normal, especially during childhood. The split increases with inspiration and decreases on expiration.
  - Additional sounds that are auscultated as a gallop, S3 and S4, can signify pathologies associated with ischemia or HF.
- The heart's conduction system is assessed using an EKG.
  - The EKG begins with the P-wave, which is atrial activation or depolarization.
  - The QRS complex represents ventricular depolarization.
  - The T-wave equates to ventricular repolarization.
  - EKG changes associated with ischemia include ST-segment depression or T-wave inversion.
  - EKG changes associated with infarction include ST elevation, ST depression, and the development of Q waves.

Key Takeaways

- Understanding the structure and function of the cardiovascular and peripheral vascular systems provides the foundation for evidence-based assessment.
- Completing a comprehensive, evidence-based history and physical examination when an individual presents with concerns, symptoms, and/or risks related to the cardiovascular and peripheral vascular systems provides a clinician with the opportunity to identify and distinguish between normal and abnormal findings.
- Early recognition of ACS, AMI, arrhythmias, heart defects, HF, and heart disease can reduce costs and improve and save lives.

REFERENCES

Aboyans, V., Criqui, M. H., Abraham, P., Allison, M. A., Creager, M. A., Diehm, C., & Treat-Jacobson, D. (2012). Measurement and interpretation of the Ankle-Brachial Index: A scientific statement from the American Heart Association. *Circulation, 126*(24), 2890–2909. doi:10.1161/CIR.0b013e318276fbcb

Agouridis, A. P., Elisaf, M. S., Nair, D. R., & Mikhailidis, D. P. (2015). Ear lobe crease: A marker of coronary artery disease? *Archives of Medical Science, 11*(6), 1145–1155. doi:10.5114/aoms.2015.56340

Allen, H. D., Shaddy, R. E., Penny, D. J., Feltes, T. F., & Cetta, F. (Eds.). (2016). *Moss and Adam's heart disease in infants, children, and adolescents* (9th ed.). Philadelphia, PA: Wolters Kluwer.

Al-Naher, A., Wright, D., Devonald, M., & Pirmohamed, M. (2018). Renal function monitoring in heart failure—What is the optimal frequency? A narrative review. *British Journal of Clinical Pharmacology, 84*(1), 5–17. doi:10.1111/bcp.13434

American Academy of Family Physicians. (2013). Don't screen for carotid artery stenosis (CAS) in asymptomatic adult patients. Retrieved from https://www.choosingwisely/org/c;omocoam-lists/american-academy-family-physicians-carotid-artery-stenosis

American College of Cardiology. (2019). Five things physicians and patients should question. Retrieved from http://www.choosingwisely.org/societies/american-college-of-cardiology

American College of Cardiology/American Heart Association Task Force on Clinical Practice Guidelines. (2018). 2017 ACC/AHA/AAPA/ABC/ACPM/AGS/APhA/ASH/ASPC/NMA/PCNA guideline for the prevention, detection, evaluation, and management of high blood pressure in adults. *Journal of the American College of Cardiology, 71*(19), e127–e248. doi:10.1016/j.jacc.2017.11.006

American Heart Association. (2015). Infective endocarditis in adults: Diagnosis, antimicrobial therapy, and management of complications: A scientific statement for healthcare professionals from the American Heart Association. *Circulation, 132,* 1435–1486. doi:10.1161/CIR.0000000000000296

American Society of Nuclear Cardiology. (2012). Five things physicians and patients should question. Retrieved from http://www.choosingwisely.org/societies/american-society-of-nuclear-cardiology

Armstrong, G. (2018). Mitral valve prolapse (MVP). In R. S. Porter (Ed.), *Merck Manual Professional Version*. Retrieved from https://www.merckmanuals.com/professional

/cardiovascular-disorders/valvular-disorders/mitral-valve-prolapse-mvp?query=mitral%20valve%20prolapse

Arnett, D. K., Blumenthal, R. S., Albert, M. A., Buroker, A. B., Goldberger, Z. D., Hahn, E. J., . . . Ziaeian, B. (2019). 2019 ACC/AHA guideline on the primary prevention of cardiovascular disease. *Journal of the American College of Cardiology, 74*(10), e177–e232. doi:10.1016/j.jacc.2019.03.010

Bates, S. M., Jaeschke, R., Stevens, S. M., Goodacre, S., Wells, P. S., Stevenson, M. D., . . . Guyatt, G. H. (2012). Diagnosis of DVT. *Chest, 141*(2 Suppl.), e351S–e418S. doi:10.1378/chest.11-2299

Betts, J. G., Young, K. A., Wise, J. A., Johnson, E., Poe, B., Kruse, D. H., . . . DeSaix P. (2013). *Anatomy and physiology.* Retrieved from https://openstax.org/books/anatomy-and-physiology/pages/19-1-heart-anatomy#fig-ch20_01_04

Budoff, M. J., Dowe, D., Jollis, J. G., Gitter, M., Sutherland, J., Halamert, E., . . . Min, J. K. (2008). Diagnostic performance of 64-multidetector row coronary computed tomographic angiography for evaluation of coronary artery stenosis in individuals without known coronary artery disease. *Journal of the American College of Cardiology, 52*(21), 1724–1732. doi:10.1016/j.jacc.2008.07.031

Catapano, A. L., Graham, I., De Backer, G., Wiklund, O., Chapman, M. J., Drexel, H., . . . Zamorano, J. L. (2016). 2016 ESC/EAS guidelines for the management of dyslipidaemias: The Task Force for the Management of Dyslipidaemias of the European Society of Cardiology (ESC) and European Atherosclerosis Society (EAS) developed with the special contribution of the European Association for Cardiovascular Prevention & Rehabilitation (EACPR). *Atherosclerosis, 253,* 281–344. doi:10.1016/j.atherosclerosis.2016.08.018

Centers for Disease Control and Prevention. (n.d.). *Public health image library (PHIL).* Retrieved from https://phil.cdc.gov/Details.aspx?pid=2457

Cheng, T. O. (2010). Upright versus supine position in examining a patient with hypertrophic cardiomyopathy. *International Journal of Cardiology, 142*(1), 1. doi:10.1016/j.ijcard.2009.11.054

Chizner, M. A. (2002). The diagnosis of heart disease by clinical assessment alone. *Disease-a-Month, 48*(1), 7–98. doi:10.1067/mda.2002.115501

Chua Chicao, J. M., Parikh, N. I., & Fergusson, D. J. (2013). The jugular venous pressure revisited. *Cleveland Clinical Journal of Medicine, 80*(10), 638–644. doi:10.3949/ccjm.80a13039

Conn, R. D., & O'Keefe, J. H. (2012). Simplified evaluation of the jugular venous pressure: Significance of inspiratory collapse of jugular veins. *Missouri Medicine, 109*(2), 150–152. Retrieved from http://www.omagdigital.com/publication/?i=108895#{%22issue_id%22:108895,%22page%22:0}

Cosford, P. A., Leng, G. C., & Thomas, J. (2007). Screening for abdominal aortic aneurysm. *Cochrane Database of Systematic Reviews,* (2), CD002945. doi:10.1002/14651858.CD002945.pub2

Criqui, M. H., & Aboyans, V. (2015). Epidemiology of peripheral artery disease. *Circulation Research, 116*(9), 1509–1526. doi:10.1161/CIRCRESAHA.116.303849

Dean, S. M. (2018). Cutaneous manifestations of chronic vascular disease. *Progress in Cardiovascular Diseases, 60*(6), 567–579. doi:10.1016/j.pcad.2018.03.004

Drazner, M. H., Rame, J. E., Stevenson, L. W., & Dries, D. L. (2001). Prognostic importance of elevated jugular venous pressure and a third heart sound in patient with heart failure. *New England Journal of Medicine, 345*(8), 574–581. doi:10.1056/NEJMoa01641

Eberhardt, R. T., & Raffetto, J. D. (2014). Chronic venous insufficiency. *Circulation, 130*(4), 333–346. doi:10.1161/CIRCULATIONAHA.113.006898

Elder, A., Japp, A., & Verghese, A. (2016). How valuable is physical examination of the cardiovascular system? *British Medical Journal, 354,* i3309. doi:10.1136/bmji3309

Ewy, G. A. (1988). The abdominojugular test: Technique and hemodynamic correlates. *Annuals of Internal Medicine, 109*(6), 456–460. doi:10.7326/0003-4819-109-6-456

Fanaroff, A. C., Rymer, J. A., Goldstein, S. A., Simel, D. L., & Newby, L. K. (2015). Does this patient with chest pain have acute coronary syndrome?: The rational clinical examination systematic review. *Journal of the American Medical Association, 314*(18), 1955–1965. doi:10.1001/jama.2015.12735

Fihn, S. D., Gardin, J. M., Abrams, J., Berra, K., Blankenship, J. C., Dallas, A. P., . . . Williams, S. V. (2012). 2012 ACCF/AHA/ACP/AATS/PCNA/SCAI/STS guideline for the diagnosis and management of patients with stable ischemic heart disease. *Journal of the American College of Cardiology, 60*(24), e44–e164. doi:10.1016/j.jacc.2012.07.013

Fleisher, L. A., Fleischmann, K. E., Auerbach, A. D., Barnason, S. A., Beckman, J. A., Bozkurt, B., . . . Wijeysundera, D. N. (2014). 2014 ACC/AHA guideline on perioperative cardiovascular evaluation and management of patients undergoing noncardiac surgery. *Journal of the American College of Cardiology, 64*(22), e77–137. doi:10.1016/j.jacc.2014.07.944

Fletcher, G. F., Ades, P. A., Kligfield, P., Arena, R., Balady, G. J., Bittner, V. A., . . . Williams, M. A. (2013). Exercise standards for testing and training. *Circulation, 128*(8), 873–934. doi:10.1161/cir.0b013e31829b5b44

Gardezi, S. K., Myerson, S. G., Chambers, J., Coffey, S., d'Arcy, J., Hobbs, R., . . . Prendergast, B. D. (2018). Cardiac auscultation poorly predicts the presence of valvular heart disease in asymptomatic primary care patients. *Heart, 104*(22), 1832–1835. doi:10.1136/heartjnl-2018-313082

Geersing, G. J., Zuithoff, N. P. A., Kearon, C., Anderson, D. R., ten Cate-Hoek, A. J., Elf, J. L., . . . Moons, K. G. M. (2014, March 10). Exclusion of deep vein thrombosis using the Wells rule in clinically important subgroups: Individual patient data meta-analysis. *BMJ, 348,* g1340–g1340. doi:10.1136/bmj.g1340

Gerhard-Herman, M. D., Gornik, H. L., Barrett, C., Barshes, N. R., Corriere, M. A., Drachman, D. E., . . . Walsh, M. E. (2017). 2016 AHA/ACC guideline on the management of patients with lower extremity peripheral artery disease: Executive summary. *Circulation, 135,* e686–e725. doi:10.1161/CIR.0000000000000470

Gewitz, M. H., Baltimore, R. S., Tani, L. Y., Sable, C. A., Shulman, S. T., Carapetis, J., . . . Kaplan, E. L. (2015). Revision of the Jones criteria for the diagnosis of acute rheumatic fever in the era of Doppler echocardiography: A scientific statement from the American Heart Association. *Circulation, 131*(20), 1806–1818. doi:10.1161/CIR.0000000000000205

Gloviczki, P., Comerota, A. J., Dalsing, M. C., Eklof, B. G., Gillespie, D. L., Gloviczki, M. L., . . . Wakefield, T. W. (2011). The care of patients with varicose veins and associated chronic venous diseases: Clinical practice guidelines of the Society for Vascular Surgery and the American Venous Forum. *Journal of Vascular Surgery, 53*(5), 2S–48S. doi:10.1016/j.jvs.2011.01.079

Goolsby, M. J. & Grubbs, L. (2019). Abdomen. In M. J. Goolsby & L. Grubbs (Eds.), *Advanced assessment: Interpreting findings and formulating differential diagnoses.* (4th ed.). (pp. 275–325). Philadelphia, PA: F. A. Davis.

Grey, J. E., Harding, K. G., & Enoch, S. (2006). Venous and arterial leg ulcers. *BMJ, 332*(7537), 347–350. doi:10.1136/bmj.332.7537.347

Hayek, E., Gring, C. N., & Griffin, B. P. (2005). Mitral valve prolapse. *Lancet, 365*(9458), 507–518. doi:10.1016/S0140-6736(05)17869-6

Heckerling, P. S., Weiner, S. L., Moses, V. K., Claudio, J., Kushner, M. S., & Hand, R. (1991). Accuracy of precordial percussion in detecting cardiomegaly. *The American Journal of Medicine, 91*, 328–334. doi:10.1016/0002-9343(91)90149-R

Heckerling, P. S., Weiner, S. L., Wolfkiel, C. J., Kushner, M. S., Dodin, E. M., Jelnin, V., . . . Chomka, E. V. (1993). Accuracy and reproducibility of precordial percussion and palpation for detecting increased left ventricular end-diastolic volume and mass. *Journal of the American Medical Association, 270*(16), 1943–1948. doi:10.1001/jama.1993.03510160061030

Herrick, A., & Muir, L. (2014). Raynaud's phenomenon (secondary). *BMJ Clinical Evidence, 2014*, 1125. Retrieved from https://www.ncbi.nlm.nih.gov/pmc/articles/PMC4200538

Herrick, A. L., & Murray, A. (2018). The role of capillaroscopy and thermography in the assessment and management of Raynaud's phenomenon. *Autoimmunity Reviews, 17*(5), 465–472. doi:10.1016/j.autrev.2017.11.036

Hoit, B. (2019). Pericarditis. In R. S. Porter (Ed.), *Merck Manual Professional Version.* Retrieved from https://www.merckmanuals.com/professional/cardiovascular-disorders/myocarditis-and-pericarditis/pericarditis?query=pericarditis

Imazio, M., Gaita, F., & LeWinter, M. (2015). Evaluation and treatment of pericarditis: A systematic review. *Journal of the American Medical Association, 314*(14), 1498–1506. doi:10.1001/jama.2015.12763

Labropoulos, N., Leon, M., Nicolaides, A. N., Giannoukas, A. D., Volteas, N., & Chan, P. (1994). Superficial venous insufficiency: Correlation of anatomic extent of reflux with clinical symptoms and signs. *Journal of Vascular Surgery, 20*, 953–958. doi:10.1016/0741-5214(94)90233-X

LeFevre, M. L. (2014). Screening for asymptomatic carotid artery stenosis: US Preventative Task Force recommendation statement. *Annals of Internal Medicine, 161*, 356–362. doi:10.7326/M14-1333

Madhero88. (n.d.). *Phonocardiograms from normal and abnormal heart sounds with pressure diagrams with location on the precordium* [Image file]. Retrieved from https://commons.wikimedia.org/wiki/File:Phonocar-diograms_from_normal_and_abnormal_heart_sounds.png#/media/File:Phonocardiograms_from_normal_and_abnormal_heart_sounds_with_pressure_diagrams_with_location_on_the_precordium.png

Maverakis, E., Patel, F., Kronenberg, D. G., Chung, L., Fiorentino, D., Allanore, Y., . . . Gershwin, M. E. (2014). International consensus criteria for the diagnosis of Raynaud's phenomenon. *Journal of Autoimmunity, 48–49*, 60–65. doi:10.1016/j.jaut.2014.01.020

McColgan, P., Bentley, P., McCarron, M., & Sharma, P. (2012). Evaluation of the clinical utility of a carotid bruit. *Quality Journal of Medicine, 105*, 1171–1177. doi:10.1093/qjmed/hcs140

McDermott, M. M., Greenland, P., Liu, K., Guralnik, J. M., Criqui, M. H., Dolan, N. C., . . . Martin, G. J. (2001). Leg symptoms in peripheral arterial disease: Associated clinical characteristics and functional impairment. *Journal of the American Medical Association, 286*(13), 1599–1606. doi:10.1001/jama.286.13.1599

McGee, S. R. (2018). *Evidence-based physical diagnosis* (4th ed., pp. 473–480, 461–468). Philadelphia, PA: Elsevier/Saunders.

Miranda, W. R., & Nishimura, R. A. (2017). The history, physical examination, and cardiac auscultation. In V. Fuster, R. Harrington, J. Narula, & Z. Eapen (Eds.), *Hurst's the heart* (14th ed., Chapter 11). New York, NY: McGraw-Hill Education. Retrieved from https://accessmedicine.mhmedical.com/book.aspx?bookID=2046

Mousa, A. Y., Broce, M., De Wit, D., Baskharoun, M., Abu-Halimah, S., Yacoub, M., & Bates, M. C. (2018). Appropriate use of venous imaging and analysis of the D-dimer/clinical probability testing paradigm in the diagnosis and location of deep venous thrombosis. *Annals of Vascular Surgery, 50*, 21–29. doi:10.1016/j.avsg.2017.12.006

Nasir, K., Michos, E. D., Blumenthal, R. S., & Raggi, P. (2005). Detection of high-risk young adults and women by coronary calcium and National Cholesterol Education Program Panel III guidelines. *Journal of the American College of Cardiology, 46*(10), 1931–1936. doi:10.1016/j.jacc.2005.07.052

Nishimura, R. A., Otto, C. M., Bonow, R. O., Carabello, B. A., Erwin, J. P., III, Guyton, R. A., . . . Thomas, J. D. (2014). 2014 AHA/ACC guideline for the management of patients with valvular heart disease: A report of the American College of Cardiology/American Heart Association Task Force on Practice Guidelines. *Circulation, 129*(23), e521–e643. doi:10.1161/CIR.0000000000000031

Norton, C. (2017). Acute coronary syndrome: Assessment and management. *Nursing Standard, 31*(29), 61–71. doi:10.7748/ns.2017.e10754

O'Gara, P. T., & Loscalzo, J. (2017). Physical examination of the cardiovascular system. In J. L. Jameson, A. S. Facui, D. L. Kasper, S. L. Hauser, D. L. Longo, & J. Loscalzo (Eds.), *Harrison's principles of internal medicine* (20th ed., Chapter 234). New York, NY: McGraw-Hill. Retrieved from https://accessmedicine.mhmedical.com/content.aspx?bookid=2129&sectionid=186950064

Park, M. (2016). *Park's the pediatric cardiology handbook* (5th ed.). Philadelphia, PA: Elsevier Saunders.

Patel, A., Tomar, N. S., Singh, N., & Bharani, A. (2016). Utility of physical examination and comparison to echocardiography for cardiac diagnosis. *Indian Heart Journal, 69*, 141–145. doi:10.1016/j.ihj2016.07.020

Pellikka, P. A., Nagueh, S. F., Elhendy, A. A., Kuehl, C. A., & Sawada, S. G. (2007). American Society of Echocardiography recommendations for performance, interpretation, and application of stress echocardiography. *Journal of the American Society of Echocardiography, 20*(9), 1021–1041. doi:10.1016/j.echo.2007.07.003

Piek, A., Du, W., de Boer, R. A., & Silljé, H. H. (2018). Novel heart failure biomarkers: Why do we fail to exploit their potential? *Critical Reviews in Clinical Laboratory Sciences, 55*(4), 246–263. doi:10.1080/10408363.2018.1460576

Pletcher, M. J., Tice, J. A., Pignone, M., & Browner, W. S. (2004). Using the coronary artery calcium score to predict coronary heart disease events. *Archives of Internal Medicine, 164*(12), 1285. doi:10.1001/archinte.164.12.1285

Pope, J. (2013). Raynaud's phenomenon (primary). *BMJ Clinical Evidence, 2013*, 1119. Retrieved from https://www.ncbi.nlm.nih.gov/pmc/articles/PMC3794700

Remick, J., Georgiopoulou, V., Marti, C., Ofotokun, I., Kalogeropoulos, A., Lewis, W., & Butler, J. (2014). Heart failure in patients with human immunodeficiency virus infection: Epidemiology, pathophysiology, treatment, and future research. *Circulation, 129*(17), 1781–1789. doi:10.1161/CIRCULATIONAHA.113.004574

Roldan, C. A., Shively, B. K., & Crawford, M. H. (1996). Value of the cardiovascular physical examination for detecting valvular heart disease in asymptomatic subjects. *American Journal of Cardiology, 77*, 1327–1331. doi:10.1016/S0002-9149(96)00200-7

Scheffold, N., Herkommer, B., Kandolf, R., & May, A. E. (2015). Lyme carditis—diagnosis, treatment and prognosis. *Deutsches Ärzteblatt International, 112*(12), 202–208. doi:10.3238/arztebl.2015.0202

Shah, S. (2017). Heart failure (HF). In R. S. Porter (Ed.), *Merck Manual Professional Version*. Retrieved from https://www.merckmanuals.com/professional/cardiovascular-disorders/heart-failure/heart-failure-hf?query=Heart%20failure

Silveira, P. C., Ip, I. K., Goldhaber, S. Z., Piazza, G., Benson, C. B., & Khorasani, R. (2015). Performance of wells score for deep vein thrombosis in the inpatient setting. *JAMA Internal Medicine, 175*(7), 1112. doi:10.1001/jamainternmed.2015.1687

Silverman, B., & Gertz, A. (2015). Present role of the precordial examination in patient care. *American Journal of Cardiology, 115*, 253–255. doi:10.1016/j.amjcard.2014.10.031

Sinsalo, J., Rapola, J., Rossinen, J., & Kupari, M. (2007). Simplifying the estimation of jugular venous pressure. *American Journal of Cardiology, 100*(12), 1779–1781. doi:10.1016/j.amjcard.2007.07.030

Sochowski, R. A., Dubbin, J. D., & Naqvi, S. Z. (1990). Clinical and hemodynamic assessment of hepatojugular reflux. *American Journal of Cardiology, 66*(12), 10002–1006. doi:10.1016/0002-9149(90)90940-3

Spentzouris, G., & Labropoulos, N. (2009). The evaluation of lower extremity ulcers. *Seminars in Interventional Radiology, 26*(4), 286–295. doi:10.1055/s-0029-1242204

Stary, H. C., Chandler, A. B., Dinsmore, R. E., Fuster, V., Glagov, S., Insull, W., Jr., . . . Wissler, R. W. (1995). A definition of advanced types of atherosclerotic lesions and a histological classification of atherosclerosis. A report from the Committee on Vascular Lesions of the Council on Arteriosclerosis, American Heart Association. *Circulation, 92*(5), 1355–1374. doi:10.1161/01.cir.92.5.1355

Sweis, R., & Jivan, A. (2018). Overview of acute coronary syndromes (ACS). In R. S. Porter (Ed.), *Merck Manual Professional Version*. Retrieved from https://www.merckmanuals.com/professional/cardiovascular-disorders/coronary-artery-disease/overview-of-acute-coronary-syndromes-acs#v934825

Thanassoulis, G., & Afshar, M. (2019). Atherosclerosis. In R. S. Porter (Ed.), *Merck Manual Professional Version*. Retrieved from https://www.merckmanuals.com/professional/cardiovascular-disorders/arteriosclerosis/atherosclerosis?query=atherosclerosis

U.S. Preventive Services Task Force. (2013). Final recommendation statement: Blood pressure in children and adolescents (hypertension): Screening. Retrieved from https://www.uspreventiveservicestaskforce.org/Page/Document/RecommendationStatementFinal/blood-pressure-in-children-and-adolescents-hypertension-screening

U.S. Preventive Services Task Force. (2014). Final update summary: Abdominal aortic aneurysm: Screening. Retrieved from https://www.uspreventiveservicestaskforce.org/Page/Document/UpdateSummaryFinal/abdominal-aortic-aneurysm-screening

U.S. Preventive Services Task Force. (2015). Final recommendation statement: High blood pressure in adults: Screening. Retrieved from https://www.uspreventiveservicestaskforce.org/Page/Document/RecommendationStatementFinal/high-blood-pressure-in-adults-screening

U.S. Preventive Services Task Force. (2018a). Final recommendation statement: Cardiovascular disease: Risk assessment with nontraditional risk factors. Retrieved from https://www.uspreventiveservicestaskforce.org/Page/Document/RecommendationStatementFinal/cardiovascular-disease-screening-using-nontraditional-risk-assessment

U.S. Preventive Services Task Force. (2018b). Final update summary: Cardiovascular disease risk: Screening with electrocardiography. Retrieved from https://www.uspreventiveservicestaskforce.org/Page/Document/UpdateSummaryFinal/cardiovascular-disease-risk-screening-with-electrocardiography

Vinayak, A. G., Levitt, J., Gehlbach, B., Pohlman, A. S., Hall, J. B., & Kress, J. P. (2006). Usefulness of the external jugular vein examination in detecting abnormal central venous pressure in critically ill patients. *Archives of Internal Medicine, 166*(19), 2132–2137. doi:10.1001/archinte.166.19.2132

Wells, P. S., Anderson, D. R., Bormanis, J., Guy, F., Mitchell, M., Gray, L., . . . Lewandowski, B. (1997). Value of assessment of pretest probability of deep-vein thrombosis in clinical management. *The Lancet, 350*(9094), 1795–1798. doi:10.1016/S0140-6736(97)08140-3

Wernovsky, G., Anderson, R. H., Kumar, K., Mussaton, K., Redington, A., & Tweddell, J. S. (Eds.). (2020). *Anderson's pediatric cardiology* (4th ed.). Philadelphia, PA: Elsevier.

Wigley, F. M., & Flavahan, N. A. (2016). Raynaud's phenomenon. *New England Journal of Medicine, 375*, 556–565. doi: 10.1056/NEJMra1507638

Yancy, C. W., Jessup, M., Bozkurt, B., Butler, J., Casey, D. E., Jr., Drazner, M. H., ... Wilkoff, B. L. (2013). 2013 ACCF/AHA guideline for the management of heart failure: A report of the American College of Cardiology Foundation/American Heart Association Task Force on Practice Guidelines. *Circulation, 128*(16), e240–e319. doi:10.1161/CIR.0b013e31829e8776

Ye, F., Winchester, D., Jansen, M., Lee, A., Silverstein, B., Stalvey, C., ... Yale, S. H. (2019). Assessing prognosis of acute coronary syndrome in recent clinical trials: A systematic review. *Clinical Medicine & Research, 17*(1), 11–19. doi:10.3121/cmr.2019.1433

7

Evidence-Based Assessment of the Lungs and Respiratory System

Alice M. Teall, Oralea A. Pittman, and Vinciya Pandian

*"Breathe deeply until sweet air extinguishes the burn of fear in your lungs
and every breath is a beautiful refusal to become anything less than infinite."*

—D. ANTOINETTE FOY

VIDEOS

- Patient Case: Adult With Cough (Pneumonia)
- Patient Case: Adolescent With Asthma Exacerbation

LEARNING OBJECTIVES

- Describe the structure and function of the respiratory system.
- Determine key assessments for evaluating the lungs and respiratory system.
- Identify assessment findings and signs and symptoms, indicating abnormalities, problems, disorders, and/or diseases of the respiratory system.

ANATOMY AND PHYSIOLOGY OF THE LUNGS AND RESPIRATORY SYSTEM

The anatomic structures of the respiratory system function to move air between the environment and the lungs and to provide for the exchange of oxygen and carbon

Visit https://connect.springerpub.com/content/book/978-0-8261
-6454-4/chapter/ch00 to access the videos.

dioxide. The processes of ventilation and diffusion are the chief functions of the pulmonary system; assessing for disruption or impairment is of prime importance.

ANATOMIC STRUCTURES OF THE THORAX
Landmarks of the Chest Wall

The region of the body designated as the **thorax** extends from the base of the neck to the diaphragm and includes the chest or thoracic cage and cavity. The thoracic cage, surrounded by muscle, skin, and fasciae, provides protection to vital organs, which include the lungs, heart, liver, and major vessels, and is able to move as the lungs expand. **Figure 7.1** illustrates the components of the chest cavity, and **Figure 7.2** illustrates the structures of the thoracic cage, which include the sternum, ribs, and cartilages.

Reference lines are used to note the anatomic landmarks of the chest wall. Assessment findings of the thoracic cage should include notation of the landmarks using directional terms as noted in **Figure 7.3**. Anterior, posterior, and lateral reference lines allow the clinician to more precisely describe, report, and interpret findings. These imagined reference lines and their locations include the following:

- *Midsternal line:* Vertical line extends down the middle of the sternum.
- *Midclavicular line:* Vertical line begins midway between the suprasternal notch and the acromioclavicular joint and extends just medial to the nipple.

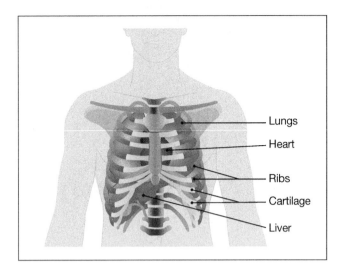

FIGURE 7.1 Chest cavity and vital organs.

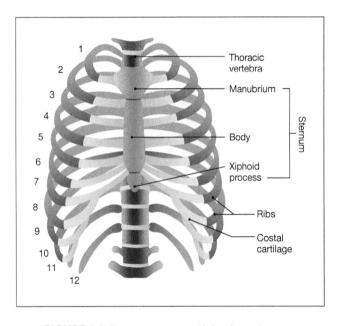

FIGURE 7.2 Bony structures of the thoracic cage.

- *Anterior axillary line:* Vertical line extends along the anterior axillary fold and is formed by the pectoralis major muscle.
- *Midaxillary line:* Vertical line extends along the lateral border of the thoracic wall.
- *Posterior axillary line:* Vertical line parallel to the anterior axillary line extends along the posterior axillary fold formed by the latissimus dorsi muscle.
- *Vertebral line:* Vertical line extends down the vertebral column.
- *Scapular line:* Vertical line extends down from the inferior angle of the scapula.

Anterior Chest Wall

Bony landmarks of the anterior chest wall allow for assessment of the clavicles, sternum, ribs, and the cartilages. These anterior chest wall structures are illustrated in **Figure 7.4**.

The two clavicles, commonly called collarbones, extend between the manubrium of the sternum and the acromion processes of the scapula. Clavicles are prominent bones typically visible under the skin that serve to attach the upper limbs to the trunk, protect the underlying neurovascular structures, and transmit force from the upper limb to the trunk.

The sternum can be differentiated into three main structures—the manubrium, body, and xiphoid process. It is important to be able to appreciate the different structures during advanced assessment for a number of reasons: (a) When patients have difficulty breathing, **retractions** in the suprasternal notch (the area immediately above the sternum) may be observed as a sinking in or pulling in of the muscles, (b) jugular venous pressure is assessed at the sternal angle or manubriosternal junction, where the manubrium and the sternal body meet, and (c) during cardiopulmonary resuscitation, the xiphoid process may be used as a bony landmark to determine the location for administering chest compressions. Pressure should not be exerted directly on the xiphoid process, as this can cause the xiphoid process to fracture and separate from the sternum, possibly puncturing the diaphragm or liver.

The thoracic cage is made up of 12 pairs of ribs and associated cartilages. The space between two ribs is called the intercostal space. Clinically, the second intercostal space is relevant to the space used for needle decompression when a patient has a pneumothorax (collapsed lung). The fourth intercostal space is used for chest tube insertion. The first seven ribs are connected to cartilages that are directly articulated with the sternum. The 8th, 9th, and 10th ribs are connected to their associated cartilages but articulate with the cartilages above them. The 11th and 12th ribs are free floating and do not connect with any cartilages.

When assessing the chest wall in women, attention needs to be directed to the presence of breast tissue. One may need to displace the breast tissue to assess the anterior chest wall more effectively.

Posterior Chest Wall

Bony landmarks of the posterior chest wall allow for assessment of the vertebral column, posterior aspects of the ribs, and the scapula. These posterior chest wall structures are illustrated in **Figure 7.5**. The thoracic vertebrae designated as T1 to T12 provide attachment for the ribs and stability for the posterior thoracic cage, which protects the heart and lungs.

Posteriorly, the 12th rib can be palpated easily and serves as a landmark to start counting the ribs upward.

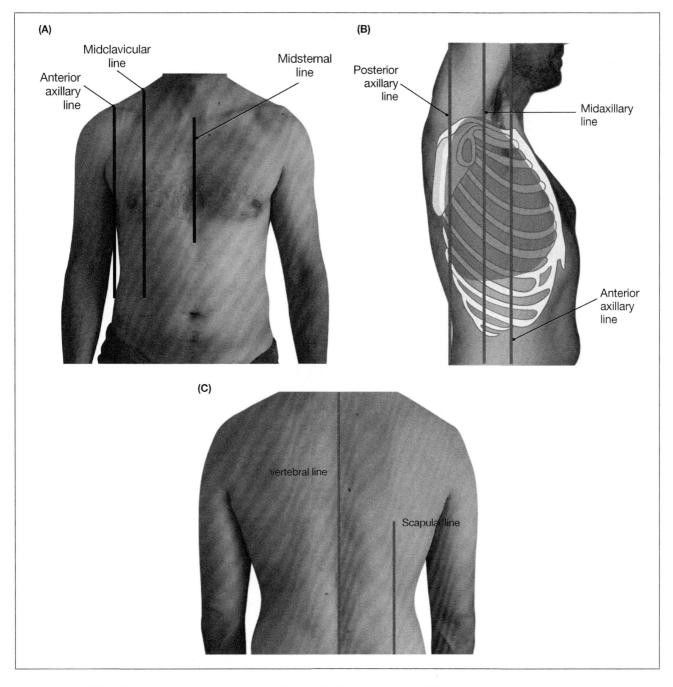

FIGURE 7.3 Landmarks of anterior (A), lateral (B), and posterior (C) chest with directional terms.

Clinically, the intercostal space between the 7th and 8th ribs typically serves as a landmark for thoracentesis as clinicians attempt to insert the needle just above the 8th rib to avoid any damage to the neurovascular bundle located below the ribs.

The scapula (shoulder blade) is a flat triangular bone located over the posterior aspect of ribs 2 to 7 bilaterally. It articulates with the humerus (glenohumeral joint [shoulder]) and acromioclavicular joint; the medial aspect is connected to the ribs and vertebral column by muscles. The function of the scapulae is to provide a wide range of movement for the upper extremities.

ANATOMIC STRUCTURES OF THE LOWER RESPIRATORY TRACT

The airway structures located in the chest wall cavity form the lower respiratory tract. The major structures of the upper respiratory tract are reviewed in Chapter 13, Evidence-Based Assessment of the Ears,

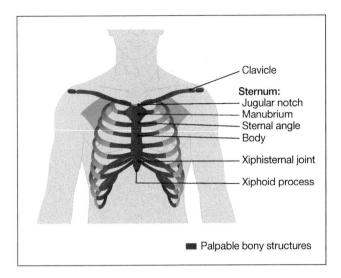

FIGURE 7.4 Anterior chest wall.

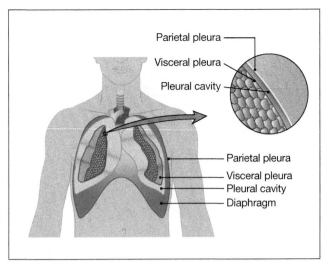

FIGURE 7.6 Pleura and diaphragm.

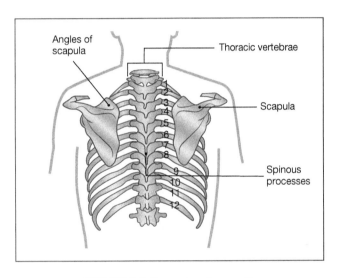

FIGURE 7.5 Posterior chest wall.

Nose, and Throat; these include the nose, nasal cavity, mouth, throat (pharynx), and larynx. The lower respiratory tract structures include the trachea, bronchi, bronchioles, alveoli, lungs, pleurae, and diaphragm.

Lungs, Pleurae, and Diaphragm

The lungs are pyramid-shaped vital organs located inside the two chambers of the thoracic cavity and connected to the trachea medially, surrounded by **pleura**, and in proximity to the **diaphragm** (a sheet of skeletal muscle) inferiorly that plays a crucial role in the inhalation process (**Figure 7.6**).

The pleura has two layers—outer parietal layer and inner visceral layer. The space between the pleura is called the pleural space, and it contains the pleural fluid.

The pleural fluid provides the required lubrication during expansion and contraction of the lungs and maintains enough surface tension to keep the lungs close to the thoracic cage. The parietal layer is in proximity to the thoracic cage, while the visceral layer is in proximity to the lungs. The amount of pleural fluid can increase because of volume overload caused by heart failure, cirrhosis, or nephrotic syndrome. An increase in the amount of pleural fluid is referred to as pleural effusion. Excess accumulation of pleural fluid can also occur in infectious processes such as pneumonia, tuberculosis, or pancreatitis. Other exudative causes of pleural effusion are blocked lymph or blood vessels, tumors, or lung injury.

The pleura folds into the lungs, forming fissures. The fissures divide the lungs into lobes. The two lungs are not identical or symmetrical as a result of these fissures. The right lung has three lobes, whereas the left lung has only two lobes. The right lung is larger but shorter than the left to accommodate the liver, which displaces the diaphragm upward. The right upper lobe is the largest lobe; the right middle lobe is the smallest; and the right lower lobe is the bottom-most lobe of the right lung. The left lung is smaller and narrower than the right lung and divided into upper and lower lobes by the oblique fissure. See **Figure 7.7** to visualize the locations of the anterior, posterior, and lateral lung fields.

Although the lungs vary in size and number of lobes, the lungs are paired and do have similar anatomic landmarks, as illustrated in **Figure 7.8**. The apices of the lungs are rounded; in adults, the apices extend anteriorly above the first rib and posteriorly to the level of T1. An indentation is present on the medial aspect of the lung and is called the cardiac notch, where it allows space for the heart. The hilum is a triangular depression above and behind the cardiac notch, where the pulmonary

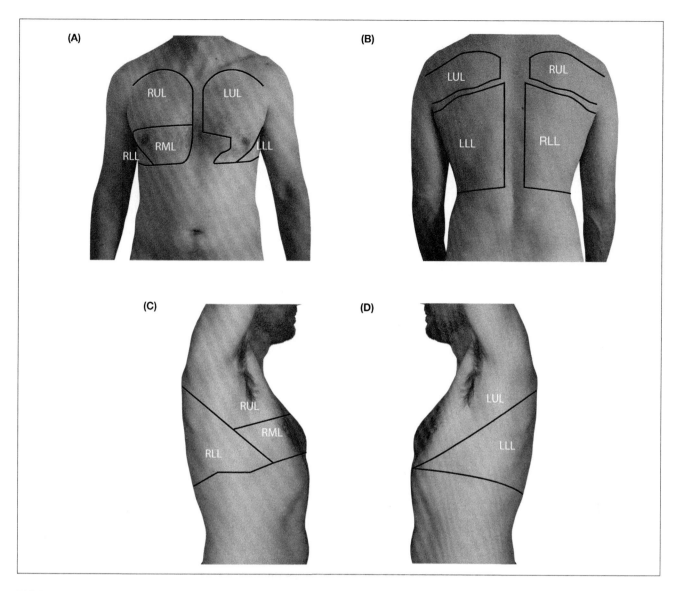

FIGURE 7.7 Lobes of the lungs. (A) Anterior lung fields. (B) Posterior lung fields. (C) Lobes of the right lung. (D) Lobes of the left lung.

LLL, left lower lobe; LUL, left upper lobe; RLL, right lower lobe; RML, right middle lobe; RUL, right upper lobe;

vein, pulmonary artery, pulmonary nerves, and the lymphatic vessels enter the lungs; this serves as the primary connection between the cardiovascular and the nervous systems. Unlike other veins and arteries in the body, the pulmonary arteries carry deoxygenated blood from the heart to the lungs, and the pulmonary veins carry oxygenated blood from the lungs to the heart. The lower borders of the lungs extend to T12 with deep inspiration, and to T9 with full expiration. The base of the lungs rests on the surface of the diaphragm.

Trachea and Bronchi

The trachea connects the upper and lower respiratory tracts, as depicted in **Figure 7.9**. The trachea

extends from the end of the larynx to the point of bifurcation (carina) in the right and left main bronchi. It is located posterior to the sternum and anterior to the esophagus. It is about 4 inches long and composed of about 20 rings made of cartilage anteriorly and smooth muscle and connective tissue posteriorly. The smooth muscle of the trachea can contract, decreasing the trachea's diameter, which forces air out and helps expel mucus. The trachea is lined with a moist mucous membrane that contains hair-like projections, called cilia, which propel foreign particles trapped in the mucus toward the pharynx. The inferior thyroid arteries primarily supply blood to the trachea.

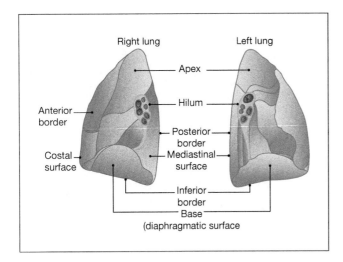

FIGURE 7.8 Landmarks of the lungs.

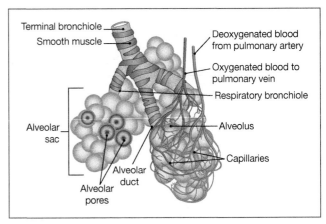

FIGURE 7.10 Alveoli.

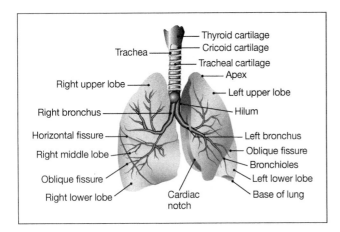

FIGURE 7.9 Lower respiratory tract.

Narrowing of the trachea, called tracheal stenosis, is caused by granulation tissue or tumors. Increased floppiness of the trachea, tracheomalacia, may result from congenital defects, smoking, or injury by artificial airways such as endotracheal or tracheostomy tubes. Abnormal connection between the trachea and esophagus is called atracheoesophageal fistula, and an abnormal connection between the trachea and the innominate (brachiocephalic) artery is called a tracheoinnominate fistula. These structural abnormalities can cause obstruction to the air moving in and out of the lungs and may result in significant respiratory compromise.

At the level of the carina, the trachea bifurcates into the right and left main bronchus. The right main bronchus extends to the segmental bronchi, which in turn extends to the right upper lobe. The segmental bronchi extend out to the right middle and lower lobes. The left main bronchus branches into two lobar bronchi, each

extending to the left upper and lower lobes. The right main bronchus is shorter, wider, and more vertical than the left, allowing foreign objects to enter the right middle and lower lobes more easily than that of the left. Right middle and lower lobes are highly susceptible to aspiration pneumonia because of the vertical nature of the right bronchus.

Alveoli

The bronchi divide into lobar bronchi; lobar bronchi divide into segmental bronchioles; segmental bronchioles divide into bronchioles; bronchioles terminate into alveolar ducts and sacs, where gas exchanges with blood. There are about 700 million **alveoli** in the lungs, and each alveolus is only one cell thick, creating the opportunity for efficient gas exchange across the large surface area created by the vast number of alveoli. The anatomic structure of the alveoli, including their capillary circulation, is illustrated in **Figure 7.10**.

The epithelial cells in the alveoli produce surfactant, a compound that lowers the surface tension of pulmonary fluids, which is vital for the maintenance of the elasticity of the lungs. Without surfactant, the alveoli would collapse during expiration. The amount of surfactant can be decreased in premature neonates, causing difficulties with lung expansion and gas exchange. The characteristics of surfactant may also be altered in the pathologic processes associated with lung diseases, including asthma, chronic obstructive pulmonary disease, chronic bronchitis, cystic fibrosis (CF), pneumonia, and interstitial lung disease.

PHYSIOLOGY OF BREATHING/RESPIRATION

Respiration, the movement of dissolved gases into and out of the lungs, occurs at the alveolar level. Alveoli are surrounded by capillary blood vessels. The space between the air and the blood averages only about one micron in thickness and allows exchange of gas molecules easily. About 5 to 8 L of air enters in and out of the lungs, and about three tenths of a liter of oxygen enters the alveoli per minute. **Diffusion** is the process by which oxygen and carbon dioxide molecules exchange within the alveoli and capillaries in the lungs. Diffusion is driven by a concentration gradient, that is, gas molecules move from a region of high concentration to one of low concentration. Oxygen molecules diffuse through the alveolar cell wall into the capillary bloodstream, where they bind to hemoglobin. Pressure gradients drive the oxygen into the cells of tissues and carbon dioxide out of tissue cells and into the capillaries. Carbon dioxide molecules diffuse from the bloodstream through the same alveolar walls into the alveoli.

Breathing involves inspiration and expiration, which is controlled by the medulla oblongata (which sends signals to the respiratory muscles to breathe) and the pons (which controls the respiratory rate). The normal respiratory rate is 12–20 breaths per minute in adults. *Ventilation* is the exchange of gases between the lungs and the external atmosphere. During inspiration, air enters the lungs from the external environment, and during expiration, air exits the lungs to the external environment. Air is a mixture of gases, primarily nitrogen (N_2; 78.6%), oxygen (O_2; 20.9%), water vapor (H_2O; 0.5%), and carbon dioxide (CO_2; 0.04%; Molnar & Gair, 2015). Oxygen and carbon dioxide flow according to their pressure and concentration gradients: Inspiration increases the oxygen pressure and concentration gradients within the alveoli, gas exchange occurs, and expiration involves the exhalation of the carbon dioxide level from the lungs.

Pulmonary ventilation is dependent on the contraction and relaxation of muscles, including the diaphragm and intercostal and accessory muscles. The inspiratory and expiratory accessory muscles, which include the sternocleidomastoid and the scalene muscles, do not play a primary role in quiet breathing but assist with additional support during conditions of high metabolic demand or respiratory dysfunction, for example, asthma exacerbation, pneumonia, or bronchitis. **Figure 7.11** depicts the muscles involved in breathing.

The movement of the diaphragm with breathing is depicted in **Figure 7.12**. Normally, inspiration occurs when the diaphragm contracts and moves downward into the abdomen, and the thoracic muscles pull the chest wall outward. As the volume of the thoracic cavity increases, the lungs expand, causing negative pressure in the lungs, which forces the air from the external environment to enter the lungs. The resultant pressure gradient created within the lungs during inspiration causes the alveoli to expand, which facilitates gas exchange. Expiration is typically a passive process and does not require much effort from the respiratory muscles. The stretch receptors in the alveoli send signals to

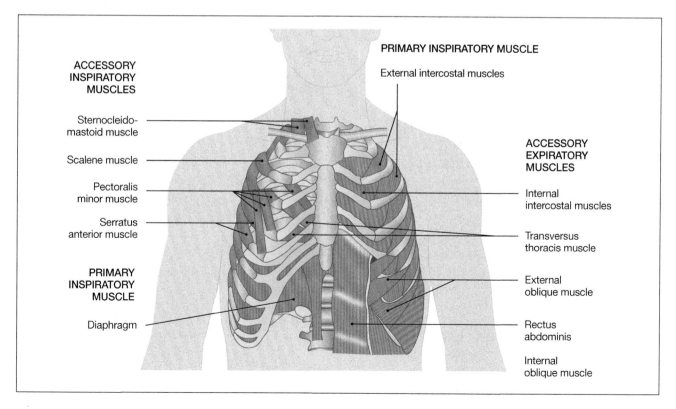

FIGURE 7.11 Muscles of ventilation.

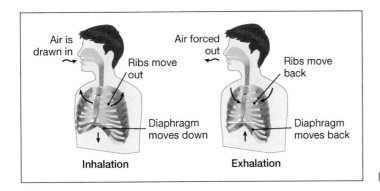

FIGURE 7.12 Diaphragm movement with breathing.

the medulla oblongata, which in turn sends signals to the diaphragm and thoracic muscles to relax. When the diaphragm and intercostal muscles relax, positive pressure is created in the lungs, which pushes air outside to the external environment.

During physical or emotional stress, with coughing and sneezing, and with alterations in breathing that occur because of certain disease processes, the use of accessory muscles becomes prominent. Altered breathing patterns change the amount of air exchanged during breathing, and the rate of exchange; this may or may not change alveolar ventilation.

LIFE-SPAN DIFFERENCES AND CONSIDERATIONS FOR THE LUNGS AND RESPIRATORY SYSTEM

Pediatric Considerations

The ribs of children are flexible and provide little structural support to the lungs. Children are more likely to use accessory muscles in times of respiratory distress. Nasal flaring and suprasternal, intercostal, substernal, and subcostal retractions are more common in small infants and children with respiratory illnesses than in adults. Young infants and children have a higher rate of oxygen consumption as well as increased metabolic rates, which increase the risk of respiratory compromise.

Pregnancy Variations

Lung capacity is affected during pregnancy. Physical adaptations include an increased thoracic diameter up to 2 cm or more, and a rise in the diaphragm up to 4 cm. Hyperventilation results from increased tidal volume and vital capacity, as well as the effects of progesterone. These changes create a notable, significant increase in ventilation, and lead to a state of respiratory alkalosis as well as frequent dyspnea. The presence of dyspnea during pregnancy commonly occurs during the first and second trimesters owing to the changes in the respiratory system; dyspnea usually remains stable during the third trimester, despite anatomic changes.

Geriatric Considerations

Physiologic and functional status vary greatly in older adults. While aging leads to predictable changes in the respiratory system, the process occurs at different rates, influenced by genetics, lifestyle behaviors, and environment. Aging does not result in pneumonia or hypoxia; however, age-related anatomic changes increase the likelihood. These include the following:

- Alveolar ducts lose collagen, resulting in decreased surface area.
- Lung tissue loses elasticity, limiting expiratory airflow.
- Dependent areas of the lung are more perfused because of circulatory changes, causing ventilation-perfusion mismatches that gradually result in lower oxygen saturation.
- The chest wall becomes stiffer and less compliant, and the diaphragm flattens, decreasing the expansion of the thoracic cage and increasing the work of breathing.
- Respiratory muscles lose strength, and the cough mechanism is less effective; this causes a decrease in mucus clearance.

KEY HISTORY QUESTIONS AND CONSIDERATIONS FOR THE LUNGS AND RESPIRATORY SYSTEM

CHIEF CONCERN

Individuals with respiratory problems or illnesses commonly present with symptoms of shortness of breath or dyspnea, cough, chest pain, and/or **hemoptysis**, the expectoration of blood/blood-tinged sputum from the respiratory tract. The most prominent or bothersome of the symptoms often becomes the reason for seeking care and should be reviewed carefully as the presenting symptom. For any individual presenting with a respiratory problem, each of these symptoms should be assessed and evaluated as part of the review of systems.

HISTORY OF PRESENT ILLNESS

Using the acronym OLDCARTS to guide history taking, ask the individual with symptoms suggestive of respiratory illness about the onset, location, duration, characteristics, aggravating and relieving factors, treatments tried, and severity of their symptoms.

Example: Shortness of Breath

- Onset: When did the shortness of breath start? What was the individual doing when they became short of breath? Did this occur suddenly, or has it been developing gradually?
- Location: Does the shortness of breath cause any chest tightness or pain? If so, where is the discomfort located?
- Duration: How long does the shortness of breath last? Over what period of time has the shortness of breath developed?
- Characteristics: Is the patient winded, unable to take air in or breathe out, or unable to catch their breath? Is there a cough associated with it?
- Aggravating factors: What actions, activities, or body positions make the symptoms worse? Has exposure to smells, dust, pollen, smoking (first or secondhand), or activities caused increased shortness of breath?
- Relieving factors: What actions, activities, or body positions decrease the shortness of breath?
- Treatment: What medications has the individual taken to help with the shortness of breath? Did the patient use any breathing treatments or inhaled respiratory medications?
- Severity: How severe is the shortness of breath on a scale of 0 to 10? Are there associated symptoms, such as itching or swelling? Is the individual feeling anxious or fearful?

PAST MEDICAL HISTORY

Past History of Illness

When obtaining past health history, the clinician should ask about the individual's history of respiratory illnesses throughout their life span, and ask adults about childhood illnesses. Assess for significant childhood health history that impacts respiratory function, including whether the individual was born prematurely; has been diagnosed with congenital lung disease(s); was previously diagnosed with asthma, bronchiolitis, bronchitis, or pneumonia; and whether they have ever been to the emergency department or hospitalized with respiratory problems. Past history of having been intubated, requiring mechanical ventilation, having had a thoracic procedure, and/or requiring respiratory resuscitation is significant. Screen young adults and adults for a chronic respiratory disease history consistent with asthma or CF, as they can have

these disorders without having ever been formally diagnosed in childhood.

The most common chronic respiratory disorder of adults and older adults is chronic obstructive pulmonary disease (COPD). Many individuals with COPD are unaware they have this disease. Ask patients who smoke or formerly smoked, individuals with recurrent bronchitis or emphysema, and individuals experiencing chronic cough about whether they are experiencing shortness of breath, wheezing, or worsening cough (The Global Initiative for Chronic Obstructive Lung Disease [GOLD], 2019; U.S. Preventive Services Task Force [USPSTF], 2016). COPD can present as emphysema, chronic bronchitis, or both. In emphysema, the walls between many of the alveoli are damaged and weak, and, as a result, the alveoli lose their shape and become floppy. Weakening of the walls can result in complete destruction of the walls of the air sacs, leading to fewer and larger alveoli. Reduction in the integrity and number of alveoli results in a decrease in the amount of gas exchanged in the lungs. In chronic **bronchitis**, the lining of the airways is constantly irritated and inflamed, causing the lining to thicken. Large amounts of thick mucus form in the airways, making it hard to breathe. Assess for increasing dyspnea and chronic productive cough.

To assess for comorbidities or risk factors related to pulmonary disease, ask the individual if they have known or suspected pulmonary, cardiac, or renal disease. Ask about recent travel, surgery, hospitalization, or immobility.

Medications

As part of the health history, ask about medications that have been prescribed and whether over-the-counter medications or supplements are being taken. Assess how often these medications are being taken. Specifically in regard to the respiratory system, assess whether the individual is using inhalers, nebulizers, and/or spacers, and how these are being used. Ask whether the individual has had recent antibiotic and/or oral steroid use.

Allergies

It is crucial to ask about allergies when collecting a history from a patient presenting with respiratory symptoms. Assess for allergies to medications, as well as seasonal, environmental, and/or food allergies. When an individual answers "yes" to being allergic to any substance or environmental trigger, clarify their reaction. Nonallergic reactions are more common than allergic reactions; these are primarily nausea and intestinal upset. Allergic reactions include skin rashes and itching. In the most severe form of immediate allergic reaction—anaphylaxis—individuals can have hives; swelling of their tongue, lips, and face; dyspnea; wheezing; dizziness; vomiting; and/or shock. Clarify whether a patient who presents with dyspnea has had previous similar symptoms and under what type of circumstances.

Immunizations

Ask all individuals whether they have been immunized, noting when they last received influenza, pertussis, and pneumococcal vaccinations. Note whether children and adults are up-to-date with their immunizations. Assess for risk factors and symptoms related to tuberculosis (reviewed later in this chapter), and ask about purified protein derivative (PPD) testing. If an individual has had a positive PPD test but has never been exposed to tuberculosis, note whether the individual received bacille Calmette-Guerin (BCG) vaccine. BCG is a vaccine given to prevent tuberculosis. It was previously administered in the United States, but is now given only in countries where the prevalence of tuberculosis is very high. BCG immunization may interfere with the PPD skin testing and may show a false positive result, which requires follow-up with chest x-ray.

Additional Pediatric Considerations

For children under 3 years of age, and for children presenting with respiratory symptoms, enquire about the child's birth history. Ask about the mother's health during pregnancy and if any fetal abnormalities were identified during the prenatal stage. Was the delivery eventful or uneventful, vaginal or C-section, prolonged or abrupt? What was the APGAR (Activity, Pulse rate, Respiration) score at birth? Low APGAR scores may indicate poorer respiratory status, use of maternal drugs, or a decrease in fetal blood supply or anoxia during birth, and these may have implications for health in later life. Ask if there was any respiratory distress after birth. Were there any apneic episodes? Did the child require oxygen, continuous pulse oximetry monitoring, or support for breathing as an infant? Neonatal ventilation, especially if multiple modes and rescue therapies were required, are suggestive of the gravity of the respiratory problems after birth.

Ask about the child's growth based on pediatric growth charts, and assess whether the child has been meeting developmental milestones, as discussed in Chapter 4, Evidence-Based Assessment of Children and Adolescents. Warning signs of suboptimal growth, including poor weight gain, may be seen in children with chronic respiratory diseases or as a temporary setback with an acute illness. Therefore, it is imperative to assess the child's eating and nutritional history. How has the child been eating? Specifically for the infant, ask the following questions: Is the infant breast- or bottle fed? Does the baby have any difficulty feeding? To clarify, difficulty feeding would include little interest

in feeding, feeling easily fatigued or perspiring during feeding, and/or any color changes, including cyanosis during feeding. Is the infant or child adequately gaining weight? Increased metabolic demand leading to inadequate weight gain can occur with chronic respiratory diseases such as asthma or bronchopulmonary dysplasia.

FAMILY HISTORY

Assess whether anyone in the family has chronic lung problems such as asthma, chronic bronchitis, tuberculosis, or lung cancer. Be careful to also ask generally whether anyone in the family has "breathing problems," as individuals may not know the name of the medical condition. Specifically for infants and children, note whether there is any history of sudden infant death in the family or if any other children have had apnea. Assess whether there is a family history of CF; reactive airway diseases; atopy or allergies; gastroesophageal reflux disease (GERD), which can trigger respiratory conditions; or congenital anomalies. Knowing the family health history provides important information regarding both inheritable and environmental factors that can contribute to the individual's respiratory condition.

SOCIAL HISTORY

Environmental Exposures

In regard to personal or social history, ask individuals about actual or potential occupational and environmental exposures. Exposure to pollutants and/or irritants in the work environment normally do not exceed threshold levels, but low-level chronic exposure to hazardous substances can trigger respiratory disorders. For individuals unsure of exposures, ask about safety/protective measures that they are expected to wear at work and the rationale for these measures. In particular, pay special attention to individuals who are miners, firefighters, chemists, silica workers, or anyone who works with any types of chemicals. Patients do not necessarily have to be scientists working with chemicals in their labs or in a chemical plant to have environmental exposures, as individuals who mix different cleaning agents to clean the house can be exposed to toxic fumes. Individuals with no history of respiratory problems are often hospitalized with an inhalational injury. Remember that pollutants disproportionately affect children and pregnant women; ask about home and work or school environments, which can be deleterious for those who live in congested urban areas. The following are also important questions: Are there any people who smoke in the home? Does anyone smoke inside the house? In the car? What are the precautions taken in regard to smoking when there are children in the home?

Lifestyle Behaviors, Including Substance Use

Asking about current health habits, including the use of substances, is a key element of an individual's social history. The use of substances, including tobacco, alcohol, prescription medications used for nonmedical purposes, illicit drugs, and over-the-counter drugs should be assessed. In regard to inhaled substances that have a significant impact on the respiratory system, tobacco products, including cigarettes, smokeless tobacco, e-cigarettes, cigars, and pipe tobacco, are the most common. Tobacco use is the leading cause of preventable death in the United States; every year, 500,000 individuals die prematurely from smoking or exposure to secondhand smoke (Centers for Disease Control and Prevention [CDC], n.d.-d). Assess exposure to secondhand smoke. Secondhand smoke causes stroke, lung cancer, and coronary heart disease in adults; children who are exposed to secondhand smoke are at increased risk for sudden infant death syndrome, acute respiratory infections, recurrent ear infections, more severe asthma, and slowed lung growth (CDC, n.d.-d).

When assessing smoking habits, calculate *pack years* to quantify smoking risks. This measure is calculated by multiplying the number of packs of cigarettes smoked per day by the number of years the individual has smoked. For example, an individual who has smoked 1.5 packs a day × 12 years has an 18 pack year history. Within this assessment, clinicians should be careful to note both the measurement of pack years and the duration of smoking in years. Smoking duration alone has been found to be correlated with the development of COPD (Bhatt et al., 2018). Because smoking cessation has a significant capacity to decrease the progression and burden of chronic disease, clinicians are encouraged to intervene in five major steps:

1. **Ask:** Identify and document tobacco use status for every patient at every visit.
2. **Advise:** Support the self-efficacy of every person who uses tobacco to quit.
3. **Assess:** Determine each individual's willingness and readiness to quit.
4. **Assist:** Individuals willing to make a quit attempt should be offered options, including counseling and pharmacotherapy as appropriate.
5. **Arrange:** Schedule follow-up, in person or by phone, within the first week of a quit date.

REVIEW OF SYSTEMS

After obtaining a history of present illness, personal and family medical history, and social history, completing a review of systems allows the clinician to appreciate other pertinent symptoms that the patient may be experiencing. Some of the common symptoms to review that are associated with the respiratory system include dyspnea, cough, hemoptysis, and chest pain.

Assess for Dyspnea

Dyspnea, or shortness of breath, is often described by an individual as difficulty with breathing; that is, a nonpainful but uncomfortable awareness of the labor of breathing beyond what is expected for the level of exertion. Begin enquiring with a broad question (e.g., "Have you had any difficulty breathing?"). Determine the severity of dyspnea based on the patient's ability to participate in daily activities. Ask if the shortness of breath is exertional, and, if so, clarify the level of exertion that results in shortness of breath.

Dyspnea on exertion is closely related to exercise tolerance. It is important to know if the patient is short of breath after running a mile versus going up a single flight of stairs or just walking from one end of the room to another. Assessing exercise tolerance is complicated and may be underestimated if the individual is sedentary to avoid exertional dyspnea. Careful interviewing is required to assess exercise intolerance, especially in older adults who may prioritize the conservation of energy. Dyspnea on exertion can indicate cardiac and/or pulmonary dysfunction, although it may not be indicative of disease if it occurs with strenuous exercise.

Ask whether the individual hears or is experiencing wheezing in addition to dyspnea. Unlike other types of breath sounds, wheezing can be loud enough to be heard without a stethoscope. Wheezing is a high-pitched whistling or musical sound made while breathing. Audible wheezing can indicate asthma, although wheezing can be heard when individuals have congestive heart failure, pneumonia, COPD, bronchiolitis, malignancies, or foreign body inhalation. Further assessment is needed for any individual with audible wheezing.

Dyspnea can be aggravated by position. Assess whether any particular position causes shortness of breath, and ask if a position change relieves it. Paroxysmal nocturnal dyspnea refers to shortness of breath that wakes an individual, often after only one or two hours of sleep; the sudden dyspnea usually leads to coughing and is relieved in the upright position. Orthopnea refers to shortness of breath when lying flat. To elicit information about orthopnea, ask about the number of pillows an individual uses at night to relieve their shortness of breath. If it is two pillows, for example, the clinician would document "two-pillow orthopnea." Orthopnea is most often caused by pulmonary congestion when supine; paroxysmal nocturnal dyspnea can also be caused by pulmonary congestion, which may be exacerbated by a decreased responsiveness of the respiratory system during sleep.

Postural dyspnea is most often associated with heart failure. Cardiac and pulmonary dysfunction can lead less commonly to trepopnea and platypnea. Trepopnea refers to dyspnea that occurs in a lateral decubitus position, which can be a sign of a pulmonary effusion, an accumulation of fluid in the pleural space. Platypnea refers to breathlessness that occurs in the upright position and is relieved by lying flat, which can be related to congenital heart defects. Individuals with postural dyspnea are likely to have dyspnea on exertion, and cough.

Assess for Cough

Cough is a reflex response to stimuli initiated by irritation of receptors in the epithelium of the upper and lower respiratory tracts, pericardium, esophagus, or stomach. Impulses from stimulated cough receptors follow a complex reflex arc that involves the vagus, phrenic, and spinal motor nerves. Cough is one of the most common symptoms of respiratory dysfunction.

Ask about the onset and duration of a cough. Acute cough for less than three weeks is commonly caused by acute respiratory tract infection or acute exacerbation of an underlying chronic pulmonary disease, pneumonia, or pulmonary embolism. Cough that has been present for three to eight weeks (subacute) or more than eight weeks (chronic) is more likely due to postnasal drip, asthma, or GERD, alone or as comorbid conditions. Chronic cough, however, can also be related to heart failure, chronic bronchitis, lung cancer, or treatment with angiotensin-converting enzyme (ACE) inhibitors.

When an individual presents with cough, clarify when the cough occurs; that is, whether it is all day, related to the time of day, at work, outdoors, during activity, or sporadically. Does the cough wake the individual at night and interfere with sleep? Does the cough worsen with activity or throughout the day? Is the cough tiring the individual and/or interfering with an individual's ability to work, attend school, or participate in daily activities?

Ask about characteristics of the cough and associated symptoms. Is the cough occurring in spasms? Can it be described as deep, barking, or whooping? Are there additional upper respiratory tract infection symptoms, such as postnasal drainage, ear pain, sore throat, hoarseness, or sinus congestion? Does the individual have a fever? Do they smoke—currently or formerly? Has the cough responded to any treatment or medications? Is the cough dry or productive? If the cough is productive, ask the individual to describe the quantity (volume of any sputum) and quality (its color, odor, and consistency). While causative agents cannot be determined by observation of the sputum alone, sputum that is frothy, foul smelling, tenacious, or that is being produced in large volumes may indicate significant disease processes that require further evaluation.

Assess for Hemoptysis

Hemoptysis is the coughing up of blood from the lungs or airways and may range from blood-streaked sputum to frank blood. Hemoptysis suggests that there is a lesion somewhere in the respiratory pathways. Expectorating sputum with blood streaks is less worrisome than the ominous sign of coughing up frank blood. When asking questions about hemoptysis, ask the individual to describe the volume of blood produced as well as other sputum attributes (i.e., quality and quantity). Try to confirm the source of the bleeding by history and examination before using the term *hemoptysis* because blood may also originate from the mouth, pharynx, or gastrointestinal tract. Blood originating in the stomach is usually darker than blood from the respiratory tract.

History questions to ask include the following: How much blood has been coughed up in the last 24 to 48 hours? Is the blood mixed with white or discolored sputum (phlegm)? Is this a new symptom? Have you ever coughed up blood before? How frequently is this happening now? Are you having shortness of breath? Do you hear yourself wheezing? What other symptoms are you having? Are you having fever, chills, or night sweats? Have you noticed any rashes? Is there blood in your urine? Are you having swelling in your hands, feet, or legs? Have you lost weight recently?

Individuals who present with a history of hemoptysis, are over the age of 50, and have more than a 30-year pack history of smoking are at high risk for malignancy.

Assess for Chest Pain

Patients with respiratory conditions may complain of chest pain. The causes of chest pain range from life-threatening to relatively benign. See Chapter 6, Evidence-Based Assessment of the Heart and Circulatory System, to review cardiac conditions that cause chest pain. Initial assessment of individuals who have a history of chest pain includes vital signs, oxygen saturation measurement, and triage for symptoms of life-threatening conditions.

Initial questions should be as broad as possible, for example, "Do you have any discomfort or unpleasant feelings in your chest?" Then, continue asking questions using the OLDCARTS tool to elicit all attributes of the patient's symptoms. The etiologies of chest pain can be cardiac, vascular, gastrointestinal, musculoskeletal, psychiatric, referred pain, or dermatologic, which creates a diagnostic challenge.

Key symptoms in individuals with pulmonary disease include pleuritic chest pain, dyspnea, and cough. Lung tissue itself has no pain fibers; therefore, pain associated with lung conditions usually arises from inflammation of the adjacent parietal pleura. Pleurisy is pain that occurs in the chest when the pleura rub together because there is not enough lubrication. Conditions that cause pleuritic chest pain, dyspnea, and cough include pneumonia, asthma, COPD, lung cancer, sarcoidosis, and pulmonary hypertension. To assess for these conditions, ask about the presence of chest pain, shortness of breath, and cough. Clarify characteristics of these symptoms, and review the individual's history of chronic lung disease and smoking.

PHYSICAL EXAMINATION OF THE LUNGS AND RESPIRATORY SYSTEM

INITIAL OBSERVATIONS

The initial assessment of an individual through a general survey provides valuable information about their physiologic stability. Consider these important initial observations of respiratory status:

- Observe the rate, rhythm, depth, and effort of breathing. Assess vital signs.
- Observe the individual's posture and position. If the patient is having respiratory distress, get the patient to lean forward with the hands on the knees in a *tripod position*. The tripod position aids in increasing the anteroposterior diameter and changing the pressure in the thoracic cavity to decrease the work of breathing.
- Note that a child with respiratory distress may also sit forward, have a muffled voice, become restless, and/or drool. These observations require an emergent response.
- Note that the ability of the patient to speak in full sentences is an indicator of their respiratory condition. The fewer the words they are able to speak before becoming dyspneic, the greater the severity of respiratory distress.
- Listen for wheezing or audible breath sounds. If the patient is exhibiting any signs and symptoms of respiratory distress, including tracheal deviation, nasal flaring, retractions, or use of accessory muscles, immediate interventions may be needed.

APPROACH TO THE PHYSICAL EXAMINATION

For the individual not in distress, the clinician completes the physical exam of the respiratory system in this order: (a) inspection, (b) palpation, (c) percussion, and (d) auscultation. Each step of the physical exam of the anterior and posterior thorax should be completed with areas of the chest reasonably exposed. Best practice for the examination of the respiratory system is avoidance of assessment over clothing. Although individuals can remain covered with a gown or drape to maintain privacy, exposure of the area being examined is required. To perform the respiratory assessment competently, thoroughly, and sensitively, clinicians can

enlist the assistance of the individual being examined. This may include asking patients to lower their gown or drape to expose their anterior or posterior chest, explaining the components of the respiratory exam, and requesting that they change positions as appropriate to allow for the exam. Completing portions of the respiratory assessment over clothing, even thin clothing, is considered poor technique. Many respiratory abnormalities are unilateral; being able to compare findings bilaterally and front to back is essential. Begin the exam with the individual seated upright, if possible.

INSPECTION

Peripheral Assessment

Evidence-based assessment of respiratory status begins with a systematic and thorough inspection. After a general survey for any indications of respiratory distress, inspection may proceed to peripheral assessment. Observe the lips, oral mucosa, and conjunctiva for cyanosis or pallor, indicating hypoxia or inadequate gas exchange. The mucosa of dark-skinned individuals can appear gray with central cyanosis. Assess the lips for pursing, a sign of increased expiratory effort.

Evaluate nail beds for color and capillary refill. Evaluate the distal fingertips for clubbing. **Clubbing** is a painless overgrowth of connective tissues and edema that result in bulbous enlargement of the ends of one or more fingers or toes and excessive sponginess or bogginess of the nail base. Clubbing results in an increase in the angle between the proximal nail fold and the nail plate. Normally, the angle between the skin and the nail bed is 160 degrees, which creates a diamond-shaped window (referred to as Schamroth's window) when two opposing fingers are held back to back; with clubbing, this space (or window) is missing (**Figure 7.13**). Clubbing is a manifestation of chronic tissue hypoxia.

Inspection of the Thoracic Cage and Chest Movement

Observe the rate, rhythm, and depth of respirations for a full minute. As reviewed in Chapter 5, Approach to the Physical Examination: General Survey and Assessment of Vital Signs, the normal rate of respirations depends on several factors, including age of the individual, recent physical activity, and level of alertness. The adult respiratory rate is normally 12 to 20 breaths/minute. The rhythm of breathing at rest should be even, with occasional sighs. The depth of breathing should not be too shallow or too deep; normal, unlabored, quiet breathing is known as eupnea. Clinicians should assess respiratory rate and rhythm without reminding the individual that they are being assessed, as awareness of breathing often changes the pattern of breathing. Variations in the rates and rhythm of breathing are reviewed in the Abnormal Findings: Variations in Patterns of Breathing

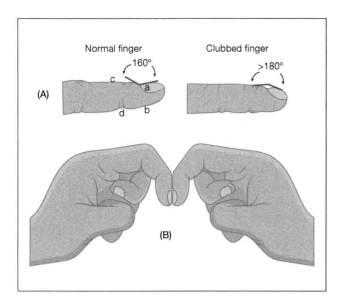

FIGURE 7.13 Assessment for clubbing. (A) Assessment of nail bed angle. (B) Schamroth's window.

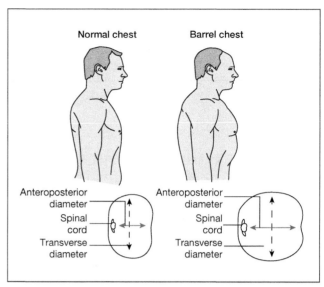

FIGURE 7.14 Barrel chest associated with chronic obstructive pulmonary disease.

section of this chapter. Assess whether the individual is using accessory muscles to breathe during the physical exam. Note nasal flaring, tracheal deviation, and suprasternal, substernal, or intercostal retractions.

Inspect the anterior and posterior chest wall. Assess for the presence of any skin lesions, masses, or discolorations; bruising may be noted over a fractured rib. Inspect the chest for shape and symmetry, noting chest or spine deformities. The anteroposterior (AP) diameter of the chest is ordinarily half of the lateral diameter, or 1:2. In other words, the thoracic cage is normally wider than deep. Assess for these variations:

- *Barrel chest:* The thoracic cage is described as being a barrel chest when the AP diameter is equal to or greater than the lateral (transverse) diameter, or 1:1. Some rounding of the rib cage can be noted in aging adults or those with arthritis. However, hyperinflation of the lungs and an increasing stiffness of the respiratory muscles associated with COPD lead to the barrel chest appearance (**Figure 7.14**).
- *Pectus excavatum:* When the anterior chest wall is depressed with a low-lying sternum, it is called pectus excavatum or sunken/funnel chest (**Figure 7.15**). The depression may be more noticeable on inspiration. This defect is usually congenital and asymptomatic. If the depression of the sternum is significant, then the reduction in lung volume and compression of the heart and great vessels may cause murmurs, palpitations, decreased exercise tolerance, and/or fatigue.
- *Pectus carinatum:* When the sternum is displaced anteriorly and protrudes outward abnormally, it is

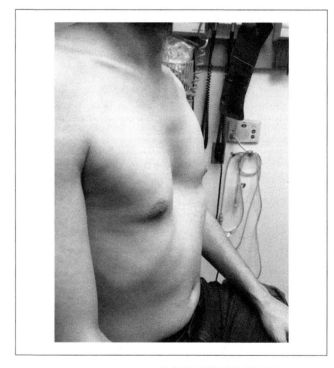

FIGURE 7.15 Pectus excavatum.

called pigeon's chest or pectus carinatum. With this less common chest wall deformity, the AP diameter will be increased. Individuals with pectus carinatum may have associated scoliosis, asthma, mitral valve prolapse, and connective tissue disorders affecting heart valves.

- *Flail chest:* When three or more ribs fracture in multiple places and a segment of the fractured ribs gets detached from the rest of the thoracic cage, the condition is known as flail chest. A late sign of this life-threatening condition is when the detached segment is in paradoxical motion with the rest of the thoracic cage; a segment is considered to be in paradoxical motion when it is pulled into the thoracic cage with inspiration and pushed out during expiration, which is the opposite of normal thoracic cage mechanics. Patients with flail chest experience chest pain and shortness of breath.

• Variations of the vertebral column include *scoliosis*, *kyphosis*, and *lordosis*. Scoliosis is an abnormal lateral curvature of the vertebral column. Kyphosis is an excessive curvature of the upper thoracic vertebral column, resulting in an exaggerated rounding of the back. Lordosis is an excessive curvature of the lumbar vertebral column. Chapter 15, Evidence-Based Assessment of the Musculoskeletal System, reviews the assessment of these spine deformities that may restrict or compromise the respiratory system. These conditions can be comorbid; kyphoscoliosis involves both lateral curvature and forward flexion of the spine and is associated with abnormal positioning and functioning of the respiratory muscles, causing increased respiratory effort and decreased reserve.

PALPATION

Using the palmar surface of the hands, palpate the posterior and anterior chest wall for tenderness, depressions, masses, deformities, or crepitus. Crepitus is the presence of air in the subcutaneous tissues, which can occur after chest injury, invasive procedures, or surgery; crepitus can be both felt and heard as crinkling, a sensation often associated with "bubble wrap." Palpate the spine to identify any tenderness. Palpate over areas of bruising to note associated tenderness or abnormalities. Note that chest wall tenderness may be associated with inflamed pleura or costochondritis.

Chest Excursion

Palpate the posterior thorax for symmetric chest expansion during respiration. With the patient sitting upright or standing with arms at the sides, place hands on the posterior chest wall, one on each side of the thorax near the level of the diaphragm, palms facing anteriorly with thumbs touching at the midline (**Figure 7.16**). Ask the patient to take a deep breath in, and then exhale. During inspiration, thumbs should separate, and each hand should rotate away from the midline equally.

Asymmetric and/or limited chest excursion is abnormal. Limited movement is associated with poor diaphragmatic excursion and hyperinflation, changes that occur with COPD. Asymmetric chest wall expansion is suggestive of unilateral lung pathology such as chronic fibrosis, lobar pneumonia, or bronchial obstruction.

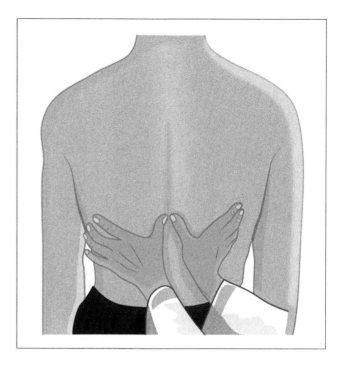

FIGURE 7.16 Palpation for symmetric chest expansion.

Asymmetry can also be caused by pleural pathology or paralysis of one side of the diaphragm.

Tactile Fremitus

Palpate the posterior and anterior chest wall for fremitus. Tactile fremitus is the palpable chest wall vibratory sensation transmitted to the surface of the chest during speech. While the patient is sitting or standing upright, place both hands firmly on either side of the vertebral column, maintaining close contact between the joints of the hands or fingers and the patient's chest wall. The bony aspects of the hands are particularly sensitive to noting vibration. Firm pressure is important to detect vibratory sensations effectively. Ask the patient to say "99" and to repeat this as the clinician assesses the entire posterior chest wall. In **Figure 7.17A**, the clinician is using the palmar aspects of both hands, keeping the metacarpal joints in contact with the skin, and in **Figure 7.17B–C**, the clinician is using the ulnar aspects of both hands, keeping the distal interphalangeal joints in contact with the skin.

Note that the techniques for assessing tactile fremitus can vary. While it is conventional to ask the patient to say "99," there is no evidence that this word is better than others. In addition, some clinicians use one hand at a time and compare side to side, while others use both hands simultaneously to appreciate any differences bilaterally. The key to the technique is to recognize increased, decreased, or absent vibrations.

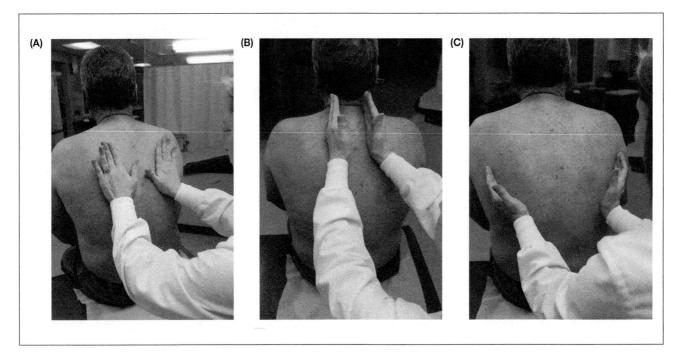

FIGURE 7.17 Palpation for tactile fremitus. (A) Technique using both hands. (B, C) Technique with ulnar aspect of both hands.

The degree of fremitus found will vary. Vibrations can be appreciated more on a thin person than on someone who is obese or muscular. Tactile fremitus is usually stronger in the anterior versus posterior thorax, stronger at the apex than at the bases, and notable in the right upper back because that area is closer to the bronchial bifurcation.

Respiratory system pathology that causes trapping of air in the lungs decreases the transmission of vocal and tactile fremitus; these include pneumothorax, emphysema, and asthma. Decreased fremitus can also be caused by thickened or scarred pleura, significant pleural edema or pleural effusion, or a tumor causing bronchial obstruction. Increased fremitus occurs with compression or consolidation of lung tissue and occurs only when the bronchus is patent and substantial consolidation extends toward the lung surfaces; examples include the presence of a tumor or pneumonia, as these conditions increase tissue density. Increased or decreased tactile fremitus is a finding that is understood to be a component of a constellation of signs and symptoms indicating respiratory disorders and is not solely diagnostic of pathology as its sensitivity and specificity are limited.

PERCUSSION

Percussion Technique and Landmarks

Percussion is a method of tapping on a surface to determine whether the underlying structure is air filled, fluid filled, or solid. When used with other methods of assessment, percussion findings can support suspicions

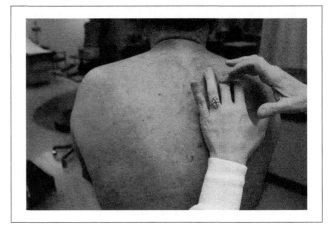

FIGURE 7.18 Percussion technique.

of underlying pathology; percussion findings are especially key when assessing an individual with dyspnea, cough, or hemoptysis.

The technique of indirect percussion is done by placing the pleximeter (nonstriking) finger of the nondominant hand on the chest wall firmly, while the remaining fingers are lifted slightly off the chest wall to avoid dampening the sound. The clinician then uses a quick, sharp wrist motion to strike the pressed finger at the midpoint between the proximal and distal interphalangeal joints with a plexor finger of the dominant hand to produce a sound (**Figure 7.18**). If the percussion sound produced is suboptimal, be sure that the finger placed on the chest wall is making firm, direct contact. Strike the finger at least twice, lightly, sharply, and consistently, to produce a clear percussion sound.

Percuss the posterior, lateral, and anterior chest wall, comparing each area bilaterally. **Figure 7.19** identifies the landmarks that are commonly used for percussion, which are the same as those that are used for auscultation. Note the pattern of the landmarks used for percussion, which begin at the upper aspect of the chest wall,

moving first from one side to the other, and then downward, a few intercostal spaces at a time. Percussion of the posterior chest wall is best completed with the patient seated, head bent forward, and arms folded, which moves the scapula laterally. Percussion of the anterior chest wall can be done when the patient is seated or supine. When percussing the anterior chest wall, avoid percussing over breast tissue, which dampens and/or obscures the sound. Ask the individual to raise their arms when percussing the lateral chest wall.

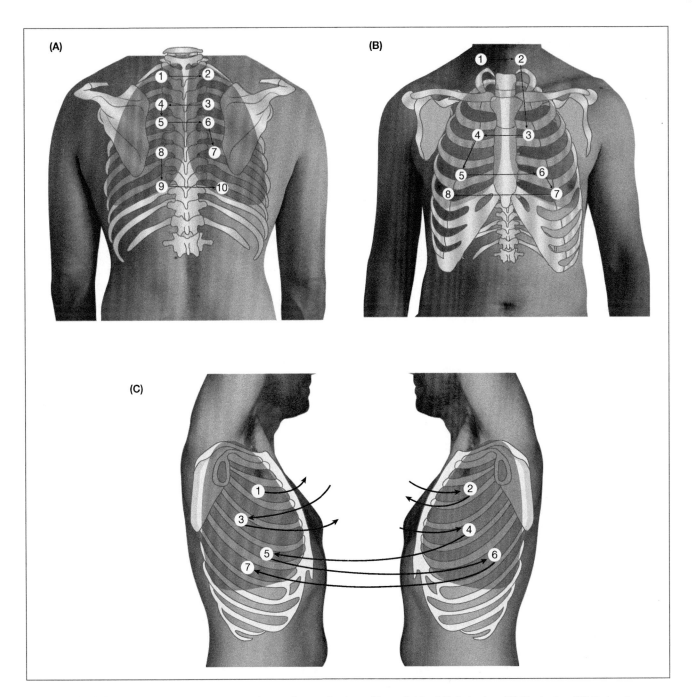

FIGURE 7.19 Landmarks for percussion and auscultation of lung fields. (A) Anterior. (B) Posterior. (C) Lateral.

Resultant percussion sounds can be resonant, hyper-resonant, dull, flat, or tympanic:

- **Resonance** is the hollow sound typically heard over normal lung tissue that is filled with air. This percussion sound is considered to be relatively loud with a low pitch.
- **Hyperresonance** is a very loud sound, lower in pitch and longer in duration than resonance. This sound is normally heard when percussing the chest wall of children or very thin adult patients. Hyperresonance also occurs when lungs are overinflated with air as a result of asthma, or COPD.
- **Dullness** is the sound heard when percussing over a dense area or solid organ, such as the heart or liver. The sound is of medium intensity, pitch, and duration. Dullness over lung tissue is an abnormal finding related to fluid or consolidation associated with pneumonia, masses or tumors, pleural effusions, hemothorax, or empyema.
- **Flatness** is lower than normal percussion sounds, soft in intensity but high in pitch and of short duration. Flatness is percussed normally over solid areas such as bones. Fluid in the pleural space from an effusion would result in flatness when percussed.
- **Tympany** is a loud and high-pitched drum-like sound that can be heard for a longer duration. Tympanic sounds are normal when percussed across the abdomen and abnormal with percussion of the chest wall. Tympanic sounds can result from excessive air in the chest caused by a pneumothorax (collapsed lung).

Diaphragmatic Excursion

Historically, clinicians have been taught to percuss for the level of the diaphragm during both deep inspiration when the diaphragm descends, and again with full expiration when the diaphragm rises. Percussion to measure diaphragmatic excursion, however, is not a reliable, evidence-based method of determining airflow limitation (Holleman & Simel, 1995, 1997; Waterer et al., 2001; Wong, Holroyd-Leduc, & Straus, 2009). When an individual has symptoms consistent with restricted airflow from pleural effusion, dullness to percussion and decreased tactile fremitus are the more reliable methods to confirm the excess pleural fluid (Wong et al., 2009). When an individual has symptoms and/or history consistent with chronic airflow limitation, spirometry is recommended to evaluate airflow limitation (GOLD, 2019; Waterer et al., 2001). Acute limitations are more often associated with pneumonia or exacerbations of asthma, and symptoms determine whether chest x-ray or spirometry are indicated. See the imaging and evidence-based recommendations listed later in this chapter for more information.

AUSCULTATION

Auscultation, listening to internal sounds of the body with a stethoscope, is an important part of the assessment of the respiratory system and aids in the diagnosis of various pulmonary pathologies. The information collected through history taking, as well as inspection, palpation, and percussion techniques prior to auscultation, inform this essential component of the physical exam. Breath sounds created by the flow of air through the airways within the lungs can be heard using a stethoscope, which amplifies and filters sounds. Because the diaphragm of the stethoscope selectively filters sounds of low frequency (and the bell filters those of high frequency), the diaphragm is best for auscultating breath sounds, which tend to be relatively higher pitched.

Auscultation Technique

The clinician should place the ear tips of the stethoscope into the patient's ears with the ear pieces facing away to create a good seal and diminish external sounds. Hold the distal end of the stethoscope by sliding the distal aspect of the index and middle fingers of the dominant hand between the bell and diaphragm. This prevents the clinician's fingers from accidentally touching the bell or diaphragm and creating extraneous sounds. Warm up the diaphragm by placing it on warm clothing. This will avoid placing cold equipment on the patient's skin. Place the diaphragm of the stethoscope directly on the skin of the chest wall using gentle pressure. Technique for auscultation is pictured in **Figure 7.20**.

Instruct the patient to sit comfortably upright and take a deep breath in and out with the mouth open. Listen to at least one full breath in each auscultatory site or location. Caution the patient to do this leisurely so as not to get fatigued or hyperventilate and to take breaks as needed for comfort. Auscultate in a systematic manner from apex to base, comparing breath sounds from side to side. Refer to **Figure 7.19** to review the anterior, posterior, and lateral landmarks.

Mistakes or pitfalls that are common for novice clinicians:

- Auscultating one side of the chest wall entirely (left or right) before moving to the opposite side. To correct this when auscultating the anterior or posterior thorax, be sure to alternate left and right before moving lower on the chest wall.
- Listening over bone. To correct this, use the intercostal spaces as anatomic landmarks, and avoid auscultating over scapula, sternum, and ribs.
- Listening over clothes, which can include shirts, gowns, or bras. To correct this, place the stethoscope directly on the skin. Uncover the patient's thorax as needed.

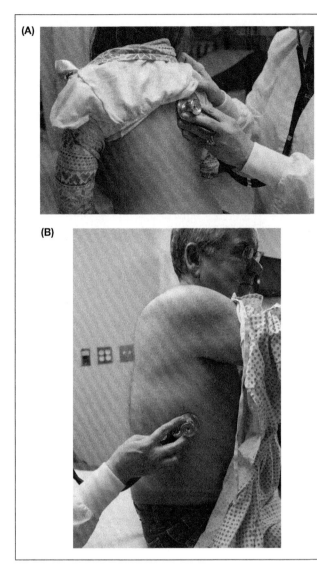

FIGURE 7.20 Auscultation technique. (A) Posterior. (B) Lateral.

- Omitting specific areas of the lungs, which may include upper, lower, or middle lobes. Remember to begin auscultating above the clavicle since the lungs extend well above the clavicle anteriorly. Be sure to listen laterally to assess right middle lobes. To assess the lower lobes of the lungs, the clinician must auscultate posteriorly.

Normal, Abnormal, and Transmitted Breath Sounds

During auscultation, the clinician can assess the rate, rhythm, and quality of breathing. The clinician can also assess the characteristics of the breath sounds. Breath sounds are typically described on the basis of intensity, pitch, duration, and location of the sounds. **Table 7.1** lists the expected breath sounds, including their location and characteristics.

Normal breath sounds can be diminished for a number of reasons. Diminished vesicular breath sounds may be heard in patients who are frail or elderly and have shallow breathing. They might also be diminished in individuals who are obese or very muscular and in whom the tissues impede the quality of the breath sounds. Obstruction related to a foreign body or thick secretions can generally decrease breath sounds, which are different than absent breath sounds. When minimal air is moving in or out of either lung, this is a worrisome sign, known as "silent chest," which signals the likelihood of severe hypoxia, respiratory distress, and/or respiratory failure. Absent breath sounds occurring on only one side of the chest can indicate pneumothorax, or a collapsed lung, which is also an emergency situation.

Respiratory conditions or pathology that decrease normal breath sounds can also create adventitious or abnormal sounds. The characteristics of these adventitious breath sounds—crackles, wheezes, rhonchi, stridor, and pleural rubs—and the associated pathophysiology are summarized in **Table 7.2**.

TABLE 7.1 Normal Breath Sounds			
Breath Sound	Description	Inspiratory:Expiratory Ratio	Depiction
Tracheal	Loudest and high pitched; usually heard over the upper aspect of the trachea; best heard on the anterior aspect of the neck	1:1	
Bronchial	Louder and higher in pitch; usually heard over the lower aspect of the trachea; best heard over the manubrium	1:2 or 1:3	
Bronchovesicular	Intermediate intensity and pitch; usually heard over the major bronchi in the midchest area anteriorly or between the scapulae posteriorly	1:1	
Vesicular	Soft intensity, low pitched, with a rustling quality during inspiration and softer with expiration; usually heard bilaterally over most of the peripheral fields	3:1	

TABLE 7.2 Abnormal Breath Sounds

Breath Sound	Description
Crackles	Crackles are classified as fine or coarse. Fine crackles are discontinuous high-pitched sounds that have a popping quality; these are usually inspiratory. Coarse crackles are discontinuous, low pitched, louder, and longer. Crackles indicate abnormalities of the lungs or airways such as pneumonia, congestive heart failure, or bronchitis. Crackles are heard as air passes through fluid-filled airways.
Wheezes	Wheezes are continuous musical sounds that can be high or low pitched. Wheezing is usually heard during expiration but may be heard during both inspiration and expiration. High-pitched wheezes sound squeaky, whereas low-pitched wheezes have a moaning quality. Wheezes are heard because of narrowing of the airways caused by asthma, COPD, or bronchitis. The tone of the wheeze varies depending on which area of the airways is affected. If the smaller airways are narrow, then the wheezes are musical in nature (polyphonic), and if the larger airways are narrow, then the wheeze sounds hoarse (monophonic).
Rhonchi	When the larger airways are obstructed with secretions, continuous low-pitched rattling sounds, called rhonchi, are heard. The rattling sounds may mimic snoring. The unique feature of rhonchi is that it clears with coughing or suctioning. Rhonchi is heard when pulmonary processes produce increased secretions (e.g., pneumonia, COPD, bronchiectasis, chronic bronchitis, or cystic fibrosis).
Stridor	Stridor is a loud and high-pitched sound caused by disrupted airflow. These abnormal breath sounds are typically during inspiration and associated with upper airway obstruction (above the thoracic cavity). When air cannot flow through the larynx, the disrupted airway creates the loud sounds. Upper airway obstruction can be caused by swelling-associated infection (croup, epiglottitis), chemical irritation (aspiration), or trauma (mechanical ventilation). Expiratory stridor may be present if the upper airway is blocked and air cannot escape through the trachea or upper airways. In rare situations, biphasic stridor may be heard when air cannot enter or leave the upper airways as subglottic stenosis due to granulation tissue. Stridor may indicate impending respiratory distress and/or failure.
Pleural Rubs	A pleural rub sound is the creaking or grating sound that can be heard during both inspiration and expiration as a result of friction (lack of lubrication or irritation) between the pleura. The sounds are comparable to that of two pieces of leather rubbing together. Pleurisy, an inflammation of the pleura, can cause pleural rubs. The pleural rub sound may not stop with coughing but will stop when the patient holds their breath. If the friction rub does not stop when the patient holds the breath, the etiology of the rub is more likely pericardial in nature.

COPD, chronic obstructive pulmonary disease.

When abnormal breath sounds are auscultated, the areas of abnormality can be further evaluated by auscultating for transmitted voice sounds. Normally, the sound of an individual's voice is muffled and difficult to understand by the clinician who is auscultating breath sounds. However, vocal sounds increase when the stethoscope is placed over denser areas of consolidation and, as a result, provide clues to pulmonary pathologies. To assess transmitted voice sounds, the clinician auscultates the anterior, posterior, and lateral thorax in the same systematic manner as auscultating for breath sounds. Clinicians can assess transmitted voice sounds using techniques known as bronchophony, egophony, or whispered pectoriloquy.

- *Bronchophony:* Ask the patient to say "99," while listening with the stethoscope. Normally, the sound of "99" will sound very faint and muffled. If

the voice sounds become clear and distinct, bronchophony is present. This occurs because sound transmits better through dense consolidation than through air.
- *Egophony:* Ask the patient to repeatedly say the sound "ee," while listening with the stethoscope. Normally, it will sound muffled but unchanged. If the sound changes to "aaay" while the patient is saying "ee," then egophony is present. This indicates the presence of consolidation or fluid in the lungs. The "aaay" sound will also be louder in the presence of consolidated tissue.
- *Whispered pectoriloquy:* For the whispered pectoriloquy test, ask the patient to whisper a few numbers or a short phrase and continue to repeat it. For example, "1, 2, 3, 1, 2, 3, 1, 2, 3, ..." Auscultate while the patient is whispering. Normally, the whispered voice will be distant, muffled, and not intelligible. If there

is consolidation in an area of the lung, the whispered voice will sound unusually clear and loud.

Systematically and thoroughly auscultating the chest for normal, abnormal, and transmitted breath sounds provides the clinician with key information about the integrity of the respiratory system.

PEDIATRIC PHYSICAL EXAMINATION CONSIDERATIONS

For infants and children, the order of physical exam can be modified depending on their state of wakefulness and/or cooperativeness. Chapter 4, Evidence-Based Assessment of Children and Adolescents, explains the approach to the physical exam of children. Specifically for the respiratory system, remember that the airway in children is shorter, and, as a result, upper airway sounds are frequently transmitted to lower airways, making the respiratory assessment more challenging.

The respiratory rate of infants can vary with temperature, activity, feeding, and even with sleep. When calculating respiratory rate, be sure to count for a full minute to calculate the normal respiratory rate because of these variations. The respiratory rate and rhythm can be assessed while the infant is sleeping in a parent's arms. Infants are obligate nose breathers, and so any congestion can greatly affect their respiratory effort, as evidenced by fussiness or decreased feedings. Nose breathing can also contribute to difficulties in the respiratory assessment because of transmitted airway sounds. One way to address the difficulty with assessment is by trying to clear the nasal passages with suctioning. In infants, it is normal to find them sneezing or hiccupping; however, stridor, grunting, or periodic spasms of coughing may indicate distress.

When performing a physical exam on an infant, at some point during the exam be sure to examine the baby on the exam table, with only a diaper on so that the whole body can be viewed to get a better understanding of the infant's respiratory effort. While the infant is lying down, inspect the child's chest for size and shape. Infants are likely to have periodic, irregular breathing. Assess that the infant's color does not change and that they are not using accessory muscles to breathe, even during times of periodic breathing episodes.

GERIATRIC PHYSICAL EXAMINATION CONSIDERATIONS

As a person becomes older, the amount of mucus produced throughout the body decreases, and this can be evident with dry mucous membranes in the nares, throat, and respiratory tract. Because of changes in the respiratory system of the older adult, expect to find an increased AP diameter of the chest wall and slight hyperresonance of the lungs fields with percussion. There is also a decreased amount of chest expansion and more reliance on the diaphragm for breathing.

Older adults with pneumonia are more likely to present with atypical symptoms. Typical symptoms of pneumonia are fever, cough, chest pain, headache, muscle pain, and dyspnea. However, older adults may present with altered mental status, decreased alertness, or acute confusion and may complain of poor appetite, fatigue, and/or having had recent falls.

LABORATORY CONSIDERATIONS FOR THE LUNGS AND RESPIRATORY SYSTEMS

LABORATORY TESTS TO ASSESS FOR RESPIRATORY DISORDERS AND RESPIRATORY STATUS

The following list of lab tests is used to assess respiratory status. The list is not intended to be exhaustive; how these tests are used is discussed in more detail in the section of this text addressing the abnormal findings of common respiratory disorders.

- **Arterial blood gas** is assessed to find whether an individual is hypoxemic or hypercarbic and whether the body is compensating for the acidotic or alkalotic blood pH.
- **Complete blood count (CBC)** to detect infection, inflammation, tumor, leukemia, anemia, dehydration, vitamin deficiencies, or effects of medications is often needed as these conditions affect metabolic and respiratory needs and capacities.
- **D-dimer** is recommended as an adjunctive test to rule out venous thromboembolism (VTE) or pulmonary embolism (PE) and not as a diagnostic test to confirm PE or VTE. The test is sensitive, but not specific. It can be elevated in a variety of conditions.
- **Electrolytes** are assessed to determine the underlying pathologies. Abnormalities in potassium, magnesium, and phosphate may aggravate respiratory failure and other organ dysfunction.
- **Sputum/blood cultures** may be drawn to identify any infectious causes. Sputum for culture and sensitivity may be obtained if the patient has an acute exacerbation of a respiratory disorder and has not responded to antibiotic therapy.
- **Viral testing, allergy testing, rapid molecular testing, nucleic acid amplification testing (NAAT), and PPD testing** to screen for specific illnesses are available; the evidence-based recommendations for use of these tests are discussed in the section of this chapter addressing abnormal findings of common respiratory disorders.

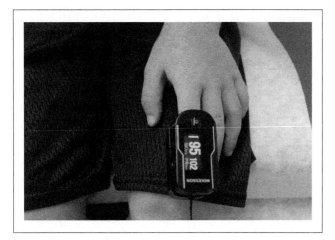

FIGURE 7.21 Pulse oximeter.

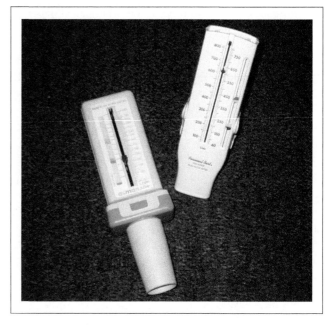

FIGURE 7.22 Peak flow meter.

TESTING TO MONITOR LUNG FUNCTION

Pulse Oximetry

A pulse oximeter is an external device that measures the oxygen saturation of arterial blood; although this test is not as accurate as the measurement done through an arterial blood gas, the test is 84.6% sensitive to hypoxemia in respiratory distress and is an easy way to estimate oxygen saturation (Amalakanti & Pentakota, 2016). The device uses a sensor that typically attaches to the finger or toe (**Figure 7.21**). The American Thoracic Society (2013) recommends the use of pulse oximetry to screen for hypoxia during acute exacerbations of respiratory disorders and cautions that the device may be inaccurate if an individual is a smoker or has chronic obstructive lung disease, because the oximeter does not identify the increased carbon dioxide levels as distinct from oxygen levels. Pulse oximetry varies in positive predictive value for individuals with chronic bronchitis or COPD from 69% to 85% (Amalakanti & Pentakota, 2016).

Peak Flow

A peak flow meter is a small, portable, hand-held device used to measure the volume of air that a person can exhale quickly after a full inspiration. Peak expiratory flow (PEF) can be measured as part of pulmonary function tests/spirometry (described in the next section) or through the use of the peak flow device (**Figure 7.22**). The value of measuring PEF using a hand-held meter is that the PEF generally correlates with airflow limitations in the individual with asthma. Expectations for peak flow measurements are based on age and height (**Figure 7.23**).

PEF is affected by the person's ability to breathe in deeply and by their ability to coordinate the use of the peak flow meter, which significantly affects the accuracy of peak flow measurement. However, accuracy and reliability can be achieved when following careful techniques for use that include directions to deeply inhale and then forcefully exhale as quickly as possible; repeating the technique three times and recording the highest of the three values also increases accuracy. Measurement of peak flow can be a component of an individual's asthma action plan; however, the optimal role for PEF monitoring has not been determined.

PULMONARY FUNCTION TESTS/SPIROMETRY

Spirometry is testing designed to detect the volume and capacity of the lungs to determine overall functioning of the respiratory system. Spirometry, or pulmonary function tests, identifies lung volumes by direct measurement. Lung capacities are calculated using two or more measures of volume. Molnar and Gair (2015) define the key volumes and capacities as including:

- *Tidal volume:* Amount of air displaced at rest between normal inhalation and exhalation
- *Residual volume:* Amount of air that remains in the lungs after a full exhalation

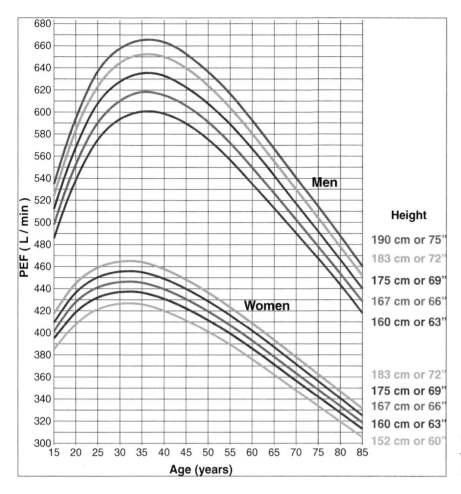

FIGURE 7.23 Peak flow chart. Normal values for peak expiratory flow (EN 13826 or EU scale).

- *Inspiratory reserve volume:* Amount of air that can be inhaled after a normal inhalation
- *Expiratory reserve volume:* Amount of air that can be exhaled after a normal exhalation
- *Inspiratory capacity:* Amount of air that can be inhaled after a normal exhalation. Inspiratory capacity is the sum of tidal volume and inspiratory reserve volume.
- *Functional residual capacity:* Amount of additional air that can be exhaled after a normal exhalation. Functional residual capacity is the sum of expiratory reserve volume and the residual volume.
- *Vital capacity:* Maximum amount of air that can be inhaled or exhaled during one respiratory cycle. Vital capacity is the sum of tidal volume, inspiratory reserve volume, and expiratory reserve volume.
- *Total lung capacity:* Total amount of air that remains in the lungs after a maximal inhalation

Additional measures taken during spirometry include the forced expiratory volume (FEV), which assesses how much air can be forced out of the lungs over a specific period, usually one second (FEV1), and the forced vital capacity (FVC), which is the total amount of air that can be forcibly exhaled (Molnar & Gair, 2015). These measures are significant because the ratio of these values (FEV1/FVC) is used to diagnose lung diseases, including asthma and COPD. If the FEV1/FVC ratio is high, this indicates that an individual was able to exhale most of their lung volume and/or that the individual's forced capacity was low, which happens in pulmonary fibrotic disorders or restrictive diseases that create noncompliant lung tissue. Conversely, when the FEV1/FVC ratio is low, there is resistance in the lung, which is characteristic of obstructive diseases that cause individuals to have difficulty moving air out of their lungs; this is reflected in less exhalation volume in one second and a much longer time needed to reach the maximal exhalation volume (Molnar & Gair, 2015).

The airflow measurements taken during pulmonary function tests/spirometry are depicted in flow volume loops or spirograms, as illustrated in **Figure 7.24**; the measures included in these specific spirograms include

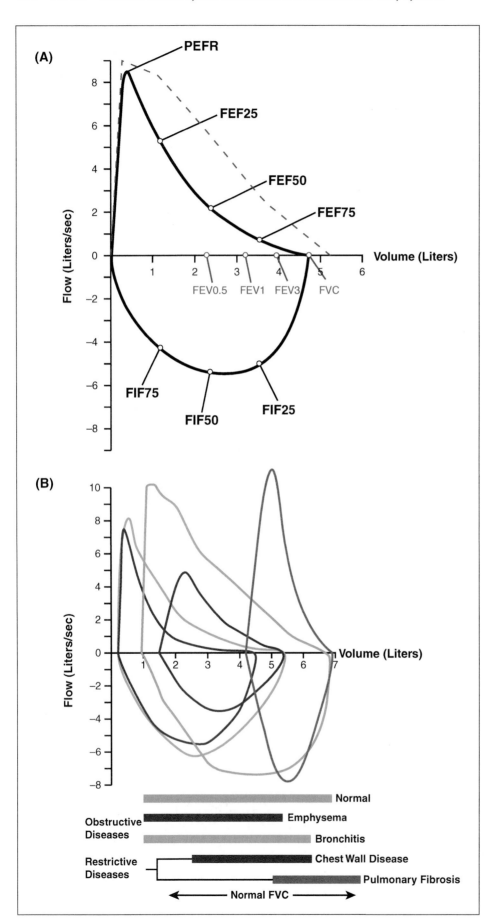

FIGURE 7.24 Normal (A) and abnormal (B) flow volume loops with pulmonary function tests.

FEF, forced expiratory flow; FEV, forced expiratory volume; FIF, forced inspiratory flow; FVC, forced vital capacity; PEFR, peak expiratory flow rate.

Source: Courtesy of Morgan Scientific, Inc.

forced inspiratory flow (FIF) and forced expiratory flow (FEF) to compare expected and abnormal findings. Flow volume loops indicate normal lung function, obstructive disease, or restrictive disease. Although pulmonary function tests include measures of peak flow, the additional measures to determine lung volume and capacity that are included in spirometry make it a reliable, effective, and powerful tool to diagnose and treat pulmonary disorders.

IMAGING CONSIDERATIONS FOR THE LUNGS AND RESPIRATORY SYSTEM

RADIOGRAPHY

Conventional chest radiographs, or chest x-rays, are imaging tests that use radiology to create images of the internal structures of the chest. Portable chest x-rays are often taken with the film placed behind the patient and the x-ray tube in front of the patient who is lying supine; the x-rays pass through the patient from front to back, that is, anterior to posterior (AP). Chest x-rays can also be completed with the patient standing, creating a posterior to anterior (PA) view, or from the side to create lateral films; when possible, PA views are preferable to AP views as the heart magnification is increased with the AP view. Whatever technique is used, interpretation of a chest x-ray requires a careful, systematic examination of the entire film. A common mnemonic to review a chest x-ray image is "ABCDEF": A for airways, B for bones, C for cardiomediastinal silhouette, D for diaphragm, E for expanded lungs/everything else, and F for foreign objects. Learning to interpret chest-x-rays requires practice and careful review. The following images are a series of normal and abnormal chest x-rays, including lateral and AP chest x-rays, that identify:

- Kyphotic curvature of the vertebral column (**Figure 7.25**)
- Fibrotic changes as a result of an empyema (**Figure 7.26**)
- Lower lobe pneumonia (**Figure 7.27**)
- Pulmonary interstitial infiltrates from *Pneumocystis* (**Figure 7.28**)
- Chickenpox pneumonia (**Figure 7.29**)
- Fibrotic changes as a result of a fungal infection (**Figure 7.30**)
- Pulmonary effusion as a sequela of lung cancer (**Figure 7.31**)

Chest x-rays are completed for individuals who present with cough, dyspnea, hemoptysis, and/or

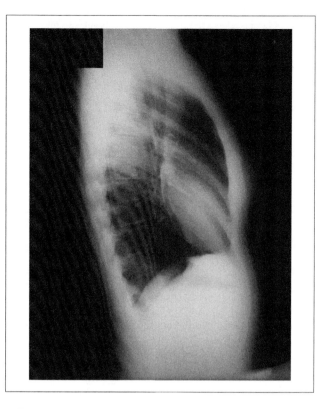

FIGURE 7.25 Kyphotic curve of the vetebral column. Normal lateral chest x-ray. The kyphotic curve of the vertebral column is on the left of the thoracic cavity, and the oblong, elliptical cardiac silhouette on the right.

Source: Image courtesy of Thomas Hooten, MD/Centers for Disease Control and Prevention.

chest pain. Evidence-based recommendations advocate against the use of routine chest x-rays for asymptomatic, low-risk individuals; avoid admission or preoperative chest x-rays for ambulatory patients with unremarkable history and physical exam (American Board of Internal Medicine [ABIM], n.d.-a). Evidence-based recommendations related to the use of chest radiographs are included in the section of this chapter that addresses common respiratory disorders.

COMPUTED TOMOGRAPHY

A computed tomography (CT) scan is a noninvasive, painless imaging test that uses multiple x-ray images from numerous angles to create cross-sectional images with greater anatomic details. Because of the higher dose of radiation (one chest CT is equivalent to almost 200 chest x-rays), careful consideration is required for the use of CT, with the awareness that a series of CT scans has more risk than one isolated scan. Additionally, CT with contrast may have additional risks for

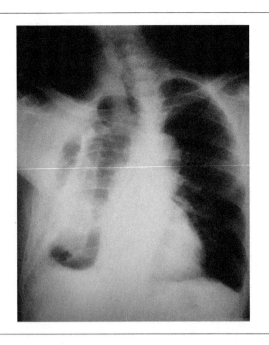

FIGURE 7.26 Significant lung tissue changes. This anteroposterior chest x-ray revealed the presence of a right fibrothorax, which was thought to be due to a previous empyema. An empyema, or pus-filled cavity, located between the two pleural membranes can give rise to fibrotic changes as the infection resolves, much like a scar formation, which appears as a denser area on x-ray.

Source: Image courtesy of Thomas Hooten, MD/Centers for Disease Control and Prevention.

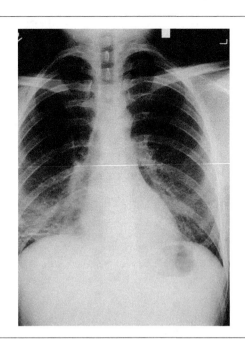

FIGURE 7.28 Pulmonary infiltrates. This anteroposterior chest x-ray revealed radiologic evidence of pulmonary pneumocystosis in the form of bilateral pulmonary interstitial infiltrates. This infection was due to the presence of an opportunistic fungal infection, by the fungal organism *Pneumocystis jirovecii.*

Source: Image courtesy of Jonathan WM Gold, MD/Centers for Disease Control and Prevention.

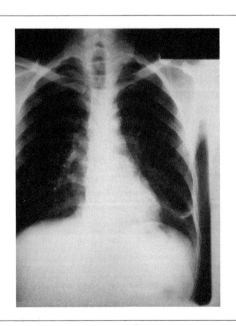

FIGURE 7.27 Early signs of pneumonia. This anteroposterior chest x-ray revealed signs of early left lower lobe pneumonia, with an unknown etiologic profile.

Source: Image courtesy of Thomas Hooten, MD/Centers for Disease Control and Prevention.

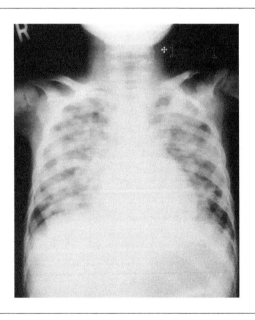

FIGURE 7.29 Chickenpox pneumonia. This anteroposterior radiograph revealed bilateral pulmonary infiltrates throughout the entirety of each lung field in the case of a child with leukemia, as well as chickenpox pneumonia. The fact that this child had leukemia made him that much more susceptible to contracting a pneumonic infection.

Source: Image courtesy of Joel D. Meyers, MD/Centers for Disease Control and Prevention.

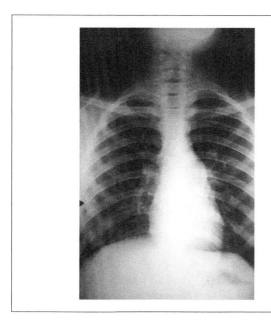

FIGURE 7.30 Fibrotic changes caused by fungal organism. This anteroposterior chest x-ray revealed pulmonary changes indicative of pulmonary fibrosis in a case of coccidioidomycosis, caused by fungal organisms. Because these changes also resemble those seen in other lung infections, including tuberculosis, the findings uncovered need to be coupled with serologic testing, as well as possible tissue biopsy. The degree of fibrotic changes indicative of scarring found on x-ray can be directly correlated with the severity of the fungal infection.

Source: Image courtesy of Lucille K. Georg, MD/Centers for Disease Control and Prevention.

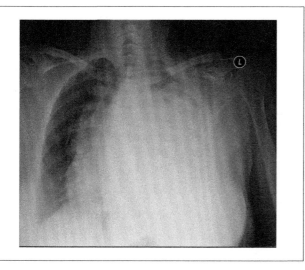

FIGURE 7.31 Pulmonary effusion. A massive left pleural effusion displacing the heart and trachea to the right; caused by pulmonary adenocarcinoma, which is obscured by the effusion and cannot be recognized in this radiograph.

Source: Image courtesy of Yale Rosen, MD.

individuals with diabetes and chronic kidney disease. Evidence-based recommendations for the use of CT are included in the section of the chapter addressing common respiratory disorders. The following images are a series of normal and abnormal CT scans that identify:

- Normal thorax taken in various views **(Figure 7.32)**
- Acute histoplasmosis **(Figure 7.33)**
- Adenocarcinoma **(Figure 7.34)**

EVIDENCE-BASED CONSIDERATIONS FOR THE LUNGS AND RESPIRATORY SYSTEM

There are a significant number of evidence-based guidelines addressing the assessment of abnormal findings in the respiratory system, although some gaps in the evidence remain. In addition to Choosing Wisely, the USPSTF, the Cochrane Library, and the CDC have many significant assessment and treatment guidelines that have been generated both nationally and internationally by professional associations and committees of experts drawn together to evaluate the evidence. Many of these organizations update their guidelines regularly. Their guidelines have been incorporated within the next section of abnormal findings related to common respiratory disorders. The following are important groups generating evidence-based guidelines and recommendations and the disease topics of those guidelines:

- American Academy of Pediatrics (bronchiolitis)
- American Academy of Sleep Medicine (obstructive sleep apnea [OSA])
- American College of Chest Physicians (CHEST; pneumonia, influenza, lung cancer, and pertussis)
- American College of Physicians (bronchitis)
- American Thoracic Society (CF)
- Infectious Disease Society of America (pneumonia and influenza)
- Global Initiative for Chronic Obstructive Lung Disease (COPD)
- Global Initiative for Asthma (asthma)
- World Health Organization (tuberculosis)

ABNORMAL FINDINGS: VARIATIONS IN PATTERNS OF BREATHING

Variations in patterns of breathing are some of the first signs and/or most significant signs of pathologic disease states. An individual's breathing pattern varies in

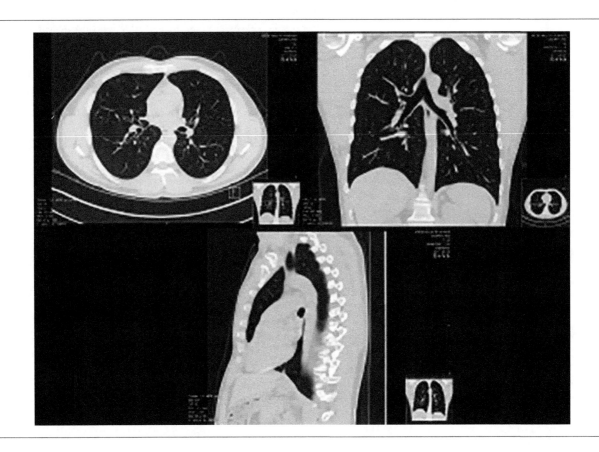

FIGURE 7.32 CT scans of normal thorax (axial, coronal, and sagittal planes). Normal thorax of a 37-year-old man who presented with unspecific breathing problems.

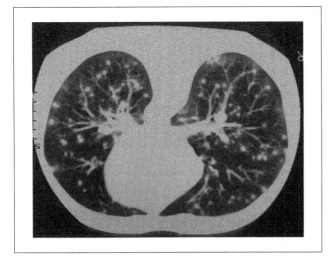

FIGURE 7.33 CT scan of lungs showing the classic snowstorm appearance of acute histoplasmosis.

Source: From the Centers for Disease Control and Prevention. Retrieved from http://www.publicdomainfiles.com/show_file. php?id=13527322819161

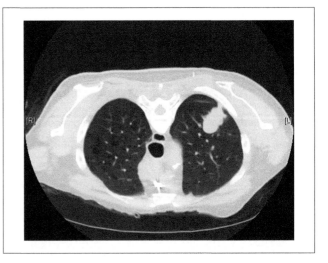

FIGURE 7.34 CT scan of lungs showing adenocarcinoma.

Source: Image courtesy of Yale Rosen, MD.

TABLE 7.3 Abnormal Patterns of Breathing

Variation	Description	Depiction
Tachypnea	Abnormally increased respiratory rate associated with shallow breaths. Patient may describe sensations of shortness of breath. Typically noted in patients with hypoxemia, hypercapnia, and fever in whom the body is compensating to maintain homeostasis. Pathological causes include pneumonia, heart failure, central nervous system abnormalities such as tumors, and salicylate intoxication.	
Hyperpnea	An increased rate and depth of breathing that is commonly associated with an increase in metabolic demand resulting from exercise, high altitude, or anemia. Also noted in patients with severe metabolic acidosis related to diabetic ketoacidosis or renal failure. The hyperpnea associated with diabetic ketoacidosis is called Kussmaul's respiration.	
Bradypnea	Abnormally slow respiratory rate that might affect alveolar ventilation. Etiology includes drug-induced respiratory depression, hypothyroidism, and neurologic conditions such as increased intracranial pressure or neuromuscular diseases such as Guillain-Barré syndrome or amyotrophic lateral sclerosis. In the United States, opioids are the primary cause of drug-induced respiratory depression and needs to be considered during history taking.	
Sighing Respiration	Normal reaction to mild emotional states or fatigue and typically nonpathologic. Respiratory rate will be normal, but certain breaths will be deeper, leading to hyperventilation during those breaths.	
Cheyne-Stokes Breathing	Abnormal breathing pattern where there are periods of progressively deeper breaths (crescendo–decrescendo) followed by periods of no breathing. Cheyne-Stokes breathing is commonly seen in patients who are in the final stages of dying. It can also be seen in patients with congestive heart failure, traumatic brain injury, carbon monoxide poisoning, hyponatremia, and medication overdoses (morphine).	
Biot's Breathing	Regular deep respirations alternating with periods of no breathing due to damage to the pons caused by cerebrovascular accident, trauma, meningitis, or brain herniation.	
Agonal	Occasional reflex-driven gasps, associated with anoxia, cardiac arrest, cerebral ischemia, or hypoxia.	
Apnea	Absence of breathing that signals a life-threatening situation resulting in death if no intervention is carried out immediately.	

response to metabolic demand or imbalance, injury to the respiratory centers of the brain, and use of medications; the impact of the variation on oxygen and carbon dioxide levels can lead to further physiologic compromise. **Table 7.3** lists common abnormal variations in breathing patterns and includes descriptions and depictions of the variations.

ABNORMAL FINDINGS: COMMON RESPIRATORY DISORDERS

ACUTE BRONCHITIS

Acute bronchitis is a lower respiratory infection most often of viral origin (Harris, Hicks, & Qaseem, 2016).

Symptoms in the first few days may appear similar to the common cold (Kincade & Long, 2016). Other common symptoms of acute bronchitis are (Kincade & Long, 2016):

- Productive cough
- Dyspnea
- Nasal congestion
- Headache
- Fever
- Substernal or chest wall pain when coughing
- Cough duration of 2 to 6 weeks

Key History and Physical Findings

- Mildly ill appearance
- Fever, usually less than 100 during the first few days of illness, then resolves
- Lung exam may be normal or reveal wheezes or rhonchi, which clears with coughing.

One of the chief concerns in evaluating acute bronchitis is differentiating bronchitis from pneumonia, which is more likely to be caused by a bacterial infection and need treatment with antibiotics. Purulent sputum is not indicative of a bacterial infection. Fever greater than 100°F should prompt evaluation for influenza and pneumonia. It is unusual for a healthy immunocompetent adult under 70 years old with normal vital signs and a normal lung exam to have pneumonia (Harris et al., 2016; Kincade & Long, 2016).

Diagnostic testing is usually not indicated for acute bronchitis. According to Cao, Choy, Mohanakrishnan, Bain, and van Driel (2013), chest x-ray does not affect the outcomes of children or adults with lower respiratory tract infection. Both procalcitonin and C-reactive protein have been studied as possible blood tests or even point-of-care tests to help differentiate between bronchitis and pneumonia. Although these tests are regarded as possibly promising and seem to have little risk, larger studies are needed before evidence-based recommendations can be made (Tonkin-Crine et al., 2017).

ASTHMA

Asthma is a disease of chronic airway inflammation with many variations. The pathology associated with asthma is depicted in **Figure 7.35**. Asthma is defined by two key features, both of which must be present to make the diagnosis (Global Initiative for Asthma, 2019):

- History of respiratory symptoms—wheeze, shortness of breath, chest tightness, and cough that vary over time and in intensity
- Variable expiratory airflow limitation

The clinician may often find through the history that the patient has more than one of the foregoing symptoms and that these may be worse at night or on waking. Symptoms are often triggered by exercise, laughter, allergens, or cold air and may occur with or worsen during viral infections. Another question that can help diagnose asthma involves occupational exposures and symptoms that improve when the patient leaves the workplace. Additional questions about family history and presence of eczema and environmental or food allergies can also help with diagnosis of some types of asthma (Global Initiative for Asthma, 2018).

The physical exam of an individual with asthma is often normal, although the most frequent finding associated with asthma is wheezing, especially on forced expiration (Global Initiative for Asthma, 2019). HEENT and skin exams may show evidence of allergies and/or eczema (Global Initiative for Asthma, 2018).

It is important to assess pregnant women and those planning to become pregnant for a history of asthma as treatment is considered safer for the fetus than repeated exacerbations (American College of Obstetricians and Gynecologists [ACOG], 2008). In children younger than 5 years of age for whom spirometry is unreliable, diagnosis is made through symptom patterns such as cough, wheeze, breathlessness manifested as activity limitation, and nocturnal worsening. These children also often have a history of allergies and eczema and respond to a trial of controller medication (Global Initiative for Asthma, 2018).

Spirometry gives evidence of the variable expiratory airflow limitation through measurement of lung volumes and flow rates. Spirometry should be used in all patients over 5 years old. The ABIM (n.d.-a) recommends that asthma should always be diagnosed and managed with spirometry. Expected spirometry findings would be as follows (Global Initiative for Asthma, 2019):

- FEV1/FVC ratio below the lower limit of normal
- Variability in lung function after inhaling a bronchodilator
- Diurnal PEF variability greater than 10% in adults and greater than 13% in children

Other tests that are sometimes used when spirometry is not diagnostic include bronchial provocation and allergy testing. Bronchial provocation tests for airway hyperresponsiveness through the inhalation of methylcholine or another possible trigger. Allergy testing may help to determine whether the patient has allergy triggers for asthma. Neither test is highly specific for asthma but can provide additional information that can help with the diagnosis (Global Initiative for Asthma, 2018). Chest x-rays are not recommended for children with uncomplicated asthma (ABIM, n.d.-a).

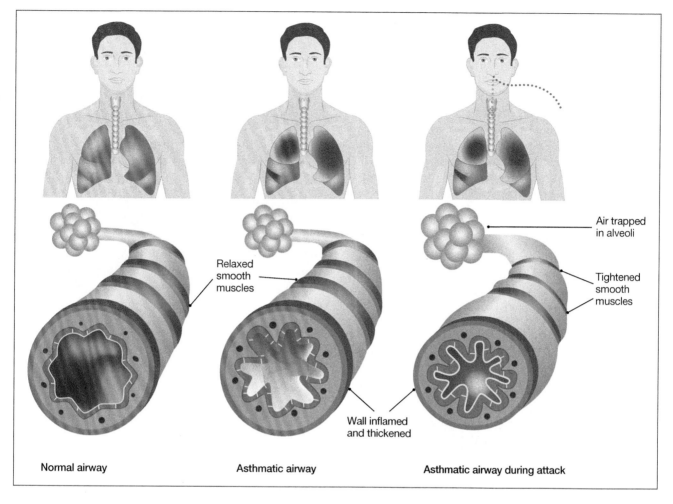

Relaxed smooth muscles

Air trapped in alveoli

Tightened smooth muscles

Wall inflamed and thickened

Normal airway   Asthmatic airway   Asthmatic airway during attack

FIGURE 7.35 Asthma pathology.

BRONCHIOLITIS

Bronchiolitis refers to a wide variety of diseases characterized by inflammation of the bronchial airways. The most common disease type of bronchiolitis is an acute viral infection that presents in children under 2 years old. Less common types of bronchiolitis in adults are characterized by an insidious onset of dyspnea and cough and can have a variety of associations, including organ and stem cell transplantation, connective tissue diseases, and exposure to toxic fumes (Chesnutt, Chesnutt, Prendergast, & Prendergast, 2019).

The young child with bronchiolitis most often presents during the winter season; the chief purpose of the history and physical exam for the child who presents with acute symptoms suggestive of this viral illness is to differentiate bronchiolitis from other disorders and to assess the severity of the disease (Ralston et al., 2014). The predicted severity has important implications in deciding whether to treat the infant as an outpatient or whether admission is necessary.

Key History and Physical Findings

- Presence of a prodromal viral upper respiratory infection followed by increased respiratory effort and wheezing
- Presence of rhinorrhea, cough
- Child's mental status and activity level
- Child's ability and interest in feeding
- Ability of the family to recognize changes in the child's condition and to return for reevaluation—transportation, funds for gas or public transportation
- Presence of underlying conditions such as prematurity, cardiac disease, chronic pulmonary disease, immunodeficiency, genetic abnormalities, in utero and current tobacco smoke exposure

Physical exam findings can include tachypnea, wheezing, and crackles. It is important to count respirations over a full minute for greatest accuracy. The clinician should also observe the child for signs of increased respiratory effort, such as grunting, nasal flaring, and intercostal and subcostal retractions (Ralston et al., 2014). There can be variability in the exam. Sometimes suctioning the nose with a bulb syringe and positioning may assist in the accuracy of the exam. At times, serial exams over time are needed (Ralston et al., 2014). Tachypnea over 70 has been associated with increased severity of illness in some studies (Ralston et al., 2014). Apnea has been observed with bronchiolitis.

History of premature birth increases the risk of bronchiolitis and associated apnea. Full-term infants over 1 month of age or preterm infants 48 weeks post conception with no previous apnea are considered at low risk for apnea (Ralston et al., 2014). However, preterm infants with a history of apnea who were born before 29 weeks' gestation are at risk for bronchiolitis. The respiratory compromise of the 28-week infant pictured in **Figure 7.36** increased his vulnerability to bronchiolitis through the first year of his life. Most bronchiolitis is caused by respiratory syncytial virus (RSV). Premature infants may qualify for monthly RSV vaccine prophylaxis. **Figure 7.37** depicts the infant with a history of prematurity while hospitalized in his first year with bronchiolitis;

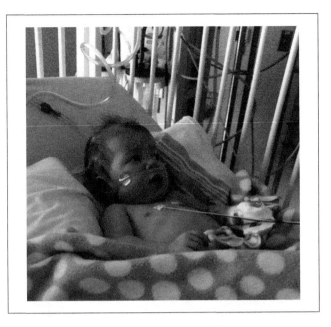

FIGURE 7.37 Infant with bronchiolitis. Infant with history of prematurity hospitalized with bronchiolitis caused by respiratory synctial virus. Note intercostal retractions.

the course of his illness did include apnea that was quickly recognized and treated with a positive outcome.

Bronchiolitis is complicated in children with a history of prematurity. In uncomplicated bronchiolitis, neither chest x-ray nor viral testing is recommended (ABIM, n.d.-b; Ralston et al., 2014).

CHRONIC OBSTRUCTIVE PULMONARY DISEASE

COPD is a common, chronic, and treatable disease characterized by respiratory symptoms and airflow limitation. The pathology of COPD has to do with small airway disease; lung tissue destruction, also called emphysema; and loss of alveolar attachments to the small airways. Chronic inflammation and decreased elasticity of the lungs are also part of the picture of COPD (GOLD, 2019).

Important history to collect from patients includes both risk factors for the development of COPD and symptoms of COPD. The biggest risk factor for the development of COPD is current or former tobacco smoking. Household exposure also contributes to COPD worldwide, especially exposure to wood smoke used in cooking and heating. This is especially a problem for women worldwide. Prevalence of COPD also increases with age. Never-smokers can also develop COPD, but their disease tends not to be as severe. Lung growth and development also play a role. Birthweight, early childhood lung infections, in utero smoke exposure, and home overcrowding in early life can affect later lung function. Genetics also plays a role in disease development (GOLD, 2019). The alpha-1 antitrypsin deficiency (AATD) and some single-gene correlations are

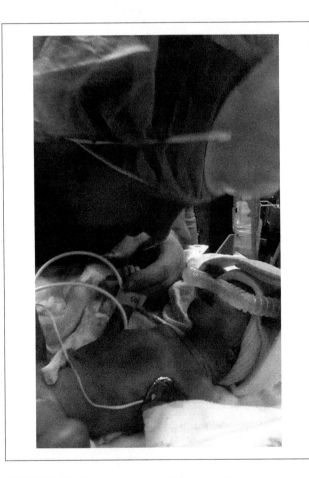

FIGURE 7.36 Premature infant. Twenty-eight-week premature infant taking first breaths with support from father. Suprasternal, substernal, and intercostal retractions related to lung immaturity.

implicated in the development and severity of COPD. Asthma may also be a risk factor (GOLD, 2019).

Symptoms of COPD include the following although they may not all be present in every patient (GOLD, 2019; USPSTF, 2016):

- Chronic cough
- Dyspnea
- Sputum production
- Recurrent lower respiratory tract infections
- Chest tightness—especially after exercise

Key History and Physical Findings

In severe disease, both characteristic history and physical exam findings may be present. These include fatigue, weight loss, and anorexia. COPD can lead to right heart failure, the only sign of which may be ankle edema. Rib fractures and syncope from prolonged cough may also be present in severe disease (GOLD, 2019). Widespread inspiratory and expiratory wheezes may be present on physical exam, but this may not be present in early disease. Decreased lung sounds due to destruction of lung tissue is also common. The absence of physical exam findings in COPD does not exclude the diagnosis (GOLD, 2019).

Diagnostic Considerations

The most important diagnostic test for COPD is spirometry. The definition of airflow limitation is an FEV1/FVC less than 0.70 (GOLD, 2019; USPSTF, 2016). If a patient has an FEV1/FVC between 0.6 and 0.8, repeat spirometry on a separate occasion is recommended (GOLD, 2019). COPD severity is staged using the FEV1. The FEV1 in mild COPD is greater than or equal to 80% of predicted. Moderate COPD is between 50% and 80% of predicted. Severe COPD is from 30% to 50% of predicted. And very severe COPD is less than 30% of predicted (GOLD, 2019).

The severity of COPD symptoms is staged using symptom questionnaires and exacerbation history. Several symptoms questionnaires are available and have been validated. Currently, the symptom assessments recommended for use in practice are the COPD Control Questionnaire (CCQ) and the COPD Assessment Test (CAT). The risk of exacerbations is assessed in staging the severity of COPD by asking about previous exacerbations and their severity (GOLD, 2019). The FEV1 combined with the symptoms assessment and exacerbation risk give a stage that is used in pharmacologic treatment planning (GOLD, 2019).

Other tests recommended in the initial workup of COPD include blood testing for AATD and a chest x-ray to rule out other causes of the patient's symptoms. The chest x-ray is not diagnostic for COPD. Pulse oximetry is also helpful. Patients with results under 92% should have arterial blood gases (GOLD, 2019).

Although many patients may be unaware that they have COPD, even attributing symptoms to other causes, screening with spirometry or with symptom questionnaires is not recommended (USPSTF, 2016). Case finding by asking people who smoke or formerly smoked and/or those with symptoms and risk factors is recommended (GOLD, 2019; USPSTF, 2016).

CYSTIC FIBROSIS

CF is an inherited disorder caused by a mutation in the cystic fibrosis transmembrane conductance regulator (CFTR) protein. **Figure 7.38** depicts the gene transmission of this autosomal recessive trait. The gene defect causes dysfunction in the transport of chloride, sodium, and bicarbonate, which results in thick, viscous mucus within the lungs, pancreas, liver, reproductive tract, and intestines, and increased sodium content in sweat glands (Farrell et al., 2017). **Figure 7.39** depicts the structural changes in the lungs related to CF, and **Figure 7.40** depicts the anatomic changes within the airways related to CF.

In the past, most patients were diagnosed with CF after presenting with symptoms; however, because of the expansion of newborn screenings that include testing

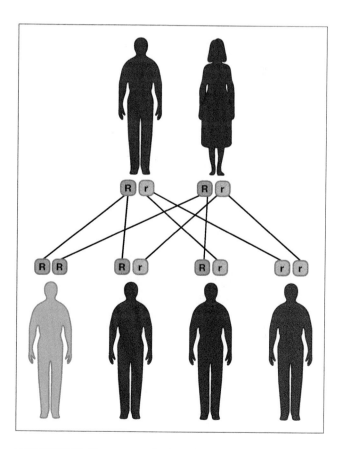

FIGURE 7.38 Gene transmission of autosomal recessive trait.

for CF, more than half of new cases are diagnosed by newborn screens (Farrell et al., 2017). Clinical presentation of CF includes positive newborn screening, signs and symptoms, and abnormal sweat chloride testing. The Cystic Fibrosis Foundation recommends that newborns with a positive CF screen should have sweat chloride testing within 4 weeks of birth and that all individuals who screen positive for both CF screening and sweat chloride testing should undergo CFTR genetic testing (Farrell et al., 2017). Although pulmonary function tests play a key role in the management of CF for children over 6 years of age, these assessments have a

limited role in the assessment and diagnosis of CF for children under 6 years of age related to the challenges of measuring lung function in young children (American Thoracic Society [ATS], 2013).

Because CFTR gene mutations can vary, symptom presentations can vary as well. Infants and children with CF may present with meconium ileus, respiratory symptoms, and failure to thrive. Symptomatic presentation in adulthood includes gastrointestinal symptoms, infertility, and diabetes. Manifestations of CF include chronic sinus congestion, pancreatic insufficiency, small bowel obstruction, cirrhosis, cholelithiasis, kyphosis, venous thrombosis, and anemia, in addition to respiratory tract involvement (Farrell et al., 2017). Common respiratory signs and symptoms of CF include the following:

- Persistent, productive cough
- Wheezing, dyspnea, tachypnea
- Hyperinflation of lungs on chest x-ray (ATS, 2013)
- Pulmonary function tests consistent with obstructive disease (ATS, 2013)
- Recurrent lung infections
- Bronchiectasis, impaired mucociliary clearance of the airway
- OSA

CF is a complex, progressive disease with a varying course. Progressive airway damage from CF is characterized by recurrent bronchiolitis, bronchopulmonary infections, deterioration of lung function, and pulmonary hypertension. Improved therapies for airway clearance, pancreatic enzyme supplements, and medication management have led to improved life expectancy for individuals with CF (Farrell et al., 2017).

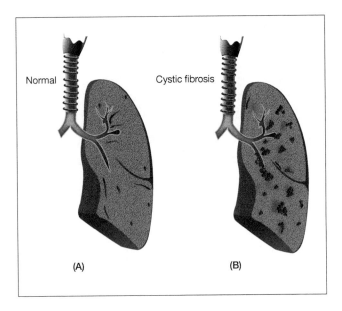

FIGURE 7.39 Structural changes in the lung related to cystic fibrosis. (A) Normal lung. (B) Lung with cystic fibrosis.

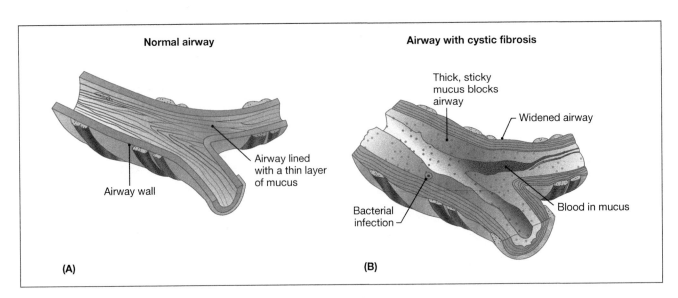

FIGURE 7.40 Anatomic changes within the airway related to cystic fibrosis. (A) Normal airway. (B) Airway with cystic fibrosis.

INFLUENZA

Influenza is a highly contagious respiratory infection that affects the nose, throat, and sometimes lungs. It can manifest as a febrile illness with cough, a worsening of a patient's chronic illness, or as confusion in the elderly (CDC, n.d.-a; Hart, 2019; Uyeki et al., 2018).

Some symptoms are highly associated with influenza but are also common to other respiratory infections (Hart, 2019). Highly associated symptoms are:

- Cough
- Fever
- Sore throat
- Myalgias
- Headache

Key History and Physical Findings

This combination of highly associated symptoms is most likely to be influenza when there is a community outbreak in progress (Hart, 2019). Even though fever is considered one of the main symptoms of influenza, some patients may present without fever, including infants, the elderly, and immunocompromised adults. Influenza can still occur if the patient has had the seasonal influenza vaccine.

Another category of patients who may have influenza are those who present first with flu complications. In children, these complications may include otitis media, acute myositis presenting as refusal to walk, sepsis, croup, bronchiolitis, or pneumonia. Adult complications from influenza can include sinusitis, otitis media, myositis, sepsis, pneumonia, myocarditis, encephalitis, multiorgan failure, and exacerbations of chronic diseases.

The physical exam in influenza is nonspecific, appearing similar to many other upper respiratory illnesses except for the likelihood of fever. Abnormal lung findings would generally point to another illness or a complication of influenza.

Diagnostic Considerations

Diagnostic testing is not necessary to make the diagnosis of influenza, especially in the midst of a community outbreak, but it can be helpful if it will change treatment (Uyeki et al., 2018). If the patient has no link to an influenza infection, testing may help make the diagnosis (Uyeki et al., 2018). Beyond the rapid tests outlined in the text that follows, other tests would be done only if necessary to diagnose complications or monitor exacerbations of chronic disease.

There are a variety of lab tests available for influenza. Because antiviral treatment is best if given early in the illness, usually started within the first 2 days, rapid testing with molecular tests and reverse transcriptase tests has become the norm for clinical management both in the inpatient and outpatient settings (Hart, 2019; Uyeki et al., 2018). These tests are also called NAATs. Rapid tests for influenza need to be done within 4 days of symptom onset (Hart, 2019). Results using nasopharyngeal swabs in the outpatient setting are available in about 30 minutes. Rapid influenza diagnostic tests (RIDTs) and immunofluorescence tests have fallen out of favor with the development of rapid molecular testing because of their low sensitivity (Uyeki et al., 2018). Viral cultures take 1 to 3 days for results to be available and are useful only to confirm negative RIDTs and immunofluorescence tests (CDC, n.d.-a; Uyeki et al., 2018). Serological testing is used only by public health and reference labs for research (CDC, n.d.-a).

LUNG CANCER SCREENING

Although multiple groups now recommend lung cancer screening, controversies still exist about whom to screen, how often, the ratio of benefits and harms to screening, and the design of effective screening programs (American Geriatrics Society, 2015; Manser et al., 2013; Mazzone et al., 2018). The most recent screening guidelines from the CHEST (Mazzone et al., 2018) are based on moderate- to low-quality evidence. The only strong recommendations made are that smoking cessation treatment be included in any screening program and that persons with comorbidities that adversely influence their ability to tolerate further evaluation of abnormal screening or treatment of early stage lung cancer not be screened. The USPSTF guidelines from 2013 are currently under review.

The most recent guideline recommends that annual screening with low-dose CT be offered between the ages of 55 and 77 to asymptomatic smokers who have smoked 30 pack years and who continue to smoke or quit within the last 15 years (Mazzone et al., 2018). Other important recommendations include the following:

- Do not screen those who do not meet the age and smoking criteria, even if they seem high risk (Mazzone et al., 2018).
- If the patient has comorbidities that limit their ability to tolerate screening or treatment or that limit their life expectancy, do not screen (American Geriatrics Society, 2015; Mazzone et al., 2018).
- Smoking cessation treatment is recommended as part of a screening program (Mazzone et al., 2018).
- If patients have symptoms of lung cancer, they should have a diagnostic evaluation rather than a screening (Mazzone et al., 2018).

Patients who are being considered for screening need to be evaluated carefully and involved in shared decision-making regarding the screening (Mazzone et al., 2018). Issues to consider in the evaluation include comorbidities, ability to tolerate further evaluation and cancer surgery and treatment, and any symptoms of lung cancer (Mazzone et al., 2018). Symptoms of lung cancer that should prompt diagnostic evaluation instead of screening include the following (Mazzone et al., 2018):

- Cough that is poorly explained
- Hemoptysis
- Shortness of breath
- Chest pain
- Unintentional weight loss
- Hoarseness
- Bone pain
- Headaches
- Vision changes
- Confusion
- Nausea
- Constipation
- Weakness
- Clubbing

OBSTRUCTIVE SLEEP APNEA

OSA is a syndrome in which patients suffer from either repeated episodes of reduced airflow during sleep or the temporary complete cessation of airflow during sleep (Qaseem et al., 2014). This is due to repeated collapse and reopening of the airways (Kapur, 2010). **Figure 7.41** depicts the positioning of the tongue, soft palate, and uvula during sleep for the individual with OSA. When the airways collapse, the increased work of breathing causes arousal, and the upper airway muscles are activated to reopen the airway (Kapur, 2010). These repeated arousals from sleep can result in daytime sleepiness, impaired concentration, and risk for falling asleep while driving (Qaseem et al., 2014). OSA is also

associated with other poor health outcomes such as cardiovascular disease, hypertension, metabolic abnormalities such as type 2 diabetes, and an increased risk of postoperative cardiac and respiratory complications (Qaseem et al., 2014).

Although the USPSTF does not recommend screening for OSA owing to insufficient evidence of benefit, clinicians should be alert to the presentations of undiagnosed patients who present to their practice (USPSTF, 2017). The most common symptom of sleep apnea is unexplained daytime sleepiness (Qaseem et al., 2014). Other symptoms include (Qaseem et al., 2014):

- Loud snoring
- Frequent arousals
- Disruption of sleep
- Presence of associated adverse clinical outcomes

Key History/Physical Findings and Diagnostic Considerations

The most common physical finding is obesity (Qaseem et al., 2014). The best diagnostic testing is polysomnography (PSG) observed in a sleep lab. This may elicit signs of hypoxemia and lower limb movements in addition to measuring hypopnea and apnea episodes. One result of the PSG is reported as an apnea–hypopnea index/hour (AHI). An AHI of greater than 15 episodes without symptoms and greater than five with symptoms is diagnostic of OSA (Qaseem et al., 2014). Another test to consider is testing for thyroid disease (Qaseem et al., 2014).

PERTUSSIS

Pertussis, commonly known as whooping cough, is a contagious bacterial respiratory disease caused by *Bordetella pertussis*. In its worst stage, it is characterized by paroxysmal coughing. It is most serious in infants, but also affects children, adolescents, and adults. Incubation can take from 5 days to 3 weeks (CDC, n.d.-c). Cases can occur year-round but peak in late summer to autumn. Neither infection nor vaccination produces lifetime immunity, although vaccinated persons may have less severe disease (CDC, n.d.-c).

Pertussis has a three-stage course, with changing symptoms in each course. In the first stage, called the catarrhal stage, which lasts 1 to 2 weeks, pertussis is characterized by the following (CDC, n.d.-c; Rivard & Viera, 2014):

- Runny nose and sneezing
- Mild cough
- Low-grade fever—often not present in adults (Moore, Harnden, Grant, Patel, & Irwin, 2019)
- Apnea or cyanosis in infants (Moore et al., 2017)

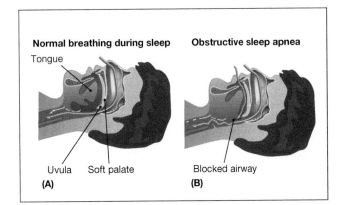

FIGURE 7.41 Obstructive sleep apnea (OSA). (A) Open airway during sleep. (B) Blocked airway associated with OSA.

The second stage, the paroxysmal stage, lasts 1 to 6 weeks and is characterized by severe coughing paroxysms that may leave the patient devoid of air in the lungs. When the patient breathes in to refill the lungs, the characteristic whoop is produced. Most adolescents and adults do not produce the whoop. The cough is often worse at night and can induce vomiting either during or after the paroxysm (CDC, n.d.-c; Rivard & Viera, 2014). Adults are more likely than children to have posttussive vomiting (Moore et al., 2017). In adults with the cough, the whoop and the posttussive vomiting are considered the most specific clinical indicators of pertussis (Moore et al., 2019). In children with the cough, three clinical symptoms are considered the most specific: paroxysms of coughing, whoop, and posttussive vomiting (Moore et al., 2019).

The final stage is convalescence. It lasts about 2 to 3 weeks. The cough gradually improves, but it may return with further respiratory infections for several months (CDC, n.d.-c; Rivard & Viera, 2014).

Key History/Physical Findings and Diagnostic Considerations

Besides symptoms and timing and course of the illness, important questions in the history are about immunization history and contacts with known cases of pertussis.

The main focus of the physical exam is observation of the patient for the coughing paroxysms. This disease is not diagnosed clinically. Diagnostic testing is required when the history indicates a possible infection with pertussis (American Academy of Pediatrics [AAP], 2018a; Rivard & Viera, 2014). Currently, the recommended testing is NAAT, including polymerase chain reaction (PCR), which can be done up to 3 weeks into the illness (AAP, 2018a). Culture is also used but must be collected in the first 2 weeks of the illness. False-negative cultures can occur if the patient has been vaccinated or has started antibiotics (AAP, 2018a). Elevated WBC counts with lymphocytosis may also occur, especially in infants (Moore et al., 2017).

PNEUMONIA

Pneumonia is a bacterial infection of the lower respiratory tract characterized by cough, abnormal vital signs, and abnormal lung exam findings. The key signs and symptoms are depicted in **Figure 7.42**. Common symptoms include:

- Cough
- Dyspnea
- Pleural pain
- Sweating and night sweats
- Fever greater than 100.6°F
- Chills
- Myalgias

Key History and Physical Findings

Additional important patient historical factors that may help in predicting the course and severity of the illness include the following (Reuben et al., 2019):

- Age-related changes in pulmonary reserve
- Alcoholism
- Altered mental status
- Aspiration
- COPD
- Heart disease
- Diabetes
- Malnutrition
- Medications like immunosuppressants, sedatives, inhaled corticosteroids, antipsychotics, anticholinergics, antacids, proton pump inhibitors, and H2 blockers
- Intubation
- Nasogastric tubes
- Oral care
- Problems swallowing
- Supine positioning

Common physical exam findings are (Harris et al., 2016):

- Tachycardia greater than 100 beats per minute
- Tachypnea greater than 24 breaths per minute
- Fever greater than 100.6°F
- Crackles
- Egophony
- Tactile fremitus

In patients over age 65, the CURB-65 Pneumonia Severity Scale is a severity scoring model that can assist in decision-making regarding inpatient and outpatient treatment (Reuben et al., 2019). This scoring system gives one point for each sign/symptom that is present and zero points if the sign/symptom is not present. The signs/symptoms that contribute to the score are as follows:

- **C**onfusion
- **B**UN greater than or equal to 19 mg/dL
- **R**espiratory rate greater than 30
- Systolic **B**P less than 90 mmHg or diastolic BP less than 60 mmHg
- Age greater than or equal to **65**

The CURB-65 is scored as 1 point = outpatient treatment, 2 points = consider hospitalization or outpatient treatment, 3 points = hospitalize, 4–5 points = hospitalize and consider ICU treatment (Reuben et al., 2019). In a small retrospective study, the CURB-65 was considered an adequate predictive tool. Although it has some limitations compared with other models tested, it was the easiest for the clinician to use (Xiao et al., 2013).

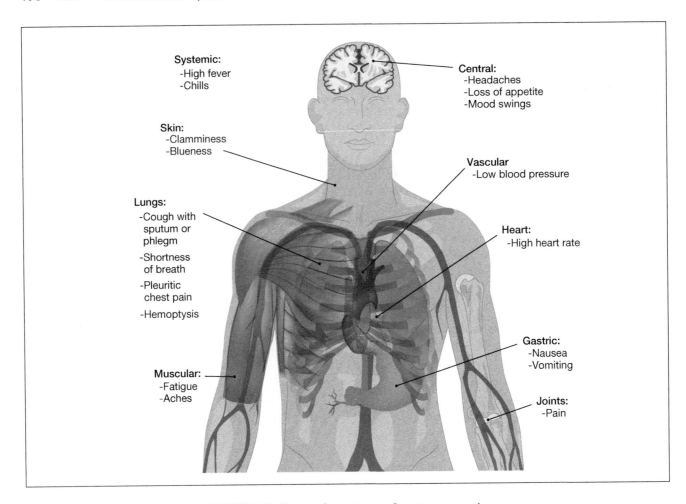

Systemic:
-High fever
-Chills

Central:
-Headaches
-Loss of appetite
-Mood swings

Skin:
-Clamminess
-Blueness

Vascular
-Low blood pressure

Lungs:
-Cough with sputum or phlegm
-Shortness of breath
-Pleuritic chest pain
-Hemoptysis

Heart:
-High heart rate

Gastric:
-Nausea
-Vomiting

Muscular:
-Fatigue
-Aches

Joints:
-Pain

FIGURE 7.42 Signs and symptoms of acute pneumonia.

Diagnostic Considerations

Diagnostic testing in a suspected case of pneumonia varies with the age and condition of the patient as well as the need, at times, to confirm the need for antibiotics. Most guidelines are aimed at using diagnostic testing judiciously to avoid overuse of antibiotics. Although the Cochrane Database of Systemic Reviews does not recommend chest x-rays routinely for pneumonia, because there is no evidence of improved outcomes (Cao et al., 2013), other guidelines recommend that a chest x-ray be done to confirm the diagnosis, although the guideline acknowledges that chest x-rays do not change the outcome for most patients (Hill et al., 2019).

If a CURB-65 is needed to make decisions about an older adult, a BUN is necessary to complete the scoring model. C-reactive protein (CRP) greater than 30 mg/L can help make the diagnosis of pneumonia in addition to the signs and symptoms listed earlier. In the patient with acute cough, pneumonia is less likely to be present if the CRP is less than 10 mg/L. In the patient without dyspnea and fever, pneumonia is less likely when the

CRP is 10–50 mg/L as well. Procalcitonin is not recommended (Hill et al., 2019; Schuetz et al., 2017). In hospitalized patients with ventilator-associated pneumonia, endotracheal aspiration is recommended for microbiological specimens. In hospitalized patients who are not on ventilators, samples should also be obtained noninvasively through cough, sputum induction, or nasotracheal suctioning, and treatment should be based on the microbiological results. Clinical criteria are recommended for diagnosis rather than use of procalcitonin, CRP, bronchoalveolar lavage fluid, and clinical decision models (Kalil et al., 2016).

TUBERCULOSIS

Tuberculosis (TB) is an infectious disease primarily caused by *Mycobacterium tuberculosis* (AAP, 2018b, p. 829). Signs and symptoms of active infection can include (CDC, n.d.-e):

- Cough, possibly productive of blood or sputum
- Chest pain
- Fatigue

- Weight loss or, in children, growth delay
- Anorexia
- Chills
- Fever
- Night sweats

Extrapulmonary disease can include meningitis, as well as granulomatous inflammation of the lymph nodes, bones, joints, skin, middle ear, and mastoid. Gastrointestinal and kidney tuberculosis can occur as well. In neonates, sepsis, pneumonia, and hepatosplenomegaly can occur (AAP, 2018b, p. 829). No single symptom, physical finding, or chest x-ray result can diagnose active TB by itself.

In latent tuberculosis, infected patients have no symptoms and are not contagious to others (CDC, n.d.-b). Five to ten percent of persons with latent TB will progress to active TB. The risk is highest among those who are immunocompromised and in children under 5 (World Health Organization [WHO], 2018).

In patients who may have tuberculosis, two different issues arise in assessment. The first is determining who should be screened for latent TB infection, and the second is the assessment for active TB. According to the USPSTF guidelines (USPSTF, 2016), the following adults over age 18 should be tested with either the Mantoux tuberculin skin test (TST) or the interferon-gamma release assays (IGRA):

- Persons who were born in or are former residents of countries with increased tuberculosis prevalence, including Mexico, Philippines, Vietnam, India, China, Haiti, and Guatemala
- Persons who live in or lived in high-risk congregate settings, including homeless shelters, prisons, and long-term care facilities

The WHO (2018) adds to this list to include persons who are immunocompromised who do not have active TB. According to the WHO algorithms, preventive treatment for TB can be given to those who do not have cough, fever, weight loss, and night sweats, especially where testing with TSTs or IGRAs is unavailable or difficult to access. The WHO would recommend preventive treatment without testing (if not easily available) in the following populations:

- Adults, adolescents, and children over 12 months old living with HIV
- Infants with HIV who are in contact with a case of TB
- Household contacts (especially children under 5 years of age, and older children/adults who can be evaluated with TSTs or IGRAs)
- Patients initiating anti-TNF treatment, receiving dialysis, preparing for an organ or hematologic transplant, and patients with silicosis

Key History and Physical Findings

Assessment for active TB includes assessing for the signs and symptoms of active TB. The history should also include the following (CDC, 2013):

- History of previous diagnosis or treatment
- Immunocompromising conditions
- Countries of origin or travel to countries with a high prevalence of TB
- Previous living conditions and possible contacts with TB
- A review of symptoms for extrapulmonary TB such as back pain, hematuria, headache, confusion, and hoarseness

Diagnostic Considerations

The physical exam cannot be used solely to confirm or rule out active TB but can give clues to the patient's overall condition (CDC, 2013). Diagnostic testing after the TST or IGRA should include a chest x-ray, although in settings where that is difficult to obtain, the chest x-ray should not delay treatment if the risk factors and history indicate TB (WHO, 2018). Chest x-ray findings can be nonspecific but may include lymphadenopathy, especially in children; nodular and fibrotic lesions; infiltrates; pleural effusions; and cavitations. The chest x-ray may also be normal, but that does not rule out TB in a person with other signs and symptoms (CDC, 2013).

Other necessary diagnostic tests are done on sputum or urine or cerebrospinal fluid if the patient is suspected of having extrapulmonary disease (CDC, 2013). Sputum should be collected in an airborne infection isolation room or in an isolated, well-ventilated area like outdoors. Three sputum specimens collected 8 to 24 hours apart are recommended. They can be collected through cough or sputum induction. Sputum induction, or inducing a deep sputum-producing cough, is completed by having the patient inhale an aerosol of warm, sterile, hypertonic saline. Gastric aspiration of swallowed sputum is sometimes used if sputum cannot be collected in any other way. Gastric aspiration must be done first thing in the morning. Bronchoscopy can be used if no other method is successful at obtaining sputum but is very invasive and requires anesthesia (CDC, 2013). It is recommended that NAAT be done on at least one specimen of sputum (AAP, 2018b). Although NAAT does not replace culture, its benefits include earlier lab confirmation of TB, improved outcomes due to earlier treatment, and earlier identification of drug-resistant TB (AAP, 2018b; CDC, 2013). Microscopy is also often done on sputum, but lack of TB bacilli on microscopy does not mean that TB is not present (CDC, 2013).

CASE STUDY: Shortness of Breath

Reason for Seeking Care

JJ is a 14-year-old African American female who is experiencing shortness of breath. Her mom is here with her today in the urgent care. Mom shares that she thinks JJ is "having an asthma attack."

History of Present Illness

The following is the dialogue between the clinician (in italics) and the adolescent:

When did the "asthma attack" start?
I think that the attack started about an hour ago at home. I couldn't find my inhaler because I haven't used it in a long time.

Are you having pain?
Yes, I am having some tightness in my chest. Not terrible pain, but I cannot take a deep breath in. I feel like I am breathing through a straw.

Are your symptoms getting worse?
This asthma attack does seem to be getting worse over the last hour, which is why we came here to the urgent care. (Mom shares that if her daughter had not been getting worse, they would have called the pediatric office and gotten a refill on her inhaler. Mom also states that her daughter is probably worse than she is sharing, and that she heard her daughter wheezing this morning.)

Describe your symptoms to me:
I had a lot of coughing last night, and now I am having trouble breathing.

Do you know what might be making this worse?
I am not exactly sure, but I stayed overnight with a friend last night. My mom doesn't know this, but my friend's mom smokes cigarettes. I think that is why I started coughing last night and this morning.

Have you tried anything to make it better?
I usually get relief when I use my inhaler, but I don't have one at home.

Are you having any other symptoms?
I feel a little dizzy.

Describe the timing of your symptoms to me:
Yesterday and this morning I was coughing a lot. Then I started wheezing this morning. Right now I am not hearing myself wheeze, but I am having trouble getting air in my lungs.

Can you rate the severity of this on a scale of 1 to 10?
9/10; I think this is the worst asthma attack that I have ever had.

General Survey

Because the adolescent has significant respiratory distress, the clinician completes a general survey and notes that the teen is awake and alert; she is speaking more in phrases than with long sentences. She is afebrile, with a pulse and blood pressure within normal limits. Her respiratory rate is 18 breaths/minute, and her pulse oximeter reading is 94. While her mucosa is pink, she is having shallow breathing with slight intercostal retractions. Breath sounds are diminished in the bases, with faint scattered wheezes bilaterally. The clinician makes a decision to begin a nebulizer treatment and completes the remainder of the patient's history.

Differential Diagnoses

Asthma exacerbation; dyspnea

Past Medical, Family, Social, and Cultural History

As JJ receives her aerosol treatment, the mom shares the following history: JJ is rarely ill. She has never been to the urgent care before. She has no history of hospitalizations or surgeries. Her vaccines are up-to-date. She was not ill prior to this asthma exacerbation. She was diagnosed with asthma as a preschooler, just after the family moved to a home with a wood-burning fireplace. Smoke has always been a trigger for her asthma. One of the reasons that JJ could not find her inhaler is that she rarely has to use it, except during soccer season, when she uses an albuterol inhaler before games and practices. She is not allergic to any medications, and she is not taking any routine medications. Her only prescribed medication is her inhaler, which is used as needed, and which has

(continued)

CASE STUDY: Shortness of Breath (*continued*)

never been used more than prior to exercise for the past few years. She does not typically wake at night with coughing.

JJ denies headache, nausea, vomiting, itching, or discomfort anywhere other than her chest, which is generalized. She denies eye drainage, ear pain, throat pain, or fatigue. She does agree that she felt worried and anxious on her way in to the urgent care today and states that the breathing treatment is "making me feel a little jittery."

JJ lives with her family, which consists of mom, grandmother, sister, and brother. Her mother and grandmother have hypertension and diabetes; her father is deceased as a result of a motor vehicle accident, which happened several years ago. Her mother states that she had asthma as a young child and "grew out of it." Her younger brother is healthy. JJ does well in school and hopes to eventually play college soccer.

Physical Examination

After the nebulizer treatment, JJ is actively coughing in short spasms. Her cough is nonproductive. She is no longer retracting with her breathing, but both her heart rate and respiratory rate are elevated. Her mucosa is pink. No noted skin lesions or rashes. Exam of her eyes, ears, nose, mouth, and throat are all within normal limits. Her breath sounds with auscultation reveal scattered expiratory wheezes bilaterally; she is now moving air in the bases of her lungs. Inspiration-to-expiration ratio is 1:2, and movement of the chest wall is symmetrical. No tactile fremitus or egophony are noted on exam. JJ has resonant lung fields with percussion anteriorly and posteriorly. Current pulse oximeter reading is 99.

Final Diagnoses

Asthma exacerbation; history of mild intermittent asthma

CASE STUDY: Cough and Fatigue

Reason for Seeking Care

MS is a 66-year-old male who presents to the primary care office with complaints of fatigue and cough. Vital signs: Temperature 101.2°F, Pulse 85/min, Respirations 18/min, and BP 138/78. He appears nontoxic but fatigued. His pulse oximeter reading is 96. His BMI is 35.

History of Present Illness, Review of Symptoms, and Health History

MS begins the visit by sharing that he owns his own landscaping business and works outside; he loves his job and has been "really busy." He has been married for 35 years with three sons who are involved in the business with him (ages 33, 30, and 27). His stress level is very high, and "he doesn't have time to be sick!"

This illness started 3 days ago with a scratchy throat and body aches and is getting progressively worse. Yesterday, he had fever and chills. He is "exhausted" and has spent the last 2 days in bed or on the couch trying to sleep. He has a significant cough that is deep, harsh, and productive of discolored mucus in small amounts. MS explains that when he

coughs, he has spasms of coughing and feels like he just cannot stop. The cough is waking him up at night.

MS has been taking two extra-strength acetaminophen three times daily for the past 2 days without relief. He tried taking a cough medicine "safe for people with high blood pressure" at bedtime for the past two nights without relief. He has eaten very little, but has been drinking water, hot tea, and soup broth. He notes that he has not been on an antibiotic since his bronchitis a year ago. He wonders if this is a very bad bronchitis. MS denies having ever been hospitalized; he has no surgical history and no recent travel outside of the country. He is a former smoker, but quit smoking 10 years ago after having been a 1/2 pack/day smoker for over 30 years. He has no history of using medications not prescribed to him and has one or two beers after work daily.

MS has a history of hypothyroidism, hypertension, and osteoarthritis. He denies ever receiving a flu shot and has not had a vaccine since childhood. Although he has fatigue currently, he states that he typically does not have energy loss; problems concentrating;

(*continued*)

CASE STUDY: Cough and Fatigue (*continued*)

or feelings of sadness, worry, insomnia, or hopelessness. He occasionally has heartburn, and denies nausea, vomiting, recent change in appetite, abdominal pain, chest pain, or headaches. He takes his blood pressure at home weekly, and it is usually less than 130/80. His medication list includes:

- Acetaminophen prn
- Levothyroxine 100 mcg daily
- Losartan 50 mg daily
- Omeprazole OTC 20 mg daily

MS does have a family history of respiratory disorders. His mother has COPD and smokes cigarettes. His father has hypertension. Both of his parents and an older brother are still living. His brother also has hypertension. His wife and children are healthy, and he attributes this to the fact that he quit smoking a decade ago and that he has never smoked in their home.

Differential Diagnoses

Pneumonia; bronchitis; influenza; COPD exacerbation; pneumonitis from environmental exposure

Physical Examination

- General: Mucosa pink, no skin rashes, capillary refill brisk, no edema, no clubbing
- HEENT: PERRLA (pupils equal, round, reactive to light and accommodation), tympanic membranes pearly gray, +nasal congestion, tenderness noted over sinuses bilateral, pharynx with erythema and thick posterior nasal drainage; tonsils absent

- Head/neck: No carotid or temporal bruits. +Anterior cervical lymphadenopathy with tenderness to palpation
- Heart: Heart rate and rhythm regular with no murmurs, clicks, or gallops
- Lungs: Symmetric expansion with no retractions noted. Dullness to percussion in the area of the left lower lobe. In the same area, increased tactile fremitus, +egophony. Lungs auscultated bilaterally—faint crackles noted in lower left lobe
- Neurologic/psychiatric: Speech is clear and distinct; gait is smooth and even. Appearance, behavior, and cognition appropriate for the circumstances
- Abdomen: Nontender, nondistended. No abdominal bruits

Laboratory and Imaging

- Chest x-ray (confirmed pneumonia)
- CBC with differential (elevated WBC count)
- Rapid influenza test (negative for influenza A or B)

Note that the BUN was not ordered, as this patient does not have confusion, respiratory rate greater than 20, systolic BP less than 90, or diastolic BP less than 60. His CRB-65 score is 1, which indicates that the BUN is not indicated to determine if outpatient treatment is appropriate.

Final Diagnoses

Left lower lobe pneumonia; community-acquired pneumonia

Clinical Pearls

- The assessment of respiratory status is a key factor in determining extent or severity of illness.
- Best practice for the examination of the respiratory system is avoidance of assessment over clothing.
- Pulmonary function tests are essential to the diagnosis of asthma and COPD.
- Ask about smoking status and exposure to secondhand smoke. Advise individuals that it is never too late to quit smoking.

Key Takeaways

- History related to respiratory problems or disorders commonly includes symptoms of shortness of breath or dyspnea, cough, hemoptysis, and/or chest pain.
- Physical exam of the respiratory system includes inspection, auscultation, percussion, and palpation.

REFERENCES

Amalakanti, S., & Pentakota, M. R. (2016). Pulse oximetry overestimates oxygen saturation in COPD. *Respiratory Care, 61*, 423–427. doi:10.4187/respcare.04435

American Academy of Pediatrics. (2018a). Pertussis. In D. W. Kimberlin, M. T. Brady, M. A. Jackson, & S. S. Long (Eds.), *Red book: 2018 report of the Committee on Infectious Diseases* (31st ed., pp. 620–634). Itasca, IL: American Academy of Pediatrics.

American Academy of Pediatrics. (2018b). Tuberculosis. In D. W. Kimberlin, M. T. Brady, M. A. Jackson, & S. S. Long (Eds.), *Red book: 2018 report of the Committee on Infectious Diseases* (31st ed., pp. 829–853). Itasca, IL: American Academy of Pediatrics.

American Board of Internal Medicine. (n.d.-a). *Clinician lists: Asthma.* Retrieved from https://www.choosingwisely.org/clinician-lists/#keyword=asthma

American Board of Internal Medicine. (n.d.-b). *Clinician lists: Bronchiolitis.* Retrieved from https://www.choosingwisely.org/clinician-lists/#keyword=bronchiolitis

American College of Obstetricians and Gynecologists. (2008). Clinical management guidelines for obstetrician-gynecologists: Asthma in pregnancy. *Obstetrics and Gynecology, 111*, 457–464. doi:10.1097/AOG.0b013e3181665ff4

American Geriatrics Society. (2015). Breast, colorectal and prostate cancer screening in older adults. Retrieved from https://www.choosingwisely.org/clinician-lists/american-geriatrics-society-breast-colorectal-prostate-cancer-screening-in-older-adults

American Thoracic Society. (2013). An official American Thoracic Society workshop report: Optimal lung function tests for monitoring cystic fibrosis, bronchopulmonary dysplasia, and recurrent wheezing in children less than 6 years of age. *Annals of the American Thoracic Society, 10*(2), S1–S11. doi:10.1513/AnnalsATS.201301-017ST

Bhatt, S. P., Kim, Y. Il, Harrington, K. F., Hokanson, J. E., Lutz, S. M., Cho, M. H., … Bailey, W. C. (2018). Smoking duration alone provides stronger risk estimates of chronic obstructive pulmonary disease than pack-years. *Thorax, 73*, 414–421. doi:10.1136/thoraxjnl-2017-210722

Cao, A. M. Y., Choy, J. P., Mohanakrishnan L. N., Bain, R. F., & van Driel, M. L. (2013). Chest radiographs for acute lower respiratory tract infections. *Cochrane Database of Systematic Reviews*, (12), CD009119. doi:10.1002/14651858.CD009119.pub2

Centers for Disease Control and Prevention. (2013). *Core curriculum on tuberculosis* (6th ed., pp. 75–108). Retrieved from https://www.cdc.gov/tb/education/corecurr/pdf/chapter4.pdf

Centers for Disease Control and Prevention. (n.d.-a). *Influenza (flu): Key facts about influenza (flu).* Retrieved from https://www.cdc.gov/flu/about/keyfacts.htm

Centers for Disease Control and Prevention. (n.d.-b). *Latent TB infection and TB disease.* Retrieved from https://www.cdc.gov/tb/topic/basics/tbinfectiondisease.htm

Centers for Disease Control and Prevention. (n.d.-c). *Pertussis: Signs and symptoms.* Retrieved from https://www.cdc.gov/pertussis/about/signs-symptoms.html

Centers for Disease Control and Prevention. (n.d.-d). *Smoking & tobacco use: Secondhand smoke.* Retrieved from https://www.cdc.gov/tobacco/basic_information/secondhand_smoke/index.htm

Centers for Disease Control and Prevention. (n.d.-e). *Tuberculosis: Signs and symptoms.* Retrieved from https://www.cdc.gov/tb/topic/basics/signsandsymptoms.htm

Chesnutt, A. N., Chesnutt, M. S., Prendergast, N. T., & Prendergast, T. J. (2019). Pulmonary disorders. In M. A. Papadakis, S. J. McPhee, & M. W. Rabow (Eds.). *Current medical diagnosis and treatment 2019* (58th ed., Chapter 9). New York, NY: McGraw Hill. Retrieved from https://accessmedicine.mhmedical.com/book.aspx?bookID=2449

Farrell, P. M., White, T. B., Ren, C. L., Hempstead, S. E., Accurso, F., Derichs, N., . . . Sosnay, P. R. (2017). Diagnosis of cystic fibrosis: Consensus guidelines from the Cystic Fibrosis Foundation. *Journal of Pediatrics, 181*(Suppl.), S4–S15. doi:10.1016/j.jpeds.2016.09.064

Global Initiative for Asthma. (2018). *Global strategy for asthma management and prevention.* Retrieved from https://ginasthma.org/wp-content/uploads/2018/04/wms-GINA-2018-report-V1.3-002.pdf

Global Initiative for Asthma. (2019). *Pocket guide for asthma management and prevention (for adults and children older than 5 years): A pocket guide for health professionals.* Retrieved from https://ginasthma.org/wp-content/uploads/2019/04/GINA-2019-main-Pocket-Guide-wms.pdf

The Global Initiative for Chronic Obstructive Lung Disease. (2019). *Global strategy for the diagnosis, management and prevention of chronic obstructive pulmonary disease 2019 report.* Retrieved from https://goldcopd.org/wp-content/uploads/2018/11/GOLD-2019-v1.7-FINAL-14Nov2018-WMS.pdf

Harris, A. M., Hicks, L. A., & Qaseem, A. (2016). Appropriate antibiotic use for acute respiratory tract infection in adults: Advice for high-value care from the American College of Physicians and the Centers for Disease Control and Prevention. *Annals of Internal Medicine, 164*, 425–433. doi:10.7326/M15-1840

Hart, A. M. (2019). Influenza: A clinical update following a century of influenza science. *The Journal for Nurse Practitioners, 15*, 429–433. doi:10.1016/j.nurpra.2018.12.026

Hill, A. T., Gold, P. M. El Solh, A. A., Metlay, J. P., Ireland, B., & Irwin, R. S. (2019). Adult outpatients with acute cough due to suspected pneumonia or influenza. *Chest, 155*(1), 155–167. doi:10.1016/j.chest.2018.09.016

Holleman, D. R., & Simel, D. L. (1995). Does the clinical examination predict airflow limitation? *The Journal of the American Medical Association, 273*(4), 313–319. doi:10.1001/jama.1995.03520280059041

Holleman, D. R., & Simel, D. L. (1997). Quantitative assessments from the clinical examination: How should clinicians integrate the numerous results? *Journal of General Internal Medicine, 12*(3), 165–171. doi:10.1046/j.1525-1497.1997.012003165.x

Kalil, A. C., Metersky, M. L., Klompas, M., Muscedere, J., Sweeney, D. A., Palmer, L. B., . . . Brozek, J. L. (2016). Management of adults with hospital-acquired and ventilator-associated pneumonia: 2016 clinical practice guidelines by the Infectious Diseases Society of America and the American Thoracic Society. *Clinical Infectious Disease, 63*(1), e61–e111. doi:10.1093/cid/ciw353

Kapur, V. K. (2010). Obstructive sleep apnea: Diagnosis, epidemiology, and economics. *Respiratory Care, 55,* 1155–1167. Retrieved from http://rc.rcjournal.com/content/55/9/1155

Kincade, S., & Long, N. A. (2016). Acute bronchitis. *American Family Physician, 94*(7), 560–565. Retrieved from https://www.aafp.org/afp/2016/1001/p560.html

Manser, R., Lethaby, A., Irving, L. B., Stone, C., Byrnes, G., Abramson, M. J., & Campbell, D. (2013). Screening for lung cancer. *Cochrane Database of Systematic Reviews,* (6), CD001991. doi:10.1002/14651858.CD001991.pub3

Mazzone, P. J., Silvestri, G. A., Patel, S., Kanne, J. P., Kinsinger, L. S., Wiener, R. S., . . . Detterbeck, F. C. (2018). Screening for lung cancer: CHEST Guideline and Expert Panel report. *Chest, 153,* 954–985. doi:10.1016/j.chest.2018.01.016

Molnar, C., & Gair, J. (2015). *Concepts of biology* (1st Canadian ed.). Victoria, BC, Canada: BCcampus. Retrieved from https://opentextbc.ca/biology

Moore, A., Ashdown, H. F., Shinkins, B., Roberts, N. W., Grant, C. C., Lasserson, D. S., . . . Harnden, A. (2017). Clinical characteristics of pertussis-associated cough in adults and children. *Chest, 152,* 353–367. doi:10.1016/j.chest.2017.04.186

Moore, A., Harnden, A., Grant, C. C., Patel, S., & Irwin, R. S. (2019). Clinically diagnosing pertussis-associated cough in adults and children. *Chest, 155,* 147–254. doi:10.1016/j.chest.2018.09.027

Qaseem, A., Dallas, P., Owens, D. K., Starkey, M., Holty, J. E. C., & Shekelle, P. (2014). Diagnosis of obstructive sleep apnea in adults: A clinical practice guideline from the American College of Physicians. *Annals of Internal Medicine, 161,* 210–220. doi:10.7326/M12-3187

Ralston, S. L., Lieberthal, A. S., Meissner, H. C., Alverson, B. K., Baley, J. E., Gadomski, A. M., . . . Hernandez-Cancio, S. (2014). Clinical practice guideline: The diagnosis, management, and prevention of bronchiolitis. *Pediatrics, 134,* e1474–1502. doi:10.1542/peds.2014-2742

Reuben, D. B., Herr, K. A., Pacala, J. T., Pollock, B. G., Potter, J. F., & Semla, T. P. (2019). *Geriatrics at your fingertips* (20th ed.). New York, NY: The American Geriatrics Association.

Rivard, G., & Viera, A. (2014). Staying ahead of pertussis. *The Journal of Family Practice, 63*(11), 658–659, 666–669. Retrieved from https://www.mdedge.com/familymedicine/article/88224/infectious-diseases/staying-ahead-pertussis

Schuetz, P., Wirz, Y., Sager, R., Christ-Crain, M., Stolz, D., Tamm, M., . . . Mueller, B. (2017). Procalcitonin to initiate or discontinue antibiotics in acute respiratory tract infections. *Cochrane Database of Systematic Reviews,* (10), CD007498. doi:10.1002/14651858.CD007498.pub3

Tonkin-Crine, S. K. G., Tan, P. S., van Hecke, O., Wang, K., Roberts, N. W., McCullough, A., . . . Del Mar, C. B. (2017). Clinician-targeted interventions to influence antibiotic prescribing behaviour for acute respiratory infections in primary care: An overview of systematic reviews. *Cochrane Database of Systematic Reviews,* (9), CD012252. doi:10.1002/14651858.CD012252.pub2

U.S. Preventive Services Task Force. (2016). Screening for chronic obstructive pulmonary disease: U.S. Preventive Services Task Force recommendation statement. *The Journal of the American Medical Association, 315,* 1372–1377. doi:10.1001/jama.2016.2638

U.S. Preventive Services Task Force. (2017). Screening for obstructive sleep apnea in adults: U.S. Preventive Services Task Force recommendation statement. *The Journal of the American Medical Association, 317,* 407–414. doi:10.1001/jama.2016.20325

Uyeki, T. M., Bernstein, H. H., Bradley, J. S., Englund, J. A., File, T. M., Fry, A. M., & Pavia, A. T. (2018). Clinical practice guidelines by the Infectious Diseases Society of America: 2018 update on diagnosis, treatment, chemoprophylaxis, and institutional outbreak management of seasonal influenza. *Clinical Infectious Disease, 68*(6), e1–e47. doi:10.1093/cid/ciy866

Waterer, G. W., Wan, J. Y., Kritchevsky, S. B., Wunderink, R. G., Satterfield, S., Bauer, D. C., . . . Crapo, R. O. (2001). Airflow limitation is under recognized in well-functioning older people. *Journal of the American Geriatrics Society, 49*(8), 1032–1038. doi:10.1046/j.1532-5415.2001.49205.x

Wong, C. L., Holroyd-Leduc, J., & Straus, S. E. (2009). Does this patient have a pleural effusion? *Journal of the American Medical Association, 301*(3), 309–317. doi:10.1001/jama.2008.937

World Health Organization. (2018). *Latent tuberculosis infection: Updated and consolidated guidelines for programmatic management.* Geneva, Switzerland: Author.

Xiao, K., Su, L. X., Han, B. C., Yan, P., Yuan, N., Dent, J., & Xie, L. X. (2013). Analysis of the severity and prognosis assessment of aged patients with community-acquired pneumonia: A retrospective study. *Journal of Thoracic Disease, 5,* 626–633. doi:10.3978/j.issn.2072-1439.2013.09.10

8

Approach to Evidence-Based Assessment of Body Habitus (Height, Weight, Body Mass Index, Nutrition)

Emily Hill Guseman, Kate Gawlik, and Alice M. Teall

> *"Symptoms are not enemies to be destroyed, but sacred messengers who encourage us to take better care of ourselves."*
>
> —Jon Gabriel

LEARNING OBJECTIVES

- Understand the basic biological aspects of nutrient and physical activity requirements of children and adults.
- Recognize the linkages between nutrients, physical activity, and disease processes, body size, mental ability, and performance.

NUTRITION PHYSIOLOGY

DIET

The human body needs energy in order to grow, function, and survive. As such, adequate and balanced nutrition is a vital component of overall health. Optimal functioning of biological systems requires a delicate balance of vitamins, minerals, and nutrients to complete various functions and to maintain homeostasis. When dietary intake is not matched to energy demand, the resulting nutritional imbalance can lead to a variety of diseases and conditions.

The U.S. Department of Health and Human Services (DHHS) releases updated Dietary Guidelines for Americans on a 5-year schedule. The DHHS recommendations provide guidance on achieving a well-balanced and nutrient-dense diet.

The Balanced Diet

The components of a healthy eating pattern include fruits, vegetables, protein, dairy, grains, and oils. These components provide the macronutrients (carbohydrates, proteins, and fats) and micronutrients (vitamins and minerals) necessary for growth, metabolic demands, and repair of the body. These nutrients should be balanced in a way that daily requirements for these macro- and micronutrients are met at a caloric intake that is appropriate for the individual's age, sex, and lifestyle.

Carbohydrates include fiber, starches, and sugars. *Dietary fiber* refers to carbohydrates that are not digestible and not absorbed in the gastrointestinal tract. Fiber can include nondigestible carbohydrates and lignins that naturally occur in foods and fiber that is synthetically manufactured or extracted from natural sources and added to foods or supplements. Certain types of fiber can pull water into the gastrointestinal tract, increasing the bulk of feces and shortening intestinal transit time. Fibers can also absorb cholesterol so that it is excreted rather than absorbed. Fruits and vegetables are good sources of fiber, and individuals should be encouraged to eat a variety of plant-based foods to obtain adequate intake of all fiber types. *Sugars* provide readily accessible energy and provide a sweet flavor to foods but should be limited in the diet to reduce risk of unhealthy weight gain and development of chronic health conditions. The World Health

Organization (WHO) and U.S. Department of Agriculture (USDA) recommend limiting sugar intake to less than 10% of total calories and further reduction to less than 5% of calories for additional health benefits. Individuals may limit sugar intake by consuming fresh fruits and vegetables, limiting processed foods, and limiting intake of sugar-sweetened beverages (DHHS & USDA, 2015; WHO, 2015).

Proteins provide the amino acids that are essential for healthy tissue growth and repair. Each amino acid consists of carbon, a carboxyl group, a functional R group, and an amino group that includes nitrogen. After ingestion, proteins are broken down into their component amino acids, and these amino acids provide the building blocks to synthesize body proteins. These body proteins form structural components of cells, enzymes, hormones, and other important functional units. Amino acids are classified as *essential*, meaning they cannot be synthesized in the human body and must be obtained through dietary intake, or *nonessential*, which can be synthesized in the body (DHHS & USDA, 2015).

Fats are both an essential part of the diet and a macronutrient that should be consumed in limited quantities. *Unsaturated fats*, which include mono- and polyunsaturated fatty acids, are typically liquid at room temperature and found primarily in plant-based sources, fish, and shellfish. *Saturated fats* are solid at room temperature and found primarily in animal products and tropical oils. *Trans fats* are present naturally in some dairy products and are also synthesized and found in processed foods. Fats provide a significant source of energy and are important for absorption of fat-soluble vitamins, for cellular structure and function, and for hormone synthesis. Saturated fat intake should be limited to less than 10% of calories per day. Trans fats are not a necessary component of the diet and should be limited as much as possible (DHHS & USDA, 2015).

Vitamins are found primarily in fruits, vegetables, and some animal products and are important for optimal cellular function. *Fat-soluble* vitamins include vitamins A, D, E, and K, while *water-soluble* vitamins include vitamin C (ascorbic acid), thiamin, riboflavin, niacin, vitamin B6, vitamin B12, choline, and folate. Dietary sources of vitamins and their major functions are outlined in **Table 8.1**. Recommended dietary allowances (RDA) and adequate intakes (AI) are outlined by the USDA and vary according to age, sex, and life stage (e.g., pregnancy or lactation; DHHS & USDA, 2015).

TABLE 8.1 Vitamins: Functions, Dietary Sources, and Recommended Daily Value

Vitamin	Functions	Dietary Sources	Daily Value*
Biotin	• Energy storage • Protein, carbohydrate, fat metabolism	• Avocados • Cauliflower • Eggs • Fruits (e.g., raspberries) • Liver • Pork • Salmon • Whole grains	300 mcg
Folate/folic acid *Important for pregnant women and women capable of becoming pregnant*	• Prevention of birth defects • Protein metabolism • Red blood cell formation	• Asparagus • Avocados • Beans and peas • Enriched grain products (e.g., bread, cereal, pasta, rice) • Green leafy vegetables (e.g., spinach) • Orange juice	400 mcg
Niacin	• Cholesterol production • Conversion of food into energy • Digestion • Nervous system function	• Beans • Beef • Enriched grain products (e.g., bread, cereal, pasta, rice) • Nuts • Pork • Poultry • Seafood • Whole grains	20 mg

(continued)

TABLE 8.1 Vitamins: Functions, Dietary Sources, and Recommended Daily Value (*continued*)

Vitamin	Functions	Dietary Sources	Daily Value*
Pantothenic acid	• Conversion of food into energy • Fat metabolism • Hormone production • Nervous system function • Red blood cell formation	• Avocados • Beans and peas • Broccoli • Eggs • Milk • Mushrooms • Poultry • Seafood • Sweet potatoes • Whole grains • Yogurt	10 mg
Riboflavin	• Conversion of food into energy • Growth and development • Red blood cell formation	• Eggs • Enriched grain products (e.g., bread, cereal, pasta, rice) • Meats • Milk • Mushrooms • Poultry • Seafood (e.g., oysters) • Spinach	1.7 mg
Thiamin	• Conversion of food into energy • Nervous system function	• Beans and peas • Enriched grain products (e.g., bread, cereal, pasta, rice) • Nuts • Pork • Sunflower seeds • Whole grains	1.5 mg
Vitamin A	• Growth and development • Immune function • Reproduction • Red blood cell formation • Skin and bone formation • Vision	• Cantaloupe • Carrots • Dairy products • Eggs • Fortified cereals • Green leafy vegetables (e.g., spinach and broccoli) • Pumpkin • Red peppers • Sweet potatoes	5,000 IU
Vitamin B6	• Immune function • Nervous system function • Protein, carbohydrate, and fat metabolism • Red blood cell formation	• Chickpeas • Fruits (other than citrus) • Potatoes • Salmon • Tuna	2 mg
Vitamin B12	• Conversion of food into energy • Nervous system function • Red blood cell formation	• Dairy products • Eggs • Fortified cereals • Meats • Poultry • Seafood (e.g., clams, trout, salmon, haddock, tuna)	6 mcg

(*continued*)

TABLE 8.1 Vitamins: Functions, Dietary Sources, and Recommended Daily Value (*continued*)			
Vitamin	**Functions**	**Dietary Sources**	**Daily Value***
Vitamin C	• Antioxidant • Collagen and connective tissue formation • Immune function • Wound healing	• Broccoli • Brussels sprouts • Cantaloupe • Citrus fruits and juices (e.g., oranges and grapefruit) • Kiwifruit • Peppers • Strawberries • Tomatoes and tomato juice	60 mg
Vitamin D *Nutrient of concern for most Americans*	• Blood pressure regulation • Bone growth • Calcium balance • Hormone production • Immune function • Nervous system function	• Eggs • Fish (e.g., herring, mackerel, salmon, trout, and tuna) • Fish liver oil • Fortified cereals • Fortified dairy products • Fortified margarine • Fortified orange juice • Fortified soy beverages (soymilk)	400 IU
Vitamin E	• Antioxidant • Formation of blood vessels • Immune function	• Fortified cereals and juices • Green vegetables (e.g., spinach and broccoli) • Nuts and seeds • Peanuts and peanut butter • Vegetable oils	30 IU
Vitamin K	• Blood clotting • Strong bones	• Green vegetables (e.g., broccoli, kale, spinach, turnip greens, collards, Swiss chard, mustard greens)	80 mcg

*The Daily Values are the amounts of nutrients recommended per day for Americans 4 years of age or older.
Source: From U.S. Food and Drug Administration. (2016). *Vitamins and minerals chart.* Retrieved from https://www.accessdata.fda.gov/scripts/interactivenutritionfactslabel/factsheets/vitamin_and_mineral_chart.pdf

Minerals are also abundant in whole foods and necessary for cellular function, including transmission of neural impulses, muscle contraction, and bone strength. As with vitamins, the USDA provides RDA and AI guidance and, in the case of sodium, an upper limit (UL; DHHS & USDA, 2015). Dietary sources of minerals and their primary functions are outlined in **Table 8.2**.

Water is the major component of the human body and is essential for maintenance of cellular function, blood volume, and thermoregulation. Daily water intake recommendations for Americans issued by the USDA consider water in beverages as well as that obtained through food intake. An individual's actual daily water requirement varies with age, sex, lifestyle, and environmental conditions. Most American adults should consume between 2.7 and 3.7 L of water per day, while children require less (Institute of Medicine, 2005).

METABOLISM

Maintenance of a healthy body weight requires matching energy intake and energy expenditure. When energy intake exceeds energy expenditure, weight gain results; conversely, weight loss occurs when energy expenditure exceeds intake. Total daily energy expenditure (TDEE; kilocalories per day) is dictated by a combination of an individual's resting metabolic rate (RMR, or resting energy expenditure—REE), physical activity energy expenditure (PAEE), and the thermic effect of food (TEF; the energy required to digest and store nutrients taken in from food; **Figure 8.1**). RMR is the largest component of TDEE in most people and is primarily influenced by individual characteristics, including age and sex, while TEF makes up a small fraction of TDEE and is influenced by dietary composition. PAEE is the most variable component of TDEE and is heavily influenced by individual behaviors.

Daily energy requirements are dictated by an individual's sex, age, height, weight, and also by their lifestyle habits. Individuals desiring to gain or lose weight need to make further adjustments to their energy intake and/or energy expenditure to achieve the desired energy balance (i.e., net deficit for weight loss or a net surplus for weight gain). The Dietary Guidelines for Americans recommend a target energy intake of 1,600 to 2,400 kcal/day for adult women or 2,000 to 3,000 kcal/day for adult men (DHHS & USDA, 2015). Sedentary

TABLE 8.2 Minerals: Functions, Dietary Sources, and Recommended Daily Value

Mineral	Functions	Dietary Sources	Daily Value*
Calcium *Nutrient of concern for most Americans*	• Blood clotting • Bone and teeth formation • Constriction and relaxation of blood vessels • Hormone secretion • Muscle contraction • Nervous system function	• Almond, rice, coconut, and hemp milks • Canned seafood with bones (e.g., salmon and sardines) • Dairy products • Fortified cereals and juices • Fortified soy beverages (soymilk) • Green vegetables (e.g., spinach, kale, broccoli, turnip greens) • Tofu (made with calcium sulfate)	1,000 mg
Chloride	• Acid–base balance • Conversion of food into energy • Digestion • Fluid balance • Nervous system function	• Celery • Lettuce • Olives • Rye • Salt substitutes • Seaweeds (e.g., dulse and kelp) • Table salt and sea salt • Tomatoes	3,400 mg
Chromium	• Insulin function • Protein, carbohydrate, fat metabolism	• Broccoli • Fruits (e.g., apple and banana) • Grape and orange juice • Meats • Spices (e.g., garlic and basil) • Turkey • Whole grains	120 mcg
Copper	• Antioxidant • Bone formation • Collagen and connective tissue formation • Energy production • Iron metabolism • Nervous system function	• Chocolate and cocoa • Crustaceans and shellfish • Lentils • Nuts and seeds • Organ meats (e.g., liver) • Whole grains	2 mg
Iodine	• Growth and development • Metabolism • Reproduction • Thyroid hormone production	• Breads and cereals • Dairy products • Iodized salt • Potatoes • Seafood • Seaweed • Turkey	150 mcg
Iron *Nutrient of concern for young children, pregnant women, and women capable of becoming pregnant*	• Energy production • Growth and development • Immune function • Red blood cell formation • Reproduction • Wound healing	• Beans and peas • Dark green vegetables • Meats • Poultry • Prunes and prune juice • Raisins • Seafood • Whole grain, enriched, and fortified cereals and breads	18 mg

(continued)

TABLE 8.2 Minerals: Functions, Dietary Sources, and Recommended Daily Value (*continued*)

Mineral	Functions	Dietary Sources	Daily Value*
Magnesium	• Blood pressure regulation • Blood sugar regulation • Bone formation • Energy production • Hormone secretion • Immune function • Muscle contraction • Nervous system function • Normal heart rhythm • Protein formation	• Avocados • Bananas • Beans and peas • Dairy products • Green leafy vegetables (e.g., spinach) • Nuts and pumpkin seeds • Potatoes • Raisins • Wheat bran • Whole grains	400 mg
Manganese	• Carbohydrate, protein, cholesterol metabolism • Cartilage and bone formation • Wound healing	• Beans • Nuts • Pineapple • Spinach • Sweet potato • Whole grains	2 mg
Molybdenum	• Enzyme production	• Beans and peas • Nuts • Whole grains	75 mcg
Phosphorus	• Acid–base balance • Bone formation • Energy production and storage • Hormone activation	• Beans and peas • Dairy products • Meats • Nuts and seeds • Poultry • Seafood • Whole grain, enriched, and fortified cereals and breads	1,000 mg
Potassium *Nutrient of concern for most Americans*	• Blood pressure regulation • Carbohydrate metabolism • Fluid balance • Growth and development • Heart function • Muscle contraction • Nervous system function • Protein formation	• Bananas • Beet greens • Juices (e.g., carrot, pomegranate, prune, orange, and tomato) • Milk • Oranges and orange juice • Potatoes and sweet potatoes • Prunes and prune juice • Spinach • Tomatoes and tomato products • White beans • Yogurt	3,500 mg
Selenium	• Antioxidant • Immune function • Reproduction • Thyroid function	• Eggs • Enriched pasta and rice • Meats • Nuts (e.g., Brazil nuts) and seeds • Poultry • Seafood • Whole grains	70 mcg

(continued)

TABLE 8.2 Minerals: Functions, Dietary Sources, and Recommended Daily Value (*continued*)

Mineral	Functions	Dietary Sources	Daily Value*
Sodium *Nutrient to get less of*	• Acid–base balance • Blood pressure regulation • Fluid balance • Muscle contraction • Nervous system function	• Breads and rolls • Cheese (natural and processed) • Cold cuts and cured meats (e.g., deli or packaged ham or turkey) • Mixed meat dishes (e.g., beef stew, chili, and meat loaf) • Mixed pasta dishes (e.g., lasagna, pasta salad, and spaghetti with meat sauce) • Pizza • Poultry (fresh and processed) • Sandwiches (e.g., hamburgers, hot dogs, and submarine sandwiches) • Savory snacks (e.g., chips, crackers, popcorn, and pretzels) • Soups • Table salt	2,400 mg
Zinc	• Growth and development • Immune function • Nervous system function • Protein formation • Reproduction • Taste and smell • Wound healing	• Beans and peas • Beef • Dairy products • Fortified cereals • Nuts • Poultry • Seafood (e.g., clams, crabs, lobsters, oysters) • Whole grains	15 mg

*The Daily Values are the amounts of nutrients recommended per day for Americans 4 years of age or older.
Source: From U.S. Food and Drug Administration. (2016). *Vitamins and minerals chart.* Retrieved from https://www.accessdata.fda.gov/scripts/interactivenutritionfactslabel/factsheets/vitamin_and_mineral_chart.pdf

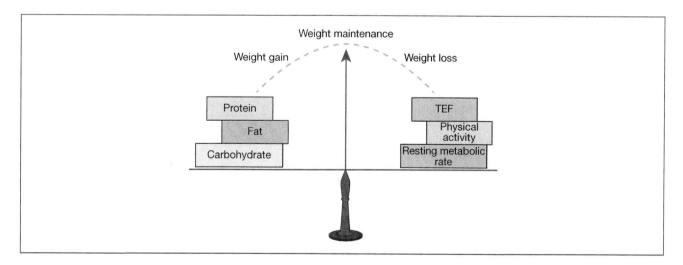

FIGURE 8.1 Energy balance equation.

TEF, thermic effect of food.

individuals should be near the bottom of the recommended range, while physically active individuals will require progressively more as activity increases. RMR tends to decline with aging; as such, older adults do not require the same level of energy intake as younger adults. Similarly, young children require fewer calories per day than do adolescents and adults. Numerous online calculators are available to estimate individual needs.

PHYSICAL ACTIVITY

Physical activity can be defined as movement produced by skeletal muscle that raises energy expenditure significantly above resting levels (Caspersen, Powell, & Christenson, 1985). Insufficient physical activity and/or excessive sedentary behavior increases the risk of death from all causes and also of noncommunicable diseases. Any physical activity is good, but more is generally better. The most recent Physical Activity Guidelines for Americans, released by the DHHS in late 2018, state that adults should participate in aerobic exercise (e.g., walking, running) that is continuous in nature and involves movement of major muscle groups throughout the week and should minimize time spent sedentary (see **Figure 8.2**). Exercise should be at least moderate in intensity, which is often described as the intensity at which an individual can talk but not sing. Activities are considered vigorous if the individual is able to speak only a few words before pausing to take a breath. Additionally, adults should strive to participate in resistance training for all major muscle groups on at least 2 days weekly. Meeting these guidelines is expected to promote overall health and to reduce the risk of diseases, including hypertension, cardiovascular disease, diabetes, osteoporosis, and some types of cancer. Adults engaging in sufficient activity can also expect improved quality of life, reduced risk of anxiety and depression, improved sleep, easier weight management, and improved cognition, among other benefits. Additional guidance exists for adults with chronic health conditions, older adults, and children. The full guidelines, scientific report, and fact sheets are available at https://health.gov/paguidelines/second-edition.

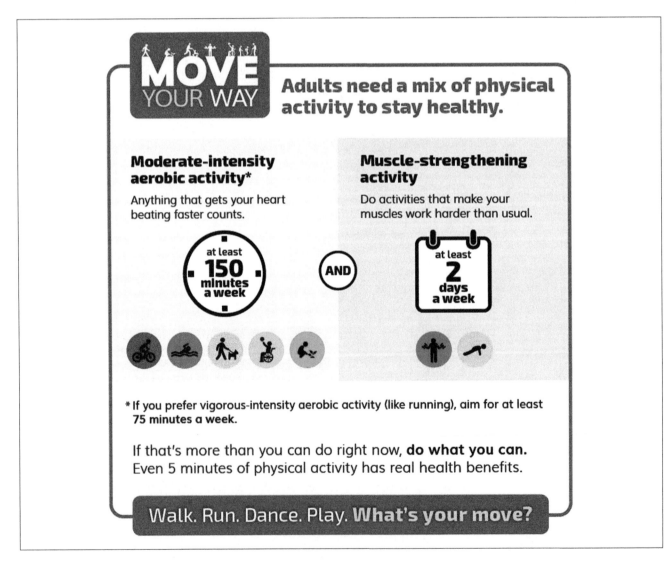

FIGURE 8.2 Move Your Way campaign. Recommended exercise guidelines for adults.

Source: From U.S. Department of Health and Human Services. (2018). *Physical activity guidelines for Americans* (2nd ed.). Retrieved from https://health.gov/paguidelines/second-edition/pdf/Physical_Activity_Guidelines_2nd_edition.pdf

LIFE-SPAN DIFFERENCES AND CONSIDERATIONS IN ANATOMY AND PHYSIOLOGY

Infants

The American Academy of Pediatrics (AAP) and the WHO advocate that infants should be exclusively breastfed for the first 6 months of life (AAP, 2012; WHO, 2001). Food can be introduced after 6 months, and breastfeeding should continue for at least 1 to 2 years (AAP, 2012; WHO, 2001). In addition, the United States Preventive Services Task Force (USPSTF, 2016a) recommends supporting breastfeeding by providing interventions both during pregnancy and after birth (Grade B).

Children

Adequate nutrient intake and healthy physical activity are crucial to support healthy growth and development. Although children require fewer calories per day than adolescents and adults, the demands associated with growth mean that children can become malnourished quickly. As such, it is vital to pay close attention to growth parameters and monitor lifestyle behaviors. Close monitoring of a child's growth history allows a clinician to spot early signs of malnourishment and/or accelerated growth.

Physical activity recommendations for children differ from those for adults. Preschool-aged children (3–5 years) should be active throughout the day and limit sedentary activities. Caregivers should encourage a variety of activities, including structured and unstructured play. Activities that include hopping, skipping, jumping, and tumbling encourage bone health. Older children (6–17 years) should achieve at least 60 minutes (1 hour) of physical activity each day and should engage in muscle and bone strengthening activities at least 3 days a week. Additionally, they should engage in vigorous activities on at least 3 days a week.

Adolescents

Adolescence is a time of rapid growth, and puberty is a dynamic period of change that varies in timing and tempo between individuals. It can be greatly affected by nutritional status, and adequate nutrition is crucial for achieving full growth potential. Appetite increases during adolescence, and total nutritional requirements are likely greater than any other period in life (Das et al., 2017). Clinicians should monitor stages of sexual maturation as described by Tanner and Marshall (i.e., Tanner Stages; Emmanuel & Bokor, 2019). Body composition naturally changes during puberty, and significant differences between boys and girls begin to emerge during this time. However, puberty is also a critical period of risk of developing obesity; as such, growth curves should be monitored closely.

Elderly

Older adults are at risk for a variety of nutritional problems because of a variety of environmental, behavioral, social, and economic factors. Physiological changes, including the presence of disease, can reduce appetite and/or make it hard to eat, resulting in malnutrition. The National Institute on Aging (n.d.) suggests being sure an older patient's diet includes at least two servings of milk or dairy products, two servings of high-protein foods, four servings of fruits and vegetables, and four servings of bread or grain products daily. Older adults benefit from the same daily level of physical activity as is recommended for younger adults but should take extra care in the case of osteoporosis, musculoskeletal disorders, or other chronic health conditions.

KEY HISTORY QUESTIONS AND CONSIDERATIONS FOR BODY HABITUS

HISTORY OF PRESENT ILLNESS

Common Presenting Symptoms

- Overweight/obesity
- Underweight
- Weight gain
- Weight loss
- Malnutrition
- Nutritional deficiencies

Example: Overweight/Obesity

- Chief concern: Overweight/obesity
- Onset: Sudden or insidious; age of onset
- Duration: Recent or chronic issue; progressive versus stagnant
- Character: Awareness or concerns about weight or weight gain
- Associated symptoms: Hyperphagia, physical or mental health symptoms, thoughts about body/weight
- Aggravating factors: Caloric intake, sedentary lifestyle, exercise habits, food preparation
- Relieving symptoms: Previous failed or successful attempts at weight loss
- Temporal factors: Recent or current physical or mental health comorbidities

Differential Diagnoses

Overweight, obese, diabetes, prediabetes, depression, hypothyroidism, hypertension, dyslipidemia, edema, heart failure, weight gain related to medication use

Example: Weight Loss

- Chief concern: Weight loss
- Onset: Recent, chronic; sudden versus insidious; when the patient first noticed they were losing weight

- Duration: Recent or chronic issue; progressive versus stagnant
- Character: Intentional versus unintentional
- Associated symptoms:
  - Intentional weight loss: Weight goal, dietary and exercise patterns, fruit and vegetable intake, support group participation, health promotion lifestyle changes
  - Unintentional weight loss: Fever, night sweats, recent illness or trauma, vomiting, diarrhea, depressive symptoms, new medications
- Aggravating factors: Caloric intake, exercise habits, food preparation
- Relieving factors: Previous failed or successful attempts at weight gain
- Temporal factors: Recent or current physical or mental health comorbidities

Differential Diagnoses

Malignancy, hyperthyroidism, anorexia, Addison's disease, celiac disease, weight loss due to dietary/exercise lifestyle modifications, depression, diabetes, weight loss due to medications, peptic ulcer disease, heart failure, substance use disorder, ulcerative colitis, HIV/AIDS, chonic obstructive pulmonary disease (COPD), heart failure

PAST MEDICAL HISTORY

- Chronic diseases, including cardiovascular disease, hypertension, diabetes, renal disease(s), thyroid disorders, liver disease(s), HIV, inflammatory bowel disease, celiac disease, growth hormone deficiency, rheumatologic conditions
- Cancer
- Chemotherapy
- Tuberculosis
- Anemia (iron deficiency or pernicious)
- Lactose intolerance
- Eating disorders, including anorexia nervosa, bulimia nervosa, binge eating disorder, orthorexia
- Depression
- Osteoarthritis
- Dementia
- Sleep apnea
- Surgeries (bariatric surgery—gastric bypass, lap band)

MEDICATIONS

- Chemotherapy
- Laxatives
- Diet pills
- Creatinine
- Steroid use
- Antipsychotic medications
- Appetite suppressants
- Over-the-counter vitamins and herbal supplements

- Diuretics
- Antiseizure medications
- Insulin
- Diabetes medications
- Thyroid medications
- Anticholinesterase inhibitors

FAMILY HISTORY

- Obesity
- Thyroid disease
- Eating disorders
- Diabetes
- Cardiovascular disease
- Depression
- Cancer (particularly gastrointestinal, lung, lymphoma, renal, and prostate cancers)

SOCIAL HISTORY

- Nicotine addiction
- Alcohol intake
- Use of laxatives (current or past)
- IV drug use/drug use prescribed, not prescribed (e.g., cocaine, amphetamines)
- Consumption of sweetened beverages (amount, frequency)
- Consumption of fast food (frequency, type)
- Diet (e.g., vegetarian, vegan, gluten-free)
- Food insecurity
- Recent travel out of the country
- Stress and coping
- Breastfeeding
- Athletes (specifically, long-distance runners, dancers, gymnasts, wrestlers, weight lifters)

REVIEW OF SYSTEMS

- General: Anorexia, fatigue, fever, pain, weakness
- Head, Eyes, Ears, Nose, Throat (HEENT): Dysphagia, ill-fitting dental wear
- Cardiovascular and respiratory: Tachycardia, chest pain, shortness of breath
- Gastrointestinal (GI)/Genitourinary (GU): Abdominal pain, early satiety, dysphagia, odynophagia, diarrhea, steatorrhea, black stools, hematochezia, abdominal distention, nausea, vomiting, hyperphagia
- Neurologic: Weakness, numbness, dizziness
- Endocrine: Changes to skin, hair; temperature intolerance
- Hematologic/metabolic: Hypercalcemia
- Integumentary: Acrodermatitis enteropathica (zinc), purpura (vitamins C and K), glossitis (vitamin B), hair loss and brittle nail (protein), acanthosis nigricans
- Psychiatric: Depression, sadness, worry, insomnia; behaviors suggestive of anorexia/bulimia, self-induced vomiting

PREVENTIVE CARE CONSIDERATIONS

- Dental problems (e.g., pain, cavities, ill-fitting dental devices, gum disease)
- Dietary behaviors, including salt intake, sugar intake, sugary beverage consumption; balance of carbohydrate, protein, and fat intake
- Exercise (frequency, duration, intensity, excessive tendencies)
- Strength training (frequency, duration, intensity)
- Age-appropriate cancer screenings

PHYSICAL EXAMINATION OF BODY HABITUS

INSPECTION

The most recent national surveillance data indicate a high prevalence of obesity among American adults (39.6%) and children (18.5%), with severe obesity found in 7.7% of adults (body mass index [BMI] >40 kg/m²) and 5.6% of children (BMI >120% of the 95th percentile; Hales, Fryar, Carroll, Freedman, & Ogden, 2018). Various visual indicators of obesity exist, and the clinician should be aware of these and other visual indicators of growth abnormalities. Clinicians should watch for apparent changes in body weight and body proportions, posture, and signs of endocrine disorders. Beyond apparent weight gain or loss, visual indicators may include gynecomastia, the presence of a cervicodorsal hump (a soft mound of tissue at the posterior nape of the neck), changes in gait, lordosis, knee valgus or varus, hirsutism and acne, and other skin changes.

Changes in body proportions may also indicate other growth disorders. Marfan's syndrome may be visually apparent by above-average height, long limbs, and a very long arm span. Giantism is characterized by rapid linear growth and coarse facial features, which progress with increasing age. Cushing's syndrome may be indicated by rapid weight gain, particularly around the abdomen, and the presence of a cervicodorsal hump.

Height

Height (stature) is defined as the distance from the plantar surface of the foot to the crown of the head. It is measured in the standing position once an individual reaches 2 years of age and is able to stand independently. Measurement is completed using a *stadiometer*, which typically consists of a vertical ruler and a sliding horizontal piece with a flat bottom. It is important to be familiar and practice with the equipment prior to measuring patients as each stadiometer may be a little different. The stadiometer should be precise enough to measure in increments of 1 mm. Make sure the patient's shoes, any excess or bulky clothing, and any hats are removed prior to measurement as these things can skew measurement results. Height is measured by asking the patient to stand straight with feet together and heels and back against the vertical measuring surface (**Figure 8.3**). Adjust the head so that it is in the Frankfort plane (the outer canthus of the eye is horizontal with the external auditory canal; **Figure 8.4**).

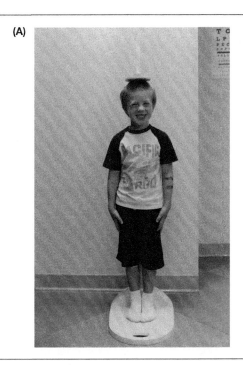
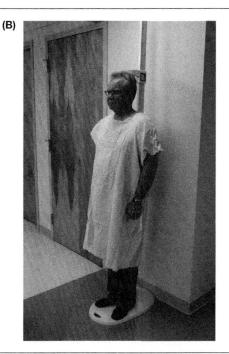

FIGURE 8.3 Correct measurement of height using a stadiometer. (A) Child. (B) Adult.

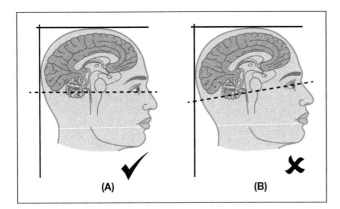

(A) **✔** **(B)** **✗**

FIGURE 8.4 Head positioning when measuring height. (A) Correct position. (B) Incorrect position.

Weight

Weight represents the total body mass. Alone, body weight is a poor predictor of health because it is strongly correlated with height and not reflective of body composition. To evaluate the appropriateness of a patient's weight, it must be considered in relation to height. Assessment of body composition may be of additional benefit in some cases, as discussed later.

Scales for measuring body weight must be placed on a solid, flat surface and should be balanced appropriately (consult the operating manual for the device). Similar to using a stadiometer for the first time, be familiar and practice with the scale prior to weighing patients. Weight should be measured to the nearest 0.1 kg (or nearest 0.1 lb). Make sure the patient's shoes and any excess or heavy clothing are removed. Ask the patient to remove any belongings from their pockets, including wallets, keys, and phones. Have the patient place both feet in the center of the scale and avoid movement while measurement is occurring.

Body Mass Index Calculation

Weight may be evaluated relative to height by calculating the body mass index (BMI), sometimes referred to as Quetelet's Index. An accurate height and weight are needed in order to calculate a BMI. Height and weight can be self-reported if a stadiometer and scale are not available but most patients over-report height and under-report weight (Opichka & Smith, 2018; Pursey, Burrows, Stanwell, & Collins, 2014).The BMI is calculated by dividing weight in kilograms by height in meters squared. It is expressed as kg/m^2 (if measuring in inches and pounds, BMI may be calculated as [lb/in^2] × 703; **Figure 8.5**). Adult patients' weight status may then be classified according to standard cut-points outlined by the National Heart, Lung, and Blood Institute (NHLBI; **Table 8.3**). For children, weight status should be evaluated according to age- and sex-specific percentiles

determined by the appropriate growth chart. BMI is not used for children under 2 years of age. There are many BMI charts that can be printed and/or electronic BMI calculators that can be accessed online (https://www.nhlbi.nih.gov/health/educational/lose_wt/BMI/bmi-m.htm). Despite its widespread use in clinical practice, the BMI metric does have limitations. BMI is a poor indicator of percentage of body fat and does not capture information on the mass of fat distribution in different body sites (Nuttall, 2015).

Waist Circumference

Measurement of circumferences can be useful for further assessment of body composition without requiring specialized equipment or imaging. Most commonly used are waist circumference and waist:hip ratio. The presence of elevated waist circumference and/or elevated waist:hip ratio is an indicator of proportionally more adipose tissue distribution around the abdomen compared with the hip and thigh. This distribution of adiposity around the abdomen is also referred to as an android (or apple) distribution, as opposed to a gynoid (or pear) distribution (**Figure 8.6**). The android pattern of adiposity is associated with increased risk of adverse health outcomes, including cardiovascular diseases and diabetes, and remains so even after statistically accounting for BMI.

To measure a waist circumference, have the patient remove any constricting clothing from their waistline. Tell the patient to breathe normally and avoid "sucking it in." The clinician should then use the hands to walk up both sides of the patient's hips. When the top of the iliac crest is felt, this is the correct place to put the tape measure (**Figure 8.7**). Use a flexible tape measure that measures in inches or centimeters. Make sure that the tape measure is snug but does not compress the skin and that the tape measure lies parallel to the floor. Have the patient relax and exhale.

It is not necessary to do a waist circumference on any patient with a BMI of 35 or greater or any individual with a height under 5 feet because of inaccuracies. A high waist circumference is associated with an increased risk for type 2 diabetes, dyslipidemia, hypertension, and cardiovascular disease in patients with a BMI in a range between 25 and 34.9 kg/m^2 (NHLBI, n.d.). Monitoring changes in waist circumference over time may be helpful, in addition to measuring BMI, since it can provide an estimate of increased abdominal adipose tissue even in the absence of a change in BMI. Furthermore, in obese patients with metabolic complications, changes in waist circumference are useful predictors of changes in cardiovascular risk factors.

The value of waist circumference is limited in cases of patients who are unable to stand, are pregnant, have had certain abdominal surgeries, or are especially lean

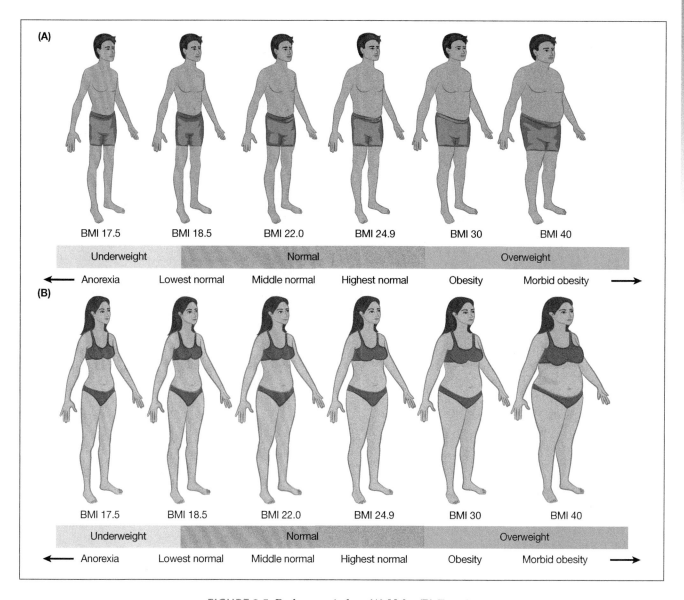

FIGURE 8.5 Body mass index. (A) Male. (B) Female.

Classification	Adults	Children (2–20 years)
TABLE 8.3 Classification of Body Mass Index in Adults and Children		
Underweight	<18.5 kg/m^2	<5th percentile
Normal	18.5–24.9 kg/m^2	5th–84.9th percentile
Overweight	25.0–29.9 kg/m^2	85th–94.9th percentile
Obesity	≥30.0 kg/m^2	≥95th percentile

Adult obesity may be further classified in increments of 5 kg/m^2: Class I 30.0 to 34.9 kg/m^2, Class II 35.0 to 39.9 kg/m^2, Class III >40.0 kg/m^2.
Sources: Centers for Disease Control and Prevention. (n.d.). About child & teen BMI. Retrieved from https://www.cdc.gov/health
yweight/assessing/bmi/childrens_bmi/about_childrens_bmi.html#percentile; National Heart, Lung, and Blood Institute. (n.d.). Classification of
overweight and obesity by BMI, waist circumference, and associated disease risks. Retrieved from https://www.nhlbi.nih.gov/health/
educational/lose_wt/BMI/bmi_dis.htm

or underweight. Waist circumference cut-points that are specific to different ethnicities and countries of origin have been published by the International Diabetes Federation (Alberti, Zimmet, & Shaw, 2007).

Other Circumferences

In certain circumstances, it may be necessary to measure the circumference of other body areas. When using this method to assess nutritional status, it is important

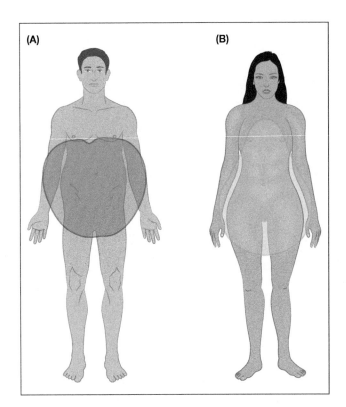

FIGURE 8.6 Weight distribution. (A) Android (apple) distribution. (B) Gynoid (pear) distribution.

that trained clinicians perform the measurements to ensure accuracy and consistency for long-term comparisons (**Figure 8.8**). In pediatric patients aged 6 to 59 months, the mid-upper arm circumference (MUAC) is also an independent anthropometric assessment tool used to determine undernutrition. MUAC has been correlated with BMI in children and can be a helpful measure when children have certain conditions like fluid overload or lower extremity edema (Becker et al., 2015). MUAC is also the most capable in predicting 12-month follow-up mortality risk in older adults. Calf circumference is also used to assess nutritional status in adults and has been shown to have good diagnostic capacity (Bonnefoy, Jauffret, Kostka, & Jusot, 2002; Hsu, Tsai, & Wang, 2016; Tsai, Lai, & Chang, 2012).

SPECIAL TESTS

Nutritional Assessments

The primary determinants of nutritional status are food and nutrient intake. This can be assessed by estimating the energy and protein intake of an individual. Estimates can be obtained through the history (verbal report, food diary, food tracking app, etc.) or, when feasible, by direct observation. Ideally, indirect calorimetry should be used to estimate energy requirements. This is a noninvasive test that uses the patient's breath to determine their RMR. When this option is unavailable, the Food and Agriculture Organization (FAO)/WHO and

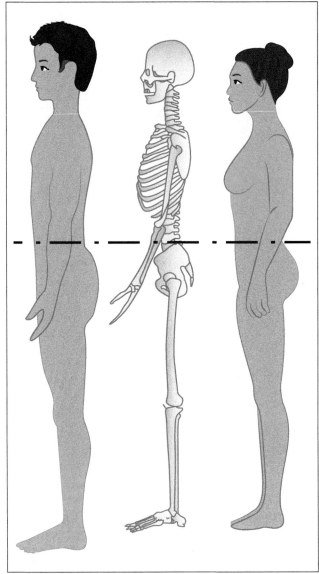

FIGURE 8.7 Correct placement for measuring waist circumference.

Schofield equations can be utilized to estimate energy expenditure of a healthy adult or child, although there are limitations to these equations (Becker et al., 2015).

The Academy of Nutrition and Dietetics (the Academy) and the American Society for Parenteral and Enteral Nutrition (ASPEN) have developed a set of evidence-based diagnostic criteria to identify and document pediatric undernutrition in routine clinical practice. These criteria, outlined in **Tables 8.4** and **8.5**, are intended for use in children and adolescents aged 1 month to 18 years and can be used across multiple populations, including primary care, inpatient, and residential care settings (Hurt & McClave, 2016).

There are many valid and reliable nutritional assessment tools available to screen for malnutrition in adults,

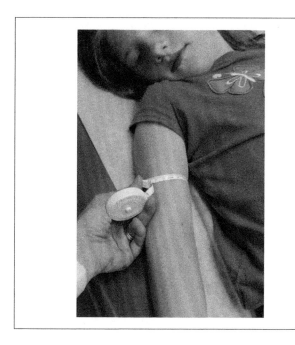

FIGURE 8.8 Measuring mid-upper arm circumference.

and they are typically used in the nursing home and rehabilitation settings. The malnutrition screening tool (MST; **Exhibit 8.1**) and the Mini Nutritional Assessment (MNA®; www.mna-elderly.com/forms/mini/mna_mini_english.pdf) are two screening tools that are well known and should be considered if a patient presents with recent weight loss, recent poor intake/appetite, and/or a low BMI. Both tools have a high sensitivity and specificity—MST sensitivity 93%, specificity 93%; MNA sensitivity 97.9%, specificity 100% (Guigoz, 2006).

Percent Body Fat

Assessment of body composition accounts for not only an individual's body weight, or mass under the influence of gravity, but also the proportion of weight that is made up of fat and lean tissue (e.g., muscle, connective tissues, and nerve tissues). The most widely utilized term to reflect fat content of the body is **percent body fat (% BF)**, calculated by dividing fat body weight by total body weight. Body weight is not a good reflection of body composition because the densities of lean and fat tissues vary. Lean tissue is composed primarily of

TABLE 8.4 Indicators for Identification of Pediatric Undernutrition: Single Data Point Available

	Mild Malnutrion	Moderate Malnutrion	Severe Malnutrion
Weight-for-height z score	−1 to −1.9 z score	−2 to −2.9 z score	−3 or greater z score
BMI-for-age z score	−1 to −1.9 z score	−2 to −2.9 z score	−3 or greater z score
Length/height-for-age z score	No data	No data	−3 z score
Mid-upper arm circumference	Greater than or equal to −1 to −1.9 z score	Greater than or equal to −2 to −2.9 z score	Greater than or equal to −3 z score

Source: Republished with permission of John Wiley and Sons, Inc., from Becker, P., Carney, L. N., Corkins, M. R., Monczka, J., Smith, E., Smith, S. E., . . . White, J. V. (2015). Consensus statement of the Academy of Nutrition and Dietetics/American Society for Parenteral and Enteral Nutrition: Indicators recommended for the identification and documentation of pediatric malnutrition (undernutrition). *Nutrition in Clinical Practice, 30*(1), 147–161. doi:10.1177/0884533614557642. Permission conveyed through Copyright Clearance Center, Inc.

TABLE 8.5 Indicators for Identification of Pediatric Undernutrition: Two or More Data Points Available

	Mild Malnutrion	Moderate Malnutrion	Severe Malnutrion
Weight gain velocity (<2 years of age)	Less than 75% of the norm for expected weight gain	Less than 50% of the norm for expected weight gain	Less than 25% of the norm for expected weight gain
Weight loss (2–20 years of age)	5% usual body weight	7.5% usual body weight	10% usual body weight
Deceleration in weight for length/height z score	Decline of 1 z score	Decline of 2 z score	Decline of 3 z score
Inadequate nutrient intake	51%–75% estimated energy/protein need	26%–50% estimated energy/protein need	≤25% estimated energy/protein need

Source: Republished with permission of John Wiley and Sons, Inc., from Becker, P., Carney, L. N., Corkins, M. R., Monczka, J., Smith, E., Smith, S. E., . . . White, J. V. (2015). Consensus statement of the Academy of Nutrition and Dietetics/American Society for Parenteral and Enteral Nutrition: Indicators recommended for the identification and documentation of pediatric malnutrition (undernutrition). *Nutrition in Clinical Practice, 30*(1), 147–161. doi:10.1177/0884533614557642. Permission conveyed through Copyright Clearance Center, Inc.

EXHIBIT 8.1 Malnutrition Screening Tool

	Answer	Points
Have you recently lost weight without trying?	No	0
	Unsure	1
If yes, how much weight have you lost? (Answer this question only if *unsure* was marked on above question)	2–13 lb	1
	14–23 lb	2
	24–33 lb	3
	34 lb or more	4
	Unsure	2
Have you been eating poorly due to a decreased appetite?	No	0
	Yes	1

Total Points

Interpretation of Score for Malnutrition Screening Tool

Risk Category	Total Score
Not at risk	0 or 1
At risk	2+

Source: Reprinted from Ferguson, M., Capra, S., Bauer, J., & Banks, M. (1999). Development of a valid and reliable malnutrition screening tool for adult acute hospital patients. *Nutrition, 15,* 458–464. doi:10.1016/S0899-9007(99)00084-2, with permission from Elsevier.

skeletal muscle, which is more dense than fat. Therefore, two individuals of the same body weight can vary greatly in body composition. This variation explains the limited utility of the BMI among athletic populations, those with comparatively low muscle mass (i.e., sarcopenia), and variation by ethnicity.

Some of the more popular techniques used to estimate % BF include hydrostatic (underwater) weighing, dual-energy x-ray absorptiometry (DEXA or DXA) scans, and skinfold thickness. Of these techniques, hydrostatic weighing and DEXA are considered the most accurate, but can be prohibitively costly (Madden & Smith, 2016).

Hydrostatic Weighing

The hydrostatic weighing (underwater weighing) technique is based on the densities of body tissues. The densities of bone and muscle tissue are higher than that of water, while the density of fat is less than that of water. Therefore, a person with more bone and muscle mass than fat mass will sink in water. Various experiments on cadavers allow for the difference between air weight and underwater weight to be converted to body density and then % BF.

Dual-Energy X-Ray Absorptiometry

While hydrostatic weighing has long been considered the gold standard in body fat assessment, DEXA is now recognized as one of the most accurate means of assessment. A DEXA scan works by passing x-ray beams of two intensities (attenuations) through the body. Because different tissue types will absorb dissimilar amounts of radiation, the technique can differentiate between lean tissue, adipose tissue, and bone. DEXA is frequently used in clinical settings to evaluate bone mineral density and can also be used to evaluate the composition of specific body regions, but cannot differentiate between subcutaneous and visceral adipose tissue (Shepherd, Ng, Sommer, & Heymsfield, 2017).

Skinfold Thicknesses

Skinfold thicknesses involve the measurement of the thickness of a fold of skin and the underlying subcutaneous adipose tissue at multiple body sites. Several methods and body density equations exist, including methods that assess as few as three body sites to as many as seven sites. The clinician locates the site to be measured, lifts the skin firmly by grasping between the thumb and forefinger, and uses specialized calipers to measure the thickness of the fold in millimeters. The clinician should rotate through all of the measurement sites until two consistent measurements are obtained at each site. Then, the sum of skinfolds is used to calculate body density and % BF using sex-, age-, and ethnicity-specific equations (American College of Sports Medicine, 2018).

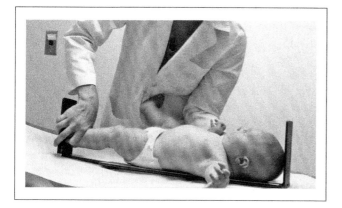

FIGURE 8.9 Obtaining length measurement in an infant.

LIFE-SPAN CONSIDERATIONS FOR PHYSICAL EXAMINATION

Infants

For children under 2 years of age, recumbent length is assessed in place of standing height. The child should be laid on the back with the head in the Frankfort plane against a fixed plate, the hips and knees fully extended, and soles of the feet against a sliding board (**Figure 8.9**). Infants should be weighed in as little clothing as possible, preferably nude. As with older children, it is best to use the same scale at each visit to accommodate for device-specific measurement error.

Head circumference reflects the growth of the cranium and its contents and should be assessed at each well visit during the first 2 years. It should be measured with a flexible, but nonstretchable, measuring tape placed at the greatest circumference of the head, typically around the occipital and frontal bones (**Figure 8.10**). In the case of small or large head circumferences, additional assessments may be necessary.

Children and Adolescents

Children and adolescents should undergo anthropometric assessment at each well child visit since growth is the primary outcome measure of nutritional status in children. Regular assessment should include height, weight, BMI (beginning at age 2), and associated percentiles. Circumferences, growth velocity, and food/nutrient intake may be additionally assessed if indicated (i.e., suspected over- or undernutrition). The same stadiometer and scale should be used at each visit, if possible, to accommodate for device-specific measurement error. Serial measurements are necessary to adequately follow growth.

Older Adults

Changes in nutritional status, environmental influences, and hormonal status in older adults may complicate measures of body size. Loss of height occurs in later adulthood and results from a combination of compression of

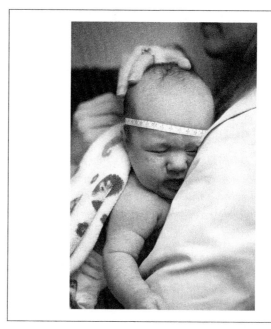

FIGURE 8.10 Measuring the head circumference of an infant.

the intervertebral discs and loss of bone mineral leading to osteoporosis. Further, older adults may experience *kyphosis*, a curvature of the upper spine, and illnesses that may make standing straight difficult. As with children, serial measures are particularly important.

LABORATORY CONSIDERATIONS FOR BODY HABITUS

Laboratory considerations will vary depending on the chief concern. Laboratory parameters often remain normal for a period of time after malnutrition has begun; therefore, physical examination is a better tool for diagnosing malnutrition (Becker et al., 2015; Bharadwaj et al., 2016). Historically, laboratory markers like serum albumin and prealbumin have been used as markers of undernutrition, but evidence supporting these are generally weak (Bharadwaj et al., 2016). These types of laboratory markers should be used to augment the physical examination.

If unintentional weight loss is the primary concern and there is no suspected diagnosis based on the history and physical exam, the following tests should be considered: complete blood count with differential, complete metabolic panel, hemoglobin A1c, thyroid stimulating hormone (TSH), stool hemoccult, erythrocyte sedimentation rate (ESR), C-reactive protein, HIV, hepatitis C, and any age-appropriate screenings (Gupta & Evans, 2019). If malignancy is suspected, C-reactive protein (CRP), hemoglobin, lactate dehydrogenase, and albumin should also be considered.

EVIDENCE-BASED PRACTICE CONSIDERATIONS FOR BODY HABITUS

The USPSTF has several published guidelines that discuss body habitus, exercise, and nutrition. Clinicians should be aware of these evidence-based guidelines and use them to guide practice.

- "The USPSTF concludes that the current evidence is insufficient to assess the balance of benefits and harms of the use of multivitamins for the prevention of cardiovascular disease or cancer" (Grade I Recommendation; 2016c, "Recommendation Summary").
- "The USPSTF recommends offering or referring adults who are overweight or obese and have additional cardiovascular disease (CVD) risk factors to intensive behavioral counseling interventions to promote a healthful diet and physical activity for CVD prevention" (Grade B Recommendation; 2016c, "Recommendation Summary").
- "The USPSTF recommends that clinicians screen for obesity in children and adolescents 6 years and older and offer or refer them to comprehensive, intensive behavioral interventions to promote improvements in weight status" (Grade B Recommendation; 2017, "Recommendation Summary").

ABNORMAL FINDINGS OF BODY HABITUS

MALNUTRITION

According to the WHO (2016), malnutrition is defined as "deficiencies, excesses or imbalances in a person's intake of energy and/or nutrients." This can be due to one of two conditions: undernutrition or being overweight/obese. Malnutrition can lead to adverse effects on body composition, function, and clinical outcomes (Saunders, Smith, & Stroud, 2019). Malnutrition increases the risk of death, length of hospital stay, and healthcare costs.

Undernutrition

Undernutrition is due to lack of adequate nutrition. This can be caused by not having enough food or by not eating enough foods that contain the nutrients needed for proper growth and development. Chronic undernutrition can lead to stunting (low height for age of reference population), wasting (low weight for height of reference population), underweight (low weight for age of reference population), developmental delays in children, poor immune function, and micronutrient deficiencies or insufficiencies (a lack of important vitamins and minerals). Undernutrition can also result from a chronic condition that causes malabsorption, psychosocial circumstances, effects

of illness or injury, an eating disorder, organ failure, severe infection, or physical trauma (Saunders et al., 2019).

Key History and Physical Findings

- Very young and very old are more at risk
- History of functional decline, dementia, or Alzheimer's disease in an elderly person
- Resident of a nursing home or rehabilitation facility
- Lack of specific nutrients in the diet (even the lack of one vitamin can lead to malnutrition)
- An unbalanced diet
- History of a malabsorption syndrome(s) and/or cancer(s)
- Loss of appetite
- Dental pain or problems
- Weight loss
- Stunting
- Wasting
- Symptoms specific to the nutrient(s) that is lacking (**Table 8.6**)

Overweight/Obesity

Obesity is a multifactorial disease. Obesity is classified as a BMI of 30 or greater in adults (**Figure 8.11**), and overweight is classified as a BMI of 25 to 29.9. Children are classified as overweight if they are in the 85th to less than 95th percentile for BMI-for-age weight and classified as obese if they are in the 95th percentile or greater. It can be possible to be both overweight and micronutrient deficient. Overweight/obesity results from a combination of genetics, behavioral and environmental factors, and other idiosyncratic causes like medications and other chronic conditions. Contributory behavioral factors include such things as sedentary lifestyle, physical inactivity, and dietary patterns. Obesity contributes to many chronic conditions, including cardiovascular disease, diabetes, cancer, stroke, sleep apnea, and mental illnesses.

Key History and Physical Findings

- Imbalance in caloric intake and caloric expenditure
- Reported diet high in sugar, trans fats, saturated fats
- Sedentary lifestyle
- Little to no exercise
- BMI of 25 or greater (overweight) or 30 or greater (obese; adults)
- BMI from 85th to 94th percentile (overweight) and at or above the 95th percentile (obese) for children and teens of the same age and sex

WEIGHT GAIN

Similar to obesity, weight gain may arise from one of many causes. Unplanned weight gain may be explained by lifestyle changes, including reduced physical activity

TABLE 8.6 Signs and Symptoms of Macro- and Micronutrient Deficiencies

Deficiency	Clinical Features	Laboratory Findings
Calories	Weight loss with normal appetite	
Fat	Pale and voluminous stool, diarrhea without flatulence, steatorrhea	Fractional fat excretion (% of dietary fat not absorbed) >6%
Protein	Edema, muscle atrophy, amenorrhea	Hypoalbuminemia, hypoproteinemia
Carbohydrates	Watery diarrhea, flatulence, acidic stool pH, milk intolerance, stool osmotic gap	Increased breath hydrogen
Vitamin B12	Anemia, subacute combined degeneration of the spinal cord (early symptoms are paresthesias and ataxia associated with loss of vibration and position sense)	Macrocytic anemia, vitamin B12 decreased, abnormal Schilling test, serum methylmalonic acid and homocysteine increased
Folic acid	Anemia	Macrocytic anemia, serum and RBC folate decreased; serum homocysteine increased
Vitamin B, General	Cheilosis, painless glossitis, acrodermatitis, angular stomatitis	
Iron	Microcytic anemia, glossitis, pagophagia	Serum iron and ferritin decreased, total iron binding capacity increased
Calcium and Vitamin D	Paresthesia, tetany, pathologic fractures due to osteomalacia, positive Chvostek and Trousseau signs	Hypocalcemia, serum alkaline phosphatase increased, abnormal bone densitometry
Vitamin A	Follicular hyperkeratosis, night blindness	Serum retinol decreased
Vitamin K	Hematoma, bleeding disorders	Prolonged prothrombin time, vitamin K-dependent coagulation factors decreased

Source: Mason, J. B. (2019). Approach to the adult patient with suspected malabsorption. In S. Grover (Ed.), *UpToDate.* Retrieved from https://www.uptodate.com/contents/approach-to-the-adult-patient-with-suspected-malabsorption

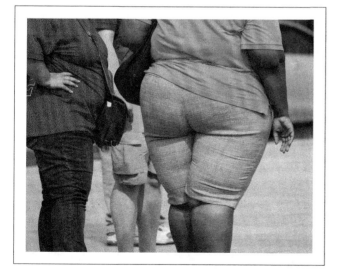

FIGURE 8.11 Overweight/obese adults.

and/or increased energy intake, and other causes, including medication changes, metabolic, endocrine, and/or psychosocial factors.

Key History and Physical Findings

- Imbalance in caloric intake and caloric expenditure
- Reported diet high in sugar, trans fats, saturated fats
- Reduction in physical activity/increase in sedentary behavior
- Certain medications

WEIGHT LOSS

Weight loss results from energy expenditure that is in excess of energy intake. This may result from a simple change in dietary habits and/or physical activity, or more complex causes, including medications, endocrine factors, psychosocial factors, and other illnesses.

Key History and Physical Findings

- Imbalance in caloric intake and caloric expenditure
- Reported reduction in energy intake; diet low in fats, protein, calories
- Reported increase in physical activity
- Medications
- Gastrointestinal symptoms
- Poor dentition

- Decreased appetite (anorexia)
- Generalized muscle wasting
- Decreased hand/grip strength

CACHEXIA

Cachexia is a multiorgan syndrome that is characterized by anorexia, a dramatic loss of skeletal muscle mass and adipose tissue, substantial weight loss, and inflammation. It is often associated with certain disease states such as advanced cancers, AIDS, certain autoimmune diseases, and other chronic conditions like heart failure and chronic kidney disease. Cancer data strongly suggests that cachexia hinders treatment responses and patients' ability to tolerate treatment. Inflammatory cytokines, in particular, have been closely associated with cachexia and mortality in cancer patients (Argiles, Busquets, Stemmler, & Lopez-Soriano, 2015).

Key History and Physical Findings

- Weight loss in adult or growth failure in children
- Anorexia
- Inflammation

- Insulin resistance
- Increased muscle protein breakdown
- Decreased muscle strength
- Fatigue
- Low free fat mass index (FFMI)
- Increased inflammatory markers (CRP >5.0 mg/L, IL-6 >4.0 pg/mL)
- Anemia (<12 g/dL)
- Low serum albumin (<3.2 g/dL)

SARCOPENIA

Sarcopenia is a complex and multifaceted process that involves the degenerative loss of skeletal muscle mass, quality, and strength. It is often the result of healthy aging. It can, however, affect balance, gait, and overall ability to perform activities of daily living (ADLs).

Key History and Physical Findings

- Loss of muscle mass, strength, and function
- Most commonly seen in inactive people but can also affect those who remain physically active throughout their lives
- Difficulty performing ADLs

CASE STUDY: Wellness Visit

Reason for Seeking Care

A 10-year-old male, Jae Sean, presents to the clinic with his mother for a routine well visit.

Review of Wellness

He has no general concerns about his health. He feels good but does note that he does not feel like he can always keep up the pace of other kids when he plays sports. He reports being "fairly active" on recess. He does not currently participate in any extracurricular sports or activities. When asked about other hobbies, he says that he likes to play video games and spends about 3 to 5 hours/day playing. When asked about his diet, he says that he often has frozen waffles for breakfast, the school lunch, and whatever his mom cooks for dinner. His favorite snacks are tortilla chips and buttered popcorn. He reports consuming about one fruit daily and rarely any vegetables. He eats fast food 4 to 5 times/week. He consumes sports drinks and soda about 3 to 4 days/week. He usually sleeps 10 hours per night. He feels well connected to his family; his mother reports that he is happy at home and that there have been no recent changes in their home life. He has a history of asthma that is well controlled with only a rescue inhaler that he uses as needed. He has one to two good friends at school and feels

safe at home and at school. He says his grades "are fine." He has no other chronic illnesses and takes no other medications. His mother has hypertension and is obese. His father has hypertension, diabetes, hyperlipidemia, and obesity. He is up to date on his vaccines. Parents have stable jobs, and mother denies food insecurity or transportation issues. They live in a safe neighborhood.

Vital signs

Temperature 98.4°F, respirations 14, blood pressure 110/74, pulse 82, weight 102 lbs, height 56 inches

Physical Examination

- Patient is alert and oriented × 3. Patient is articulate and makes eye contact.
- Heart rate and rhythm are regular.
- Lungs are clear to auscultation bilaterally without adventitious breath sounds.
- Abdomen is soft, nontender in all four quadrants.

Questions to Consider

1. What are some things you would like to address at this well visit?
2. What is Jae Sean's BMI? What classification is he?
3. What are some recommendations to consider for Jae Sean today?

Clinical Pearls

- Help children stand straight and still while measuring their height by getting down to their level and having a parent stand behind you.
- Some stadiometers include a digital display that reports the height measured. If this is not available, it is important to complete the reading in the same horizontal plane to avoid measurement error; as such, it is often useful to keep a stool next to the stadiometer.
- The key to achieving and maintaining a healthy weight is not short-term dietary changes; it is about a lifestyle that includes healthy eating and regular physical activity.
- If a patient needs to improve nutrition, it is important to educate the individual who is in charge of meal preparation and cooking on healthy eating and healthy food preparation.
- Children and adolescents can also serve as healthy change agents for their parents when it comes to improving diet and exercise habits within the family unit.

Key Takeaways

- Nutrition and exercise are important parts of the overall health and well-being of individuals and families and should be routinely addressed and emphasized.
- It is important to be accurate and precise in the measurement and recording of biometric measures, including height and weight.
- Being overweight/obese is a modifiable risk factor that is associated with multiple chronic diseases and illnesses.
- Prevention through early intervention is the key to avoiding obesity.
- BMI does not account for increased muscle mass.

REFERENCES

Alberti, K. G., Zimmet, P., & Shaw, J. (2007). International Diabetes Federation: A consensus on Type 2 diabetes prevention. *Diabetic Medicine*, *24*(5), 451–463. doi:10.1111/j.1464-5491.2007.02157.x

American Academy of Pediatrics. (2012). Breastfeeding and the use of human milk. *Pediatrics*, *129*(3), e827–e841. doi:10.1542/peds.2011–3552

American College of Sports Medicine. (2018). *ACSM's guidelines for exercise testing and prescription* (10th ed.). Philadelphia, PA: Wolters Kluwer.

Argiles, J., Busquets, S., Stemmler, B., & Lopez-Soriano, F. (2015). Cachexia and sarcopenia: Mechanisms and potential targets for intervention. *Current Opinion in Pharmacology*, *22*, 100–106. doi:10.1016/j.coph.2015.04.003

Becker, P., Carney, L. N., Corkins, M. R., Monczka, J., Smith, E., Smith, S. E., . . . White, J. V. (2015). Consensus statement of the Academy of Nutrition and Dietetics/American Society for Parenteral and Enteral Nutrition: Indicators recommended for the identification and documentation of pediatric malnutrition (undernutrition). *Nutrition in Clinical Practice*, *30*(1), 147–161. doi:10.1177/0884533614557642

Bharadwaj, S., Ginoya, S., Tandon, P., Gohel, T. D., Guirguis, J., Vallabh, H., . . ., Hanouneh, I. (2016). Malnutrition: Laboratory markers vs nutritional assessment. *Gastroenterology Report*, *4*(4), 272–280. doi:10.1093/gastro/gow013

Bonnefoy, M., Jauffret, M., Kostka, T., & Jusot, J. F. (2002). Usefulness of calf circumference measurement in assessing the nutritional state of hospitalized elderly people. *Gerontology*, *48*, 162–169. doi:10.1159/000052836

Caspersen, C. J., Powell, K. E., & Christenson, G. M. (1985). Physical activity, exercise, and physical fitness: Definitions and distinctions for health-related research. *Public Health Reports (Washington, D.C.: 1974)*, *100*(2), 126–131. doi:10.1093/nq/s9-IX.228.365-f

Centers for Disease Control and Prevention. (n.d.). About child & teen BMI. Retrieved from https://www.cdc.gov/healthy weight/assessing/bmi/childrens_bmi/about_childrens _bmi.html#percentile

Das, J. K., Salam, R. A., Thornburg, K. L., Prentice, A. M., Campisi, S., Lassi, Z. S., . . . Bhutta, Z. A. (2017). Nutrition in adolescents: Physiology, metabolism, and nutritional needs. *Annals of the New York Academy of Sciences*, *1393*(1), 21–33. doi:10.1111/nyas.13330

Emmanuel, M., & Bokor, B. R. (2019). Tanner stages. In *StatPearls* [Internet]. Treasure Island, FL: StatPearls Publishing. Retrieved from https://www.ncbi.nlm.nih.gov/books/NBK470280

Ferguson, M., Capra, S., Bauer, J., & Banks, M. (1999). Development of a valid and reliable malnutrition screening tool for adult acute hospital patients. *Nutrition*, *15*, 458–464. doi:10.1016/S0899-9007(99)00084-2

Guigoz, Y. (2006). The Mini-Nutritional Assessment (MNA®) review of the literature—What does it tell us? *The Journal of Nutrition, Health and Aging*, *10*, 466–487.

Gupta, R., & Evans, A. T. (2019). Approach to the patient with unintentional weight loss. In J. Elmore (Ed.), *UpToDate* Retrieved from https://www.uptodate.com/contents/approach -to-the-patient-with-unintentional-weight-loss

Hales, C. M., Fryar, C. D., Carroll, M. D., Freedman, D. S., & Ogden, C. L. (2018). Trends in obesity and severe obesity prevalence in US youth and adults by sex and age, 2007–2008 to 2015-2016. *The Journal of the American Medical Association*, *319*(16), 1723–1725. doi:10.1001/jama.2018.3060

Hsu, W., Tsai, A., & Wang, J. (2016). Calf circumference is more effective than body mass index in predicting emerging care-need of older adults—Results from a national cohort study. *Clinical Nutrition, 35*(3), 735–740. doi:10.1016/j .clnu.2015.05.017

Hurt, R. T., & McClave, S. A. (2016). Nutritional assessment in primary care. *Medical Clinics of North America, 100*(6), 1169–1183. doi:10.1016/j.mcna.2016.06.001

Institute of Medicine. (2005). *Dietary Reference Intakes for water, potassium, sodium, chloride, and sulfate* (pp. 73–185). Washington, DC: National Academies Press. Retrieved from http://www.nap.edu/openbook.php?record_id=10925

Madden, A. M., & Smith, S. (2016). Body composition and morphological assessment of nutritional status in adults: A review of anthropometric variables. *Journal of Human Nutrition and Dietetics, 29*(1), 7–25. doi:10.1111/ jhn.12278

Mason, J. B. (2019). Approach to the adult patient with suspected malabsorption. In S. Grover (Ed.), *UpToDate.* Retrieved from https://www.uptodate.com/contents/ approach-to-the-adult-patient-with-suspected-malabsorption

National Heart, Lung, and Blood Institute. (n.d.). Classification of overweight and obesity by BMI, waist circumference, and associated disease risks. Retrieved from https://www .nhlbi.nih.gov/health/educational/lose_wt/BMI/bmi_dis .htm

National Institute on Aging. (n.d.). Know your food groups. Retrieved from https://www.nia.nih.gov/health/ know-your-food-groups

Nuttall, F. Q. (2015). Body mass index: Obesity, BMI, and health: A critical review. *Nutrition Today, 50*(3), 117–128. doi:10.1097/NT.0000000000000092

Opichka, K., & Smith, C. (2018). Accuracy of self-reported heights and weights in a predominately low-income, diverse population living in the USA. *American Journal of Human Biology, 30*, e23184. doi:10.1002/ajhb.23184

Pursey, K., Burrows, T. L., Stanwell, P., & Collins, C. E. (2014). How accurate is web-based self-reported height, weight, and body mass index in young adults? *Journal of Medical Internet Research, 16*(1), e4. doi:10.2196/jmir.2909

Saunders, J., Smith, T. R., & Stroud, M. A. (2019). Malnutrition and undernutrition. *Medicine, 47*(3), 152–158. doi:10.1016/j.mpmed.2018.12.012

Shepherd, J. A., Ng, B. K., Sommer, M. J., & Heymsfield, S. B. (2017). Body composition by DXA. *Bone, 104*(2017), 101–105. doi:10.1016/j.bone.2017.06.010

Tsai, A., Lai, M., & Chang, T. (2012). Mid-arm and calf circumference (MAC and CC) are better than body mass index (BMI) in predicting health status and mortality risk in institutionalized elderly Taiwanese. *Archives of Gerontology and Geriatrics, 54*(3), 443–447. doi:10.1016/j.archger.2011.05.015

U.S. Department of Health and Human Services. (2018). *Physical activity guidelines for Americans* (2nd ed.). Retrieved from https://health.gov/paguidelines/second -edition/pdf/Physical_Activity_Guidelines_2nd_edition .pdf

U.S. Department of Health and Human Services and U.S. Department of Agriculture. (2015). *2020 Dietary guidelines for Americans 2015–2020* (8th ed.). Retrieved from https://health.gov/dietaryguidelines/2015/guidelines/

U.S. Food and Drug Administration. (2016). *Vitamins and minerals chart.* Retrieved from https://www.accessdata .fda.gov/scripts/interactivenutritionfactslabel/factsheets/ vitamin_and_mineral_chart.pdf

U.S. Preventive Services Task Force. (2016a). Final recommendation statement: Breastfeeding: Primary care interventions. Retrieved from https://www.uspreventiveservices taskforce.org/Page/Document/final-recommendation -statement154/breastfeeding-primary-care-interventions

U.S. Preventive Services Task Force. (2016b). Final recommendation statement: Healthful diet and physical activity for cardiovascular disease prevention in adults with cardiovascular risk factors: Behavioral counseling. Retrieved from https://www.uspreventiveservicestaskforce .org/Page/Document/RecommendationStatementFinal/ healthy-diet-and-physical-activity-counseling-adults-with -high-risk-of-cvd

U.S. Preventive Services Task Force. (2016c). Final recommendation statement: Vitamin supplementation to prevent cancer and CVD: Preventive medication. Retrieved from https://www.uspreventiveservicestaskforce.org/Page/ Document/RecommendationStatementFinal/vitamin -supplementation-to-prevent-cancer-and-cvd-counseling

U.S. Preventive Services Task Force. (2017, June). Final update summary: Obesity in children and adolescents: Screening. Retrieved from https://www.uspreventiveservicestask force.org/Page/Document/UpdateSummaryFinal/obesity -in-children-and-adolescents-screening1

World Health Organization. (2001). The World Health Organization's infant feeding recommendation. Retrieved from http://www.who.int/nutrition/topics/infantfeeding_recom -mendation/en/index.html

World Health Organization. (2015). *Guideline: Sugars intake for adults and children.* Geneva, Switzerland: Author. Retrieved from https://apps.who.int/iris/bitstream/handle/ 10665/149782/9789241549028_eng.pdf

World Health Organization. (2016). What is malnutrition? Retrieved from https://www.who.int/features/qa/ malnutrition/en

9

Evidence-Based Assessment of Skin, Hair, and Nails

Lisa E. Ousley and Retha D. Gentry

*"Sun protection doesn't need to be complicated or expensive—
it needs to be consistent. Keep it simple, but do it forever!"*

—HILLARY FOGELSON (2015)

 VIDEO

- Patient Case: Infant With Rash

LEARNING OBJECTIVES

- Review the anatomy and describe the life-span variances of the skin, hair, and nails.
- Develop a systematic approach to performing a comprehensive history and physical examination of the integumentary system.
- Analyze key history and physical examination findings of common skin disorders.

ANATOMY AND PHYSIOLOGY OF SKIN, HAIR, AND NAILS

Understanding the structure and the function of the skin complements evidence-based physical assessment of the integumentary system. A competent clinician must have fundamental knowledge of the skin's functions, topography, and major components. The **skin** functions to protect and contain, secrete and excrete, and regulate body

Visit https://connect.springerpub.com/content/book/978-0-8261 -6454-4/chapter/ch00 to access the videos.

temperature and sensation. The structure of the skin varies depending on the anatomic location, an individual's dermatoglyphics, and the Langer's lines. The layers of the skin include the epidermis, dermis, and hypodermis. The other major components of the skin are the adnexal structures: (a) the hair, (b) the nails, (c) the sebaceous glands, (d) the eccrine glands, and (e) the apocrine sweat glands.

The skin, the body's largest organ, accounts for approximately 20% of the body's weight (McCann & Huether, 2019). The skin and the accessory structures (hair, nails, and glands) collectively form the **integumentary system**. As a protective barrier, the skin has several vital functions that include defending the body and internal structures from pathogens, ultraviolet (UV) radiation, loss of fluids and electrolytes, and physical trauma. The skin is also responsible for thermoregulation, immune surveillance, synthesis of vitamin D, and sensory input from the environment.

The skin is composed of three layers: the epidermis, the dermis, and the hypodermis or subcutaneous tissue (**Figure 9.1**). The epidermis is the most superficial layer of the skin and is composed of stratified squamous epithelium (Wilson & Giddens, 2013). The epidermis consists of five strata (layers). The stratum corneum, the outermost, waterproof layer, is a continuously renewing layer and lies atop the stratum lucidum, stratum granulosum, stratum spinosum, and stratum basale.

There are three types of branched cells within the epidermis. The melanocytes synthesize melanin, the Langerhans cells provoke skin immune reactions, and the Merkel cells are associated with touch receptors (Habif, 2010; McCann & Huether, 2019).

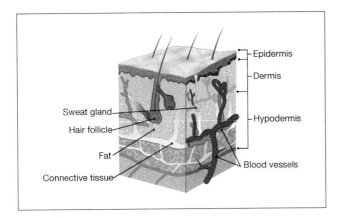

FIGURE 9.1 Anatomy of the skin.

The dermis is composed of vascular connective tissue, including collagen, elastin, and reticulum, which supports and separates the epidermis from the hypodermis. Elastin and collagen provide strength, stability, and mobility of the skin. The dermis holds nerves, blood and lymph vessels, hair follicles, sweat and oil glands, and sensory receptors. The sensory nerve fibers, responsible for the sensation of pain, touch, and temperature, are contained within the dermis (Ball, Dains, Flynn, Solomon, & Stewart, 2015).

The hypodermis, or the subcutaneous layer, is composed of loose connective tissue combined with subcutaneous fat (Wilson & Giddens, 2013). This adipose layer generates heat, provides insulation, cushions the body against trauma, and stores fat for energy (Ball et al., 2015; D'Amico & Barbarito, 2016; Lyons & Ousley, 2015).

The accessory structures, or appendages, of the skin include eccrine and apocrine sweat glands, sebaceous (oil) glands, and the hair and nails. The **eccrine glands** are widely distributed over the body, with the greatest numbers in the palms of the hands, soles of the feet, and the forehead (Ball et al., 2015; D'Amico & Barbarito, 2016; McCann & Huether, 2019). Eccrine glands produce clear perspiration of water and salt and regulate the body's temperature through evaporation (Ball et al., 2015; Bickley, 2017; D'Amico & Barbarito, 2016; McCann & Huether, 2019). The **apocrine sweat glands** are located primarily in the axillary and anogenital areas. Remaining dormant until puberty, these glands secrete water, salt, fatty acids, and proteins, which are released into hair follicles (D'Amico & Barbarito, 2016; Wilson & Giddens, 2013). Apocrine sweat mixed with bacteria on the skin's surface creates body odor. Sebaceous glands secrete sebum, a lipid substance, into the hair follicles that prevents the hair and skin from drying (Ball et al., 2015). Although the greatest distribution is found on the face and scalp, sebaceous glands are present on all surfaces of the skin, except the palms and soles. The enlargement of sebaceous glands indicates early signs of puberty (McCann & Huether, 2019).

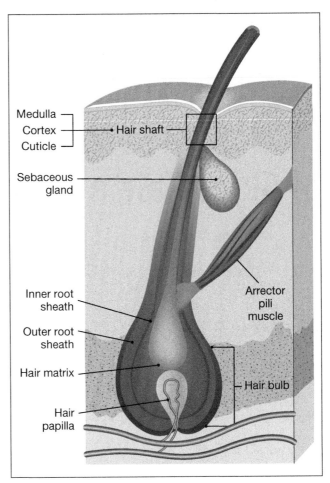

FIGURE 9.2 Anatomy of a hair follicle.

Hairs are dead keratinized fibers that insulate the body, protect against UV and infrared rays, perceive movement and touch, and protect the eyes from sweat and the nasal passages from foreign particles (D'Amico & Barbarito, 2016; Swartz, 2010). Hair consists of a root, a shaft, and a follicle (**Figure 9.2**). Variations in hair color, density, and the pattern of distribution vary considerably as a result of age, gender, race, and hereditary factors (Wilson & Giddens, 2013). The melanocytes in the hair shaft provide color. Males and females have the same amount of hair follicles (Ball et al., 2015; Lyons & Ousley, 2015).

Adults have both vellus and terminal hair. Vellus hair is short, fine, soft, and nonpigmented and is located on the margin of the lips, nipples, palms, and soles. Terminal hair is coarse, longer, thicker, and usually pigmented and is located on the scalp, eyebrows, face (men only), axilla, and in the pubic region. Each hair goes through a cycle of growth, atrophy, and rest, after which the hair is shed (Ball et al., 2015). The lower end of the hair shaft consists of actively proliferating epithelial cells (Swartz, 2010). These epithelial cells are some of the most rapidly growing and dividing cells in the human body. This explains why chemotherapy causes hair loss as it often targets the rapidly dividing cells (Swartz, 2010).

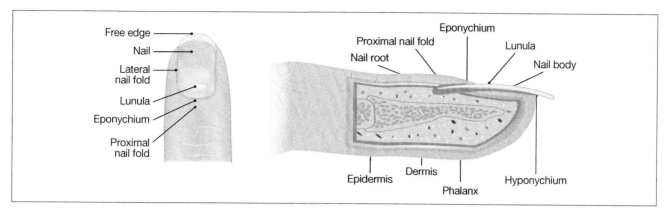

FIGURE 9.3 Anatomy of the nail.

Nails are epidermal cells that convert to hardened keratin and grow continually. The nails function to protect the ends of the fingers and toes, and aid in picking up small items, grasping, and scratching (D'Amico & Barbarito, 2016). The six structural components of the nail are: the proximal nail fold, the cuticle (eponychium), the matrix that supports nail growth and the nail root, the nail bed (hyponychium), the nail plate, and the lateral nail fold (paronychium; McCann & Huether, 2019; **Figure 9.3**). The site of nail growth can be marked past the proximal nail fold. This white semilunar area is called the lunula. Daily fingernail growth equals approximately 1 mm or less (Bickley, 2017; McCann & Huether, 2019). The tissue beneath the nail is extremely vascular. This tissue provides vital physical assessment data related to the patient's oxygen status and vascular perfusion (Wilson & Giddens, 2013).

LIFE-SPAN DIFFERENCES AND CONSIDERATIONS IN ANATOMY AND PHYSIOLOGY OF SKIN, HAIR, AND NAILS

The anatomy and physiology of the skin vary across the life span. Knowledge of the internal and external structure between the skin's layers allows the clinician to have a better understanding of these life-span variations. It is imperative that the clinician comprehends the vital functions of the skin throughout the life cycle.

Premature Infants

The structural integrity of the outermost layer of skin is related to the gestational age (Visscher, Adam, Brink, & Odio, 2015). Premature infant skin structure is immature. It has a poor epidermal barrier with few cornified layers, and a deficiency of structural proteins in the dermal layer. In a very premature infant, the underdeveloped stratum corneum may have less than 2 to 3 layers, compared with 10 to 20 layers in the full-term infant skin (Johnson, 2016). There are fewer fibrils to provide cohesiveness of the epidermis to the dermis. The pH of the premature

infant's skin is altered, provoking an extended alkaline surface environment. These characteristics increase the risk for permeability to exogenous materials, water loss, electrolyte imbalance, thermal instability, additional skin damage, delayed barrier maturation, and infection (Visscher et al., 2015). Infants born before 28 weeks' gestation do not have vernix (Visscher et al., 2015). Vernix caseosa is a white substance that covers the skin of the fetus during the last trimester of pregnancy. It protects the newborn skin and facilitates extra-uterine adaptation of skin following birth. The time for barrier maturation for the premature infant may be as long as 9 weeks postnatal age (Visscher et al., 2015).

Sweat glands are underdeveloped in premature infants. The secretory coils of the glandular segment and the sweating response to external stimuli are limited (Oranges, Dini, & Romanelli, 2015). Formation of the sebum glands occurs between 16 and 18 weeks and peaks in the third trimester (Jurica et al., 2016). By 22 weeks, the first sweat glands to develop are the palmoplantar sweat ducts, followed by the other eccrine sweat glands at 24 to 36 weeks (Jurica et al., 2016). The ability to sweat is associated with gestational age, and there is a propensity for anhidrosis in the premature infant a few days after birth (Oranges et al., 2015).

Fine, silky hair, called lanugo, is more common in preterm infants and is usually present on the back and shoulders. This hair is usually shed within approximately 10 to 14 days (Ball et al., 2015).

Infants and Children

There is controversy related to the development and integrity of the epidermis of the newborn. Some authors insist the newborn skin is immature at birth, whereas others believe an infant is born with a proficient epidermal layer that mimics adult skin (Visscher et al., 2015). In utero, during the last trimester, vernix caseosa begins to coat the entire skin surface, which aids in skin development. The vernix caseosa has antimicrobial properties, protects the epidermis from amniotic fluid, and facilitates the development of the stratum corneum. New evidence promotes retention of the vernix rather than removal at birth. The stratum corneum and the epidermis of the full-term infant skin are well developed and functional at birth (Visscher et al., 2015). Subcutaneous tissue in newborns is poorly developed and predisposes the infant to problems with thermoregulation (Ball et al., 2015).

Desquamation of the stratum corneum may be present shortly after birth, ranging from slight peeling to shedding of large areas of cornified epidermis (Ball et al., 2015). Skin cracking, dryness, and peeling are more common in postterm infants (41–42 weeks' gestation) owing to the lower amounts of vernix at birth (Ball et al., 2015; Visscher et al., 2015).

After the first month of life, the eccrine glands begin to function. The apocrine glands are not yet active, thus giving the skin a less oily texture and inoffensive perspiration (Ball et al., 2015). Lanugo may cover the newborn's body, particularly the shoulders and back, and is also shed within 10 to 14 days (Ball et al., 2015). Some newborns have large amounts of hair on their head, whereas others may be bald. At approximately 2 to 3 months of age, most hair is shed and replaced with new permanent hair with a different texture and often a new color (Ball et al., 2015).

Adolescents

Throughout childhood, skin undergoes significant maturational development. This includes epidermal thickening, increase in pigmentation, and increased subcutaneous fat deposits, especially in females during puberty (D'Amico & Barbarito, 2016).

Apocrine glands mature, leading to increased axillary perspiration and the potential for body odor (D'Amico & Barbarito, 2016). Increased hormone levels, primarily androgen, cause sebaceous glands to increase sebum production, giving the skin an oily appearance and increasing the risk of acne in this age group (Ball et al., 2015; D'Amico & Barbarito, 2016).

In response to changes to androgen levels, coarse terminal hair appears. The hair grows in the pubic and axillae during this developmental stage in males and females, and on the face and chest of males (Ball et al., 2015; D'Amico & Barbarito, 2016).

Pregnant Women

During pregnancy, there is an increase in blood flow to the skin caused by peripheral vasodilation and increased capillaries. Blood flow is increased throughout the body. Diffuse redness, resulting from increased blood flow and increased production of estrogen, may be present on the hands and feet. Sweat and sebaceous gland activity is increased. Both increased blood flow and sebaceous gland activity assist in dispersing the additional heat caused by accelerated pregnancy metabolism. The skin thickens, and fat is deposited below the epidermal layers. The skin stretches due to weakened connective tissues and may stretch and create separation. Hormonal changes cause the oil and sweat glands to become more active in pregnancy. This increased secretion may worsen acne in the first trimester with improvement of acne in the third trimester (D'Amico & Barbarito, 2016). During pregnancy, the growing phase of hair is prolonged, and hair loss is decreased due to circulating hormones (Ball et al., 2015). With the increase of hairs in the growth phase, more than a normal amount of hairs reach maturity and are shed between months 1 to 5 postpartum. Most of the hair grows back between 6 and 15 months postpartum (D'Amico & Barbarito, 2016).

Older Adults

In the older adult, a decrease in collagen and elastin fibers of the skin and a lifetime of sun exposure causes the epidermis to thin, stretch, and take on a wrinkled appearance (Ball et al., 2015; D'Amico & Barbarito, 2016). There is an earlier onset and greater skin wrinkling with Whites than other races. The skin may appear pale in older adults with light skin and dull, gray, or darker in dark-skinned elderly due to the decreased vascularity of the dermis (Ball et al., 2015; D'Amico & Barbarito, 2016). Due to decreased subcutaneous tissue, the skin may appear to hang from the frame. The joints may appear sharp with deepening of the hollows in the thoracic, axillary, and supraclavicular areas. Decreased sebaceous and sweat gland activity leads to drier skin and hair (Ball et al., 2015; D'Amico & Barbarito, 2016).

A decrease in functioning melanocytes causes hair to turn gray. The amount of axillary and pubic hair declines due to decreased hormone production. Hair thickness and growth decrease with aging. Hair follicles change in size. Terminal scalp hair transitions into vellus hair, thus producing baldness in both men and women. The opposite change, from vellus to terminal, occurs in the hair of the nares and on the tragus of the ears in males.

The result of increased androgen and decreased estrogen produces coarse facial hair in women. Males and females experience hair loss of the trunk and extremities (Ball et al., 2015). Due to decreased peripheral circulation, nail growth slows. The nails may become thick and hard and appear yellowed or opaque (Ball et al., 2015; D'Amico & Barbarito, 2016). They are more susceptible to breaking, splitting, brittleness, and peeling (Ball et al., 2015; D'Amico & Barbarito, 2016).

KEY HISTORY QUESTIONS AND CONSIDERATIONS FOR SKIN, HAIR, AND NAILS

Taking a comprehensive history is one of the most important tools in determining an accurate diagnosis. It is estimated that approximately 80% of the information needed for diagnosis is obtained through history questions (Muhrer, 2014). A thorough history is fundamental to competent skin care. This includes collecting subjective data, both general and specific, about the patient's present and past health (Wilson & Giddens, 2013). The patient's current health status, past medical history, family history, and personal and psychosocial history as well as home, occupational, and travel history may all affect the condition of their skin, hair, and nails. The clinician must also consider the patient's age, gender, race, culture, and environment.

The following are general questions related to the patient's skin that should be included in the well exam: Describe your skin, hair, and nails today. Have they changed compared with 1 month and 1 year ago? Do you have any concerns about your skin, hair, and nails? Have you noticed any changes to existing lesions? What are your usual bathing practices (skin, hair, and nails)? Have you ever been diagnosed with a skin disorder? If so, what was the diagnosis? Have you been diagnosed with any other chronic illnesses? What is your occupation? Do you have a history of sunburns? How do you protect your skin while in the sun (e.g., sunscreen, sunglasses, hat, and clothing)?

HISTORY OF PRESENT ILLNESS

The history of present illness allows the clinician to obtain more information about the chief concern or presenting symptoms. Specific questions are asked when the patient has a skin concern or condition.

Skin

- Describe the concerns about your skin.
- Have you noticed any changes in your skin?
- When did you first notice these changes?
- Did the changes occur slowly or suddenly?
- Has it changed since onset?
- Are there any symptoms with these changes? Itching? Drainage? Tenderness or pain? Bleeding? Changes in color? Variations related to weather/season? Fever?
- Can you relate the changes to stress?
- Where have the changes occurred? Are these changes in more than one area of your skin?
- Does anyone you have been in contact with have a similar skin disorder?
- What do you think caused this skin disorder?
- How have you been treating the problem (e.g., medications such as steroids or antifungals)? Have any treatments helped? What makes this worse or better?
- How has this skin condition affected you (physically, psychologically, or socially)?
- Are you currently taking antibiotics or new medications, including over-the-counter (OTC) medications?
- Have you started using new skin care products or new household cleaning products?

- Have you traveled recently? If so, where, when, how long did you stay? Are you aware of any exposures (e.g., hot tubs, pools, lakes)?
- Are you aware of any exposure to toxins or chemicals (environmental or occupational)?
- Do you use tanning beds?

Hair

- Have you had any changes to your hair? Loss? Growth (slow or excessive)? Texture? Color?
- If so, when did this occur? Was it sudden or gradual? One-sided or both sides of your head?
- Has this occurred before?
- Are there any other symptoms? Pain? Itching? Lesions? Recent stress? Hair pulling?
- Are you aware of any exposure to drugs, toxins, or chemicals (environment or occupation), or commercial hair care products?
- Have there been any changes to your diet?
- How have you been treating the problem (e.g., steroids or antifungals)? Have these treatments helped?
- Does anything make these hair changes worse or better?
- Has this problem with your hair affected you? If so, how?
- Are you taking any medications or remedies for hair loss?

Nails

- Have you noticed any changes in your nails?
- Are these changes related to a recent illness, trauma, or stress?
- Are there any other symptoms? Tenderness or pain? Swelling? Drainage?
- When did these changes occur? Were they sudden or gradual?
- How have you been treating the problem? Have these treatments helped? What makes this worse or better?
- Have you injured your nails or fingers?
- Are you currently taking any medications, specifically chemotherapy, psoralens, retinoids, tetracyclines, or antimalarials (Ball et al., 2015)?
- Are you aware of any exposure to toxins or chemicals (environmental or occupational)?
- Are your hands frequently in water?

PAST MEDICAL HISTORY
Skin

- Have you had any skin conditions in the past?
- Is your skin sensitive?
- Have you had allergic reactions? How were these conditions treated?
- Do you have a history of skin cancer, dysplastic nevi, or suspicious lesions?

- Does your skin burn easily in the sun? Have you had any serious sunburns?
- Do you have any chronic illnesses?
- Do you have a history of tanning bed use?

Hair

- Have you had any problems with your hair in the past?
- Have you lost hair? Has your hair thinned? Does your hair break easily? Were these problems treated? If so, how?
- Have you had too much hair growth? If so, where?
- Do you have any chronic illnesses?

Nails

- Have you had any problems with your nails (injury or infection)?
- Do your nails grow fast?
- Are your nails brittle or thin?
- Are your nails thickening or changing in color?
- Have you noticed any discoloration in your nails?
- Do you have any chronic illnesses?

FAMILY HISTORY

- Does your family have a history of any skin disorders (skin cancer, psoriasis, eczema, hives, or hay fever)? If so, who has these disorders?
- Are there any significant allergies or asthma in your family?
- Have any of your family members lost hair (receding hairline, baldness)?

SOCIAL HISTORY

- Describe your skin care routine.
- Do you apply any products to your skin?
- Have there been any recent changes to your routine?
- How much sun exposure have you had (recreational or occupational)?
- Have you had any sunburns?
- How do you protect your skin from the sun?
- Do you perform a skin self-examination?
- Do you have an annual total body skin examination (TBSE) by a healthcare clinician?
- How do you care for your hair and nails?
- Have there been any changes to this routine?
- Do you color your hair or have permanents?
- Do you pull or twist your hair?
- How do you trim your nails?
- Do you bite, peel, or pick your nails or surrounding skin?
- Do you paint your nails or apply artificial nails?
- Does your occupation place you at risk for chemical exposure to skin, hair, and nails? If so, how?
- Are your hands frequently in water?

- Do you use personal protective equipment at work?
- Do you practice any cultural rituals that may affect your skin, hair, or nails?
- Have you experienced any recent stress?
- Do you use alcohol, tobacco, or recreational drugs?
- Have you ever been diagnosed with a sexually transmitted infection or disease?

PREVENTIVE CARE CONSIDERATIONS

- Are your immunizations up to date (measles, mumps, and rubella [MMR], varicella, zoster, and human papillomavirus [HPV])?
- Do you consistently wear sunscreen and reapply? If so, how much sun protection factor (SPF) and how often?
- Do you wear sun-protective clothing, including hats and sunglasses?
- Do you have a TBSE completed by a clinician?
- Do you perform skin self-examinations?
- Do you work in an environment with chemical, water, or sun exposure?
- Do you wear personal protective equipment? If yes, which ones?
- Do you consistently wear condoms during sexual encounters?

LIFE-SPAN CONSIDERATIONS FOR HISTORY
Infants

- Is the infant breast or formula fed? If formula, what type?
- Have foods been introduced? If so, what has been introduced and when?
- What is the skin-cleansing routine with diaper changes? What type of diapers are used? What types of laundry products are used?
- What types of soaps, oils, and lotions are applied to the infant's skin?
- Does the infant have a new blanket or new clothing?
- How do you dress your child during the change in seasons?
- What type of heating and cooling systems are in the home?

Children and Adolescents

- What types of food does your child eat? What are their usual eating habits?
- Does your child have any food allergies?
- Are you aware of any infectious diseases to which your child may have been exposed?
- Does your child have any of the following conditions: eczema, urticaria, pruritis, hay fever, asthma, or other chronic respiratory disorders?
- Are there any pets/animals in the home or your child's usual environment?

- Is your child exposed to outdoor areas or activities such as playgrounds, hiking, camping, picnics, or gardening?
- Has your child had any recent skin injuries? Frequent/recent falls or abrasions? Unexplained injuries?
- Does your child pull or twist their hair?
- Does your child bite or pick their nails or surrounding skin?

Pregnant Women

- How many weeks' gestation? How many weeks postpartum?
- Do you regularly moisturize your breasts and abdomen?
- Are you aware of any exposure to potential skin irritants?
- Did you have any skin disorders or issues prior to pregnancy? If so, how has pregnancy affected these?

Older Adults

- Do you have any lesions or rashes?
- Does your skin itch?
- Do you have increased or decreased sensation to touch?
- Ask about relevant childhood illnesses.
- What is your level of lifetime sun or irritant exposures? Occupational exposure?
- Do you have a history of skin cancer?
- Have you recently traveled? If so, where?
- Do you fall frequently?
- Do you have any limitations in your mobility?
- Do you have hair loss?
- Do you have thickened nails?
- Ask about current and chronic medication use.
- Are you taking any anticoagulants?
- Have you had the herpes zoster (shingles) vaccine?
- Are you incontinent of bowel or bladder?
- Complete a focused nutritional assessment.
- Do you have a history of diabetes mellitus (DM) or peripheral vascular disease?

UNIQUE POPULATION CONSIDERATIONS FOR HISTORY

Three distinctive patient populations are being considered when completing a patient history and skin assessment: (a) patients of various races and ethnicities, (b) patients with behavioral health disorders, and (c) patients in occupations that pose increased skin risks. Evidence-based rationale and the clinical relevance for physical exam techniques and strategies are included.

Ethnicity and Race

- How do you care for your skin?
- Do you have any cultural practices, customs, and/or beliefs that would help me to take better care of you?

Behavioral Health

- Have you been diagnosed with a mental health disorder? If so, do you take medication for this? What medication?
- Are you now experiencing, or have you ever experienced, intermittent or prolonged anxiety, depression, or emotional upset?
- How would you describe your stress level? Has it changed in the past few weeks? Few months? Describe.
- Can you describe your current living situation (whom do you live with and type of residence)?
- Do you recall what you have eaten and drunk in the past 24 hours? Describe.
- Do you ever twist or pull your hair, bite nails, or pick your skin?

Occupation

- Are you required to wear a specific type of helmet, hat, goggles, gloves, or shoes?
- Does your work require you to perform repetitive tasks?
- Do you work with or around chemicals? If so, which ones?
- Do you work outdoors? Do you wear sunscreen or sun-protective clothing? What is the SPF of the sunscreen and how often do you apply?

REVIEW OF SYSTEMS

The review of systems (ROS) is a vital part of evidence-based skin assessment. This portion of the patient encounter allows the clinician to create a list of questions arranged by systems to aid the clinician in discovering clinical problems that may be the cause of the skin disease process (Phillips, Frank, Loftin, & Shepherd, 2017). Systemic diseases often have cutaneous manifestations; therefore, the ROS can serve as a guide to help identify underlying disease.

- General: Fatigue; malaise; fever; weight loss or gain; pain anywhere in the body
- Head, eyes, ears, nose, throat (HEENT): Hair loss or excessive growth; change of hair texture; ringing in the ears; decreased hearing; changes in vision; photosensitivity; blurred vision; dry eyes; runny nose; altered smell; sinus congestion; sore throat; hoarseness; dry mouth; changes in teeth or gums; enlarged lymph nodes on the head or neck
- Respiratory: Shortness of breath; cough (productive or dry); painful or altered breathing
- Cardiovascular: Chest pain; shortness of breath; palpitations; arrhythmias; hair loss on the lower extremities; swelling of hands, legs, or feet
- Gastrointestinal (GI): Abdominal pain; bloating or distention; changes in bowel movements; heartburn; nausea; vomiting

- Genitourinary (GU): Painful urination; urinary frequency, retention, or urgency; incontinence; difficulty starting urine stream; blood in urine; vaginal or penile discharge, pain, or swelling
- Musculoskeletal: Single or multiple joint pain; swelling of joints; decreased movement or strength; muscle pain and/or muscle weakness; skin changes over bony prominences
- Neurologic: Headaches; change in thinking or cognition; memory loss; tingling or numbness
- Hematologic: Easy bruising; bleeding; spider, prominent, or painful blood vessels
- Integumentary: Changes in skin color, texture, thickness or thinning; excessive sweating or dryness; new lesions or rashes; temperature change; scar or nail changes; any loss of tissue in face, arms, legs, or buttocks
- Psychiatric: Increased or persistent anxiety and/or depression; scratching or picking skin or nails; pulling of the hair; self-harm behaviors

PHYSICAL EXAMINATION OF SKIN, HAIR, AND NAILS

A skin assessment should be part of every patient encounter, whether during a complete physical examination, a problem-focused assessment, or an integrated exam. The components of the examination include inspection, palpation, and olfaction of the skin, hair, and nails. Comprehensive assessment of the skin should include color, consistency, thickness, symmetry, hygiene, lesions, and odors (Ball et al., 2015).

TOTAL BODY SKIN EXAMINATION

TBSE is the best screening test for skin cancer. With the patient disrobed, the entire skin surface must be systematically examined, including the scalp, nails, palms of the hands and soles of the feet, and mucous membranes (Bickley, 2017). Incorporating the total body skin assessment into the head-to-toe physical exam can decrease examination time and increase effectiveness.

Inspection

The assessment should begin with the patient in a gown. The patient should be given an explanation of the technique and purpose of the skin assessment. The skin assessment can be performed with the patient seated or supine, then prone. Inspect the skin in a head-to-toe sequence with the breast and genitalia examined last. Use the same assessment technique and order to maintain consistency and avoid omitting any portion of the patient's skin. Start with a general survey of the skin,

including color, pigmentation, vascularity, bruising, lesions, color variations, and general hygiene (Ball et al., 2015; Wilson & Giddens, 2013). During the skin assessment, note distribution, texture, and quantity of hair. Inspect the fingernails and toenails, noting color and shape. Nail polish should be removed.

Palpation

Palpation of the skin offers valuable assessment findings. Throughout the TBSE, palpate the skin and note the temperature, texture, moisture, and turgor. Palpate fingernails and toenails for texture and note capillary refill time (CRT).

INTEGRATED SKIN EXAM

An integrated skin exam can be incorporated into any physical exam. During this exam, the clinician would assess the skin on any area examined. If a body part is uncovered or exposed, a skin examination should be integrated simultaneously; for example, inspecting the skin of the head, face, ear, and neck as the otoscopic exam is performed.

LESION-FOCUSED EXAMINATION

The lesion-focused exam is an assessment of a specific lesion or rash. These exams are typically completed with the naked eye with appropriate lighting. Dermatoscopes can improve a clinician's ability to recognize skin lesions; however, training is required for proficiency (**Figure 9.4**; Marghoob, Usatine, & Jaimes, 2013). All characteristics of the lesion or rash are considered. See **Tables 9.1** and **9.2** for primary and secondary lesions.

Inspection and Palpation

During inspection of the skin using the naked eye, the light is reflected off the stratum corneum, making it

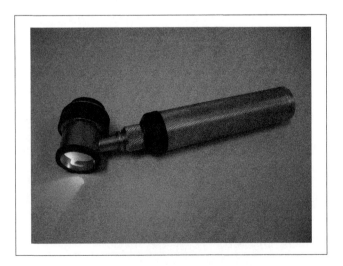

FIGURE 9.4 Dermatoscope.

TABLE 9.1 Primary Skin Lesions

Lesion	Description	Examples	Visual With Diagnosis
Macule	• Flat, nonpalpable • Smaller than 1 cm	• Freckles • Flat moles (nevi) • Measles • Petechiae	Leukocytoclastic Vasculitis
Patch	• Flat, nonpalpable • Larger than 1 cm	• Vitiligo • Mongolian spots • Port-wine stains • Chloasma • Café au lait patch	Tinea Versicolor
Papule	• Elevated, solid palpable • Smaller than 0.5 cm	• Elevated moles • Warts • Insect bites • Lichens planus	Bedbug Bites
Plaque	• Groups or papules • Larger than 5 cm	• Psoriasis • Seborrheic and actinic keratosis • Lichen planus	Psoriasis

(continued)

TABLE 9.1 Primary Skin Lesions (*continued*)

Lesion	Description	Examples	Visual With Diagnosis
Pustule	• Elevated, pus-filled vesicle or bullae • Size varies	• Acne • Impetigo • Carbuncles	**Pustules Resulting From Fire Ant Bites**
Cyst	• Elevated, encapsulated, fluid- or semisolid-filled, or solid mass in dermis or subcutaneous layers • 1 cm or larger	• Sebaceous cyst • Epidermoid cyst • Acne	**Inflamed Sebaceous Cyst**
Vesicle	• Elevated, fluid-filled, round or oval-shaped with thin, translucent walls • Smaller than 0.5 cm	• Herpes simplex or zoster • Early chicken pox • Poison ivy • Small burn blister	**Herpes Zoster**
Bullae	• Elevated, fluid-filled, round or oval-shaped with thin, translucent walls • Larger than 0.5–1 cm	• Contact dermatitis • Friction or fracture blister • Large burn blister • Pemphigus vulgaris	**Fracture Blister**

(continued)

TABLE 9.1 Primary Skin Lesions (*continued*)

Lesion	Description	Examples	Visual With Diagnosis
Nodule	• Elevated, solid, hard or soft, palpable mass deeper in the dermis • Smaller than 2 cm	• Small lipoma • Squamous cell carcinoma • Fibroma • Nevi • Erythema nodosum	Nodular Melanoma
Tumor	• Elevated, solid, hard or soft, palpable mass deeper in the dermis with irregular borders • Larger than 2 cm	• Lipomas • Carcinoma • Hemangioma • Benign tumor	Basal Cell Carcinoma
Wheal	• Elevated, often reddish area with irregular borders caused by diffuse fluid in tissues (cutaneous edema) • Size varies	• Insect bites • Hives (urticarial) • Allergic reaction	Urticarial Drug Reaction

impossible to see structures below (Marghoob et al., 2013). For the trained clinician, the dermatoscope allows the visualization of structures below the skin's surface (see **Figure 9.4**). Inspect and measure all skin lesions. Describe the findings, noting number, location, size, color, shape, morphology, distribution, and configuration. Palpate appropriate lesions, assessing the texture of the lesion, presence of tenderness or pain, temperature of lesion and surrounding skin, fluidity, and blanching capacity.

LIFE-SPAN CONSIDERATIONS FOR PHYSICAL EXAM

A thorough and comprehensive history and physical assessment of the body's largest organ, the skin, requires knowledge of the stages of human development. Competent physical assessment skills mandate that the clinician consider the age of the patient when assessing the skin.

Preterm Infants

The skin of preterm and full-term newborns and infants undergoes a specific process of maturation, and, therefore, skin care delivered to these young patients needs to be individualized (Oranges et al., 2015). Unlike adults, the physical exams of children are conducted with the least invasive procedures first. The infant should be completely undressed except for the diaper, which will remain in place until assessment

TABLE 9.2 Secondary Skin Lesions

Lesion	Description	Examples	Visual With Diagnosis
Atrophy	• Thinning or wasting of skin due to loss of collagen and elastin	• Striae • Aged skin	Pruritic Urticarial Papules and Plaques of Pregnancy (PUPPP) Rash
Excoriation	• Absence of superficial epidermis, causing a moist, shallow depression	• Scratch marks • Abrasion • Scabies	Abrasion (bike wreck on asphalt)
Keloid	• Elevated area of excessive scar tissue that extends beyond the site of original injury (caused by excessive collagen formation during healing)	• Keloid for ear piercing or following surgery	Keloids from Folliculitis Barbae
Scale	• Flakes of greasy keratinized skin tissue • May be white, gray, or silver • Texture may be fine or thick • Varies in size	• Dry skin • Dandruff • Psoriasis • Eczema	Psoriasis

(continued)

TABLE 9.2 Secondary Skin Lesions (*continued*)

Lesion	Description	Examples	Visual With Diagnosis
Crust	• Dried blood, serum, or pus on the epidermis from ruptured vesicles or pustules • Slightly elevated • May be red, brown, orange, or yellow • Size varies	• Eczema • Impetigo • Herpes • Scabs following an abrasion	Early Impetigo
Fissure	• Linear crack or break with sharp edges extending into the dermis • May be moist or dry	• Cracks at corner of the mouth, on the fingers, or feet (athlete's foot)	Fissure Caused by Finger Eczema
Lichenification	• A rough, thickened, hardened area of the epidermis resulting from chronic irritation such as scratching or rubbing (often involves flexor surfaces)	• Chronic dermatitis	Chronic Dermatitis
Scar	• Elevated, irregular area of connective tissue left after a lesion or wound has healed • New scars may be red or purple • Old scars may be silvery or white	• Healed surgical wound or injury • Healed acne	Surgical Scar: Knee Replacement

(continued)

TABLE 9.2 Secondary Skin Lesions (*continued*)			
Lesion	Description	Examples	Visual With Diagnosis
Ulcer	• Irregularly shaped area of skin loss that extends into the dermis or subcutaneous tissue; concave • Depth varies	• Stasis and decubiti ulcers • Aphthous ulcers	Aphthous Ulcer

of the genitalia and buttocks. While the skin exam is being performed, it is important not to allow the infant to become chilled. The color of the skin depends on the amount of subcutaneous tissue present. Days immediately after delivery, preterm infants' skin often appears ruddy, gelatinous, and almost transparent due to the decreased presence of stratum corneum and the small amount of fat present (Johnson, 2016; Jurica et al., 2016; Wilson & Giddens, 2013). The skin is less elastic. Fine, silky hair called lanugo is more common (Ball et al., 2015) in preterm infants and is usually present on the back and shoulders. This hair is usually shed within approximately 10 to 14 days (Ball et al., 2015). The preterm and full-term infant's nails are soft and flexible. Postterm infants may be born with longer nails.

Newborns, Infants, and Children

The newborn's skin may appear reddened immediately after birth due to vasomotor instability; however, this coloration should fade within the first few days of life. Also, during this time, the newborn's lips, nail beds, and feet may appear dusky. Once the newborn is warmed, this dusky color should fade, and the skin should take on a well-oxygenated tone (Wilson & Giddens, 2013). Newborns with skin of color may appear hypopigmented for the first 2 to 3 months of life.

Approximately 50% of newborns experience physiological jaundice, which is a normal phenomenon resulting from increased hemolysis of red blood cells following birth (Wilson & Giddens, 2013). The skin, mucous membranes, and sclerae may have a yellow hue. The newborn's body may be covered in fine, soft hair called lanugo. Lanugo can be present anywhere on the body but is common on the scalp, ears, shoulders, and back (Wilson & Giddens, 2013). This lanugo is replaced

within a few months with vellus hair (D'Amico & Barbarito, 2016). The hair of an infant should be fine and soft. Seborrheic dermatitis (cradle cap) may be present on the scalp of infants and appears as a scaly crust (Wilson & Giddens, 2013).

There may be various harmless markings on newborns (D'Amico & Barbarito, 2016). They may have tiny, white facial papules (milia), which result from sebum collecting in the openings of hair follicles. These papules usually fade without intervention within the first few weeks of life. Newborn skin may also have vascular markings (salmon patches/stork bites; **Figure 9.5**). These markings appear as irregular red or pink patches, are most commonly found on the back of the neck, and resolve within the first year. Mongolian spots (congenital dermal melanocytosis) appear as irregularly shaped, dark (gray, blue, or purple), flat areas on the sacrum and buttocks and usually disappear by age 3 years (**Figure 9.6**). These harmless skin markings are most

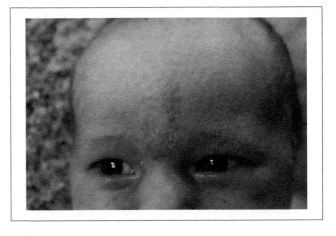

FIGURE 9.5 Salmon patch on the forehead of a newborn.

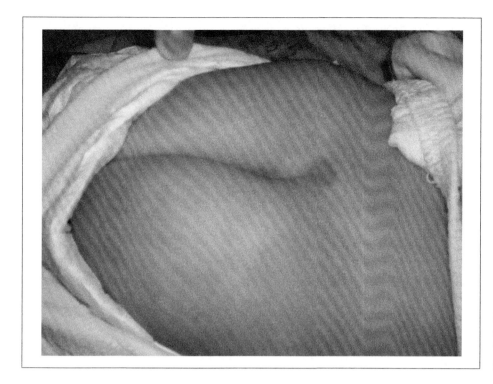

FIGURE 9.6 Mongolian spot on the lower back of a 6-month-old Taiwanese infant.

Source: Image courtesy of Abby Lu.

common in African American, Hispanic, Native American, and Asian children (Wilson & Giddens, 2013). These can be misdiagnosed as bruises or child abuse.

The skin of infants and children should be smooth and soft with appropriate color for ethnicity and no lesions. Turgor should be brisk. Bruising to lower legs may be present as the child becomes mobile. Infants and children should have very little body and facial hair. The nails should be smooth and intact. Clinicians should always assess for nail biting (Wilson & Giddens, 2013). There are a variety of different rashes that typically occur only in childhood. See **Table 9.3** for more information on common childhood rashes.

Adolescents

The skin assessment of an adolescent should be completed in the same sequence as that in the case of an adult. Although the assessment of skin is direct, adolescents may be more sensitive due to maturational changes and the development of body hair. Throughout adolescence, the presence and characteristics of facial hair (males) and body hair (males and females) change considerably. By the end of this developmental stage, the skin, hair, and nails acquire adult characteristics (Wilson & Giddens, 2013). Increased perspiration, oiliness, and acne are common in this age group due to increased sebaceous activity (Wilson & Giddens, 2013).

Pregnant Women

It is important for the clinician to distinguish the skin changes of pregnancy from abnormal skin changes.

Several normal variations or changes can be identified during examination of the pregnant woman. During the second trimester, as the skin over the abdomen stretches to accommodate the fetus, purplish stretch marks (striae gravidarum) may present on the abdomen, thighs, and breasts (Ball et al., 2015; Bickley, 2017). The stretching of skin may result in itching of the abdomen and breasts. Palms of the hands and soles of the feet may have diffuse redness due to increased vascularity and increased estrogen production (Ball et al., 2015; Wilson & Giddens, 2013). The nails may become thin and brittle; however, some women report fast-growing, strong nails when taking prenatal vitamins (Wilson & Giddens, 2013).

Approximately 70% of women may develop hyperpigmentation on the face, referred to as chloasma, melasma, or "the mask of pregnancy" (**Figure 9.7**). Although sometimes permanent, this normal condition usually disappears after pregnancy (D'Amico & Barbarito, 2016). Skin darkening of the face, nipples and areolae, axillae, vulva, perianal skin, and umbilicus is common in pregnancy (Ball et al., 2015). A dark, brownish-black pigmented, vertical line (linea nigra) may be present on the abdomen of the pregnant woman, extending midline from the symphysis pubis to the top of the fundus (Ball et al., 2015; Bickley, 2017; **Figure 9.8**). Existing nevi may increase in size and appear darker, and new nevi may form.

Older Adults

Skin assessment technique is the same for the older adult as it is for the younger adult. The clinician must

TABLE 9.3 Common Childhood Rashes

Disease State	History and Physical Findings	Visual
Fifth's Disease • Also called erythema infectiosum • Caused by parvovirus B19 • Transmitted through respiratory secretions and blood	• Incubation period is 4–14 days • Often have fever, rhinorrhea, myalgias, and a headache • Facial rash that has a "slapped cheek" appearance • Can get a second itchy rash a few days after the facial rash that appears on the chest, back, buttocks, or arms and legs	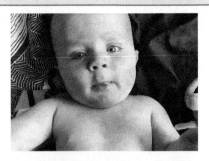
Hand, Foot, Mouth Disease • Caused by a virus called coxsackievirus A16 • Transmitted through respiratory secretions, fecal–oral route, or vesicle fluid	• Usually affects infants and children 5 years old or younger • Typically occurs in summer and early fall • Starts with fever, malaise, sore throat, and anorexia • Painful macular or vesicular lesions can develop in the mouth several days after the fever starts • Rash on the palms of the hands and soles of the feet may also develop over 1 or 2 days as a macular and/or vesicular red rash; it may also appear on the knees, elbows, buttocks, or genital area	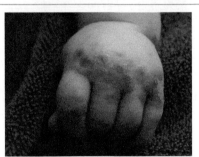 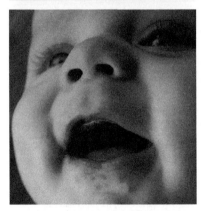
Impetigo • Usually caused by *Staphylococcus aureus* or *Streptococcus pyogenes* • Bacteria is introduced through a break in the skin • There are three types of impetigo: **bullous** (large blisters), **non-bullous** (crusted), and **ecthyma** (ulcers)	• Most common in children between the ages of 2 and 6 • Lesions can be anywhere, but usually occur on the face, around the mouth and nose, and on the hands/feet • Lesions are vesicular, burst, and develop honey-colored crusts • Can be spread to other areas of the body by fingers, clothing, and towels • Bullous impetigo has larger blisters that are more likely to be on the trunk • Ecthyma impetigo can form deep, painful ulcers	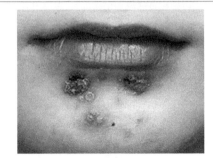

(continued)

TABLE 9.3 Common Childhood Rashes (*continued*)

Disease State	History and Physical Findings	Visual
Infantile Seborrheic Dermatitis • Commonly referred to as "cradle cap" when it is found on the scalp • Noncontagious	• Affects the oily areas of the body, including the scalp, face, sides of the nose, eyebrows, ears, eyelids, and chest • Typically presents with erythema and greasy scales • Usually benign and self-limited • Typically resolves within several weeks to several months	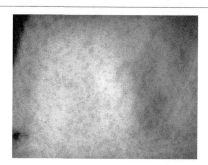
Measles (Rubeola) • Caused by the virus Rubeola • Spread to others through respiratory secretions • Highly contagious • Vaccination available	• Incubation period is 7–14 days after a person is infected • Maculopapular rash that starts on the head and moves down the body • Other symptoms include malaise, high fever, cough, rhinorrhea, conjunctivitis, koplik spots (tiny white spots inside the mouth) • Conjunctivitis is the main symptom that distinguishes it from influenza	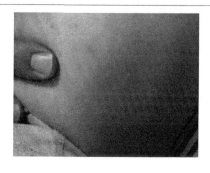
Molluscum contagiosum • Caused by a virus called the poxvirus • Transmitted from direct person-to-person physical contact and through contaminated fomites	• White, pink, or flesh-colored papules that are umbilicated • They often have a pearly appearance • Usually smooth and firm • Lesions range from about 2–5 millimeters in diameter • They may become pruritic, painful, erythematous, and/or swollen • May occur anywhere on the body, including the face, neck, arms, legs, abdomen, and genital area • They can occur alone or in groups	
Mumps • Caused by the mumps virus, which belongs to a family of viruses known as paramyxoviruses • Transmitted through direct contact with saliva or respiratory droplets from the mouth, nose, or throat • Vaccination available	• Symptoms typically appear 16–18 days after infection • Puffy cheeks and a tender, swollen jaw due to swollen salivary glands on one or both sides (parotitis) • Other symptoms include fever, headache, myalgias, malaise, and anorexia • Can be asymptomatic in some	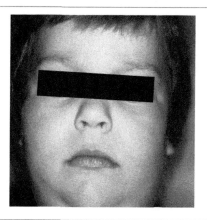

(*continued*)

TABLE 9.3 Common Childhood Rashes (*continued*)

Disease State	History and Physical Findings	Visual
Roseola • Caused by a virus called human herpesvirus 6 (HHV-6) • Transmitted by oral and respiratory secretions and direct person-to-person contact • Vaccination available	• Incubation period is 9–10 days • Common in children aged 3 months to 4 years (most commonly, 6 months to 1 year) • Initial symptoms include acute onset high fever, eye redness, sore throat, irritability, rhinorrhea • Once the fever resolves (after 2–4 days), a pinkish red, maculopapular rash presents • Rash starts on trunk and spreads peripherally	
Rubella • Also called German Measles • Caused by the rubella virus (Genus *Rubivirus* in the family *Togaviridae*) • Transmitted via direct or droplet contact with respiratory secretions • Vaccination available	• Symptoms that may occur 1–5 days before the rash appears include low-grade fever, headache, conjunctivitis, lymphadenopathy, cough, and/or rhinorrhea • Rash generally first appears on the face and then spreads to the rest of the body and lasts about 3 days • Can be asymptomatic • Typically, mild presentation	
Scarlet Fever • Also known as scarlatina • Caused by *group A hemolytic streptococcus* • Rash caused by an erythrogenic exotoxin emitted by the streptococci	• Most common in children 5–15 years • Most commonly seen in conjunction with strep pharyngitis • Typically starts with a high fever and sore throat • Rash appears after 1–2 days • Maculopapular exanthematous rash that looks like a sunburn and feels like sandpaper • Rash initially appears on the neck and chest, then spreads over the body • Pastia's sign (linear bright red coloration of the creases in the axillary and inguinal folds) • Tongue may appear white, with red, swollen papillae (white strawberry tongue), but by the fourth or fifth day, it becomes bright red (red strawberry tongue) • Other symptoms include headache, chills, flushed face, nausea, and vomiting • Rash usually fades in 4–5 days and is followed by diffuse desquamation	

(*continued*)

TABLE 9.3 Common Childhood Rashes (*continued*)

Disease State	History and Physical Findings	Visual
Varicella • Caused by the varicella-zoster virus • Transmitted mainly through close contact with someone who has chicken pox • Highly contagious disease • Vaccination available	• Incubation period is from 10–21 days • Rash first appears on the chest, back, and face and then spreads over the entire body • Initial appearance of rash is vesicular, followed by simultaneous occurrence of papular and macular rashes with crusting • Rash is highly pruritic • Other symptoms include fever, malaise, anorexia, and headache • Last 5–6 days • Disease is contagious until crusting appears	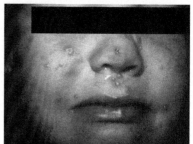

Sources: Centers for Disease Control and Prevention (roseola; rubella; scarlet fever; varicella); Centers for Disease Control and Prevention and Heinz F. Eichenwald, MD (measles [rubeola]); Centers for Disease Control and Prevention, Patricia Smith, and Barbara Rice (mumps).

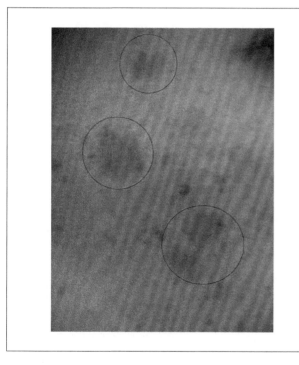

FIGURE 9.7 Melasma on the face—the "mask of pregnancy."
Source: Image courtesy of Elord.

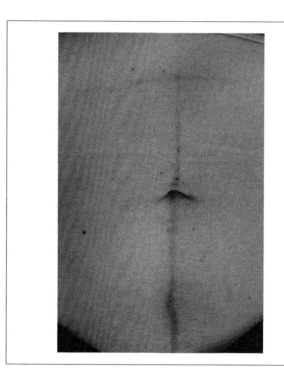

FIGURE 9.8 Linea nigra present on the abdomen of a pregnant woman.

be cognizant of signs of maltreatment by assessing for bruising, lacerations, pressure ulcers, dehydration, and poor hygiene. Skin may appear pale and to hang from the frame. Normal older adult skin variations may include solar lentigo (liver spots; **Figure 9.9**), seborrheic keratosis (**Figure 9.10**), and acrochordon (skin tag;

Figure 9.11). Skin tears may also be present due to the fragility of the skin (Kennedy-Malone, 2019; Wilson & Giddens, 2013).

The hair may be thin, gray, and coarse with symmetric balding in men. The amount of body hair decreases (body, pubic, and axillary hair). Men have an increase in

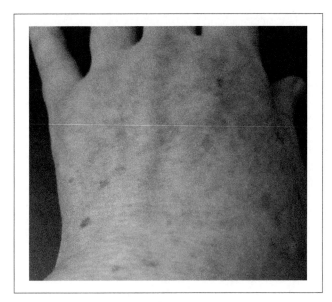

FIGURE 9.9   Solar lentigo (liver spots) on the hand of a 63-year-old Caucasian man.
Source: Image courtesy of BM Ken.

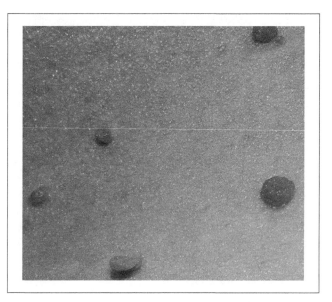

FIGURE 9.11   Several acrochordons (skin tags) on the skin of the lower neck.
Source: Image courtesy of Jmarchn.

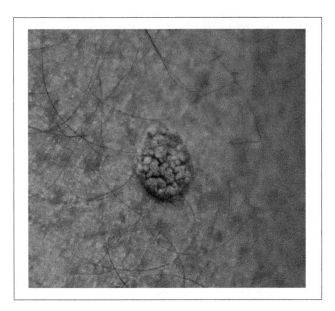

FIGURE 9.10   Seborrheic keratosis.

the amount and coarseness of nasal and eyebrow hair, and women may develop coarse facial hair (Wilson & Giddens, 2013).

UNIQUE POPULATION CONSIDERATIONS FOR EXAMINATION

Race and Ethnicity

Culturally competent assessment skills are required to examine, diagnose, manage, and care for people with skin of different ethnicities, skin of color, and persons classified as IV, V, or VI on the Fitzpatrick Skin Phototype scale (Czerkasij, 2013). Hispanics, Asians, American Indians (including Pacific Islanders), Africans, and Black Americans have unique skin presentations.

A predisposition to scarring and pathogenesis of skin disorders are unique and common to these groups. The dermis of dark skin is thicker and more compact, with prominent and abundant fiber fragments (Czerkasij, 2013). In Blacks, collagen is extremely compact and more numerous below the epidermis as compared with white skin. Ethnic skin is susceptible to dyschromia, especially hypopigmentation, or a loss of skin color (Czerkasij, 2013; Kundu & Patterson, 2013). Conversely, black skin may experience hyperpigmentation, a darkening of skin. Hispanics, Asians, and Blacks have a tendency to form melasma, a common skin disorder that causes gray and brown patches on sun-exposed areas, particularly the face, earlier (during the first 10 years of life), as opposed to lighter skin individuals, who form melasma at the onset of puberty or later (Czerkasij, 2013; **Figure 9.12**).

Skin of color is 15 times more likely to form a scar as compared with white skin (Czerkasij, 2013). Darker skin tends to form excessive scars called keloids. These benign lesions tend to be larger than the site of trauma and are often distressing to patients that form them.

Related to the compact stratum corneum of black skin, vesicles and bulla remain intact longer compared with white skin (Czerkasij, 2013). This fact is significant when diagnosing disorders such as eczema. Eczematous black skin presents with papules and appears

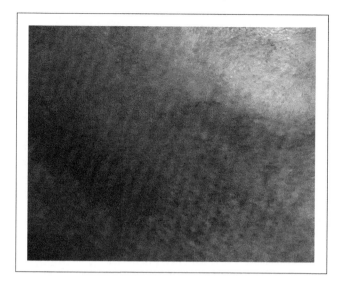

FIGURE 9.12 Melasma on the face of an African American woman.

lichenified. Eczema may also present as soft ivory, light lavender, or faint brown with a scale (Czerkasij, 2013). Although Blacks have a higher rate of eczema than Whites, the diagnosis is often delayed, and the disorder can be complicated by infection.

Any skin condition that presents in persons of color is compounded by the color of the skin. Discoid lupus erythematous is three times more common in Blacks (Czerkasij, 2013). This autoimmune disorder has significant cutaneous manifestations, resulting in the formation of granulomas. Sarcoidosis affects Black women disproportionately and often has early, nonspecific cutaneous symptoms that include irregular pink to red lesions that can coalesce (Czerkasij, 2013).

Special clinical considerations and key features related to skin of color and skin cancer exist. Skin cancer occurs at a lower rate in ethnic skin compared with the case in Whites; however, the morbidity and mortality are significantly higher in persons of color due to late diagnosis (Czerkasij, 2013; Kundu & Patterson, 2013).

Basal cell carcinomas (BCC) are often pigmented and pearly, arising from scars and ulcers. BCCs are most common in Hispanics and Asians, favor the head and neck, and present with multiple lesions (Czerkasij, 2013). Clinicians often mistake BCC for seborrheic keratosis (Czerkasij, 2013).

Squamous cell carcinomas (SCC) are the most common skin cancer in Blacks (Skin Cancer Foundation, 2019). SCC are responsible for 75% of skin cancer deaths in persons of black color (Czerkasij, 2013). SCC often presents as a nonhealing sore and occurs in areas not frequently exposed to the sun. SCC also arises from chronic scarring and inflammation or discoid lupus erythematous lesions, which are prone to metastasize.

Although melanomas are less common in Blacks, Asians, and American Indians, melanomas more frequently present on non–sun-exposed areas, such as the palms, soles, nail beds, and in the mouth (Czerkasij, 2013; Kundu & Patterson, 2013). Melanomas typically present as a single, fast-evolving hyperpigmented macule, papule, or nodule commonly on the back or lower legs (Kundu & Patterson, 2013). It is evidenced that Hispanic and Black patients present with advanced lesions, which implies a poorer prognosis with increased mortality (Czerkasij, 2013; Kundu & Patterson, 2013).

Behavioral Health

Assessing the psychological burden of skin disease should be included when taking the patient's history and performing a physical assessment. Mental health influences skin health, and, conversely, skin health influences emotional well-being. A significantly higher prevalence of clinical depression, anxiety disorder, and suicidal ideation among patients with common skin diseases have been identified (Dalgard et al., 2015). The Dalgard et al. (2015) study reported higher depression in patients with leg ulcers, hand eczema, atopic dermatitis, psoriasis, and infections of the skin; higher anxiety in patients with psoriasis, leg ulcers, hand eczema, and acne; and statistically significant suicidal ideation in patients with psoriasis.

Understandably, hygiene and grooming practices, as well as proper nutrition and hydration, influence the condition of the skin, hair, and nails (D'Amico & Barbarito, 2016). Altered emotional stress may exacerbate existing skin disorders such as rashes, nail biting, hair twisting or pulling, and skin picking (D'Amico & Barbarito, 2016). Recognizing disorders related to the skin, hair, and nails should provoke consideration of psychological health status as well as the presence and effect of common skin conditions.

Occupation

A patient's employment can affect the health of the skin, hair, and nails (D'Amico & Barbarito, 2016). There are multiple external irritants and allergens in work environments that can provoke an inflammatory skin disease. The skin absorbs chemicals used in industries (e.g., acetone, dry-cleaner fluids, dyes, formaldehyde, paint thinner, and other various chemicals). Excessive exposure to irritants and toxic plants, frequent immersion of hands in water, and frequent sun exposure can cause rashes, skin reactions, and skin cancers (Ball et al., 2015; D'Amico & Barbarito, 2016). Contact dermatitis is the most common occupational skin disease and is responsible for seven to nine out of ten workers' skin dermatosis (Martin et al., 2018). Additionally, required occupational wear (i.e., helmets, hats, goggles, gloves, or shoes) for work can be ill-fitting and cause skin abrasions (Centers for Disease Control and Prevention [CDC], n.d.-d).

Multiple occupations require outdoor work. Frequent sun exposure increases the risk of sun damage and sun cancers. Unfortunately, there is no single strategy to protect people completely from the sun. Adequate application and frequency of sunscreen 30 SPF or higher is a small portion of needed protection. Additional protective measures should include seeking shade and wearing sun-protective clothing, which includes wide-brimmed hats and appropriate sunglasses (Skin Cancer Foundation, 2018).

LABORATORY CONSIDERATIONS FOR SKIN, HAIR, AND NAILS

LESION CULTURES

Identifying microorganisms is a common diagnostic strategy in primary care. Culture testing of the skin is performed to identify bacteria, virus, and fungi. Dermatitis, of a noninfectious cause, can become secondarily infected with bacteria. Specific culture media are required for bacterial, viral, and fungal testing. The lesion's top is opened, if not already, and swabbed in the lesion center or an area of suitable drainage with a cotton-tipped applicator. The applicator is then inserted into a container with an appropriate holding solution. The clinician must be knowledgeable of the handling requirements of specific specimens (i.e., temperature and time to transport) and should check with the lab to ensure appropriate requirements are met.

MICROSCOPY

A microscope with 10× and 40× magnification is appropriate for most primary care office skin evaluations. Potassium hydroxide (KOH) is used to assess the stratum corneum for superficial fungal disease. The alkaline KOH solution separates and eventually destroys cells of the stratum corneum, permitting hyphae and spores of dermatophytes to become more clearly visible. The technique for a suspected fungus lesion is to gently scrape the lesions' active border with the edge of a microscope slide or scalpel. Flakes are collected on another slide. A drop of 10% to 20% KOH is applied over the specimen, and a cover slide is placed on top. Diagnosis of fungus is confirmed when the clinician identifies the fungal hyphae, which appear cylindrical, uniform in diameter, and branched. Microscopy is also used to assess bacteria, parasites, and nasal, fecal, and urine sediment (CDC, 2016).

PUNCH BIOPSY

With appropriate training, many primary care clinicians perform incisional or punch skin biopsies. Biopsies allow the clinician to evaluate the tissue pathology in the deeper layers of the dermis. The technique is not difficult; however, the decision of which lesion will give the most diagnostic accuracy requires skill. This testing is particularly helpful in a vesiculobullous disorder like pemphigoid. The technique requires the specimen to be obtained with a 2 to 8 mm cylindrical punch biopsy instrument. Select the site that is the most representative of newly active disease (Consultant 360, 2012). Outline the area prior to the procedure. Administer an anesthetic (e.g., lidocaine) of choice. After preparing the site, stretch the skin perpendicular to the Langer's lines. While holding the skin taut, insert the instrument vertically with a smooth, twisting motion until the desired depth is reached. Withdraw the instrument, and gently retract the specimen with forceps and cut the specimen using small, curved scissors, being sure not to crush the specimen. Place the specimen in the appropriate media for lab analysis. Once the specimen is removed, close the wound with hemostasis or a suture (Prather, 2018). If a cutaneous malignancy (e.g., melanoma) is suspected, the patient should be referred to a dermatologist.

EVIDENCE-BASED PRACTICE CONSIDERATIONS FOR SKIN, HAIR, AND NAILS

Competent clinicians utilize evidence-based clinical guidelines in primary care practice. Evidence-based clinical guidelines related to skin assessment are contained within two general categories. The first category is directed toward skin cancer screening and skin cancer prevention (i.e., U.S. Preventive Services Task Force [USPSTF]). The USPSTF recommendation for a visual skin inspection by a clinician to screen for skin cancer is a Grade I. A Grade I recommendation states that current evidence is insufficient to assess the balance of benefits and harms (USPSTF et al., 2016). The American Cancer Society (2019b) does not have guidelines for the early detection of skin cancer but supports self-exams and exams by clinicians for patients' skin concerns. When evidence-based guidelines are not available, as in the case of adult skin exams, clinicians can integrate evidence into practice with appropriate systematic reviews and randomized controlled studies.

The second category provides evidence-based guidelines of care for various dermatological conditions. An example is the current American Academy of Dermatology Association's (AAD's) clinical practice guidelines, which include acne, atopic dermatitis, melanoma, nonmelanoma skin cancer, office-based surgery, and psoriasis. The AAD evidence-based guideline, *Guidelines of Care for the Management of Acne Vulgaris*, addresses important clinical questions in the management of acne vulgaris (Zaenglein et al., 2016). The guideline includes grading of the disease using the skin assessment findings, and the topical and systemic management of acne vulgaris (Zaenglein et al., 2016).

The AAD, via the *Choosing Wisely* initiative, has listed 10 evidence-based dermatological recommendations that can support conversations between patients and clinicians about evidence-based treatments, tests, and procedures. One example recommendation, Statement #1, supports not prescribing an oral antifungal therapy for suspected nail fungus without confirmation of a fungal infection through a nail culture (AAD, 2018b).

Similarly, the U.S. Cochrane Center (https://us .cochrane.org) provides reliable and relevant sources of evidence from research to help practitioners and patients make informed decisions about skin health. Some of the evidence includes: *Interventions for BCC of the Skin; Treatment of Acne Scars;* and *Creams, Lotions and Gels (Topical Treatments) for Fungal Infections of the Skin and Nails of the Foot.* This type of evidence addresses specific skin disorders and their management, which includes the skin assessment process, but it does not specifically separate skin physical assessment.

ABNORMAL FINDINGS OF SKIN, HAIR, AND NAILS

ACNE

Acne is a chronic inflammatory dermatosis affecting the pilosebaceous follicles of the skin. Acne is one of the most common chronic skin diseases presenting in primary care. An estimated 50 million people in the United States have acne vulgaris (Zaenglein et al., 2016). Largely, acne affects 80% to 85% of adolescents and young adults but is fairly common in adults aged 25 to 34 (8%) and 35 to 44 (3%) and occurs in children (Zaenglein et al., 2016).

The AAD reports that acne is more common in adolescent males but higher in adult women, with approximately 15% affected (as cited in Tanghetti et al., 2014). Caucasians experience more nodulocystic acne (Davis & Callender, 2010). Even though acne is not life-threatening, it often creates profound physical and psychological injury. The inflammatory lesions can be painful, create permanent scarring, alter self-image, and provoke depression and anxiety in people (Zaenglein et al., 2016).

The pathogenesis of acne involves follicular hyperkeratinization, microbial colonization (*propionibacterium acnes*), sebum production, and follicular inflammation and rupture (Zaenglein et al., 2016). If pores become clogged with excess sebum and keratinous material, they form closed comedones (whiteheads) or may open to create open comedones (blackheads). Further extension forms inflammatory papules, pustules, nodules, and cysts. Papules and pustules are painful lesions that are larger than comedones but less than 5 mm in diameter. Pustules are filled with pus and nodules, and cysts are 5 to 10 mm in diameter, deep, and frequently painful.

The acne vulgaris diagnosis is based on clinical findings. There are numerous acne assessment tools available. Assessment and examination should focus on the extent and severity of acne lesions, number of lesions, anatomic location of acne, scarring, and quality of life and other psychosocial metrics. Grading and classification systems may also be useful in acne patient care by specifically classifying acne (mild, moderate, or severe), directing treatment options, and assessing patient response to therapy (Zaenglein et al., 2016). Microbiologic testing is generally unnecessary in acne patients (AAD, 2018b).

Key History and Physical Findings

- Adolescents
- Closed and open comedones (noninflammatory acne; **Figure 9.13**)
- Papules, pustules, nodules, or cysts (inflammatory acne; see **Figure 9.13**)
- May affect only the face, but the chest, back, and upper arms are frequently involved due to the density of sebaceous glands
- Postinflammatory hyperpigmentation and/or atrophic scars (moderate to severe acne)

ACTINIC KERATOSIS

Actinic keratosis (AK), or solar keratosis, is a condition in which premalignant skin lesions form from an abnormal production of keratinocytes after excessive prolonged ultraviolet exposure. Light-skinned people are at the greatest risk for developing AKs, but there is

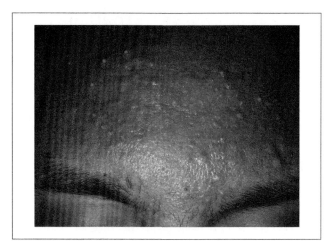

FIGURE 9.13 Adolescent male with moderately severe acne vulgaris.

Source: Image courtesy of Roshu Bangal.

also an elevated risk of immunocompromised individuals developing AKs. AKs have the potential to transform into SCC. Even though the risk of an individual AK lesion developing into SCC is low, the lesion provides an indicator of sun damage and skin cancer risk (Dodds, Chia, & Shumack, 2014). AKs are most frequently seen in people over 50 but are also identified in patients in their twenties and thirties who have had excessive UV exposures. A history of sunburns increases AK risk. Human papillomavirus is associated with an increased risk for AKs (Lyons & Ousley, 2015). Immunosuppressed individuals are at a higher risk for SCC and AKs. Men form actinic keratosis more often than women, and the prevalence of AKs increases as a person ages (Lyons & Ousley, 2015). Any single AK lesion will either remit, remain stable, or transform into SCC (Dodds et al., 2014).

Key History and Physical Findings

- Erythematous, hyperkeratotic scaly macules, papules, and plaques on sun-damaged skin (**Figure 9.14**)
- Typically located on the face, ears, scalp, neck, and extremities
- The average number of lesions identified is 6 to 8 (Dodds et al., 2014)
- Lesions range in size from a few millimeters to 2 centimeters (Lyons & Ousley, 2015)
- The lesions range in color from white, yellow, pink, or red
- Rough feeling on palpation

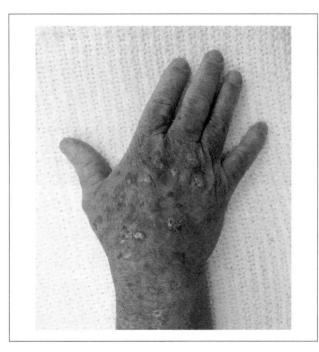

FIGURE 9.14 Actinic keratosis on the back of hand.
Source: Image courtesy of James Heilman, MD.

BED BUGS

Bed bugs (*Cimex lectularius*) are small, parasitic insects that feed on the blood of people and animals while they sleep. Bed bugs do not transmit diseases but do cause pruritic bites and can be difficult to eradicate once an infestation occurs. Bed bug infestations usually occur around or near the areas where people sleep. The bed bug injects a local anesthesia into the person, so they do not feel the bite when it occurs (CDC, n.d.-a).

Key History and Physical Findings

- Bite marks appear anywhere from one to several days after the initial bite.
- Bite marks can occur in a random distribution, a straight line, or in groups of three (commonly referred to as breakfast, lunch, and dinner; **Figure 9.15A**).
- Bites are mildly erythematous and pruritic (**Figure 9.15B**).
- Bites can cause insomnia, anxiety, and additional skin problems, like secondary infections, that arise from intense scratching of the bites.

CELLULITIS

Cellulitis is a bacterial infection of the deeper dermis and subcutaneous tissues predominantly caused by group A streptococcus, *S. aureus* in adults, and *Haemophilus influenza* type B in children under 3 years old (Habif, 2010; Sullivan & de Barra, 2018). The pathogen enters through nonintact skin (Buttaro, Trybulski, Polgar-Bailey, & Sandberg-Cook, 2017). The skin's surface is usually compromised by local trauma, abrasions, ulcers, or at psoriatic, eczematous, or tinea lesions (Habif, 2010). Cellulitis typically affects the skin on the lower legs but can occur on any skin surface area. Patients with a history of lymphedema, venous insufficiency, a previous history of cellulitis, tinea pedis, and obesity are at increased risk for cellulitis (Sullivan & de Barra, 2018). Comorbidities of diabetes and peripheral vascular disease also place these individuals at a higher risk of developing cellulitis. In a nonimmunocompromised patient, the erythema may be localized, in contrast to spreading erythema and fulminant sepsis seen with necrotizing fasciitis (Sullivan & de Barra, 2018).

Key History and Physical Findings

- Erythema
- Color
- Edema of the skin (**Figure 9.16**)
- Pain
- Fever
- Leukocytosis
- Mildly elevated sedimentation rate
- Unilateral
- Has indistinct borders

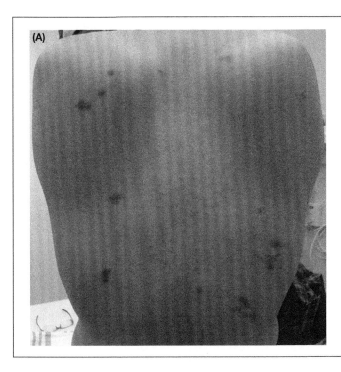

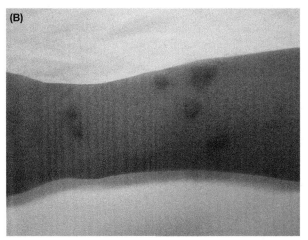

FIGURE 9.15 Bed bug bites. A. Random distribution on back with characteristic grouping of three (breakfast, lunch, and dinner). B. Mildly erythematous bites.

Source: Images courtesy of James Heilman, MD.

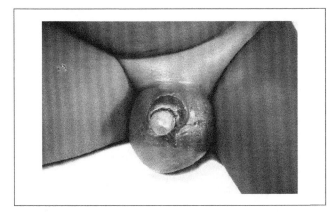

FIGURE 9.16 Cellulitis on the scrotum of an infant.

Source: Centers for Disease Control and Prevention/Robert S. Craig.

CONTACT DERMATITIS

Contact dermatitis is an eczematous inflammatory skin condition. Dermatitis of this form is generally caused by contact with toxins that have an external, noninfectious, immunological, chemical, or physical effect; however, it can be triggered by an endogenous or exogenous allergen (Brasch et al., 2014). There are two forms of contact dermatitis: irritant and allergic (Rashid & Shim, 2016).

Irritant dermatitis accounts for 80% of contact dermatitis cases, is a nonimmunologic response, and is caused by direct damage to the skin from an irritant (i.e., chemical, frequent use of hand soaps/cleaners, or toxic chemicals; Aneja, 2018). Allergic dermatitis accounts for the other 20% of the disorder and is an immunologic response to an allergen in which the patient has developed a sensitivity (Helm, 2019; Rashid & Shim, 2016). Clinical symptoms frequently do not help classify the dermatitis as contact or allergic (Brasch et al., 2014). Approximately 80% of occupational skin disorders are a form of contact dermatitis (Rashid & Shim, 2016). Older adults have an increased risk of irritant dermatitis due to dry skin (Walsh & Deligiannidis, 2019).

Key History and Physical Findings

- Dryness and scaling
- Pruritic papules, vesicles, and/or bullae with an erythematous base (**Figure 9.17**)
- Crusting and oozing may be present.
- Chronic presentation may include lichenification, scaling, and fissuring.
- Can occur on any part of the body that has come in contact with the offending agent.
- Skin areas more vulnerable to contact dermatitis include hands, face, eyelids, neck, scalp, lower extremities, feet, and the anogenital region (Rashid & Shim, 2016).

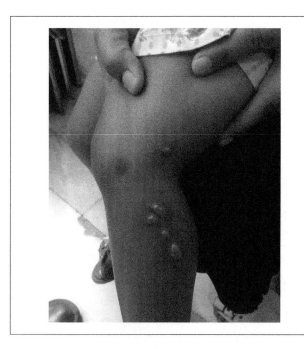

FIGURE 9.17 Contact dermatitis after contact with poison ivy.
Source: Images courtesy of Alborz Fallah.

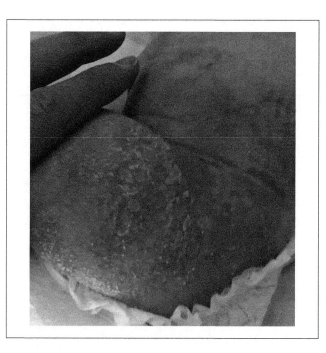

FIGURE 9.18 Atopic dermatitis (eczema) on the abdomen and thigh of an infant.
Source: Image courtesy of GZ.

- Areas with thinner epidermis are at increased risk (Walsh & Deligiannidis, 2019).
- Some cases require a patch test (Rashid & Shim, 2016).

ECZEMA

Eczema, or atopic dermatitis, is an inflammatory skin disorder characterized by pruritus and exacerbation and remission of dry, itchy, erythematous skin (Buttaro et al., 2017). This skin disease has no known etiology but is correlated with other atopic diseases such as asthma, allergic rhinitis, urticaria, or acute allergic reactions to certain foods (Buttaro et al., 2017).

The onset of eczema occurs most commonly in infants 3 to 6 months of age. Eczema affects 1 in 10 children and 1 in 10 to 14 adults. Eczema occurs in 85% of children by 5 years of age (Lyons & Ousley, 2015). The occurrence of eczema is higher in females (4:1).

Key History and Physical Findings
Hallmark Signs
- Pruritis
- Erythematous lesions
- Xerosis
- Lichenification
- Excoriation
- Possible erosions

Infantile Eczema
- Presents as generalized xerosis and erythematous, scaly plaques affecting the cheeks, forehead, scalp, and extensor extremities (diaper area is usually spared; **Figure 9.18**).
- As the child ages, the lesions move to the flexor areas (antecubital and popliteal fossae; creases of buttocks and thighs; **Figure 9.18**).
- May include pityriasis alba of the face

EPIDERMOID CYSTS

Epidermoid cyst, also known as a sebaceous cyst, is a benign encapsulated, subepidermal keratin–filled nodule (Zito & Scharf, 2018). Epidermoid cysts, the most common cutaneous cysts, develop within the follicular infundibulum. The prevalence of the cysts are a 2:1 male-to-female ratio, with no race or ethnic prevalence identified.

Most epidermoid cysts develop sporadically in patients during their thirties and forties. Rarely do epidermoid cysts form before puberty. Obtaining a thorough history assists in determining whether the cyst is an isolated case, caused by medications, or part of a genetic syndrome (Zito & Scharf, 2018). Epidermoid cysts are most commonly located on the face, neck, and trunk; however, epidermoid cysts can develop anywhere (including the scrotum, genitalia, fingers, and within the buccal mucosa). Cyst development is usually slow, and a cyst may be present for years (Zito & Scharf, 2018). In neonates, milia (small epidermal cysts) are common (Zito & Scharf, 2018). In the elderly, epidermoid cysts can be related to chronic sun damage (Zito & Scharf, 2018). One percent of epidermoid cysts may transform into SCC or BCC. Epidermoid cysts are associated with autosomal dominant Gardner syndrome (familial adenomatous polyposis), Gorlin syndrome (basal cell nevus syndrome), and pachyonychia congenita (Lyons & Ousley, 2015; Zito & Scharf, 2018). Imiquimod and cyclosporine can cause epidermal inclusion cysts (Zito & Scharf, 2018).

Key History and Physical Findings

- Typically slow growing
- An asymptomatic mobile nodule, 0.5 cm to several centimeters in size, nonfluctuant, compressible, smooth, and shiny (**Figure 9.19**)
- A central, dark comedone opening is frequently present.
- If the cyst ruptures, it may look like a furuncle with tenderness, erythema, and swelling.
- A foul-smelling, yellowish cheese-like discharge.

ERYTHEMA MIGRANS

Lyme disease is a bacterial infection caused by the bacterium *Borrelia burgdorferi*. It is transmitted to humans through the bite of an infected blacklegged tick. There are three stages of Lyme disease. The classic bulls-eye rash associated with Lyme disease, erythema migrans (EM), occurs in Stage 1. In this stage, the bacteria have not yet spread throughout the body. During Stages 2 and 3, the bacteria start to disseminate, causing multiple signs and symptoms if not treated (CDC, n.d.-b).

Key History and Physical Findings

- EM rash: Typically occurs at the site of the tick bite
- Appears 3 to 30 days after the bite occurred (average is about 7 days)
- Has a distinct bull's-eye appearance (**Figure 9.20**)
- Expands in size gradually over a period of days reaching up to 12 inches or more (30 cm) across
- May have mild calor
- Nonpruritic, nonpainful
- Can also be associated with fever, myalgias, lymphadenopathy, fatigue, and malaise

FOLLICULITIS

Folliculitis is an infection of the hair follicles caused by damage to the hair follicle or blockage of the follicle. It can occur anywhere on the skin. It can mimic the appearance of acne pustules or can present as nonhealing ulcers with crusts. An acute eruption is typically due to *Staphylococcus aureus* bacteria and can be treated with either topical or oral antibiotics. Folliculitis can also be caused by *Pseudomonas aeruginosa* and commonly takes the name "hot tub folliculitis" since this type of bacteria commonly grows in hot tubs, whirlpools, and swimming pools (Laureano, Schwartz, & Cohen, 2014; **Figure 9.21**).

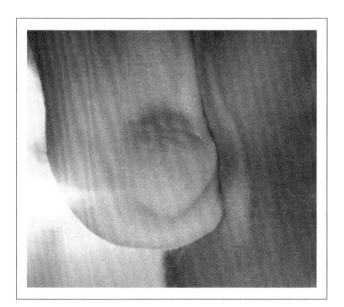

FIGURE 9.19 Epidermoid cyst of the ear.

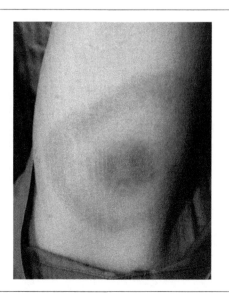

FIGURE 9.20 Erythema migrans. Distinct bull's-eye appearance denotes Stage 1 of Lyme disease.

Source: Centers for Disease Control and Prevention.

Key History and Physical Findings

- Use of razor in affected area
- Papules or pustules around a hair follicle
- Can cause itching or soreness

HERPES ZOSTER (SHINGLES)

Herpes zoster (shingles) is a cutaneous viral infection caused by the reactivation of the varicella-zoster virus, the same virus that causes varicella (chicken pox; Buttaro et al., 2017; Lyons & Ousley, 2015). The varicella virus remains dormant in the body for decades, and reactivation depends on the individual's immune status (Lyons & Ousley, 2015).

The incidence of herpes zoster is thought to be often, but not always, dependent on the person's ability to mount an immune response (Lyons & Ousley, 2015). One third of Americans carry a lifetime risk of developing herpes zoster (CDC, n.d.-c). Persons at greatest risk for herpes zoster include older adults and immunosuppressed individuals (John & Canaday, 2017).

Key History and Physical Findings

Diagnosis of herpes zoster can be made clinically. There are two phases of clinical presentation: prodromal (a sensory change over the involved dermatome prior to the rash) and acute.

Prodromal Phase

- Tingling
- Pruritus
- Burning, throbbing, or stabbing ("knife-like") pain in the dermatomal area

Acute Phase

- Fatigue
- Malaise
- Headache
- Low-grade fever
- Dermatomal rash (thoracic and lumbar areas are the most common sites)
- Unilateral lesion eruption that is initially erythematous and maculopapular and then develops into clusters of clear vesicles (**Figure 9.22**)
- Regional lymphadenopathy may be present.
- The lesions crust within 7 to 10 days of eruption.

MELANOMA

Melanoma is a malignancy of the pigment-producing melanocytes in the basal layer of the epidermis. Most melanomas are black or brown, but can be skin colored, pink, red, purple, blue, or white (Skin Cancer Foundation, 2018; **Figure 9.23**). Depending on the stage of the melanoma, the lesion may resemble other skin cancers.

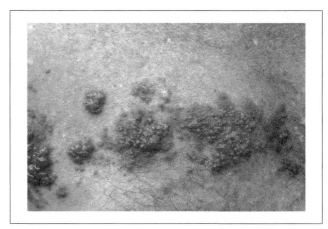

FIGURE 9.22 Herpes zoster.

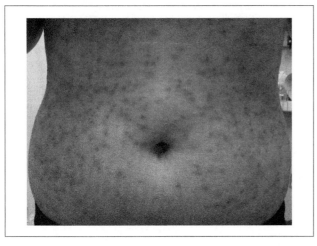

FIGURE 9.21 "Hot tub" folliculitis.
Source: Image courtesy of James Heilman, MD.

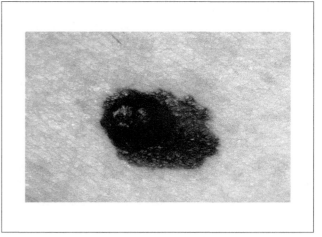

FIGURE 9.23 Nodular melanoma.

Although the least common of skin cancers in adults, melanoma is aggressive and has a great potential to metastasize. Melanoma is the most common skin cancer in children and accounts for 3% of all pediatric cancers (Dean, Bucevska, Strahlendorf, & Verchere, 2017; St. Jude, 2018). Treatment of childhood melanoma is delayed 40% of the time due to misdiagnosis (Skin Cancer Foundation, 2019). Although rare in young children, approximately 7% of cancers in children aged 15 to 19 are melanomas (St. Jude Children's Research Hospital, n.d.). Melanoma affects approximately 2% of the U.S. population (American Cancer Society, 2019a). Over 10,000 people die from melanoma each year in the United States, and every hour one American dies from melanoma (American Cancer Society, 2019a).

In African Americans, Asians, Filipinos, Indonesians, and Native Hawaiians, melanoma can occur on nonexposed skin with less pigment; 60% to 75% of lesions present on the palms, soles, mucous membranes, and nails. Melanoma is often diagnosed in later stages in Hispanics and African Americans, leading to poorer survival rates (Skin Cancer Foundation, 2019). Clinicians must be aware of these specific ethnic presentations.

Key History and Physical Findings

- A history of the following may indicate a melanoma lesion: (a) an open sore that does not heal for 3 weeks; (b) a spot or sore that burns, itches, stings, crusts, or bleeds; and (c) any mole or spot that changes in size or texture, develops irregular borders, or appears pearly, translucent, or multicolored (Buttaro et al., 2017)
- *Lesion ABCDE:* **A**symmetry, **B**order irregularity, **C**olor variegation, **D**iameter larger than 6 mm, and **E**volution or timing of the lesion's growth
- Most commonly located in sun-exposed areas
- Satellite lesions, which are new moles that grow near an existing mole
- Lesions may be present on palms of hands, soles of feet, under the nails, and on mucous membranes (specifically skin of color).
- In the pediatric population, melanomas may be whitish, yellowish, or red and may be misdiagnosed as warts (Dana-Farber Cancer Institute, 2015).

NONGENITAL WARTS

Verruca vulgaris, or warts, are benign epidermal growths that are caused by various types of human papillomavirus (HPV). Warts may occur anywhere on the epidermis (Lyons & Ousley, 2015). Although primarily transmitted by skin-to-skin contact, HPV can be transmitted indirectly or through autoinoculation (Shenefelt, 2018). Diagnosis of warts is typically confirmed clinically (Buttaro et al., 2017). Individuals with diseases that compromise the barrier of the skin, such as atopic dermatitis or immunosuppression, are prone to verruca vulgaris.

Key History and Physical Findings

- Hyperkeratotic papules with a rough irregular surface
- May vary in size from 1 mm to more than 1 cm
- Commonly occur on the hands and knees but can occur anywhere on the body (Shenefelt, 2018)

NONMELANOMA SKIN CANCER

Skin cancer is the most common cancer in the United States with nonmelaoma skin cancer (BCC and SCC) rates of 3.3 million Americans each year (AAD, 2018). BCC is the most common malignancy in humans (Bichakjian et al., 2018). SCC is the second most common form of cancer and poses a substantial risk for morbidity, mortality, and impact on quality of life (Alam et al., 2018).

BCC evolves from the basal cells found in the lower layer of the epidermis. BCC most commonly develops on sun-exposed skin areas, is slow growing, and usually does not metastasize. All ethnicities, races, and skin types are affected by BCC, but fair skin patients are disproportionately affected. Males have a 2:1 ratio when compared with females.

SCC arises from the epidermal keratinocytes. Lesions may develop on scars and skin areas exposed to past radiation but are most common on sun-exposed areas of the skin (Gonzalez & Goodheart, 2019). SCC is the most common skin cancer in Blacks. In elderly Black women, they are most commonly found on the legs (Skin Cancer Foundation, 2019). Untreated SCC can invade the deeper skin layers, disfigure, and metastasize (Lyons & Ousley, 2015). SCC lesions develop from flat, scale-like skin cells, called keratinocytes, that lie beneath the top layer of the epidermis (Lyons & Ousley, 2015). Patients who had radiation therapy as children are at increased risk for SCC (Firnhaber, 2012). BCC have greater prevalence in persons 55 to 75 years of age. The highest incidence of SCC is in males and the elderly.

Key History and Physical Findings
Basal Cell Carcinoma
- Slow growing
- Usually on an area of sun-exposed skin
- A nonhealing sore that is friable and umbilicated (Lyons & Ousley, 2015)
- Waxy papules with central depression, pearly, erosion, or ulceration (**Figure 9.24**)
- Bleeds with trauma
- Crusting
- Rolled border
- Translucency
- Surface telangiectasia

Squamous Cell Carcinoma

- Generally slow growing
- A raised, firm, skin-colored or pink, hyperkeratotic papule or plaques (**Figure 9.25**)
- Normally situated on an area of sun-damaged skin
- The lesion can be isolated, or there can be multiple lesions.
- Most lesions occur on the head and upper extremities on sun-exposed areas.

ONYCHOMYCOSIS

Onychomycosis is a disease of the nail(s) caused by yeast, dermatophytes, and nondermatophyte molds. Candida is the most common type of yeast species involved. Risk factors for onychomycosis include diabetes,

human immunodeficiency virus, immunosuppression, obesity, smoking, and older age. Diagnosis is based on a variety of methods, but direct microscopic examination with KOH or culture is the gold standard. Microscopy, although an inexpensive option, has a low sensitivity (48%) and a high rate of false negatives. Onychomycosis can be difficult to treat (Gupta, Versteeg, & Shear, 2017).

Key History and Physical Findings

- Typically affects the toenails but can also be on the fingernails
- Discoloration of the nail(s) (whitish, yellow, brown in color; **Figure 9.26**)
- Thickened and brittle nail(s)
- Distortion of shape (ragged, crumbly)
- Onycholysis
- Can have an associated foul odor, pain, or paresthesia

PITYRIASIS ROSEA

Pityriasis rosea (PR) is an acute exanthematous disease. It is associated with the endogenous systemic reactivation of human herpesvirus (HHV)-6 and/or HHV-7. The disease is typically mild and self-limiting (Drago, Ciccarese, Rebora, Broccolo, & Parodi, 2016).

- It begins with a single, circular, erythematous patch called a herald patch (**Figure 9.27**).
- Herald patch is followed by a secondary eruption with smaller patches on the cleavage lines of the trunk (configuration of a "Christmas tree").
- The duration may vary from 2 weeks to a few months.
- Rash usually disappears on its own without treatment.

PSORIASIS

Psoriasis is a complex, inflammatory, multisystem disease characterized by hyperproliferation of

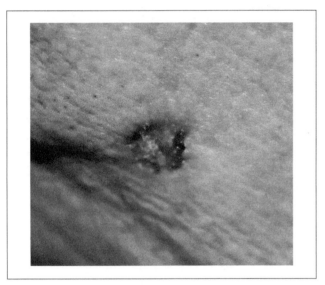

FIGURE 9.24 Basal cell carcinoma.

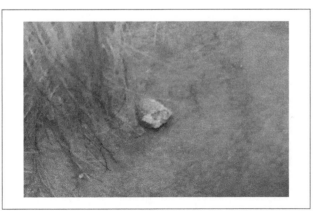

FIGURE 9.25 Squamous cell carcinoma.
Source: National Cancer Institute/Kelly Nelson, MD.

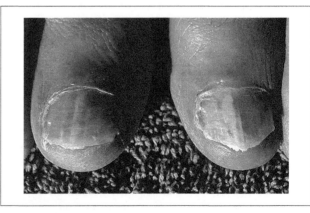

FIGURE 9.26 Onychomycosis of the toenails.
Source: Centers for Disease Control and Prevention/Edwin P. Ewing, Jr, MD.

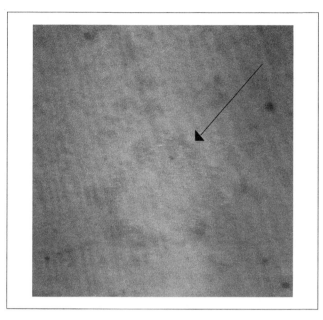

FIGURE 9.27 Pityriasis rosea and associated erythematous "herald patch."

Source: Image courtesy of James Heilman, MD.

the keratinocytes in the epidermis (Habashy, 2019; Menter et al., 2019). This chronic skin disease of adults and children is multifactorial and appears to be induced by genetic, environmental, and immunologic factors (Habashy, 2019). Psoriasis is a common inflammatory disease of adults and children (Menter et al., 2019). Prevalence peaks between ages 20 to 30 and 50 to 60 (Needham & Matz, 2019). Skin lesions are often the most prominent and the only recognized feature of the disease. Psoriasis flares may result from systemic, psychological, infectious, and environmental influences (Needham & Matz, 2019). Afflicted patients are undiagnosed, undertreated, and frequently not treated (Menter et al., 2019). Skin involvement varies depending on the type of psoriasis. The most common type of psoriasis is psoriasis vulgaris.

Key History and Physical Findings

- Reddish pink, well-demarcated macules, papules, and plaques with a silvery scale (Habashy, 2019; Menter et al., 2019; Needham & Matz, 2019; **Figure 9.28**)
- The Auspitz sign, pinpoint bleeding with removal of scales, is a hallmark sign (Needham & Matz, 2019).
- Psoriasis vulgaris is common on the scalp, behind the ears, and on extensor surfaces, genitals, umbilicus, and lower back (Habashy, 2019; Needham & Matz, 2019).
- Plaque psoriasis is common on extensor surfaces of the knees, elbows, scalp, and trunk (Habashy, 2019).

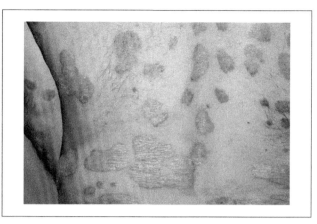

FIGURE 9.28 Psoriasis.

ROSACEA

Rosacea (sometimes referred to as acne rosacea) is a common, chronic, and relapsing inflammatory skin condition involving the face and, less often, the neck and chest (Buttaro et al., 2017). Rosacea may coexist with acne vulgaris and often mimics it. A difference between rosacea and acne is the absence of comedones in rosacea (Buttaro et al., 2017). Although the etiology is not fully known, there are certain triggers of rosacea. Triggers may include ultraviolet light (most common), stress, exercise, wind, heat, spicy foods, dairy, and alcohol (Oge, Muncie, & Phillips-Savoy, 2015).

The incidence of rosacea is estimated at 1.5%, and it disproportionately affects persons of fair-skinned European and Celtic origin (Dahl, 2019). Rosacea is rare in children and adolescents and is most common in women ages 30 to 50 who are fair-skinned (Marai, 2015).

A thorough history should be obtained with suspected rosacea to determine the triggering factors. People with rosacea may have a history of facial flushing in childhood or adolescence (Lyons & Ousley, 2015). Diagnosis of rosacea is based solely on history and clinical presentation, because there is no diagnostic testing needed (Oge et al., 2015).

Key History and Physical Findings

- Symptoms vary among patients, depending on the type of rosacea.
- Prior history of facial flushing
- Nontransient erythema, telangiectasia, roughness of the skin, or papulopustular lesions (Oge et al., 2015; **Figure 9.29**)
- Comedones are absent.
- Neck and upper chest may also have erythema or flushing (Lyons & Ousley, 2015).
- Thickening of the skin of the nose (rhinophyma)
- Ocular involvement may be present.

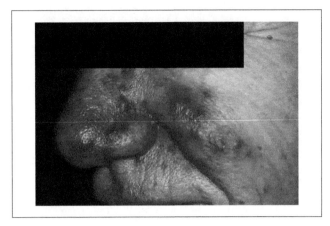

FIGURE 9.29 Rosacea.

Source: Image courtesy of Michael Sand, Daniel Sand, Christina Thrandorf, Volker Paech, Peter Altmeyer, and Falk G. Bechara.

SCABIES

Scabies is a skin infestation caused by *Sarcoptes scabiei*, which are tiny parasites that burrow into the skin and lay eggs. Scabies is highly contagious. It is spread by direct, prolonged, skin-to-skin contact with another person who harbors the mites but can also be spread indirectly by sharing articles such as clothing, towels, or bedding used by an infested person. Symptoms can take 2 to 6 weeks to appear after exposure. People can be contagious even when they do not have symptoms. There is a more severe type of scabies known as Norwegian or crusted scabies. This form of scabies typically occurs only in institutionalized people, and indirect spread occurs more frequently.

Key History and Physical Findings

- Intense, pruritic rash (**Figure 9.30**)
- Pruritus worsens at night
- Maculopapular rash that can be found anywhere but tends to occur between the fingers and toes, under jewelry or watches on the wrist, and in armpits, skin folds, and genitalia
- Lesions can arrange in linear patterns.
- The rash can also resemble pimples, eczema, and insect bites.
- Infants and young children with scabies may appear irritable, not wanting to eat or sleep, and have the rash in less common areas, including on their palms or the soles of their feet, face, scalp, and neck.

TINEA CORPORIS

Tinea corporis is a dermatophyte (fungal) infection of the face, trunk, and/or extremities. Tinea corporis has similar characteristics as other skin disorder presentations; therefore, clinical diagnosis is unreliable. Tinea corporis is gender neutral, occurs in all, and has the

highest prevalence in children. Within 1 to 3 weeks of exposure, the fungus invades the epidermis in an annular pattern, which creates the raised, scaly border (Lyons & Ousley, 2015). Diagnosis should be confirmed with potassium hydroxide (KOH) preparation microscopy and/or culture (Ely, Rosenfeld, & Stone, 2014).

Key History and Physical Findings

- A red, scaly patch with distinct annular borders and central clearing (Backer, 2019)
- Lesions may be pruritic or asymptomatic, occasionally burn, and vary in number.
- The size of lesions ranges from 1 to 5 cm, but varying size and distribution may occur (Ely et al., 2014).
- At the lesions' border, inflammation, scale, crusts, papules, vesicles, and bullae can develop (Lyons & Ousley, 2015; **Figure 9.31**).

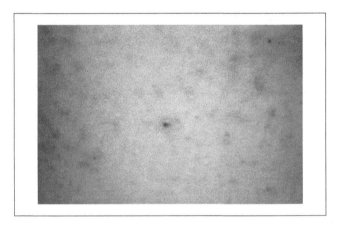

FIGURE 9.30 Scabies.

Source: Centers for Disease Control and Prevention/Joe Miller.

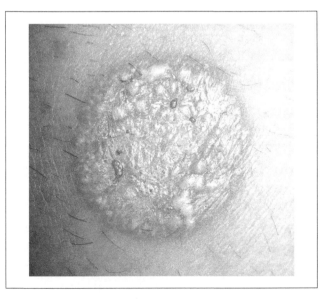

FIGURE 9.31 Tinea corporis.

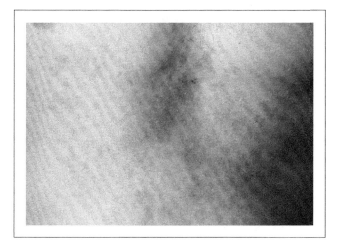

FIGURE 9.32 Tinea versicolor.

Source: Centers for Disease Control and Prevention/Lucille K. George, MD.

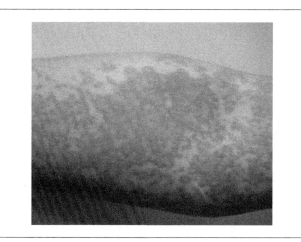

FIGURE 9.33 Urticaria.

Source: Image courtesy of James Heilman, MD.

TINEA VERSICOLOR

Tinea versicolor is a benign fungal infection of the skin caused by the fungus Malassezia furfur. Most cases occur in healthy patients, but patients who are immunocompromised may be predisposed. It is often diagnosed in summer, when the patches become more noticeable due to having tan skin with patches that do not tan (Hu & Bigby, 2010).

Key History and Physical Findings

- Multiple tan, brown, salmon, pink, or white scaling patches on the trunk, neck, abdomen, and, occasionally, face (**Figure 9.32**)
- Patches may coalesce.
- Budding and hyphae noted on a KOH wet mount.

URTICARIA

Urticaria (hives) is the most frequent skin disorder seen in the United States urgent cares and emergency departments. Urticaria carries a lifetime prevalence of approximately 20% of the U.S. population (Lyons & Ousley, 2015). Urticaria (hives) is caused by the release of histamine and other inflammatory mediators from mast cells and basophils in the dermis (Schaefer, 2017).

This skin condition may be acute or chronic and is often self-limited and benign; however, it may cause significant pruritus (as a result of the histamine released in the dermis) and discomfort. Urticaria that is recurrent is frequently associated with sun exposure, exercise, emotional or physical stress, and exposure to water (Lyons & Ousley, 2015). The most frequently identified cause of urticaria is infection (Lyons & Ousley, 2015). The clinician must assess for angioedema and other systemic signs and symptoms and rule out anaphylaxis with any presentation of hives. Hives can be triggered by pregnancy, usually in the third trimester, and typically resolve spontaneously shortly after delivery (Lyons & Ousley, 2015).

Key History and Physical Findings

- Raised wheals that blanch with palpation (**Figure 9.33**)
- May appear on any part of the body
- Can be linear, annular (circular), or arcuate (serpiginous; Wong, 2018)
- Lesions are typically temporary on the affected skin and are usually mobile (Lyons & Ousley, 2015).
- Usually resolve within 24 hours; however, they may persist depending on underlying etiology

CASE STUDY: Acne

History of Present Illness

Jackie is a 25-year-old female who visits your office because she has developed acne over the last 6 months. She describes recent acne flare-ups, primarily affecting her face and sometimes upper back. Jackie is distressed about the effect of her acne on her appearance; she is confused as to why she has developed acne now, considering she did not have acne as a teenager. She has tried a number of OTC remedies, with little to no success so far.

Specific History Questions

- Can you describe your skin?
- Have you had acne in the past? If so, describe.
- When did you begin to break out?
- Can you think of anything that would have triggered breaking out?
- Can you describe where the lesions started? Can you describe the lesions? Are they pink or red?
- Are your lesions tender or painful?
- When did you start your menstrual period?
- Can you relate the acne with your menstrual cycle?
- Are you using birth control? If so, what type?
- Have you tried any OTC or home remedies to treat your acne? If so, what have you tried? Did it improve your acne? Did you have any SE?
- Can you describe your daily skin care routine? What products are you using?
- Can you explain your history of sun exposure? How much sun exposure do you get currently?
- Do you use sunscreen? What SPF? How often do you reapply?
- Do you have a family history of skin cancer, atopy, atopic dermatitis, rhinitis, or asthma?
- What about psoriasis, autoimmune diseases, or acne?

Past Medical History

- Surgical history: Tonsillectomy age 7; no known allergies

- Medications: Depo-Provera 150 mg IM every 3 months; zinc 50 mg orally each day for acne

Family History

- Parents: Mother, DM II; Father, Hypertension (HTN). history of cystic acne; no siblings
- Maternal grandparents: Grandmother (GM), DM II; Grandmother (GF), deceased from cerebrovascular accident (CVA) age 67
- Paternal grandparents: GM, HTN; GF, alive and well

Social History

Jackie is married, has no children, and works full time as a graphic designer. She is an athlete who runs five times weekly in the morning before work and competes in marathon runs on weekends. She typically wakes early, runs, and then showers before work.

Physical Examination

- Vital signs: Blood pressure (BP) 110/70; pulse 56; respirations 16; temperature 98.0°F; weight 111 lbs; height 5′6″
- 10 to 20 open and closed comedones on her forehead, cheeks, chin, and nose
- 20 to 30 papules and pustules, mostly on her cheeks and forehead near the hairline
- 10 to 15 papules and lesions on her upper back
- Chest and arms are clear of lesions

Differential Diagnoses

- Bacterial folliculitis (Titus & Hodge, 2012)
- Drug-induced acne (Titus & Hodge, 2012)
- Miliaria (Titus & Hodge, 2012)
- Perioral dermatitis (Titus & Hodge, 2012)

Diagnosis

Acne is diagnosed by identification of lesions (Titus & Hodge, 2012). Final diagnosis is moderate papulopustular acne vulgaris.

CASE STUDY: Atypical Skin Lesions

History of Present Illness

A 77-year-old African American woman presents to clinic today with a chief concern of a "dark flakey place" on her left lower leg for the past 6 months. She says the place on her leg itches and will bleed if she scratches it. She reports that while she is there she wants the clinician to check a bump on her right forehead "that's been there a very long time" but does not bother her.

Specific History Questions

- When did you notice the place on your leg?
- Describe if and how the place on your leg has changed.
- Besides itching, is the place on your leg tender or painful? Does the place ever drain or bleed? If so, when?
- Have you put any medicines on the place on your leg?
- Have you ever seen a clinician for this same problem?
- When did you notice the lesion on your forehead? Please try to estimate the time when you first noticed it?
- Describe if and how the place on your forehead has changed.
- Does the lesion on your forehead cause itching, tenderness, or pain?
- Do you have any other lesions or skin problems?
- Can you describe your skin concerns?
- What is your history of sun exposure?
- Did your occupation expose you to sun? Describe.
- Have you ever had a sunburn?
- Do you protect your skin from the sun? If so, describe.
- Do you have a personal or family history of skin cancers?
- How do you care for your skin?

Past Medical History

- Hypertension (diagnosed age 45)

- Obstetric history: G3P3A0; last menstrual period at age 52

Social History

- Retired air-traffic controller in Atlanta, GA
- Married for 45 years
- Active in church, walks 3 days a week

Family History

- Parents: Mother, deceased, age 78, HTN, renal failure; Father, deceased, age 55, CVA
- Brother: Age 72, diabetic; adult children are alive and well

Physical Examination

- Vital signs: BP, 140/78; pulse, 68; respirations 14; temperature 98.6°F; weight 165 lbs; height 5′4″
- General: Well-developed, well-nourished 77-year-old Black female who appears younger than her stated age in no acute distress
- Left lower extremity (LLE): The physical examination revealed a 2-cm black, hyperkeratotic plaque on the patient's left lower lateral leg. The plaque is nontender and is not draining any fluid. Lower extremities have no edema or noted varicosities. Inguinal, popliteal, dorsalis pedis, and posterior tibialis pulses are + 2 and symmetrical. No left inguinal adenopathy noted.
- Right forehead: The exam revealed at approximately 1″ below hairline, a 5-mm smooth firm translucent pearly papule, with a 1-mm central ulceration noted. The lesion is not mobile or tender.

Differential Diagnoses

- Nonmelanoma skin cancer
- Squamous cell carcinoma
- Basal cell carcinoma
- Actinic keratosis

Final diagnosis

Suspicious for BCC (forehead) and SCC (lower leg)

Clinical Pearls

- A thorough skin history provides approximately 80% of data needed to make a diagnosis.
- Be sure to ask about the patient's occupational history (exposure to chemicals, water, sun, etc.).
- Be consistent in the order that the comprehensive skin exam is conducted. This will ensure a skin region is not missed.
- Integrate an exam of the surrounding skin when examining a specific body area.
- Include palpation of the skin in an attempt to feel abnormal areas on the skin that may be visually missed.
- During a TBSE, include an assessment of the mucous membranes of the oral cavity.
- There is assessment value in the use of smell during a skin exam to identify varied skin disorders.
- If acne-like lesions are centered in the perioral and nasal areas and are unresponsive to conventional acne treatments, consider bacterial culture and sensitivities to evaluate for gram-negative folliculitis.

consumption of carotene-rich foods such as carrots, yams, pumpkin, and butternut squash (Ball et al., 2015).
- No sunscreen use before age 6 months. Infants should be protected from the sun at all times.
- Adolescent assessment is best performed with clothes on to increase their privacy (Bickley, 2017).
- Be aware that nevi may darken and increase in number during pregnancy (Ball et al., 2015).
- Hair loss in women may indicate underlying conditions such as anemia, nutritional deficiencies, or hypothyroidism.
- Because skin turgor is normally reduced as a person ages, it is not a good indicator of hydration. It is important to use other assessment findings such as saliva, urine output, and specific gravity to assess hydration (Ball et al., 2015).
- SCC is the most common skin cancer in Blacks. In elderly Black women, SCCs are found most commonly on the legs (Skin Cancer Foundation, 2019).

Key Takeaways

- Skin cancer screening with a TBSE is the safest, easiest, and probably the most cost-effective screening test in healthcare; however, there is no national consensus regarding its benefit or implementation (Johnson et al., 2017).
- The risk for melanoma more than doubles if an individual has had five or more sunburns (Skin Cancer Foundation, 2019).
- The majority of nonmelanoma skin cancers (BCC and SCC) occur most often on sun-exposed areas, including the head, neck, face, and ears (Kundu & Patterson, 2013; Skin Cancer Foundation, 2019 [stats and facts]).
- Women experience more skin cancer on the legs (Apalla, Lallas, Sotiriou, Lazaridou, & Ioannides, 2017; Mayo Clinic, 2019).
- Patients who use sunscreen generally do not use enough and do not reapply every 2 hours (Ball et al., 2015).
- Risk factors for skin cancer include age, sun-exposure history, and genetics.
- Infants' palms of hands may have an orange or yellow color (carotenemia). Ask about

REFERENCES

Alam, M., Armstrong, A., Baum, C., Bordeaux, J., Brown, M., Busam K. J., . . . Eisen D. (2018). Guidelines of care for the management of cutaneous squamous cell carcinoma. *Journal of the American Academy of Dermatology, 78*(3), 560–578. doi:10.1016/j.jaad.2017.10.007

American Academy of Dermatology Association. (2018a). *Skin conditions by the numbers*. Retrieved from https://www.aad.org/media/stats/conditions/skin-conditions-by-the-numbers

American Academy of Dermatology Association. (2018b). *Ten things physicians and patients should question*. Retrieved from https://www.choosingwisely.org/wp-content/uploads/2015/02/AAD-Choosing-Wisely-List1.pdf

American Cancer Society. (2019a). *Cancer facts and figures 2019*. Retrieved from https://www.cancer.org/research/cancer-facts-statistics/all-cancer-facts-figures/cancer-facts-figures-2019.html

American Cancer Society. (2019b). *How to do a skin self-exam*. Retrieved from https://www.cancer.org/content/cancer/en/healthy/be-safe-in-sun/skin-exams.html

Aneja, S. (2018). Irritant contact dermatitis. In W. D. James (Ed.), *Medscape*. Retrieved from https://emedicine.medscape.com/article/1049353-overview

Apalla, Z., Lallas, A., Sotiriou, E., Lazaridou, E., & Ioannides, D. (2017). Epidemiological trends in skin cancer. *Dermatology Practical & Conceptual, 7*(2), 1–6. doi:10.5826/dpc.0702a01

Backer, E. L. (2019). Tinea (capitis, corporis, cruris). In F. J. Domino (Ed.), *The 5-minute clinical consult 2019* (pp. 986–987). Philadelphia, PA: Wolters Kluwer.

Ball, J. W., Dains, J. E., Flynn, J. A., Solomon, B. S., & Stewart, R. W. (2015). *Seidel's guide to physical exam* (8th ed.). St. Louis, MO: Mosby/Elsevier.

Bichakjian, C., Armstrong, A., Baum, C., Bordeaux, J., Brown, M., Busam K., … Eisen, D. (2018). Guidelines of care for the management of basal cell carcinoma. *Journal of the American Academy of Dermatology, 78*(3), 540–559. doi:10.1016/j.jaad.2017.10.006

Bickley, L. S. (2017). *Bate's guide to physical examination and history taking* (12th ed.). Philadelphia, PA: Wolters Kluwer.

Brasch, J., Becker, D., Aberer, W., Bircher, A., Kränke, B., Jung, K., … Schnuch, A. (2014). Guideline contact dermatitis: S1-Guidelines of the German Contact Allergy Group (DKG) of the German Dermatology Society (DDG), the Information Network of Dermatological Clinics (IVDK), the German Society for Allergology and Clinical Immunology (DGAKI), the Working Group for Occupational and Environmental Dermatology (ABD) of the DDG, the Medical Association of German Allergologists (AeDA), the Professional Association of German Dermatologists (BVDD) and the DDG. *Allergo Journal International, 23*(4), 126–138. doi:10.1007/s40629-014-0013-5

Buttaro, T. M., Trybulski, J., Polgar-Bailey, P., & Sandberg-Cook, J. (2017). *Primary care: A collaborative practice* (5th ed.). St. Louis, MO: Elsevier.

Centers for Disease Control and Prevention. (n.d.-a). Bed bugs FAQs. Retrieved from https://www.cdc.gov/parasites/bedbugs/faqs.html

Centers for Disease Control and Prevention. (n.d.-b). *Lyme disease.* Retrieved from https://www.cdc.gov/lyme/index.html

Centers for Disease Control and Prevention. (n.d.-c). Shingles (herpes zoster). Retrieved from https://www.cdc.gov/shingles/index.html

Centers for Disease Control and Prevention. (n.d.-d). *The National Institute for Occupational Safety and Health (NIOSH): Skin exposures & effects: Recommendations and resources.* Retrieved from https://www.cdc.gov/niosh/topics/skin/recommendations.html

Centers for Disease Control and Prevention. (2016). *Provider-performed microscopy procedures: A focus on quality practices.* Retrieved from https://www.cdc.gov/clia/docs/15_258020-A_Stang_PPMP_Booklet_FINAL.pdf

Consultant 360. (2012). Skin biopsy techniques: When and how to perform punch biopsy. *Consultant, 52*(6). Retrieved from https://www.consultant360.com/article/skin-biopsy-techniques-when-and-how-perform-punch-biopsy

Czerkasij, V. (2013). Skin of color: A basic outline of unique differences. *The Nurse Practitioner, 38*(5), 34–40. doi:10.1097/01.NPR.0000428813.26762.66

Dahl, M. (2019). Rosacea: Pathogenesis, clinical features, and diagnosis. In A. O. Ofori (Ed.), *UpToDate.* Retrieved from http://www.uptodate.com/contents/rosacea-pathogenesis-clinical-features-and-diagnosis

D'Amico, D., & Barbarito, C. (2016). *Health & physical assessment in nursing* (3rd ed.). Hoboken, NJ: Pearson.

Dalgard, F. J., Gieler, U., Tomas-Aragones, L., Lien, L., Poot, F., Jemec, G., … Kupfer, J. (2015). The psychological burden of skin diseases: A cross-sectional multicenter study among dermatological out-patients in 13 European countries. *The Journal of Investigative Dermatology, 135*(4), 984–991. doi:10.1038/jid.2014.530

Dana-Farber Cancer Institute. (2015). *Melanoma in children and teens.* Retrieved from http://www.danafarberbostonchildrens.org/conditions/solid-tumors/pediatric_melanoma.aspx

Davis, E. C., & Callender, V. D. (2010). A review of acne in ethnic skin: Pathogenesis, clinical manifestations, and management strategies. *The Journal of Clinical and Aesthetic Dermatology, 3*(4), 24–38. Retrieved from http://jcadonline.com/a-review-of-acne-in-ethnic-skin-pathogenesis-clinical-manifestations-and-management-strategies

Dean, P., Bucevska, M., Strahlendorf, C., & Verchere, C. (2017). Pediatric melanoma: A 35-year population-based review. *Plastic and Reconstructive Surgery–Global Open, 5*(3), e1252. doi:10.1097/GOX.0000000000001252

Dodds, A., Chia, A., & Shumack, S. (2014). Actinic keratosis: Rationale and management. *Dermatology Therapy, 4*(1), 11–31. doi:10.1007/s13555-014-0049-y

Drago, F., Ciccarese, G., Rebora, A., Broccolo, F., & Parodi, A. (2016). Pityriasis rosea: A comprehensive classification. *Dermatology, 232*, 431–437. doi:10.1159/000445375

Ely, J. W., Rosenfeld, S., & Stone, M. S. (2014). Diagnosis and management of tinea infections. *American Family Physician, 90*(10), 702–711. Retrieved from https://www.aafp.org/afp/2014/1115/p702.html

Firnhaber, J. M. (2012). Diagnosis and treatment of basal cell and squamous cell carcinoma. *American Family Physician, 86*(2), 161–168. Retrieved from https://www.aafp.org/afp/2012/0715/p161.html

Fogelson, H. (2015, May 27). The 10 best quotes about sun protection. *Summerskin.* Retrieved from https://yoursummerskin.com/blogs/news/75511557-the-10-best-quotes-about-sun-protection

Gonzalez, M. E., & Goodheart, H. P. (2019). Squamous cell carcinoma, cutaneous. In F. J. Domino (Ed.), *The 5-minute clinical consult 2019* (pp. 940–941). Philadelphia, PA: Wolters Kluwer.

Gupta, A. K., Versteeg, S. G., & Shear, N. H. (2017). Onychomycosis in the 21st century: An update on diagnosis, epidemiology, and treatment. *Journal of Cutaneous Medicine and Surgery, 21*(6), 525–539. doi:10.1177/1203475417716362

Habashy, J. (2019). Psoriasis. In W. D. James (Ed.), *Medscape.* Retrieved from https://emedicine.medscape.com/article/1943419-overview

Habif, T. (2010). *Clinical dermatology: A color guide to diagnosis and therapy* (5th ed.). St. Louis, MO: Mosby/Elsevier.

Helm, T. N. (2019). Allergic contact dermatitis. In W. D. James (Ed.), *Medscape.* Retrieved from https://emedicine.medscape.com/article/1049216-overview

Hu, S. W., & Bigby, M. (2010). Pityriasis versicolor: A systematic review of interventions. *Archives of Dermatological, 146*(10), 1132–1140. doi:10.1001/archdermatol.2010.259

John, A. R., & Canaday, D. H. (2017). Herpes zoster in the older adult. *Infectious Disease Clinics of North America, 31*(4), 811–826. doi:10.1016/j.idc.2017.07.016

Johnson, D. (2016). Extremely preterm infant skin care: A transformation of practice aimed to prevent harm. *Advances in Neonatal Care, 16*(Suppl. 5S), S26–S32. doi:10.1097/ANC.0000000000000335

Johnson, M. M., Leachman, S. A., Aspinwall, L. G., Cranmer, L. D., Curiel-Lewandrowski, C., Sondak, V. K., . . . Wong, M. K. (2017). Skin cancer screening: Recommendations for data-driven screening guidelines and a review of the US Preventive Services Task Force controversy. *Melanoma Management, 4*(1), 13–37. doi:10.2217/mmt-2016-0022

Jurica, S., Colic, A., Gveric-Ahmetasevic, S., Loncarevic, D., Filipovic-Grcic, B., Stipanovic-Kastelic, J., . . . Resic, A. (2016). Skin of the very premature newborn—Physiology and care. *Paediatria Croatica, 60,* 21–6. doi:10.13112/pc.2016.4

Kennedy-Malone, L. (2019). Skin and lymphatic disorders. In L. Kennedy-Malone, L. Martin-Plank, & E. Duffy (Eds.), *Advanced practice nursing in the care of older adults* (2nd ed., pp. 96–126). Philadelphia, PA: F.A. Davis Company.

Kundu, R., & Patterson, S. (2013). Dermatologic conditions in skin of color: Part I. Special considerations for common skin disorders. *American Family Physician, 87*(12), 850–856. Retrieved from https://www.aafp.org/afp/2013/0615/p850.html

Laureano, A. C., Schwartz, R. A., & Cohen, P. J. (2014). Facial bacterial infections: Folliculitis. *Clinics in Dermatology, 32*(6), 711–714. doi:10.1016/j.clindermatol.2014.02.009

Lyons, F., & Ousley, L. (2015). *Dermatology for the advanced practice nurse.* New York, NY: Springer Publishing Company.

Marai, M. (2015). *A clinico-pathological investigation of rosacea with particular regard to systemic diseases* (Doctoral dissertation). The University of Leeds School of Medicine, Leeds, UK.

Marghoob, A., Usatine, R., & Jaimes, N. (2013). Dermoscopy for the family physician. *American Family Physician, 88*(7), 441–450. Retrieved from https://www.aafp.org/afp/2013/1001/p441.html

Martin, S. F., Rustemeyer, T., & Thyssen, J. P. (2018). Recent advances in understanding and managing contact dermatitis. *F1000Research, 7,* (F1000 Faculty Rev), 810. doi:10.12688/f1000research.13499.1

Mayo Clinic. (2019). *Skin cancer.* Retrieved from https://www.mayoclinic.org/diseases-conditions/skin-cancer/symptoms-causes/syc-20377605

McCann, S. A., & Huether, S. E. (2019). Structure, function, and disorders of the integument. In V. Brashers & N. Rote (Eds.), *Pathophysiology: The biologic basis for disease in adults and children* (8th ed., pp. 1496–1529). St. Louis, MO: Elsevier.

Menter, A., Strober, B., Kaplan, D., Kivelevitch, D., Prater, E., Stoff, B., . . . Elmets, C. A. (2019). Joint AAD-NPF guidelines of care for the management and treatment of psoriasis with biologics. *Journal of the American Academy of Dermatology, 80*(4), 1029–1072. doi:10.1016/j.jaad.2018.11.057

Muhrer, J. C. (2014). The importance of the history and physical in diagnosis. *The Nurse Practitioner, 39*(4), 30–35. doi:10.1097/01.NPR.0000444648.20444.e6

Needham, M., & Matz, R. (2019). Psoriasis. In F. J. Domino (Ed.), *The 5-minute clinical consult 2019* (pp. 838–839). Philadelphia, PA: Wolters Kluwer.

Oge, L., Muncie, H., & Phillips-Savoy, A. (2015). Rosacea: Diagnosis and treatment. *American Family Physician, 92*(3), 187–196. Retrieved from https://www.aafp.org/afp/2015/0801/p187.html

Oranges, T., Dini, V., & Romanelli, M. (2015). Skin physiology of the neonate and infant: Clinical implications. *Advances in Wound Care, 4*(10), 587–595. doi:10.1089/wound.2015.0642

Phillips, A., Frank, A., Loftin, C., & Shepherd, S. (2017). A details review of systems: An educational feature. *Journal for Nurse Practitioners, 13*(10), 681–686. doi:10.1016/j.nurpra.2017.08.012

Prather, C. (2018). Skin biopsy technique. In D. M. Elston (Ed.), *Medscape.* Retrieved from https://emedicine.medscape.com/article/1997709-technique

Rashid, R. S., & Shim T. N. (2016). Contact dermatitis. *British Medical Journal, 353*(i3299), 1–12. doi:10.1136/bmj.i3299

Schaefer, P. (2017). Acute and chronic urticaria: Evaluation and treatment. *American Family Physician, 95*(11), 717–724. Retrieved from https://www.aafp.org/afp/2017/0601/p717.html

Shenefelt, P. D. (2018). Nongenital warts clinical presentation. In W. D. James (Ed.), *Medscape.* Retrieved from https://emedicine.medscape.com/article/1133317-clinical#showall

Skin Cancer Foundation. (2009). Ask the expert: Is there a skin cancer crisis in people of color? Retrieved from https://skincancer.org/blog/ask-the-expert-is-there-a-skin-cancer-crisis-in-people-of-color

Skin Cancer Foundation. (2018). Ask the expert: Does a high SPF protect my skin better? Retrieved from https://www.skincancer.org/skin-cancer-information/ask-the-experts/does-a-higher-spf-sunscreen-always-protect-your-skin-better

Skin Cancer Foundation. (2019). *Skin cancer facts & statistics.* Retrieved from https://www.skincancer.org/skin-cancer-information/skin-cancer-facts

St. Jude Children's Research Hospital. (n.d.). Melanoma. Retrieved from https://together.stjude.org/en-us/about-pediatric-cancer/types/melanoma.html

Sullivan, T., & de Barra, E. (2018). Diagnosis and management of cellulitis. *Clinical Medicine (London), 18*(2), 160–163. doi:10.7861/clinmedicine.18-2-160

Swartz, M. H. (2010). *Textbook of physical diagnosis: History and examination* (6th ed.). Philadelphia, PA: Saunders/Elsevier.

Tanghetti, E., Kawata, A., Daniels, S., Yeomans, K., Burk, C., & Callender, V. (2014). Understanding the burden of adult female acne. *The Journal of Clinical and Aesthetic Dermatology, 7,* 22–30. Retrieved from https://www.ncbi.nlm.nih.gov/pmc/articles/PMC3935648

Titus, S., & Hodge, J. (2012). Diagnosis and treatment of acne. *American Family Physician, 86*(8), 734–740. Retrieved from https://www.aafp.org/afp/2012/1015/p734.html

U.S. Preventive Services Task Force. (2016). Screening for skin cancer: U.S. Preventive Services Task Force recommendation statement. *The Journal of the American Medical Association, 316*(4), 429–435. doi:10.1001/jama.2016.8465

Visscher, M. O., Adam, R., Brink, S., & Odio, M. (2015). Newborn infant skin: Physiology, development, and care. *Clinics in Dermatology, 33,* 271–280. doi:10.1016/j.clindermatol.2014.12.003

Walsh, A., & Deligiannidis, K. E. (2019). Dermatitis, contact. In F. J. Domino (Ed.), *The 5-minute clinical consult 2019* (pp. 270–271). Philadelphia, PA: Wolters Kluwer.

Wilson, S., & Giddens, J. (2013). *Health assessment for nursing practice* (5th ed.). St. Louis, MO: Mosby|Elsevier.

Wong, H. K. (2018). Urticaria. In D. M. Elston (Ed.), *Medscape.* Retrieved from https://emedicine.medscape.com/article/762917-overview

Zaenglein, A. L., Pathy, A. L., Schlosser, B. J., Alikhan, A., Baldwin, H. E., Berson, D. S., … Bhushan, R. (2016). Guidelines of care for the management of acne vulgaris. *Journal of the American Academy of Dermatology, 74*(5), 945–973. doi:10.1016/j.jaad.2015.12.037

Zito, P., & Scharf, R. (2018). *Cyst, epidermoid (Sebaceous cyst).* Treasure Island, FL: StatPearls [Internet]. Retrieved from https://www.ncbi.nlm.nih.gov/books/NBK499974

10

Evidence-Based Assessment of the Lymphatic System

Kate Gawlik and Alice M. Teall

"Your body can stand almost anything. It is your mind that you have to convince."

—AUTHOR UNKNOWN

LEARNING OBJECTIVES

- Describe the structure and function of the lymphatic tissue (lymph fluid, vessels, ducts, and organs).
- Discuss the cells of the immune system, how they function, and their relationship with the lymphatic system.
- Understand the key components of a comprehensive, evidence-based history and physical exam of the lymphatic system.
- Distinguish between normal and abnormal findings in the lymphatic system.

ANATOMY AND PHYSIOLOGY OF THE LYMPHATIC SYSTEM

The lymphatic system is a complex network of vessels, tissues, and organs. The one-way network of lymphatic vessels regulates and maintains fluid balance, helps large molecules enter the blood, delivers nutrients, removes wastes, and provides an immunological surveillance and defense against infections, abnormal body cells, and foreign proteins. The lymphatic system has a vital supporting role toward both the cardiovascular and the immune systems. Lymph vessels are found in all tissues except the central nervous system and tissues without blood vessels, like the cartilage.

The lymphatic system consists of lymph, lymphatic vessels, lymphatic organs, and lymphocytes. Lymph is a clear fluid made up primarily of lymphocytes. Lymph travels around the body in much the same way as blood travels around the body through the blood vessels. The lymph vessels are as extensive as the vessels of the circulatory system. Lymph flow is constantly circulating. Lymph travels from the major lymphatic vessels to the small lymphatic vessels to the lymphatic capillaries, which are present in almost every tissue in the body and assist in screening out harmful things discovered in the body.

FLUID BALANCE

One of the primary functions of the lymphatic system is to regulate and maintain fluid balance in the body. Every day, 20 L of fluid, water, and protein leak out of the capillaries and become part of interstitial fluid between the cells. Seventeen of those twenty liters gets quickly reabsorbed back into capillaries, leaving approximately 3 L in the tissues. In order to keep the body's interstitial fluid volume and blood volume constant over time, the lymphatic vessels collect the excess interstitial fluid and return it to the blood (**Figure 10.1A**). Once the interstitial fluid is in the lymphatic vessels, it is called lymph. Unlike the circulatory system, the lymphatic system is not a closed loop because fluid and proteins make their way into lymphatic capillaries. Lymphatic capillaries are the smallest lymphatic vessels, and they are located throughout the interstitial space (**Figure 10.1B**). Lymphatic capillaries are extremely permeable because

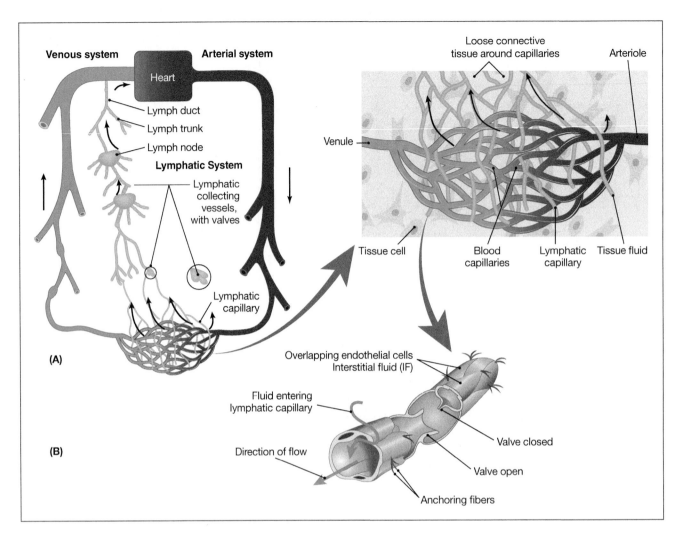

FIGURE 10.1 The lymphatic system. (A) Lymphatic vessels collect excess interstitial fluid and return it to the blood. (B) Lymphatic capillaries.

their walls are made of endothelial cells that loosely overlap, forming one-way mini-valves. When pressure in the interstitial space is greater than in the lymphatic capillary, the endothelial mini-valves open up, allowing fluid to enter. When the pressure in the interstitial space is less than the pressure in the lymphatic capillary, the mini-valves are pushed shut, keeping the lymph fluid inside.

Once the lymph fluid is inside the capillaries, it is deposited into the lymphatic veins, then the lymphatic trunks, and, finally, the lymphatic ducts (**Figure 10.2A**). Smooth muscles in lymph vessels react to the pulsing of nearby arteries by propelling the lymph forward. External pressure from surrounding tissue and skeletal muscle keeps lymph moving along until it has reached a lymphatic trunk. One-way valves in the vessels keep lymph from flowing backward. There are nine lymphatic trunks that drain lymph from a particular area of the body. There are two lumbar, two bronchomediastinal,

two subclavian, two jugular, and one intestinal trunk. Once lymph has filtered through the trunks, it then moves to the ducts. There are only two ducts, a thoracic duct and a right lymphatic duct. The right lymphatic duct is much smaller and collects lymph from the right arm, right head, neck, and chest and dumps it into the right jugular and subclavian vein. The thoracic duct is much larger and collects lymph from the rest of the body. It then dumps the lymph into the left side of body with an entry point of the jugular and subclavian veins. The pressures in the jugular and subclavian veins are low, allowing the lymph tissue to easily enter the circulation (**Figure 10.2B**).

LYMPHATIC ORGANS AND TISSUES

Lymphatic organs are classified into primary and secondary organs (**Figure 10.3**). There are two primary lymphatic organs: the red bone marrow and the thymus

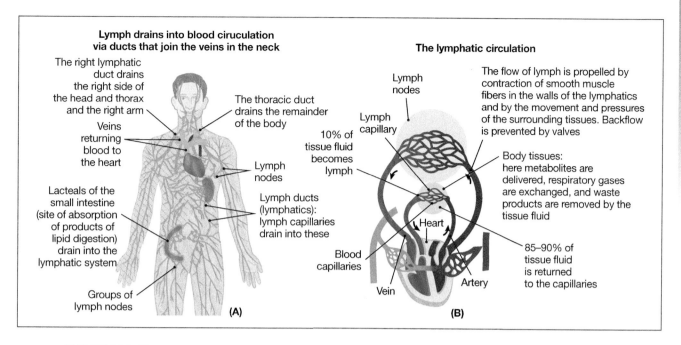

FIGURE 10.2 The role of the lymphatic system. (A) Lymphatic drainage patterns. (B) Lymphatic circulation.

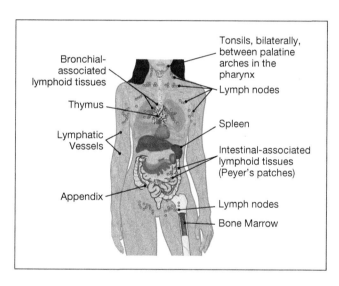

FIGURE 10.3 Lymphatic organs.

gland. The lymphocytes, primarily B and T cells, originate in the bone marrow. B cells mature in the bone marrow, but T cells migrate and mature in the thymus. The thymus is located in the mediastinum, posterior to the sternum. The thymus contains lobules with a cortex (outer region) and medulla (inner region). The thymus is very active in the neonatal and preadolescent years. After puberty, it slowly atrophies and is replaced by fat. Hormones from this gland produce maturation of the T cells.

Secondary lymphatic organs include the lymph nodes, lymphoid tissues, the spleen, the tonsils, and the

appendix. The lymph vessels drain fluid from the tissues and transport it to the lymph nodes. The lymph nodes are collections or gland-like masses of tissue. There are over 600 lymph nodes in the body, most of which are not palpable. Lymph nodes are composed of lymphoid cells and proteins. They are scattered throughout the body but are mostly concentrated in the neck, axillae, and groin, where lymphatic vessels branch. They act as checkpoints for the body and function similar to a kitchen water filter, purifying the lymph before it enters the veins. All substances that are transported through the lymph must pass through at least one lymph node. When lymph nodes are enlarged, they should be classified into generalized lymphadenopathy (more than two involved regions) or localized lymphadenopathy (one region is involved). Generalized lymphadenopathy is more suspicious for systemic illness or malignancy. Localized lymphadenopathy often indicates an infection or disease associated with the region involved according to lymphatic drainage patterns (**Figure 10.4**).

Diffuse lymphoid tissues are loose aggregates of lymphoid tissue with no distinct demarcation from surrounding tissues (**Figure 10.5**). They are found in various submucosal membrane sites of the body, such as the gastrointestinal (GI) tract, oral passage, nasopharyngeal tract, and the lungs. This tissue is also referred to as mucosa-associated lymphoid tissue or MALT. MALT constitutes about 50% to 70% of the lymphoid tissue in the human body. The GI tract has its own lymphoid tissue, which is termed gut-associated lymphoid tissue, or GALT. An example of GALT is Peyer's patches. Peyer's patches are found on the mucosa of the small intestines

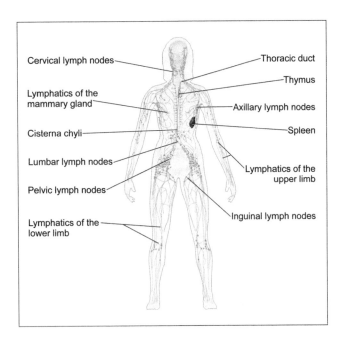

FIGURE 10.4 Lymphatic drainage patterns.

Source: Image courtesy of Bruce Blaus.

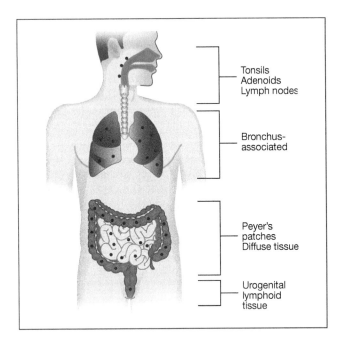

FIGURE 10.5 Mucosa-associated lymphoid tissues (MALT).

and are highly concentrated with B cells. This lymphoid tissue facilitates an immune response when pathogens are detected.

The spleen is an organ that is below the diaphragm on the left side. It lies lateral to the stomach between ribs nine and eleven. It is responsible for the regulation of both innate and adaptive immune homeostasis. The spleen has two areas called pulps. The red pulp is composed of red blood cells (RBC). It keeps RBC and platelets available for release in case of an emergency. The white pulp is like a giant lymph node. Antibody-coated bacteria are filtered out of the body, and antibodies are generated by B cells. The spleen can be removed for various reasons. Although it is not an essential organ for body functioning, more frequent and severe infections can occur in people without a spleen owing to its contribution to immune function.

Two smaller secondary lymphatic organs are the tonsils and the appendix. The tonsils include the adenoid, tubal, palatine, and lingual tonsils. Together, they form a ring of lymphoid tissue around the throat and trap pathogens from food that is ingested and air that is inhaled. The appendix, once thought to be useless in the body, is a finger-shaped pouch that projects from the colon on the lower right side of the abdomen. It is now known that it contains lymphoid tissue similar to tissue found in Peyer's patches, is the primary site for the production of IgA, and serves to stimulate and act as a reservoir for beneficial gut bacteria.

LYMPHOCYTES

There are two main types of lymphocytes found in the body, the B cells and the T cells (**Figure 10.6**). They are made in the bone marrow. The B cells remain in the bone marrow for maturation, whereas the T cells move to the thymus to mature.

The T cells are responsible for cell-mediated immunity. This means the T cells are not based on an antibody response. There are three main functional types of T cells: cytotoxic T cells, also called CD8+ cells; helper T cells, also called CD4+ cells; and T regulatory cells, also called suppressor T cells. Cytotoxic T (CD8+) cells kill target cells. They migrate into areas where infection is present. To be activated, T cells must be exposed to an antigen. They then attack or destroy any foreign bodies that are present. They do this by releasing lysosomes that contain enzymes that destroy the infections. They will only kill cells with antigens that present with a certain molecule. These molecules, called major histocompatibility complex molecules (MHC), are what allow the body to identify friendly cells versus abnormal cells. The molecules will present foreign antigens to T cells. This process flags or signals other cells that there is a problem, and the antigen is tagged as an invader. There are two distinct types of MHC molecules, MHC I and MHC II. The CD8+ cells will bind to class I MHC, and the CD4+ cells will bind to class II MHC.

Helper T cells (CD4+) are like the generals on the battlefield. They secrete cytokines that coordinate the efforts of a variety of immune cells. As noted previously, they only see antigens if they are presented on

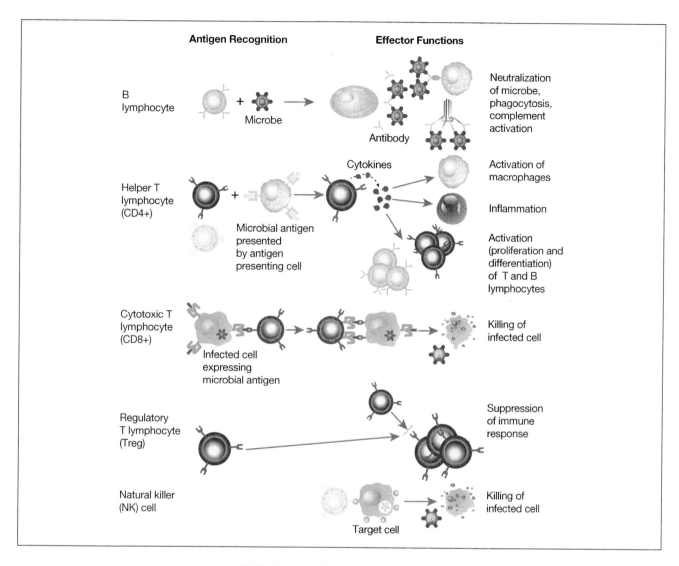

FIGURE 10.6 Classes of lymphocytes.

an MHC II protein. There are four classes of helper T cells, two of which will be discussed here, the Th1 and Th2 cells. These cells are distinguished by the different cytokines they secrete. Th1 cells are cytokine-secreting cells that regulate the immunological activity and the development of a variety of cells, including macrophages and other types of T cells. Th2 cells, on the other hand, secrete cytokines that act on B cells to drive their differentiation into plasma cells that then make antibodies. This is explained in more detail later.

The regulatory T cells (Treg) turn off or suppress other T cell immune responses. Less is known about this subset of T cells. Suggested functions for Treg cells include prevention of autoimmune diseases by maintaining self-tolerance; suppression of allergy, asthma, and pathogen-induced immunopathology; fetomaternal tolerance; and oral tolerance.

The B cells are responsible for antibody-mediated immunity. Antibodies develop when B cells turn into plasma cells. They are activated to turn into plasma cells when they receive a signal from a helper T cell. When the T cell is activated, it helps the B cells turn into a plasma cell. The plasma cell will then divide, differentiate, and start secreting massive amounts of antibodies. This can take a few weeks to peak. Each plasma cell has its own antibody molecules that only react to particular antigens. There is also a type of B cell called a memory B cell. This type of B cell retains a memory on how to make antibodies for particular antigens. Approximately 40% of human B cells in adults are memory B cells. Memory B cells generate a stronger and faster secondary response when compared with the primary B cell response.

There are five different classes of antibodies, also called immunoglobulins (Ig). These antibodies include

TABLE 10.1 Immunoglobulin Functions

Immunoglobulin	Function
IgG	Predominant isotype found in the body; four subclasses; activate effector cells, such as NK cells or monocytes, to destroy the antibody-coated target; activation of the complement cascade; neutralization of toxins and viruses; participation in the secondary immune response; transplacental transport
IgE	Potent immunoglobulin. It is associated with hypersensitivity and allergic reactions as well as the response to parasitic worm infections
IgD	Function remains unclear; can react with specific bacterial proteins
IgM	The first immunoglobulin expressed during B cell development; associated with a primary immune response
IgA	Two subclasses; protecting mucosal surfaces from toxins, virus, and bacteria by direct neutralization or by prevention of binding to the mucosal surface

IgA, immunoglobulin A; IgD, immunoglobulin D; IgE, immunoglobulin E; IgG, immunoglobulin G; IgM, immunoglobulin M; NK, natural killer.

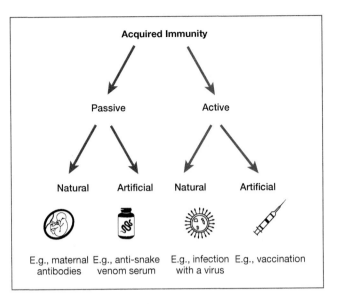

FIGURE 10.7 Acquired immunity: passive and active.

IgG, IgE, IgD, IgM, and IgA. Each antibody type has a different and synergistic function. See **Table 10.1** for associated functions. These antibodies float freely and circulate in the serum. When they identify a specific pathogen that is foreign to the body, they hold onto that antigen so it cannot do further damage in the body. This is called acquired immunity because the cells are primed. This is a specific defense of the immune system.

IMMUNE FUNCTION

In acquired immunity, the cells are primed through the processes already noted. It is a coordinated activity by the T and B cells. There are two types of acquired immunity, passive and active, also referred to as the specific defenses of the immune system (**Figure 10.7**).

Passive immunity is immunity that is produced from the transfer of antibodies from one person to another. For example, naturally occurring passive immunity occurs when babies get antibodies from their mother through both the placenta connection and breast milk. Passive immunity can also be induced. This is where a naive individual is given prepared antibodies via an injection to protect against a recent exposure to some type of disease organism. Protection from passive immunity diminishes in a relatively short time, usually a few weeks or months. Active immunity is naturally acquired. For example, it occurs after an individual is exposed to something in their environment. When pathogenic microorganisms are introduced, it allows antibodies to develop so the body will recognize these microorganisms in the future. Similar to passive immunity, active immunity can also be acquired through vaccines. Vaccines introduce a killed or weakened form of the disease organism, which stimulates the body to build its own immune response.

As part of the immune response, the body also has nonspecific defenses against pathogens. In this case, the immune response is fast and has the same response regardless of what's invading. There is no memory unlike the specific defenses noted previously. Some examples of these nonspecific defenses are physical barriers, phagocytic cells, natural killer (NK) cells, interferons, inflammation, and fever. An example of a physical barrier would be nasal hair. When a person breathes in air, dust and pathogens can get caught in the nasal hair, thereby stopping these foreign bodies from entering the body and the bloodstream. Phagocytic cells, such as monocytes, surround and engulf foreign modules. Another cell type, called the NK cells, is not nearly as specific in regard to whom they kill, unlike the CD8+ and CD4+ cells. NK cells are lymphocytes in the same family as T and B cells, coming from a common progenitor, except they do not need an MHC protein in order to kill a foreign cell. NK cells will kill a person's own body cells that are morphing and becoming abnormal. Interferons are chemicals (peptides/proteins) that make it harder for a virus to spread by making cells in the region where the virus is less susceptible to the virus entering them; regardless of what kind of infections one is exposed to, these secretions will make it more likely that the virus is defeated. Inflammation responds to a pathogen by expanding blood vessels in the affected area so more lymphocytes and white blood cells (WBC) can penetrate the area and get rid of the infection. Lastly, a fever makes it harder for the pathogen to spread owing to the elevated body temperature.

LIFE-SPAN DIFFERENCES AND CONSIDERATIONS IN ANATOMY AND PHYSIOLOGY OF THE LYMPHATIC SYSTEM

Infancy, Childhood, and Adolescence

The innate immune system is subdued at birth, making the newborn, and particularly the premature baby, relatively susceptible to bacterial and viral infections. During the last 3 months of pregnancy, the mother transfers IgG antibodies through the placenta. After birth, these antibodies continue to be transferred through breast milk. Although temporary, these antibodies provide critical protection against many infectious diseases. The type and amount depend on the mother's immunity. Protection starts to decrease weeks to months after birth. The risks to the infant of infectious disease have been greatly reduced by vaccinations. The immune system gradually matures during infancy and childhood. Immunological memory is acquired over time; this is why young adults suffer fewer infections than children.

Older Adults

Immunological memory starts to fade with older age, and the overall immune system starts to experience a decline in function. This puts elderly patients at a higher risk of acquiring acute viral and bacterial infections and having increased severity of symptoms. Mortality from these infections is much higher compared with younger adult patients who acquire the diseases. This immune senescence causes elderly patients to experience diminished efficacy of vaccines and reactivation of latent viruses, such as the varicella-zoster virus. Older adults also begin to have more proinflammatory cytokines circulating, putting them in a chronic inflammatory state. This chronic inflammation leads to the onset or exacerbation of diseases such as cancer, atherosclerosis, and dementia.

KEY HISTORY QUESTIONS AND CONSIDERATIONS FOR THE LYMPHATIC SYSTEM

HISTORY OF PRESENT ILLNESS
Common Presenting Symptoms
- Enlargement of lymph nodes
- Edema of limb (lower legs, feet, hands; peripheral edema)
- Painful, swollen lymph node(s)
- Fever and fatigue
- Infected bite

Example: Enlargement of Lymph Nodes
- Chief concern: Enlargement of lymph nodes (generalized or regional lymphadenopathy)
- Onset: Recent, intermittent, and/or chronic
- Location: One lymph node versus one region of lymph nodes versus multiple regions of lymph nodes, unilateral versus bilateral
- Duration: Increasing in enlargement or intermittent
- Character: Painful, size, mobile, fixed, soft, hard, matted, discrete, erythema, red streaks
- Associated symptoms: Fever, chills, fatigue, night sweats, sore throat, abdominal pain, nausea/vomiting, arthralgias, rashes, recent infection/illness, exposure to cats
- Aggravating factors: Recent illness, stressors, sleep problems
- Relieving symptoms: Pharmacologic treatment, including over-the-counter (OTC) pain relief, nonpharmacologic treatment, including application of heat, cold
- Temporal factors: Enlargement of lymph node in the past, recent or current illness/infection
- Differential diagnoses: MIAMI mnemonic (**M**alignancies, **I**nfections, **A**utoimmune disorders, **M**iscellaneous/Unusual conditions, and **I**atrogenic causes)

Example: Edema of Limb
- Chief concern: Edema of limb
- Onset: Recent, chronic; sudden versus insidious
- Location: Area of the body, unilateral versus bilateral
- Duration: Increasing, persistent, or intermittent
- Character: Pitting, warmth or coolness to touch
- Associated symptoms: Heaviness, skin changes, pain, pain with walking/activity, systemic symptoms, recent illness or injury
- Aggravating factors: Limb dependency, medication history
- Relieving factors: Elevation, diuretics, compression
- Temporal factors: Recent or past illness/infection, surgery, or travel

- Differential diagnoses: (Unilateral) lymphedema, chronic venous insufficiency, deep vein thrombosis, cellulitis, compartment syndrome, iliac vein obstruction; (bilateral) medication induced, lipedema, obstructive sleep apnea, congestive heart failure, pulmonary hypertension, chronic renal or hepatic disease, severe malnutrition or other diseases causing protein loss, cat scratch disease

PAST MEDICAL HISTORY

- Chronic diseases (including cancers, congenital disorders, autoimmune disorders, cardiac disease, renal diseases, HIV)
- Anemia
- Surgeries (including lymph node dissection/removal)
- Blood transfusions
- Radiation therapy
- Recent injury, trauma, or skin infection
- Recent strep throat or mononucleosis
- Allergies
- Allergic reactions
- Chronic venous insufficiency
- Tuberculosis (recent testing)

FAMILY HISTORY

- Cancer
- Infectious disease
- Immune disorders
- Anemia
- Tuberculosis or positive TB reading

SOCIAL HISTORY

- Smoking history/history of tobacco use
- Intravenous (IV) drug use/drug use prescribed, not prescribed
- Recent travel out of the country
- Sleep history
- Sexual history (including risk factors for HIV exposure)
- Animal or food contact
- Exposure to cat feces
- Insect bites
- Stress and coping

REVIEW OF SYSTEMS

- General: Weight loss or gain, fatigue, fever, pain
- Head, Eyes, Ears, Nose, Throat (HEENT): Headache, ear pain, nasal congestion, sinus pain, sore throat
- Cardiovascular/respiratory: Shortness of breath at rest or with exertion, cough, chest pain, orthopnea
- GI/Genitourinary (GU): Abdominal pain, nausea, vomiting, difficulty swallowing, black or tarry stools, dysuria, vaginal/penile discharge, dyspareunia
- Neurologic: Weakness, numbness, dizziness

- Endocrine: Changes to skin, hair; temperature intolerance
- Hematologic: Bruising, bleeding, jaundice, paleness
- Integumentary: Itching, rashes, lesions changing shape, size, or color, nonhealing sores/wounds
- Psychiatric: Depression, sadness, worry, insomnia; changes in memory, concentration, or mood

PREVENTIVE CARE CONSIDERATIONS

- Healthy lifestyle behaviors
- Immunization history, including yearly flu vaccination
- Regular handwashing
- Proper food handling and cooking
- Washing of fruits and vegetables
- Consumption of raw or unpasteurized foods/drinks

Unique Population Considerations for History

Individuals with weakened immune systems are very susceptible to infections. Weakened immune systems can occur with a variety of illnesses, including cancer, hyposplenia, and asplenia. Certain medications, including chemotherapy, tumor necrosis factor (TNF) inhibitors, and corticosteroids, can also weaken the immune system, making an individual more likely to experience severe and frequent infections. As a component of their assessment, ask individuals who are immunocompromised about the precautions being taken to prevent infection, including handwashing, safe food handling and storage, limiting exposure to environmental toxins, handling animals safely, practicing safe sex, and taking extra care when traveling.

PHYSICAL EXAMINATION

INSPECTION

The clinician should start the lymphatics exam as they would any exam. Conduct a general survey, and note the patient's vital signs. A height, weight, and body mass calculation should be completed and compared with previous visits, if possible, to help identify any signs of chronic disease or weight loss. This is especially important to note with children as it can signify poor growth or failure to thrive. A complete visual inspection, including axillae and groin, should take place at the beginning of the exam. Lymph nodes and lymphatic organs should never be visible on inspection. If a lymph node or the spleen is visible in an adult, this is cause for concern and requires further investigation and a clinical work-up. Note any edema, as well as redness, including erythematous lines along nodal tracks, lesions/rashes, or indications of trauma on the skin. Note any areas of localized edema in the limbs.

PALPATION

When palpating for the lymph nodes, it is important to remember what part of the body a particular lymph node drains into so the clinician can also examine this particular area to look for local signs of infection or abnormality. Seventy-five percent of all peripheral lymphadenopathy are localized to one area; over half of these cases involve lymph nodes in the head and neck, 1% involve the supraclavicular lymph nodes, 5% involve the axillary nodes, and 14% involve the inguinal nodes. The location of the lymphadenopathy needs to be taken into consideration when conducting the exam. If there is concern for a throat infection, palpation of the lymph nodes in the head and neck should be a priority. If there is concern for a GU infection, palpation to detect enlargement of lymph nodes in the inguinal region would be most appropriate. With certain chief concerns and conditions, the clinician would want to palpate the lymph nodes in all regions to look for generalized lymphadenopathy.

When palpating for lymph nodes, the hands should be clean, dry, and warm, and fingernails should be short. The clinician's fingers should be placed firmly in alignment and against one another to provide a large surface area and better coverage for detection of enlargement or abnormalities. The pads of the fingers should be used for palpation (**Figure 10.8**). Palpation should be completed using a fluid, circular motion. Soft palpation should be followed by a deeper palpation in order to feel for any hidden enlargement. Too much pressure can cause a mobile lymph node to move out of the clinician's line of palpation. Care should be taken to ensure the entire surface area of the lymphatic region is palpated.

BOX 10.1
LYMPH NODE CHARACTERISTIC RED FLAGS THAT REQUIRE FURTHER INVESTIGATION
Hard
Fixed
Matted
>1 cm in size
Located in supraclavicular, infraclavicular, iliac, popliteal, or epitrochlear regions
Generalized
Unilateral
Associated with systemic symptoms of weight loss, fever, and/or night sweats

If a lymph node is palpated, the clinician should note the size, consistency, discreteness, mobility, tenderness, warmth, and border edges of the lymph node. It is also important to palpate the surrounding tissues since lymph nodes are often found in chains. Lymph nodes can also adhere to one another (termed matted) so they can appear as a large lump. Shotty lymph nodes are a clustering of multiple, small, contiguous lymph nodes that are often benign and associated with a recent viral infection. The description of lymph nodes as "shotty" refers to their similarity to "buckshot or pellets" that are also small, hard, and round.

Lymph nodes greater than 1 cm in diameter, or about the size of the top of the fifth finger (pinkie), are considered to be abnormal. Any palpable supraclavicular, infraclavicular, iliac, epitrochlear, or popliteal lymph nodes should be considered abnormal, regardless of size. Hard, matted, fixed, nontender, or irregular lymph node(s) are more suspicious for pathogenicity and require further investigation into the etiology. See **Box 10.1** for other red flags.

Lymph Nodes of the Head and Neck Region (Figure 10.9)

Cervical lymph nodes are more often enlarged than other lymphatic regions. To be thorough in examining the superficial cervical nodes, ask the individual to remove all clothing from the regions of the head, neck, and upper shoulders. The approach should be systematic. When palpating the head and neck, start by asking

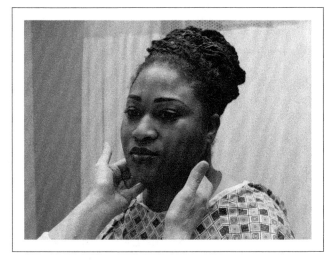

FIGURE 10.8 Proper hand placement for palpation of anterior cervical lymph nodes.

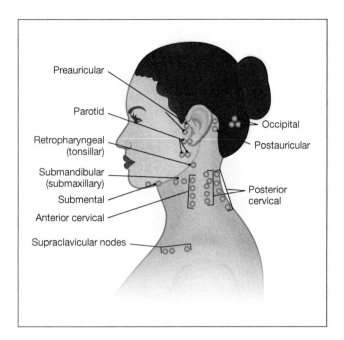

FIGURE 10.9 Lymph nodes of the head and neck.

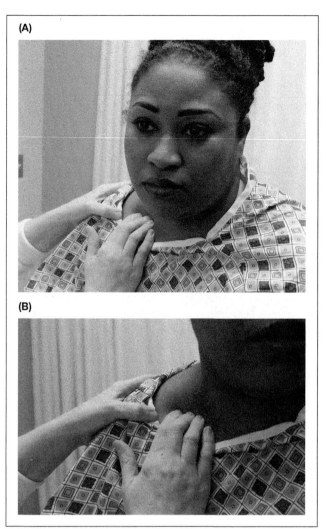

FIGURE 10.11 Palpation of supraclavicular lymph nodes.

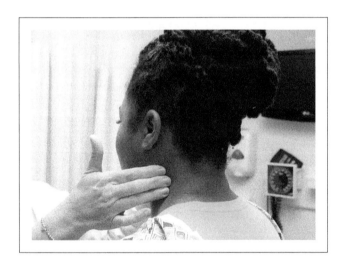

FIGURE 10.10 Palpation of the posterior cervical lymph node chain.

the patient to tilt the head slightly down and relax the neck and shoulder muscles. Using both hands, palpate the occipital and posterior cervical lymph nodes (**Figure 10.10**). Have the patient return their neck to its upright position and ask the patient to raise their chin. Palpate the submental, submandibular, retropharyngeal, tonsillar, preauricular, postauricular, and anterior cervical lymph nodes. Ask the patient to move their shoulders slightly forward, and palpate the supraclavicular fossa for supraclavicular lymph nodes

(**Figure 10.11**). Then palpate below the clavicles to feel for any infraclavicular lymph nodes. Evaluate for symmetry. Clinically significant lymph nodes often present asymmetrically (**Figure 10.12**).

Lymph Nodes of the Axillary Region (Figure 10.13)

When palpating the axilla, make sure clothing has been removed from the area. It is best to have the patient lie supine and raise their arm over their head (**Figure 10.14**). Axillary palpation can occur with the patient sitting in an upright position, but this method can be limiting, both for visual inspection and for palpation. If the clinician is doing axillary palpation with the patient in a seated position, raise the patient's arm slightly to the side, and use the other hand to palpate the axilla (**Figure 10.15**). Use the same circular motion, and ensure the entire surface has been palpated; then move the hand slowly down toward the elbow until the epitrochlear notch has been located (**Figure 10.16**).

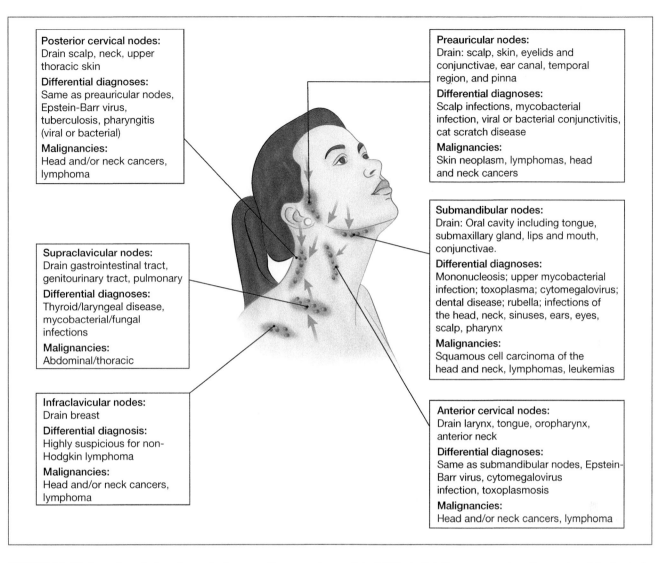

Posterior cervical nodes:
Drain scalp, neck, upper thoracic skin
Differential diagnoses:
Same as preauricular nodes, Epstein-Barr virus, tuberculosis, pharyngitis (viral or bacterial)
Malignancies:
Head and/or neck cancers, lymphoma

Preauricular nodes:
Drain: scalp, skin, eyelids and conjunctivae, ear canal, temporal region, and pinna
Differential diagnoses:
Scalp infections, mycobacterial infection, viral or bacterial conjunctivitis, cat scratch disease
Malignancies:
Skin neoplasm, lymphomas, head and neck cancers

Supraclavicular nodes:
Drain gastrointestinal tract, genitourinary tract, pulmonary
Differential diagnoses:
Thyroid/laryngeal disease, mycobacterial/fungal infections
Malignancies:
Abdominal/thoracic

Submandibular nodes:
Drain: Oral cavity including tongue, submaxillary gland, lips and mouth, conjunctivae.
Differential diagnoses:
Mononucleosis; upper mycobacterial infection; toxoplasma; cytomegalovirus; dental disease; rubella; infections of the head, neck, sinuses, ears, eyes, scalp, pharynx
Malignancies:
Squamous cell carcinoma of the head and neck, lymphomas, leukemias

Infraclavicular nodes:
Drain breast
Differential diagnosis:
Highly suspicious for non-Hodgkin lymphoma
Malignancies:
Head and/or neck cancers, lymphoma

Anterior cervical nodes:
Drain larynx, tongue, oropharynx, anterior neck
Differential diagnoses:
Same as submandibular nodes, Epstein-Barr virus, cytomegalovirus infection, toxoplasmosis
Malignancies:
Head and/or neck cancers, lymphoma

FIGURE 10.12 Lymph node locations, drainage patterns, and associated differential diagnoses and malignancies: (clockwise) preauricular, submandibular, anterior cervical, infraclavicular, supraclavicular, posterior cervical, and preauricular.

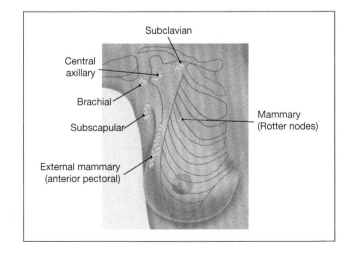

Subclavian
Central axillary
Brachial
Subscapular
External mammary (anterior pectoral)
Mammary (Rotter nodes)

FIGURE 10.13 Axillary lymph nodes.

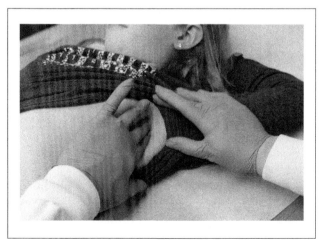

FIGURE 10.14 Palpation of axillary lymph nodes in supine position.

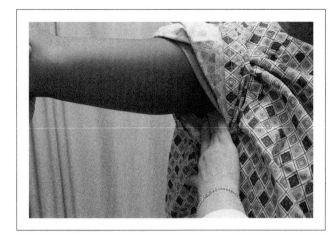

FIGURE 10.15 Palpation of axillary lymph nodes in sitting position.

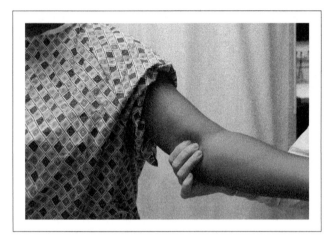

FIGURE 10.16 Palpation of epitrochlear lymph node.

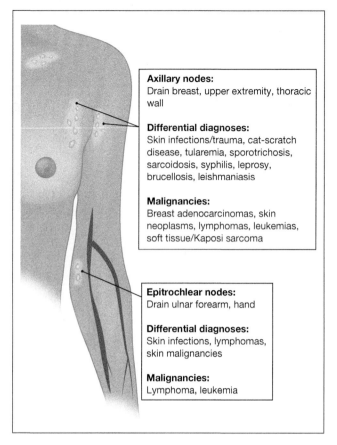

Axillary nodes:
Drain breast, upper extremity, thoracic wall

Differential diagnoses:
Skin infections/trauma, cat-scratch disease, tularemia, sporotrichosis, sarcoidosis, syphilis, leprosy, brucellosis, leishmaniasis

Malignancies:
Breast adenocarcinomas, skin neoplasms, lymphomas, leukemias, soft tissue/Kaposi sarcoma

Epitrochlear nodes:
Drain ulnar forearm, hand

Differential diagnoses:
Skin infections, lymphomas, skin malignancies

Malignancies:
Lymphoma, leukemia

FIGURE 10.17 Lymph node locations, drainage patterns, and associated differential diagnoses and malignancies: axillary and epitrochlear.

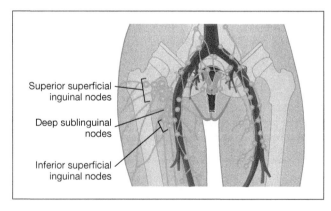

Superior superficial inguinal nodes

Deep sublinguinal nodes

Inferior superficial inguinal nodes

FIGURE 10.18 Inguinal lymph nodes.

The epitrochlear nodes are found on the medial aspect of the elbow, about 4 to 5 cm above the humeral epitrochlea. Repeat on the other side. See **Figure 10.17** for clinically significant lymph nodes.

Lymph Nodes of the Inguinal Region (Figure 10.18)

When palpating for inguinal lymph nodes, have the patient lie supine. Remove all clothing from the area, but maintain a modest environment for the patient by keeping them covered before and after the exam. Locate the iliac crest. The clinician should move their hand toward midline, and then palpate downward in a diagonal line, remaining parallel to the crease separating the upper thigh from the abdomen (**Figure 10.19**). Be sure to cover the entire region using a firm, circular motion. With the patient already lying supine, this is a good opportunity to palpate for the spleen if needed. See **Figure 10.20** for clinically significant lymph nodes.

Life-Span Considerations for Physical Examination of the Lymphatic System

Infancy and Childhood

Palpable lymph nodes in children are common. Roughly 50% of healthy children have palpable lymph nodes at any one time that are either benign or infectious in

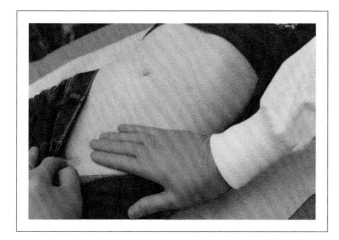

FIGURE 10.19 Palpation of inguinal lymph nodes with the patient in supine position.

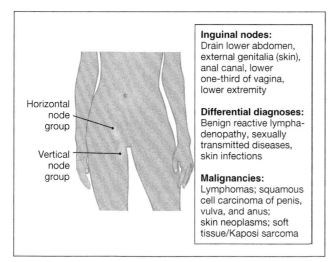

Inguinal nodes:
Drain lower abdomen, external genitalia (skin), anal canal, lower one-third of vagina, lower extremity

Differential diagnoses:
Benign reactive lymphadenopathy, sexually transmitted diseases, skin infections

Malignancies:
Lymphomas; squamous cell carcinoma of penis, vulva, and anus; skin neoplasms; soft tissue/Kaposi sarcoma

Horizontal node group

Vertical node group

FIGURE 10.20 Inguinal lymph node locations, drainage patterns, and associated differential diagnoses and malignancies.

etiology; up to 90% of children aged 4 to 8 have palpable cervical lymph nodes. The lymphadenopathy is typically self-limiting and does not require further work-up or treatment. Similar to adults, both large and supraclavicular lymph nodes in children need further investigation especially in the presence of systemic symptoms.

Malformations of the lymphatic system may present at birth, during infancy, or during childhood. These malformations are also referred to as lymphangiomas or cystic hygromas. Most lymphatic malformations are identified before the age of 2. They most commonly occur in the head and neck regions. The presentation can vary drastically in the associated severity of symptoms and complications based on the location and extent of

the malformation. Some present as a tiny blue or red spot, while others can affect an entire limb. Some diagnoses occur during the prenatal ultrasound, while others may need an ultrasound, MRI, or computed tomography (CT) scan for diagnosis when the child is older.

LABORATORY CONSIDERATIONS FOR THE LYMPHATIC SYSTEM

The complete blood count (CBC) is a blood test commonly used to look at immune system function. CBC testing measures the cells that circulate in the blood and provides information about RBC, WBC, and platelets. The WBC count with differential provides a percentage of each type of WBC. Only mature cells should be circulating in the blood. An elevation or depression of the WBC count can indicate pathology and provide evidence or clues to support a clinical diagnosis. The CBC with differential is commonly used to provide information on infections, inflammatory processes, bone marrow alterations, and immune disorders.

Other laboratory tests to consider when evaluating immune function and lymphadenopathy include a chemistry panel; tests to evaluate for specific infections (e.g., chest x-ray, urinalysis); erythrocyte sedimentation rate (ESR); and/or C-reactive protein (CRP).

More specific tests, such as bone marrow biopsy, HIV antibody test, peripheral blood smear, or a fine needle aspiration biopsy, are often necessary for definitive diagnosis and are components of individualized (and often specialized) patient management.

IMAGING CONSIDERATIONS FOR THE LYMPHATIC SYSTEM

When the diagnosis of lymphadenopathy is thought to be a more severe diagnosis (cancer metastasis versus mononucleosis), accurate assessment is imperative. In studies comparing lymph node palpation with ultrasonography, ultrasonography is superior and is the recommended choice. The sensitivity of lymph node palpation ranged from 23.1% to 85.4%, whereas ultrasonography's sensitivity ranged from 87.5% to 99.1%. Specificity ranged from 63.2% to 99.7% for palpation and 96.8% to 99.7% for ultrasonography.

Ultrasound, Doppler, CT, or MRI may be used to distinguish lymph nodes from other surrounding structures or identify other pathological processes such as malignancies. Special imaging tests may be required to rule out or rule in specific diagnoses. For example, if an older woman presents with axillary lymphadenopathy, a mammogram, ultrasound or breast MRI may be indicated. The most appropriate imaging modality will be used on the basis of the specific characteristics of the lymph node enlargement, location of the lymph node, individualized patient needs, and current evidence.

Lymphoscintigraphy is another imaging test used when looking specifically at the lymphatic system (**Figure 10.21**). It is used to determine lymphatic malformations and lymph drainage patterns and reveal relevant primary and subsequent lymphatic basins. This imaging test is most commonly used to locate the sentinel node for biopsy to determine whether a patient's cancer has spread. If cancer cells have not spread to the sentinel node, there is a high likelihood that subsequent lymph nodes will also be negative for malignancy. Lymphoscintigraphy consists of a radioisotope being injected into the patient followed by dynamic imaging. This allows for the sentinel node's location to then be marked for the surgeon who will perform the biopsy. Lymphoscintigraphy is also a sensitive and specific test used to confirm diagnosis of lymphedema when uncertainty exists.

ABNORMAL FINDINGS OF THE LYMPHATIC SYSTEM

CAT SCRATCH DISEASE (FEVER)

Cat scratch disease is a bacterial infection caused from the organism *Bartonella henselae*. Cats typically acquire the bacteria from fleas or flea dirt (droppings). The way the disease spreads to the human is when an infected cat licks a person's open wound or bites or scratches hard enough to break the surface of the skin.

Key History and Physical Findings

- Erythema, edema, and/or purulent discharge at the site of the bite or scratch
- Fever
- Headache
- Anorexia
- Persistent regional lymphadenopathy (if bite is on arm, axillary lymphadenopathy, etc.)
- Positive *Bartonella henselae* immunofluorescence assay (IFA) blood test

HIV/AIDS

Human immunodeficiency virus (HIV) is a virus that enters the body and invades helper T cells (**Figure 10.22**). It is a retrovirus, meaning it is a type of virus that integrates its viral DNA into the DNA of the host cell by converting its RNA to DNA. HIV destroys the T cells, making it hard for the body to fight infection or infection-related cancers. If left untreated, HIV can lead to acquired immunodeficiency syndrome (AIDS). By the time an individual has progressed to AIDS, the immune system is so weak that opportunistic infections and cancers easily develop.

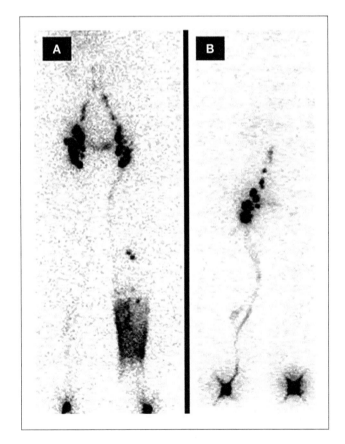

FIGURE 10.21 Sample lymphoscintigraphy image.
Source: Image courtesy of Ekim H.

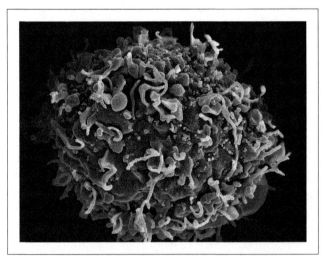

FIGURE 10.22 HIV (yellow) infecting a human cell.
Source: Seth Pincus, Elizabeth Fischer, and Austin Athman, National Institute of Allergy and Infectious Diseases, National Institutes of Health.

Key History and Physical Findings

Stage 1 – Acute HIV Infection:
- High-risk sexual activity (multiple partners, unprotected sexual activity, prostitution, anal intercourse, sexual activity with an HIV-infected individual or IV drug user)
- IV drug use (exposure to contaminated needles or syringes, sexual activity with IV drug users)
- Flulike symptoms within 2 to 4 weeks after infection
- Fever, chills, lymphadenopathy, fatigue, myalgias, night sweats, sore throat
- Some individuals are asymptomatic
- High-risk period for transmission to other people
- Positive HIV test (will not be positive for 3 to 12 weeks after initial exposure)

Stage 2 – Chronic HIV Infection (Clinical Latency; Can Last Up to 10 Years):
- Often asymptomatic
- Lasts an average of 10 years

Stage 3 – AIDS (Late Stage):
- Rapid weight loss
- Lymphadenopathy
- Chronic diarrhea
- Mouth, anus, and/or genital sores
- Night sweats
- Opportunistic infections (pneumonia, tuberculosis, etc.)
- Cancers (Kaposi's sarcoma, cervical cancer; **Figure 10.23**)
- Memory loss, depression, and other neurologic disorders
- Decreasing CD4+ lymphocytes and increasing viral load levels (CD4+ count is <200 cells/mm^3)

LYMPHANGITIS

Lymphangitis is an inflammation or infection of the lymphatic vessels that commonly develops after cutaneous inoculation of microorganisms into the lymphatic vessels through a wound in the skin. It can also occur as a complication of a distal infection. It most often results from an acute streptococcal or staphylococcal infection of the skin.

Key History and Physical Findings
- Fever, malaise
- Enlarged lymph nodes (often in the axillae, groin, or epitrochlear regions)
- Abrasion, wound, or coexisting infection (cellulitis) of the skin
- Red streaking extending proximally from a wound or site of infection toward regional lymph nodes **(Figure 10.24)**
- Leukocytosis

LYMPHADENITIS

Lymphadenitis is inflammation or infection of one or more lymph nodes. It most often results from an acute streptococcal or staphylococcal infection. Pain and tenderness typically distinguish lymphadenitis from lymphadenopathy.

Key History and Physical Findings
- Often unilateral
- Lymph node enlargement
- Pain/tenderness in lymph node
- Lymph node filled with exudate
- Can have erythema or red streaking over lymph nodes
- Fever, malaise

LYMPHEDEMA

Lymphedema is edema or enlargement due to localized lymphatic fluid retention. It generally occurs in a single limb (arm or leg). It can be primary or secondary in origin. Primary lymphedema is due to a

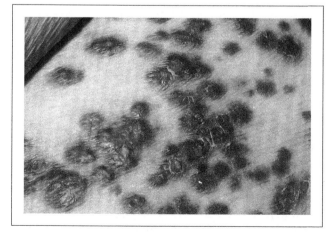

FIGURE 10.23 Kaposi's sarcoma lesions on the skin of an AIDS patient.
Source: National Cancer Institute.

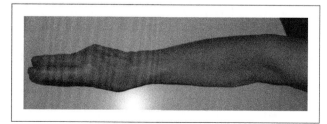

FIGURE 10.24 Lymphangitis. Red streak extending proximally from site of infection on second finger to lymph nodes.
Source: Image courtesy of Jmarchn.

TABLE 10.2 International Society of Lymphology Lymphedema Staging Criteria

Stage	Description
0	Latent stage; there is lymphatic dysfunction and transport but no signs or symptoms. May exist months to years before progression.
1	Early accumulation of fluid with possible pitting in the early stage. Will improve with limb elevation.
2	Tissue fibrosis occurs. Limb elevation does not improve swelling. May or may not pit.
3	Lymphostatic elephantiasis is present with significant skin changes (e.g., thickened skin, deposition of further fibrosis and fat deposits, acanthosis, and warty overgrowths). Pitting is absent.

Source: International Society of Lymphology. (2016). The diagnosis and treatment of peripheral lymphedema: 2016 consensus document of the International Society of Lymphology. *Lymphology, 49,* 170–184. Retrieved from https://journals.uair.arizona.edu/index.php/lymph/article/view/20106/19734

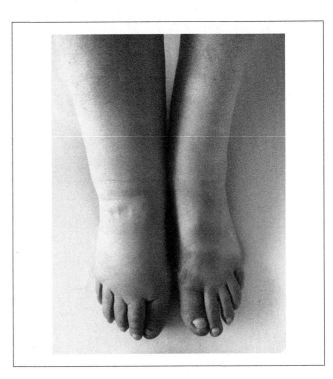

FIGURE 10.25 Lymphedema.
Source: Image courtesy of Abdullah Sarhan.

TABLE 10.3 International Society of Lymphology Functional Severity Assessment

Classification	Volume Difference
Minimal	>5 to <20% increase in limb volume
Moderate	20%–40% increase in limb volume
Severe	>40% increase in limb volume

Source: International Society of Lymphology. (2016). The diagnosis and treatment of peripheral lymphedema: 2016 consensus document of the International Society of Lymphology. *Lymphology, 49,* 170–184. Retrieved from https://journals.uair.arizona.edu/index.php/lymph/article/view/20106/19734

congenital malformation or dysfunction of the lymphatic system. Secondary lymphedema is an acquired condition due to injury, removal, or damage to the lymphatic vessels from surgery, radiation, infection, malignancy, or lymph node dissection. Symptoms can vary from mild to severe, depending on the extent of damage and fluid retention. See **Table 10.2** for staging and **Table 10.3** for functional severity assessment criteria.

Key History and Physical Findings

- Swelling of part or all of the arm or leg, including fingers or toes (**Figure 10.25**)

- A feeling of heaviness, fullness, or tightness in the affected area
- Restricted range of motion and decreased flexibility in nearby joints
- Aching, tingling, or discomfort in the affected area
- Recurring infections
- Changes in skin texture or appearance, such as tightness, redness, or hardening
- Noticeably tighter clothing or jewelry in the affected area
- May or may not pit
- Diuretics do not improve the swelling
- Elevation of the limb may improve swelling in the early stages but not as the condition progresses.

LYMPHATIC FILARIASIS (ELEPHANTIASIS)

Lymphatic filariasis is a parasitic disease that is transmitted through mosquitos. Infected mosquitos deposit mature parasite larvae onto the skin of people they bite, providing an entry for the parasite into the body. The larvae migrate to the lymphatic system and mature into adult nematodes (roundworms). The adult roundworms embed themselves in the lymphatic vessels and produce millions of microscopic worms. The worms impair the normal function of the lymphatic system, causing edema and impaired immune function. *Wuchereria bancrofti* is responsible for 90% of cases.

Key History and Physical Findings

- Travel to endemic areas: Asia, Africa, the Western Pacific, Haiti, the Dominican Republic, Brazil, Guyana, and parts of the Caribbean
- Can be asymptomatic and never develop symptoms
- Gross edema of an entire limb or body area (most commonly affects the legs but can occur in arms, breasts, vulva, or scrotum; **Figure 10.26**)
- Hardening and thickening of the skin in the affected extremity
- Increased infections in the skin and lymph systems
- Elevated levels of antifilarial IgG$_4$ in serum
- Microfilariae in a blood smear by microscopic examination

LYMPHOMA

Lymphoma is a form of cancer that originates in the lymphatic system. The two main types are Hodgkin lymphoma and non-Hodgkin lymphoma (NHL), although many different subtypes exist. In lymphomas, tumors develop from the T cells or B cells.

Key History and Physical Findings

- Family history of lymphoma
- Personal history of the Epstein-Barr Virus (EBV)
- Generalized, painless lymphadenopathy (with the exception of the inguinal region)
- Fatigue
- Fever
- Night sweats
- Unexplained weight loss

- Severe pruritus
- Chest or abdominal pain

MONONUCLEOSIS

Mononucleosis (or Mono) is a contagious illness caused by the EBV. The EBV invades the body's B cells and is spread through saliva. It is most common in children and young adults. Children typically do not have it as a dramatic presentation, so it is often missed. Most people will get mononucleosis at some point in their life.

Key History and Physical Findings

- Fever (children may not have)
- Anterior/posterior cervical lymphadenopathy (other lymph nodes can be enlarged as well)
- Severe pharyngitis
- White exudate on posterior pharynx and tonsillar area (**Figure 10.27**)
- Swollen uvula
- Extreme fatigue (can last for months)
- Petechiae on the soft and hard palates
- Evanescent nonpruritic maculopapular rash (often occurs early in the illness)
- Headaches
- Myalgias
- Palpebral edema (**Figure 10.28**)
- Splenomegaly (50% of cases)
- Hepatomegaly (10% of cases)
- Jaundice (5% of cases)
- Elevated liver enzymes
- Positive mononucleosis spot blood test

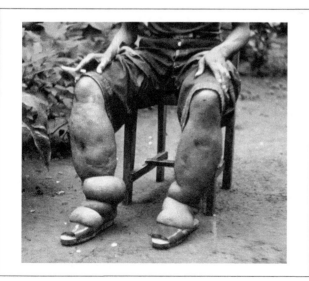

FIGURE 10.26 Lymphatic filariasis (elephantiasis) that manifested in severed edema of lower legs.
Source: Centers for Disease Control and Prevention.

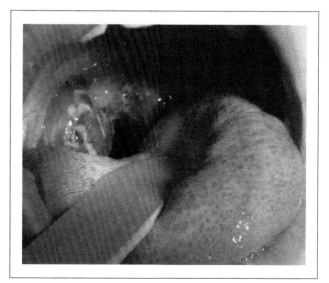

FIGURE 10.27 Tonsillar exudate seen in a patient with mononucleosis.
Source: Image courtesy of James Heilman, MD.

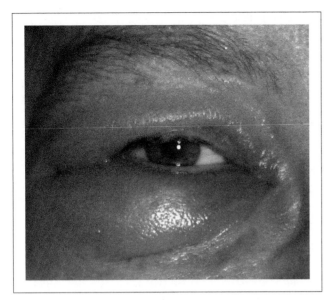

FIGURE 10.28 Palpebral edema.
Source: Image courtesy of Klaus, P. D.

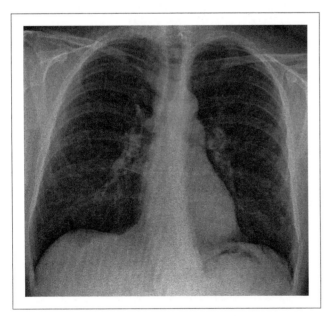

FIGURE 10.29 Sarcoidosis of the lung.

SARCOIDOSIS

Sarcoidosis is an inflammatory disease in which granulomas develop and form in organs of the body, most commonly the lung, lymph nodes, eyes, and skin (**Figure 10.29**). Granulomas are tiny pockets of inflammatory cells. When granulomas are present in a particular organ, it does not function as efficiently and can cause long-term complications depending on the extent of disease present. The cause of sarcoidosis remains unknown.

Key History and Physical Findings

- Weight loss
- Fatigue
- Night sweats
- Fever
- Shortness of breath, wheezing, or dry cough (if lungs are affected)
- Persistent regional or generalized lymphadenopathy (if the lymph nodes are affected)
- Painful and tender bumps or ulcers (if the skin is affected)
- Burning, itching, tearing, erythema, dryness, photophobia, or blurry vision (if the eyes are affected)

TOXOPLASMOSIS

Toxoplasmosis is a disease caused from a parasite called *Toxoplasmosis gondii*. The infection is typically transmitted when eating contaminated meat or shellfish, drinking contaminated water, accidentally consuming the parasite after contact with cat feces or coming into contact with contaminated soil, and through congenital transmission.

Key History and Physical Findings

- Often asymptomatic
- Generalized lymphadenopathy
- Myalgias

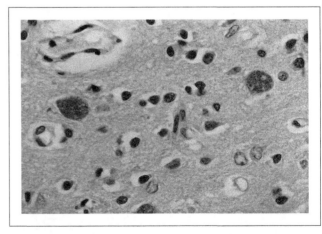

FIGURE 10.30 Toxoplasmosis. Photomicrograph of a brain tissue sample reveals some of the cytoarchitectural details associated with a case of neurotoxoplasmosis. *T. gondii* organisms are visible in the field of view.
Source: Jonathan W.M. Gold, M.D./Centers for Disease Control and Prevention.

- Fatigue
- Severe cases can affect the brain, eyes, or other organs causing such complications as reduced vision, blurred vision, and eye pain

- Positive IFA and enzyme immunoassay (EIA) tests for IgG and IgM antibodies
- Observation of parasites in patient specimens **(Figure 10.30)**

CASE STUDY: Fever, Sore Throat, Fatigue, and Lymphadenopathy

History

A previously healthy 17-year-old female presents to her primary care office owing to fever, sore throat, fatigue, and cervical lymphadenopathy. Symptoms started 5 days ago and have been increasingly worse. Has been taking ibuprofen 200 mg every 6 to 8 hours, which she states improves the fever and sore throat. She rates her current pain as 8/10. She reports her brother had similar symptoms about 1 month ago. She denies weight loss, night sweats, other sites of lymph node enlargement, cough, rhinorrhea, abdominal pain, diarrhea, constipation, or rash. She has allergic rhinitis and takes Loratadine 10 mg PO daily. She has no drug allergies. She had a tonsillectomy at age 8. She has no significant family history. She denies smoking, recent travel, exposure to cats, or IV drug use. She is not sexually active and denies ever having intercourse. She is a high school student who is currently running track. She has had to miss practice owing to illness.

Physical Examination

She appears ill. Her temperature is 101.8°F (38.7°C). Her pulse is 93 and respirations are 18. Her weight is stable based on her previous visit. On physical examination, the clinician finds anterior cervical, posterior cervical, and axillary lymphadenopathy. Lymph nodes are bilateral, soft, mobile, and tender to palpation. Size of lymph nodes is estimated at 8 to 10 mm. She has no other superficial lymphadenopathy or splenomegaly on examination. Her posterior pharynx is erythematous without exudate. Tonsils are surgically removed. Her skin is clean, dry, and intact without any rashes, abrasions, or signs of infections. Heart rate and rhythm are regular, and lungs are clear to auscultation bilaterally.

Differential Diagnoses

Mononucleosis, strep pharyngitis, acute viral pharyngitis

Laboratory and Imaging

A rapid strep and mono spot test were completed in the office. The rapid strep was negative, and the mono spot test was positive.

Final Diagnosis

Mononucleosis

CASE STUDY: Flu-Like Symptoms

History

A previously healthy 25-year-old female presents to her primary care office with flu-like symptoms (fever, myalgias, fatigue) and left-sided lymphadenopathy of the supraclavicular and anterior cervical regions of the neck. She denies weight loss, night sweats, or other sites of lymph node enlargement. She has no significant personal or family medical history. She denies ever having mononucleosis. She does not take any medications and does not have any drug allergies. She denies recent infection. She denies smoking, recent travel, unprotected intercourse,

or IV drug use. She does have an indoor cat and changes the litter box.

Physical Examination

She appears tired but alert and oriented × 3. Her temperature is 99.4°F (37.4°C). Her pulse is 87 and respirations are 16. Her weight is stable based on her previous visit. On physical examination, the clinician finds several fixed lymph nodes of hard consistency in the left anterior cervical and supraclavicular regions. Size of lymph nodes is estimated at 2.5 cm and are nontender to palpation.

(continued)

CASE STUDY: Flu-Like Symptoms (*continued*)

She has no other superficial lymphadenopathy or splenomegaly on examination. Her posterior pharynx is nonerythematous. Tonsils are 0+ without exudate. Heart rate and rhythm are regular, and lungs are clear to auscultation bilaterally. Her skin is clean, dry, and intact without any rashes, abrasions, or signs of infections.

Differential Diagnoses

Hodgkin lymphoma, non-Hodgkin lymphoma, mononucleosis, HIV, toxoplasmosis

Laboratory and Imaging

The following laboratory tests were ordered: CBC with differential, protein electrophoresis; lactate dehydrogenase (LDH); comprehensive metabolic panel; protein electrophoresis; serology tests for EBV, toxoplasmosis, HIV, and ESR; and CRP inflammatory tests. All labs were insignificant except for an increased ESR and CRP as well as a neutrophilic leukocytosis of approximately 14,000 leukocytes per microliter.

A chest x-ray and neck ultrasound were also ordered. The neck ultrasound confirmed the left supraclavicular lymphadenopathy (2.3 × 1.2 cm) of the neck, with pathological aspects that were consistent with a lymphoproliferative disorder. The chest x-ray showed a left mediastinal enlargement.

Subsequent chest CT scan revealed enlarged lymph nodes in the left supraclavicular and cervical regions, in the upper mediastinum, including paratracheal prevascular, subcarinal, bilateral lung hilum sites, and bilaterally in the axillae.

Final Diagnosis

Lymph node biopsy and histological examination led to the diagnosis of Hodgkin lymphoma (nodular sclerosis subtype).

Clinical Pearls

- In both adults and children, enlarged lymph nodes that are present less than 2 weeks or greater than 12 months without changing in size have a very low likelihood of being neoplastic.
- Lymph nodes do not pulsate.
- Both edema and lymphedema can exist in the same patient.
- Virchow's node is a palpable left supraclavicular lymph node and is highly suspicious for thoracic or abdominal malignancy.

Key Takeaways

- The lymphatic system has many functions in the body and plays a large role in immune system function.
- Palpable lymph nodes can be a normal part of an infectious process or can be a sign of underlying pathology.
- Multiple disease processes can cause lymphadenopathy.
- Lymph nodes greater than 1 cm in diameter or in the supraclavicular region should be further investigated.

REFERENCES

Butte, M. J., & Stiehm, E. R. (2019). Laboratory evaluation of the immune system. In A. M. Feldweg (Ed.), *UpToDate*. Retrieved from https://www.uptodate.com/contents/laboratory-evaluation-of-the-immune-system

Cheson, B. D., Fisher, R. I., Barrington, S. F., Cavalli, F., Schwartz, L. H., Zucca, E., & Lister, T. A. (2014). Recommendations for initial evaluation, staging, and response assessment of Hodgkin and non-Hodgkin lymphoma: The Lugano classification. *Journal of Clinical Oncology*, *32*(27), 3059–3068. doi:10.1200/JCO.2013.54.8800

Cunnane, M., Cheung, L., Moore, A., di Palma, S., McCombe, A., & Pitkin, L. (2016). Level 5 lymphadenopathy warrants heightened suspicion for clinically significant pathology. *Head and Neck Pathology*, *10*(4), 509–512. doi:10.1007/s12105-016-0733-6

Gaddy, H. L., & Reigel, A. M. (2016). Unexplained lymphadenopathy: Evaluation and differential diagnosis. *American Family Physician*, *94*(11), 896–903. Retrieved from https://www.aafp.org/afp/2016/1201/p896.html

Gay, G., & Parker, K. (2003). Understanding the complete blood count with differential. *Journal of Perianesthesia Nursing*, *18*(2), 96–114. doi:10.1053/jpan.2003.50013

Girard-Madoux, M. J. H., Gomez de Agüero, M., Ganal-Vonarburg, S. C., Mooser, C., Belz, G. T., Macpherson, A. J., & Vivier, E. (2018). The immunological functions of the appendix: An example of redundancy? *Seminars in Immunology*, *36*, 31–44. doi:10.1016/j.smim.2018.02.005

Gradidge, E. (2013). Fever, lymphadenopathy, and splenomegaly: Did the cat do it? *Clinical Pediatrics*, *52*(11), 1072. doi:10.1177/0009922813501224

Grywalska, E., Pasiarski, M., Gozdz, S., & Rolinkski, J. (2018). Immune checkpoint inhibitors for combating T-cell dysfunction in cancer. *OncoTargets and Therapy, 11*, 6505–6524. doi:10.2147/OTT.S150817

Hassanein, A. H., Maclellan, R. A., Grant, F. D., & Greene, A. K. (2017). Diagnostic accuracy of lymphoscintigraphy for lymphedema and analysis of false-negative tests. *Plastic and Reconstructive Surgery Global Open, 5*(7), e1396. doi:10.1097/GOX.0000000000001396

International Society of Lymphology. (2016). The diagnosis and treatment of peripheral lymphedema: 2016 consensus document of the International Society of Lymphology. *Lymphology, 49*, 170–184. Retrieved from https://journals.uair.arizona.edu/index.php/lymph/article/view/20106/19734

Iwasaki, A., & Medzhitov, R. (2015). Control of adaptive immunity by the innate immune system. *Nature Immunology, 16*, 343–353. doi:10.1038/ni.3123

Moncayo, V. M., Aarsvold, J. N., & Alazraki, N. P. (2015). Lymphoscintigraphy and sentinel nodes. *Journal of Nuclear Medicine, 56*(6), 901–907. doi:10.2967/jnumed.114.141432

Moore, J. E., & Bertram, C. D. (2018). Lymphatic system flows. *Annual Review of Fluid Mechanics, 50*(1), 459–482. doi:10.1146/annurev-fluid-122316-045259

National Center for Advancing Translational Sciences. (2017). *Lymphatic malformations.* Retrieved from https://rarediseases.info.nih.gov/diseases/9789/lymphatic-malformations

Padera, T. P., Meijer, E. F., & Munn, L. L. (2016, September 5). The lymphatic system in disease processes and cancer progression. *Annual Review of Biomedical Engineering, 18*(1), 125–158. doi:10.1146/annurev-bioeng-112315-031200

Pettmann, J., Santos, A. M., Dushek, O., & Davis, S. J. (2018). Membrane ultrastructure and T cell activation. *Frontiers in Immunology, 9*, 2152. doi:10.3389/fimmu.2018.02152

Poultsidi, A., Dimopoulos, Y., He, T.-F., Chavakis, T., Saloustros, E., Lee, P. P., & Petrovas, C. (2018). Lymph node cellular dynamics in cancer and HIV: What can we learn for the follicular CD4 (Tfh) cells? *Frontiers in Immunology, 9*, 2233. doi:10.3389/fimmu.2018.02233

Rajasekaran, K., & Krakovitz, P. (2013). Enlarged neck lymph nodes in children. *Pediatric Clinics, 60*(4), 923–936. doi:10.1016/j.pcl.2013.04.005

Randolph, G. J., Ivanov, S., Zinselmeyer, B. H., & Scallan, J. P. (2017). The lymphatic system: Integral roles in immunity. *Annual Review of Immunology, 35*(1), 31–52. doi:10.1146/annurev-immunol-041015-055354

Restrepo, R., Oneto, J., Lopez, K., & Kukreja, K. (2009). Head and neck lymph nodes in children: The spectrum from normal to abnormal. *Pediatric Radiology, 39*(8), 836–846. doi:10.1007/s00247-009-1250-5

Simon, A. K., Hollander, G. A., & McMichael, A. (2015). Evolution of the immune system in humans from infancy to old age. *Proceedings of the Royal Society B: Biological Sciences, 282*(1821), 20143085. doi:10.1098/rspb.2014.3085

Takeuchi, Y., & Nishikawa, H. (2016). Roles of regulatory T cells in cancer immunity. *International Immunology, 28*(8), 401–409. doi:10.1093/intimm/dxw025

Zolla, V., Nizamutdinova, I. T., Scharf, B., Clement, C. C., Maejima, D., Akl, T., . . . Santambrogio, L. (2015). Aging-related anatomical and biochemical changes in lymphatic collectors impair lymph transport, fluid homeostasis, and pathogen clearance. *Aging Cell, 14*(4), 582–594. doi:10.1111/acel.12330

Evidence-Based Assessment of the Head and Neck

Alice M. Teall and Kate Gawlik

"Never bend your head. Always hold it high. Look the world straight in the eye."

—Helen Keller

LEARNING OBJECTIVES

- Review the anatomy and physiology of the head and neck.
- Determine key assessments for evaluating disorders, injuries, and diseases of the head, face, neck, thyroid, and parathyroid glands.
- Evaluate normal and abnormal findings of the exam of the head, face, and neck.

ANATOMY AND PHYSIOLOGY OF THE HEAD AND NECK

SKELETAL STRUCTURE OF THE HEAD

The **skull** is the skeletal structure of the head that supports and protects the brain, sensory organs, nerves, and vasculature of the head and provides an anchor for the musculature of the face and scalp. Of the 22 individual bones that comprise the skull, 21 are immobile and form a single unit. The only movable bone of the skull is the mandible. The skull, or **cranium**, can be divided into two sections: the neurocranium, composed of cranial bones and sutures, and the viscerocranium, formed by the bones of the face. The bones of the skull that comprise the neurocranium have numerous foramina, or openings, through which cranial nerves, arteries, veins, and other structures pass.

Regions of the head are defined by the eight bones of the neurocranium (**Figure 11.1**). One bone establishes the *frontal* region, which forms the forehead, anterior cranial floor, and part of the orbit of the eye. The *parietal* region is formed from two bones that create the top and upper sides of the cranium. The *occipital* region is the base and back of the cranium formed from one bone. Two *temporal* bones form the base and sides of the cranium, or the temporal region. The *sphenoid* region formed from one bone is located at the anterior base of the skull and forms part of the walls of the orbit. The *ethmoid* bone also forms part of the orbit and the floor of the cranium.

The cranial bones are separated by narrow fibrous joints known as sutures (**Figure 11.2**). The sutures of the skull consist of dense connective tissue; these immovable joints, with little elasticity, offer vital protection for the brain and underlying structures. At birth, numerous skull bones are unfused, and sutures attach to fibrous, membrane-covered gaps called fontanels. Timing of closure of the fontanels, ossification of cranial bones, and fusion of sutures vary greatly, with some sutures closing during childhood and most fusing during early adulthood. The main sutures in adulthood are *coronal*, which fuses the frontal bone with the two parietal bones; *sagittal*, which fuses the two parietal bones; and *lambdoid*, which fuses the occipital bone to the two parietal bones.

Fourteen facial bones form the viscerocranium, or facial skeleton (**Figure 11.3**). Six of the facial bones are paired; the paired bones are the *zygomatic*, which form the cheekbones of the face; *lacrimal*, which form

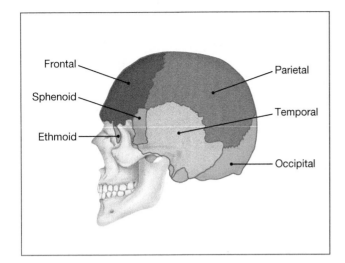

FIGURE 11.1 Regions of the head defined by eight bones of the neurocranium. Bone counts for the regions are as follows: frontal region, one bone; parietal region, two bones; occipital region, one bone; temporal region, two bones; sphenoid region, one bone; ethmoid region, one bone.

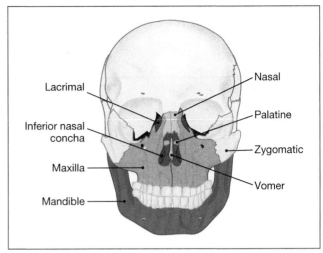

FIGURE 11.3 Fourteen facial bones form the facial skeleton. Six of the facial bones are paired; the paired bones are the zygomatic, the lacrimal, the nasal, the inferior nasal conchae, the palatine, and the maxilla. The unpaired facial bones are the vomer and the mandible.

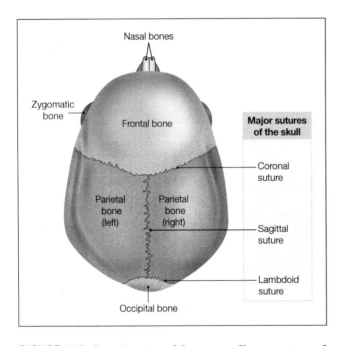

FIGURE 11.2 Superior view of the narrow fibrous sutures of the adult cranium.

the walls of the orbit and nasal cavity; *nasal*, located at the bridge of the nose; *inferior nasal conchae*, located in the nasal cavity; *palatine*, which form part of the hard palate in the oral cavity; and *maxilla*, which comprise part of the upper jaw and hard palate. The unpaired facial bones are the *vomer*, which forms part of the nasal septum, and the *mandible*, which articulates with the base of the cranium at the temporomandibular joint.

The shape and appearance of the face are determined largely by the viscerocranium and neurocranium. The facial skeleton contains four openings—a nasal, an oral, and two orbital apertures. The anatomy of the face includes superficial and deep fat compartments, muscles of facial expression and mastication innervated by the trigeminal and facial cranial nerves, and retaining ligaments. The skin and soft tissue of the face primarily receive their arterial supply from branches of the facial, maxillary, and superficial temporal arteries. Facial landmarks assessed for size, shape, position, and prominence include forehead, hairline, cheeks, midface, palpebral fissures, nasolabial folds, and chin.

STRUCTURES OF THE NECK

Neck structures, including cervical vertebrae, nerves, muscles, ligaments, and tendons, allow for head movement and stability. The bony structures of the neck include the seven vertebral segments of the cervical spine that connect the base of the skull to the thoracic spine. Back and neck muscles that move the vertebral column allow for flexion, extension, rotation, and lateral bending of the head and neck. The muscles of the neck facilitate speech and swallowing, in addition to providing stabilization of the head.

The anatomic areas of the neck, designated as "triangles," are useful in assessing superficial structures (**Figure 11.4**). The sternocleidomastoid muscle (attached to the sternum, clavicle, and mastoid process of the temporal bone) provides a visible landmark that separates the anterior and posterior triangles of the neck. The posterior triangle of the neck includes the

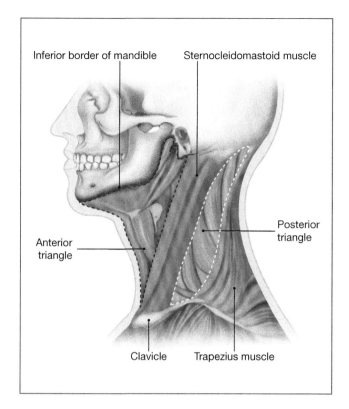

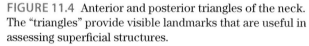

FIGURE 11.4 Anterior and posterior triangles of the neck. The "triangles" provide visible landmarks that are useful in assessing superficial structures.

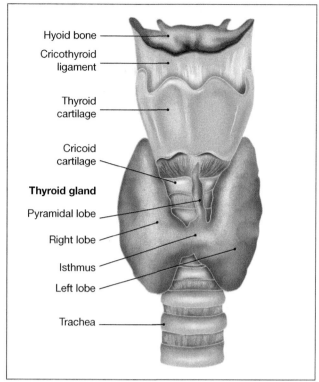

FIGURE 11.5 Midline structures of the neck within the anterior triangle.

external jugular vein, posterior cervical lymph nodes, and the accessory cranial nerve. The anterior triangle of the neck includes the bifurcation of the common carotid artery; anterior cervical lymph nodes; and the facial, glossopharyngeal, vagus, accessory, and hypoglossal cranial nerves. Underlying structures located within the anterior triangle form the midline of the neck; these structures include the hyoid bone, thyroid cartilage, cricoid cartilage, trachea, and **thyroid** and **parathyroid** glands (**Figure 11.5**).

STRUCTURE AND FUNCTION OF THE THYROID AND PARATHYROID GLANDS

The butterfly-shaped thyroid gland, located anterior to the trachea, is composed of the medial isthmus region and two lobes; the thyroid gland weighs 10 to 20 g in adults. Thyroid volume increases with age and body weight, decreases with iodine intake, and is slightly greater in men than women. The tissues of the thyroid gland are formed by thyroid follicular cells surrounding a lumen filled with colloid; when the thyroid gland is stimulated, these follicular cells become columnar cells, which causes the lumen to be depleted of the thyroglobulin-containing colloid. When the thyroid gland function is suppressed, the follicular cells become flat, and

colloid accumulates. The regulation of thyroid hormone synthesis and secretion is sensitive to small changes in circulating hormone levels. In thyroid follicular cells, iodine diffuses rapidly and is transported, oxidized, and bound to tyrosine residues of thyroglobulin, which makes iodine ready for thyroid hormone synthesis.

Thyroid hormones stored in the circulation and in the thyroid gland are critical to metabolism and organ function. The two biologically active thyroid hormones are thyroxine (T4) and triiodothyronine (T3). While the production and metabolism of T4 occurs primarily in the thyroid gland, approximately 80% of T3 is produced outside of the thyroid gland by de-iodination of T4. The thyroid gland contains large quantities of T4 and T3 incorporated in thyroglobulin, the protein within which the hormones are both synthesized and stored. More than 99% of T4 and T3 are bound to serum proteins (primarily thyroglobulin), which allows for immediate secretion when needed, storage within tissues and organs, and precise maintenance of serum levels of free T4 and T3 concentrations. Thyroid hormone production is regulated within the thyroid by the pituitary thyroid-stimulating hormone (TSH); the secretion of TSH is increased in response to the thyrotropin-releasing hormone, and is inhibited by serum T3 and T4 concentrations, creating a negative feedback loop. Very

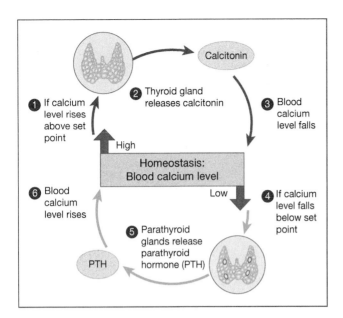

FIGURE 11.6 Feedback loops that regulate serum calcium levels include hormone release from thyroid and parathyroid glands.

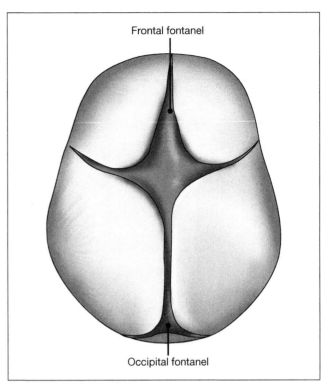

FIGURE 11.7 Anterior and posterior fontanels of the newborn's skull.

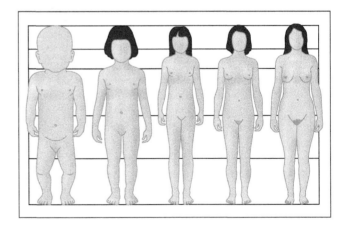

FIGURE 11.8 Proportions of head and body across the life span. At birth, the head of a newborn is one fourth the total body length, whereas in the adult it is one seventh.

small changes in serum free T4 prompt large reciprocal changes in serum TSH concentrations.

Parathyroid glands are endocrine glands located on the posterior surfaces of the thyroid gland. Despite their proximity, these glands function independently of the thyroid gland and are closely aligned with formation of the thymus. Parathyroid glands are approximately the size of a lentil or grain of rice; most individuals (84%) have four parathyroid glands. The location of the parathyroid glands can vary greatly. These glands produce parathyroid hormone (PTH), which regulates the body's calcium level by direct action on bone and the kidneys. To increase serum calcium, PTH stimulates bone resorption by osteoclasts, decreases calcium clearance within the kidney, and stimulates synthesis of vitamin D, causing calcium absorption in the GI tract. As with other endocrine glands, parathyroid gland function is controlled by a negative feedback loop; PTH production and secretion occur in response to serum calcium and vitamin D levels (**Figure 11.6**). The function of the parathyroid glands is critical in maintaining homeostasis of serum calcium.

LIFE-SPAN DIFFERENCES AND CONSIDERATIONS

Infancy, Childhood, and Adolescence Variations in Cranium and Neck

The skull of a newborn is considerably pliable as six fontanels and unfused skull bones allow for molding, or overlap of cranial bones, during passage through the birth canal (**Figure 11.7**). Molding usually resolves within 3 to 5 days after birth. The small posterior fontanel, where the two parietal bones join the occipital bone, usually closes during the first 2 months of life. The larger anterior fontanel, where the two frontal and two parietal bones join, can remain open for 2 years, but usually closes by 15 months, and can vary in size during that time.

Infants and children have considerable variations in the size, shape, and structure of their skulls as their brains grow and develop (**Figure 11.8**). At birth, the head of a newborn is one fourth the total body length, whereas in the adult it is one seventh. Infant head shape also differs significantly from that of the adult; the infant's skull is much more elongated, with large frontal and parietal prominences. Head circumference increases markedly during the child's first year of life. Because infants and children have greater head mass and less strength of the neck muscles, ligaments, and vertebrae until adolescence, they are especially prone to injury of the head, neck, and spine.

Pregnancy Variations in Thyroid Function

Pregnancy causes hormonal and physiologic changes in thyroid function. The presence of human chorionic gonadotropin hormones can stimulate the thyroid gland, which may result in subclinical or overt hyperthyroidism. In addition, the thyroid can increase in size during pregnancy, especially in iodine-deficient environments. During the first 10 to 12 weeks of pregnancy, the fetus is dependent on maternal thyroid hormone for brain development, which necessitates close monitoring of maternal thyroid function to avoid adverse outcomes. Pregnant and postpartum women are at increased risk for thyroid dysfunction, including hypothyroidism and thyroiditis (Tingi, Syed, Kyriacou, Mastorakos, & Kyriacou, 2016).

KEY HISTORY QUESTIONS AND CONSIDERATIONS FOR THE HEAD AND NECK

HISTORY OF PRESENT ILLNESS

Common Presenting Symptoms

For each sign or symptom, targeted history of present illness (HPI) questions are required to determine the needed physical exam and differential diagnoses. Table 11.1 lists presenting signs and symptoms that may indicate a concern related to the head, neck, or thyroid gland. One of the most common presenting symptoms, headache, is listed in detail in this section.

Example: Headache

- Onset: Time of onset, manner in which symptoms began, presence of prodrome or aura
- Location: Site of pain; unilateral versus bilateral, generalized area versus specific location
- Duration: Progression and persistence of headache since onset
- Character: Intensity, quality, and radiation of pain
- Associated symptoms: Presence or absence of numbness, tingling, weakness, vision changes, eye pain, lacrimal discharge, nausea, vomiting, fever, neck pain

TABLE 11.1 Presenting Signs or Symptoms: Head and Neck	
Subjective symptoms (acute, episodic, chronic)	• Headache • Facial pain • Neck pain • Difficulty or pain with chewing • Difficulty swallowing; sense of lump in throat with swallowing • Systemic symptoms of constipation, fatigue, irritability, temperature intolerances
Objective signs (acute, episodic, chronic)	• Head injury or trauma • Hoarseness, change in voice • Limited mobility of neck or jaw • Lump in neck (masses or nodule(s)) • Skin or hair changes • Nonhealing lesion • Weight loss, rapid heartbeat • Weight gain

- Aggravating factors: Sensitivity to light or sound; exacerbation with changes in position or activity; recent illness, stressors, or trauma; recent changes in sleep, weight, or diet
- Relieving symptoms: Pharmacologic, including over-the-counter (OTC) analgesics (use and rebound after use); nonpharmacologic, including withdrawal to dark room or lying flat
- Timing or temporal factors: Number of headaches per month; personal/family history of headaches; known triggers such as food, alcohol, stressors, medications, environment; for women: association with menstrual cycle or change in method of birth control
- Red flag symptoms indicating need for emergency evaluation: See Table 11.2.

Differential Diagnoses

Primary headache (tension-type headache, migraine, cluster headache) or secondary headache (as determined by red flags outlined in Table 11.2).

For any individual who presents with symptoms or signs related to the head, neck, or thyroid, reviewing past medical history; family and social history; systems; and history of primary care preventive practices are appropriate.

PAST MEDICAL HISTORY

- Headache
- Injury or trauma to the head or neck
- Cancer

TABLE 11.2 Red Flags Indicating Secondary Headache Disorders

Mnemonic SNOOP		
S	Systemic symptoms or conditions	Unexplained fever, weight loss, myalgia, fatigue, and new onset of headache when immunocompromised can indicate tumor, malignancy, metastasis, or meningitis
N	Neurologic signs or symptoms	Altered consciousness, motor weakness, sensory loss, ataxia, diplopia, pulsatile tinnitus, and/or nuchal rigidity can indicate malignant, inflammatory, and/or vascular disorders of the brain
O	Onset	Sudden onset like a "clap of thunder" or "in a split second" can indicate critical vascular events: subarachnoid hemorrhage, costovertebral angle, carotid dissection, venous thrombosis
O	Older age	New onset of migraine-type headaches in those over age 50 can indicate inflammatory, infectious, or neoplastic processes
P	Pattern change	The "4Ps" of pattern change: (1) progressing to daily, (2) precipitated by valsalva, (3) postural aggravation, and (4) papilledema can indicate malignant, vascular, or inflammatory disorders

- HIV
- Hypertension
- Depression, anxiety, or mental health disorder
- Osteoarthritis or rheumatoid arthritis
- Constitutional changes (weight loss/gain, fatigue: see Review of Systems (ROS) section)
- Use of medications
- Allergies to medications or other allergies, asthma
- Past surgical history
- Past history of radiation therapy
- Smoking history
- Recent motor vehicle accident

FAMILY HISTORY

- Migraine or recurrent headaches
- Neck or thyroid cancer

- Thyroid disorders
- Endocrine disorders
- Arthritis

SOCIAL HISTORY

- Tobacco use
- Alcohol intake
- Drug use including prescribed/not prescribed
- Environmental exposures
- Stress
- Sleep
- Nutrition
- Social support system
- Sports participation (specifically, contact sports like football)

REVIEW OF SYSTEMS

- Neurologic: Weakness, numbness, loss of consciousness, headache, recent fall, dizziness
- Musculoskeletal: Injury history, pain with movement; neck pain, stiffness, or swelling
- Endocrine: Changes to skin, hair; temperature intolerance, weight changes, fatigue
- Eyes, Ears, Nose, Throat (EENT): Ear pain, eye redness or drainage, nasal congestion, sinus pain, sore throat
- Psychiatric: Sadness, worry, insomnia; changes in memory, concentration, or mood
- Lymphatic: Bruising, bleeding, lymphadenopathy

PREVENTIVE CARE CONSIDERATIONS

- Healthy lifestyle behaviors, including exercise
- Human papillomavirus (HPV) vaccination
- Recent lab work, screenings, or imaging

PHYSICAL EXAMINATION OF THE HEAD AND NECK

The evidence-based physical exam begins with a general survey. Assess vital signs. Talk to the individual to assess mental status. Begin the assessment of the head and neck with a thorough inspection.

INSPECTION OF HEAD, FACE, AND NECK

The assessment of the head and neck begins with observation. Note the position of the head. Observe for tremor, lesions, or signs of trauma. Inspect the cranium for symmetry; note the quality and condition of the skin of the scalp. Systematically parting the hair may be needed for a thorough assessment if the individual has itching of the scalp, dandruff, or concerns regarding infestation or infection in their history. Assessment of the head includes observing the hair of the head for texture and distribution, specifically assessing for coarseness, thinning hair, and areas or patterns of hair loss.

Assessment of the face includes noting symmetry, shape, features, and facial expression. An accurate assessment of symmetric alignment of the eyebrows, eyes, ears, nose, and mouth, and position of facial features relative to the face, including palpebral fissures and the nasolabial fold, can reveal genetic, endocrine, or neurologic disorders. Prominence or depression of the forehead, cheeks, and chin should be noted. Asking individuals to raise their eyebrows, smile, frown, and puff their cheeks to observe symmetry in movements is a component of the complete neurologic exam. Inspection of the face includes assessing for skin integrity, lesions, discoloration, or edema.

While an individual holds the head in a neutral position, inspect the neck, noting deformities, asymmetry, or pulsations, and assessing for areas of edema or discoloration. A thorough, complete physical exam includes assessing for limitation or pain with movement; ask the individual to tip the chin to the chest, turn the head to each side, and tip the head toward each shoulder.

PALPATION OF HEAD AND NECK

For the individual who presents with signs or symptoms of head/neck concerns, palpation of the head may be warranted. Palpate the head gently for areas of edema or tenderness. Note any tenderness of the mastoid process. Palpate directly over the temporomandibular joint while the patient opens and closes the mandible to assess for smooth, symmetric movement and full range of motion. Note any clicking of the jaw or if the patient reports any pain while performing this movement. Palpation of the head and neck includes lymph node assessment, thyroid assessment, and neurologic assessment for sensation.

Palpating the thyroid gland to assess for nodules and enlargement begins with identifying the structures and landmarks of the neck (**Figure 11.9**). An anterior or posterior approach can be used for thyroid palpation (**Figure 11.10**). Clinicians should note that the thyroid gland is less palpable as individuals age and that physical findings of a single nodule and/or enlargement are not indicative of cancer, goiter, or thyroid disease based solely on physical findings.

To begin the anterior approach to thyroid assessment, ask the individual to tip the head back slightly, and use the landmarks of the notched thyroid cartilage and the cricoid cartilage to locate the thyroid. (In men, the thyroid cartilage is commonly called the "Adam's apple," and is more easily seen than in women.) Palpate the region below the cricoid cartilage to identify the contours of the thyroid (see **Figure 11.10A**). Modifying this approach to include simultaneously moving

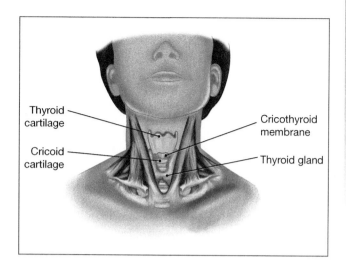

FIGURE 11.9 Anatomic structures and landmarks of the neck used to assess thyroid gland.

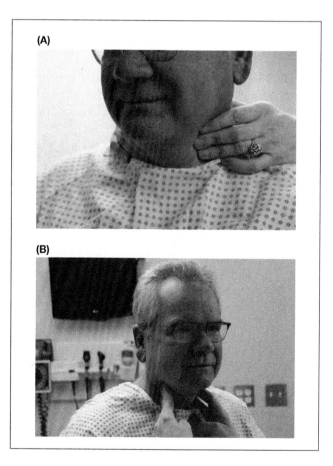

FIGURE 11.10 Palpation of the thyroid. (A) Posterior approach. (B) Anterior approach.

the sternocleidomastoid muscles further apart causes the skin to be taut over the thyroid gland and can enhance the anterior inspection and palpation techniques (Chung, Patrone, & Lariccia, 2015). To verify the location of the thyroid gland, ask the individual to swallow, as the thyroid gland moves during swallowing. With palpation, the thyroid gland is normally soft, without distinctly palpable nodules.

To palpate the thyroid gland using a posterior approach, ask the individual to tip their chin slightly forward; the clinician should stand behind the individual and place their fingers on the individual's neck just below the cricoid cartilage (see **Figure 11.10B**). Ask the individual to swallow while keeping fingers steady in this position, and the thyroid isthmus can be felt rising under the pads of the fingers as the person swallows. To palpate the lobes of the thyroid, the clinician can (1) ask the individual to tip their chin to their chest, (2) displace the individual's trachea slightly and gently to the right with their left hand, and (3) in this position, palpate the right thyroid lobes with their right hand. Repeat this technique on the other side, by displacing the trachea to the left with the right hand, and palpating the left thyroid lobes.

PERCUSSION AND AUSCULTATION OF HEAD AND NECK

Auscultation and percussion of the head and neck are not components of the routine head and neck exam for asymptomatic, healthy individuals, but may be components of the assessment of the head and neck related to specific concerns or conditions.

PEDIATRIC PHYSICAL EXAMINATION CONSIDERATIONS

Inspection and Palpation of Head and Neck

Inspect the head of a newborn, infant, or child to assess size, shape, and form, including presence of fontanels and suture ridges. An accurate head circumference measurement, using a nonstretchable measuring tape to measure above the eyebrows and ears, should be compared with expected size on the growth chart (**Figure 11.11**). Inspect for symmetry or asymmetry of an infant or child's head from above and from all angles. Unusual or asymmetric head shapes can be positional or can result from early closure of sutures and fontanels. Confirm that the line of the eyes is horizontal and that the child's ears are in alignment, to confirm head symmetry (**Figure 11.12**).

During the first days of life, expect that the newborn will have cranial molding. Inspect and palpate the head, noting overlapping suture ridges. A newborn's scalp that is diffusely soft and swollen, a condition called *caput succedaneum*, is a result of the pressure on the baby's head during vaginal birth. Caput succedaneum resolves in a few days and crosses the midline, distinguishing it from a *cephalohematoma*, which is a collection of blood beneath the periosteum that does

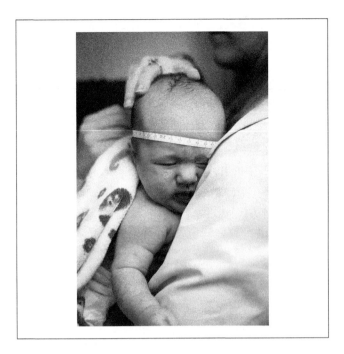

FIGURE 11.11 Measurement of head circumference.

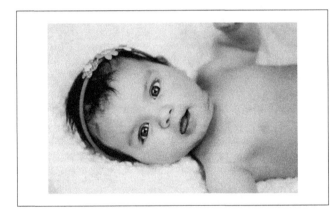

FIGURE 11.12 A newborn head/face that is symmetric without molding post C-section delivery and with molding postvaginal delivery.

not cross suture lines, can take months to resolve, and needs close monitoring to assess for significant bleeding (**Figure 11.13**).

Inspect and palpate the fontanels of infants and children under age 2. While the posterior fontanel is often not palpable beyond 2 months of age, the anterior fontanel can be palpable up to the age of 2 years. Fontanels should be flat, not depressed or bulging, when palpated; the average size of the anterior fontanel is 2 cm. Begin the exam while the infant is calm. Palpate the fontanels while the child is held in both supine and upright positions. Palpation of the anterior fontanel in the upright position may reveal a normal, slight pulsation. If the

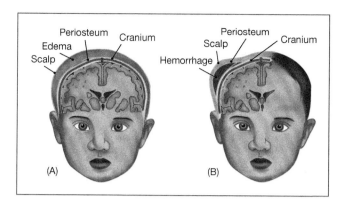

FIGURE 11.13 Caput and cephalohematoma. (A) Caput results from diffuse swelling. (B) Cephalohematoma results from bleeding beneath the periosteum.

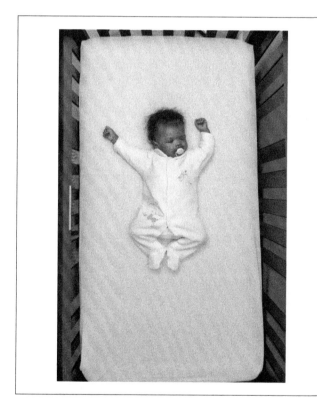

FIGURE 11.14 Infant in safe sleep environment.
Source: From the National Institutes of Health.

anterior fontanel has closed prematurely, percuss the skull near the junction of the frontal, temporal, and parietal bones to assess for Macewen's sign, an unusually resonant, "cracked-pot" sound, that indicates increased intracranial pressure. Infants with an asymmetrical shape of the cranium that has resulted from positioning, a condition known as plagiocephaly, will have normal cranial suture lines and flat fontanels, which is distinguished from craniosynostosis, asymmetry of the head and a wide anterior fontanel caused by premature

closure of one or more cranial sutures (Kiesler & Ricer, 2003). Ask the parent to clarify the position and environment in which the infant sleeps; see **Figure 11.14**, which illustrates a safe sleep position and environment for an infant. While positioning an infant on their back to sleep increases the likelihood of some degree of positional plagiocephaly, safe sleep recommendations have decreased the incidence of sudden infant death syndrome.

Observe the infant or child's neck control, head movement, and position. Palpate the neck for masses and/or lymphadenopathy. To more easily assess the neck of a newborn, elevate the upper back of the infant to allow the head to extend slightly. Infants and children should have full and easy range of motion of the neck. Nuchal rigidity, or resistance to flexion of the neck, is associated with meningeal irritation. Postural torticollis, twisting of the neck muscles, is relatively common in newborns related to positioning in utero; associated physical exam reveals a preference for tilting the head in one direction.

LABORATORY CONSIDERATIONS FOR THE HEAD AND NECK

ASSESSMENT OF THYROID FUNCTION

Thyroid function is assessed by measuring the serum concentration of TSH, total T4, total T3, and/or free T4 concentration. Age-based normal values are important to note, as TSH concentrations shift higher in older populations. Thyroid function tests are used in combination to screen for thyroid disorders and monitor treatment for thyroid disease.

Serum TSH concentration provides a measure of thyroid function. An elevated TSH is associated with hypothyroidism, and a low TSH is associated with hyperthyroidism. Some experts recommend including a measurement of free T4 in addition to TSH when assessing thyroid function, as this will screen for unsuspected pituitary disease. Laboratory considerations for thyroid function as recommended by the American Thyroid Association (2018) are:

- When the serum TSH is normal, no further lab testing is needed.
- If serum TSH is high, measure free T4 to determine degree of hypothyroidism.
- If serum TSH is low, measure free T4 and T3 to determine degree of hyperthyroidism.
- When pituitary disease is suspected, measure both serum TSH and free T4.
- If serum TSH is normal *and* the patient has convincing symptoms of hypo- or hyperthyroidism, measure free T4.

Serum TSH also provides important clinical information when individuals are being treated for thyroid dysfunction. For those who have primary hypothyroidism and are taking thyroid replacement hormone, if the TSH is high, the dose may need to be increased, and if the TSH is low, the dose may need to be decreased. For individuals with hyperthyroidism, T3 concentrations may be disproportionately elevated; to monitor response to treatment of hyperthyroidism, lab evaluation may need to include TSH, serum T3, and free T4.

Laboratory assessments and results are expected to be different for individuals taking medication to suppress TSH in order to prevent recurrence of thyroid cancer. For these individuals, the TSH concentration should be undetectable or subnormal.

ASSESSMENT OF PARATHYROID FUNCTION

Parathyroid disorders most commonly present with serum calcium abnormalities. Serum concentration of PTH is assessed to determine the cause of calcium imbalance. In addition to the needed history and physical exam when individuals present with a calcium imbalance, assessments should include measures of serum PTH, magnesium, creatinine, phosphorus, 25-hydroxyvitamin D, and 1,25-dihydroxyvitamin D. Measuring 1,25-dihydroxyvitamin D is needed only when an individual has abnormal calcium levels, PTH levels, or decreased kidney function, in order to identify underlying causes. The measurement of serum 25-hydroxyvitamin D levels measures the stores of vitamin D, indicating deficiency, and may be indicated for individuals who have normal serum calcium levels. In combination, these measures evaluate parathyroid function and may indicate absence or presence of kidney disease, bone disorders, vitamin D deficiency, or toxicity.

IMAGING CONSIDERATIONS FOR THE HEAD AND NECK

HEADACHE OR HEAD INJURY

The American College of Radiology (2017) recommends that imaging is not necessary for individuals who present with uncomplicated headaches. If there are no red flags for structural disorders, then imaging is not likely to change management or improve outcomes and may actually lead to additional medical procedures and expense for incidental findings (American College of Radiology, 2017).

For individuals who present with mild headache related to recent injury or trauma, the American Medical Society for Sports Medicine (2014) does not recommend imaging (computed tomography [CT] or magnetic resonance imaging [MRI]); additional imaging is not necessary to evaluate for acute concussion unless there are worsening neurologic symptoms or focal neurologic findings or there is concern for skull fracture. Concussion is a clinical diagnosis that is not reliant on CT or MRI abnormalities. These studies *should* be ordered if more severe brain injury is suspected. CT is best used to evaluate for skull fracture and intracranial bleeding; MRI is indicated for prolonged symptoms, worsening symptoms, or other suspected structural pathology (American Medical Society for Sports Medicine, 2014).

DISCRETE THYROID LESIONS (NODULES)

According to the American Thyroid Association (2018), the finding of incidental thyroid nodules is common; in addition to a careful history and physical exam, evaluation of a thyroid nodule should begin with measuring TSH (Tamhane & Gharib, 2016). If the TSH is low, thyroid scintigraphy/radionuclide thyroid scan should be done; if the TSH is normal or high, thyroid ultrasound should be performed to evaluate the nodule(s) and assess for suspicious nodules. The next step in the evaluation of thyroid nodule, depending on evaluation of risk, is a fine-needle aspiration biopsy (American Thyroid Association, 2018; Tamhane & Gharib, 2016).

EVIDENCE-BASED PRACTICE CONSIDERATIONS FOR THE HEAD AND NECK

HEADACHE OR HEAD INJURY

Evidence-based recommendations regarding imaging of the head and neck from the Choosing Wisely® (n.d.) campaign include:

1. Avoid CT of the head in asymptomatic adult patients who present in the emergency department with syncope, insignificant trauma, and a normal neurologic evaluation. In the absence of head injury or signs of stroke, CT scans rarely find abnormalities and expose patients to radiation and undue costs (American College of Emergency Physicians, 2018).

2. CT scans are not necessary in the immediate evaluation of minor head injuries in children; clinical observation criteria should be used to determine whether imaging is indicated (American Academy of Pediatrics, 2018).

THYROID DISORDERS

Recommendations from the U.S. Preventive Services Task Force (USPSTF) regarding screenings for thyroid dysfunction:

1. USPSTF (2017) recommends against screening for thyroid cancer in asymptomatic adults.
2. "[E]vidence is insufficient to assess the balance of benefits and harms of screening for thyroid dysfunction in nonpregnant, asymptomatic adults." (USPSTF, 2015, "Recommendation")

Recommendations from the Choosing Wisely (n.d.) campaign regarding lab testing and imaging for disorders of the thyroid:

1. Clinicians should not routinely order thyroid ultrasound in patients with abnormal thyroid function tests if there is no palpable abnormality of the thyroid gland. Thyroid ultrasound is used to identify and characterize thyroid nodules (Endocrine Society, 2018).
2. No evidence supports recommending ultrasound for incidental thyroid nodules found on CT, MRI, or non–thyroid-focused neck ultrasound in low-risk patients unless the nodule meets age-based size criteria or has suspicious features. Imaging of the neck often reveals thyroid nodules, and most are not malignant (American College of Radiology, 2017).
3. Avoid routinely ordering thyroid ultrasounds in children who have simple goiters or autoimmune thyroiditis. Limit the use of ultrasounds to children who have asymmetric thyroid enlargement, palpable nodules, or concerning cervical lymphadenopathy (American Academy of Pediatrics, 2018).
4. Avoid routinely measuring thyroid function and/or insulin levels in children with obesity. Slightly elevated TSH levels are a consequence of obesity and are rarely true hypothyroidism. These tests are not necessary to establish a management plan for children with obesity (American Academy of Pediatrics, 2018).

ABNORMAL FINDINGS OF THE HEAD AND NECK

HEADACHE

Headache pain is one of the most common physical concerns. The International Headache Society (IHS) Classification of Headache Disorders divides headaches into two categories: primary and secondary. Primary headaches are those that have no identifiable cause on exam; the diagnosis of a primary headache is made based on recognizing a pattern (International Headache Society, 2018). Migraine with and without aura, tension-type, and cluster headaches are primary headaches.

Secondary headaches are those with an underlying cause; for example, tumor, trauma, infection, or inflammation. While less than 10% of headaches have a secondary cause, the higher likelihood of serious complications with secondary headaches warrants a comprehensive history and exam. Completing a thorough patient history is the key to differentiating whether a headache is primary or secondary. **Table 11.2**, Red Flags Indicating Secondary Headache Disorders, outlines key history questions.

IHS classifications include more than 300 types and subtypes of headaches (International Headache Society, 2018). **Table 11.3** outlines the key assessment findings related to primary headaches.

HEAD INJURY OR TRAUMA

Epidural Hematoma

An epidural hematoma is believed to result from the severing of the middle meningeal artery owing to blunt trauma or traumatic injury of the skull. Patients typically experience a brief loss of consciousness after the trauma, regain consciousness, then experience progressively worsening headache and become obtunded. An epidural hematoma is a neurosurgical emergency since the bleeding is under arterial pressure.

Facial Fractures

Facial fractures are common and generally trauma related (e.g., road traffic collisions, fights, and falls). They are often associated with clinical features such as profuse bleeding, swelling, deformity, and anesthesia of the skin. The nasal bones are most frequently fractured, owing to their prominent position at the bridge of the nose.

Skull Fractures

Fractures of the skull base should be considered, especially in high-impact motor vehicle accidents. The type of fracture and the impact that it has on the contents of the skull are determined by the location of the fracture and the mechanism of injury. Thin-slice CT has become an integral part of the diagnosis of subtle skull base fractures.

There are four major types of cranial fracture:

- Depressed fracture from skull indentation as a result of a direct blow
- Linear fracture that traverses the full thickness of the bone and is likely to have radiating (stellate) fracture lines away from the point of impact but does not move the cranial bones; this is the most common type of skull fracture

TABLE 11.3 Key Assessment Findings That Indicate Primary Headache Disorders

	Migraine Headache	Tension-Type Headache	Cluster Headache
Onset	Gradual in onset, then builds in intensity	Gradual onset	Quick onset, pain intense within minutes
Location	Unilateral in most adults; bilateral in children, teens	Bilateral; general or localized	Unilateral, begins around the eye, temple
Duration	From 4 to 72 hours may be recurrent	30 minutes to 1 week; can be infrequent, frequent, or chronic	Recurrent, short, painful attacks of 15 minutes to few hours
Characteristics	Moderate to severe intensity; throbbing; may have aura or prodrome; recurrent	Pressure, heaviness, or band-like tightness	Severe or very severe burning, piercing, or stabbing
Associated symptoms	Nausea, vomiting, photophobia, phonophobia	No nausea or vomiting; may have feelings of stress, anxiety, or fatigue	Ipsilateral lacrimation and redness of the eye, congestion, pallor, sweating, or ptosis
Relieving factors	Prefers dark, quiet setting	May need relaxation or rest	Can remain active
Timing	Triggers include stress, food, alcohol, hunger, weather, menstrual cycle, hormones, environment, and sleep disturbances	May be related to stress and tension in neck and back; can be precipitated or co-occur with migraine	Abrupt onset can happen at night; attacks occur 1–8 times daily for weeks, followed by remission

Source: International Headache Society. (2018). Headache Classification Committee of the International Headache Society (IHS): The international classification of headache disorders, 3rd edition. *Cephalalgia, 38*(1), 1–211. doi:10.1177/0333102417738202

- Basal skull fracture that affects the base of the skull and characteristically causes bruising behind the ears, known as Battle's sign (mastoid ecchymosis; **Figure 11.15**), and/or bruising around the eyes/orbits, known as "Raccoon eyes," and can include clear fluid drainage from eyes or nose; this is one of the most serious skull fractures and requires close observation
- Diastatic fracture that occurs along a suture line, causing a widening of the suture, which is more likely to occur in infants and children

Acute Mild Traumatic Brain Injury (Concussion)

Mild traumatic brain injuries (TBI) occur as a result of motor vehicle accidents, falls, occupational accidents, assaults, and contact sports. Mild TBI results from direct external contact forces or from acceleration/deceleration forces. The diagnosis of concussion refers to the characteristic symptoms and signs that an individual may experience after a mild TBI, including:

- Incoordination, delayed verbal expression
- Inability to focus; blank stare or stunned appearance
- Disorientation; slurred and incoherent speech
- Headache, dizziness
- Emotionality and memory deficits

Individuals who experience mild TBI require acute evaluation that includes a neurologic exam and mental status testing. Prolonged unconsciousness, persistent

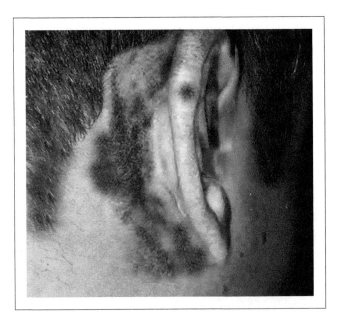

FIGURE 11.15 Battle's sign.

Source: Image courtesy of S. Bhimji. © 2019 StatPearls Publishing LLC.

mental status alterations, or abnormalities on neurologic examination require urgent imaging and neurologic consultation, as these assessments indicate more severe TBI. Key assessments include:

- History of the incident: Individuals should be asked to describe the incident in detail, including what led to the event and what happened after the injury. Information from an observer or bystander can provide key information as individuals often experience posttraumatic amnesia.
- Current symptoms including mental status: Use of a symptom checklist is invaluable. One evidence-based example is the Standardized Assessment of Concussion (Grubenhoff, Kirkwood, Gao, Deakyne, & Wathen, 2010). Commonly reported symptoms include fatigue, drowsiness, neck pain, difficulty concentrating, and difficulty remembering. Simple questions of orientation have inadequate sensitivity to detect mild TBI after head injury; assess short-term memory as well as attention and concentration. (See Chapter 5, Approach to the Physical Examination: General Survey and Assessment of Vital Signs, to review mental status exam techniques.)
- Neurologic exam: Assess cranial nerves III through VII (extraocular movements, pupillary reactivity, face sensation, and movement) as well as limb strength and coordination and gait. (See Chapter 14, Evidence-Based Assessment of the Nervous System, to review techniques).

Some form of ongoing assessment and observation is recommended for at least 24 hours after a mild TBI because of the risk of intracranial complications. Follow-up imaging is indicated for those who experience deterioration and may be appropriate for high-risk individuals (see Imaging section). The assessment of children and adolescents who experience concussion requires similar neurologic and mental status assessments and conservative follow-up.

PARATHYROID DISORDERS

Hypoparathyroidism

Hypoparathyroidism is a relatively uncommon condition related to decreased secretion or activity of PTH that leads to hypocalcemia. The most common cause is accidental removal of parathyroid glands during surgery of the thyroid or neck. Key signs and symptoms include paresthesia in fingertips, toes, and lips; myalgia; muscle spasms; fatigue; dry skin; and fatigue.

Hyperparathyroidism

In hyperparathyroidism, enlargement of one of more of the parathyroid glands causes excess production of

PTH, which results in hypercalcemia. Key assessments include kidney stones, abdominal pain, joint or bone pain, osteoporosis, fatigue, and depression symptoms. This condition is more likely in the older adult population. While parathyroid cancer is rare, hyperparathyroidism can be an early sign of malignancy.

THYROID DISORDERS

Hypothyroidism

Disorders and conditions that cause subclinical or overt hypothyroidism include:

- Primary hypothyroidism, a condition in which the thyroid gland is not responding to elevated TSH levels; primary hypothyroidism is often linked to iodine deficiency
- Hashimoto's thyroiditis, which is the most common cause of hypothyroidism in iodine-sufficient areas of the world, like the United States; also known as chronic autoimmune thyroiditis, this disorder leads to gradual loss of thyroid function
- Thyroid dysfunction caused by medications, which include lithium and immunotherapies
- Hypothyroidism as a result of radioactive iodine therapy and/or thyroidectomy to treat hyperthyroidism
- Transient hypothyroidism caused by postpartum thyroiditis

Key assessments indicating hypothyroidism are related to metabolic changes that result from lack of thyroid hormone. These signs and symptoms include:

- Fatigue, weakness, dyspnea on exertion
- Intolerance of cold temperatures
- Weight gain
- Constipation
- Cognitive dysfunction, slow movement, and slow speech
- Bradycardia, diastolic hypertension
- Delayed relaxation of tendon reflexes
- Carpal tunnel syndrome
- Dry, coarse skin; hair loss
- Periorbital edema and enlargement of the tongue
- Nonpitting edema (myxedema)
- Decreased hearing
- Hoarseness
- Myalgia, arthralgia
- Heavy menstrual bleeding (women)

Hyperthyroidism

Disorders and conditions that cause subclinical or overt *hyperthyroidism* include:

- Graves' disease, an autoimmune disease that causes hyperthyroidism (elevated thyroid hormone synthesis), goiter (thyroid enlargement), eye disease, and localized myxedema

- Toxic adenoma and toxic multinodular goiter, which are caused by hyperplasia of thyroid follicular cells
- Iodine-induced hyperthyroidism, an uncommon condition that can develop after administration of contrast agents used for CT scan, or iodine-rich medications like amiodarone

Older adults and individuals with milder hyperthyroidism often have isolated symptoms that warrant evaluation, including unexplained weight loss, decreased appetite, weakness, and new onset of atrial fibrillation. Most individuals with overt hyperthyroidism have a dramatic constellation of symptoms. These include:

- Increased perspiration and heat intolerance
- Hyperpigmentation, itching, and thinning of hair
- Stare and lid lag, impairment of eye muscle function
- Proptosis or exophthalmos, and periorbital edema (Graves' disease)
- Tachycardia, systolic hypertension, atrial fibrillation
- Dysphagia due to goiter; weight loss
- Urinary frequency and nocturia
- Amenorrhea or oligomenorrhea (women)
- Anxiety, emotional lability
- Weakness, tremor, and palpitations

Thyroid Nodules and Thyroid Cancer

Thyroid nodules can be incidental findings during routine physical exam or imaging tests. Their clinical importance is primarily related to the need to exclude thyroid cancer, yet history and physical exam related to the evaluation of the thyroid and thyroid nodules have low accuracy for predicting malignancy. Key physical exam findings of a fixed hard mass, symptoms of dysphagia and hoarseness, cervical lymphadenopathy, or vocal cord paralysis all suggest the need to evaluate for thyroid cancer. (See Laboratory Considerations for the Head and Neck and Imaging Considerations for the Head and Neck sections for additional assessments related to thyroid nodules.) Individuals at risk for thyroid cancer are patients with a history of childhood head or neck irradiation, adults under 30 years of age, and individuals with a family history of thyroid cancer. While the majority of cystic nodules are benign, malignant nodules may be cystic. See **Figure 11.16** for an individual with a scar related to thyroidectomy.

PEDIATRIC CONSIDERATIONS

CRANIOFACIAL DISORDERS

Children with craniofacial disorders, or abnormalities of the face or skull, may have disfigurement as a

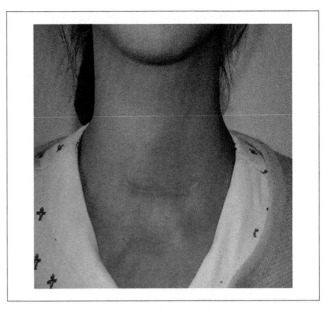

FIGURE 11.16 Thyroidectomy scar.

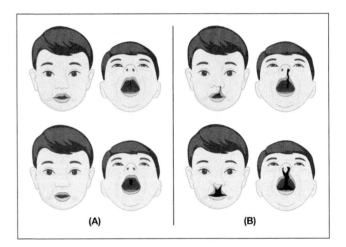

FIGURE 11.17 Cleft lip. (A) A cleft lip may be minimal or extend past the upper border of the lip, or (B) may be unilateral or bilateral and extend into the nares.

Source: From Chiocca, E. M. (2015). *Advanced pediatric assessment* (2nd ed.). New York, NY: Springer Publishing Company.

result of genetic disorders, trauma, and/or disease processes. Craniofacial disorders may or may not have associated musculoskeletal, neurologic, cardiac, and/or brain disorders; prompt assessment and identification is necessary for maximizing health and wellness. Some of the more common disorders and/or syndromes include:

- *Cleft lip and palate* abnormalities in which the lip and/or hard/soft palate do not completely form; degree varies from mild notch to severe large opening extending to the nasal cavity (**Figure 11.17**)

- *Craniosynostosis*, early fusion of the bones of the skull, results in increased intracranial pressure and/or skull abnormalities; differs from plagiocephaly, which is a flat area on the head or side of the infant's head resulting from positioning, that is, pressure from being repeatedly in a supine position can cause the back of the skull to flatten
- *Down syndrome*, a genetic disorder caused by an extra chromosome (Trisomy 21); associated craniofacial abnormalities include flattened nasal bridge, shortened neck, small low-set ears, and slanted epicanthal folds
- *Fetal alcohol syndrome*–associated facial abnormalities include smooth philtrum, thin upper lip, flat nasal bridge, short or upturned nose, and wide set eyes with epicanthal folds (**Figure 11.18**)
- *Hemangioma*, an abnormal collection of blood vessels in the skin that is faint at birth, then appears larger and darker in the first few months after birth; also known as port wine stain, salmon patch, or strawberry hemangioma
- *Treacher Collins* genetic disorder that causes maxillary hypoplasia and auricular deformities, in addition to a smaller skull or microcephaly
- *Turner syndrome*, a genetic disorder that affects development in females; appearance can include thickened neck, low hairline, prominent earlobes, and crowding of teeth (**Figure 11.19**)

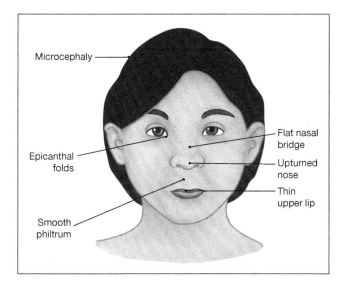

FIGURE 11.18 Facial abnormalities associated with fetal alcohol syndrome.

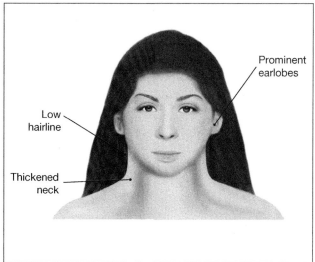

FIGURE 11.19 Facial abnormalities associated with Turner syndrome.

CASE STUDY: Recurrent Headaches

History

A 32-year-old woman presents with concerns of recurrent headaches. The headaches occur at the beginning of her menstrual cycles and can last up to 24 hours. She describes the pain as unilateral, sharp, and having moderate intensity rated as a "6" on a 1 to 10 scale. She has tried OTC pain medications without relief. The only thing that she has found to relieve the headache pain is to be in a dark, quiet room. She experiences nausea but not vomiting with these headaches. She denies visual changes before or during the headache and states that her mother had similar headaches associated with her menstrual cycles as well. The individual shares that she does have a stressful job and that she misses work almost once monthly because of her headaches. While she is not overweight, she notes that her diet would not be described as "healthy." She is married, has three children, and sleeps approximately 6 hours a night. She is a nonsmoker who drinks two to three glasses of wine most evenings. She has no diagnosed comorbidities and has an intrauterine device for contraception.

(continued)

CASE STUDY: Recurrent Headaches (*continued*)

Differential Diagnoses

Migraine with or without aura, tension-type headache, secondary headache

Physical Examination

- Blood pressure, heart rate, temperature, and body mass index within normal limits
- No obvious or palpable abnormalities of the skull base, temporomandibular joints, temporal arteries, cervical spine, or neck musculature
- No carotid or temporal bruits

- No abnormalities in neurologic exam: Speech is clear and distinct, patient is easily understood, gait is smooth and even, cranial nerves II to XII are intact, upper and lower extremity reflexes are 2+, strength 5/5 all extremities

Laboratory and Imaging

No lab work or imaging are required for this patient (Dodick, 2010).

Final Diagnosis

Migraine without aura (triggered by menstrual cycle)

CASE STUDY: Constellation of Symptoms and Comorbidities

History

A 62-year-old man presents with a constellation of symptoms that include fatigue, weight gain, dry skin, and constipation. These symptoms have been slowly worsening over the last 3 months. He has a 5-year history of type 2 diabetes, hyperlipidemia, and hypertension. He states that he has been struggling with his weight, despite efforts to limit carbohydrates and increase intake of fruits and vegetables. He also states that he has had difficulty with controlling his blood sugars; his home blood glucose monitoring results range from 140 to 260 mg/dL. His current medications include lovastatin, metformin, and lisinopril.

Differential Diagnoses

Hypothyroidism, goiter, myxedema, subacute thyroiditis, polyglandular autoimmune syndrome

Physical Examination

- Blood pressure 140/90; heart rate, temperature, and respiratory rate within normal limits
- General survey: BMI 40, pleasant, awake and alert
- Head: Coarse, brittle, thinning hair; periorbital puffiness, hoarseness, macroglossia; no obvious lesions or rashes
- Neck: Diffuse, nodular goiter; no lymphadenopathy, full range of motion

- Heart: Regular rate and rhythm, distinct S1 and S2 without murmur or gallop
- Lungs: Clear to auscultation bilaterally
- Abdomen: Soft, nontender, no palpable hepatosplenomegaly
- No abnormalities in neurologic exam: Speech is clear and distinct, patient is easily understood, gait is smooth and even, cranial nerves II to XII are intact, upper and lower extremity reflexes are 2+, strength 5/5 all extremities
- Skin is dry; generalized nonpitting edema of upper and lower extremities
- Exam of feet bilaterally reveals ability to sense touch and vibration without limitation

Laboratory and Imaging

For this individual, lab work included blood glucose, HbA1c, renal panel, lipid profile, TSH, and free T4. Results indicated dramatic elevation of triglycerides (above 500 mg/dL), elevated LDL level (above 180 mg/dL), elevated TSH (above 4.0 mU/L), decreased T4 levels (below 3 mcg/dL), elevated HbA1c (13%), and elevated blood glucose level (350 mg/dL).

Final Diagnosis

Primary hypothyroidism (in addition to type 2 diabetes, obesity, HTN, hyperlipidemia)

Clinical Pearls

- Pertinent review of systems relative to assessment of the head and neck will include review of neurologic, musculoskeletal, and vascular systems.
- Expose the neck and clavicles to fully view the head and neck for symmetry, obvious masses, or lesions.
- Infants and children with craniofacial abnormalities may have an underlying genetic syndrome.

Key Takeaways

- Physical exam of the patient begins with a general survey, observation, and inspection of the head and neck.
- More than 90% of individuals who present with a headache have a primary headache disorder, and their physical exam will be normal.
- Maintain a high index of suspicion for hypothyroidism because signs and symptoms can be mild, nonspecific, and varied.
- Symptoms of depression and anxiety often accompany thyroid dysfunction.

REFERENCES

American Academy of Pediatrics. (2018). *Ten things physicians and patients should question.* Retrieved from http://www.choosingwisely.org/societies/american-academy-of-pediatrics

American College of Emergency Physicians. (2018). *Ten things physicians and patients should question.* Retrieved from http://www.choosingwisely.org/societies/american-college-of-emergency-physicians

American College of Radiology. (2017). *Ten things physicians and patients should question.* Retrieved from http://www.choosingwisely.org/societies/american-college-of-radiology

American Medical Society for Sports Medicine. (2014). *Five things physicians and patients should question.* Retrieved from http://www.choosingwisely.org/societies/american-medical-society-for-sports-medicine

American Thyroid Association. (2018). *American Thyroid Association (ATA) guidelines and surgical statements.* Retrieved from https://www.thyroid.org/professionals/ata-professional-guidelines

Chiocca, E. M. (2015). *Advanced pediatric assessment* (2nd ed.). New York, NY: Springer Publishing Company.

Choosing Wisely. (n.d.). *Clinician lists.* Retrieved from http://www.choosingwisely.org/clinician-lists

Chung, M. K., Patrone, C. C., & Lariccia, P. J. (2015). A modified approach to thyroid exams. *The Journal of Family Practice, 64*(2), 83. Retrieved from https://www.mdedge.com/familymedicine/article/96821/endocrinology/modified-approach-thyroid-exams

Dodick, D. W. (2010). Pearls: Headache. *Seminars in Neurology, 30*(1), 74–81. doi:10.1055/s-0029-1245000

Endocrine Society. (2018). *Five things physicians and patients should question.* Retrieved from http://www.choosingwisely.org/societies/endocrine-society

Grubenhoff, J. A., Kirkwood, M., Gao, D., Deakyne, S., & Wathen, J. (2010). Evaluation of the standardized assessment of concussion in a pediatric emergency department. *Pediatrics, 126*(4), 688–695. doi:10.1542/peds.2009-2804

International Headache Society. (2018). Headache Classification Committee of the International Headache Society (IHS): The international Classification of headache disorders, 3rd edition. *Cephalalgia, 38*(1), 1–211. doi:10.1177/0333102417738202

Kiesler, J., & Ricer, R. (2003). The abnormal fontanel. *American Family Physician, 67*(12), 2547–2552. Retrieved from https://www.aafp.org/afp/2003/0615/p2547.html

Tamhane, S., & Gharib, H. (2016). Thyroid nodule update on diagnosis and management. *Clinical Diabetes and Endocrinology, 2*, 17. doi:10.1186/s40842-016-0035-7

Tingi, E., Syed, A. A., Kyriacou, A., Mastorakos, G., & Kyriacou, A. (2016). Benign thyroid disease in pregnancy: A state of the art review. *Journal of Clinical & Translational Endocrinology, 6*, 37–49. doi:10.1016/j.jcte.2016.11.001

U.S. Preventive Services Task Force. (2015). *Thyroid dysfunction: Screening.* Retrieved from https://www.uspreventiveservicestaskforce.org/Page/Name/recommendations

U.S. Preventive Services Task Force. (2017). *Thyroid cancer: Screening.* Retrieved from https://www.uspreventiveservicestaskforce.org/Page/Name/recommendations

12

Evidence-Based Assessment of the Eye

John Melnyk, Rosie Zeno, and Alice M. Teall

"I never questioned the integrity of an umpire. Their eyesight, yes."

—LEO DUROCHER

LEARNING OBJECTIVES

- Review the anatomy and physiology of the eye.
- Discuss common signs and symptoms related to ocular disorders.
- Identify components of the adult and pediatric eye exam.
- Consider the evidence-based screening recommendations for abnormal ocular conditions.

ANATOMY AND PHYSIOLOGY OF THE EYE

The eyes are complex sensory organs with components that are neurologic (retina, optic nerve), vascular (central retina arteries and veins), and optical (cornea and lens). **Figure 12.1** depicts the anatomy of the ocular system, the eye, cornea, lens, and fluids. The eyeball sits in the orbit, the bony cavity within the skull, which is, technically speaking, outside the body; however, only one sixth of the eyeball is exposed to the outside air because of the protection offered by the orbit (see **Figure 12.2**). The components of the ocular system and the complexity of the neurophysiology of vision operate to create a sensitive sensory system. More than half of the sensory receptors in the human body are located in the eyes, and a significant portion of the cerebral cortex is used to interpret visual information (Rehman, Mahabadi, & Ali, 2019).

Changes in vision and/or ocular pain, in and around the eye, may be some of the first indicators of systemic as well as ocular disease. Early detection and treatment of these conditions may make the difference between long-term disabling effects on the body and/or the vision. The goal of early detection is to be able to restore fully functioning life and vision and to successfully treat many of these conditions. This is why it is so critical for the clinician, who may be the first to assess an individual's concerns, to be aware of signs and symptoms of ocular changes that indicate urgent or emergent concerns.

ACCESSORY STRUCTURES OF THE EYE

External, accessory structures protect the eye; eyebrows, eyelids and eyelashes, the conjunctiva, lacrimal apparatus, and extrinsic eye muscles are all considered accessory structures. The coarse hairs of the eyebrows and the fine hairs of the eyelashes protect the eye from small particles and irritants. Sensitive to the external environment, eyelashes are a component of the blink response to threats to the eye.

The eyelids, or palpebrae, are the movable folds of skin that cover the eyes during sleep; protect the eyes from excess light, particles, and irritants; and spread lubricating secretions over the eyeball. The tarsal plate, composed of connective tissue, provides support to the eyelids. The upper eyelid exhibits greater movement than the lower eyelid because it contains the levator palpebrae superioris muscle (see **Figure 12.3**). The opening between the upper and the lower eyelids that exposes the eye is the **palpebral fissure**, where the eyelids meet medially and laterally form the medial and lateral canthus. The lacrimal caruncle, the small, pink,

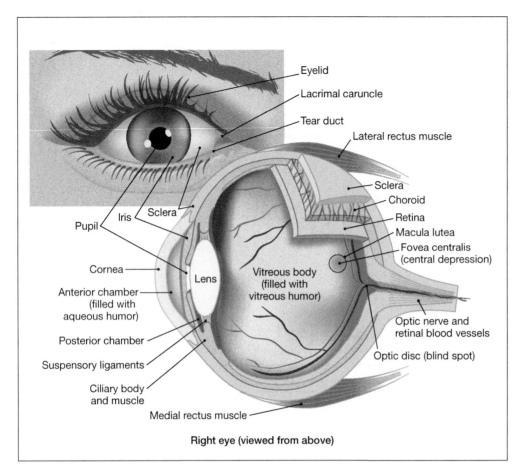

Right eye (viewed from above)

FIGURE 12.1 Anatomy of the eye.

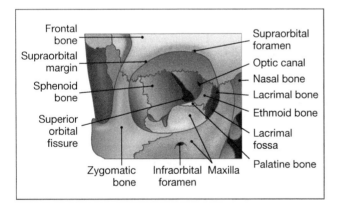

FIGURE 12.2 Bones of the orbit.

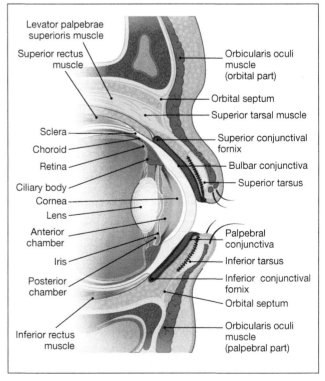

FIGURE 12.3 Eyelid.

nodule at the inner corner, or medial canthus, of the eye contains both oil and sweat glands. The eyelids also contain sebaceous glands, known as accessory lacrimal glands or meibomian glands, which produce lipid and mucin to lubricate the eyes and eyelids.

The conjunctiva is a thin, protective mucous membrane that lines the interior of the eyelids (palpebral conjunctiva), continues over the anterior surface of the eye (bulbar conjunctiva), and meets, but does not

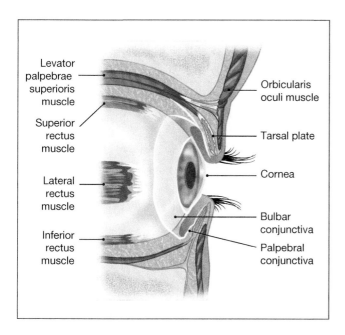

FIGURE 12.4 Conjunctiva and muscles of the eye.

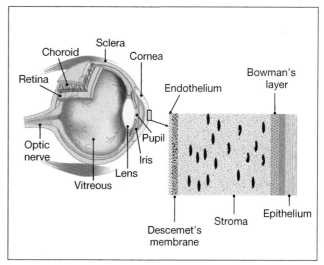

FIGURE 12.5 Internal eye anatomy.

cover, the cornea. The goblet cells of the conjunctiva also produce mucin, which aids in lubricating and protecting the eye and eyelids (see **Figure 12.4**). The lacrimal apparatus produces and drains lacrimal fluid, or tears, onto the surface of the conjunctiva; this physiologic system includes the lacrimal gland (found superotemporally in the lacrimal fossa of the frontal bone), which is an exocrine gland, similar to the salivary or mammary glands. The lacrimal apparatus produces the aqueous portion of the tear film. The "puncta" are openings in the superior and inferior nasal portion of the lids that drain lacrimal fluid, or tears, through the nasolacrimal ducts to the back of the nose. Narrowing or obstruction of the lacrimal duct system is reviewed in the Abnormal Findings of the Eye section of this chapter.

Each eye has six extrinsic or **extraocular muscles (EOMs)** that are innervated by three cranial nerves: the oculomotor (III), trochlear (IV), and abducens (VI). The six EOMs are the lateral rectus, medial rectus, superior rectus, inferior rectus, inferior oblique, and superior oblique muscles; together, the EOMs are capable of moving the eye in almost any direction. The EOMs allow the eyes to move smoothly as an individual shifts their gaze to focus left, right, upward, downward, near, or far.

PRINCIPAL STRUCTURES OF THE EYE

The adult eyeball measures approximately 2.5 cm (1 inch) in diameter. The outermost layer consists of the **cornea** anteriorly and the **sclera** posteriorly. The cornea is transparent and allows light to enter the eye. The density of pain receptors in the cornea makes it sensitive and responsive to touch, temperature, chemicals, and

particles. Although transparent, the tissues and layers of the cornea are organized and structured to carry oxygen and nutrients from tears and aqueous humor. The cornea contributes significantly to the eye's ability to focus.

The sclera is the dense fibrous membrane that covers the entire eyeball except for the cornea. The sclera maintains the shape of the eye and is the white fibrous component that is visible anteriorly. The internal eye anatomy, including the five tissue layers of the cornea, are depicted in **Figure 12.5**.

The middle layer of the eye includes the choroid and the iris. The choroid is a vascular, pigmented layer that lines the internal surface of the sclera and provides nutrients to the retina. The choroid contains melanocytes that produce the pigment melanin, which absorbs excess light and prevents reflection and scattering of light within the eyeball. The **iris** is the flat, colored, ring-shaped membrane located between the cornea and the lens; the amount of melanin in the iris determines eye color (see **Figure 12.6**). In the anterior portion of this vascular layer, the choroid becomes the ciliary body, which includes ciliary processes and ciliary muscle. The iris is attached to these ciliary processes; its main function is to regulate how much light passes through the **pupil**, or circular opening in the center of the iris. The choroid, iris, and ciliary body of the middle layer of the eye are referred to as the uveal tract (Spalton, Hitchings, & Hunter, 2002).

The lens is located in the cavity of the eyeball, behind the pupil and iris (see **Figure 12.7**). The transparent, flexible tissue of the lens is made up of about 65% water and 35% protein and traces of minerals. In a manner similar to the cornea, the lens refracts light to be focused on the retina. The lens divides the interior of the eye into two cavities: the anterior cavity and the vitreous cavity. The anterior cavity is divided into

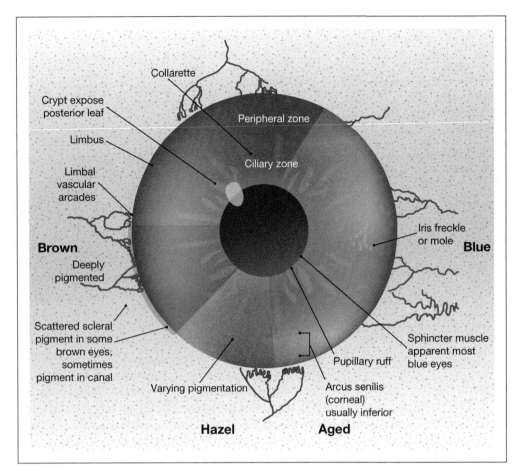

FIGURE 12.6 Iris.

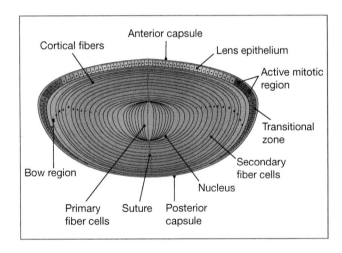

FIGURE 12.7 Lens.

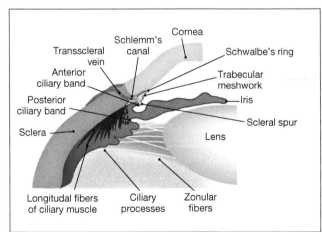

FIGURE 12.8 Anterior chamber.

the anterior chamber and the posterior chamber. The anterior chamber is located between the cornea and the iris. The posterior chamber is located behind the iris and lens. Both chambers of the anterior cavity are filled with aqueous humor, a watery fluid produced by the outer nonpigmented epithelium of the ciliary body (see **Figure 12.8**).

The purpose of aqueous humor is to nourish the endothelium of the cornea and the lens, and maintain intraocular pressure (IOP). Aqueous humor is secreted at a rate of approximately 2.75 μL/minute, which allows it to be replaced every 90 minutes (Brubaker, 1996). To work as it should, the production of aqueous humor must be balanced by a drainage system to maintain a

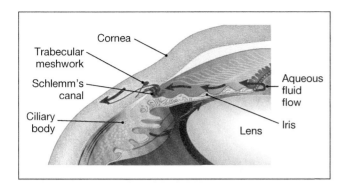

FIGURE 12.9 Flow of aqueous humor.

stable amount of fluid in the anterior chamber. If the balance is not maintained, this may be an indication of **glaucoma**, a condition that results in damage to the optic nerve, vision loss, and/or blindness. The "normal" IOP is generally accepted to be no greater than 21 mmHg; although it is possible to have IOPs greater than 21 mmHg that are benign. The presence of elevated fluid pressure inside the eye with no signs of optic nerve damage (increased cupping) and no visual field defects is referred to as ocular hypertension. Another condition in which the IOP is normal but there are visual field losses and optic nerve cupping is normal tension (or low tension) glaucoma. These conditions are reviewed in the Abnormal Findings of the Eye section of this chapter.

The normal flow of aqueous humor is depicted in **Figure 12.9**. The trabecular meshwork is porous tissue, located near the cornea, through which aqueous humor flows into Schlemm's canal and out of the eye into systemic circulation; Schlemm's canal is a unique structure that is thought to have both vascular and lymphatic characteristics (Abu-Hassan, Acott, & Kelley, 2014; Karpinich & Caron, 2014). Serious ocular pathology is associated with increased resistance to drainage of aqueous humor through the conventional outflow system, which involves the trabecular meshwork and the Schlemm's canal.

Vitreous humor fills the cavity of the posterior chamber of the eye, between the lens and the retina. The transparent vitreous humor is a fluid and gelatinous substance that is approximately 99% water; the other constituents are hyaluronic acid and collagen fibrils, whose viscoelastic properties help to maintain the shape of the eye and hold the retina against the choroid. Unlike the aqueous humor, the vitreous body does not undergo rapid replacement; it contains phagocytic cells that remove debris to maintain unobstructed vision (Rehman et al., 2019). Age-related changes and eye disorders can lead to debris within the vitreous humor, casting a shadow on the field of vision; these floaters can be benign or can signify infection, inflammation, or deterioration.

NEUROLOGIC COMPONENTS OF THE OCULAR SYSTEM

The innermost layer of the eyeball is the retina, a neurosensory layer that is attached to the posterior pole of the eye. The retina is composed of several layers of specialized cells that work in a coordinated fashion to absorb light, process visual data, and transmit neural-visual impulses to the brain. **Figure 12.10** depicts the anatomy of the retina, including the specialized pigmented and neural layers.

Light enters the eye; is refracted or deflected by the cornea, aqueous humor, lens, and vitreous humor; and then passes through both the ganglion and bipolar cell layers of the retina before it reaches the photoreceptor layer, where photoreceptor cells convert light rays into nerve impulses. The two types of photoreceptor cells are rods and cones. Each retina contains about 6 million cones and more than 100 million rods (Rehman et al., 2019). Rods function in dim light and are more numerous in the periphery of the retina. Cones function in bright light and are predominant in the

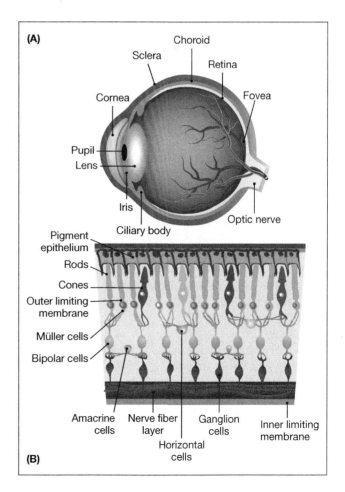

FIGURE 12.10 Anatomy of the retina. (A) Location within the eye. (B) Specialized pigmented and neural layers.

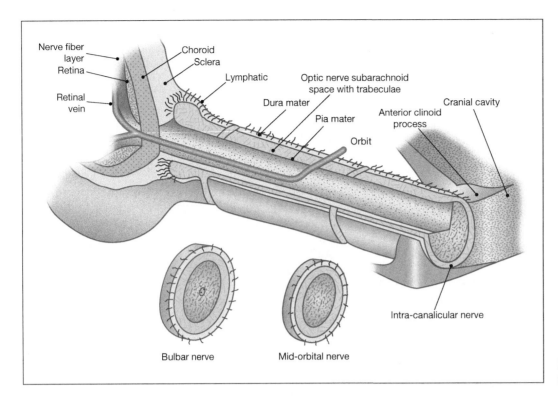

Nerve fiber layer
Retina
Retinal vein
Choroid
Sclera
Lymphatic
Dura mater
Optic nerve subarachnoid space with trabeculae
Pia mater
Orbit
Anterior clinoid process
Cranial cavity
Intra-canalicular nerve

Bulbar nerve
Mid-orbital nerve

FIGURE 12.11 Optic nerve anatomy.

central region of the retina. **Color vision** results from the stimulation of different combinations of blue, green, and red cones.

The **optic nerve** is the sensory nerve (cranial nerve II) that transmits the neural-visual impulses from the retina to the brain. The pathway and anatomic features of the optic nerve in relation to the eye are depicted in **Figure 12.11**. The impulses travel along the fibers of the optic nerve that join the temporal fibers from the opposite eye at the optic chiasm; this optic tract encircles the brain, and the impulse is transmitted to the occipital lobe for interpretation.

The fundus of the eye is the interior surface visible by ophthalmoscopic exam. (See the Physical Examination of the Eye section to review information about direct ophthalmoscopy.) The normal fundoscopic exam is pictured in **Figure 12.12**. Anatomic structures viewed by **fundal exam** include:

- *Peripheral retina:* The fundal background should be a deep red color, without exudate or hemorrhages. Damage to the retina caused by microinfarctions associated with diabetes, hypertension, severe anemia, and other disorders may appear as cotton wool spots, plaques, or lesions within the peripheral retina. Proliferative lesions can indicate diabetic retinopathy. Patchy areas of hyperpigmentation or depigmentation scattered throughout may indicate macular degeneration.

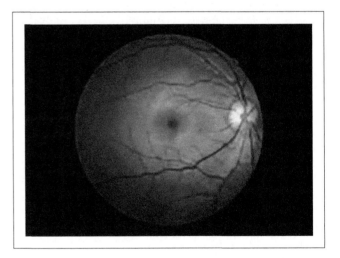

FIGURE 12.12 Normal fundal exam.

- *Optic nerve:* The optic nerve is seen as a round sphere with sharp margins. The physiologic cup is contained within the optic disc and is usually less than half the diameter of the disc. Optic disc edema (papilledema) is a serious sign of increased intracranial pressure. The elevated IOP caused by glaucoma may cause the central cup of the optic disc to deepen and widen so it occupies greater than half of the disc diameter; this pathology is known as optic cupping.

- *Macula:* The macula is a dark, flat spot located in the exact center of the posterior portion of the retina. The fovea centralis is located in the center of the macula, contains only cones, and is the area of highest visual acuity or resolution. No vessels should be noted around the macula.
- *Vasculature:* Vessels emerge from the nasal side of the optic disc. Arteries are narrower and lighter in color than veins. Central retinal arteries and veins and branch retinal arteries and veins are the only blood vessels in the human body that can be directly inspected. The vasculature should not be tortuous. No hemorrhages should be noted. If an individual has chronic hypertension, causing arteries to stiffen and thicken, the arteries may indent and displace veins at their crossing points, which is known as arteriovenous (AV) nicking.

KEY HISTORY QUESTIONS AND CONSIDERATIONS FOR THE EYE

Thorough history taking provides the clinician with key information on which to base their physical exam and diagnosis. The clinician's role includes asking an individual to clarify or elaborate on symptoms. Clinicians familiar with urgent/emergent disorders of the eye will recognize the significance of symptoms, personal health history, and/or family history that indicate the need for immediate, specialized visual exam.

HISTORY OF PRESENT ILLNESS

Common Presenting Symptoms

- Eye pain (assessments related to history of eye pain are provided in the example that follows)
- Eye swelling and/or itching
- Eye redness and/or drainage
- Decreased visual acuity or vision loss
- Blurry vision or floaters, cloudy vision, diplopia (double vision)
- Photophobia (painful spasm on exposure to bright light)

Example: Eye Pain

- Onset: Recent, intermittent, and/or chronic
- Location: Unilateral or bilateral; part of the eye most bothersome
- Duration: Persistent or transitory, increasing or unchanged
- Character: Itching, tearing, burning, foreign body sensation, photophobia, deep pain, pain on eye movement, or tenderness to touch, flashing lights in vision, floaters
- Associated symptoms: Acute decrease in visual acuity or loss of vision (alarm symptoms), double vision, blurry vision, or eye discharge
- Aggravating factors: Eye injury, foreign body or chemical substance in eye, recent illness, stressors, sleep problems, overuse of digital devices/computer screens
- Relieving symptoms: Pharmacologic treatment, including over-the-counter (OTC) pain relief and nonpharmacologic treatment, including application of heat, cold, flushing of the eye with water
- Temporal factors: Recent or current illness/infection
- Severity: Pain rating on 1 to 10 scale
- Differential diagnoses: Conjunctivitis, corneal abrasion, glaucoma, orbital cellulitis, scleritis, sty, uveitis

PAST MEDICAL HISTORY

- Recent injury, trauma, or infection
- Medications currently prescribed, OTC, herbs, supplements
- Allergies; allergic reactions, including history of anaphylaxis, reactions to medications
- Past history of eye problems, disorders, diseases, injury, surgery
- If contact wearer, current practices: Daily cleaning, sleeping/napping in contacts, change contacts as prescribed
- Prescription eyewear, glasses, contacts; myopia, astigmatism

History of systemic disease/disorder with ocular signs and symptoms:

- Metabolic endocrine: Diabetes with most recent HbA1c level, thyroid disorders
- Vascular: Hypertension, stroke, migraines, clotting disorders, sickle cell anemia
- Autoimmune: Systemic lupus erythematosus (SLE), sarcoidosis, temporal (giant cell) arteritis, rheumatoid arthritis (RA), Sjögen's syndrome, myasthenia gravis
- Inflammatory bowel disease: Crohn's, ulcerative colitis
- Idiopathic disorders: Multiple sclerosis (MS)
- Infective disorders: Cytomegalovirus (CMV), human immunodeficiency virus (HIV), acquired immunodeficiency syndrome (AIDS)
- Neoplastic disorders: Melanoma, pituitary adenoma, metastatic carcinoma, lymphoma
- Congenital disorders: Marfan syndrome, Down syndrome, neurofibromatosis

FAMILY HISTORY

- Ocular history: Glaucoma, cataracts, retinal detachment, blindness
- Visual history: Poor visual acuity, macular degeneration
- History of diseases impacting vision: Diabetes, hypertension, migraines, RA, MS, thyroid or clotting disorders

SOCIAL HISTORY

- Smoking history/history of tobacco use
- Sleep history
- Risk factors for HIV exposure
- Stress and coping
- Occupational/educational/recreational vision requirements

REVIEW OF SYSTEMS

- General: Weight loss or gain, fatigue, fever, pain
- Head/Neck: Acute or recurrent headache, neck pain, lymphadenopathy
- Ears, Nose, Throat (ENT): Ear pain, nasal congestion, rhinorrhea, sinus pain, sore throat, itchy ears, nose, or throat
- Eyes: Additional symptoms of redness, discharge, blurry vision, eye pain, vision loss
- Cardiovascular/Respiratory: Shortness of breath at rest or with exertion, cough, chest pain, orthopnea
- Gastrointestinal (GI)/Genitourinary (GU): Nausea, vomiting; likelihood of pregnancy
- Musculoskeletal: Inflamed joints, arthritis, weakness, gait or posture defects, need for assistive devices
- Neurologic: Numbness, dizziness, light sensitivity, asymmetric facial movements
- Endocrine: Polyuria, polydipsia, polyphagia
- Integumentary: Itching; rashes; lesions changing shape, size, or color; nonhealing sores/wounds
- Psychiatric: Depression, sadness, worry, insomnia; changes in memory, concentration

PREVENTIVE CARE CONSIDERATIONS

- Diet includes fruits, vegetables high in vitamin A, antioxidants
- Use of sunglasses to limit sun exposure/damage
- Regular handwashing and avoidance of touching the eye
- Proper handling of contact lenses and/or glasses
- Routine eye exams as recommended related to age, chronic disease, and/or visual acuity
- Use of protective eyewear for occupational/sports safety

- Limitations on screen time, and/or strategies to avoid eye strain

PHYSICAL EXAMINATION OF THE EYE

While comprehensive clinical examination of the eye is not typically performed as part of routine adult wellness exams, a thorough exam should be performed for any individual presenting with acute or chronic eye concerns, such as eye pain, eye injury, red eye, vision loss, eye discharge, double vision, dry eye, or floaters. As noted in the Key History Questions and Considerations of the Eye section, individuals with certain conditions such as diabetes, hypertension, multiple sclerosis, and lupus are at higher risk for eye disease. These individuals should have a comprehensive eye examination performed by an optometrist or ophthalmologist on a routine basis (see the Evidence-Based Considerations for the Eye section.) Examination of the eye by the generalist or primary care clinician involves inspection in conjunction with various clinical techniques that incorporate careful observation.

INSPECTION

Begin the eye exam by inspecting eyelids, eyelashes, conjunctivae, sclera, corneas, and irises for abnormal lesions, rashes, redness, swelling, or drainage. Note any asymmetry of the eyelids (ptosis) or pupils (anisocoria). One eyelid drooping lower than the other or a difference in pupil size may be a benign finding, but may also be a sign of a serious neurologic condition.

ASSESSMENT OF CORNEAL LIGHT REFLEX

Assess for a symmetric corneal light reflex (Hirschberg's test) by shining a light directly in front of the patient who is focusing on an object across the room, as demonstrated in **Figure 12.13**. Observe where the light reflects back within the pupil of both eyes simultaneously. An asymmetric corneal light reflex may indicate a misalignment of the eyes, or **strabismus**. See the Abnormal Findings of the Eye section of this chapter to review the distinction between strabismus and pseudostrabismus.

ASSESSMENT OF PUPILLARY LIGHT REFLEX, ACCOMMODATION, AND CONVERGENCE

If possible, perform the pupillary exam in a dimly lit room. Have the patient focus on an object across the room. Shine a light in each pupil, and note the size, position, shape, equality of the pupils, and their response to bright light (constrict to direct illumination). See

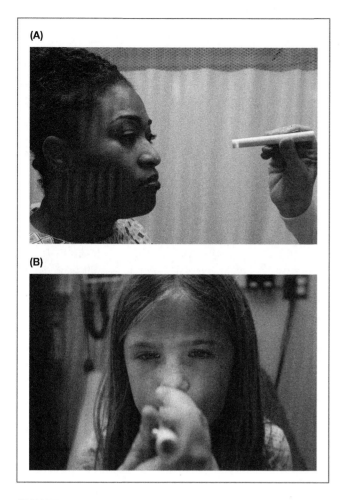

FIGURE 12.13 Hirschberg test to assess corneal light reflex: (A) Adult. (B) Child.

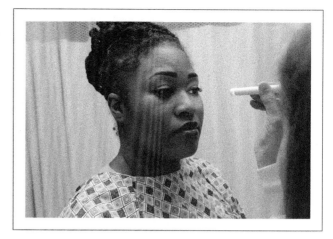

FIGURE 12.14 Assessing direct response to light.

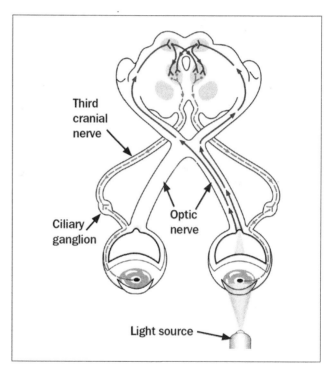

FIGURE 12.15 Pupil reflex pathway.
Source: Image courtesy of John Yaw-Jong Tsai, Touro University.

Figure 12.14 which depicts the clinician eliciting direct response to light. Shining a light in one pupil should also cause the other pupil to constrict (consensual response). The reflex arc that results in the consensual response is depicted in **Figure 12.15**. Assess direct and consensual response for each eye; appropriate pupillary response reflects the integrity of CN III, IV, and VI.

Pupils should change in size when the eyes change focus on near and far objects. To assess this accommodation reflex, have the patient focus on a distant object, then focus on a penlight and slowly move the penlight toward the patient's nose (**Figure 12.16**). Both eyes should turn inward (convergence), and both pupils should constrict (accommodation). These functions are necessary for binocular vision.

VISUAL FIELDS TESTING

Confrontation visual field testing is used as a screening for integrity of the optic nerve (CN II), visual field defects, scotomas (blind spots), and early signs of serious ocular disorders. To test **visual fields** by confrontation, the clinician should sit (or stand) approximately 2 feet away from the patient; the clinician and patient should face one another. Both cover one eye (as a mirror image) and maintain eye contact. The clinician should extend an arm and raise a finger. Starting from the periphery, slowly advance the finger into the patient's field of vision. Ask the patient to say "now" when

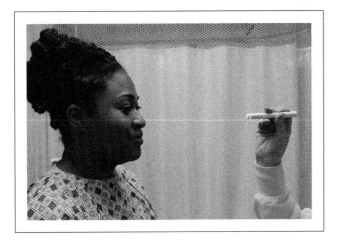

FIGURE 12.16 Assessment of accommodation and convergence.

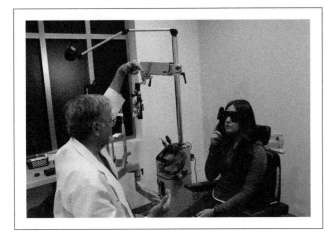

FIGURE 12.17 Simultaneous visual field testing by confrontation.

the finger becomes visible. Assuming the clinician has normal peripheral vision, the patient should be able to see the finger at the same time the clinician does. A delay in seeing the finger would indicate impaired peripheral vision. This should be repeated on both sides and can include all fields of vision. Because the visual fields of both eyes overlap, each eye should be tested independently.

Alternatively, the clinician can hold up a certain number of fingers peripherally, equidistant between themselves and the patient. The patient is asked to correctly identify the number of fingers. All quadrants (upper and lower, temporal and nasal) should be tested.

Confrontation visual field testing is highly specific but has limited sensitivity (Anderson, Shuey, & Wall, 2009). To improve identification of any defects in central processing, the clinician may perform additional

testing with both eyes open, presenting stimuli in the right and left visual fields simultaneously, as demonstrated in **Figure 12.17**. The gold standard for identification of visual field defects, however, is automated static perimetry, which is discussed in the section of this chapter that addresses ocular assessment as completed by a specialist.

TESTING MOVEMENT OF THE EXTRAOCULAR MUSCLES

Smooth and coordinated eye movement requires the use of the EOMs of each eye that are innervated by CN III, IV, and VI. Eye movement occurs in six cardinal fields of gaze. To assess the EOMs, the clinician stands in front of the patient and asks the patient to follow the clinician's finger with their eyes while keeping the head still and steady in a neutral position. If the clinician uses their finger to trace an "H" or rectangular shape in front of the patient, all EOMs will be required by the patient to follow their finger smoothly (**Figure 12.18**). Note the importance of moving the finger far enough out laterally and vertically to elicit all appropriate eye movements, and remembering to assess the movement across the entire "H." EOMs tested by specific eye movements are listed in **Table 12.1**.

ASSESSMENT OF THE RED REFLEX

The "red reflex" refers to the red or reddish-orange reflection of light from the fundus. This can commonly be seen in photographs as "red eye." To best elicit this reflex, use an ophthalmoscope to visualize the pupil. Look through the ophthalmoscope while shining the light into the pupil. This technique works best in a dimly lit room. The clinician may need to view at different angles to elicit the reflex. Any asymmetry in red reflex, dark spots, or leukocoria (white reflex) is abnormal and may be indicative of cataracts, retinal disease, or ocular tumor. See the Abnormal Findings of the Eye section of this chapter for additional information.

DIRECT OPHTHALMOSCOPY

Direct ophthalmoscopy, or fundoscopy, is used to assess concerns related to the retina, macula, optic nerve, or vasculature of the eye. In most cases, eye concerns in the primary care setting present with sufficient signs and symptoms (by history and physical exam) to guide clinical decision-making without the reliance on the results of the fundoscopic exam to determine the need for referral to ophthalmology. Signs, symptoms, and/or history that are concerning for serious eye disease or increased intracranial or IOP should be urgently referred. A dilated fundoscopic exam (facilitated by mydriatic

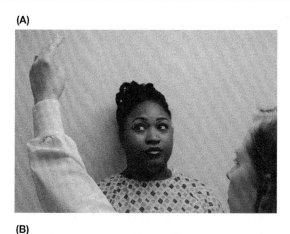

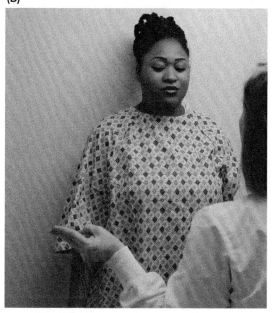

FIGURE 12.18 Assessment of extraocular muscles. (A) Assess upward gaze (top of the "H" on patient's right side). (B) Assess downward gaze (bottom of the "H" on patient's right side).

| TABLE 12.1 Clinical Testing of Extraocular Muscles | |
Muscle Being Tested	Movement to Assess
Superior rectus	Looks laterally and upward
Inferior rectus	Looks laterally and downward
Lateral rectus	Looks laterally
Medial rectus	Looks medially
Inferior oblique	Looks medially and upward
Superior oblique	Looks medially and downward

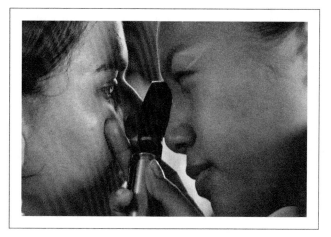

FIGURE 12.19 Direct ophthalmoscopy.

drops) should be performed by an ophthalmologist or optometrist for diagnostic purposes. Clinical considerations related to dilated and undilated eye exams are reviewed in the Evidence-Based Considerations for the Eye and Clinical Pearls sections of this chapter.

Inspection of the peripheral retina, optic nerve, macula, and vasculature of the eye using direct ophthalmoscopy is a particularly difficult technique because of the small field of view and magnification adjustments required for the individual who has poor visual acuity. It is even more challenging when the pupils are not dilated. To perform the exam as effectively as possible, darken the room and ask the patient to focus on an object far away to help dilate the pupil. The clinician should place the ophthalmoscope firmly against their own cheek. The clinician and ophthalmoscope should move as one unit. Use the right hand/eye to assess the patient's right eye. Look through the ophthalmoscope to determine if it is in focus and adjust the diopter setting if needed. Direct the light of the ophthalmoscope into the pupil at a medial angle, and watch for the red reflex. Slowly move toward the patient while following the red reflex. (If the red reflex is lost, start over.) Follow the red reflex all the way in until the vasculature is seen. Follow the direction of the blood vessels in until the optic disc is visualized. At this point, the clinician is approximately nose-to-nose with the patient, as seen in **Figure 12.19**, and can pivot the ophthalmoscope to view the remainder of the retina, macula/fovea, and blood vessels.

MEASUREMENT OF VISUAL ACUITY

Visual acuity is not assessed on a routine basis as a component of wellness or screening exams in most cases, except for children. (See the Life-Span Considerations for the Eye section of this chapter for pediatric considerations.) However, assessing visual acuity can provide useful data when individuals present with clinical

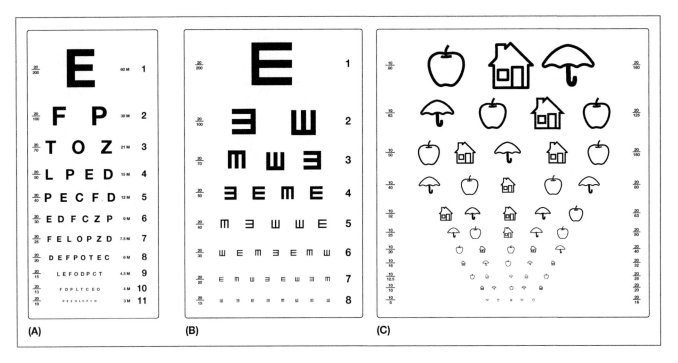

FIGURE 12.20   Vision charts. (A) Snellen vision chart. (B) Tumbling E's vision chart. (C) Pediatric picture vision chart.

concerns. **Visual acuity** is defined as the ability of the visual system to detect spatial changes (Rosenfield & Logan, 2009). Essentially, it is the ability of the eye to detect and resolve the different components of an object. This is similar to the resolving power of a telescope, used to magnify and clarify the view of distant stars. Several charts are used to measure visual acuity; acute change in visual acuity may be a worrisome sign. Visual acuity may be assessed using handheld acuity cards for both far and near vision.

The Snellen visual acuity charts are widely used to assess visual acuity; they have been modified over the years for different languages, and to include numbers and pictures for children and others who cannot read the letters. These charts, shown in **Figure 12.20**, are best used as a screening tool rather than a diagnostic test for corrective vision needs. Patients with poor or declining vision should be referred to an optometrist or ophthalmologist.

Testing visual acuity with a Snellen chart involves requiring the patient to stand at a distance of 20 feet. Each eye is tested independently; that is, one eye is covered, while the other is used to read. The patient should be allowed to wear their glasses and the results documented as "best corrected vision." Ask the patient to read the line with the smallest characters that they can see. The numbers at the end of the line provide an indication of the patient's acuity compared with those who have normal vision. The larger the denominator, the worse the acuity. For example, 20/200 indicates that the patient can see at 20 feet what an individual with normal vision can see at 200 feet. If the patient is unable to read any of the lines on the chart, an estimate of what they are capable of seeing should be assessed, for example, ability to count fingers, detect motion, or perceive light.

Visual acuity is reliant on the function of CN II and on the shape and clarity of the cornea and lens. **Myopia** (nearsightedness) is a refractive error that results when light is not bent or refracted properly. When the acuity with the Snellen chart is less than 20/20, the clinician can verify that the results are related to refractive error (and thus correctable with prescription lenses) by using a pinhole test. Ask the patient to hold a pinhole occluder, or a paper with a small hole in it. Reassess visual acuity with the Snellen chart. This maneuver allows light to enter only the central part of the lens, which will improve visual acuity when the focus was distorted by refractive error by at least one line on the chart. Individuals with vision loss not related to refractive error will show limited to no improvement with the pinhole and will require more urgent evaluation.

INTRAOCULAR PRESSURE TESTING

Elevated IOP is often asymptomatic unless severely elevated. Severely elevated IOPs are usually indicative of angle-closure glaucoma or may indicate uveitis, in some cases. These conditions will usually be associated with significant eye pain, head pain, nausea, or vomiting. IOP is measured by tonometry. A tonometer is an instrument that measures IOP by measuring the resistance of the cornea to indentation. It is measured in millimeters of mercury (mmHg). IOP measurements are usually not performed in general practice. They are often found in emergency departments and ophthalmologic or optometric practices.

LIFE-SPAN CONSIDERATIONS FOR THE EYE

PEDIATRIC CONSIDERATIONS

The pediatric eye exam has few physical differences from that pertaining to the older adolescent and adult; however, visual development is rapidly taking place in the first few years of life. It is essential for all children to have a regular eye examination and vision assessment to ensure early detection and prompt referral for any abnormalities. The American Academy of Pediatrics (AAP) recommends that formal vision screening be performed at ages 4 and 5 years, and then every other year beginning at age 6 years (Hagan, Shaw, & Duncan, 2017). Normal visual acuity in the newborn ranges from 20/100 to 20/400 and gradually develops to 20/20 by 5 to 6 years of age; this development of vision is known as emmetropization. The clinician should refer children to ophthalmology for an abnormal visual acuity for age, or more than a two-line difference between eyes; for example, right eye 20/20 and left eye 20/30. Instrument-based screening uses automated technology that essentially photographs a child's eyes to provide information regarding strabismus, refractive errors (myopia, hyperopia, and/or astigmatism), opacities (cataracts), or retinal abnormalities (retinoblastoma). It can be performed on children as young as 12 to 24 months and is especially helpful for screening nonverbal, speech delayed, or preliterate children.

At each routine wellness visit, the following assessments should be performed on all children aged newborn to 3 years:

- Vision assessment, including visual fixation, tracking, visual interest, and attentiveness
- Inspection of eyes, including lids, eyelashes, conjunctiva, corneas, sclera, irises, pupils
- Assessment of corneal light reflex and movement of the eyes (EOMs)
- Pupillary function, including reaction to light, accommodation, convergence
- Red reflex (may appear gray or cream colored in infants with darker-pigmented skin)

Normal findings will vary depending on age. The pupillary light reflex is underdeveloped until 5 months of age, and transient nystagmus can be a normal finding in infants younger than 6 months. EOM function is not well established in the first 6 months of age; therefore, intermittent phorias/strabismus may be observed. Poor muscle coordination and abnormal ocular alignment

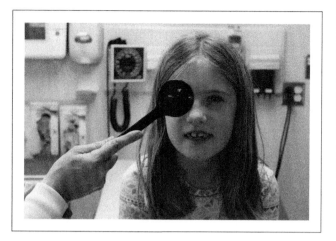

FIGURE 12.21 Pediatric binocular assessment with cover test.

after 6 months of age may warrant referral and further evaluation.

Corneal light reflex and observation are the primary methods for assessing eye alignment in infants. In young cooperative children, the cover test can be used. To perform the cover test, have the child focus on an object straight ahead. Check for deviation in either eye. Cover one eye for 3 seconds, as demonstrated in **Figure 12.21**. The tested, uncovered eye is observed for movement out of (or back into) its original position. The untested eye is uncovered, while the tested eye is again observed for any deviation out of (or into) alignment. Repeat for the other eye.

For children aged 3 years and older, age-appropriate visual acuity screening and an attempt at ophthalmoscopy should be routinely included as components of the pediatric eye exam. Clinicians should complete these screening exams when children are able to be cooperative, and not when children are experiencing illness or fatigue.

PREGNANCY CONSIDERATIONS

Numerous physiologic effects occur within the body during pregnancy, and the eye is no exception. Normal physiologic changes that resolve during postpartum may include:

- Decrease in corneal sensitivity
- Slight increase in corneal thickness
- Changes in corneal curvature
- Contact lens intolerance as a result of a change in corneal curvature, increased corneal thickness/edema, or an altered tear film
- Decreased or transient loss of accommodation

Preeclampsia, a complication of pregnancy characterized by hypertension and proteinuria, can affect the ocular system. The most commonly associated concern early in preeclampsia is blurry vision. However, severe preeclampsia can lead to retinopathy, optic neuropathy, and retinal detachments; retinopathy associated with preeclampsia may be more severe with underlying diabetes, chronic hypertension, and renal disease (Alizadeh Ghavidel, Mousavi, Bagheri, & Asghari, 2018). The visual prognosis for ocular involvement in mild preeclampsia is excellent in most cases because of the transient nature of preeclampsia and high rate of spontaneous recovery (Alizadeh Ghavidel et al., 2018).

CONSIDERATIONS FOR THE OLDER ADULT

Changes associated with structures of the eye include (Salvi, Akhtar, & Currie, 2006):

- Eyelid laxity and deepening of the lines of expression
- Changes in corneal curvature and decreased corneal luster
- Increased resistance to the outflow of aqueous humor in the trabecular network
- Hardening (nuclear sclerosis) of the lens
- Less collagen causes liquefaction of vitreous humor
- Decline in visual function, including function of the lens, results in presbyopia, far-sightedness
- Decreased contrast sensitivity resulting in reduced depth perception
- Increased susceptibility to age-related diseases (e.g., macular degeneration)

OCULAR ASSESSMENTS COMPLETED BY SPECIALISTS

Individuals who are not experiencing acute or emergent eye problems or disorders but who are at risk related to family health history, personal health history, or recent changes in their health may have questions about the type of screenings or assessments offered by eye specialists, that is, ophthalmologists and optometrists. Clinicians should explain that a comprehensive ocular assessment as completed by an eye professional includes more than a visual acuity exam. The comprehensive eye exam offered by specialists begins with "entrance exams," or screening assessments and functional tests that include:

- Inspection of the external eye
- Visual acuity measurement
- Pinhole visual acuity
- Amplitude of accommodation, or the maximum potential increase in optical power that an eye can achieve in adjusting its focus

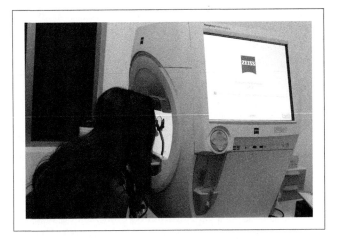

FIGURE 12.22 Humphrey perimeter (visual field perimeter).

- Color vision
- Stereopsis, or depth perception
- Near point of convergence to assess the ability to converge the eyes smoothly
- Functional tests of accommodation and systems needed to achieve binocular vision
- Pupil testing
- EOM testing
- Testing of visual fields

While some of the previously noted assessments are performed at a screening level by the general practice clinician, the ophthalmologist and/or optometrist has the ability to assess and evaluate these exams as diagnostic components of a more comprehensive exam. One example is the assessment of visual fields: Rather than performing a screening test, the specialist can measure the visual fields through a process known as static perimetry. **Figure 12.22** depicts a visual field perimeter, which may be used to assess the individual with glaucoma, optic neuropathies, or severely reduced visual acuity. Assessment of the structure and function of the eye by the specialist may also include assessment of color vision, refraction, and fundoscopy.

TESTING OF COLOR VISION

While some forms of color blindness are congenital, an ophthalmologist may assess color vision to diagnose retinal or optic nerve disorders. Assessment of color vision includes:

- **Ishihara color test**—Hue discrimination test to assess for red–green color blindness (**Figure 12.23A**)
- **Hardy–Rand–Rittler**—Test to assess for color blindness associated with optic neuropathies (**Figure 12.23B**)

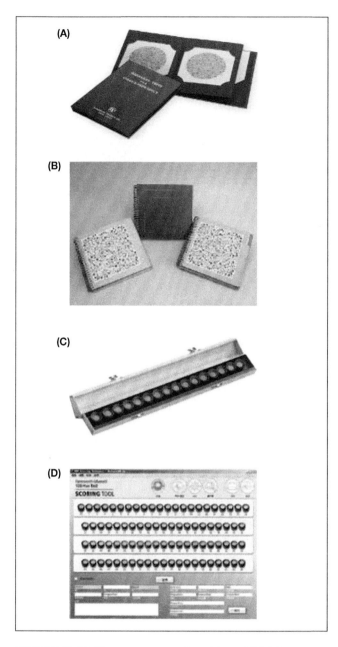

FIGURE 12.23 Tests to assess color vision. (A) Ishihara color blindness plates. (B) Hardy–Rand–Rittler (HRR) plates. (C) Farnsworth D-15 test. (D) FM 100-Hue test.

- **Farnsworth D-15**—Arrangement test for congenital and acquired color defects (**Figure 12.23C**)
- **Farnsworth–Munsell 100-Hue test**—Arrangement test requires hue discrimination (**Figure 12.23D**)

ASSESSMENT OF REFRACTION

An ophthalmologist's or optometrist's assessment of refraction is a multistep process using a series of ophthalmic lenses to arrive at a correction that will provide the clearest image that the patient's eye is

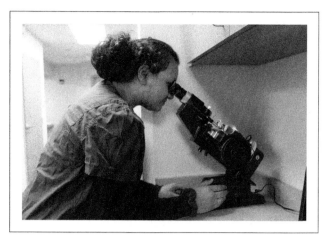

FIGURE 12.24 Lensometer.

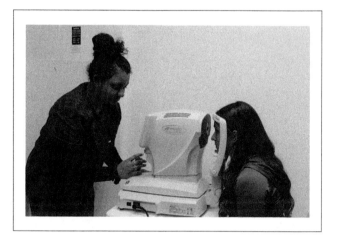

FIGURE 12.25 Keratometer and autorefractor.

capable of producing. This assessment is indicated either if there are initial patient concerns of blurred vision or if the clinician measures significantly decreased vision during the examination (Carlson & Kurtz, 2004). The process of refraction assessment includes:

- Lensometry: Use of an instrument (lensometer) to determine measurements of the current lenses, including the spherical and cylindrical power, axis, and prismatic power. A lensometer is pictured in **Figure 12.24**.
- Keratometry: Use of an instrument (keratometer) to measure the curvature of the anterior surface of the cornea; used to fit contact lenses, and assess the integrity of the corneal surface. A keratometer is pictured in **Figure 12.25**.
- Retinoscopy: Process of initially determining the spherical and cylindrical power and axis of the eye. Often, the final prescription will be close to the

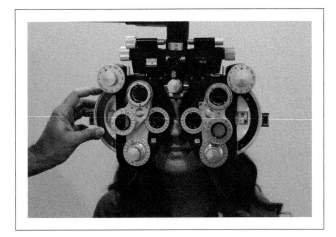

FIGURE 12.26 Retinoscopy: Phoropter use.

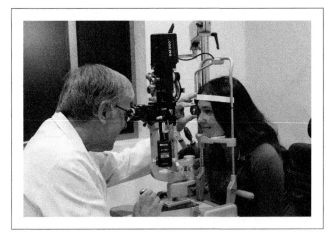

FIGURE 12.28 Fundoscopy using the slit lamp biomicroscope.

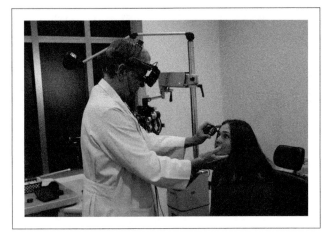

FIGURE 12.27 Binocular indirect ophthalmoscopy.

results of retinoscopy, but refinement steps are usually needed. Retinoscopy with the use of a phoropter is pictured in **Figure 12.26**. An automated version of performing retinoscopy, with an autorefractor, can be done using the keratometer with autorefractor pictured in **Figure 12.25**.

DILATED FUNDOSCOPY

The dilated fundal exam is a priority for individuals who have a high risk of retinopathy and retinal detachment. See the Abnormal Findings of the Eye section for more information about these disorders. Two techniques are used in the dilated eye by specialists. The first is the use of binocular indirect ophthalmoscopy (BIO; **Figure 12.27**). The second is fundoscopy using the slit lamp biomicroscope (**Figure 12.28**). The advantages of using BIO and fundoscopy with the slit lamp biomicroscope are that they are binocular techniques that allow the specialist to appreciate raised lesions of the retina, choroid, and optic nerves.

LABORATORY CONSIDERATIONS FOR THE EYE

Testing or labs to support specific diagnoses associated with ocular diseases or disorders are warranted, depending on the patient's history and presentation of symptoms; lab results provide clues to underlying clinical conditions. Considerations would include:

- Complete blood count (CBC) to assess for bacterial or viral infections; note immunosuppression, anemia
- Blood glucose to assess for diabetes or prediabetes
- Inflammatory markers, including erythrocyte sedimentation rate (ESR), C-reactive protein (CRP), antinuclear antibodies (ANA), IgG, and/or rheumatoid factor (RF) to support the diagnosis of an inflammatory disorder associated with ocular changes
- Polymerase chain reaction (PCR) testing for viral pathogens, including human herpes virus
- Venereal Disease Research Laboratory (VDRL) or fluorescent treponemal antibody-absorption (FTA-ABS) to consider ocular signs of syphilis, particularly in cases of uveitis as syphilis can mimic other conditions

IMAGING CONSIDERATIONS FOR THE EYE

Similar to laboratory considerations, imaging is determined by patient's history and presentation of symptoms. For example, individuals presenting with signs and symptoms of increased intracranial pressure and pupil abnormalities associated with head trauma may be candidates for CT evaluation. Individuals who present with signs of tumor or malignancy may be candidates for an MRI.

Ultrasonography is widely used to measure the length of the eye for refractive or cataract surgery. Ultrasound is also used to assess eye lesions, specifically melanomas. There is specialized ultrasound imaging that can be used to evaluate angle-closure glaucoma, although the imaging is not widely available. Gonioscopy is the gold-standard method of diagnosing angle-closure glaucoma. This technique involves using a special lens for the slit lamp, which allows the ophthalmologist to visualize the angle.

A few notes of caution from the Choosing Wisely® initiative:

- Do not "routinely order imaging tests for patients without symptoms or signs of significant eye disease" (American Academy of Ophthalmology, 2013, #2).
- Do not "order retinal imaging for patients without symptoms or signs of eye disease" (American Association for Pediatric Ophthalmology and Strabismus, 2019, #5).
- Do not routinely order neuroimaging for all patients with double vision (American Association for Pediatric Ophthalmology and Strabismus, 2019).

EVIDENCE-BASED CONSIDERATIONS FOR THE EYE

- For newborns: The U.S. Preventive Services Task Force (USPSTF, 2019, Grade A recommendation) recommends prophylactic ocular topical medication for all newborns to prevent gonococcal neonatal conjunctivitis. Erythromycin 0.5% ophthalmic ointment is currently the only available prophylactic treatment in the United States.
- For young children: The USPSTF (2017, Grade B recommendation) recommends universal vision screening for all children at least once between the ages of 3 and 5 years to assess for amblyopia or its risk factors. Current evidence is insufficient to recommend vision screening in children younger than age 3 years.
- For school-aged children: The American Optometric Association (AOA, 2017, Grade B recommendation) recommends that school-aged children should receive an in-person comprehensive eye and vision examination before beginning school to diagnose, treat, and manage any eye or vision conditions. School-aged children should receive an in-person comprehensive eye and vision examination annually to diagnose, treat, and manage any eye or vision problems.
- For adults: The AOA (2015, Grade B recommendation) recommends comprehensive eye and vision examinations at least every 2 years for asymptomatic, low-risk persons 40 through 64 years of age to evaluate changes in eye and visual function and provide for the early detection of eye diseases, which may lead to significant vision loss, and systemic conditions that may affect health or vision.
- For older adults: The USPSTF (2016, Grade I recommendation) determined that current evidence is insufficient to assess the risks and benefits of screening for impaired visual acuity in older adults.
- Specific disease-related recommendations: The USPSTF (2013, Grade I recommendation) determined that current evidence is insufficient to assess the risks and benefits of screening for primary open-angle glaucoma in adults.
- Specific patient populations: The American Diabetes Association (ADA) recommendations from 2017 are summarized in **Table 12.2** (Solomon et al., 2017).

ABNORMAL FINDINGS OF THE EYE

CATARACTS

Cataracts are cloudy changes to the lens of the eye due to protein buildup. The incidence of cataracts increases with age. Other risk factors include diabetes, smoking, alcohol use, and prolonged exposure to ultraviolet sunlight. With the exception of a traumatic cause, cataracts progress slowly over a period of years, even decades, causing a decrease in vision if untreated. Key signs and symptoms include cloudy, blurry vision; poor night vision; double vision; and/or seeing a halo around lights. Surgery is usually required.

Cataracts in children are much less common than cataracts in older adults. Pediatric cataracts are either present at birth (congenital) or develop in early childhood. In children, cataracts are caused by a genetic predisposition, metabolic disorders like diabetes, or eye trauma that damages the lens. Unfortunately, infants and young children are unable to verbalize vision disturbances. A missing or irregular red reflex often leads to the discovery of cataracts in children (see **Figure 12.29**).

CONJUNCTIVITIS

Conjunctivitis is a hyperemic (reddening due to increased blood flow) reaction of the conjunctiva due to inflammation or infectious processes. Common signs and symptoms of conjunctivitis include redness and swelling of the conjunctiva, burning, itching, foreign body sensation, crusting of the lashes or lids, and/or eye drainage. The etiology of conjunctivitis needs to be differentiated to ensure appropriate treatment.

TABLE 12.2 American Diabetes Association Screening Recommendations	
Population	Recommendation
Type 1 diabetes	Comprehensive, dilated examination by ophthalmologist or optometrist within 5 years after the onset of diabetes (Grade B)
Type 2 diabetes	Comprehensive, dilated examination by ophthalmologist or optometrist at the time of diabetes diagnosis (Grade B)
Type 1 or Type 2 diabetes	If there is no evidence of retinopathy for one or more annual eye exams, then exams every 2 years may be considered. If any level of diabetic retinopathy is present, subsequent dilated retinal examinations for patients with type 1 or type 2 diabetes should be repeated at least annually by an ophthalmologist or optometrist. If retinopathy is progressive or sight threatening, then examinations will be required more frequently (Grade B)
Women with preexisting diabetes who are planning pregnancy or are pregnant	Review and discuss the risk of development and/or progression of diabetic retinopathy. Eye examinations should occur before pregnancy or in the first trimester in patients with preexisting type 1 or type 2 diabetes, and then these patients should be monitored every trimester and for 1 year postpartum as indicated by the degree of retinopathy (Grade B)

Source: From Solomon, S. D., Chew, E., Duh, E. J., Sobrin, L., Sun, J. K., VanderBeek, B. L., … Gardner, T. W. (2017). Diabetic retinopathy: A position statement by the American Diabetes Association. *Diabetes Care, 40*(3), 412–418. doi:10.2337/dc16-2641

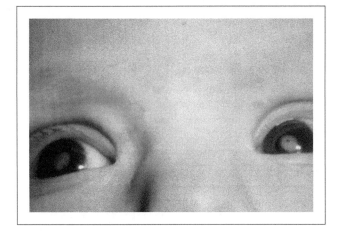

FIGURE 12.29 Infant with cataracts from congenital rubella syndrome.
Source: Centers for Disease Control and Prevention.

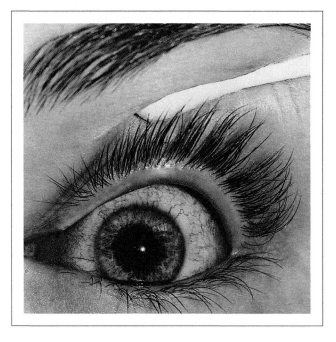

FIGURE 12.30 Viral conjunctivitis.
Source: Image courtesy of Joyhill09.

Viral Conjunctivitis

Viral conjunctivitis usually occurs concomitantly with symptoms of a viral respiratory infection like adenovirus or influenza. Symptoms of reddened sclera and watery drainage usually begin in one eye and may spread to the other (**Figure 12.30**). However, other viruses like measles or herpes simplex virus (HSV) can also infect the conjunctiva. These types of viral conjunctivitis would present with additional extraocular, cutaneous lesions consistent with the causative organism.

Bacterial Conjunctivitis

Bacterial conjunctivitis is an acute bacterial infection of the eye, commonly referred to as "pink eye."

Key signs and symptoms include scleral erythema, lid swelling, purulent eye discharge, and crusting/matting of the lashes and lids, especially first thing in the morning (**Figure 12.31**). Bacterial conjunctivitis is more common in children than in adults. In children, bacterial conjunctivitis can occur concomitantly with an ear infection (otitis media). While the infection may be unilateral, it is contagious and often spreads to both eyes.

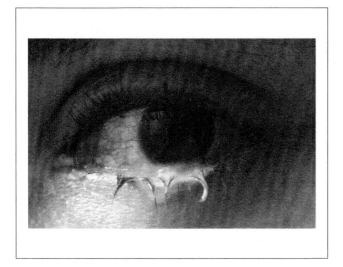

FIGURE 12.31 Bacterial conjunctivitis.
Source: Image courtesy of Tanalai.

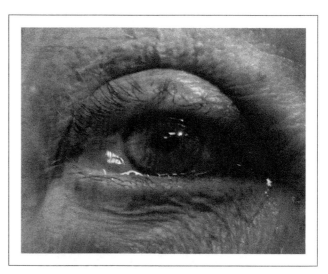

FIGURE 12.33 Allergic conjunctivitis.
Source: Image courtesy of James Heilman, MD.

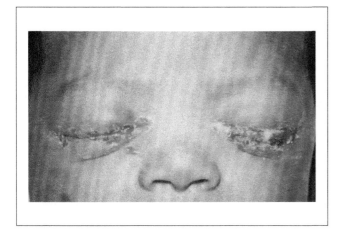

FIGURE 12.32 Neonatal conjunctivitis.
Source: Centers for Disease Control and Prevention/J. Pledger.

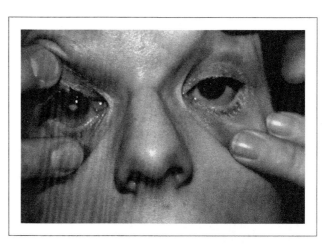

FIGURE 12.34 Fungal conjunctivitis.
Source: Centers for Disease Control and Prevention/Brinkman.

Neonatal Conjunctivitis

Neonatal conjunctivitis (ophthalmia neonatorum) describes a bacterial conjunctivitis in the newborn that is caused by a bacterial organism from the birth canal, most often gonorrhea or chlamydia. Gonococcal conjunctivitis appears about 2 to 4 days after birth, while chlamydial conjunctivitis appears 5 to 12 days after birth. Key symptoms include red, swollen eyelids and thick, purulent eye discharge (**Figure 12.32**). If gonorrhea or chlamydia is suspected, the newborn may require hospitalization for treatment to prevent corneal perforation, blindness, and neonatal sepsis.

Allergic Conjunctivitis

Allergic conjunctivitis presents as a result of the body's reaction to allergens such as pollen, ragweed, dust

mites, molds, pet dander, medicines, or cosmetics. Allergic conjunctivitis is not contagious and occurs more commonly in people with other allergic conditions like asthma and eczema. Key signs and symptoms include reddened sclera, itchy eyes, and watery or clear mucoid drainage (**Figure 12.33**).

Fungal Conjunctivitis

Similar to viral and bacterial conjunctivitis, fungal organisms can also infect the conjunctiva. Key signs and symptoms include reddened sclera, mucopurulent drainage, and blepharitis (infections of the eyelid). Fungal conjunctivitis is less common than other types. Culture of the eye drainage may be needed to determine the causative organism. Note in **Figure 12.34** that the right eye has a large corneal ulcer, often characteristic of fungal infections.

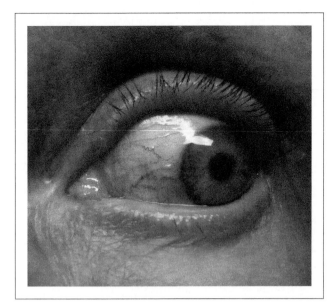

FIGURE 12.35 Irritant conjunctivitis.
Source: Image courtesy of Rosmarie Voegtli.

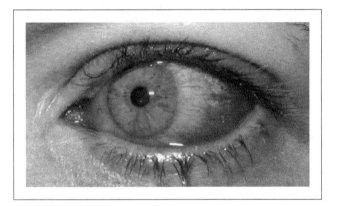

FIGURE 12.36 Keratoconjunctivitis.
Source: Image courtesy of Marco Mayer.

Irritant Conjunctivitis

Irritant conjunctivitis describes a conjunctivitis caused by any type of irritant to the eye such as a foreign body; exposure to smoke, dust, fumes, or chemicals; or wearing of contact lenses longer than recommended. Key signs and symptoms include scleral erythema, watery drainage, and history of preceding event (**Figure 12.35**).

Keratoconjunctivitis

Keratoconjunctivitis is an inflammatory and/or infectious condition that affects both the conjunctiva and the cornea (keratitis). Key signs and symptoms include a foreign body sensation, scleral erythema, photophobia, and/or mucopurulent discharge in association with a corneal opacity (**Figure 12.36**).

Common causes include viral (measles, adenovirus, and HSV) and bacterial organisms (Staphylococcus, Streptococcus, and Pseudomonas). Contact wearers are at highest risk for keratoconjunctivitis. If keratoconjunctivitis is suspected, an urgent ophthalmologic referral is warranted.

CORNEAL ABRASION

A corneal abrasion is defined as a defect in the epithelial surface of the cornea caused by a mechanical trauma, including:

- Foreign body (e.g., rust, sand, mulch)
- Contact lens related (e.g., overworn, ill-fitting)
- Traumatic (e.g., fingernail, tree branch)

The corneal epithelium is richly innervated with sensory pain fibers. Key signs and symptoms include excruciating eye pain that precludes normal daily activities and an inability to open the eye due to a "foreign body sensation." The clinician should perform a penlight exam to evaluate the eye structures and pupil function and rule out any penetrating trauma (ruptured globe), as evidenced by clear drainage of the aqueous humor. If a foreign body is suspected, the clinician may perform a lid eversion, "flipping" the lid inside out to inspect for a retained foreign body.

To confirm the diagnosis, the fluorescein-staining technique may be performed: apply the fluorescein (yellow-orange) dye with a blotting paper to the outer surface of the eye beneath the lower lid, and have the patient blink a few times. Dim the lights and view the eye through a cobalt blue light source. Corneal abrasions will appear as a green abrasion on the surface of the cornea (see **Figure 12.37**). The abrasion lines appear this way because of the up-and-down movement of the lids during blinking. If symptoms persist longer than 24 to 48 hours, or if discharge develops, the patient should be referred to an ophthalmologist.

DACRYOSTENOSIS AND DACRYOCYSTITIS

Dacryostenosis, also called congenital lacrimal duct obstruction, describes a narrowing (stenosis) of the tear duct (lacrimal canal). See lacrimal duct in **Figure 12.38**. Dacryostenosis is usually noted shortly after birth. Key signs and symptoms include persistent tearing and clear eye discharge without a reddened sclera. The condition typically resolves spontaneously by age 6 to 12 months. Management includes nasolacrimal canal massage and close observation. If the condition persists beyond age 6 months, a referral to ophthalmology is warranted. Surgical intervention may be required.

Dacryocystitis, an infection of the nasolacrimal duct system, is a rare complication of dacryostenosis. Key signs and symptoms include erythema, swelling,

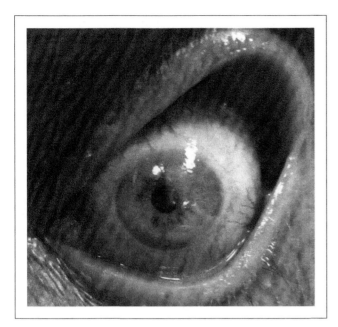

FIGURE 12.37 Corneal abrasion with fluorescein staining.
Source: Image courtesy of James Heilman, MD.

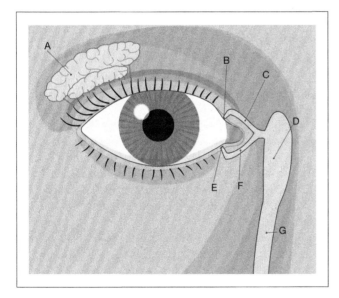

FIGURE 12.38 Tear system. (A) Tear/lacrimal gland.
(B) Superior lacrimal punctum. (C) Superior lacrimal
canal. (D) Lacrimal duct. (E) Inferior lacrimal punctum.
(F) Inferior lacrimal canal. (G) Nasolacrimal canal.

warmth, and tenderness of the nasolacrimal sac, and/
or purulent eye drainage. This condition should be
treated promptly to prevent orbital cellulitis, sepsis, or
meningitis.

DIPLOPIA

Diplopia describes the condition of double vision.
Causes of diplopia depend primarily on whether the
diplopia is monocular or binocular. Binocular diplopia
is present when both eyes are open and absent when
one eye is closed. Monocular diplopia persists even
when one eye is closed.

Monocular Diplopia

Monocular diplopia is suggestive of local unilateral eye
disease or refractive error. An ophthalmologist should
manage most cases of monocular diplopia. The most
likely cause is that of mature cataracts. This type of
diplopia is easily corrected with surgery. Other causes
of monocular diplopia include:

- High astigmatism error, which is an abnormal curvature of the frontal surface of the cornea. This type
  of diplopia is often correctable with eyeglasses or
  contact lenses.
- Keratoconus, which is a collagen vascular condition
  that results as fibers in the cornea begin to proliferate in a disorderly fashion, causing a very steep cornea. Scleral contact lenses or corneal cross-linking
  are useful treatments.
- Displacement of the lens, also known as a subluxation of the lens or ectopia lentis. This is a common
  occurrence found in Marfan's syndrome. Ectopia lentis is also commonly found in cases of ocular trauma.
- Ectopia Lentis et Pupillae is a rare genetic disorder
  in which there is a pupil that is displaced in the opposite direction of the lens displacement. The pupils
  in ectopia lentis et pupillae are usually asymmetric,
  poorly reactive, and oval (Cross, 1979).

Binocular Diplopia

Binocular diplopia is a problem of ocular misalignment,
which may occur for a number of reasons. Three pairs
of EOMs are responsible for moving each eye vertically,
horizontally, and torsionally (diagonally). It is important to determine which eye muscles are affected by determining which field of gaze is affected.

Some common causes of binocular diplopia include:

- Strabismus
- Neurologic cranial lesion
- Palsy of CN III, IV, or VI
- Myasthenia gravis or Graves' disease
- Trauma to the eye muscles

Sudden development of binocular diplopia should be
evaluated as soon as possible to rule out neurologic disorders, vascular pathologies, or mass/lesion etiologies.

GLAUCOMA

Glaucoma is an optic neuropathy usually characterized by either unequal or elevated IOP from insufficient
drainage or excessive production of aqueous humor.

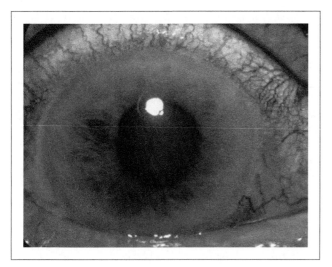

FIGURE 12.39 Acute angle-closure glaucoma.
Source: Image courtesy of Jonathan Trobe, M.D.

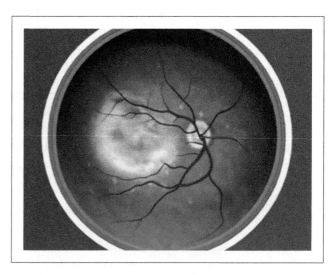

FIGURE 12.40 Macular degeneration.
Source: National Institutes of Health and National Eye Institute.

The elevated IOP leads to optic nerve damage, vision loss, and blindness if untreated. There are two primary types of glaucoma: open-angle and acute angle-closure (**Figure 12.39**). These terms refer to the angle between the iris and the cornea in the respective types. Secondary types of glaucoma can be caused by trauma or certain medications.

Unfortunately, open-angle glaucoma is missed by most patients. This is why it is given the name "the Silent Blinder." Characteristic signs of open-angle glaucoma include patchy blind spots in the peripheral or central vision or tunnel vision in advanced stages. Often (although not always), there are asymmetric IOPs. While it is generally found (on exam) in one eye, it frequently occurs in both eyes.

Key signs and symptoms of acute angle-closure glaucoma include severe headache, eye pain, severely elevated and/or asymmetric IOPs, blurred vision, eye redness, light halos, and/or nausea and vomiting. Acute angle-closure glaucoma is uncommon and should be treated as a medical emergency.

MACULAR DEGENERATION

Macular degeneration is an age-related degenerative disease of the macula (central portion of the retina) that results in loss of central vision. It is the most common ocular disorder in people over 50. Key signs and symptoms can include reduced central vision in one or both eyes, increased difficulty adapting to low light levels, increased blurriness of printed words, and difficulty recognizing faces. **Figure 12.40** depicts advanced macular degeneration on exam, and **Figure 12.41** depicts an Amsler grid, a tool that can be used by individuals at

risk for macular degeneration to detect changes in their vision, and the changes that the individual might notice with macular degeneration.

OPTIC NEURITIS AND RETROBULBAR NEURITIS

Optic neuritis is an inflammatory condition of the optic nerve characterized by a sudden onset of unilateral visual loss. The loss may be mild to profound. Retrobulbar neuritis indicates that the posterior part of the optic nerve is involved, which may lead to complete or partial loss of vision in one or both eyes. Neuritis of the optic nerve occurs most often in ages 18 to 45 years.

Critical signs and symptoms include unilateral orbital pain, loss of color vision in the affected eye, afferent pupillary defect (APD), and one of several field defects (central, cecocentral, arcuate, or altitudinal). Many cases will include papilledema, flame-shaped hemorrhages, and vitreous cells. Causes include multiple sclerosis, infective organisms (including viruses), granulomatous inflammatory conditions, tuberculosis, syphilis, sarcoidosis, and autoimmune disorders.

ORBITAL AND PERIORBITAL CELLULITIS

Orbital cellulitis is an infection of the tissue in the orbit (eye socket; **Figure 12.42**), while periorbital (or preseptal) cellulitis is an infection of the anterior portion of the eyelid (**Figure 12.43**). The globe is not affected in either condition. Periorbital cellulitis rarely leads to serious complications; however, orbital cellulitis may lead to abscess, vision loss, or intracranial spread of infection, resulting in meningitis or death.

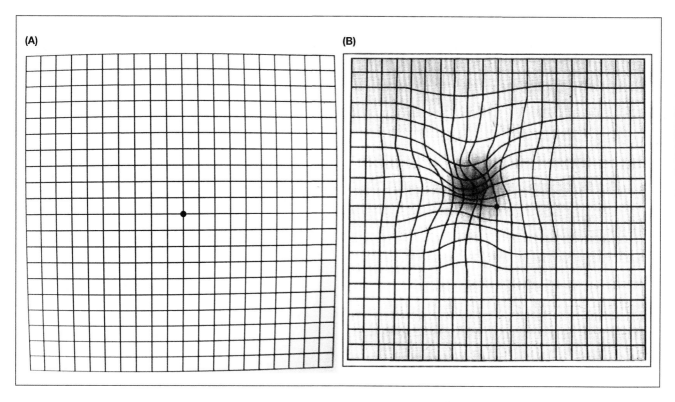

FIGURE 12.41 Amsler grid. (A) Amsler grid to detect changes in vision. (B) Distorted Amsler grid.

Source: (A) Image courtesy of Rosmarie Voegtli. (B) National Institutes of Health and National Eye Institute.

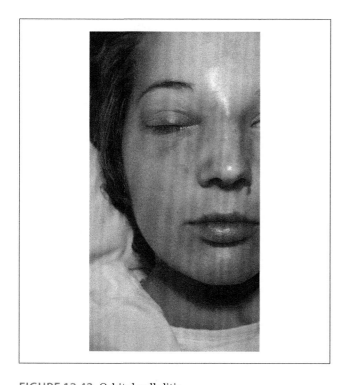

FIGURE 12.42 Orbital cellulitis.

Source: Centers for Disease Control and Prevention/Dr. Thomas F. Sellers, Emory University.

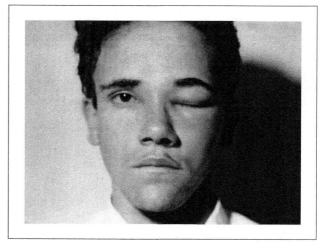

FIGURE 12.43 Periorbital cellulitis.

Source: Centers for Disease Control and Prevention/M. A. Parsons. Donated by G. Rosenfeld, MD.

These infections can be difficult to distinguish on exam, especially in infants and young children. Key signs and symptoms include eye pain with eyelid swelling and erythema. However, orbital cellulitis generally presents with more severe clinical features: pain with

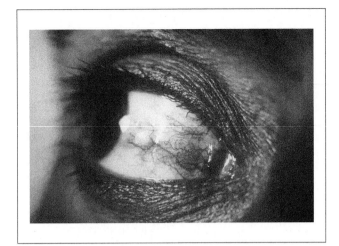

FIGURE 12.44 Pinguecula.
Source: Centers for Disease Control and Prevention.

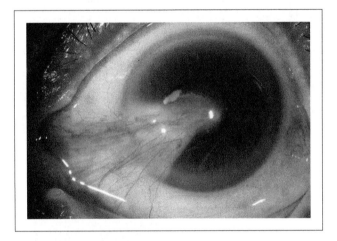

FIGURE 12.45 Pterygium.
Source: Image courtesy of Jmvaras.

eye movements, ophthalmoplegia (impaired eye movement), and proptosis (forward displacement of the globe). The most common cause of periorbital cellulitis is infection secondary to local skin trauma. The most common causes of orbital cellulitis include acute sinusitis, ophthalmic surgery, and orbit trauma. Cases that are difficult to distinguish may require an orbital CT.

PINGUECULUM AND PTERYGIUM

Pinguecula and pterygium are benign growths of the conjunctiva. Pinguecula is a growth that appears as a yellow bump on the inner canthus of the conjunctiva (**Figure 12.44**). Pterygium is a growth of fleshy tissue that often arises from the pinguecula (**Figure 12.45**); it can potentially obstruct vision by causing an astigmatic

distortion of the cornea. These conditions are thought to be from chronic dry eyes and chronic exposure to wind, dust, and ultraviolet light or sunlight.

RETINAL TEARS, FLOATERS, AND RETINAL DETACHMENT

"Floaters" describes a condition in which specks, black spots, or threads "float about" in a person's vision. Floaters move as the eyes move, and they are most noticeable to people when looking at a plain, bright background. Some common causes include:

- Age-related changes in the vitreous: The vitreous becomes more liquefied in some areas and more condensed and stringy in others. These changes are seen as floaters.
- Posterior vitreous detachment: As the vitreous liquefies over time, it can become detached from the retina. Many patients do not experience symptoms, while other patients experience flashes or new floaters.
- Retinal tear: In some cases of posterior vitreous detachment, the vitreous can pull away hard enough to tear the retina. A torn retina may result in a torn retinal vessel, which results in blood leaking into the vitreous (vitreous hemorrhage). Any case of floaters should be evaluated for retinal tear.

Retinal detachment occurs when the retinal cells separate from the layer of blood vessels that supply the retina. Signs and symptoms include acute onset of floaters, flashes of light (photopsia), blurred vision, and impaired peripheral vision. Any acute visual changes are concerning for a serious condition and should be evaluated urgently by an ophthalmologist. Infants and young children that present with suspicion of abusive head trauma should be evaluated emergently for retinal tears, hemorrhage, or detachment.

RETINOPATHY

Retinopathy describes a condition in which damage to the retina causes visual impairment. Symptoms may include floaters, blurry vision, poor night vision, impaired color vision, and blank/dark areas in the field of vision. There are different types of retinopathy.

- Diabetic retinopathy occurs when chronic elevated blood-sugar levels damage the blood vessels of the retina (**Figure 12.46**). This retinopathy occurs in two basic forms: proliferative and nonproliferative, which refers to whether there is growth of abnormal blood vessels on the retina. Both eyes are typically affected. It occurs more often in patients with chronic diabetes (>5 years) and history of uncontrolled blood sugar (HbA1c significantly above 7.0).

- Hypertensive retinopathy occurs as a result of chronic uncontrolled hypertension, which damages the small blood vessels of the retina (**Figure 12.47**). Visual changes can occur with advanced disease, and, although uncommon, blindness can occur.
- Retinopathy of prematurity (ROP) occurs in a small percentage of premature infants born less than 31 weeks' gestation. These babies often require intensive respiratory support, including oxygen therapy. The condition is thought to be a result of disorganized growth of retinal blood vessels, which can cause retinal scarring and detachment. Oxygen toxicity and hypoxia may also contribute to the development of ROP.

SCLERITIS AND EPISCLERITIS

Scleritis is the inflammation of the sclera or choroid of the eye (**Figure 12.48**). Episcleritis is inflammation of the episclera (outer covering of the sclera). It is made up of collagen and elastic fibers. Because of this makeup, the sclera is subject to many of the same conditions that affect connective tissue found in other parts of the body, particularly systemic lupus erythematous (SLE) or rheumatoid arthritis (RA).

Episcleritis results in a localized area of inflammation of the episcleral tissues, which may be diffuse or wedge shaped and may have an associated nodule, in the form known as nodular episcleritis. This condition is benign with mild discomfort and is self-limited over the time frame of a few weeks.

Scleritis is less common than episcleritis but more serious as it affects deeper tissues of the sclera. Key signs and symptoms include "boring" pain, watery discharge, photophobia, and blurred vision. This condition can permanently affect vision and is often associated with other systemic conditions, such as RA, SLE, ankylosing spondylitis, inflammatory bowel disease (IBD), and infectious diseases. Scleritis may be diffuse or nodular, necrotizing, or posterior. Diffuse, nodular, and posterior are potentially serious, but fairly successfully treated, while necrotizing scleritis is often associated with life-threatening RA in older female patients.

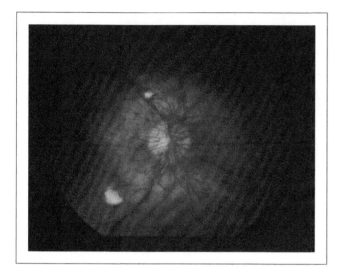

FIGURE 12.46 Proliferative diabetic retinopathy.
Source: National Institutes of Health and National Eye Institute.

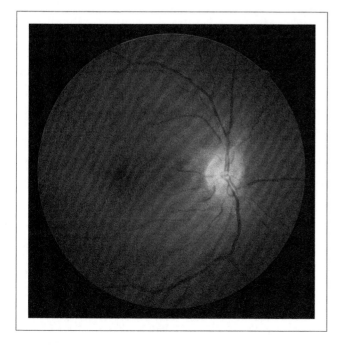

FIGURE 12.47 Hypertensive retinopathy.
Source: Image courtesy of Frank Wood.

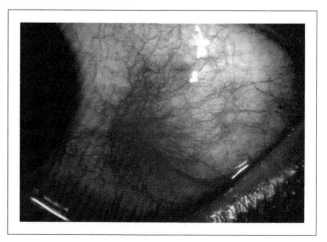

FIGURE 12.48 Scleritis.
Source: Image courtesy of Kribz.

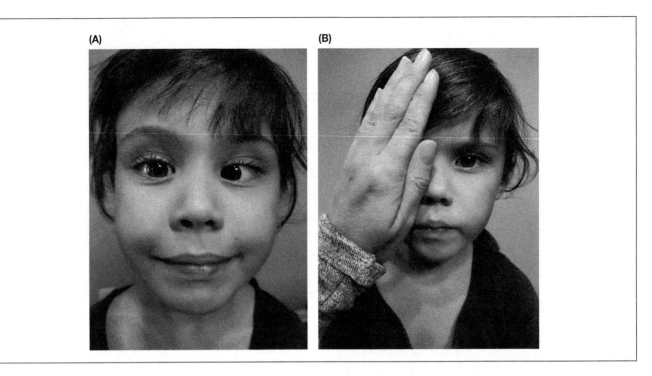

FIGURE 12.49 Esotropia. (A) Uncorrected. (B) Corrected during exam.

STRABISMUS

Strabismus is a misalignment of the eyes that is often congenital and occurs with various degrees of severity. The misalignment occurs because of an imbalance in EOM function. The axis of misalignment can occur in one of several directions. As one eye fixates, the other eye may deviate inward (esotropia), outward (exotropia), upward (hypertropia), or downward (hypotropia). Strabismus is more common in children than adults, and particularly more common in children with neurologic disorders like cerebral palsy. In **Figure 12.49**, the corneal light reflex cannot be appreciated symmetrically because the left eye deviates inward (**Figure 12.49A**); when the clinician covers the unaffected right eye, the affected eye returns to alignment (**Figure 12.49B**).

Pseudostrabismus describes a condition in which the eyes appear to be misaligned when in fact they are not. This is thought to be a result of undeveloped facial features of infants and young children, and/or may be the result of variation in the slant of palpebral fissures. The key physical finding is a symmetric corneal light reflex. True strabismus will exhibit an asymmetric corneal light reflex. In **Figure 12.50**, the left eye appears to be esophoric; however, the corneal light reflexes are symmetric between both pupils.

Strabismus can lead to amblyopia (reduced vision) or blindness, as the child's developing brain prioritizes vision in the aligned eye and disregards the visual stimulus in the deviated eye, adversely affecting visual development. Persistent loss of visual stimulation in the

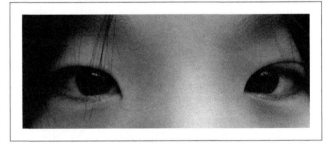

FIGURE 12.50 Pseudostrabismus.

affected eye eventually leads to the amblyopia. Early intervention and treatment are crucial to prevent vision loss. Acute onset of strabismus in an older adult can be indicative of a more serious condition, for example, a CN VI or CN III palsy, and should be considered a medical emergency.

STY

A sty, or hordeolum, is an acute pustular infection of the eyelid margin (**Figure 12.51**). An external hordeolum arises from an eyelash follicle or tear gland of the lid margin. An internal hordeolum is an acute inflammation of a meibomian gland just under the conjunctival side of the eyelid. The key sign/symptom is a red, tender papule/pustule on the eyelid margin. An internal hordeolum may evolve into a chronic inflammatory lesion (chalazion), which presents as a firm, rubbery

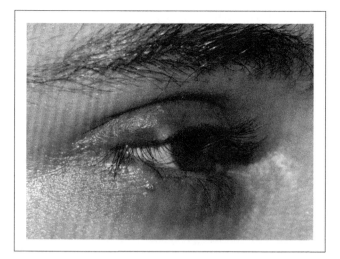

FIGURE 12.51 Sty of upper eyelid.

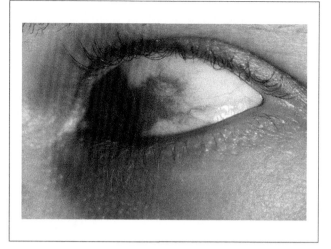

FIGURE 12.52 Subconjunctival hemorrhage.
Source: Image courtesy of Daniel Flather.

nodule within the eyelid. These conditions are self-limited and will not affect vision.

When an individual presents with redness and crusting but not tearing, the condition is more likely blepharitis, inflammation of the eyelids, which can be caused by infection or systemic illnesses, such as seborrheic dermatitis, rosacea, or dry eye syndromes.

SUBCONJUNCTIVAL HEMORRHAGE

Subconjunctival hemorrhage describes a demarcated area of ruptured blood vessels just beneath the surface of the eye (**Figure 12.52**). It can be seen as a distinct collection of blood within the sclera and differs in appearance from a more generalized hyperemia associated with acute conjunctivitis. The condition is asymptomatic and can be diagnosed by clinical appearance. It can be caused by traumatic injury to the head or eye, but may also occur with Valsalva-associated coughing, straining, or vomiting; from anticoagulant therapy; or with contact lens insertions or removal. If the patient presents with a history of head trauma, the clinician must evaluate for a ruptured globe.

UVEITIS

Uveitis is an inflammatory condition of the uveal tract (**Figure 12.53**). Physical findings vary depending on the portion of the uveal tract affected—anterior chamber, ciliary body, or posterior chamber. Uveitis usually appears suddenly, with nonspecific symptoms of eye pain, redness, and severe photophobia.

Uveitis can be widely disseminated throughout the uveal tract (panuveitis) or localized to a specific

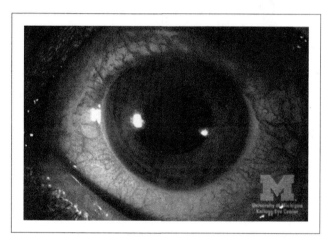

FIGURE 12.53 Uveitis.
Source: Image courtesy of Jonathan Trobe, M.D.

chamber: the anterior chamber (iritis), ciliary body (cyclitis), or the posterior chamber (retinitis or choroiditis). The cause of uveitis varies depending on the etiology of the inflammation.

- Infectious causes include herpes; CMV; toxoplasmosis; syphilis; tuberculosis; and West Nile, Ebola, and Zika viruses.
- Systemic or immune conditions include spondyloarthritis, sarcoidosis, juvenile idiopathic arthritis, psoriatic arthritis, IBD, MS, Vogt–Koyanagi–Harada syndrome (VKH), Behçet syndrome, Sjögren's syndrome, and SLE.

CASE STUDY: Eye Pain and Swelling

History

J.P. is an otherwise healthy 28-year-old male who presents to the clinic with recent onset of left eye pain and swelling that has worsened over the past 2 days. He first noticed his symptoms when he returned from a camping trip 3 days ago. He is now unable to open his eye. He reports eye watering with crusting and matting of the lashes this morning. He denies fevers, nausea, vomiting, headaches, or recent history of head trauma. He has washed his eye several times and has been using cool compresses. He reports having had a recent upper respiratory tract infection approximately 1 week ago, but denies wearing glasses or contact lenses.

Physical Examination

- On exam, J.P. is alert and in no acute distress. His temperature is 100.4°F. Heart rate is 100 and blood pressure is 120/70.
- Right eye: No lid swelling, conjunctival injection, or exudate. Red reflex intact, pupil is 3 mm, round, and reactive. EOMs intact.

- Left eye: Significant periorbital swelling and erythema. Small amount of mucoid exudate at the inner canthus. Unable to independently open eye. Tender to touch. Minimal eye opening with manual traction. Hyperemic sclera. Pupil round and reactive. Unable to obtain full EOM assessment.

Differential Diagnoses

Acute conjunctivitis (bacterial, viral, or fungal), keratoconjunctivitis, periorbital cellulitis, orbital cellulitis, corneal abrasion with retention of foreign body

Laboratory and Imaging

CT of the orbit revealed no evidence of sinus infection or orbital involvement.

Final Diagnosis

Periorbital (preseptal) cellulitis

Clinical Pearls

- The fundoscopic exam (direct ophthalmoscopy) in the undilated eye yields assessment findings that are limited. Because the pupils are neurologically designed to close significantly when light is shown in the eye, using an ophthalmoscope to view the posterior retina is restricted.
- Dilating an individual's pupils in the primary care setting has risks and challenges. Those with cataracts or small pupils or who are unable to cooperate will not benefit from a dilated eye exam. Dilated exams are unsafe for small children, infants, anyone who is hyperopic, and anyone who has had previous acute angle-closure glaucoma. There is a risk of precipitating acute angle-closure glaucoma when dilating an individual's pupils.
- Clinicians should inform patients that any exam of an undilated eye is limited by the small field of view, despite the high magnification.
- Clinicians should recommend to individuals who are at high risk for retinopathy (e.g., individuals with diabetes, hypertension, and/or diseases that have associated ocular symptoms), that they would benefit from vision screening,

as recommended by the AOA, ADA, or USPSTF. For these individuals, the authors of this chapter recommend that clinicians defer completing an undilated eye exam; often, individuals who have had an undilated eye exam believe that they have had the exam as recommended and forgo the specialist evaluation by dilated eye exam. The consequences of failing to have recommended dilated eye exams for these populations can be significant vision loss.
- Timing is everything. Do not hesitate to refer individuals for ophthalmology for abnormal findings associated with ocular assessment and vision.

Key Takeaways

- Changes in vision and/or ocular pain, in and around the eye, may be some of the first indicators of systemic as well as ocular disease.
- Early detection and treatment of these conditions may make the difference between long-term disabling effects on the body and/or vision.

REFERENCES

Abu-Hassan, D. W., Acott, T. S., & Kelley, M. J. (2014). The trabecular meshwork: A basic review of form and function. *Journal of Ocular Biology, 2*(1), 9. doi:10.13188/2334-2838.1000017

Alizadeh Ghavidel, L., Mousavi, F., Bagheri, M., & Asghari, S. (2018). Preeclampsia induced ocular change. *International Journal of Women's Health and Reproduction Sciences, 6*(2), 123–126. doi:10.15296/ijwhr.2018.20

American Academy of Ophthalmology. (2013). *Five things physicians and patients should question.* Retrieved from http://www.choosingwisely.org/societies/american-academy-of-ophthalmology

American Association for Pediatric Ophthalmology and Strabismus. (2019). *Five things physicians and patients should question.* Retrieved from http://www.choosingwisely.org/societies/american-association-for-pediatric-ophthalmology-and-strabismus

American Optometric Association Evidence-Based Optometry Guideline Development Group. (2015). *Evidence-based clinical practice guideline—Comprehensive adult eye and vision examination.* Retrieved from http://aoa.uberflip.com/i/578152-aoa-clinical-practice-guidelines-adult-eye-exam

American Optometric Association Evidence-Based Optometry Guideline Development Group. (2017). Evidence-based clinical practice guideline: Comprehensive pediatric eye and vision examination. Retrieved from http://aoa.uberflip.com/i/807465-cpg-pediatric-eye-and-vision-examination

Anderson, A. J., Shuey, N. H., & Wall, M. (2009). Rapid confrontation screening for peripheral visual field defects and extinction. *Clinical and Experimental Optometry, 92*(1), 45–48. doi:10.1111/j.1444-0938.2008.00280.x

Brubaker, R. (1996). Measurement of aqueous flow by fluorophotometry. In R. Ritch, M. B. Shields, & T. Krupin (Eds.), *The glaucomas* (pp. 447–454). St. Louis, MO: Mosby.

Carlson, N., & Kurtz, D. (2004). *Clinical procedures for the ocular examination* (3rd ed.). Boston, MA. McGraw-Hill.

Cross, H. E. (1979). Ectopia lentis et pupillae. *American Journal of Ophthalmology, 88,* 381–384. doi:10.1016/0002-9394(79)90637-8

Hagan, J. F., Shaw, J. S., & Duncan, P. (Eds.). (2017). *Bright futures: Guidelines for health supervision of infants, children and adolescents* (4th ed.). Elk Grove Village, IL: American Academy of Pediatrics.

Karpinich, N. O., & Caron, K. M. (2014). Schlemm's canal: More than meets the eye, lymphatics in disguise. *Journal of Clinical Investigation, 124*(9), 3701–3703. doi:10.1172/JCI77507

Rehman, I., Mahabadi, N., & Ali, T. (2019). *Anatomy, head and neck, eye fovea.* Treasure Island, FL: StatPearls. Retrieved from https://www.ncbi.nlm.nih.gov/books/NBK482428

Rosenfield, M., & Logan, N. (2009). *Optometry: Science, techniques and clinical management* (2nd ed.). Oxford, UK: Butterworth Heinemann/Elsevier.

Salvi, S. M., Akhtar, S., & Currie, Z. (2006). Ageing changes in the eye. *Postgraduate Medical Journal, 82,* 581–587. doi:10.1136/pgmj.2005.040857

Solomon, S. D., Chew, E., Duh, E. J., Sobrin, L., Sun, J. K., VanderBeek, B. L., … Gardner, T. W. (2017). Diabetic retinopathy: A position statement by the American Diabetes Association. *Diabetes Care, 40*(3), 412–418. doi:10.2337/dc16-2641

Spalton, D. J., Hitchings, R. A., & Hunter, P. A. (Eds.). (2002). *Atlas of clinical ophthalmology* (2nd ed.). Philadelphia, PA: Mosby.

U.S. Preventive Services Task Force. (2013). Glaucoma: Screening. Retrieved from https://www.uspreventiveservicestaskforce.org/Page/Document/UpdateSummaryFinal/glaucoma-screening

U.S. Preventive Services Task Force. (2016). Final recommendation statement: Impaired visual acuity in older adults: Screening. Retrieved from https://www.uspreventiveservicestaskforce.org/Page/Document/RecommendationStatementFinal/impaired-visual-acuity-in-older-adults-screening

U.S. Preventive Services Task Force. (2017). Final recommendation statement: Vision in children ages 6 months to 5 years: Screening. Retrieved from https://www.uspreventiveservicestaskforce.org/Page/Document/RecommendationStatementFinal/vision-in-children-ages-6-months-to-5-years-screening

U.S. Preventive Services Task Force. (2019). Ocular prophylaxis for gonococcal ophthalmia neonatorum: Preventive medication. Retrieved from https://www.uspreventiveservicestaskforce.org/Page/Document/UpdateSummaryFinal/ocular-prophylaxis-for-gonococcal-ophthalmia-neonatorum-preventive-medication1

13

Evidence-Based Assessment of the Ears, Nose, and Throat

Maria Colandrea and Eileen M. Raynor

"The words of the tongue should have 3 gatekeepers;
Is it true? Is it kind? Is it necessary?"

—ARABIAN PROVERB

VIDEOS

- Patient Case: Child With Ear Pain (Otitis Media)
- Patient Case: Young Adult With Upper Respiratory Infection Symptoms
- Patient History: Child With Sore Throat

LEARNING OBJECTIVES

- Identify anatomy of the ear, nose, paranasal sinuses, mouth, and throat.
- Discuss the physiology and pathophysiology of hearing and common problems related to the nose, paranasal sinuses, mouth, and throat.
- Elicit a comprehensive history and perform a thorough exam of the ears, nose, mouth, and throat.
- Identify differential diagnoses for frequent patient concerns related to the ears, nose, mouth, and throat.

ANATOMY AND PHYSIOLOGY OF EARS, NOSE, AND THROAT

The anatomy of the head and neck is one of the most complex in the human body. This region is home to four of the five senses, the smallest bones in the body, and the only area where cranial nerve endings (CNI) are open to the environment. A great many vital structures pass through this region providing blood supply and neurologic information to and from the cranium. Humans interact with their environment through hearing, smell, taste, touch, and speech, and any pathology within this area can significantly affect breathing, communication, swallowing, and other important functions.

THE EAR

The **ear** consists of three compartments: the **external ear**, the **middle ear**, and the **inner ear**. The external ear consists of the pinna and the external auditory canal (ear canal). The pinna is made up of cartilage, covered by skin. The helix is the top curvature of the ear, with the antihelix just beneath it. The concha is the bowl-like area right before the ear canal. The purpose of the auricle is to funnel sound into the ear canal. Anatomic landmarks of the external or outer ear are shown in **Figure 13.1**.

Visit https://connect.springerpub.com/content/book/978-0-8261 -6454-4/chapter/ch00 to access the videos.

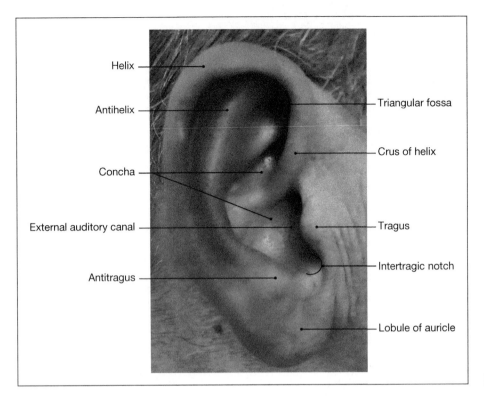

FIGURE 13.1 Right outer ear.

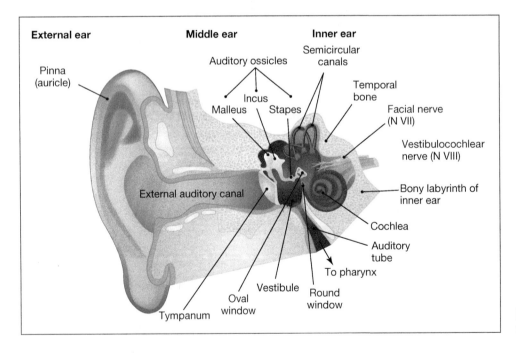

FIGURE 13.2 Anatomy of the ear.

The external auditory canal (EAC) is approximately 2.5 cm long and ends at the tympanic membrane (eardrum). In adults, the first one-third of the EAC is cartilaginous and has hair follicles and cerumen glands, which produce cerumen (ear wax). The last two-thirds of the ear canal lies within the temporal bone and lacks hair follicles and cerumen glands. The ear canal is lined with skin throughout, and the purpose of the EAC is to direct sound toward the middle ear. Behind and below the ear canal sits the mastoid part of the temporal bone. The mastoid process is palpated behind the ear lobule. Anatomic landmarks of the internal ear are shown in **Figure 13.2**.

The **tympanic membrane** is a thin, cone-shaped membrane that separates the external ear from the middle ear. Its purpose is to send vibratory sound to

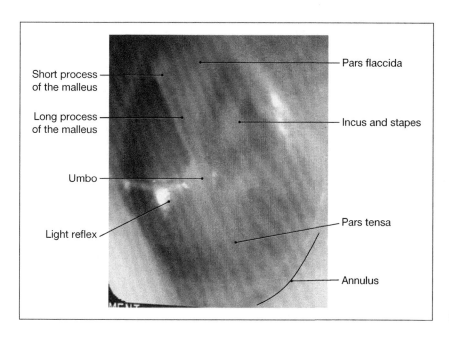

- Short process of the malleus
- Long process of the malleus
- Umbo
- Light reflex
- Pars flaccida
- Incus and stapes
- Pars tensa
- Annulus

FIGURE 13.3 Left tympanic membrane.

the **ossicles** and middle ear. The landmarks of the tympanic membrane include the main portion, the pars tensa, the superior portion, and the pars flaccida. The short process of the malleus separates these portions of the tympanic membrane. The bone extending down to the middle of the ear is the manubrium (handle) of the malleus, which ends at the umbo. The cone of light is usually beneath the umbo. Anatomic landmarks of the tympanic membrane are shown in **Figure 13.3**.

The middle ear is not directly visibly accessible for an examination unless there is a perforation within the tympanic membrane. To measure the function of the middle ear, audiograms or pneumatic otoscopy is completed.

The middle ear is an air-filled cavity that contains the three ossicles. The ossicles amplify the vibrations of the tympanic membrane to send signals into the cochlea (inner ear) and produce hearing. **Figure 13.4** depicts the ossicles within the space of the middle ear.

The middle ear space ends laterally by the tympanic membrane and medially by the lateral wall of the inner ear. It has communication with the mastoid air cells and the nasopharynx via the eustachian tube. The eustachian tube's purpose is to keep the external and middle ear pressure equalized. The angle of the eustachian tube is straighter and shorter in length, which allows for microorganisms from the nasopharynx to enter the middle ear. This anatomic difference predisposes certain children to frequent ear infections. After age 7, the eustachian tube angle becomes less acute, and ear infections become less frequent. **Figure 13.5** depicts the anatomic differences of eustachian tubes in children and adults.

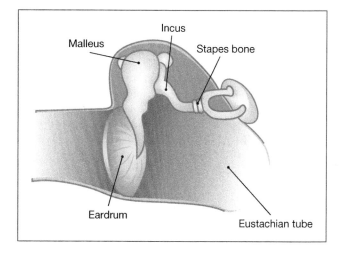

- Malleus
- Incus
- Stapes bone
- Eardrum
- Eustachian tube

FIGURE 13.4 Ear ossicles.

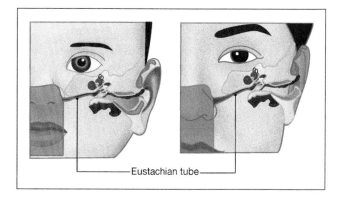

- Eustachian tube

FIGURE 13.5 Eustachian tube in an adult (right) and a child under 7 years old (left).

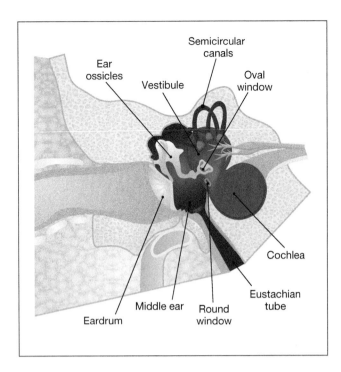

FIGURE 13.6 Anatomy of the inner ear.

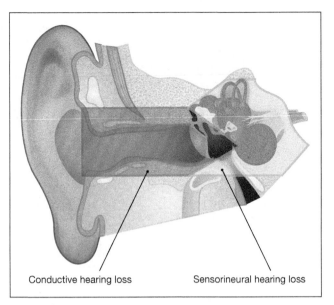

FIGURE 13.7 Conductive and sensorineural hearing loss. Conductive hearing loss occurs when sound waves do not reach the inner ear. Sensorineural hearing loss occurs when sound waves are not processed correctly.

The inner ear contains the cochlea (auditory end organ). The function of the cochlea is to detect sound. The vestibular end organs (utricle, saccule, and semicircular canals) are responsible for balance and sense acceleration along with gravitational forces. Anatomy of the inner ear is shown in **Figure 13.6**.

Physiology of Hearing

There are two phases of **hearing**: the conductive phase and the sensorineural phase. The conductive phase begins when sound waves are funneled by the external ear to the EAC and cause vibration of the eardrum. The eardrum then causes the ossicles to vibrate, and the stapes bone pushes on the oval window, allowing sound to transmit to the cochlea. If there is something that creates a barrier for the sound waves within the external ear or the middle ear, this causes a **conductive hearing loss**. Common causes of conductive hearing loss include fluid, otitis media, eustachian tube dysfunction, perforation of the tympanic membrane, cerumen impaction, otitis externa, or a foreign body in the ear canal.

Once the sound is transmitted into the cochlea, the sensorineural phase begins. In this phase, sound waves are passed into the cochlea, which is a hard, shell-like organ filled with fluid and hair cells. The fluid (endolymph and perilymph) vibration stimulates the hair cells, which then send signals to the temporal cortex of the brain via the vestibulocochlear nerve (CN VIII). Common causes of **sensorineural hearing loss** include aging, ototoxic medications, hereditary hearing loss, trauma, secondary causes due to various illnesses/conditions, and the result of listening to loud noises or explosions. See **Figure 13.7** to review the differences between conductive and sensorineural hearing loss.

THE NOSE

The function of the **nose** is to warm, humidify, and filter the air before it enters into the lungs. The upper third of the nose is supported by bone and the lower two-thirds is made of cartilage. Air enters the vestibule of the nose and passes through the nasal cavity to the nasopharynx. The medial wall of the nose is called the **septum**, which is made up of both cartilage and bone. The septum separates the left and right sides of the nasal cavity. It is covered by mucous membranes and is rich in blood supply. The nasal vestibule is lined with hair and skin. Anatomic landmarks of the nose are shown in **Figure 13.8**.

The anterior septum is made of cartilage, and posterior septum is made of bone. The septum is covered by a vascular mucous membrane. The majority of nosebleeds occur from the anterior aspect of the septum owing to a rich plexus of blood vessels called the Keisselbach's plexus. **Figure 13.9** depicts bones of the nose, and **Figure 13.10** depicts its vasculature.

Inside the nose, there are three bony structures called the **nasal turbinates** or nasal conchae. The turbinates are named on the basis of their anatomic location in the nasal cavity and include the inferior turbinate, the middle turbinate, and the superior turbinate. The turbinates provide increased surface area to warm, humidify, and filter the air. They are covered

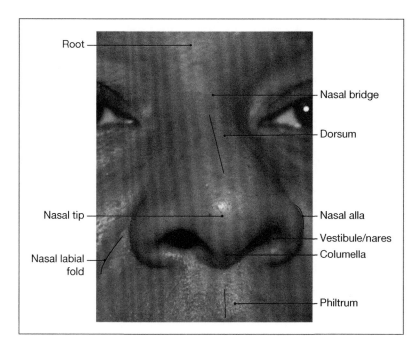

FIGURE 13.8 Anatomy of the external nose.

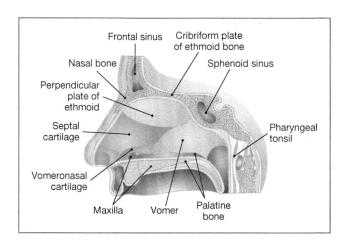

FIGURE 13.9 Bones of the nose.

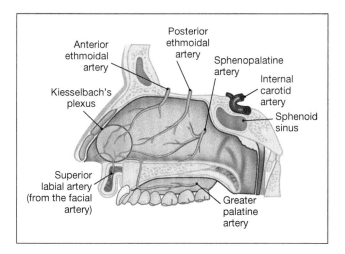

FIGURE 13.10 Vasculature of the nasal cavity.

with mucous membrane and are rich in blood supply. Beneath each nasal turbinate lies an aligning meatus or nasal passage termed the inferior meatus, middle meatus, and superior meatus. The nasal meatuses help to facilitate facial drainage. The inferior turbinate drains the nasolacrimal duct. The middle meatus drains the frontal, maxillary, and anterior ethmoidal sinuses. The superior meatus, the smallest of the three meatuses, drains the posterior ethmoidal sinuses and the sphenoidal sinuses. Anatomic landmarks of the internal nasal cavity are shown in **Figure 13.11**.

The **paranasal sinuses** are air-filled cavities within the skull and include the frontal, maxillary, ethmoid, and sphenoid sinuses; the anatomy of the sinuses is depicted in **Figure 13.12**. The sinuses are named according to their anatomic position in relation to the surrounding facial bones. The sinuses are lined with respiratory epithelium, which contains cilia. The cilia transport mucus from the sinuses through the ostium into the nasopharynx. Their functions include lightening the weight of the cranium, humidifying and filtering inhaled air, providing resonance to the voice, assisting in immune function, and providing a bony framework for the face and eyes.

THE MOUTH AND PHARYNX

The complexity of the anatomy of the pharynx is depicted in **Figure 13.13**. The **lips** are muscular folds that begin the entrance of the mouth. The lips play an important role in facial expression, phonation, sensation, and mastication. Inside the lips lie the **teeth** and **gingiva**. The lips are attached to the gingiva by the upper and lower frenulum (**Figure 13.14A**). The inner

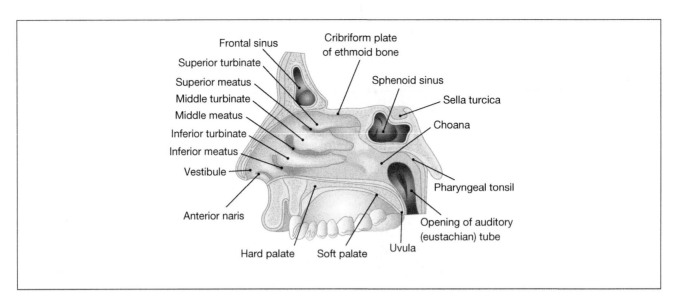

FIGURE 13.11 Anatomy of the internal nasal cavity.

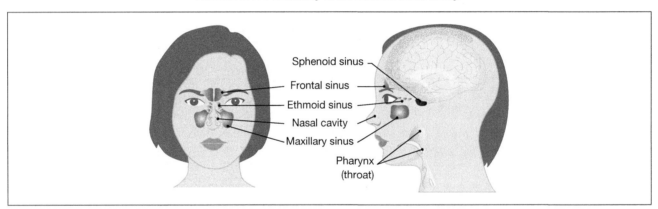

FIGURE 13.12 Paranasal sinuses.

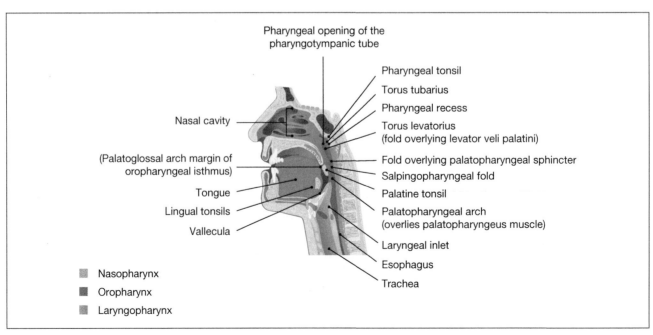

FIGURE 13.13 Anatomy of the pharynx.

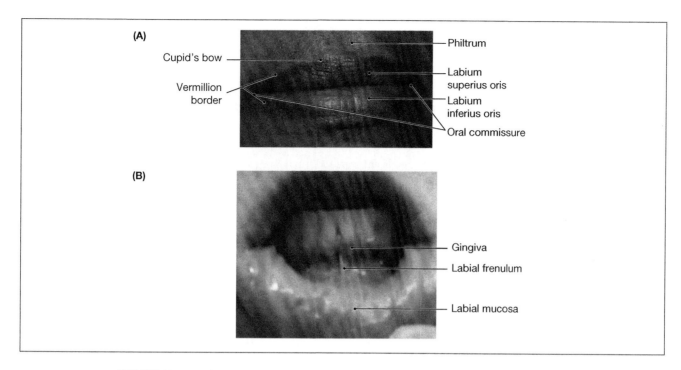

FIGURE 13.14 (A) Anatomy of the lips. (B) Anatomy of the labial mucosa and frenulum.

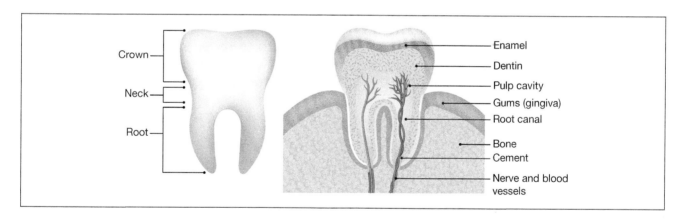

FIGURE 13.15 Anatomy of a tooth.

side of the lips is called the labial mucosa. Above the labial frenulum is the gingiva (**Figure 13.14B**).

The gingiva houses the roots of the teeth. The adult has 32 teeth, 16 in each jaw. Infants are born without teeth, and at about 10 months, teeth start to erupt. Children have 20 teeth in their mouth, 10 on top and 10 on the bottom. Each tooth is made up of dentin with an outer layer of enamel. The tooth root lies within the bone of the mandible or maxilla. Small blood vessels enter the tooth through the apex and then extend into the pulp chamber. The teeth are responsible for the breakdown of food via mastication. The anatomy of a single tooth is shown in **Figure 13.15**, and the anatomy and number of teeth in adults and children are depicted in **Figure 13.16**.

The **tongue** is a muscular organ covered with small papillae, giving it a rough surface (**Figure 13.17**). There are five basic tastes that these papillae can sense: sweet, salty, sour, bitter, and savory. The role of the tongue is for **taste** perception, to aid with mastication, and to assist with swallowing (deglutition). The tongue is also important in speech and articulation. Under the tongue, the lingual frenulum attaches to the floor of the mouth. Along the lingual frenulum, the submandibular salivary duct (Wharton's duct) provides an entrance for saliva into the mouth from the submandibular gland. This initiates the first phase of food digestion.

Posterior and superior to the tongue lies the anterior and posterior pharyngeal pillars. The palatine tonsils sit between these pillars. The **tonsils** consist of

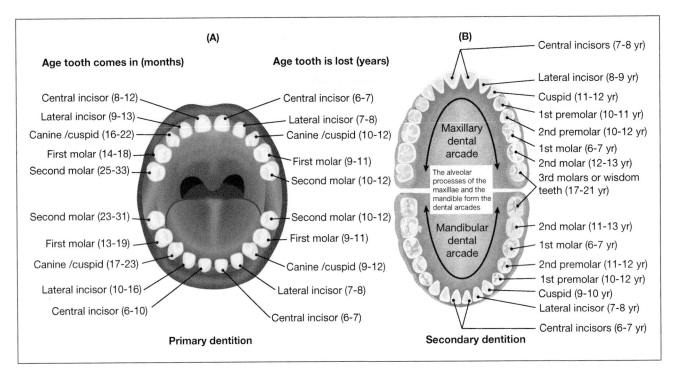

FIGURE 13.16 (A) Primary dentition. (B) Secondary dentition.

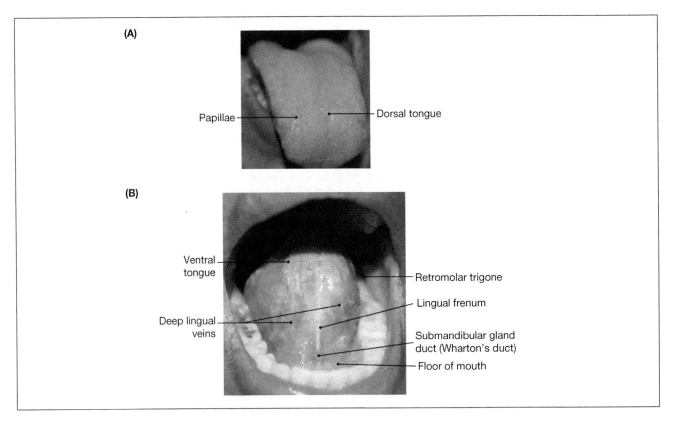

FIGURE 13.17 Anatomy of the tongue. (A) Dorsal surface. (B) Ventral surface.

lymphatic tissue, and they play a role in immune function. Waldeyer's ring consists of lymphoid tissue around the entrance of the aerodigestive tract (palatine tonsils, lingual tonsils, and adenoids). The uvula hangs down midline from the soft palate. The uvula and soft palate prevent food from entering the nasopharynx. The oral mucosa is lined with minor salivary glands, which produce lubrication, keeping the oral cavity moist. Saliva

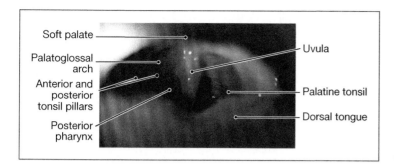

FIGURE 13.18 Oropharynx.

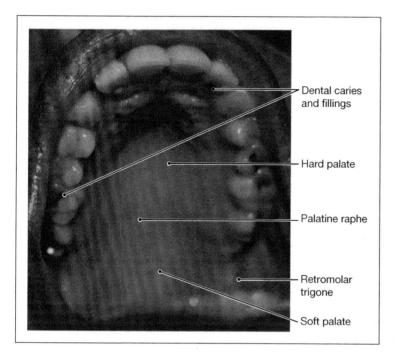

FIGURE 13.19 Hard palate.

also contains IgA to protect harmful bacteria from entering the body. The buccal mucosa lines the cheeks. The parotid ducts are located along the upper second molar, bilaterally, and allow for saliva to enter the mouth from the parotid gland. The anatomic landmarks of the oropharynx and the hard palate are shown in **Figures 13.18** and **13.19**.

Physiology of Smell and Taste

The sense of **smell** is a function of the olfactory receptors and the olfactory nerve or cranial nerve I (CN I). The olfactory epithelium is located in the superior and posterior nasal cavities, which have olfactory receptors. Olfactory receptors can detect thousands of odorants. These receptors transmit signals through the olfactory nerve and olfactory tract, where the signals are then processed by the brain. When pathology exists in the neurologic system, the sense of smell can be affected. Anosmia describes the complete absence of olfactory function. Hyposmia describes a decreased sense of smell. Phantosmia is the perception of odor when it is not present. Smell disorders occur in 1%

to 2% of the population and increase to 24% to 48% of patients over the age of 50. Causes of smell disorders include upper respiratory infection, head trauma, sinonasal disease, medications, and chemical exposure (Gould & Ramakrishnan, 2016).

The sense of **taste** is the function of taste receptors found on the tongue papillae. The anterior two-thirds of the tongue contains fungiform papillae that are innervated by the facial nerve (CN VII). The posterior aspect of the tongue has circumvallate and foliate papillae, which are innervated by the glossopharyngeal nerve (CN IX). There are also taste buds in the palate, larynx, pharynx, and epiglottis that are innervated by the vagus nerve (CN X). CN VII, IX, and X send signals through the brainstem to the thalamus and end in the gustatory cortex. Disorders of the sense of taste can be described as ageusia, which is the absence of taste; dysgeusia, which is a change in taste quality; and hypogeusia, which is a decreased taste sensation.

Chemosensation is the perception of chemicals and is an important function of taste and smell. Chemosensation is important to guide us in making decisions

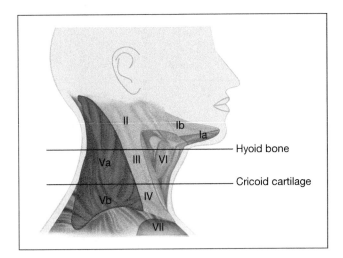

FIGURE 13.20 Lymph node levels. Diagram of the cervical lymph node levels as they relate to location and drainage areas.

related to food ingestion and detection of unsafe food choices or environments. For example, it can detect fire or spoiled foods. Smell and taste are linked, which means patients who present with taste impairments often have olfactory dysfunction. Some patients who have lost their sense of taste experience a decreased desire to enjoy foods. This could result in weight loss, depression, and decreased quality of life.

LYMPHATIC SYSTEM

The head and neck contain an extensive lymphatic network with over 300 lymph nodes and their intermediate channels. These are responsible for drainage from the head, scalp, sinuses and nasopharynx, salivary glands, oral cavity, oral pharynx, larynx, and hypopharynx. The locations of the lymph nodes in relation to the areas that they drain are shown in **Figure 13.20.** Since the nasal and oral cavity are often the first line of entry for foreign materials (bacteria, viruses, antigens), these lymphatics are important for immunologic defense. Abnormalities of the lymphatic system may indicate a variety of disorders from a common viral upper respiratory infection to head and neck cancer.

KEY HISTORY QUESTIONS AND CONSIDERATIONS FOR THE EARS, NOSE, AND THROAT

HISTORY OF PRESENT ILLNESS

Chief Concern: Hearing Loss

- Onset of symptoms: Gradual or sudden
- Location: Unilateral or bilateral

- Duration: Hours, days, months, years
- Severity: Complete hearing loss or decrease in hearing, fluctuating
- Exacerbating or relieving factors
- History of noise exposure
- Recent trauma, head injury, traumatic noise exposure (blast/explosion)
- Associated symptoms: Presence of tinnitus, ear fullness, vertigo, otalgia, otorrhea
- Change or recent medication that caused hearing loss: Chemotherapy, antibiotics
- Currently taking doses of aspirin; nonsteroidal anti-inflammatory (NSAIDs) medications, including BC powder®, naproxen, and/or ibuprofen

Chief Concern: Otalgia

- Onset of symptoms: Sudden, gradual, progressive
- Location: Unilateral or bilateral
- Duration: Days, months, years
- Severity of pain: Scale 0 to 10
- Intensity: Aching, sharp pain, throbbing
- Associated symptoms: Hearing loss, muffled hearing, tinnitus, disequilibrium, vertigo, otorrhea
- Upper respiratory infection concerns: Cough, fevers, chills, rhinorrhea, postnasal drip
- Recent trauma to head or ear
- Presence of neck masses, throat pain, trismus, odynophagia, dysphagia, weight loss
- Teeth grinding or history of temporomandibular joint disorders (TMD or TMJ)
- Neck pain, cervical spine issues
- Dental pain or caries

Chief Concern: Allergic Rhinitis

- Onset of symptoms: sudden, gradual, progressive
- Location: Unilateral or bilateral
- Duration: Days, months, years
- Severity of pain: Scale 0 to 10
- Intensity: Aching, sharp pain, throbbing
- Pruritis involving the nose, eyes, palate (distinguishes the diagnosis of allergic versus nonallergic rhinitis)
- Presence of fevers, chills, shortness of breath, wheezing
- Associated symptoms: Watery, itchy eyes; itchy nose; rhinorrhea, clear or colored; sneezing; nasal congestion; postnasal drip; frequent throat clearing; cough, malaise, and fatigue may be present in children
- Exacerbating factors: Seasonal versus perennial; exacerbated by environmental stimuli (plants, animals, perfumes); symptoms with irritants, including smoke exposure or chemicals
- Alleviating factors: Improved with antihistamines, nasal corticosteroids, avoidance of environmental factors, past history of allergy testing or allergy shots

Chief Concern: Epistaxis

- Duration of symptoms: Days, months, years
- Frequency of bleeding episodes: Multiple times per day, daily, weekly, monthly
- Duration of nosebleed
- Bleeding from one or both nares
- Bleeding from anterior nose or posterior nose
- Volume of blood: Can you fill a cup, or do you see blood on your tissue?
- History of trauma: Nose picking or injury
- Dry environment, use of humidifiers
- Intranasal illicit drug use (e.g., cocaine)
- Use of prescription or over-the-counter (OTC) medications, including warfarin, aspirin and so on
- Associated symptoms: Lightheadedness, fatigue, dyspnea, nasal obstruction, pain, numbness in parts of the face or teeth, headaches, visual or orbital concerns, hearing loss, enlarged lymph nodes, weight loss

Chief Concern: Acute Rhinosinusitis

- Three cardinal symptoms:
  - ○ Up to 4 weeks of purulent nasal drainage
  - ○ Nasal obstruction: Unilateral or bilateral
  - ○ Facial pain or pressure
- Location of symptoms: Maxillary or frontal facial pain/pressure, maxillary dental pain
- Duration of symptoms: Days, months, years
- Severity of symptoms: 0 to 10 scale
- Presence of upper respiratory infection symptoms: Fevers, chills, cough, malaise, fatigue, headache
- Anosmia or hyposmia
- Ear fullness
- Symptoms worsen within 10 days after initial improvement (double worsening)
- Recurrent symptoms: Number of sinus infections within the past year
- Allergy symptoms: Sneezing, itchy/watery eyes, itchy nose
- Known deviated septum, nasal trauma
- Symptoms that indicate malignant process, invasive fungal sinusitis, or meningitis:
  - ○ Hyponasal speech, indicating nasal obstruction
  - ○ Orbital cellulitis
  - ○ Facial cellulitis
  - ○ Neck stiffness
  - ○ Abnormal eye movement

Chief Concern: Oral Lesion

- Location and duration of lesion
- Changes in size or color of lesion
- Recent oral trauma such as hot foods, biting, chemicals
- Recent oral surgery or dental work
- Unintentional weight loss

- Dental pain or signs of infection
- Severity of pain: Scale 0 to 10
- Associated symptoms: Burning, bleeding, sore throat, dysphagia, odynophagia, otalgia, decreased tongue movement, trismus, neck mass, fever, chills
- Dry mouth
- Dental care regimes: Brush teeth once or twice a day, floss
- Neck mass/lymphadenopathy

Chief Concern: Sore Throat/Pharyngitis

- Onset of symptoms: Gradual, sudden, intermittent
- Location: Unilateral or bilateral
- Duration: Hours, days, months, years
- Severity of pain: Scale 0 to 10
- Associated symptoms: Dysphagia, odynophagia, changes in voice, otalgia, hemoptysis, weight loss, lymphadenopathy, trismus, fever
- Exacerbating and alleviating factors: What makes symptoms better or worse?
- Sick contacts: Exposure to cold, mononucleosis, streptococcus, influenza, sexually transmitted infections
- Presence of upper respiratory infection symptoms: Fever, chills, cough, rhinitis, malaise
- Coughing: Productive or nonproductive
- Allergic rhinitis (AR), postnasal drip
- Burning in throat after eating or lying down: Gastroesophageal reflux symptoms
- Change in voice (i.e., "hot potato voice")
- Sniffing or tripod position—may indicate epiglottis in children
- Stridor, wheezing, shortness of breath may indicate airway restriction/obstruction
- Halitosis

Chief Concern: Hoarseness

- Onset of symptoms: Gradual, sudden, progressive
- Duration: Hours, days, months, years
- Severity: Complete hearing loss or decrease in hearing, fluctuating
- Quality of voice: Coarse, breathy, aphonia
- Associated symptoms: Sore throat, hemoptysis, neck mass, otalgia, dysphagia, odynophagia
- Choking or aspirating with eating or drinking
- Exacerbating or alleviating symptoms: What makes it better or worse? Is it worse with prolonged speaking or straining voice?
- Symptoms of upper respiratory infection that precipitated symptoms
- Constant throat clearing
- Postnasal drip
- Gastroesophageal reflux symptoms
- Shortness of breath with speaking
- Stridor, upper airway wheeze

- Globus sensation
- Weight loss
- Overuse of voice (screaming, excessive speaking, singing)
- Neck mass
- Recent surgeries or intubation

PAST MEDICAL HISTORY

- Chronic medical conditions, including:
  - Liver disease
  - Cardiovascular disease
  - Hematologic disorders
  - High blood pressure
  - Asthma
  - Eczema
  - Migraines
  - Recent or past strokes
  - Cancer (specifically head and neck)
  - Cystic fibrosis
  - Ciliary dyskinesia
  - Sleep-disordered breathing
  - Autoimmune disorders, including inflammatory bowel disease, Sjögren's syndrome
  - Anemia
  - Gastroesophageal reflux disease (GERD)
  - Parkinson's disease
- Viral diseases such as Epstein-Barr virus, meningitis, or recent viral upper respiratory infection
- History of frequent ear infections as child/adult, sudden hearing loss, eardrum rupture, deviated or perforated septum, recurrent sinus infections, nasal polyps, conjunctivitis, vitamin deficiencies, lichen plantus, frequent strep throat/tonsillitis, tonsilliths, sexually transmitted infections
- Birth weight less than 3.3 pounds
- Anatomic malformation of the head or neck
- Craniofacial abnormalities (e.g., cleft palate)
- Birth complications such as severe asphyxia or low Apgar scores
- Prior surgeries on ears, nose, sinuses, tonsils, adenoids, or neck
- History of myringotomy with tympanostomy tubal placement
- History of allergy testing and results
- Exposure to radiation
- Frequency of routine dental exams and cleanings

Medications

- Current or past medications, including:
  - NSAIDs
  - Antibiotic use (aminoglycosides)
  - Oxymetazoline
  - Anticoagulants (both prescribed and OTC)
  - Chemotherapy
  - Human papillomavirus (HPV) vaccination
  - Steroids, including oral steroid inhalers
  - Bisphosphonates
  - Hormones
  - OTC saline rinses or saline irrigations

FAMILY HISTORY

- Hearing loss, especially in childhood
- Head and neck cancers
- AR
- Asthma
- Eczema
- Sinus disease
- Bleeding disorders
- Ethnicity (those of Asian descent have higher risk of nasopharyngeal cancer)
- Ciliary dyskinesia
- Autoimmune disorders
- Genetic malformations
- Human immunodeficiency virus (HIV)
- Laryngeal disorders
- Thyroid disorders
- Perinatal viral infections such as cytomegalovirus (CMV), rubella, herpes, toxoplasmosis, or syphilis

SOCIAL HISTORY

- Tobacco use, including chewing tobacco, snuff, e-cigarettes, cigarettes, and cigars
  - Pack years (or equivalent)
  - Secondary exposure
  - Quitting history and attempts
  - Current desire to quit
- Alcohol use: Frequency, quantity, type
- Illicit drug use, especially intranasal use
- Use of headphones, gun use, attendance at loud music concerts, playing in a band
- Occupation: Operation of heavy machinery, exposure to loud noises; exposure to wood dust, chemicals, asbestos, nickel; teachers, speakers, singers, or professionals who use their voice often
- Use of paan (Betel quid)
- High-risk sexual behavior or exposure to human papillomavirus (HPV)

REVIEW OF SYSTEMS

- General: Fatigue, fevers, weight loss, weakness
- Eyes: Eye pain, double vision, blurry vision
- Ears, Nose, Throat: See "History of Present Illness"
- Lymphatic: Lymphadenopathy
- Cardiovascular: Chest pain, palpitations
- Respiratory: Shortness of breath, cough, wheezing
- Gastrointestinal: Abdominal pain, gastroesophageal reflux, diarrhea, constipation, blood in stool
- Neurologic: Headaches, facial palsies, dizziness, numbness
- Integumentary: Rashes, ulcers, sores, lumps

PREVENTIVE CARE CONSIDERATIONS

Oral Health

Health promotion should include daily brushing of teeth with fluoride toothpaste and flossing to reduce caries and periodontal disease. According to the American Dental Association (ADA), recommendations for optimal oral health include brushing teeth twice a day using fluoride toothpaste, flossing teeth daily, eating healthy foods and snacks with limited sugar intake, tobacco cessation, and yearly dental exams (ADA, 2019). In the pediatric populations, clinicians should prescribe oral fluoride supplementation, starting at age 6 months, for children whose water supply is deficient in fluoride, and fluoride varnish should be applied to the primary teeth of infants and children starting at the age of primary tooth eruption (United States Preventive Services Task Force [USPSTF, 2014, Grade B Recommendations]). There is currently not enough evidence to support routine oral cancer screening in asymptomatic adults (USPSTF, 2013, Grade I Recommendation).

Tobacco Cessation

Tobacco dependence currently affects over 40 million Americans and has caused premature death in over 20 million people since the 1964 Surgeon General's report (U.S. Department of Health and Human Services, 2014). Smoking is estimated to kill about a half a million people a year (Centers for Disease Control and Prevention [CDC], 2014). Research has linked smoking directly to damage altering DNA molecules, which increases the incidence of cancer mutations, especially in tissues directly exposed to nicotine (Alexandrov et al., 2016). It is incumbent on healthcare clinicians to discuss this healthcare epidemic and provide patients with the education and resources they need to quit. At every visit, tobacco use should be assessed, cessation should be encouraged, and both behavioral and/or pharmacotherapy should be offered (USPSTF, 2015, Grade A Recommendation). The use of e-cigarettes has increased in the teenage and young-adult population. According to Soneji et al. (2017), there is an increased risk of progression from e-cigarette use to cigarette use. The CDC has published best practices for comprehensive tobacco control programs, giving all 50 states recommendations on how to tackle the tobacco crisis (CDC, 2014).

Hearing Loss

Hearing loss affects 48 million people in the United States and 360 million people globally (Carroll et al., 2017; Olusanya, Neumann, & Saunders, 2014). The leading cause of hearing loss is age (presbycusis), with noise exposure coming in second. According to the USPSTF (2018) draft statement on hearing loss screening, adults over the age of 50 should be screened for hearing loss using the whispered voice test, finger rub test, watch tick test, hearing loss questionnaire, and screening audiometry (if available). An audiogram is recommended for those adults with subjective concerns of hearing loss. Preventive interventions should be discussed with patients to decrease the risk of hearing loss. Asking patients if they experience hearing-loss symptoms can help to detect hearing loss early on and provide opportunities to discuss further harmful noise exposure prevention strategies. Avoiding prolonged exposure to loud noise and using hearing protection can help decrease hearing loss in patients (Carroll et al., 2017). See **Tables 13.1** and **13.2** for common causes of hearing loss.

Head and Neck Cancer Screening

Squamous cell carcinoma is the most common type of head and neck cancers. Cancers of the head and neck involve the nasopharynx, lips, oropharynx, hypopharynx, and larynx. Other malignancies include salivary gland malignancy, Kaposi's sarcoma, other sarcomas, melanoma, and lymphoma. Head and neck cancers account for approximately 4% of all cancers (about 65,000 men and women) in the United States. These cancers are diagnosed more commonly in men than women (2:1) and usually occur in patients over 50. With the prevalence of HPV, head and neck cancers are now being diagnosed earlier in people without a smoking or alcohol history and are affecting younger people as early as 30 (Goddard, 2016; National Cancer Institute, n.d.-a). Tobacco use (cigarettes, chewing tobacco, snuff, and vaporized tobacco) and heavy alcohol use are significant risk factors for cancers of the head and neck. Certain strains of the HPV (HPV 16 and HPV 18) are also a significant risk factor for cancers of the tonsils and base of tongue and usually affect the younger population who lack the risk factors of heavy alcohol and tobacco use. In the United States, the incidence of HPV-associated cancers of the oropharynx is rising (National Cancer Institute, n.d.-b). It is projected that 70% of oropharyngeal cancers in the United States are caused by HPV, making oropharyngeal cancers the most common HPV-related cancer in the United States. There are, however, no FDA-approved tests to detect HPV infections or HPV-caused cell changes in the oropharyngeal tissues (National Cancer Institute, 2019). Other risk factors for head and neck cancers include paan (Betel quid); occupational exposure, such as wood dust, asbestos, synthetic fibers, nickel, formaldehyde; Epstein-Barr virus; genetics (Asian ancestry is a risk factor for nasopharyngeal cancer); and radiation exposure in salivary and thyroid cancers (National Institute on Deafness and Other Communication Disorders, 2019). Early diagnosis and treatment are essential to improve patient outcomes, morbidity, and mortality. There is evidence that the HPV combivalent vaccine can help reduce the incidence of head and cancer along with cessation of risky behaviors such as tobacco and alcohol use.

TABLE 13.1 Conductive Hearing Loss: Causes and Physical Examination Findings

Causes of Conductive Hearing Loss	Physical Examination Findings
Cerumen	Yellow, orange, brown waxy substance in the ear canal blocking visualization of the TM. Symptoms include muffled hearing, aural fullness, decreased hearing, Weber lateralizes to affected ear.
Otitis media with effusion (most common in children)	Usually painless with amber fluid behind the TM. Usually can see air bubbles. Symptoms include aural fullness, muffled hearing, decreased hearing, Weber lateralizes to the affected ear.
Acute otitis media	On inspection, bulging tympanic membrane with purulent material behind TM. Often precipitated by an upper respiratory infection. Symptoms include pain with palpation over the mastoid; decreased, muffled hearing; otalgia.
TM perforation	Hole in the TM with view into the middle ear. Disrupts the vibration of the TM onto the ossicles. Symptoms may include otorrhea, pain with spontaneous rupture followed by relief of pain, muffled hearing.
Otosclerosis	Calcifications on the hearing bones, specifically the stapes, which does not allow the oval window to open and allow sound into the cochlear. Not visible on exam but will demonstrate conductive hearing loss.
Otitis externa	Erythema, edema, exudate within the ear canal. Can have white, yellow debris or purulent drainage. Can be difficult to visualize the TM. Pain on pulling on the helix and pressing the tragus.
Ear canal mass/middle ear mass (glomus tumor, osteomas)	White hard round masses within the ear canal (osteomas) or red pulsating mass within the middle ear, which could extend through the TM.
Tympanosclerosis	Scarring on the TM. Usually white in color.
Cholesteatoma	White skin debris or hard cerumen that usually occurs in the pars flaccida. There is usually a history of chronic ear infections and could be some scutum erosion, TM perforation.

TM, tympanic membrane.

TABLE 13.2 Sensorineural Hearing Loss: Causes and Physical Examination Findings

Causes of Sensorineural Hearing Loss	Physical Examination Findings*
Presbycusis (National Institute on Deafness and Other Communication Disorders, 2019)	Gradual, symmetric, high-frequency, permanent hearing loss that occurs over the age of 60. Patient often complains of tinnitus, aural fullness.
Noise exposure (National Institute on Deafness and Other Communication Disorders, 2019)	Exposure to loud noise typically over 85 dB. The louder the sound, the shorter the time it takes to cause hearing loss. Symptoms may be loud tinnitus and a subjective decrease in hearing.
Hereditary	In infants, this can affect between 1–3 children per 1,000. Newborn hearing screening can detect this hearing loss.

(continued)

TABLE 13.2 Sensorineural Hearing Loss: Causes and Physical Examination Findings (*continued*)	
Causes of Sensorineural Hearing Loss	Physical Examination Findings*
Ototoxicity (Cabrera-Muffly, 2016)	Drugs known to cause ototoxic effects in the cochlear: Aminoglycoside antibiotics, platinum-based chemotherapeutic medications, loop diuretics, salicylates/NSAIDs. Symptoms include symmetric, bilateral hearing loss. If high doses of foregoing medications occur, there could be sudden hearing loss. Other symptoms include vestibular imbalance, oscillopsia.
Sudden idiopathic hearing loss (Stachler et al., 2012)	A medical emergency that needs to be identified early in order to preserve hearing. Symptoms include sudden, most of the time, unilateral hearing loss. May be accompanied by vertigo, tinnitus, aural fullness. Physical exam reveals normal ear exam and Weber lateralizes away from affected ear. Treatment with high-dose steroids and MRI brain internal auditory canal protocol to rule out acoustic schwannoma. Immediate referral to otolaryngologist is indicated.
Autoimmune hearing loss	Very rare. Symptoms include fluctuating hearing loss and possibly vertigo.
Ménière's disease	Inner ear disorder believed to be caused by too much endolymph inside the cochlea. Symptoms include fluctuating hearing loss associated with vertigo lasting 20 minutes or more, roaring tinnitus, and aural fullness; recurrent. Treatment includes diuretics, antihistamines, or possibly surgery. Can be debilitating. Usually unilateral, but can be bilateral.
Vestibular schwannoma (Stachler et al., 2012)	Rare, affecting 1–2 per 100,000 people; slow-growing, benign tumor. Symptoms include slow, progressive hearing loss, usually unilateral. May be associated with aural fullness and/or vertigo. Some people may present with a sudden hearing loss. Physical exam findings reveal normal otoscopy. If tumor is large, patient may have facial paresis due to compression of CN VII (facial nerve).
Infections (meningitis, viral labyrinthitis)	In meningitis, patient may have severe headache, fevers, cranial nerve palsies, and decreased hearing. In viral labyrinthitis, some patients may have precipitating viral upper respiratory infection causing vertigo, decreased hearing, or sudden hearing loss.

*In all of these situations, otoscopy is normal. Weber would lateralize away from the affected ear. AC should be louder than BC.
AC, air conduction; BC, bone conduction; MRI, magnetic resonance imaging; NSAIDs, nonsteroidal anti-inflammatory drugs.

PHYSICAL EXAMINATION OF THE EARS, NOSE, AND THROAT

INSPECTION AND PALPATION OF THE EAR

Prepare equipment needed for ear examination (**Figure 13.21**). Start with inspection of the outer ear. Look for erythema, edema, tissue deformity, lesions, or masses. Palpating on the tragus and mastoid or pulling up on the pinna can provide information as to whether there is an ongoing, infective process as these maneuvers will generally produce pain if inflamed.

In order to see the ear canal and tympanic membrane, an otoscope will need to be used. If the patient is experiencing ear pain, pull up on the ear. Palpate the tragus and mastoid process to see if this elicits pain. When getting ready to use the otoscope, the clinician should place the nondominant hand on the helix and pull up and back. In children under the age of 3, the angle of the ear canal is less acute, so the clinician will need to pull back and down on the posterior helix. This allows for proper placement of the speculum into the external ear canal. It is helpful to have a parent or assistant stabilize the head for the clinician.

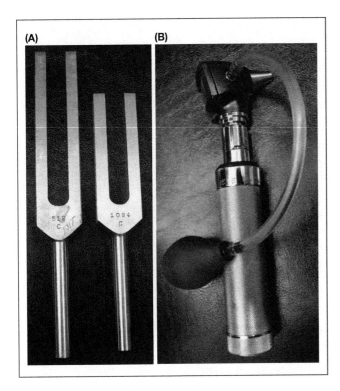

FIGURE 13.21 Equipment needed for ear examination.
(A) Tuning forks: 512 Hz (left) and 1,024 Hz (right).
(B) Otoscope with or without pneumatic otoscopy and speculums.

The clinician should place the otoscope in their dominant hand. The otoscope can be held several different ways according to the preference and comfort of the clinician. One way is to put the handle between the thumb and the fingers, wrapping the hand around the handle, with the handle pointing toward the floor. This works well when adult patients are being examined and not much movement of the head is expected. When examining children or someone who may not be able to stay still, the clinician should stabilize the otoscope by using the side of their hand against the patient's head. Hold the handle of the otoscope between the thumb and the fingers, with the handle facing upward. Place the side of the hand against the patient's cheek to stabilize the otoscope. This will help prevent jerky movements and prevent trauma from sudden patient head movements. In many cases, the parent or an assistant can help stabilize the child's head.

Pneumatic otoscopy is a method of examining the middle ear by using an otoscope with an attached rubber bulb to change the pressure in the ear canal. Changing the pressure in the ear helps the clinician to determine whether the tympanic membrane moves. If the middle ear is well aerated, the tympanic membrane will move from the pressure exerted with the rubber bulb. If an ear has an effusion, the tympanic membrane cannot move because fluid is pushing against it from the other side. According to the American Academy of Otolaryngology—Head and Neck Surgery's (OOA-HNS) clinical practice guideline on otitis media, pneumatic otoscopy is recommended to evaluate for effusion in the middle ear (Rosenfeld et al., 2016). If a rubber bulb is not available, ask the patient, while looking into their ear with an otoscope, to autoinsufflate. This means asking the patient to blow gently against pinched nostrils and a closed mouth, as when the patient is popping their ears on a plane. This technique provides the same mechanism of action as the rubber bulb and will allow the clinician to see movement (or lack thereof) of the tympanic membrane. **Figure 13.22** shows the techniques of the otoscopic exam, including otoscopy.

ASSESSING AUDITORY ACUITY

Whisper Test

The clinician should explain to the patient that three words will be whispered to them, and the patient should repeat those words back to the clinician. The patient will be asked to occlude one ear canal. If the patient cannot do this, the clinician can press on the tragus occluding the ear canal. The clinician should stand behind the patient or cover their mouth to ensure that the patient does not read the clinician's lips. Standing about 1 to 2 feet away, the clinician should exhale fully and whisper softly three words or numbers toward the unoccluded ear. The words or numbers should be equally accented syllables like baseball or ninety-nine. If the patient responds correctly, the hearing is considered normal. If the patient does not respond correctly, repeat using three different words or numbers. The patient is considered to have passed if they repeat three out of six answers correctly.

Finger-Rub Test

Standing in front of the patient, the clinician should place the hands on the side of the patient's head. Gently rub the fingers on one side together, asking if the patient hears the sound. Repeat on the other side. Wait for the patient's response. Repeat with both hands, asking if the patient hears them equally on both sides.

ASSESSING AIR AND BONE CONDUCTION

The tuning fork exam should be used in addition to the physical exam when evaluating hearing. This provides valuable information and can assist in distinguishing diagnoses that are consistent with a conductive or sensorineural hearing loss. These are screening tests and do not replace formal audiometry.

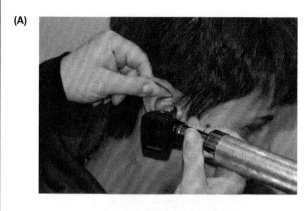

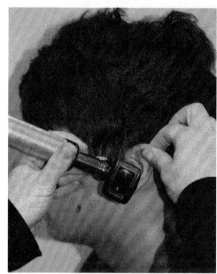

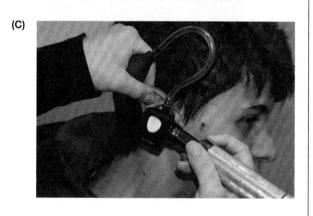

FIGURE 13.22 Performing an otoscopic examination. (A) When looking in the right ear, stabilize the otoscope with the right hand, placing the fifth digit against the patient's cheek, while pulling up and back on the helix with the other hand. (B) When looking in the left ear, use the left hand, stabilize the otoscope on the cheek using the fifth digit, while pulling up on the helix. (C) When using pneumatic ostoscopy, have the bulb in the hand that is pulling up on the helix and, while looking through the otoscope, compress the bulb and view the tympanic membrane move with the addition of air into the ear canal.

Weber Screening Test

In a quiet room, lightly hit the fork to start a light vibration. The clinician can do this by hitting the tuning fork on the knuckles/elbow or stroking the forks between the fingers. Once vibration is felt, lightly place the 512-Hz tuning fork on the patient's scalp at midline. Ask the patient if they hear the tone louder in the left ear or the right ear or if it is equally loud in both ears. The exam is considered normal if the sound is heard equally in each ear (**Figure 13.23A**). In unilateral conductive hearing loss, the sound lateralizes to the affected ear (it will be heard louder in the affected ear). In unilateral sensorineural hearing loss, the sound lateralizes away from the affected ear (it will be heard louder in the normal ear). If nothing is heard, try again, or move the turning fork onto the upper front teeth. This cannot be done if the patient is edentulous or has false teeth (**Figure 13.23B**).

Rinne Test

Place a lightly vibrating 512-Hz tuning fork on the mastoid bone behind the ear. Ask the patient to cover the opposite ear with one hand. When the patient can no longer hear the sound, move the vibrating tuning fork in front of the same ear canal. Avoid touching the ear. The "U" portion of the tuning fork should face forward in order to maximize the sound for the patient. The patient should report when the vibratory sound is no longer being heard. The test is considered normal if the patient continues to hear the vibratory sound for twice the amount of time when the tuning fork is held next to their ear as when it was placed on their mastoid bone. This indicates that air conduction (AC) is greater than bone conduction (BC), signifying a normal test. The Rinne test would detect unilateral conductive hearing loss if the vibratory sound is heard through the bone as long as or longer than through the air (AC < BC or AC = BC; **Figure 13.24**).

AUDIOMETRY

Testing Recommendations

- Tympanometry should be done in a patient with suspected otitis media. This can be available in some medical offices or performed by a licensed audiologist.
- In patients with a concern of hearing loss, an audiogram by a licensed audiologist is recommended. In **Figure 13.25**, an audiometry exam is being demonstrated for a child.
- Any abnormal tuning fork exam findings should prompt a referral for an audiologic evaluation.

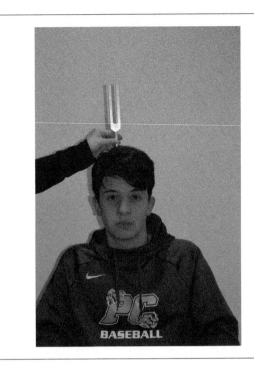
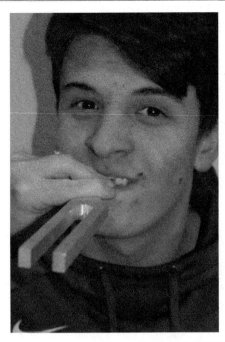

FIGURE 13.23 Weber exam.

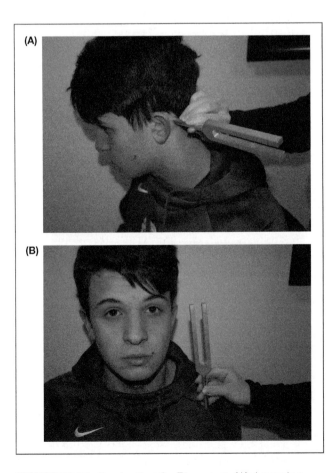

(A)

(B)

FIGURE 13.24 Conducting the Rinne test. (A) Assessing bone conduction. (B) Assessing air conduction.

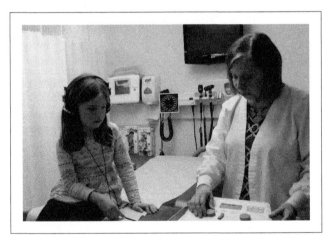

FIGURE 13.25 Conducting an audiometry exam.

INSPECTION AND PALPATION OF THE NOSE AND SINUSES

Inspect the outside of the nose. Look for shape, deformity, lesions, asymmetry, and deviation. Assess the nares as the patient breathes in and out of the nostrils. To assess for nasal obstruction, press on one naris at a time, asking the patient to breathe in and out, assessing airflow through the nasal vestibules. Palpate the sinuses to evaluate for tenderness. Palpate the frontal sinuses, which are located under the eyebrows, without pressing on the eyes. Palpate the maxillary sinuses, which are located approximately 1 cm lateral to the nasal

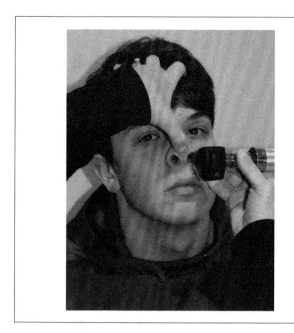

FIGURE 13.26 The proper way to use an otoscope to perform anterior rhinoscopy.

bridge bilaterally. Inspect the inside of the nose with an otoscope and the largest ear speculum available. Have the patient tilt the head back and press the nasal tip up to open the nasal vestibule. Grabbing the otoscope between the thumb and the index finger, brace the otoscope using your fifth digit against the patient's cheek. This will stabilize the scope and prevent sudden jerking movements in the nose. Look posteriorly and superiorly to visualize the anterior septum, anterior inferior turbinate, and, possibly, the middle turbinate. Evaluate the septum for deviation, lesions, perforation, bleeding, and/or crusting. Assess the nasal cavity and mucosa for color, lesions, drainage, ulcerations, and polyps. Assess the turbinates for color, size, polyps, lesions, and ulcerations. Nasal polyps tend to look like grapes. They are mucin-filled balls with a translucent mucosal lining. **Figure 13.26** depicts the use of the otoscope to perform anterior rhinoscopy.

INSPECTION OF THE MOUTH AND POSTERIOR PHARYNX

Lips

Inspection of the oral cavity first starts with the lips. Ensure the lips are symmetrical at the oral commissure. Asymmetry can indicate stroke or facial nerve palsies. Assess the lips for color, lesions, and closure. Nonhealing lesions on the lip can indicate cancer.

Mouth

Inspect the mouth with a light source and tongue depressor. Inspect the gingiva and dentition for caries,

abscesses, periodontal disease, and lesions. Note the condition of the teeth, and provide education on oral hygiene if poorly maintained. Look at the floor of the mouth under the tongue for pooling of saliva or ulcerations that could indicate cancer.

Tongue

Inspect the buccal mucosa, dorsal tongue, ventral tongue, floor of the mouth, retromolar trigone, hard palate, and soft palate. Use the tongue blade to help pull back the buccal mucosa, lift the tongue, or depress the tongue to get good visualization. Cancer of the tongue is common in the older male population, especially in tobacco users. Obtaining a good view of the posterior tongue, lateral sides of the tongue, ventral tongue, and floor of the mouth is essential for evaluation of masses, ulcerations, and discolorations (red or white patches). Document the color of mucous membranes, locations of discolorations, swelling, ulcerations, and masses. Ask the patient to stick out the tongue and move it from side to side, assessing for fasciculations, symmetry, and function of CN XII. In infants and young children, have the patient sit on a parent's or adult's lap. The parent/adult should hold the head stable while the clinician examines the mouth with a tongue blade and light source. Inspect the frenulum of the tongue. In some patients, this can be short and thick, causing ankyloglossia or tongue tie, as depicted in **Figure 13.27**.

Posterior Pharynx

Inspect the **posterior pharynx** by asking the patient to say "Ahh." Watch the soft palate elevate. This examines the function of CN X. Assess the uvula for deviation. Deviation can indicate peritonsillar abscess or

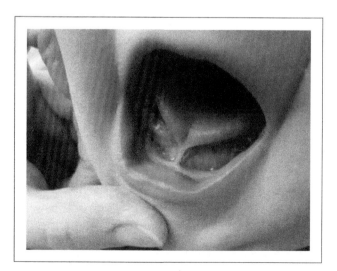

FIGURE 13.27 Ankyloglossia (tongue tie).

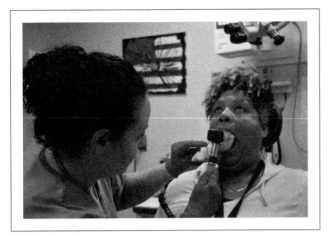

FIGURE 13.28 Inspection of oral cavity and posterior pharynx.

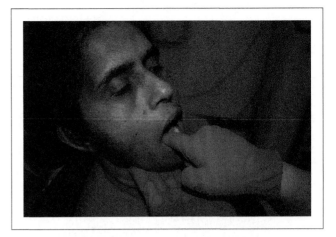

FIGURE 13.30 Palpation during the oral examination.

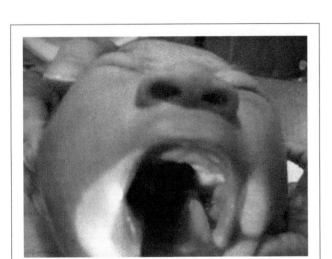

FIGURE 13.29 Inspection of oral cavity in a child with cleft palate (secondary).

CN X paralysis. Inspect the posterior pharynx, tonsillar pillars, retromolar trigone, soft palate, and uvula. Document if there are any discolorations, masses, or white or red discolorations. Inspect the tonsils for symmetry, size, crypts, exudates, white spots (tonsilliths), and/or masses.

It may be difficult to see the posterior pharynx in an infant. It is best visualized when the infant is crying. If you cannot get good visualization, listen to the quality of infant crying, as this can indicate whether there is any obstruction or restriction of the airway. Look at the palate for a bifid uvula or a cleft. Cleft can be submucosal and appear as a thin line within the soft palate (zona pellucida). **Figure 13.28** depicts how to inspect the oral cavity in an adult, and **Figure 13.29** depicts this exam for a child with cleft palate.

PALPATION OF THE MOUTH AND JAW

Palpation is a very important part of an oral examination. It can provide more information than just inspection. Lesions can be submucosal, causing the exam to "look" normal, when, in fact, there is a pathologic condition occurring. With gloved hands, ask the patient to stick out their tongue. Move it side to side, assessing for color, lesions, asymmetries, rough texture/smooth texture, and/or white/red patches, as shown in **Figure 13.30**.

Next palpate the entire tongue-lateral surfaces, dorsal surface, ventral surface, and floor of mouth. Bimanual palpation of the floor of the mouth is helpful to rule out masses and evaluate salivary glands for masses or sialadenitis. If there is asymmetry of the tonsils or a concern of a sore throat in a patient who is a tobacco user, palpate the tonsils and base of the tongue. Explain to the patient that this may cause the patient to gag. Oral or tonsillar lesions can cause referred pain to the ear (**Figure 13.31**).

TEMPORAL MANDIBULAR JOINT

Palpate and examine the TMJ. Assess the patient opening and closing the mouth, and palpate the TMJ joint with adduction and abduction of the jaw, as shown in **Figure 13.32**. Patients with TMJ arthritis may have pain that radiates to the ear, causing ear pain. The clinician can also feel for crepitus or shifting of the joint when affected patients open their mouth.

LIFE-SPAN CONSIDERATIONS FOR PHYSICAL EXAMINATION OF THE EARS, NOSE, AND THROAT

Pediatric Considerations

According to the CDC, 1.6 per 1,000 infants tested will have hearing loss. Of those patients with hearing

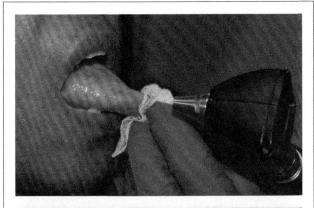

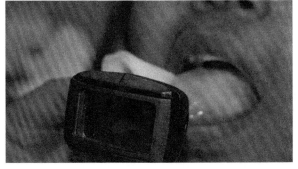

FIGURE 13.31 Inspection and palpation of the tongue.

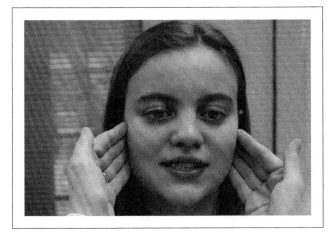

FIGURE 13.32 Assessing the temporal mandibular joint.

loss, genetic conditions are responsible for 50% to 60% of those children. Infections during pregnancy and complications from birth or other environmental causes are responsible for 30% of those children with hearing loss, the most common etiology being congenital CMV (CDC, n.d.). Hearing evaluation in infants is a screening requirement implemented by the Early Hearing Detection and Intervention (EHDI)

Act. Hearing screenings are implemented to detect hearing loss and deafness in infants in order to provide early intervention and services for the infant and family. Two types of hearing screenings in newborns are used, otoacoustic emissions (OAE) and auditory brainstem response.

OAE measure the infant's response to sound using a small microphone and earphone. Both microphone and earphone are placed in the infant's ear, and sounds are played. The microphone picks up an echo reflected back into the ear canal, which reveals normal hearing. If there is no echo, there may be a loss of hearing. If this first test is abnormal, auditory brainstem response (ABR) is done to measure the auditory nerve function. Electrodes are placed on the infant's head, and a small microphone is placed in the ear. The electrodes pick up the response from the sounds. Brainwaves from the auditory pathway are followed to identify the hearing level in each ear.

Otitis media with effusion (OME) can also cause significant hearing problems in children, resulting in speech and learning delays. According to the 2016 revised AAO-HNS's clinical practice guidelines on OME, clinicians should assess children between the ages of 2 and 12 who exhibit speech or learning problems. Subtle symptoms of poor balance, behavioral problems, school performance issues, or speech delay may also point to an underlying hearing problem. It is important to rule out OME in these children as management can improve hearing outcomes. Those patients who are at particularly increased risk for OME are those with Down syndrome, cleft palate, chronic ear infections, poor eustachian tube function, and children with stenotic ear canals (Rosenfeld et al., 2016). Ear tubes should not, however, be placed "in otherwise healthy children who have had a single episode of ear fluid lasting less than 3 months" (AAO-HNS Foundation, 2019, #6).

An additional consideration in the pediatric population is the heightened activity of the tonsil and adenoid tissue from the ages of 4 to 10. The most common bacterial infection that affects this area is *Group A Beta-Hemolytic Streptococcus* (GABHS), which causes tonsillitis. Other common bacterial organisms include *Staphylococcus aureus*, *Moraxella catarrhalis*, non-GABHS bacteria, and beta-lactamase producing organisms, *Hemophilus* species and *actinomycosis*. Viral pathogens such as adenovirus, coxsackievirus, parainfluenza, enteroviruses, Epstein-Barr virus, herpes simplex, and respiratory syncytial virus can also be responsible for tonsillitis. Guidelines from the AAO-HNS recommend tonsillectomy in children who have had seven or more tonsil infections within 1 year, five or more infections within 2 years, or three tonsil infections within 3 years. The Paradise criteria for tonsil infection include a sore throat plus at least one of the following features: temperature over 38.3°C (101°F), adenopathy, tonsil exudate, or a positive culture for GABHS (Mitchell et al., 2019).

LABORATORY CONSIDERATIONS FOR THE EARS, NOSE, AND THROAT

For a concern of epistaxis, typically lab work is not indicated unless the patient has lost a significant amount of blood or continues to have recurrent episodes despite conservative therapy. If large blood loss is suspected, complete blood count should be drawn to assess the hemoglobin and hematocrit. If the patient is on anticoagulants or a coagulopathy is suspected, coagulation studies can be drawn, including an assessment for Von Willebrand's disease.

When patients present with a severe sore throat and fever and have obvious tonsillar exudate, rapid strep testing is often beneficial to know whether to start antibiotics. In some milder cases or if the symptoms have gone on for more than 48 hours, the rapid strep may be negative, in which case a culture swab can help with the diagnosis. For oral lesions that appear vesicular and desquamate and do not resolve within 7 to 10 days on their own or are recurrent, a viral culture can help with the diagnosis of herpes simplex virus (HSV) or other pathologies. To determine whether rapid strep testing is needed, consider the Centor Criteria outlined in **Box 13.1**.

If symptoms of AR are refractory to medical management, allergy testing should be done to solidify the diagnosis. There are two forms of allergy testing—blood and skin testing. Please see **Table 13.3** for a description and considerations of each form of testing.

BOX 13.1
CENTOR CRITERIA

Centor criteria used to determine if rapid strep testing is needed:

- Fever
- Anterior cervical lymphadenopathy
- Tonsillar exudate
- Absence of cough

Each symptom is worth 1 point. For scores ≥3, complete a rapid strep. Scores <3 are unlikely to be group A *Streptococcus* and do not require testing or treatment.

IMAGING CONSIDERATIONS FOR THE EARS, NOSE, AND THROAT

WHEN TO IMAGE
- Computed tomography (CT) scan without contrast should be performed in patients with suspected temporal bone trauma.
- CT scan or magnetic resonance imaging (MRI) without contrast should be performed in patients with suspected cholesteatoma.
- MRI with and without contrast with fine cuts through the internal auditory canal should be ordered in a patient with sudden sensorineural hearing loss or if the individual has asymmetric sensorineural hearing loss to rule out acoustic schwannoma.
- CT sinus without contrast should be considered if the patient presents with three or more sinus infections within a 6-month period or unresolved symptoms after maximal medical therapy, including antibiotics, intranasal steroids, saline lavages, and antihistamines, as indicated.
- CT neck with contrast should be used to evaluate a patient with a hard, fixed mass of the oropharyngeal cavity as this is suspicious for cancer.
- MRI with and without contrast can evaluate the soft tissue and nerves if CN palsies are noted.

WHEN NOT TO IMAGE
- Do not obtain sinonasal imaging in patients with isolated AR (AAO-HNS, 2019).
- Do not obtain paranasal imaging for uncomplicated acute rhinosinusitis (AAO-HNS, 2019).
- In chronic, uncomplicated sinusitis, do not order more than one CT scan of the paranasal sinuses within 90 days (AAO-HNS, 2019).
- Do not obtain imaging studies for patients who present with nonpulsatile bilateral tinnitus, symmetric hearing loss, and a normal history/physical exam (AAO-HNS, 2019).
- Do not obtain a CT scan of the head/brain for sudden hearing loss unless there are focal neurologic findings, history of trauma, and/or chronic ear disease (AAO-HNS, 2019).
- Do not order imaging studies in a patient with hoarseness until after performing laryngoscopy (AAO-HNS, 2019).

EVIDENCE-BASED PRACTICE CONSIDERATIONS FOR THE EARS, NOSE, AND THROAT

The evidence-based practice guidelines used within this chapter and used to analyze advanced assessment findings are listed in **Box 13.2**.

TABLE 13.3 Allergy Testing: Types, Descriptions, and Considerations

Blood Testing	Skin Testing

Blood tests use immunoassays to measure the level of IgE in the blood specific to an antigen:
• RAST: Radioallergosorbent test uses a fluorescent antibody that binds to IgE, and reaction is determined by level of fluorescence. Not very sensitive compared with other technologies. They have a low rate of false-positive results and a fair number of false-negative results.
• ELISA: Enzyme-linked immunosorbent assay uses a polymer that binds to IgE in the blood and measures the antibody reaction. They have have variability per testing facility, no standards for testing.
• Sensitivity ranges from 60% to 95% with specificity ranges from 30% to 95%.
• No medical contraindications for blood tests
• Advantages of blood testing:
  ○ Do not need to stop medication prior to testing
  ○ Can test in patients with uncontrolled asthma, eczema, dermatographism, or significant medical conditions
  ○ Will not cause anaphylaxis
• Drawbacks: More expensive, takes longer to get results back, not as sensitive with low rate of false positives but fair number of false negatives
	Considered gold standard
	• Highly specific and sensitive (over 80%)
	• Introduces specific allergen into the skin, allowing for direct observation of the body's reaction
	• Reaction is caused by histamine release and causes wheal to form within 15–20 minutes
	• Contraindicated in patients with uncontrolled asthma or any condition that could compromise the patient
	• Must hold medications 3–5 days before testing:
	  ○ Oral antihistamines
	  ○ Intranasal antihistamines
	  ○ Tricyclic antidepressants
	  ○ H1 antagonists
	  ○ Selective serotonin reuptake inhibitors
	  ○ Selective norepinephrine reuptake inhibitors
	  ○ Benzodiazepines
	  ○ Atypical antidepressants
	  ○ Antipsychotics
	  ○ Hypnotics
	  ○ Proton pump inhibitors
	  ○ H2 antagonists
	• Advantages of skin testing include fast results, cheaper than blood testing
	• Drawbacks: Medication can interfere with testing, risk of reaction to reagent

BOX 13.2
EVIDENCE-BASED PRACTICE RESOURCES

Ears

American Academy of Audiology. (2011). *Childhood hearing screening guidelines.* Retrieved from https://www.cdc.gov/ncbddd/hearingloss/documents/AAA_Childhood-Hearing-Guidelines_2011.pdf

Rosenfeld, R., Shin, J., Schwartz, S., Coggins, R., Gagnon, L., Hackell, J. M., … Corrigan, M. D. (2016). Clinical practice guideline: Otitis media with effusion (update). *Otolaryngology—Head and Neck Surgery, 154*(1, Suppl.), S1–S41. doi:10.1177/0194599815623467

Stachler, R., Chandrasekhar, S., Arcer, S., Rosenfeld, R., Schwartz, S., Barrs, D. M., … Robertson, P. J. (2012). Clinical practice guideline: Sudden hearing loss. *Otolaryngology—Head and Neck Surgery, 146*(3, Suppl.), S1–S35. doi:10.1177/0194599812436449

Tunkle, D., Bauer, C., Sun, G., Rosenfeld, R., Chandrasekhar, S., Cunningham, E. R., Jr., … Whamond, E. J. (2014). Clinical practice guideline: Tinnitus. *Otolaryngology—Head and Neck Surgery, 151*(2, Suppl.), S1–S40. doi:10.1177/0194599814545325

U.S. Department of Health and Human Services. (2017). *Newborn screening contingency plan version II.* Retrieved from https://www.cdc.gov/ncbddd/documents/Screening-Contingency-Plan-Version-II.pdf

U.S. Preventive Services Task Force. (2019). Final research plan for hearing loss in older adults: Screening. Retrieved from https://www.uspreventiveservicestaskforce.org/Page/Document/final-research-plan/hearing-loss-in-older-adults-screening1

(continued)

BOX 13.2
EVIDENCE-BASED PRACTICE RESOURCES (*continued*)

Nose

Rosenfeld, R. M., Piccirillo, J. F., Chandrasekhar, S. S., Brook, I., Ashok Kumar, K., Kramper, M., ... Corrigan, M. D. (2015). Clinical practice guideline (update): Adult sinusitis. *Otolaryngology—Head and Neck Surgery, 152*(2, Suppl.), S1–S39. doi:10.1177/0194599815572097

Seidman, M. D., Gurgel, R. K., Lin, S. Y., Schwartz, S. R., Baroody, F. M., Bonner, J. R., ... Nnacheta, L. C. (2015). Clinical practice guideline: Allergic rhinitis. *Otolaryngology—Head and Neck Surgery, 152*(1, Suppl.), S1–S43. doi:10.1177/0194599814561600

Lips, Mouth, Throat

Centers for Disease Control and Prevention. (2014). *Best practices for comprehensive tobacco control programs.* Atlanta, GA: U.S. Department of Health and Human Services, Centers for Disease Control and Prevention, National Center for Chronic Disease Prevention and Health Promotion, Office on Smoking and Health. Retrieved from https://www.cdc.gov/tobacco/stateandcommunity/best_practices/pdfs/2014/comprehensive.pdf

Mitchell, R., Archer, S., Ishman, S., Rosenfeld, R., Coles, S., Finestone, S., Friedman, N., ... Nnacheta, L. (2019). Clinical practice guideline: Tonsillectomy in children (Update). *Otolaryngology—Head and Neck Surgery, 160*(1, Suppl.), S1–S42. doi:10.1177/0194599818801757

National Institute for Health and Center Excellence. (2017). *Head and neck cancers* (NICE Quality Standard No. 146). Retrieved from https://www.nice.org.uk/guidance/qs146

Pynnonen, M., Gillespie, B., Roman, B., Rosenfeld, R., Tunkel, D., Bontempo, L., ... Corrigan, M. (2017). Clinical practice guidelines: Evaluation of the neck mass in adults. *Otolaryngology—Head and Neck Surgery, 157*(2, Suppl.), S1–S30. doi:10.1177/0194599817722550

Stachler, R., Francis, D., Schwartz, S., Damask, C., Digoy, G., Krouse, H., ... Nnacheta, L. (2018). *Clinical practice guideline: Hoarseness (dysphonia). Otolaryngology—Head and Neck Surgery, 158*(1, Suppl.), S1–S42. doi:10.1177/0194599817751030

U.S. Preventive Services Task Force. (2016). Final update summary: Dental caries in children from birth through age 5 years: Screening. https://www.uspreventiveservicestaskforce.org/Page/Document/UpdateSummaryFinal/dental-caries-in-children-from-birth-through-age-5-years-screening

ABNORMAL FINDINGS OF THE EARS, NOSE, AND THROAT

ABNORMAL FINDINGS OF THE EAR

Otitis Media

Otitis media is infection or inflammation involving the middle ear. It can be purulent and symptomatic with otalgia and fever, or there can be serous or mucoid fluid behind the tympanic membrane that may or may not cause hearing impairment and rarely other associated symptoms. See **Figure 13.33**, which depicts the bulging tympanic membrane.

Key History and Physical Findings
- Otalgia (typically unilateral)
- Fever
- Difficulty hearing typically described as muffled hearing
- May have additional symptoms of upper respiratory infection concurrent with or prior to symptoms
- Bulging, erythematous tympanic membrane (TM)
- Posterior to TM, purulent fluid noted inside middle ear

- Weber lateralization to the affected ear
- No movement of TM with pneumatic otoscopy or autoinsufflation

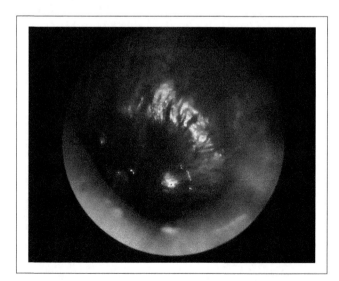

FIGURE 13.33 Otitis media.
Source: Image courtesy of B. Welleschik.

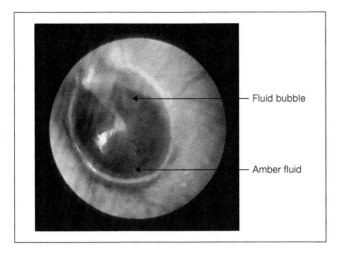

FIGURE 13.34 Otitis media with effusion.
Source: Image courtesy of Michael Hawke, MD.

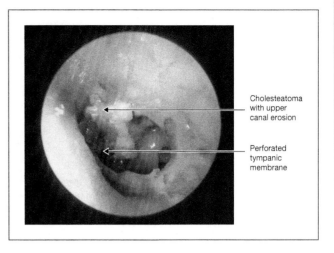

FIGURE 13.35 Cholesteatoma with upper canal erosion.
Source: Image courtesy of Michael Hawke, MD.

Differential Diagnoses
- Otitis media with effusion
- Otitis externa

Otitis Media With Effusion

OME is fluid that accumulates behind an intact TM (**Figure 13.34**). The fluid is generally nonpurulent in nature. The fluid can occur with or without signs of an acute otitis media (AOM). OME may occur spontaneously because of poor eustachian tube function or as an inflammatory response following an AOM. Between 60% and 70% of OME will resolve spontaneously within 3 months.

Key History and Physical Findings
- Hearing loss often described as muffled hearing
- Tinnitus
- Aural fullness/pressure
- May have vertigo
- Often following an upper respiratory infection or with seasonal allergies
- Amber fluid behind the TM
- Bubbles behind the TM
- Weber lateralizes to the affected ear
- Audiogram will reveal conductive or mixed hearing loss of affected ear

Cholesteatoma

Cholesteatoma occurs when squamous epithelium becomes entrapped either behind the ossicles or within the crevices of the temporal bone and causes bony erosion, hearing loss, and TM perforations (**Figure 13.35**). It is due to long-term eustachian tube dysfunction and/or repeated middle ear infections. This results in severe retraction of the TM around these osseous structures. If cholesteatomas are left untreated, they can cause hearing loss, infections, dizziness, and injury to the facial nerves.

Key History and Physical Findings
- Difficulty hearing
- Chronic ear infections and/or eustachian tube dysfunction
- Chronic otorrhea
- May experience vertigo and tinnitus
- Accumulation of debris most of the time in the upper ear above the malleus (pars flaccida); debris can resemble white skin and/or mixed with cerumen
- Bony erosion of the upper ear canal (scutum erosion)

Differential Diagnoses
- Otitis externa
- Cerumen impaction

Eustachian Tube Dysfunction

Eustachian tube dysfunction occurs when there is negative pressure in the middle ear and the TM is pulled into the middle ear cavity (**Figure 13.36**). Blockage of the eustachian tube isolates the middle ear space from the outside environment, creating a negative pressure that pulls the TM inward, causing pressure, pain, and accumulation of fluid.

Key History and Physical Findings
- Difficulty hearing usually described as muffled hearing
- Difficulty popping or equalizing pressure in ear
- Otalgia
- Tinnitus
- Aural fullness in affected ear
- History of frequent ear infections
- TM is sucked into the middle ear space, creating a pocket.
- Weber lateralizes to affected ear.

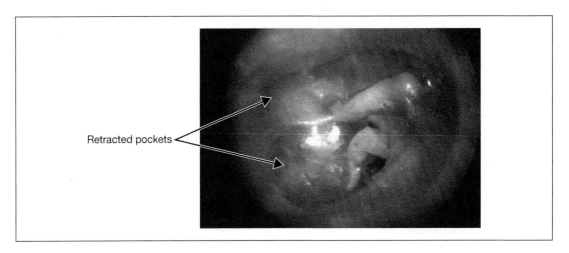

FIGURE 13.36 Retracted tympanic membrane.

Differential Diagnosis
- TM perforation

Osteomas

Osteomas are smooth, skin-lined bony lesions involving the EAC (**Figure 13.37**). They are usually asymptomatic but can interfere with cerumen cleaning or use of hearing aids. They are felt to be a result of long-term swimming in cold water (<70°F).

Key History and Physical Findings
- Patients may have no symptoms if the osteomas are small
- May obstruct the ear or cause cerumen to lodge behind the osteomas, causing impaction if osteomas are large
- Difficulty hearing, likely reported as muffled hearing
- Aural fullness

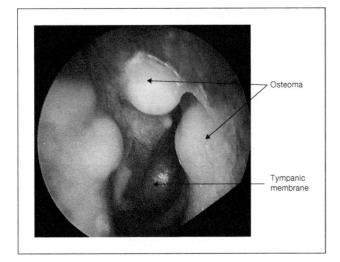

FIGURE 13.37 Osteomas.
Source: Image courtesy of Didier Descouens.

- Reported discomfort or pain
- Round, symmetric lesions in the ear canals that are hard on palpation
- Typically bilateral
- If ear canal is occluded, may have Weber lateralized to affected ear

Differential Diagnoses
- Squamous cell cancer
- Cholesteatoma

Tinnitus

Tinnitus is usually referred to as ringing in the ears but can be any type of sound one hears that is not external. This is frequently described as a ringing, whining, pulsating, humming, or electrical type of sound and is a common concern in adults. It is a subjective perception of sound that originates in the brain and is not an outside source. It can occur in one or both ears and may be either intermittent or constant. About 85% of patients with hearing loss have tinnitus. If the patient reports a pulsatile quality to the sound, a vascular origin should be investigated. See **Box 13.3** for the clinical evaluation of tinnitus.

Key History and Physical Findings
- Subjective sound reported as hissing, ringing, buzzing, humming, or chirping in one or both ears
- Can be reported as pulsatile (sound like heartbeat is in the ear)
- Causes interference with concentration and hearing
- Heard constantly or intermittently
- Can lead to decreased quality of life
- Otoscopic exam is typically normal.
- Audiogram typically shows hearing loss.

Tinnitus
- Thorough history of symptoms, past medical history
- Complete otologic exam
- Audiometric evaluation by licensed audiologist
- Referral to otolaryngologist

Pulsatile Tinnitus
- Audiogram
- If vascular abnormality is seen on physical exam, MRI/MRA or CT to evaluate soft tissue, nerve, and bone destruction
- Auscultate carotids for bruit, and, if heard, order carotid ultrasound

CT, computed tomography; MRA, magnetic resonance angiography; MRI, magnetic resonance imaging.

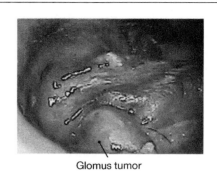
Glomus tumor

FIGURE 13.38 Glomus tumor.

Malignant Otitis Externa

Malignant otitis externa is the sequela of a severe outer ear infection, mostly from *Pseudomonas aeruginosa* or *S. aureus*. It is most commonly seen in patients who have uncontrolled diabetes or who are immunocompromised. The infection begins as an external otitis media and progresses into an osteomyelitis of the temporal bone.

Key History and Physical Findings
- Otalgia
- Otorrhea
- Change in hearing
- Facial weakness in severe cases
- Immunocompromised status or uncontrolled diabetes
- Granulation at the bony cartilaginous junction of the ear canal
- Pain with manipulation of the auricle
- Culture from otorrhea is positive for *P. aeruginosa*.
- Osteomyelitis is noted on CT temporal bone or gallium scan.

Glomus Tumor

Glomus tumor is a vascular lesion that involves the middle ear and petrous bone. It can be visible within the middle ear cavity (glomus tympanicum) or may not be visible unless imaging is done (glomus jugulare; **Figure 13.38**).

Key History and Physical Findings
- Pulsatile tinnitus (heart beat) in affected ear
- Hearing loss

- Muffled hearing
- Aural fullness
- Pulsating mass in the middle ear
- Weber would lateralize to the affected ear.
- Audiogram would show conductive or mixed hearing loss.
- CT temporal bone shows a mass with bony deformation (moth-eaten appearance of the bone) in either the middle ear or the petrous bone along the jugular bulb. If enlarged, it will enhance with contrast.
- MRI or magnetic resonance angiography (MRA) shows very bright lesion on T2 images with a salt-and-pepper type of appearance; low signal on T1, but this will still demonstrate the salt-and-pepper appearance.

Differential Diagnosis
- Squamous cell carcinoma

Microtia and Anotia

Microtia is a smaller-than-normal ear and may be of varying severity. It is commonly classified as Type 1, 2, or 3. Type 1 is a smaller but otherwise normal appearing ear. Type 2 has most of the elements of the ear but is not normal, and Type 3 generally contains a few ear remnants such as a lobule or small cartilaginous ridge.

Anotia is the absence of an external ear. These are often, but not always, associated with canal atresia, where the EAC is either completely closed off or has a pinhole-type appearance.

Key History and Physical Findings
- Hearing loss on the affected side if canal is atretic
- Abnormal appearance of ear, may only have small cartilaginous or skin remnant

ABNORMAL FINDINGS OF THE NOSE
Allergic Rhinitis

AR is a very common chronic disease in the United States. According to the 2017 Summary Health Statistics,

AR affects about 20 million adults and 6 million children aged 18 and younger (CDC: National Center for Health Statistics, 2017a). AR can also be associated with other conditions such as atopic dermatitis, eczema, asthma, sleep-disordered breathing, conjunctivitis, rhinosinusitis, and otitis media. It is an inflammatory, IgE-mediated disease triggered by exposure to allergens. Boggy, pale, cyanotic nasal mucosa may signify allergy in all populations. Additionally, nasal polyps or polypoid changes may indicate AR, allergic fungal sinusitis, or cystic fibrosis (Finkas & Katial, 2016).

Key History and Physical Findings
- Sneezing
- Itchy eyes, nose, or throat
- Nasal congestion
- Postnasal drip
- Clear, watery, bilateral rhinorrhea
- Pale, boggy nasal mucosa
- Swelling of turbinates
- Puffiness/darkening around eyes or "allergic shiners"
- Posterior pharynx cobblestoning
- Nasal polyps (occasional)

Differential Diagnosis
- Vasomotor rhinitis
- Nonallergic rhinitis
- Viral upper respiratory infection

Nonallergic Rhinitis

Nonallergic rhinitis can resemble AR, but allergy testing is negative for IgE with this condition. Usually, environmental irritants will trigger it, but it can be triggered by medications or pregnancy.

Key History and Physical Findings
- Postnasal drip
- Congestion
- Sneezing
- Lack of nasal itching
- Edematous turbinates
- Rhinorrhea (clear)

Acute Sinusitis

According to the CDC National Center for Health Statistics (2018) survey, **acute sinusitis** is diagnosed in over 28.9 million people in the United States. Despite clinical practice guidelines, antibiotics are prescribed in 86% of patients with a diagnosis of sinusitis, regardless of source (Smith et al., 2013). Acute viral rhinosinusitis (AVRS) is a self-limiting condition that peaks at 3 days and gradually declines within 10 to 14 days. According to the evidence-based clinical practice guideline on sinusitis, antibiotic therapy does not decrease the length of time of sinus symptoms and has the potential to cause side effects such as a rash, allergic reaction,

upset stomach, and diarrhea (Rosenfeld et al., 2015). AVRS is distinguished from acute bacterial rhinosinusitis (ABRS) when symptoms of AVRS persist over 10 days or symptoms worsen after an initial improvement, although they are the same. Chronic sinusitis is typically diagnosed when symptoms have persisted longer than 12 weeks, cause a change in the sense of smell or loss of the sense of smell, or cause headaches, periorbital pressure, and cough (Hauser & Kingdom, 2016; Chain, 2016).

Key History and Physical Findings (AVRS and ABRS)
- Duration of symptoms less than 4 weeks
- Three core symptoms:
  ○ Purulent nasal drainage
  ○ Facial pain/pressure
  ○ Nasal obstruction
- Additional symptoms:
  ○ Cough
  ○ Headache
  ○ Maxillary dental pain
  ○ Aural fullness
  ○ Anosmia
  ○ Purulent nasal drainage
  ○ Edematous, erythematous nasal mucosa
  ○ Injected throat, with purulent mucus in posterior pharynx
  ○ Possible head and neck lymphadenopathy

Chronic Sinusitis

Key History and Physical Findings
- Symptoms persist over 12 weeks
- Same symptoms as AVRS/ABRS
- History of AR and allergies
- Purulent nasal drainage
- Sinus tenderness
- Erythematous nasal mucosa
- Anatomic findings such as deviated septum, turbinate hypertrophy
- Nasal mass
- Nasal polyps

Epistaxis

Epistaxis is caused by a ruptured blood vessel. It is common among children between ages 2 and 10 and adults between 50 and 80. Anterior epistaxis is most common (90%–95%) in the Kiesselbach's plexus (Connelly & Ramakrishnan, 2016). Less common and more serious are posterior bleeds that occur from the sphenopalatine artery or Woodruff's plexus. Local causes include use of intranasal medications, digital trauma, inhaled illicit drugs, dry environment, deviated septum, and nasal and canula oxygen use. Systemic causes include uncontrolled hypertension, alcoholism, coagulopathies, medications that affect coagulation, and vascular malformations.

Key History and Physical Findings
- Bleeding of nose either anteriorly or posteriorly
- Nasal obstruction
- Blood clots inside the nose
- Prominent vasculature on anterior septum
- Modifiable risk factors:
  - Digital trauma
  - Medication
  - Dry environment
  - Elevated blood pressure
- Nonmodifiable risk factors:
  - Upper respiratory infection
  - AR
  - Septal deviation
  - Trauma
  - Malignant neoplasm
  - Vascular abnormalities
  - Coagulopathies

Differential Diagnoses
- Angiofibroma
- Carcinoma

Nasal Polyp

Nasal polyps are mucus-filled lobular lesions that occur within the nose and paranasal sinuses. They are typically found in conditions like cystic fibrosis or allergic fungal sinusitis but can also be seen in chronic AR or incidentally. They have a "grape"-like appearance and can cause nasal symptoms (**Figure 13.39**).

Key History and Physical Findings
- Nasal congestion
- Nasal obstruction
- Postnasal drip

- Rhinorrhea
- Will likely have allergy symptoms such as itchy watery eyes, itchy nose, sneezing
- May have chronic sinus infections because of the obstruction
- Boggy pale, enlarged turbinate
- Round, symmetric, pale grape-like mass

Differential Diagnoses
- Carcinoma
- Papilloma

Verruca of Nasal Septum

Verrucous lesions have a warty appearance and can look similar to papillomas (**Figure 13.40**). A dry crust often overlies the mucosal lesion. They are often seen along the septum or inferior turbinate as a result of nasal trauma.

Key History and Physical Findings
- Hard crusting lesion intranasally
- May cause bleeding
- Nasal obstruction
- History of digital manipulation
- Pedunculated, wart-like papule in the anterior nose

Differential Diagnoses
- Squamous cell carcinoma
- Papilloma

Deviated Septum

Deviated septum is when the septum that separates the nasal cavity is bent into one or both sides of the nose. This may be an incidental finding or a result of trauma or surgical manipulation. The septum can have

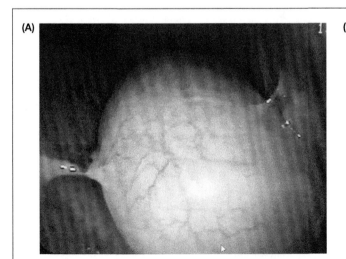
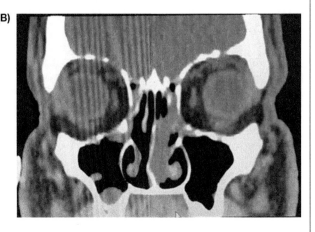

FIGURE 13.39 Nasal polyp. (A) Nasal polyp left nares between the inferior turbinate and septum. (B) Computed tomography (CT) scan without contrast to evaluate nasal polyp (A).

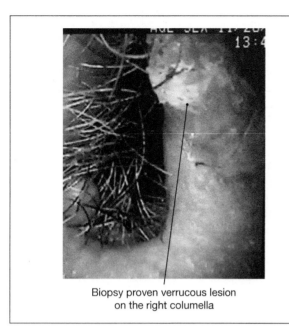

Biopsy proven verrucous lesion
on the right columella

FIGURE 13.40 Verruca of nasal septum.

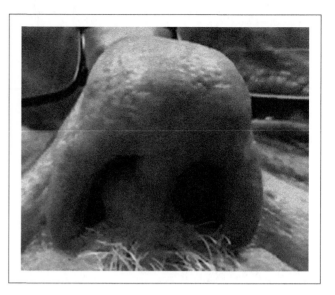

FIGURE 13.41 Deviated septum. Anterior septal deviation to the right causing decrease of the nasal valve on right.

a C shape and obstruct one nostril or an S shape and cause obstruction on both sides. Septal spurs are bony outcroppings at the level of the bony cartilaginous junction that can protrude into the nasal cavity and cause obstruction and/or epistaxis.

- Nasal obstruction (likely unilateral)
- Can be caused by nasal trauma
- Deviation of the dorsum/nasal bone
- Deviation off the columella
- Internal deviation of the septum causing narrowing of the nares on one or both sides (**Figure 13.41**)

Septal Perforation

A septal perforation is a hole within the septum. It can be tiny or involve the majority of the septum. They may cause a whistling noise when breathing through the nose, or they may be entirely asymptomatic. Large septal perforations can cause saddle nose deformity where the nasal dorsum appears sunken into the face.

Key History and Physical Findings
- Epistaxis
- Crusting
- Malodorous smell in nose
- Hole in the septum

Differential Diagnoses
- Postsurgical trauma
- Trauma
- Iatrogenic (nose picking, cocaine)

ABNORMAL FINDINGS OF THE THROAT
Tonsil Cancer

Squamous cell carcinoma of the tonsils is often seen in conjunction with the same risk factors as those found in most head and neck cancers: tobacco, alcohol use, and HPV. This may present as a yellowish/white or ulcerated lesion on the tonsil or tonsillar fossa with or without associated bleeding (**Figure 13.42**).

Key History and Physical Findings
- Persistent sore throat
- Unilateral otalgia
- Odynophagia
- Weight loss
- Trismus
- Unilateral neck mass
- Erythema
- Erythroleukoplakia

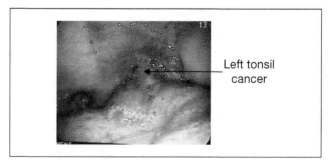

Left tonsil cancer

FIGURE 13.42 Tonsil cancer.

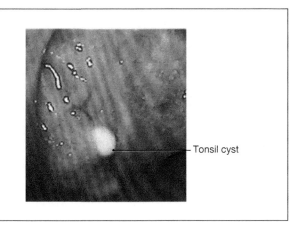

FIGURE 13.43 Tonsil cyst.

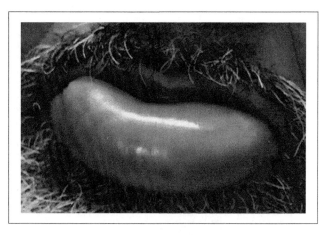

FIGURE 13.44 Angioedema of the lip.

- Exophytic mass firm to palpation
- Normal ear exam despite ear pain; may have OME
- May present with neck mass

Differential Diagnoses
- Erythroleukoplakia
- Candida
- Tonsillar abscess

Tonsil Cyst

Tonsil cysts are usually mucosal-lined soft lesions that contain a thick fluid (**Figure 13.43**). These are usually salivary in origin and can become large enough to produce symptoms. They are often seen incidentally during a physical or dental visit.

Key History and Physical Findings
- Globus sensation
- Cough
- Scratchy throat
- Halitosis
- Small, smooth, well-circumferential cyst on the tonsil
- Soft to palpation

Differential Diagnoses
- Tonsillith/tonsil stone
- Tonsil mass

Angioedema

Angioedema is swelling of the deeper layers of the skin in response to an allergen (**Figure 13.44**). It commonly affects the eyes, cheeks, and lips. Common causes include medications, foods, insect stings, latex, environmental factors, and underlying medical conditions. Rarely, it can be a hereditary disorder. If not treated, severe cases can be life threatening owing to risk of airway compromise.

Key History and Physical Findings
- History of certain medications known to cause reactions (e.g., angiotensin-converting [ACE] inhibitors, antibiotics)
- History of allergies (e.g., certain foods, latex, insect venom)
- Sudden swelling of the face, lips, and/or tongue but can occur in any part of the body
- Swelling of the airway
- Sudden, severe shortness of breath or trouble breathing
- Voice changes
- Stridor
- May have other allergic reaction such as pruritus or rash
- Edema of lips
- Edema around the eyes
- May cause edema of oral mucosa and tongue

Differential Diagnoses
- Anaphylaxis
- Cellulitis

Tongue Papilloma

Papilloma are wart-type lesions that are a result of the HPV virus. These lesions may occur on any mucosal surface and are often seen on the tongue, palate, or tonsillar fossae (**Figure 13.45**).

Key History and Physical Findings
- Papule that increases in size
- History of HPV
- Can grow anywhere in the oropharynx, pharynx, hypopharynx, larynx
- Firm, pedunculated, with an irregular surface, and sometimes appears as a cauliflower
- Can grow in clusters
- Wart appearance

(A)

(B)

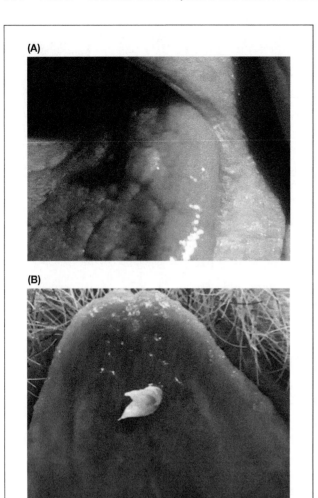

FIGURE 13.45 Tongue papilloma.

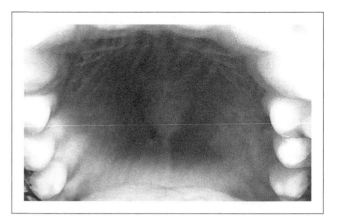

FIGURE 13.46 Palatine torus.
Source: Image courtesy of dozenist.

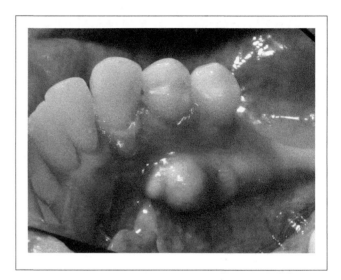

FIGURE 13.47 Mandibular tori.
Source: Image courtesy of D. Rosenbach.

Differential Diagnoses
- Squamous cell carcinoma
- Verruca

Palatine Torus

Torus palatine is a benign, hard bony lesion that is covered by normal mucosa that arises from cortical bone (**Figure 13.46**). This condition is usually asymptomatic but may interfere with wearing dentures or oral appliances. Heredity, lifestyle, and traumatic causes are considered risk factors for the development of palatine torus.

Key History and Physical Findings
- Asymptomatic
- Slow-growing benign lesion
- Hard bone growth on the hard palate, usually midline

Differential Diagnoses
- Squamous cell carcinoma
- Vascular malformation
- Fibroma

Mandibular Tori

Similar to palatal tori, mandibular tori are bony lesions covered by normal mucosa (**Figure 13.47**). They occur on the lingual surface of the mandible and may interfere with use of dentures. They are generally asymptomatic.

Key History and Physical Findings
- Slow-growing hard mass
- Asymptomatic
- Hard bony growth off the mandible on the lingual surface

Differential Diagnoses
- Fibromas
- Squamous cell cancer
- Sialocele

Aphthous Ulcer

Aphthous ulcers are frequently referred to as cold sores and are small, painful lesions that occur inside the lips, on the tongue, buccal or palatal mucosa, and floor of the mouth (**Figure 13.48**). They normally appear during an immunocompromised state (such as during an upper respiratory infection) and self-resolve.

Key History and Physical Findings
- Painful, burning, or tingling sensation
- May have fever
- Duration about 1 to 2 weeks
- Can occur on ventral tongue, gingiva, or buccal mucosa
- Shallow ulcer with white or yellow center surrounded by erythema

Differential Diagnoses
- Leukoplakia
- Squamous cell cancer
- Lichen planus

Leukoplakia

Leukoplakia is a thin white lesion on the mucosal surface anywhere within the oral cavity. It is usually not painful and does not brush or rub off. It can be a premalignant lesion in some cases. It is associated with heavy alcohol use, chewing tobacco, and heavy smoking and is diagnosed with a biopsy.

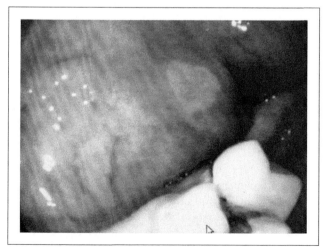

FIGURE 13.48 Aphthous ulcer.

Key History and Physical Exam
- History of smoking or chewing tobacco
- Often asymptomatic
- White, thick patches on mucosa and/or tongue
- Can be thickened or hardened
- Can be seen along with raised, red lesions
- Does not rub off

Differential Diagnoses
- Thrush
- Carcinoma in situ

Oral Candidiasis

Candidiasis (or thrush) is due to a fungal infection involving the mucosal surfaces. It may be painful and affect feeding. It is a white lesion that will leave an erythematous base when scraped off and generally has a flaky appearance involving several areas.

Key History and Physical Findings
- Often seen in infants and the elderly
- Immunocompromised status
- Use of an inhaled steroid
- Wears dentures
- History of diabetes, HIV, or cancer
- Soreness around area
- Difficulty eating or swallowing
- Loss of taste
- Burning or redness in mouth
- White lesion that rubs off with red underlying
- Patches are typically found on tongue or inner cheek.
- Can spread to roof of mouth, gingiva, tonsils, or posterior pharynx.

Differential Diagnosis
- Leukoplakia

Oral Cancer

Typically, oral cancers are squamous cell carcinomas. These can look like ulcerations, white or reddish areas that contain nonhealing sores around the edges. They may have firm nodules under their surface and be painful to palpation. They may also have a wart-like appearance owing to the potential for HPV-associated malignancy. When examining the oral mucosa or oropharynx for a suspicious lesion, palpation should be utilized to assess whether the mass is firm and fixed. If the lesion is fixed and firm, there should be suspicion for squamous cell carcinoma, which should be ruled out as a diagnosis. For more information on head and neck cancers, see **Table 13.4**. An example of a head and neck cancer, tongue cancer, is depicted in **Figure 13.49**.

TABLE 13.4 Head and Neck Cancers

Oropharyngeal Cancers	Nasopharyngeal Cancers	Hypopharyngeal and Laryngeal Cancers
These include cancers of the: • Tongue • Tonsils • Base of tongue • Soft/hard palate • Floor of mouth • Retromolar trigone	These include cancers of the: • Nasal cavity • Sinus • Nasopharynx	These include cancers of the: • Supraglottis • Glottis • Subglottis • Pyriform sinus • Postcricoid space • Posterior pharyngeal wall
Risk Factors: • Tobacco (cigarettes, snuff, chewing tobacco, vaping) • Heavy alcohol use • Paan (Betel quid) • HPV 16, 18	Risk Factors: • Tobacco use cigarettes/vapor tobacco • Heavy alcohol use • Occupational exposure (e.g., wood dust, industrial fumes, nickel, leather, formaldehyde, asbestos) • Epstein-Barr virus • Asian ancestry • Inverting papilloma	Risk Factors: • Tobacco use cigarettes/vapor tobacco • Heavy alcohol use • Laryngopharyngeal reflux
Symptoms: • Throat pain • Dysphagia • Odynophagia • Unilateral ear pain • Hearing loss/OME • Change in voice • Trismus • Difficulty with tongue mobility • Unintentional weight loss • Neck mass	Symptoms: • Unilateral nasal obstruction • Unilateral nasal discharge • Unilateral sinus infections • Unilateral epistaxis • Unilateral orbital symptoms • Pain or numbness along the maxillary nerve • Cheek swelling • Cranial nerve neuropathies • Unintentional weight loss • Neck mass	Symptoms: • Hoarseness • Dysphagia • Odynophagia • Unilateral otalgia • Globus sensation • Airway obstruction: difficulty breathing when lying flat • Stridor • Hemoptysis • Unintentional weight loss • Neck mass
Primary lymphatic drainage of the oropharynx to level II, III, IV with the most common to level II.*	Primary lymphatic drainage pathway of the nasopharynx to level IA/IB.*	Primary lymphatic drainage pathway of the hypopharynx and larynx II and III and can occur bilaterally.*

*See **Figure 13.14** for lymphatic levels.
OME, otitis media with effusion.
Source: From Eustaquio, M., & Quattlebaum, C. (2016). Cancer of the hypopharynx, larynx and esophagus. In M. Scholes & V. Ramakrishnan (Eds.), *ENT secrets* (4th ed., pp. 87–93). Philadelphia, PA: Elsevier.

Key History and Physical Findings
- History of HPV
- History of smoking or chewing tobacco
- History of heavy alcohol use
- Poor oral hygiene
- Bleeding
- Pain
- Dysphagia
- Odynophagia
- Red or white, unresolving patch or ulcer on the lips, tongue, cheeks, floor of the mouth, hard and soft palate, sinuses, and pharynx (throat)
- Tender with palpation
- May be firm to palpation
- Loose teeth
- Adenopathy

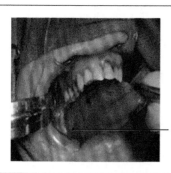

FIGURE 13.49 Tongue cancer.

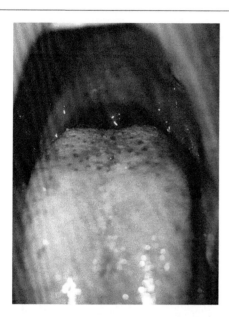

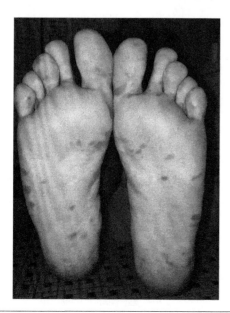

FIGURE 13.50 Herpangina.

Differential Diagnoses
- Fibroma
- Traumatic injury

Herpangina

Herpangina is a contagious illness most often caused by Coxsackie group A viruses (**Figure 13.50**). It is typically found in young children (ages 3 to 10) but adults can also get it. Herpangina is most commonly spread through contact with respiratory secretions or via the fecal–oral route. It is seen more frequently in the summer and fall months. It is similar to hand, foot, and mouth disease (HFMD; see Chapter 9, Evidence-Based Assessment of Skin, Hair, and Nails, for more information).

Key History and Physical Findings
- High Fever
- Headache
- Anorexia
- Sore throat
- Odynophagia
- Ulcerative lesions in the mouth and throat
- Similar lesions on feet, hands, and buttocks
- Vomiting

Acute Pharyngitis

Pharyngitis is edema, odynophagia, or scratchiness in the pharynx. It is commonly associated with many different viral and bacterial illnesses and can be hard to differentiate between the various types of illnesses. Pharyngitis is often accompanied by other symptoms, including rhinorrhea, cough, fever, fatigue, malaise, and/or myalgia. Viral pharyngitis is self-limiting; bacterial (or streptococcal) pharyngitis should be treated with antibiotics to prevent complications such as rheumatic fever and glomerulonephritis. See **Box 13.1** for the Centor Criteria, which can help to discriminate streptococcal pharyngitis from other types of pharyngitis.

Clinical Pearls

- When evaluating a patient with hearing loss, utilize tuning forks to confirm diagnosis.
- If a patient presents with otalgia with a normal exam, consider other pathology such as TMJ, cervical pain, dental abscess, or cancer of the oropharynx and larynx. Make sure a thorough history is obtained.
- In children, if a child presents with unilateral purulent nasal drainage, suspect a foreign body. This is common among preschool children, as they like to stick small items into orifices.

- For patients with compromised immune systems and chronic sinus concerns, the clinician should think about invasive fungal sinusitis.
- Viruses are responsible for the majority of acute rhinosinusitis, yet most sinus concerns are treated with antibiotics. Obtain a thorough history and assess the time frame of symptoms. If symptoms have been present for less than 10 days without worsening, recommend watchful waiting and symptom relief.
- In patients with unilateral nasal obstruction, epistaxis, and unilateral chronic sinusitis, a differential diagnosis of intranasal mass or foreign body should be excluded.
- In a patient with recurrent unilateral epistaxis, nasal obstruction, facial pain, and chronic sinusitis, nasal carcinoma should be considered a differential diagnosis.
- Modifiable risk factors for epistaxis are digital trauma, dry environment/lack of humidity, and medication use. Nonmodifiable risk factors include inflammation within the nose caused by infection/allergies, trauma, septal deviation, coagulopathies, malignant process, or vascular abnormalities.
- Tobacco cessation should be discussed at every appointment. Tobacco use puts the patient at risk for poor oral health, head and neck cancers, and many other diseases.
- When performing an oral exam, have the patient remove their dentures to ensure all of the oral mucosa is evaluated.
- If you cannot get a good view of the posterior pharynx because the patient is guarding, have the patient pant in and out or yawn. This will elevate the soft palate, while relaxing the tongue.
- In a patient who had recent sinus surgery, recurrent meningitis, or a history of head trauma, excessive clear, watery fluid draining from the nose could be indicative of a cerebrospinal leak.

Key Takeaways

- The head and neck are a complex area that are responsible for many vital functions.
- Hearing loss has many underlying causes and should be thoroughly evaluated to maximize communication potential.
- Proper diagnosis of infectious versus allergic causes of sinonasal symptoms can help avoid

inappropriate antibiotic use and decrease the amount of money spent on OTC medications.
- Head and neck cancer should be considered in patients who have enlarging or ulcerative lesions that are not responding to appropriate medical therapy within an appropriate time frame (2 weeks).
- If there is any doubt as to the diagnosis or management, refer to an ear, nose, and throat clinician for further evaluation.

REFERENCES

Alexandrov, L., Seok, Y., Haases, K., Van Loo, P., Martincorena, I., Nik-Zainal, S., . . . Stratton, M. (2016). Mutational signatures associated with tobacco smoking in human cancer. *Science, 354*(6312), 618–622. doi:10.1126/science.aag0299

American Academy of Otolaryngology—Head and Neck Surgery Foundation. (2019). *Ten things physicians and patients should question.* Retrieved from http://www.choosingwisely.org/societies/american-academy-of-otolaryngology-head-neck-surgery-foundation

American Dental Association. (2019). *Oral health topics.* Retrieved from https://www.ada.org/en/member-center/oral-health-topics/home-care

Cabrera-Muffly, C. (2016). Hearing loss and ototoxicity. In M. Scholes & V. Ramakrishnan (Eds.), *ENT secrets* (4th ed., pp. 213–220). Philadelphia, PA: Elsevier.

Carroll, Y., Eichwald, J., Scinicariello, F., Hoffman, H., Deitchman, S., Radke, M., . . . Brevsse, P. (2017). Vital signs: Noise-induced hearing loss among adults—US 2011–2012. *Morbidity and Mortality Weekly Report, 66*(5), 139–144. Retrieved from https://www.cdc.gov/mmwr/volumes/66/wr/mm6605e3.htm?s_cid=mm6605e3_w

Centers for Disease Control and Prevention. (2014). *Best practices for comprehensive tobacco control programs.* Atlanta, GA: U.S. Department of Health and Human Services, Centers for Disease Control and Prevention, National Center for Chronic Disease Prevention and Health Promotion, Office on Smoking and Health. Retrieved from https://www.cdc.gov/tobacco/stateandcommunity/best_practices/pdfs/2014/comprehensive.pdf

Centers for Disease Control and Prevention: National Center for Health Statistics. (2017a). *Allergies and hay fever.* Retrieved from https://www.cdc.gov/nchs/fastats/allergies.htm

Centers for Disease Control and Prevention: National Center for Health Statistics. (2017b). *Chronic sinusitis.* Retrieved from https://www.cdc.gov/nchs/fastats/sinuses.htm

Centers for Disease Control and Prevention: National Center for Health Statistics. (2018). *Summary health statistics: National Health Interview Survey, 2018* [Table A-2a]. Retrieved from https://ftp.cdc.gov/pub/Health_Statistics/NCHS/NHIS/SHS/2018_SHS_Table_A-2.pdf

Centers for Disease Control and Prevention, National Center on Birth Defects and Developmental Disabiltie. (n.d.).

Hearing loss in children: Data and statistics about hearing loss in children. Retrieved from https://www.cdc.gov/ncbddd/hearingloss/data.html

Chain, J. (2016). Acute rhinosinusitis and infectious complications. In M. Scholes & V. Ramakrishnan (Eds.), *ENT secrets* (4th ed., pp. 242–248). Philadelphia, PA: Elsevier.

Connelly, A., & Ramakrishnan, V. (2016). Epistaxis. In M. Scholes & V. Ramakrishnan (Eds.), *ENT secrets* (4th ed., pp. 242–248). Philadelphia, PA: Elsevier.

Eustaquio, M., & Quattlebaum, C. (2016). Cancer of the hypopharynx, larynx and esophagus. In M. Scholes & V. Ramakrishnan (Eds.), *ENT secrets* (4th ed., pp. 87–93). Philadelphia, PA: Elsevier.

Finkas, L., & Katial, R. (2016). Rhinitis. In M. Scholes & V. Ramakrishnan (Eds.), *ENT secrets* (4th ed., pp. 242–248). Philadelphia, PA: Elsevier.

Goddard, J. (2016). Diseases of the oral cavity and pharynx. In M. Scholes & V. Ramakrishnan (Eds.), *ENT secrets* (4th ed., pp. 81–86). Philadelphia, PA: Elsevier.

Gould, E., & Ramakrishnan, V. (2016). Taste and smell. In M. Scholes & V. Ramakrishnan (Eds.), *ENT secrets* (4th ed., pp. 50–53). Philadelphia, PA: Elsevier.

Hauser, L., & Kingdom, T. (2016). Chronic rhinosinusitis. In M. Scholes & V. Ramakrishnan (Eds.), *ENT secrets* (4th ed., pp. 242–248). Philadelphia, PA: Elsevier.

Mitchell, R., Archer, S., Ishman, S., Rosenfeld, R., Coles, S., Finestone, S., Friedman, N., . . . Nnacheta, L. (2019). Clinical practice guideline: Tonsillectomy in children (Update). *Otolaryngology—Head and Neck Surgery, 160*(1, Suppl.), S1–S42. doi:10.1177/0194599818801757

National Cancer Institute. (n.d.-a). Cancer stat facts: Larynx. Retrieved from https://seer.cancer.gov/statfacts/html/laryn.html

National Cancer Institute. (n.d.-b). Cancer stat facts: Oral cavity and pharynx cancer. Retrieved from https://seer.cancer.gov/statfacts/html/oralcav.html

National Cancer Institute. (2019). *HPV and cancer*. Retrieved from https://www.cancer.gov/about-cancer/causes-prevention/risk/infectious-agents/hpv-and-cancer

National Institute on Deafness and Other Communication Disorders. (2019). *Noise-induced hearing loss*. Retrieved from https://www.nidcd.nih.gov/health/noise-induced-hearing-loss

Olusanva, B., Neumann, K., & Saunders, J. (2014). A global burden of disabling hearing impairment: A call to action. *Bulletin of the World Health Organization, 92*(5), 367–373. doi:10.2471/BLT.13.128728

Rosenfeld, R., Piccirillo, J., Chandrasekhar, S., Brook, I., Kumar, K., Kramper, M., . . . Corrigan, M. D. (2015). Clinical practice guideline (update) adult sinusitis. *Otolaryngology—Head and Neck Surgery, 152*(2, Suppl.), S1–S39. doi:10.1177/0194599815572097

Rosenfeld, R., Shin, J., Schwartz, S., Coggins, R., Gagnon, L., Hackell, J. M., . . . Corrigan, M. D. (2016). Clinical practice guideline: Otitis media with effusion (update). *Otolaryngology—Head and Neck Surgery, 154*(1, Suppl.), S1–S41. doi:10.177/0194599815623467

Smith, S., Evans, C., Tan, B., Chandra, R. K., Smith, S. B., & Kern, R. C. (2013). National burden of antibiotic use for adult rhinosinusitis. *Journal of Allergy and Clinical Immunology, 132*, 1230–1232. doi:10.1016/j.jaci.2013.07.009

Soneji, S., Barrington-Trimis, J., Wills, T., Leventhal, A., Unger, J., Gibson, L., . . . Dick, D. (2017). Association between initial use of e-cigarettes and subsequent cigarette smoking among adolescents and young adults: A systemic review and meta-analysis. *JAMA Pediatrics, 171*(8), 788–797. doi:10.1001/jamapediatrics.2017.1488

Stachler, R., Chandrasekhar, S., Archer, S., Rosenfeld, R., Schwartz, S., Barrs, D. M., . . . Robertson, P. J.; American Academy of Otolaryngology—Head and Neck Surgery. (2012). Clinical practice guideline: Sudden hearing loss. *Otolaryngology—Head and Neck Surgery,* 146 (3, Suppl.), S1–S35. doi:10.1177/0194599812436449

U.S. Department of Health and Human Services. (2014). *The health consequences of smoking—50 years of progress: A report of the Surgeon General*. Atlanta, GA: U.S. Department of Health and Human Services, Centers for Disease Control and Prevention, National Center for Chronic Disease Prevention and Health Promotion, Office on Smoking and Health. Retrieved from https://www.ncbi.nlm.nih.gov/books/NBK179276/pdf/Bookshelf_NBK179276.pdf

U.S. National Library of Medicine. (2019). *Nonsyndromic hearing loss*. Retrieved from https://ghr.nlm.nih.gov/condition/nonsyndromic-hearing-loss#inheritance

U.S. Preventive Services Task Force. (2013). Final recommendation statement: Oral cancer: Screening. Retrieved from https://www.uspreventiveservicestaskforce.org/Page/Document/RecommendationStatementFinal/oral-cancer-screening1

U.S. Preventive Services Task Force. (2014). Final update summary: Dental caries in children from birth through age 5 years: Screening. Retrieved from https://www.uspreventiveservicestaskforce.org/Page/Document/UpdateSummaryFinal/dental-caries-in-children-from-birth-through-age-5-years-screening

U.S. Preventive Services Task Force. (2015). Final update summary: Tobacco smoking cessation in adults, including pregnant women: Behavioral and pharmacotherapy interventions. Retrieved from https://www.uspreventiveservicestaskforce.org/Page/Document/UpdateSummaryFinal/tobacco-use-in-adults-and-pregnant-women-counseling-and-interventions1

U.S. Preventive Services Task Force. (2019). Final research plan for hearing loss in older adults: Screening. Retrieved from https://www.uspreventiveservicestaskforce.org/Page/Document/final-research-plan/hearing-loss-in-older-adults-screening1

14

Evidence-Based Assessment of the Nervous System

Leslie E. Simons

"It's not what you look at that matters, it's what you see."

—HENRY DAVID THOREAU

 VIDEOS

- Well Exam: Neurologic Exam
- Well Exam: Dix Hallpike Test
- Patient History: Adult With Headache (Migraine)
- Patient History: Adult With Dizziness

LEARNING OBJECTIVES

- Describe the structure and function of the nervous system (brain, spinal cord, central nervous system, peripheral nervous system, and cranial and spinal nerves).
- Identify the differences and considerations in the anatomy/physiology of the neurological system across the life span.
- Understand the components of a comprehensive, evidence-based history and physical examination of the nervous system.
- Distinguish between normal and abnormal findings in the nervous system.

Visit https://connect.springerpub.com/content/book/978-0-8261 -6454-4/chapter/ch00 to access the videos.

ANATOMY AND PHYSIOLOGY OF THE NERVOUS SYSTEM

The **central nervous system** (CNS) is composed of the brain and spinal cord and is responsible for control of the body. The cranial and spinal nerves and the ascending and descending pathways make up the **peripheral nervous system** (PNS), which is responsible for carrying information to and from the CNS. Coordination and regulation of the internal organs of the body (cardiac and smooth muscle) is the responsibility of the autonomic nervous system, which is divided into the sympathetic and parasympathetic divisions. The sympathetic division stimulates the body when physiologic or psychologic stress occurs and the parasympathetic division provides a protective function to conserve body resources and maintain digestion and elimination.

BRAIN

The major components of the **brain** are the cerebrum, cerebellum, and the brainstem (**Figure 14.1**). Brain tissue is gray or white. Gray matter is made up of neuronal cell bodies, which edge the surfaces of the cerebral hemispheres forming the cerebral cortex, the largest portion of the brain. White matter is made up of neuronal axons covered with myelin, which enables rapid movement of nerve impulses. The brain receives approximately 20% of

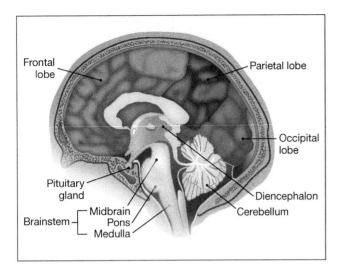

FIGURE 14.1 Brain surface anatomy. Medial view of the right half of the brain.

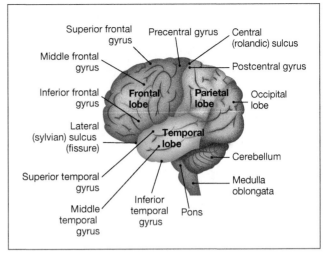

FIGURE 14.2 Cerebral cortex, cerebellum, and brainstem lobes.

the total cardiac output from the internal carotid arteries and vertebral arteries. Butterfield (2019) describes the responsibilities of the brain as "enabling a person to reason, function intellectually, express personality and mood and perceive and interact with the environment" (p. 439).

CEREBRUM

The cerebrum is composed of the right and left cerebral hemispheres, which are divided into lobes (**Figure 14.2**). The gray outer layer of the cerebral cortex receives, stores, and transmits information and controls/integrates general movement, visceral functions, perception, and behavior. Each hemisphere controls the opposite side of the body. Fibers interconnect areas in each hemisphere, allowing coordination of activities between the hemispheres. The hemispheres are divided into sections—the frontal, parietal, temporal, and occipital lobes and the basal ganglia.

The motor cortex lies within the frontal lobe and is responsible for voluntary skeletal movement, fine repetitive movement, and eye movements. Areas in the primary motor area are associated with movement of specific body parts. Cortical spinal tracts extend from the primary motor area into the spinal cord.

The parietal lobe is responsible for processing sensory data as it is received. It also assists with interpretation of tactile information such as temperature, pressure, pain, size, shape, texture, and two-point discrimination, as well as visual, taste, smell, and hearing sensations. Association fibers connect cortical areas within each cerebral hemisphere, providing communication between motor and sensory areas.

Perception and interpretation of sounds, determining their source, and integrating taste, smell, and balance are the responsibilities of the temporal lobe.

Enclosed in the temporal lobe is the Wernicke area, a sensory speech area, responsible for receiving and interpreting speech. Hippocampi, located in the medial temporal lobes, are necessary for memory storage.

The occipital lobe contains the primary vison center (Brodmann area) responsible for visual data interpretation. Located deep within the brain are basal ganglia, which function as a pathway between the cerebral motor cortex and upper brainstem. The function of the basal ganglia is to refine motor movements.

CEREBELLUM

The cerebellum is located at the base of the brain (see **Figure 14.2**). The cerebellum works in conjunction with the motor cortex of the cerebrum to assimilate voluntary movement. The cerebellum also processes sensory movement from the eyes, ears, touch receptors, and the musculoskeletal system (Ball, Dains, Flynn, Solomon, & Stewart, 2019). The cerebellum and vestibular system use sensory data for reflex control of muscle tone and balance and posture to maintain the body in an upright position. Cerebellar hemispheres have same side control of the body.

BRAINSTEM

The brainstem is composed of the midbrain, medulla, and pons and serves as a pathway between the cerebral cortex and the spinal cord (see **Figure 14.2**). The midbrain is the reflex center for eye and head movement and contains the auditory relay pathway. The medulla houses the respiratory center and controls involuntary functions such as the circulatory system as well as swallowing, coughing, and sneezing reflexes. The pons regulates respiration and is the reflex center for pupillary action and eye movement (Ball et al., 2019).

SPINAL CORD

Originating at the foramen magnum and extending to just below the medulla, the CNS continues into the **spinal cord**, which is approximately 40 to 50 cm in length. The brain and spinal cord are bathed in cerebral spinal fluid. The spinal cord lies within the **vertebral column**, ending at the first or second lumbar vertebrae. The vertebral column is divided into 33 vertebrae: seven cervical, 12 thoracic, five lumbar, five fused sacral, and four fused coccygeal vertebrae (Butterfield, 2019; **Figure 14.3**). **Spinal tracts**, fibers which run through the spinal cord, carry sensory, motor, and autonomic impulses between high brain centers to the body. Spinal cord gray matter is butterfly-shaped with anterior and posterior horns,

while the white matter of the spinal cord contains the ascending and descending spinal tracts.

CRANIAL NERVES

Twelve pairs of specialized peripheral cranial nerves arise from the cranial vault and travel from the skull foramina to structures in the head and neck. **Cranial nerves** are sequentially numbered with Roman numerals I through XII. Each nerve has motor or sensory functions, while others have specific functions for smell, vision, or hearing.

MOTOR PATHWAYS

Motor pathways, also known as motor tracts, are descending spinal tracts that transmit impulses from the brain (for cranial nerves) and in the spinal cord (for peripheral nerves; **Figure 14.4**). Motor pathways contain upper and lower motor neurons. Upper motor neurons

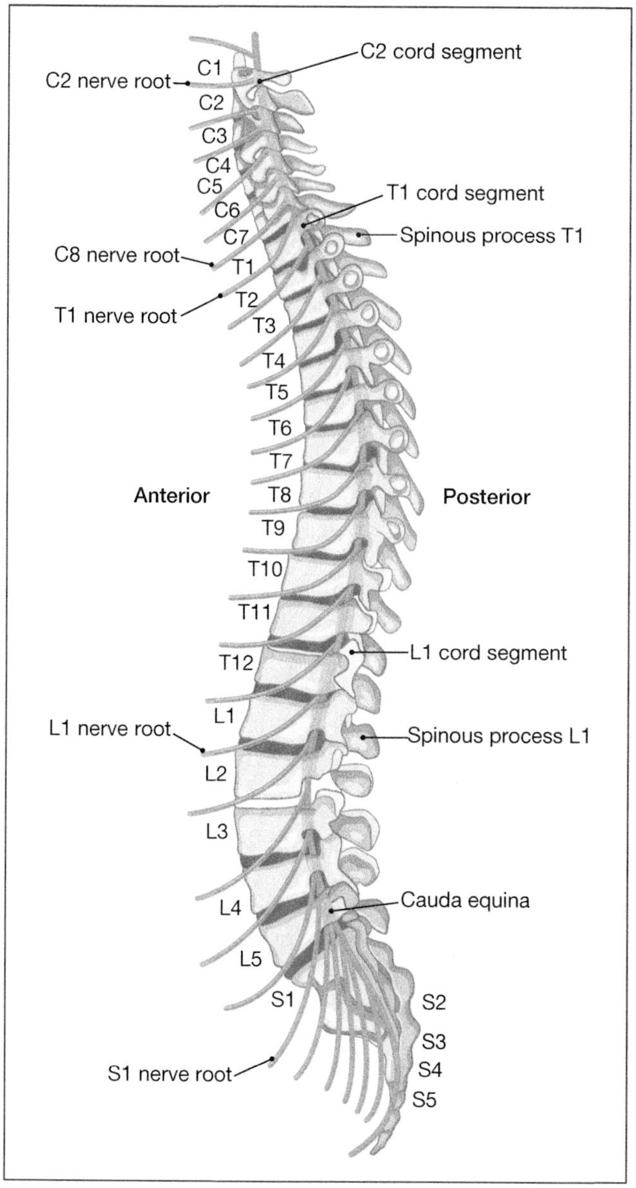

FIGURE 14.3 Lateral view of spinal cord.

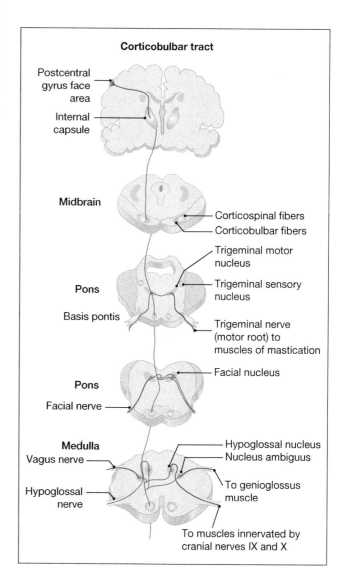

FIGURE 14.4 Corticospinal and corticobulbar motor pathways.

TABLE 14.1 Corticospinal, Basal Ganglia, and Cerebellar Motor Pathways

Pathway	Function
Corticospinal (pyramidal) tract	Mediation of voluntary movement; inhibition of muscle tone; coordination of complicated movements
Basal ganglia system	Controls muscle tone and body movements, including automatically performing a learned behavior
Cerebellar system	Coordinates muscle activity, sustains equilibrium, and maintains posture

are pathways that send impulses from the brain to the spinal cord but affect movement only through lower motor neurons. Lower motor neurons, cranial and spinal neurons, originate in the anterior horn of the spinal cord, extending to the PNS, and control muscle tone, posture, and fine movements. There are three primary motor pathways that intersect within the anterior horn cells: the corticospinal tract, the basal ganglia system, and the cerebellar system, all of which innervate movement only through lower motor neuronal systems (**Table 14.1**). Any voluntary, autonomic, or reflex movement will travel through the anterior horn cells and be converted into movement.

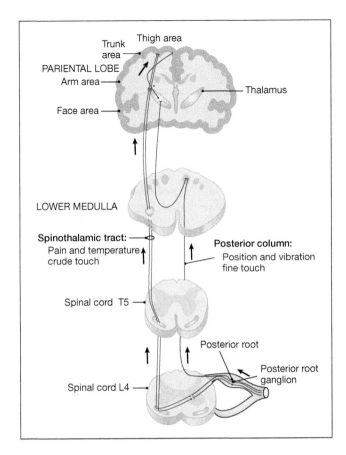

FIGURE 14.5 Spinothalamic tract and posterior columns: sensory pathways.

SENSORY PATHWAYS

Sensory pathways, also known as spinal tracts, are a system of sensory receptors that transmit impulses from the skin, mucous membranes, muscles, tendons, and viscera into the posterior root ganglia, which direct the impulses into the spinal cord (**Figure 14.5**). The sensory impulse is then relayed to the sensory brain cortex by one of two sensory pathways: the spinothalamic tract and the posterior columns.

These pathways manage sensory signals that are necessary to perform complex discrimination. The spinothalamic tract consists of small, unmyelinated sensory neurons from free nerve endings in the skin and is responsible for light and crude touch, pressure, temperature, and pain. Impulses are relayed to the spinal cord, where they then enter the dorsal horn, which relays the impulse to the opposite side where they ascend to the thalamus. Posterior columns consist of larger, unmyelinated axons that are responsible for transmitting vibration, proprioception, pressure, and fine touch from the skin to the dorsal root ganglion. These nerve impulses travel to the medulla where they cross to the opposite side and travel to the thalamus. At this level, a general distinction of the sensation is perceived. The

impulse is then sent to the sensory cortex of the brain where higher order discriminations are made.

SPINAL NERVES

There are 31 pairs of spinal nerves originating from the spinal cord and exiting at each intervertebral foramen. Eight cervical, 12 thoracic, five lumbar, and five sacral pairs of spinal nerves and one coccygeal nerve are named for the vertebral level where they exit. The first cervical nerve exits above the first cervical vertebrae with the remaining spinal nerves exiting below the corresponding cervical, thoracic, and lumbar vertebrae (**Figure 14.6**).

Spinal nerves have both sensory and motor function and supply and receive information in a specific skin distribution called a **dermatome**. Bickley and Szilagyi (2017) define dermatomes as "a band of skin innervated by the sensory root of a single spinal nerve" (p. 720; see **Figure 14.7**).

Each spinal nerve separates into anterior and posterior roots in the spinal cord. The motor fibers of the anterior root relay impulses from the spinal cord to muscles and glands. The sensory fibers of the posterior root relay impulses from sensory receptors to the spinal cord and brain. The sensory cortex of the brain

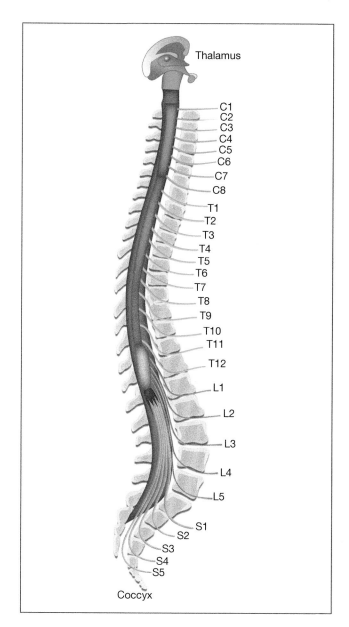

FIGURE 14.6 Relationship of exiting spinal nerves to vertebrae from a lateral view.

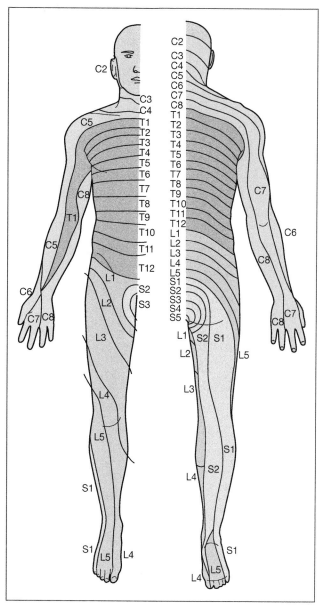

FIGURE 14.7 Dermatomal patterns from an anterior and posterior view.

Source: Adapted from Armitage, A. (2015). *Advanced practice nursing guide to the neurological exam.* New York, NY: Springer Publishing Company.

determines higher order distinction. Spinal sensory neurons may produce a reflex response when tapped in a stretched muscle (motor and sensory function).

SPINAL REFLEXES

Deep tendon reflexes (DTRs), also known as muscle stretch reflexes, occur as the result of a sensory and motor response across a single synapse. Each reflex corresponds to specific spinal segments in sequence (**Table 14.2**). Superficial or cutaneous reflexes produced by stimulation of the skin, such as lightly stroking the skin of the abdomen, may cause a localized muscular twitch. Cutaneous reflexes also correspond to spinal segments (**Table 14.3**).

LIFE-SPAN DIFFERENCES AND CONSIDERATIONS IN ANATOMY AND PHYSIOLOGY OF THE NERVOUS SYSTEM

Infancy

Major brain growth occurs in the first year of life with myelinization of the brain and nervous system. Infection, biochemical imbalance, or trauma may disrupt development and growth, producing devastating results with eventual brain dysfunction. Neurologic impulses are provided by the brainstem and spinal cord at birth.

TABLE 14.2 Deep Tendon Reflex Dermatomal Innervation

Deep Tendon Reflex	Associated Spinal Nerve
Achilles	Sacral 1 Sacral 2
Biceps	Cervical 5 Cervical 6
Brachioradial	Cervical 5 Cervical 6
Patellar	Lumbar 2 Lumbar 3 Lumbar 4
Triceps	Cervical 6 Cervical 7 Cervical 8

TABLE 14.3 Superficial Cutaneous Reflex Dermatomal Innervation

Superficial Reflex	Associated Spinal Nerve
Cremasteric	Thoracic 12 Lumbar 1 Lumbar 2
Lower abdominal	Thoracic 10 Thoracic 11 Thoracic 12
Plantar	Lumbar 5 Sacral 1 Sacral 2
Upper abdominal	Thoracic 8 Thoracic 9 Thoracic 10

Reflexes observed at this time are sucking, rooting, yawning, sneezing, hiccupping, blinking at bright lights, and withdrawing from painful stimulation, in addition to a few primitive reflexes such as the Moro, stepping, palmar, and plantar grasp reflexes. The Moro or startle reflex diminishes in strength by 3 to 4 months, disappearing by 6 months. The stepping reflex occurs at birth with disappearance at variable ages. Absence of this reflex may indicate paralysis. The palmar grasp should be strongest between 1 and 2 months, disappearing by 3 months. The plantar grasp reflex should be strong up to 8 months. These primitive reflexes diminish as the brain develops and advanced cortical functions and voluntary control become prominent.

Older Adults

In addition to decreased brain size, cerebral neurons decrease with aging. Older adults experience decreased sensory functions of smell, taste, and vision. The rate of nerve impulse conduction decreases, causing the older adult to experience slower responses to stimuli, unsteady gait, sleep disturbances, decreased level of cognition, diminished appetite, and decreased range of motion.

KEY HISTORY QUESTIONS AND CONSIDERATIONS

HISTORY OF PRESENT ILLNESS

Common Presenting Symptoms

- Headache
- Dizziness or vertigo
- Weakness or paresthesia (generalized, proximal, or distal)
- Numbness, abnormal or absent sensation
- Fainting and blacking out (near syncope)
- Seizures
- Tremors or involuntary movements
- Gait coordination
- Pain

Example: Seizure

- Chief concern: Seizure
- Frequency: Age at first seizure; total length (reported time) of seizure activity
- Onset: Recent, chronic, or sudden
- Location: Where spasm began and moved through the body, change in character of motor activity during seizure
- Duration: Increasing, persistent
- Character: Aura, irritability, tension, confusion, blurred vision, mood changes, initial focal motor seizure activity, gastrointestinal (GI) distress, muscle tone flaccidity, stiffness, tension, twitching; postictal phase: weakness, transient paralysis, drowsiness, headaches, muscle aches, and sleeping following seizure; independent observers report: Falling to ground, shrill cry, change of color of face or lips, pupil changes or eye deviations, loss of consciousness, or loss of bowel or bladder control
- Aggravating factors: Time of day, meals, fatigue, emotional stress, excitement, menses, discontinuing medications or poor compliance with medications, complementary or alternative medication that may interfere with anti-epileptic medications, alcohol, or illicit drug use
- Relieving factors: Medications, anti-epileptics
- Red Flag symptoms indicating need for emergency evaluation: Seizures from alcohol or sedative withdrawal, trauma to head with loss of consciousness

- Differential diagnoses: Focal seizures without impaired consciousness, generalized seizures, toxic or metabolic-induced seizure, drug toxicity

Example: Weakness
- Chief concern: Weakness
- Onset: Sudden, gradual or subacute, or chronic, over a long period of time
- Location: Body areas involved: proximal, distal, symmetrical or asymmetrical, generalized or focal, unilateral or bilateral, what movements are affected
- Duration: Abrupt onset, subacute onset, chronic, or gradual
- Character: Fatigue, apathy, drowsiness, or actual loss of strength; difficulty with movements such as combing hair, reaching up to a shelf, climbing stairs; worsening weakness when walking/improving after rest, decreased hand strength, tripping when walking
- Associated symptoms: Worsening weakness with effort, bilateral distal weakness with sensory loss, proximal weakness with sensation intact
- Aggravating factors: Activities of daily living, reaching, getting out of a chair, climbing stairs, opening jars
- Relieving factors: Rest, decreased activities
- Temporal factors: Recent onset of symptoms, recent/past illness/infection
- Red Flag symptoms including need for emergency evaluation: Abrupt onset of motor and sensory deficits, abrupt vision loss
- Differential diagnoses: Transient ischemic attack (TIA), stroke, Guillain-Barre syndrome, myopathy from alcohol, polyneuropathy from diabetes, and myasthenia gravis

PAST MEDICAL HISTORY
- Trauma: Concussion/brain injury, spinal cord injury or localized injury, CNS:
  - Insult, birth trauma, stroke
- Meningitis, encephalitis, lead poisoning, poliomyelitis
- Deformities, congenital anomalies, genetic syndromes
- Cardiovascular (CV) or circulatory problems: Hypertension, aneurysm, peripheral vascular disease
- Neurologic disorder, brain surgery, residual effects

FAMILY HISTORY
- Hereditary disorders: Neurofibromatosis, Huntington's chorea, muscular dystrophy, diabetes, pernicious anemia
- Alcoholism
- Intellectual disability
- Epilepsy or seizure disorder, headaches

- Alzheimer's disease or other dementia, Parkinson's disease (PD)
- Learning disorders
- Weakness or gait disorders, cerebral palsy (CP)
- Medical or metabolic disorder, thyroid disease, hypertension, diabetes

SOCIAL HISTORY
- Environmental or occupational hazards
- Hand, eye, and foot dominance; family patterns of dexterity and dominance
- Ability to care for self: Hygiene, activities of daily living, finances, communication, shopping, ability to fulfill work expectations
- Sleeping or eating pattern: Weight loss or gain
- Use of alcohol or recreational drugs, including mood-altering drugs
- Social support system
- Smoking history
- Use of cane or assistive device

REVIEW OF SYSTEMS
- General: Fever, chills, sleeplessness, fatigue, dizziness
- Head, eyes, ears, nose, throat (HEENT): Visual disturbances/visual difficulty, tearing or redness of eyes
- CV and respiratory: Respiratory irregularities, bruits, thrills
- Gastrointestinal (GI)/genitourinary (GU): Nausea, vomiting, urinary frequency, hesitancy, urgency, incontinence
- Neurologic: Weakness, numbness and tingling, change in sensation, loss of consciousness, headache, falls, dizziness
- Musculoskeletal: Headache, backache, nuchal rigidity, weakness
- Psychiatric: Depression, anxiety, changes in mentation, memory, or mood

PREVENTIVE CARE CONSIDERATIONS
- Healthy lifestyle behaviors/fall prevention
- Prevention of stroke and transient ischemic attack (TIA)
- Carotid artery screening
- Reducing risk of peripheral neuropathy, A1c within normal limits
- Herpes zoster vaccination
- Detecting delirium, dementia, and depression

Unique Population Considerations for History
Older adults may present with altered levels of cognition, not associated with or occurring as part of neurological disease. Polypharmacy occurs with many older

adults who may consume additional vitamins or herbal supplements, which may cause adverse reactions, leading to a decreased level of consciousness and gait disturbance. Alcohol, illicit drug use, or simultaneous use of opioids and benzodiazepines significantly increases risk of adverse drug reactions with resultant mentation changes or increased risk of falls. As a component of their assessment, ask individuals screening questions to assess fall risk, such as number of falls within the past year, if they feel unsteady when standing or walking, and if there are worries about falling. Depression screening is also important to determine if changes in cognition are related to depression or as part of a neurological disorder.

PHYSICAL EXAMINATION OF THE NERVOUS SYSTEM

Neurological physical assessment is critical for diagnosis and management of the neurologic patient (Lederman, 2018). Secondary to the complexity of the examination, this section is divided into five sections: mental status, cranial nerves, proprioception/cerebellar function, reflexes, and sensory function.

EQUIPMENT

- Penlight
- Tongue blade, paper clip, cotton-tipped applicator
- Tuning forks, 200 to 400 Hz and 500 to 1,000 Hz
- Familiar objects: Coins, keys, paper clip
- Cotton wisp
- 5.07 filament
- Reflex hammer
- Vials of aromatic substances: Coffee, orange, peppermint extract, oil of cloves for testing

INSPECTION

The clinician should begin the neurological examination as they would any examination. As the patient enters the room, observe gait, balance, and coordination. Listen to the patient's response to questions, which provides information regarding the patient's ability to follow directions. Conduct a general survey and document the patient's vital signs. A height, weight, and body mass calculation should be completed and compared to previous visits if possible to identify signs of chronic disease or weight loss. Assess for depression. This is important to note for older adults as depression is more common in elders and those with chronic diseases, including neurological disorders such as dementia, multiple sclerosis (MS), and PD. The Patient Health Questionnaire-2 (PHQ-2) can accurately identify major depressive disorders by asking two questions: "Over the last 2 weeks, have you been feeling down, depressed, or hopeless (depressed mood)?" and "Over the last 2 weeks, have you felt little interest or pleasure in doing things?" If the answer is yes to either or both of these questions, the entire Patient Health Questionnaire-9 (PHQ-9) should be administered. Also assess suicidality in depressed patients (Bickley & Szilagyi, 2017, p. 733).

Inspection of the face includes attention to symmetry, shape, features, and facial expression; symmetry of the eyebrows, eyes, ears, nose, and mouth; and position of facial features such as nasolabial fold and inspecting for facial muscle atrophy and tremors.

MENTAL STATUS EXAMINATION

The mental status examination should assess the patient's mood, cognition, and emotional responses. Cognition includes the patient's judgment, their ability to think and reason, and their ability to interact with their environment (Ball et al., 2019 p. 88). Mental status is typically obtained by observation of the patient and is composed of assessment of their appearance and behavior, speech and language, mood, thoughts, perceptions, and cognition.

Appearance and Behavior

- Level of consciousness
- Posture and motor behavior
- Dress, grooming, and personal hygiene
- Facial expression
- Manner/affect/relationship to people

Speech and Language

- Characteristics of patient's speech:
  - Talkative/quiet
  - Slow/rapid speech
  - Words clear
  - Nasal quality to speech
  - Articulation/fluency

Mood

- Anxiety/worry
- Contentment
- Detachment/indifference
- Euphoria
- Rage/anger
- Sad/melancholy

Thoughts and Perceptions

- Thought process:
  - Flight of ideas
  - Fabrication of facts
  - Incoherence
  - Repetition
- Thought content:
  - Anxiety
  - Delusions
  - Insight

○ Judgment
○ Obsessions
○ Phobias

Cognition

- Abstract thinking
- Attention
- Calculating ability
- Orientation
- Recent/remote memory
- Vocabulary

CRANIAL NERVES

Olfactory (I)

The olfactory nerve is tested when the patient is unable to discriminate odors. The least irritating aroma is used first so that patient perception of weaker odors is not injured. Tubes of orange or peppermint extract can be used. Before assessing, make sure the patient's nares are clear; have the patient occlude one naris at a time, and ask them to breathe in and out. Have the patient close their eyes. Holding an open vial under the nose, ask the patient to breathe deeply (**Figure 14.8**). Use a different aroma to test the other side. Repeat two to three times with two to three different odors. Patients are expected to perceive an odor on each side and to identify it.

Optic (II)

Testing for optic nerve function includes testing of distant and near vison, ophthalmoscopic examination of optic fundi, with special attention to the optic disc and testing visual fields by confrontation and extinction. When testing the visual fields, test each eye separately and both eyes together. In those patients with partial vision loss, testing of both eyes can reveal a visual field deficit; testing with one eye will miss this finding.

Oculomotor, Trochlear, and Abducens (III, IV, and VI)

The oculomotor, trochlear, and abducens nerves are tested with movement of the eyes through the six cardinal points of gaze.

Trigeminal (V)

The three divisions of the trigeminal nerve are evaluated for sharp, dull, and light touch sensations. Motor function is evaluated by observing the face for muscle atrophy, deviation of the jaw to one side, and muscle twitching. To assess, the patient should clench their teeth tightly as the muscles over the jaw are palpated, evaluating tone (**Figure 14.9**). Facial tone should be symmetric, without tremor.

The three trigeminal nerve divisions are evaluated for sharp, dull, and light touch sensations. The patient's eyes are closed, and the clinician touches each side of the face at the scalp, cheek, and chin alternately using the sharp and smooth edges of a broken tongue blade or paper clip (**Figure 14.10A**). Ask the patient to report whether each sensation is sharp or dull. Then stroke the face in the same six areas with a cotton wisp asking the patient to report sensation (**Figure 14.10B**). Discrimination of all stimuli is expected over all facial areas.

Facial (VII)

The facial nerve is tested for facial symmetry by asking the patient to form specific facial expressions (**Figure 14.11**). The clinician requests the patient to raise the eyebrows, squeeze eyes shut, wrinkle the forehead, frown smile, show their teeth, purse their lips, and puff out their cheeks. Observe for tics, unusual

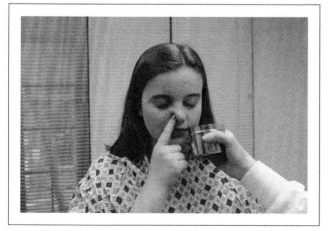

FIGURE 14.8 Olfactory nerve testing. Patient occludes one nostril while the clinician places the aroma vial under the other nostril.

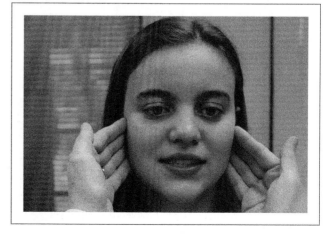

FIGURE 14.9 Motor function assessment of the trigeminal nerve.

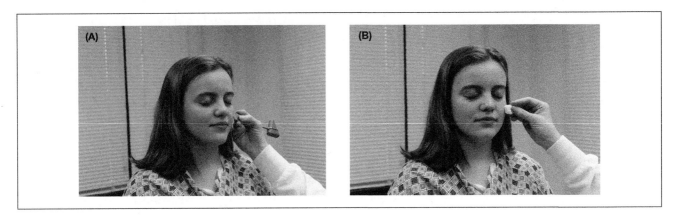

FIGURE 14.10 Evaluation of trigeminal nerve divisions.

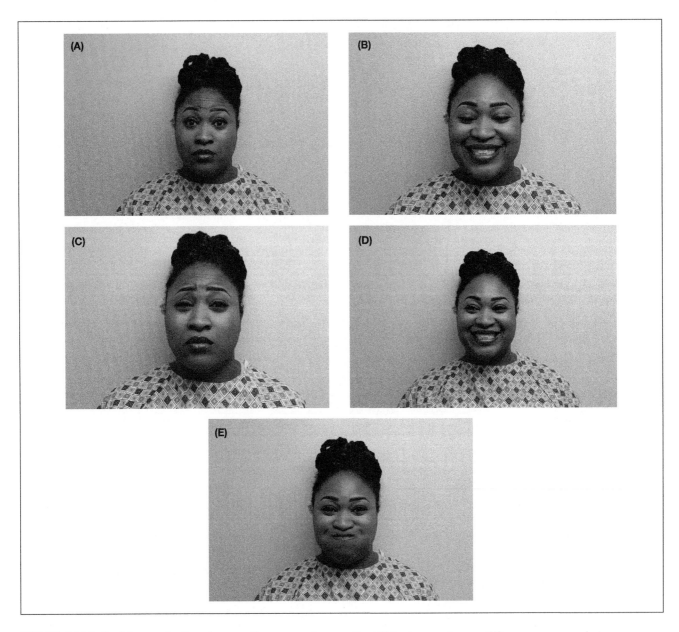

FIGURE 14.11 Facial nerve testing. Among other expressions, patient (A) raises eyebrows, (B) squeezes eyes shut, (C) frowns, (D) smiles, and (E) puffs out cheeks.

facial movements, or asymmetry. Drooping of one side of the mouth, a flattened nasolabial fold, and/or sagging of the lower eyelid are signs of muscle weakness.

Acoustic (VIII)

Assess hearing with the whispered voice test. The clinician asks the patient to repeat numbers whispered into one ear while blocking or rubbing your fingers next to the opposite ear. An audiometry examination is completed. Vestibular function is tested with the Romberg test, which tests position sense. The clinician has the patient stand with the feet together and eyes open and asks the patient to close their eyes for 30 to 60 seconds without support (**Figure 14.12**). Observe the patient's ability to maintain an upright posture. Minimal swaying is a normal finding.

Glossopharyngeal (IX) and Vagus (X)

An intact glossopharyngeal nerve gives the patient the ability to identify sour and bitter tastes on the posterior third of each side of the tongue, to gag, and to swallow. Inspect the palate and uvula, speech sounds, and gag reflex. Observe for difficulty swallowing, and assess for guttural speech sounds or hoarse voice sounds. Sensory function of taste may be completed during CN VII evaluation. Glossopharyngeal nerve function is simultaneously tested during the evaluation of the vagus nerve for nasopharyngeal sensation (gag reflex) and the motor function of swallowing. The gag reflex is initiated by touching the patient's posterior pharyngeal wall with an applicator while observing for upward movement of the palate and contraction of the pharyngeal muscles. The uvula should remain in midline. Drooping or absence of an arch on either side of the palate is abnormal. Motor function is evaluated with inspection of the soft palate for symmetry. The clinician has the patient say "ah" and observes the movement of the soft palate. If there is damage to the vagus or glossopharyngeal nerve, the palate does not rise, and the uvula will deviate from midline. To complete testing, have the patient sip and swallow water. The patient should be able to swallow easily. Listen to the patient's speech for hoarseness, nasal quality, or difficulty with guttural sounds.

Spinal Accessory (XI)

Evaluation of the spinal accessory nerve includes evaluation of the size, shape, and strength of the trapezius and sternocleidomastoid (SCM) muscles. To test the trapezius muscle, the clinician stands behind the patient and observes for atrophy or flickering movement of the skin (a symptom of disease of the nervous system). The clinician places a hand on each shoulder and asks the patient to shrug upward toward their hands and observes the strength and contraction of the muscle (**Figure 14.13**).

To test the SCM muscle, the clinician asks the patient to turn the head to each side against their hand, observing the contraction of the opposite SCM muscle and the force of movement against the hand (**Figure 14.14**).

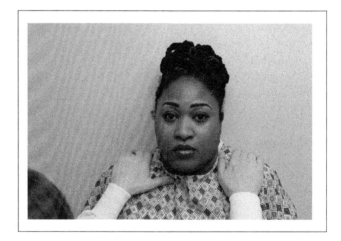

FIGURE 14.13 Testing the trapezius muscle.

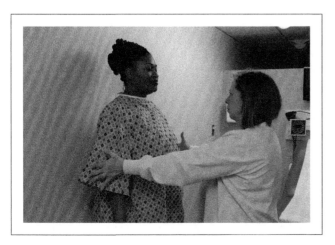

FIGURE 14.12 Romberg test.

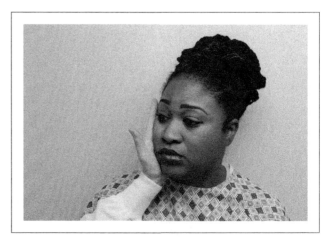

FIGURE 14.14 Testing the sternocleidomastoid muscle.

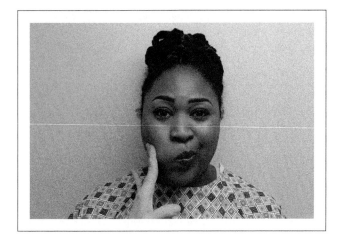

FIGURE 14.15 Testing muscle strength of the tongue.

Hypoglossal (XII)

The clinician inspects the patient's tongue while at rest on the floor of the mouth and while protruded from the mouth observing for size and shape. The patient is asked to move their tongue in and out of the mouth, side to side, and curled upward and downward. Muscle strength of the tongue is tested by asking the patient to push the tongue against the cheek as the clinician applies resistance with an index finger or hand (**Figure 14.15**). Assess lingual speech sounds (l, t, d, n) by listening to the patient's speech (**Box 14.1**).

PROPRIOCEPTION AND CEREBELLAR FUNCTION

Coordination and Fine Motor Skills

When assessing the motor system, focus on the patient's body position during movement and at rest. Look for involuntary movements (tics or tremors), muscle bulk, muscle strength, muscle tone, and the patient's coordination. Abnormal position may be due to mono- or hemiparesis from stroke.

Rapid Rhythmic Alternative Movements

The clinician asks the seated patient to pat their knees with both hands, alternately turning the palms up and down and gradually increasing the speed of movements (**Figure 14.16**). Alternatively, the clinician may request the patient to touch the thumb to each finger on the same hand from the little finger and back (**Figure 14.17**). One hand is tested at a time, gradually increasing the speed. The clinician should model the movements for the patient before having the patient complete them. The patient should be able to accomplish these movements smoothly and rhythmically. Stiff, slow, or jerky clonic movements are abnormal.

Accuracy of Movements

The clinician tests the accuracy of movements with the use of the *finger-to-nose test*, which is performed with the patient's eyes open. Ask the patient to use an index finger to touch their nose (**Figure 14.18A**), then touch the clinician's index finger which should be positioned approximately 18 inches from the patient to allow full arm extension (**Figure 14.18B**). The clinician moves their finger position several times during the test, which is then repeated on the other hand. The *heel-to-shin test* is an alternative method to test accuracy of movement. This test can be performed with the patient sitting or supine. The clinician asks the patient to run the heel of one foot up and down the shin of the opposite leg and repeat the test with the other heel. The patient should be able to move the heel up and down the shin in a straight line without deviating to the side (**Figure 14.19**).

Balance

Balance is first evaluated with the Romberg test (see **Figure 14.12**). The clinician should be prepared if the patient starts to fall. Loss of balance is a positive sign, indicating cerebellar ataxia/dysfunction or sensory loss. If the patient staggers or loses balance, postpone other tests of cerebellar function, which require balance. Other methods of evaluating balance are as follows:

- Have patient stand with feet slightly apart and push the shoulders with enough effort to throw them off balance (be ready to catch the patient, if needed). The patient should be able to quickly recover balance.
- Request the patient to close their eyes, hold their arms at the sides of the body, and stand on one foot,

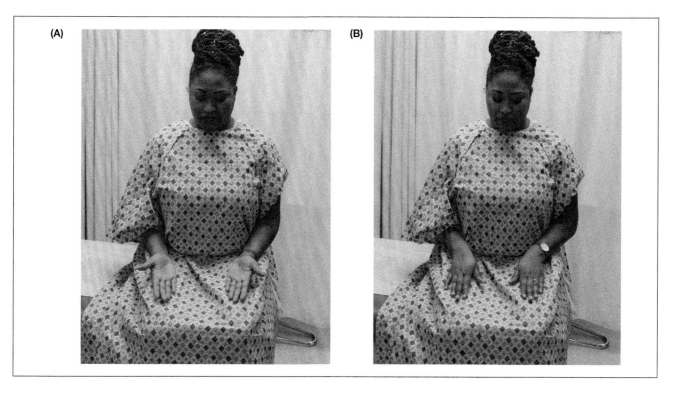

FIGURE 14.16 Testing rapid rhythmic alternative movements. Patient alternately places palms up (A) and down (B).

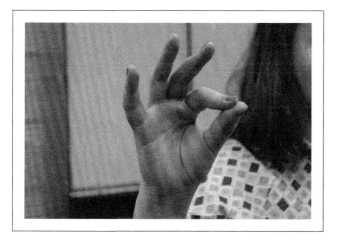

FIGURE 14.17 Testing rapid rhythmic alternative movements. Patient touches thumb to each finger.

repeating the test on the opposite foot. Slight swaying is normal, and the patient should be able to maintain balance on each foot for 5 seconds.

- With their eyes open, have the patient hop in place on one foot and then the other (tests proximal and distal muscle strength). The patient should be able to hop on one foot for 5 seconds without loss of balance. Observe for instability or need to continually touch the floor with the opposite foot or a tendency to fall.

Gait

The clinician asks the patient to:

- Walk across the room or down the hall and turn and come back, observing posture, balance, swinging of the arms, and intact movement. Walk heel-to-toe in a straight line (tandem walking; **Figure 14.20**).
- Walk on toes, then on their heels.
- Do a knee bend.

These tests assess for gait abnormalities, which increase fall risk (**Table 14.4**).

Tandem walking may reveal ataxia and distal leg weakness, and is a sensitive test for corticospinal tract damage. Difficulty hopping may be related to weakness, lack of position sense, or cerebellar dysfunction.

Testing for pronator drift should also be completed. The clinician asks the patient to stand for 20 to 30 seconds with eyes closed and both arms straight forward with palms up (**Figure 14.21A**). The patient is then instructed to keep their arms out and eyes shut. The clinician taps the arms briskly downward. The arms normally return smoothly to the horizontal position, which requires muscular strength, coordination, and good position sense. With loss of position strength, arms will drift sideward or upward, which is a positive test for pronator drift (**Figure 14.21B**). The patient may not notice the displacement.

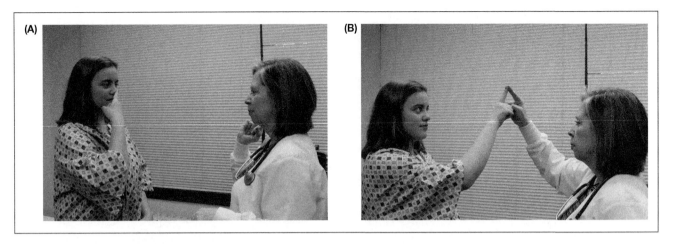

FIGURE 14.18 Finger-to-nose test.

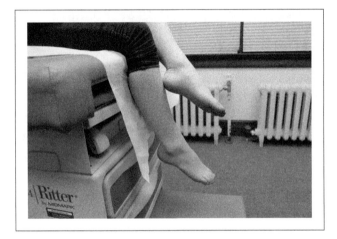

FIGURE 14.19 Heel-to-shin test.

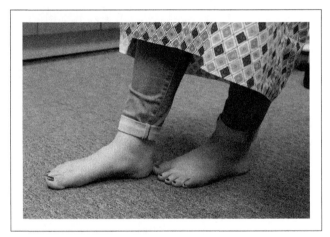

FIGURE 14.20 Assessment of gait. Tandem walking.

TABLE 14.4 Abnormal Gait Pattern Characteristics

Gait Pattern	Characteristics
Antalgic	Limited time of weight-bearing on the affected side; limping
Ataxic/cerebellar gait	Clumsy, staggering movements with wide-base gait; titubation present at rest
Choreiform/hyperkinetic gait	Nondirectional, jerky, involuntary movements in all extremities
Dystrophic/waddling gait	Legs wide apart/weight shifted side-to-side in waddling motion related to weak hip adductor muscles
Neuropathic/steppage/ equine gait	Seen in patients with foot drop (weakness of foot dorsiflexion); patient attempts to lift leg high enough so the toe does not drag on the floor
Parkinsonian	Stooped posture with head and neck forward and flexion at the knees/rigid body/short shuffling steps/difficulty initiating steps and stopping/bradykinesia

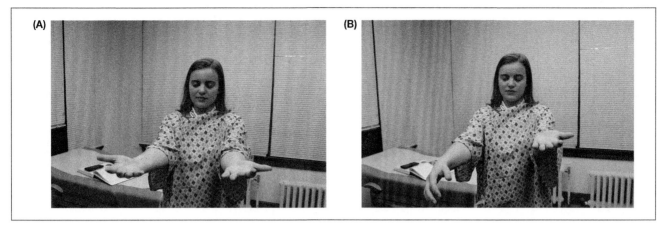

FIGURE 14.21 Testing for pronator drift. (A) Patient stands with eyes closed and arms straight forward with palms up. (B) Arms drifting sideward or upward after a brisk tap indicate a positive test.

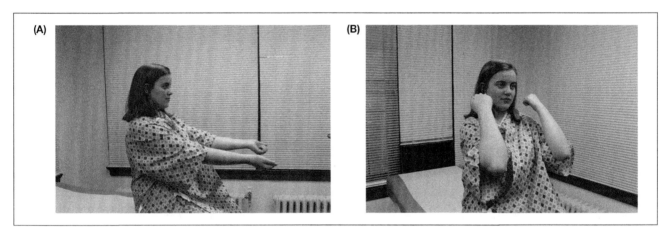

FIGURE 14.22 Elbow extension (A) and flexion (B).

Muscle Strength

Normal muscle strength varies, so the standard of normal should allow for age and sex. The patient's dominant side is usually stronger than the nondominant side, although differences may be hard to detect. Muscle strength is tested by asking the patient to actively resist the clinician's movement. The clinician should remember to give the patient the advantage as you try to overcome the patient's resistance to judge the muscle's strength. Some patients will give way during muscle strength testing secondary to pain, misunderstanding of the test, or malingering.

Muscle strength testing methods include:

- Biceps and brachioradialis at the elbow flexion and extension (**Figure 14.22**): The patient pulls and pushes against the clinician's hand.
- Extension at the wrist: The patient makes a fist and resists as the clinician presses down.

- Grip strength: The clinician asks the patient to squeeze two of their fingers as hard as possible and not let them go (**Figure 14.23**). Weak grip is seen in cervical radiculopathy, ulnar peripheral nerve disease, carpal tunnel syndrome, arthritis, and epicondylitis.
- Finger abduction: Patient's hand is positioned down with fingers spread. The clinician instructs the patient to prevent movement of fingers as the clinician tries to force them together (**Figure 14.24**). Weak finger abduction occurs in ulnar nerve disorders.
- Thumb opposition: The clinician asks the patient to touch the top of the little finger with the thumb against resistance.
- Muscle strength of the trunk: Flexion, extension, rotation, and lateral bending.
- Flexion at the hip: The clinician places their hands on the patient's mid-thigh and asks the patient to raise their leg against their hands.

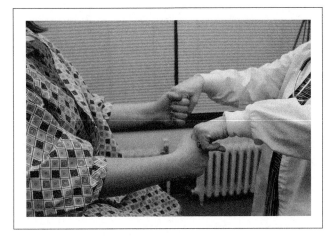

FIGURE 14.23 Testing grip strength.

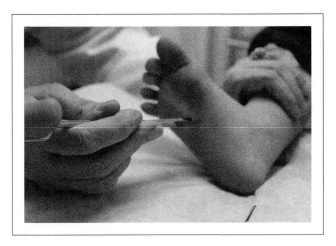

FIGURE 14.25 Plantar reflex test.

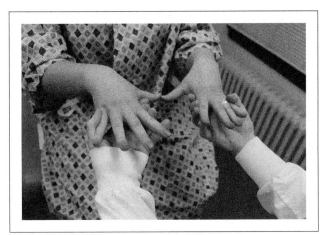

FIGURE 14.24 Finger abduction test.

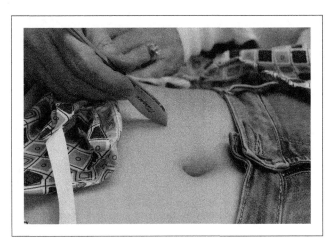

FIGURE 14.26 Abdominal reflex test.

- Adduction at the hips: The clinician puts their hands on the bed between the patient's knees and asks the patient to bring both their legs together.
- Abduction at the hips: The clinician places their hands on the outside of the patient's knees and asks the patient to spread both their legs against their hands.
- Extension at the knee: The clinician supports the knee in flexion and requests the patient to straighten the leg against their hand. Expect a forceful response as the quadriceps is the strongest muscle in the body.
- Flexion at the knee: The clinician positions the patient's leg, so the knee is flexed with the foot resting on the bed. The clinician tells the patient to keep the foot down as they try to straighten the leg.
- Foot dorsiflexion and plantar flexion at the ankle: The clinician requests the patient to pull up and push down against their hand. Heel and toe walk

assesses foot dorsiflexion and plantar flexion, respectively.

REFLEXES

Superficial Reflexes

- Plantar reflex: Using the end of a reflex hammer, the clinician strokes the lateral side of the foot from heel to ball, then across the foot to the medial side with the result of plantar flexion of the toes (**Figure 14.25**). This is a normal sign.
- Abdominal reflex: With the patient supine, the clinician strokes the four abdominal quadrants of the abdomen with the end of a reflex hammer. Stroking downward and away from the umbilicus elicits the lower abdominal reflexes, which respond with a slight movement of the umbilicus toward the area of stimulation (**Figure 14.26**). The reflex response should be equal and bilateral.

TABLE 14.5 Deep Tendon Reflex Grading	
Grade 0	No response
Grade 1+	Sluggish or diminished response
Grade 2+	Active or expected response (normal)
Grade 3+	Brisk/slightly hyperactive
Grade 4+	Brisk/hyperactive

Deep Tendon Reflexes

DTRs include the biceps, brachioradialis, triceps, patellar, and Achilles reflexes. These reflexes are tested with the patient in a seated position. Each reflex is scored as 0 to 4+. See **Table 14.5** for DTR grading. The clinician tests each reflex and compares both sides. The reflex response should be symmetric, visible, and palpable. DTRs are obtained by positioning a limb with a slightly stretched tendon and quickly tapping the tendon to be tested with a percussion hammer. The expected response is a sudden contraction of the muscle. If the tendon response is absent, consider a neuropathy. Consider upper motor neuron disorder with hyperactive reflexes. If DTRs are symmetrically diminished or absent, use a technique of isometric contraction of other muscles, which might increase reflex activity.

- Biceps reflex: With the patient's arm bent at a 45° angle at the elbow, the clinician palpates the biceps tendon and places their thumb over the tendon and their fingers under the elbow. The clinician then strikes the patient's thumb with the reflex hammer to elicit contraction of the biceps muscle (**Figure 14.27**).
- Brachioradialis reflex: With the patient's arm bent at a 45° angle at the elbow, the clinician rests the patient's arm on theirs. The patient's hand should be slightly pronated. The clinician directly strikes the brachioradial tendon 1 to 2 inches above the wrist with the reflex hammer (**Figure 14.28**). A normal response is forearm pronation and elbow flexion.
- Triceps reflex: With the patient's arm flexed at a 90° angle, the clinician supports the patient's arm just above the antecubital fossa and palpates the antecubital fossa and then directly strikes the triceps tendon with a reflex hammer just above the elbow. A normal response is extension of the elbow (**Figure 14.29**).
- Patellar reflex: With the patient's knee flexed to a 90° angle, the clinician supports the patient's upper leg with their hand to allow the patient's lower leg to hang. The clinician strikes the patellar tendon just below the patella (**Figure 14.30**). A normal response is extension of the lower leg.

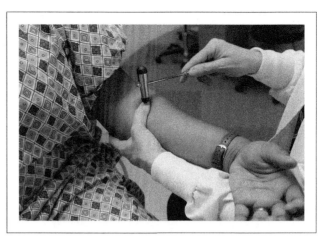

FIGURE 14.27 Biceps reflex test.

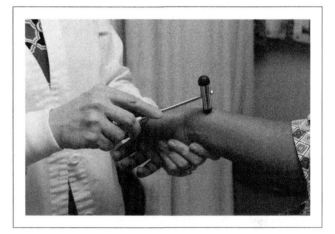

FIGURE 14.28 Brachioradialis test.

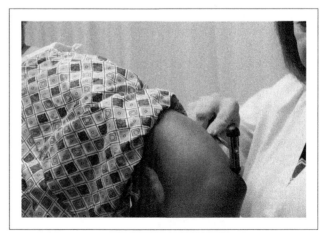

FIGURE 14.29 Triceps reflex test.

- Achilles reflex: With the patient sitting and the knee flexed to a 90° angle, keeping the ankle in a neutral position, the clinician holds the patient's foot in their hand. The clinician strikes the Achilles tendon at

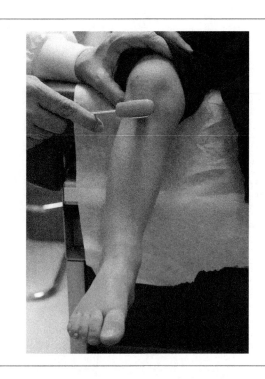

FIGURE 14.30 Patellar reflex test.

the level of the ankle malleoli. A normal response is plantar flexion of the foot.

Primitive Reflex Testing in Infancy

- Moro reflex: Supporting the infant's head, body, and legs, the clinician suddenly lowers the body, causing the arms to abduct and extend, followed by relaxed flexion; the legs should flex.
- Stepping reflex: The clinician holds the infant under the arms, allowing one of the infant's feet to touch the surface of the examination table. The clinician observes for flexion of the hip and knee. The foot should touch the table, while the other foot steps forward.
- Palmar reflex grasp: The clinician places a finger in the infant's hand pressing against the palmar surface of the hand. The infant flexes all fingers to grasp the clinician's finger. A positive grasp reflex, which lasts longer than 2 months, indicates CNS damage.
- Plantar reflex grasp: The clinician touches the sole of the infant's foot at the base of the toes, causing the toes to curl.

SENSORY FUNCTION

Evaluation of the sensory system requires testing of several kinds of sensation such as pain and temperature (spinothalamic tracts), position and vibration (posterior columns), light touch (spinothalamic tracts and posterior columns), and discriminative sensations, which depend on pain, temperature, position, vibration, and light touch (the cortex). The clinician evaluates

sensation by asking the patient to identify stimuli on the hands, distal arms, abdomen, feet, and legs. Each sensation procedure is tested with the patient's eyes closed. Contralateral areas of the body are tested, and the patient is asked to compare sensations side to side. Normal findings include:

- Minimal side-to-side differences
- Correct description of sensations (hot, cold, sharp, or dull)
- Recognition of the side of the body tested
- Location of sensation and recognition if proximal or distal to the site previously tested

When testing, the clinician focuses on the areas that have numbness, pain, or motor or reflex abnormalities. Before testing, the clinician demonstrates what they are going to do and how the patient should respond. The clinician should compare symmetric areas on two sides of the body, including arms, legs, and trunk. With pain, temperature, and touch sensation, compare distal to proximal areas of the extremities. Test fingers and toes first for vibration and sensation. If these tests are normal, the clinician can assume the more proximal areas are normal. Evaluation of light touch and superficial pain can be evaluated together.

Monofilament testing is another important sensory testing tool commonly used in the evaluation of diabetic and peripheral neuropathy. Testing with a 5.07 monofilament should be done on several sites of the foot for all patients with diabetic and peripheral neuropathy.

- Monofilament testing: With the patient's eyes closed, the clinician places the monofilament on several sites of the plantar surface of each foot and one side of the dorsal surface of the foot in a random pattern (**Figure 14.31**). The clinician applies pressure for 1.5 seconds to each site without repeating a test site. The correct amount of pressure is applied when the

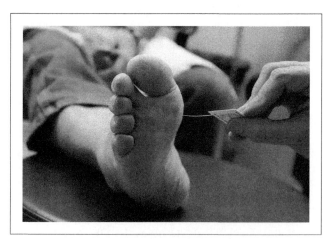

FIGURE 14.31 Monofilament test.

filament bends. Testing is positive if the patient cannot feel the monofilament.

Primary Sensory Functions

- Light touch: Clinician lightly touches the skin with a cotton wisp and asks the patient to respond when and where the sensation is felt.
- Superficial pain: Clinician alternates the sharp and smooth edges of a broken tongue blade, Wartenberg wheel (**Figure 14.32**), or paper clip to touch the skin. The patient is asked to identify each sensation as sharp or dull and where the sensation is felt.
- Temperature: Testing skin temperature is omitted if pain sensation is normal. If there are sensory deficits, use test tubes filled with hot and cold water. The patient is asked to identify if the sensation is hot or cold and where the sensation is felt.
- Vibration: Clinician uses a low-pitched tuning fork (128 Hz, which has slower reduction of vibration). Placing the stem of a vibrating tuning fork against a bony prominence at the toe or finger joint (**Figure 14.33**), the patient is asked to identify when and where the buzzing sensation is felt.
- Proprioception joint position sense: Clinician assesses the great toe of each foot and a finger on each hand. Hold the joint to be tested by the lateral aspect, in the neutral position, and move the toe up and down (**Figure 14.34**). The patient is asked to identify the joint position. Expect the patient to identify the joint position.

SPECIAL TESTS

Cortical Sensory Function

Cortical sensory or discriminatory sensory function tests assess the patient's ability to interpret sensation. Patients with lesions in the sensory cortex or posterior

spinal cord would be unable to complete these tests. The patient's eyes should be closed during testing.

- Stereognosis: Tests the patient's ability to identify a familiar object by touch. The clinician places a key or coin in the patient's hand. The patient's ability to identify the object is a normal response.

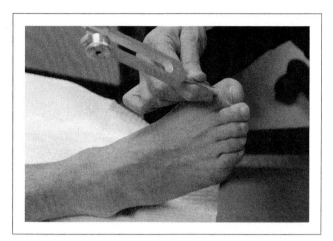

FIGURE 14.33 Testing vibration with a low-pitched tuning fork.

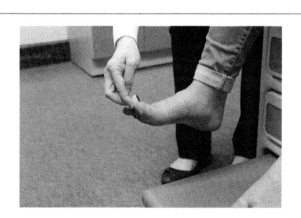

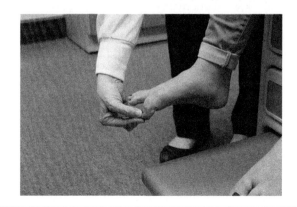

FIGURE 14.34 Testing proprioception joint position sense.

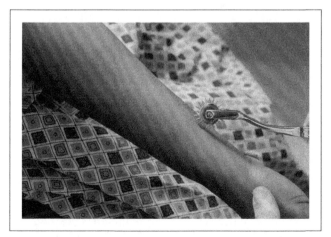

FIGURE 14.32 Testing superficial pain with a Wartenberg wheel.

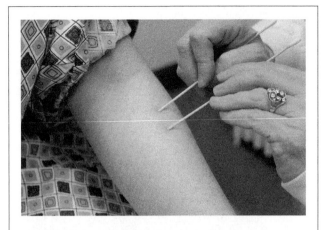

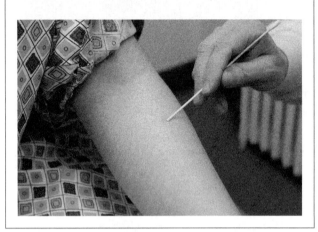

FIGURE 14.35 Two-point discrimination test.

- Two-point discrimination: Using two ends of a cotton swab or paper clip, the clinician alternates touching the patient's skin at various locations with one or two points (**Figure 14.35**).

The patient's ability to identify one- or two-point touch is a normal response.

- Extinction phenomenon: The clinician simultaneously touches two areas on each side of the body (such as the cheek or hand) with the broken end of a tongue blade. The patient should be able to discriminate the number of touches and where they are felt bilaterally.
- Graphesthesia: With the blunt end of an applicator, the clinician draws a number or shape on the palm of the patient's hand (**Figure 14.36**). The clinician then repeats the test using a different figure on the other hand. The patient should be able to identify the shape or number.

Other special tests are used when the clinician suspects meningeal irritation, which can occur with meningitis or subarachnoid hemorrhage.

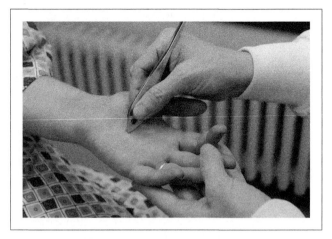

FIGURE 14.36 Graphesthesia test.

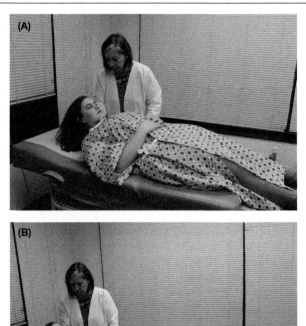

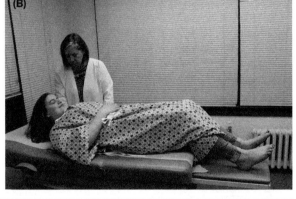

FIGURE 14.37 Brudzinski's sign test. (A) Clinician flexes the patient's neck forward. (B) Positive test is when the patient bends the hips and knees in response neck flexion.

- Brudzinski's sign: The clinician should not use this test if there is injury or fracture of the cervical vertebrae or cervical cord. With the patient lying flat, the clinician puts their hands behind the patient's head and flexes the neck forward, attempting to touch the patient's chin to their chest (**Figure 14.37A**).

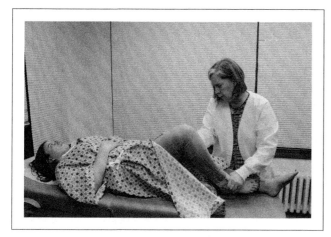

FIGURE 14.38 Kernig's sign test. The clinician flexes the patient's leg at the hip and knee, and then slowly extends the leg and straightens the knee. A positive test reveals pain with knee extension.

Normally, the patient can easily bend the head and neck forward. A positive test is when the patient bends the hips and knees in response neck flexion (**Figure 14.37B**).

- Kernig's sign: With the patient lying flat, the clinician flexes the patient's leg at the hip and knee, then slowly extends the leg, and straightens the knee (**Figure 14.38**). Normally, the patient should feel some discomfort behind the knee with extension. A positive test reveals pain with knee extension.

ABNORMAL FINDINGS OF THE NERVOUS SYSTEM

BELL'S PALSY

Bell's palsy is defined as inflammation of the facial nerve typically of unknown cause, although it has been related to herpes simplex type 1 infection and Lyme disease. The facial nerve is responsible for facial expression, taste, lacrimation, salivation, and ear sensation. Symptoms typically develop within hours, with maximum characteristics in 3 days. The patient usually recovers, but not always (Madhok et al., 2016).

Key History and Physical Findings

- Unilateral facial weakness and drooping (**Figure 14.39**)
- Eyelid weakness
- Facial pain
- Pain around the ear
- Abnormal taste
- Reduced tearing (Patel & Levin, 2015, p. 419)

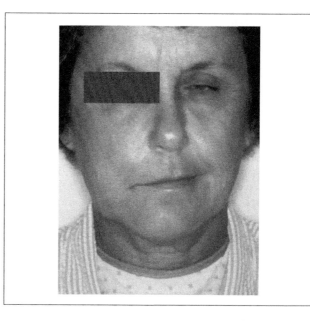

FIGURE 14.39 Bell's palsy. Unilateral facial drooping.
Source: Centers for Disease Control and Prevention.

CEREBRAL PALSY

CP is defined as a nonprogressive motor disorder secondary to damage of the fetal or infant brain. Risk factors include preterm birth, low birth weight, neonatal encephalopathy, neonatal sepsis, and meningitis (Watson & Pennington, 2015). Signs may not be evident at birth and the problems of CP continue into adulthood as those with disabilities related to the disease are living longer. Early signs may include abnormal muscle tone, abnormal motor development, and feeding difficulties. Age-related physiological changes, which occur in adults, include pain, osteoporosis, fatigue, and musculoskeletal and joint problems (Mudge et al., 2016).

Key History and Physical Findings

- Difficulty eating, drinking, and swallowing
- Poor nutrition
- Difficulty with speech, language, and communication
- Pain:
  - Musculoskeletal: Scoliosis, hip dislocation, nonspecific back pain
  - Increased muscle tone: Dystonia and spasticity
  - Muscle fatigue
  - Headache
  - Nonspecific abdominal pain
  - Dental pain
  - Dysmenorrhea
- Sleep disruption
- Mental health problems:
  - Depression
  - Anxiety disorder

- ○ Antisocial behavior
- ○ Learning disabilities
- ○ Attention deficit hyperactivity disorder
- Vision and hearing impairment
- Vomiting, regurgitation, and reflux
- Constipation
- Epilepsy

EPILEPSY

Diagnostic criteria for epilepsy are two or more unprovoked seizures occurring more than 24 hours apart. Seizures occur secondary to brief, strong surges of abnormal and disorganized activity, which may affect all or part of the brain (Brook, Hiltz, & Kopplin, 2015, p. 246). Epilepsy may be caused by perinatal anoxia, congenital brain malformation, genetic disorders, infectious disease, and traumatic brain injury and can also be triggered by sleep deprivation, dehydration, stress, alcohol, and drug use (Smith, Wagner, & Edwards, 2015). Epilepsy interferes with school, work, and driving. Children may experience physical complications from seizures and are at greater risk for negative self-image, anxiety, depression, and learning disabilities.

Epileptic seizures are either generalized, affecting both hemispheres at the same time, or focal, originating in one area of one hemisphere (typically the temporal or frontal lobe). Focal seizures are either simple or complex depending on whether the patient remains fully conscious during the seizure (simple) or has impaired consciousness (complex). Status epilepticus is a condition in which a seizure is continuous for more than 5 minutes, or two or more seizures occur without full consciousness between the seizures. Status epilepticus is considered a medical emergency due to an increased chance of death.

Key History and Physical Findings

- Description of the seizure
- Jerking movement of one or more extremities
- Nystagmus
- Abrupt movement of head to one side or the other
- Moans or cries
- Fearful or sad emotions
- Humming or buzzing noises
- Intense or unpleasant smells or tastes
- Tingling in one area or side of the body
- Flashing lights in a portion of the visual fields

HEMORRHAGIC STROKE

Hemorrhagic stroke is defined as bleeding directly into the brain tissue, caused by leakage from intracerebral arteries damaged by chronic hypertension. Hemorrhagic stroke is less common than ischemic stroke and is associated with a higher mortality rate. Patients with hemorrhagic stroke may have neurological deficits similar to ischemic stroke, but are more likely to have headache, altered mental status, seizures, nausea and vomiting, and/or pronounced hypertension. Women have a higher incidence of stroke and higher rates of hemorrhagic stroke than men, which may be due to longer life expectancy, history of preeclampsia, history of oral contraceptive use, and menopause. Risk of hemorrhagic stroke increases with advanced age, hypertension, previous stroke history, alcohol abuse, and cocaine use. Other causes include hypertension, coagulopathies, or anticoagulant therapy (Hemphil et al., 2015).

Key History and Physical Findings

- Trauma history
- General symptoms:
  - ○ Nausea, vomiting, and headache
  - ○ Altered level of consciousness
  - ○ Seizures
- Focal symptoms:
  - ○ Weakness or paralysis of an extremity, half of the body, or all extremities
  - ○ Facial droop
  - ○ Monocular or binocular blindness
  - ○ Blurred vision
  - ○ Dysarthria and trouble understanding speech
  - ○ Vertigo or ataxia
  - ○ Aphasia
- Subarachnoid symptoms may include:
  - ○ Sudden onset of severe headache
  - ○ Signs of meningitis (nuchal rigidity)
  - ○ Photophobia and eye pain
  - ○ Nausea and vomiting
  - ○ Syncope

INTRACRANIAL TUMOR

Intracranial tumor is defined as "an abnormal growth in the cranial cavity that may be primary or secondary cancer" (Ball et al., 2019, p. 598). Brain tumors include glioblastomas, meningioma, and pituitary tumors. Brainstem gliomas are one of the most common tumors in children. Brainstem glioma refers to any tumor growth in the brainstem.

Key History and Physical Findings

- Persistent headaches that wake patient from sleep
- Seizures
- Visual changes: Reduced visual acuity, loss of vision
- Appetite loss, nausea, vomiting
- Changes in behavior and personality
- Children may exhibit irritability, lethargy, cranial nerve palsies, and weight loss
- Signs vary by tumor location

- Confusion
- Papilledema
- Aphasia
- Nystagmus
- Ataxia
- Brain computed tomography (CT) scan or magnetic resonance imaging (MRI) to confirm diagnoses

ISCHEMIC STROKE

Ischemic stroke is most commonly caused by an embolus from atrial fibrillation or atherosclerotic disease, which causes a sudden loss of blood circulation to the brain. Symptoms depend on the affected brain region. Ischemic stroke can occur in adults and children. Genetic factors such as age, sex, and ethnicity can put patients at risk. Factors such as smoking, excessive alcohol use, and limited exercise increase stroke risk. History of high cholesterol, hypertension, and diabetes also cause an increased risk for stroke. Ischemic stroke symptoms most often occur concurrently (Musuka, Wilton, Traboulsi, & Hill, 2015).

Key History and Physical Findings

- Sudden severe headache with no known cause
- Abrupt onset of hemiparesis or monoparesis
- Visual field deficits
- Facial droop
- Ataxia
- Nystagmus
- Aphasia: Expressive and receptive
- Sudden numbness or weakness of the face, arm, or leg
- Abrupt decrease in level of consciousness

MENINGITIS

Meningitis is defined as inflammation of the meninges of the brain or spinal cord. Bacterial, viral, or fungal organism colonization in the upper respiratory tract are the causative organisms. Following colonization, the organism enters the bloodstream, crosses the blood–brain barrier, and infects the cerebrospinal fluid and meninges. Symptoms can develop over several hours or over 1 to 2 days. The classic triad for bacterial meningitis is fever, headache, and neck stiffness; however, patients may present with only one or two of these symptoms (Hasbun, 2019).

Key History and Physical Findings

- Fever, chills
- Headache, neck stiffness
- Lethargy, sleepiness
- Nausea
- Vomiting
- Photophobia

- Confusion
- Irritability
- Delirium
- Seizures
- Coma
- Altered mental status
- Nuchal rigidity
- Fever
- Increased blood pressure with bradycardia
- Positive Brudzinski's and Kernig's signs
- Petechial and purpura rash with meningococcal meningitis
- Infants
- Bulging fontanelle
- Paradoxical irritability (quiet when lying flat and crying when held)
- High-pitch cry
- Hypotonia

MULTIPLE SCLEROSIS

MS is defined as an inflammatory demyelinating disease characterized by episodic neurological function in the brain, spinal cord, and optic nerves.

MS is a progressive autoimmune disease. Onset is typically between 20 and 40 years of age, occurring more often in women. Patients will present with an acute neurologic episode, with multifocal symptoms lasting longer than 24 hours.

Key History and Physical Findings

- Paresthesia
- Muscle cramping due to spasticity
- Bowel, bladder, and sexual dysfunction
- Constipation
- Dysarthria, nystagmus, and intention tremor
- Lhermitte's sign (an electric shock-like sensation that occurs with flexion of the neck and goes down the spine, often going into the limbs)
- Trigeminal neuralgia (TN)
- Irregular twitching of the facial nerves
- Fatigue
- Heat intolerance
- Decreased attention span, concentration, memory loss
- Depression
- Bipolar disorder, dementia
- Localized weakness
- Focal sensory disturbances (decreasing proprioception and vibration)
- Hyper-reactive reflexes
- Increased muscle tone or stiffness in the extremities
- Optic neuritis:
  - Unilateral loss of visual acuity
  - Pain

MYASTHENIA GRAVIS

Myasthenia gravis (MG) is a common autoimmune disease affecting neuromuscular junction transmission. The etiology is unknown. Physiologic changes occur when autoantibodies are directed against the acetylcholine receptor sites destroying and blocking transmission of nerve impulses that direct muscle contraction. MG causes weakness, which worsens with activity. Ocular symptoms are most common. Young adults 30 years of age are typically affected. Diagnosis is based on history and physical examination findings and confirmed by electrodiagnostic testing and positive serum antibodies directed at proteins in the neuromuscular junction (Statland & Ciafaloni, 2013, p. 126).

Key History and Physical Findings

- Drooping eyelids
- Double vision
- Difficulty swallowing or speaking
- Fatigue or weakness
- Difficulty walking
- Facial weakness when puffing out cheeks
- Hypophonia
- Respiratory compromise or failure
- Skeletal muscle weakness

PARKINSON'S DISEASE

PD is defined as a slowly progressive neurodegenerative disorder affecting movement, muscle control, and balance caused by destruction and loss of dopaminergic neurons. Early signs and symptoms may be subtle and difficult to detect or missed secondary to slow disease progression. Nonmotor symptoms can sometimes be seen prior to motor symptoms. Diagnosis is based on signs and symptoms, patient history, physical examination, and neurological assessment.

Key History and Physical Findings

- Nonmotor symptoms:
  - Constipation
  - Depression
  - Cognitive dysfunction
  - Dementia
  - Psychosis
- Motor symptoms considered cardinal signs of PD:
  - Rest tremors
  - Slowness of movement, freezing, or inability to continue movements
  - Rigidity
  - Postural instability
- Motor symptoms:
  - Pill-rolling movement of fingers bilaterally
  - Head tremors
  - Numbness, tingling

- Muscle soreness
- Difficulty swallowing
- Drooling
- Stooped posture
- Short steps, shuffling gait, accelerating gait to maintain posture
- Slow slurred speech, softened voice

PERIPHERAL NEUROPATHY

Peripheral neuropathy is the most common type of neuropathy and is caused by nerve lesions or tissue nerve damage, which produces hyperexcitability of primary sensory neurons and cells in the dorsal root ganglia (Huether & Rodway, 2019, p. 745). This hyperexcitability causes peripheral nerve endings to become responsive to weak, normally nonpainful stimuli (allodynia) and an exaggerated response to stronger stimuli (hyperalgesia; Cohen, 2018, p. 23). Causes of peripheral neuropathy include alcohol abuse, diabetes, nutritional disorders, and neurotoxic chemotherapy.

Key History and Physical Findings

- Gradual onset of symptoms:
  - Numbness, tingling, shooting, burning, electric shock sensations
  - All sensation is painful
  - Occurs in the feet or hands
  - Night pain in one or both feet
  - Reduced touch sensation
  - Reduced sensation in feet with monofilament examination
  - Diminished posterior tibial or dorsalis pedis pulses
  - Distal muscle weakness, cannot stand on toes or heels
  - Skin ulcerations that the patient is unable to feel

TRIGEMINAL NEURALGIA

TN is a common form of neuralgia in older adults, affecting women more often than men. TN presents as recurrent paroxysmal sharp pain radiating into one or more branches of the trigeminal nerve. The trigeminal nerve (fifth cranial nerve) has motor and sensory function and is divided into three branches: ophthalmic, maxillary, and mandibular. TN can be caused by small artery compression of the trigeminal nerve, causing demyelination of the trigeminal nerve root (Puskar & Droppa, 2015).

Key History and Physical Findings

- Unilateral burning, stabbing, electric shock, excruciating facial pain in the chin or cheek
- Pain episodes may occur several times a day to several times per month

- Increased pain with:
  - Chewing, swallowing, talking, brushing teeth, cold exposure
- Intermittent pain-free periods
- Inflammation of the maxillofacial region
- Inflammation of the ear, nose, and throat

- Recent dental work
- Multiple sclerosis
- May have normal neurologic assessment
- Slight sensory impairment in painful regions
- Pain occurs in one or more divisions of the trigeminal nerve.

CASE STUDY: Facial Weakness and Drooping

History

A previously healthy 48-year-old female is seen in the primary care clinician's office for evaluation of facial weakness and drooping. Onset of symptoms was 2 to 3 days ago with progressive weakness of the left side of her face and facial pain. She has not taken any medications for pain but has used ice packs with several minutes of pain relief. The patient describes severe pain rated 8/10, which interferes with work and sleep. She denies head injury, falls, injury to face or eye, cough, rash, nasal drainage, or increased tearing. The patient denies medication, food, seasonal, or environmental allergies. She is currently taking no medications. No significant family history. Positive smoking history 1 pack per day × 20 years. Denies abnormities in taste or ear pain. Denies recent travel or sick contacts. She works in an insurance office and missed work today to be evaluated for the pain and facial drooping.

Physical Examination

She appears ill, fatigued, and anxious; she is alert, awake, and responding appropriately to questions. Vital signs: temperature, 99.6°F; pulse, 100 beats/minute; and respirations, 22 breaths/minute. Her weight is stable from previous visit. On examination: skin pink warm and dry, facial features reveal unilateral left-sided facial weakness, and drooping

left eyelid and left corner of the mouth. Otoscopic examination is normal. Palpation of preauricular, postauricular, tonsillar, submandibular, and submental nodes are soft, mobile, and nontender bilateral. Negative masses noted with neck examination. Facial examination demonstrates absent forehead wrinkling on the left side when raising eyebrows, incomplete closure of the left eye when patient attempts to close eyes, upward movement of eyes with forced eye closure, and the patient is unable to completely close the left eye. Flattening of the nasolabial fold is noted on the left. Normal strength of buccinator muscle when patient puffs out cheeks. Asymmetry of the lips on left when patient puckers lips, asymmetric grimace on the left. Positive Bell phenomenon noted. *Note: Bell phenomenon is upward and lateral deviation of the eyes with an attempt to close the eyes.*

Differential Diagnoses

Bell's palsy, ischemic stroke, TN

Laboratory and Imaging

Serologic testing and imaging should not be routinely performed for patients with new onset Bell's palsy (Baugh et al., 2013; Grade C Recommendation).

Final Diagnosis

Bell's palsy

CASE STUDY: Jaw Pain

History

A previously healthy 64-year-old female is seen in her primary care clinician's office accompanied by her husband. She was recently seen by an oral surgeon who completed a tooth implant. Two weeks later

she experienced pain in the jaw and submandibular area on the right lower jaw. She returned to the oral surgeon for reevaluation with the assessment that the implant was successful and there were no complications. Her husband states that at times

(continued)

CASE STUDY: Jaw Pain (*continued*)

the jaw pain is so intense and sharp that she cries out and is inconsolable. She describes the pain as a burning, stabbing, electric shock pain, and rates the pain as 10/10 when it occurs. The patient states washing her face or brushing her teeth is painful and, at its worst, the pain is excruciating. Currently there is no pain, but pain is sporadic and lasts for several minutes. She states pain is progressively worsening and is now occurring several times per day. Medical history is positive for hypothyroidism, anxiety, and impaired hearing in the right ear. Surgical history is positive for tooth implant. Current medications include levothyroxine 75 mcg 1 tablet daily and fluoxetine 20 mg 1 tablet daily. Denies taking medications for pain. Denies medication, food, or seasonal or environmental allergies. The patient is up-to-date on immunizations and had a flu shot this year. Mammogram completed in 2018 was negative. She wears glasses and states her last eye examination was 6 months ago. She denies smoking, alcohol intake, or illicit drug use. She and her husband have been married for 40 years. She is a homemaker. The patient denies chills, fever, night sweats, cough, nasal congestion, eye or ear drainage, nausea, vomiting, numbness or weakness of the face, or headache. Denies any falls or falls with injury in the past year.

Physical Examination

She is alert, lucid, oriented, and appropriate. She is sitting on the examination table holding her hand to her right jaw. Skin pink, warm, and dry. Vital signs: temperature, 98.7°F; pulse, 72 beats/minute; and blood pressure, 118/70 mmHg. Assessment of cranial nerves I to XII completed and negative. Otoscopic and ophthalmoscopic examination were negative. Evaluation reveals tenderness to palpation over the right lower jaw, chin, and right posterior cheek in the mandibular branch of the trigeminal nerve root distribution. Palpation of preauricular, postauricular, tonsillar, submandibular, and submental nodes are soft, mobile, and nontender bilateral.

Differential Diagnoses

TN, post-herpetic neuralgia, MS

Laboratory and Imaging

Assessment confirmed unilateral neuropathic episodic pain with a normal neurological examination. No laboratory testing is needed. Imaging should include MRI to rule out structural causes of TN or tumor. Neurology referral would be appropriate.

Final Diagnosis

TN

Clinical Pearls

- Develop a routine for the neurologic examination. Perform the examination the same way each time to ensure no portion of the examination is missed or forgotten.
- When assessing for protective sensation with use of the monofilament, do not test over calluses and do not repeat a test site.

- Older adults may present with altered levels of cognition, not associated with or occurring as part of neurological disease.
- Depression screening is also important in older adults to determine if changes in cognition are related to depression or as part of a neurological disorder.
- Sudden vision loss is a neurological emergency.

Key Takeaways

- Neurological assessment can be difficult and time-consuming but yields significant information.
- Several neurological conditions do not present with neurologic deficits.

REFERENCES

Armitage, A. (2015). *Advanced practice nursing guide to the neurological exam*. New York, NY: Springer Publishing Company.

Ball, J. W., Dains, J. E., Flynn, J. A., Solomon, B. S., & Stewart, R. W. (2019). *Seidel's guide to physical examination: An interprofessional approach* (9th ed.). St. Louis, MO: Elsevier.

Baugh, R. F., Basura, G. J., Ishii, L. E., Schwartz, S. R., Drumheller, C. M., Burkholder, R., . . . Vaughan, W. (2013). Clinical practice guideline: Bell's palsy executive summary. *Otolaryngology—Head and Neck Surgery, 149*(5), 656–663. doi:10.1177/0194599813506835

Bickley, L. S., & Szilagyi, P. G. (2017). *Bates' guide to physical examination and history taking* (12th ed., pp. 711–796). Philadelphia, PA: Wolters Kluwer.

Brook, H. A., Hiltz, C. M., & Kopplin, V. L. (2015). Increasing epilepsy awareness in schools: A seizure smart schools project. *The Journal of School Nursing, 31*(4), 246. doi:10.1177/1059840514563761

Butterfield, R. J. (2019). Structure and function of the neurological system. In K. L. McCance & S. E. Huether (Eds.), *Pathophysiology: The biologic basis for disease in adults and children* (8th ed., p. 439). St. Louis, MO: Elsevier.

Cohen, S. A. (2018). Pathophysiology of pain. In Z. H. Bajwa, R. J. Wootton, & C. A. Warfield (Eds.), *Principles and practice of pain medicine* (3rd ed., pp. 22–35). New York, NY: McGraw-Hill.

Hasbun, R. (2019). Meningitis. In M. S. Bronze (Ed.), *Medscape*. Retrieved from https://emedicine.medscape.com/article/232915-print

Hemphill, J. C., Greenberg, S. M., Anderson, C. S., Becker, K., Bendok, B., Cushman, M., . . . Woo, D. (2015). Guidelines for the management of spontaneous intracerebral hemorrhage: A guideline for healthcare professionals from the American Heart Association/American Stroke Association. *Stroke, 46*(7), 2032–2060. doi:10.1161/STR.000000000000069

Huether, S. E., & Rodway, G. W. (2019). Pain, temperature regulation, sleep, and sensory function. In K. L. McCance & S. E. Huether (Eds.), *Pathophysiology: The biologic basis for disease in adults and children* (pp. 468–503). St. Louis, MO: Elsevier.

Lederman, R. J. (2018). Is a detailed neurological physical examination always necessary? *Cleveland Clinic Journal of Medicine, 85*(6), 444–445. Retrieved from https://www.mdedge.com/ccjm/article/166652/neurology/detailed-neurologic-physical-examination-always-necessary

Luzzio, C. (2019). *Multiple sclerosis clinical presentation.* Retrieved from https://emedicine.medscape.com/article/1146199-clinical#b1

Madhok, V. B., Gagyor, I., Daly, F., Somasundara, D., Sullivan, M., Gammie, F., & Sullivan, F. (2016). Corticosteroids for Bell's palsy (idiopathic facial paralysis). *Cochrane Database of Systematic Reviews, (7)*, CD001942. doi:10.1002/14651858.CD001942.pub5

Mudge, S., Rosie, J., Stott, S., Taylor, D., Signal, N., & McPherson, K. (2016). Ageing with cerebral palsy: What are the health experiences of adults with cerebral palsy? A qualitative study. *BMJ Open, 2016*(6), e012551. doi:10.1136/bmjopen-2016-012551

Musuka, T. D., Wilton, S. B., Traboulsi, M., & Hill, M. D. (2015). Diagnosis and management of acute ischemic stroke: Speed is critical. *Canadian Medical Association Journal, 187*(12), 887–893. doi:10.1503/cmaj.140355

Patel, D. K., & Levin, K. H. (2015). Bell palsy: Clinical examination and management. *Cleveland Clinic Journal of Medicine, 82*(7), 419–427. doi:10.3949/ccjm82a.14101

Puskar, R., & Droppa, M. (2015). Trigeminal neuralgia: Pain, pricks, and anxiety. *Journal of Gerontological Nursing, 419*(3), 8–12. doi:10.3928/00989134-20150213-03

Smith, G., Wagner, J. L., & Edwards, J. C. (2015). Epilepsy update part 1: Refining our understanding of a complex disease. *American Journal of Nursing, 115*(5), 40–47. doi:10.1097/01.NAJ.0000465030

Statland, J. M., & Ciafaloni, E. (2013). Myasthenia: Five new things. *Neurology Clinical Practice, 3*(2), 126. doi:10.1212/CPJ.0b013e31828d9fec

Watson, R. M., & Pennington, L. (2015). Assessment and management of the communication difficulties of children with cerebral palsy: A UK survey of SLT practice. *International Journal of Language and Communication Disorders, 50*(2), 241–259. doi:10.1111/1460-6984.12138

15

Evidence-Based Assessment of the Musculoskeletal System

Zach Stutzman and Kate Gawlik

"To study medicine without books is to sail an uncharted sea, while to study medicine only from books is not to go to sea at all."

—WILLIAM OSLER

VIDEOS

- Patient Case: Adult With Back Pain
- Patient Case: Adult With Shoulder Pain

LEARNING OBJECTIVES

- Describe the structure and function of the musculoskeletal system.
- Identify differences and considerations in the anatomy and physiology of the musculoskeletal system across the life span.
- Understand the components of a comprehensive, evidence-based history and physical examination of the musculoskeletal system.
- Distinguish between normal and abnormal findings in the musculoskeletal system.

Visit https://connect.springerpub.com/content/book/978-0-8261 -6454-4/chapter/ch00 to access the videos.

ANATOMY AND PHYSIOLOGY OF THE MUSCULOSKELETAL SYSTEM

The musculoskeletal system provides the building blocks and the structure for the body by providing an elaborate matrix of bones, ligaments, and cartilage. It facilitates movement through the muscles, tendons, and multiple cartilaginous structures. The musculoskeletal system is the body's first line of defense, protecting the body's vital organs from numerous external forces. Additionally, the bony structure provides a storage space for minerals, and the marrow of the long bones contributes to hematopoiesis, which is the production of red blood cells (Biga et al., 2019). Owing to the diversity and variety of functions provided by this body system, injuries are common and can often be quite debilitating to a patient's health and way of life.

There are 206 **bones** in the adult human body. Infants and children have more bones until the bones fuse together later in life. Bones are made up of collagen and calcium phosphate. Collagen provides a soft framework, and calcium phosphate causes the collagen matrix to harden. There are two types of bone found in the human body—cortical and trabecular. Cortical bone is hard and compact and makes up the outer layer of the bone. Trabecular bone is the spongy matrix found in the inner portion of the bone (U.S. Department of Health and Human Services, 2018). **Figure 15.1** depicts the anatomy of bones, and **Figure 15.2** depicts the skeletal structure.

Bones come together at **joints**. These joints are typically held together by **ligaments**, or fibrous bands that

403

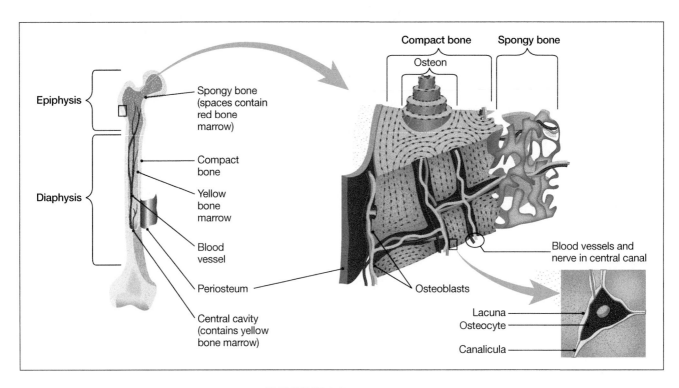

FIGURE 15.1 Bone anatomy.

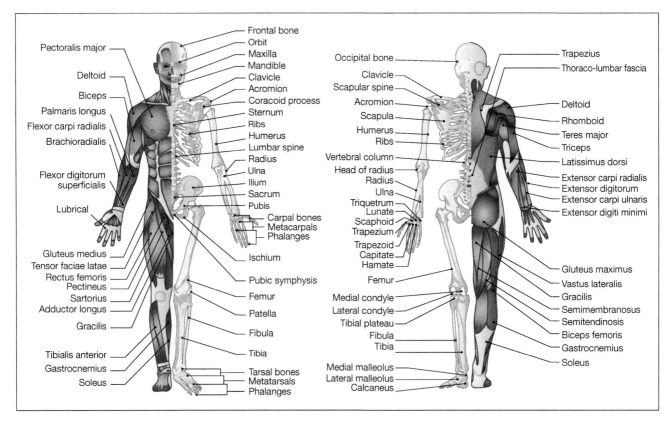

FIGURE 15.2 Human skeleton from anterior and posterior views.

hold bone to bone. The end of the bones have articular cartilage, which provides a smooth surface, allowing for the free, smooth movement of the joint. Surrounding the joint is a synovial membrane. This membrane secretes synovial fluid, further decreasing the friction in the joint space and facilitating the smooth, continuous movements (Betts et al., 2013). Owing to the tight space constrictions in joints, bursae are often situated in the spaces between bones, tendons, and ligaments. These are fluid-filled sacs meant to further reduce friction and help with the ease of motion.

Between certain joints, other fibrous cartilaginous structures form for a variety of reasons. For example, in the shoulder and hip, a labrum is present to increase the amount of surface of the joint and allow for increased stability. In the knee, the meniscus allows for a decrease of force transmission to the bone and increased stability. And, in the spine, the discs between vertebrae allow for increased force dissipation and help to provide the space to allow the nerves to move freely through a greater range of motion (Biga et al., 2019).

Tendons are connective tissues that connect the muscles to other body structures, typically bones. Skeletal **muscles** are organized into bundles of muscle fibers called fascicles. Each skeletal muscle fiber is innervated by blood vessels and an axon branch of a somatic motor neuron, which signals the muscle to contract. Skeletal muscle fibers are made up of hundreds of thousands of myofibrils. Myofibrils are made up of filamentous proteins, primarily actin and myosin. These actin and myosin filaments slide over each other to cause shortening of sarcomeres. Sarcomeres are the functional units of the skeletal muscle. Sarcomeres are made up of contractile, regulatory, and structural proteins and are linked in a series. Millions of sarcomeres work together to shorten and generate force, giving the muscle the ability to contract and produce movement (Biga et al., 2019). See **Figures 15.3** and **15.4** to review the structure and function of skeletal muscles.

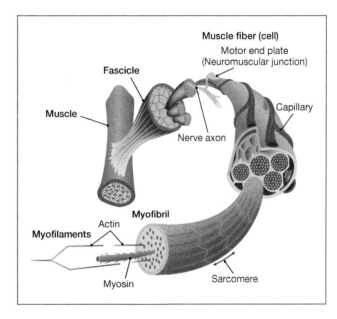

FIGURE 15.3 Skeletal muscle anatomy.

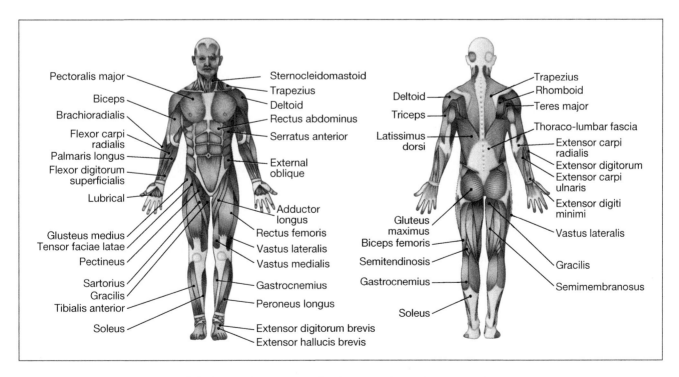

FIGURE 15.4 Skeletal muscles from anterior and posterior views.

BOX 15.1
TYPES OF MOVEMENTS

Flexion: Any joint movement that decreases the angle between two bones; bending

Extension: Any joint movement that increases the angle and straightens the joint; opposite of flexion

Rotation: Can occur within the vertebral column, at a pivot joint, or at a ball-and-socket joint

Abduction: Moving the limb or hand laterally away from the body, or spreading the fingers or toes

Adduction: Moving the limb or hand toward or across the midline of the body, or bringing the fingers or toes together

Inversion: Turning of the foot to angle the bottom of the foot toward the midline

Eversion: Turning the bottom of the foot away from the midline

Supination: Rotation of the radius that returns the bones to their parallel positions and moves the palm to the anterior facing (supinated) position

Pronation: The body movement that moves the forearm from the supinated (anatomical) position to the pronated (palm backward) position

Circumduction: Moving of the limb, hand, or fingers in a circular pattern, using the sequential combination of flexion, adduction, extension, and abduction motions; movement of a body region in a circular manner

Source: Betts, J. G., Young, K. A., Wise, J. A., Johnson, E., Poe, B., Kruse, D. H., . . . DeSaix, P. (2013). *Anatomy and physiology.* Houston, TX: OpenStax. Retrieved from http://cnx.org/contents/14fb4ad7-39a1-4eee-ab6e-3ef2482e3e22@8.24

Movements of the musculoskeletal system are defined in **Box 15.1** and are a function of joints, muscles, tendons, and multiple cartilaginous structures.

ANATOMY AND PHYSIOLOGY OF THE HEAD AND SPINE

The spine consists of 33 individual bones (vertebrae) and extends from the skull to the pelvis. It is made up of five different regions: cervical (C1–C7), thoracic (T1–T12), lumbar (L1–L5), sacral (S1–S5), and the coccyx. One of the major functions of the cervical spine is to allow freedom of movement for the head. It is important to note that flexion and extension of the head come from the interaction of the skull and C1. In contrast, rotation of the head actually comes from the interaction of C1 and C2. Between each vertebrae in the cervical, thoracic, and lumbar regions are fibrous discs. These discs provide cushioning and give space for the spinal nerves to exit at each level. The motion between

each vertebra is quite small. When all of these small motions are added together, it leads to extensive range of motion of the entire spine. The sacral spine is triangular shaped and has five bones that are fused together. The coccyx, commonly referred to as the tailbone, is the final segment of the vertebral column. It is composed of three to five coccygeal vertebrae that are also fused together. **Figures 15.5** and **15.6** depict the structure and function of the spinal column.

ANATOMY AND PHYSIOLOGY OF THE UPPER EXTREMITY

The upper extremity is attached to the trunk by the clavicle. This is the bone that allows the arms to hang away from the body and continue to function. The sternoclavicular joint attaches the clavicle to the sternum, while the acromioclavicular (AC) joint attaches it to the acromion process of the scapula. The scapula is considered a pseudojoint where it interacts with the thoracic rib cage as there is no actual joint but more of a soft tissue envelope that holds it in place. The glenohumeral joint is the articulation between the humerus and the glenoid portion of the scapula. This is a classic "ball-and-socket" joint, one of two in the body. However, it is a very shallow socket, leading to great mobility, though sacrificing stability (**Figure 15.7**). To improve on the stability, there is a cartilaginous ring around the glenoid, known as the labrum, which deepens the socket. Also providing stability are the rotator cuff muscles: the supraspinatus, infraspinatus, subscapularis, and teres minor. The supraspinatus allows for depression of the humeral head with abduction, preventing impingement on the acromion process. The subscapularis provides for anterior stability for the humeral head, while the infraspinatus and teres minor provide posterior stability (**Figure 15.8**).

The elbow is a complex hinge joint. It joins the ulna and the humerus, with the olecranon of the ulna fitting into the olecranon fossa of the humerus during full extension. At the elbow, the radial head will spin medially, allowing the radius to rotate over top of the ulna. This allows for pronation of the forearm and supination when the radius spins laterally. The proximal row of carpals interacts with the radius and ulna to allow wrist flexion and extension, while the distal row interacts with the metacarpals to allow finger opposition. The metacarpal and phalange articulations allow for the intrinsic hand motions, including finger flexion and extension and abduction and adduction (**Figure 15.9**).

ANATOMY AND PHYSIOLOGY OF THE LOWER EXTREMITY

Like the shoulder, the hip is a true "ball-and-socket" joint (**Figure 15.10**). However, here, mobility was

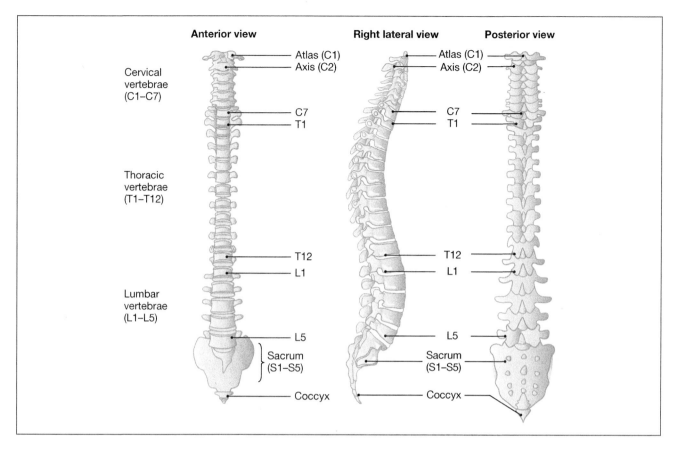

FIGURE 15.5 Spinal column.

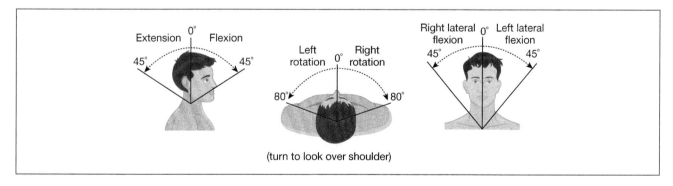

FIGURE 15.6 Rotation of cervical spine.

sacrificed for stability as the socket in the hip, the acetabulum, is much deeper than the shoulder. A labrum, though, is still present and a common structure to tear during activity. The lateral prominence at the hip, the greater trochanter, is the site for muscle attachment of the gluteals and a common place to develop bursitis related to gluteal weakness or iliotibial (IT) band tightness. The IT band forms from the distal fibers of the tensor fasciae lata and runs down the lateral leg, over the lateral femoral condyle, attaching to the lateral tibia at Gerdy's tubercle. Pain over the IT band is one of the most common sports medicine concerns.

The knee is also a hinge joint, though there is some rotational aspect when moving into full extension.

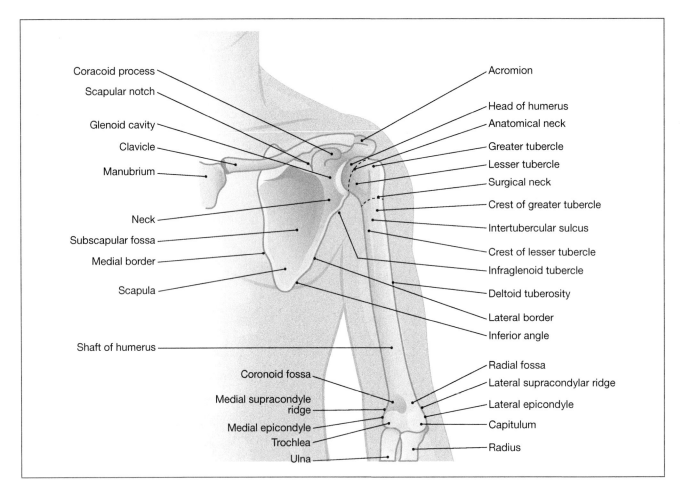

FIGURE 15.7 Bones of the shoulder.

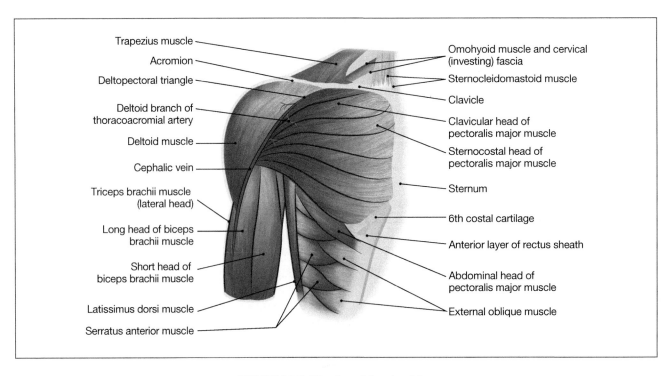

FIGURE 15.8 Muscles of the shoulder.

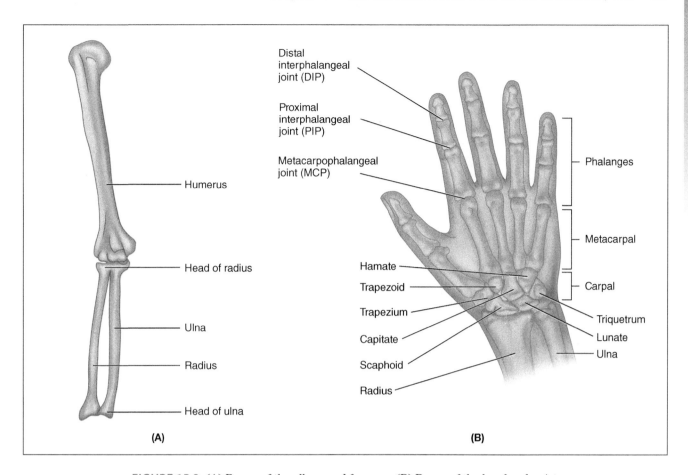

FIGURE 15.9 (A) Bones of the elbow and forearm. (B) Bones of the hand and wrist.

At the anterior knee lies the patella, a sesamoid bone, which is floating, and provides a mechanical advantage to the extensor mechanism of the knee. See **Figure 15.11** to review knee anatomy and **Figure 15.12** to review ankle anatomy. The ankle is composed of two joints: the tibiotalar and subtalar joints. The tibiotalar joint allows for plantar- and dorsiflexion. The subtalar joint, which is between the talus, navicular, and calcaneus bones, allows for eversion and inversion. The articulations between the cuboid and calcaneus bones allow for abduction and adduction. Combining inversion and adduction is known as supination of the foot, whereas the combination of eversion and abduction is known as pronation. Mobility at each of the joints allows for proper distribution of force throughout the gait cycle, leading to decreased stress at each successive level and decreased risk of injury.

LIFE-SPAN DIFFERENCES AND CONSIDERATIONS IN ANATOMY AND PHYSIOLOGY OF THE MUSCULOSKELETAL SYSTEM

Pediatric Variations

During embryogenesis, a cartilaginous skeleton develops. This skeleton is later replaced by bone via an ossification process. Ossification occurs when osteoblasts make and lay down new bone. By the time of birth, most of the cartilage has been replaced with bone. As children grow and develop, their bones have a softer structure than adults. The softer characteristic allows children's bones to fracture or break in different ways than adult bones do. The biggest difference is the presence of epiphyseal plates, or growth plates (Betts et al., 2013).

Epiphyseal plates are developing areas of cartilage tissue near the end of the long bones. An epiphyseal plate is present at the end of each long bone. On the

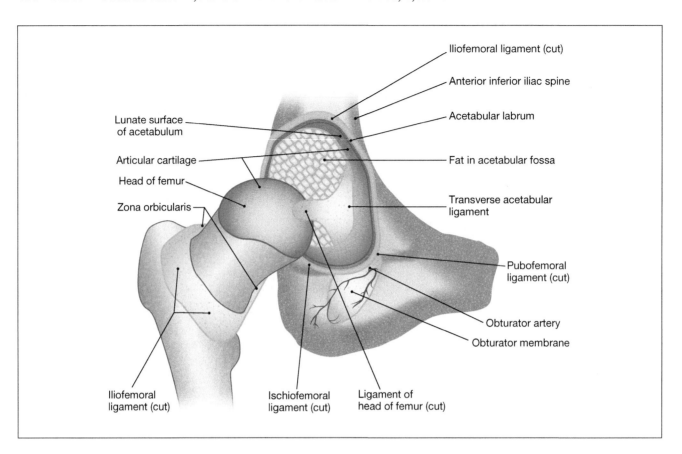

FIGURE 15.10 Hip anatomy.

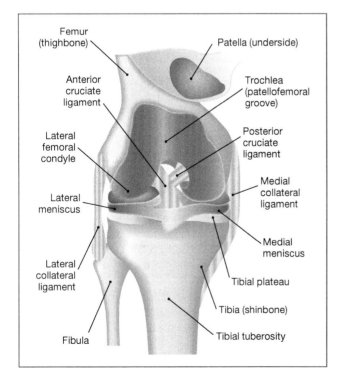

FIGURE 15.11 Knee anatomy. Frontal view of right knee (with patella reflected).

epiphyseal side of the epiphyseal plate, cartilage is formed. On the diaphyseal side, cartilage is ossified and the bone (diaphysis) grows in length. They are the weakest spots in a child's skeleton, causing frequent injuries to these areas. Roughly one-third of pediatric musculoskeletal injuries are located within or near the growth plate. These require different types of treatment compared with similar injuries in adults. When growing is complete, sometime during adolescence, the growth plate is replaced by solid bone. Bones continue to grow in length until early adulthood. The rate of growth is controlled by hormones (Betts et al., 2013).

Variations in Older Adults

As people age, they start to lose bone mass and bone density. This is especially true for women after they go through menopause. The long bones and vertebrae become more porous, making bones thinner and more brittle. For the elderly, a hip fracture can be life-threatening because of the temporary loss of mobility and its sequelae. Lean body mass decreases owing to muscle atrophy and the shrinkage of muscle fibers. This causes decreased muscle tone and more subcutaneous fat. The joints become stiffer and less flexible because

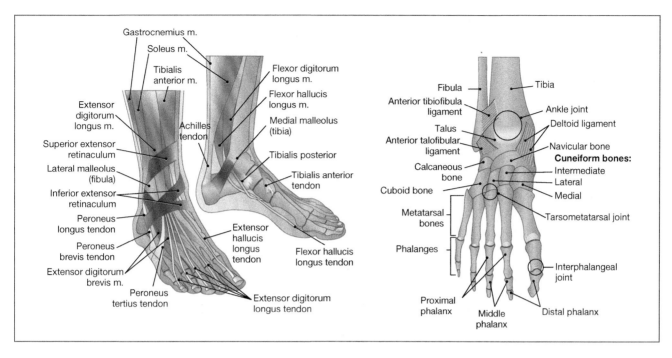

FIGURE 15.12 Ankle anatomy.

of degenerative changes in cartilage and a decrease in joint fluid. These changes put the older adult at risk for falls, injuries, and certain conditions such as osteoarthritis and osteoporosis (U.S. National Library of Medicine, n.d.).

KEY HISTORY QUESTIONS AND CONSIDERATIONS FOR THE MUSCULOSKELETAL SYSTEM

HISTORY OF PRESENT ILLNESS

Common Presenting Symptoms

- Joint pain (shoulder, elbow, wrist, hand, hip, knee, ankle, or foot pain)
- Spine (neck and back) pain
- Bone conditions (e.g., fractures, low bone density)
- Muscle conditions (e.g., myalgia, strain, sprain, sarcopenia)
- Limited mobility and/or dexterity

Example: Knee Pain

- Onset: Sudden versus insidious; associated with an injury; history of previous similar symptoms
- Location: Left or right side; medial, lateral, anterior, and/or posterior
- Duration: Acute versus chronic or intermittent
- Character: Aching, dulling, shooting, burning, sharp, locking

- Associated symptoms: Fever, weakness, inability to bear weight, clicking, popping, crunching, other joint pain (hip/ankle), stiffness, inability to straighten leg, instability or giving out, obvious deformity
- Aggravating factors: Movement, certain positions, sitting, standing, walking, running, jumping, going upstairs and downstairs
- Relieving symptoms: Pharmacologic treatment, including over-the-counter (OTC) pain relief; nonpharmacologic treatment, including application of heat, cold
- Temporal factors: Better or worse in the morning or at night, able to sleep through the night
- Mechanism of injury (if applicable): What was being done at the time of injury?

Differential Diagnoses

Ligament injury (anterior cruciate ligament [ACL], posterior cruciate ligament [PCL], medial collateral ligament [MCL], or lateral collateral ligament [LCL]), fracture, torn meniscus, bursitis, patellar tendonitis, patellofemoral syndrome, osteoarthritis, rheumatoid arthritis (RA), gout, pseudogout, septic arthritis, tibial apophysitis, patellar subluxation, medial plica syndrome, reactive arthritis

Example: Low Back Pain

- Onset: Sudden versus insidious; associated with event or trauma; history of previous or similar symptoms

- Location: Midline, right or left; radicular symptoms
- Duration: Acute versus chronic versus intermittent
- Character: Sharp, shooting, aching, stabbing, electrical
- Associated symptoms: Weakness, numbness/tingling, stiffness, fever, GI or urinary symptoms, loss of bowel/bladder, sudden erectile dysfunction
- Aggravating factors: Specific movements, sitting, standing, moving sit to stand, bending forward, or lying down
- Relieving factors: Lying, sitting, standing; leaning forward or arching backward
- Temporal factors: Able to sleep through night; change throughout the day, worse in morning or night

Differential Diagnoses
Muscle strain, degenerative disc disease, spinal stenosis, herniated disc, vertebral fracture, peripheral nerve injury, spondylolysis, spondylolisthesis, infection, tumor, kidney stone, cauda equina syndrome

PAST MEDICAL HISTORY

- Chronic diseases, including cancers, diabetes, autoimmune disorders, osteoporosis, renal diseases, thyroid disorders
- Osteoarthritis
- Anemia
- Surgeries
- Radiation therapy
- Recent or past injury, trauma, or car accidents
- Medications, including statins, steroids, antacids, antidepressants, Depo-Provera, thyroid replacement therapy, cancer chemotherapy drugs
- Supplements, including calcium and vitamin D3

FAMILY HISTORY

- Congenital diseases, including myopathies
- Autoimmune disease, including RA
- Gout
- Paget's disease of the bone
- Osteogenesis imperfecta
- Osteopenia/osteoporosis
- Muscular dystrophy (MD)

SOCIAL HISTORY

- Level of physical activity; typical exercise routines, including type of activity, frequency, warm-up/cool-down routines, stretching programs, recent changes, increases or decreases and reasoning for this change; sports participation (e.g., type, frequency of training, cross-training)
- Occupation, including how much movement during a typical workday and any repetitive motions that could put the patient at risk

- Activities of daily living (ADLs; e.g., is the patient able to dress themselves independently, brush their hair, put on their own socks, strong enough to walk stairs, carry loads, reach overhead)
- Smoking status
- Alcohol consumption
- Diet, looking for possible nutritional deficiencies

REVIEW OF SYSTEMS

- General: Fever, weight loss, fatigue
- Head, Eyes, Ears, Nose, Throat (HEENT): Conjunctivitis
- Gastrointestinal (GI)/Genitourinary (GU): Dysuria, vaginal/penile discharge, erectile dysfunction
- Neurologic: Weakness, numbness, loss of sensation, balance concerns
- Musculoskeletal: Recent falls, decreased range of motion, dropping things, decreased grip strength, changes in handwriting or fine motor movements, difficulty with completing ADLs, multiple or diffuse joint pain, early morning stiffness, past injury, or medical evaluation to affected area
- Hematologic: Anemia, bone pain
- Integumentary: Color, rash, erythema

PREVENTIVE CARE CONSIDERATIONS

- Dual-energy x-ray absorptiometry (DXA) scan
- Calcium and vitamin D supplementation
- Diet
- Physical therapy
- Occupational therapy

LIFE-SPAN CONSIDERATIONS FOR HISTORY
Pediatric History Considerations

- Birth history: Nerve or bony injuries, gestational age, interventions required after birth
- Motor skills appropriate for age
- Is the injury affecting the child's ability to play and function at school?
- Sports participation: What sports, training, frequency of participation, history of injuries

Geriatric History Considerations

- Weakness bilateral or unilateral
- Any recent falls
- Changes in handwriting/grip strength
- Vision changes

Pregnancy History Considerations

- Number of weeks of gestation
- Number of previous pregnancies
- Vaginal or Cesarean delivery
- Back pain/sciatica

PHYSICAL EXAMINATION OF THE MUSCULOSKELETAL SYSTEM

Completing the physical examination of the musculoskeletal system includes an appreciation for the techniques of the examination: (a) inspection, (b) palpation that includes noting muscle strength, (c) assessment of range of motion, and (d) use of special tests, as well as understanding of how these techniques are used to assess the integrity of the musculoskeletal system. In this section, after techniques are described, assessment of each area of the musculoskeletal system is reviewed.

INSPECTION

In the musculoskeletal examination, many clues as to pathology can be gleaned from keen observation. It is important to observe the patient throughout the examination. Observe their gait as they walk through the office, their posture, and their ability to do things (e.g., removing their shirt). Are they able to get out of a chair using only their legs, or do they need their arms? If they need their arms, do they favor one arm versus the other? Observing their handwriting and asking about changes in handwriting can be an early clue to a number of musculoskeletal or neurologic disorders.

A good inspection will identify any deformity, asymmetry, hypertrophy, or atrophy along with any skin changes, including bleeding, bruising, swelling, and previous scars. The anterior, posterior, lateral, and medial aspects of the joint should be observed. The affected joint should be compared for symmetry to the joint on the opposite side of the body. This can help identify subtle differences between corresponding joints or possible anatomical variations.

PALPATION

In the musculoskeletal examination, a solid knowledge of the bony landmarks and underlying anatomy along with precise palpation is invaluable. Tenderness over a particular bony landmark can help to determine potential differential diagnoses. Once the area of tenderness is localized, the rest of the examination can be used to narrow down differential diagnoses. The palpation portion of the examination should include range of motion and strength testing, followed by joint-specific special tests. The examination may or may not need an evaluation of deep tendon reflexes. After completing this portion of the physical examination, imaging and interventions should be considered based on current, evidence-based guidelines.

Muscle Strength

Muscle strength is graded on a scale of 0 to 5. A score of 0 indicates no movement, and a score of 5 indicates

TABLE 15.1 Muscle Strength Scale	
Grade	Level of Function
0	No movement
1	Trace movement
2	Full passive range of motion
3	Full range of motion against gravity, no resistance
4	Full range of motion with resistance, though weak
5	Full range of motion, full strength

full muscle strength. See **Table 15.1** for muscle strength grading. It is important to test strength bilaterally. Weakness can be indicative of a number of diagnoses, including neurologic injury, muscle strain, or even arthritis if the strength is limited owing to pain. If weakness is noted, it is important to investigate further, asking if the weakness is due to pain, injury, or true weakness.

RANGE OF MOTION AND SPECIAL TESTS

Range of motion is the full movement potential of a joint. Range of motion should be completed with every musculoskeletal visit. Most joints will have a contralateral joint in which to compare motion and angles. Normal range of motion values are noted in each section discussed in the text that follows. There are countless special tests described in the literature. Few though have been vigorously vetted for their efficacy. As a result, there will rarely be one test used to identify a pathology. It is more useful to use a cluster of tests to assist in identifying issues (Hegedus, Cook, Lewis, Wright, & Park, 2015). As with other examination skills, use of proper technique is essential to derive useful information from the special tests. Be sure to focus not only on proper patient positioning, but also on proper hand position and clinician position to ensure reliable and valid tests.

HEAD

The temporomandibular joint (TMJ) is the most used joint in the body, opening and closing approximately 1,500 to 2,000 times per day (Wieckiewicz, Boening, Wiland, Shiau, & Paradowska-Stolarz, 2015). The TMJ can be evaluated by having the patient open and close their mouth, move their jaw from side to side, and protract or retract their jaw. Palpate the TMJ during these movements and ask the patient about tenderness. With the patient's mouth open, the clinician's fingers should be placed below the zygomatic bone, anterior

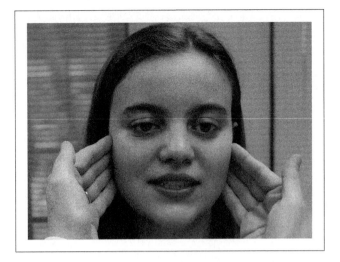

FIGURE 15.13 Palpation of the temporomandibular joint.

to the condyle (**Figure 15.13**). When the patient closes their mouth, the tip of the finger should be placed anterior to the tragus. Feel for any clicking, popping, or catching. When the patient is opening and closing the mouth, the movement should be smooth and the mandible should not have left- or right-sided deviation. When opened, there should be enough room for three fingers between the incisors.

The jaw jerk reflex can be used to evaluate for pathology along the fifth cranial nerve. This maneuver is performed by allowing the patient's mouth to relax in a slightly open position. Then place a finger over the mentum of the face and tap it with a reflex hammer. A normal response would be to see the mouth briefly close. An abnormal response would be an exaggerated closing or repeated closing, known as clonus, and could indicate an upper motor neuron lesion. An additional test used when hypocalcemia is suspected is the Chvostek test. This is performed by tapping the masseter muscle. Facial twitching or contraction of the facial muscles is considered a positive sign and indicates possible hypocalcemia.

CERVICAL SPINE

Acute cervical spine injuries can be quite devastating and can lead to significant disability or even death. A careful history and excellent examination technique in the acute setting are imperative to detection and stabilization of an acute cervical spinal injury. In the clinical setting, a variety of conditions can have cervical spine etiology, including weakness or numbness throughout the upper extremities.

When inspecting, look for deformities or asymmetries. Note the patient's posture and look for increased or decreased cervical lordosis or excessive thoracic

kyphosis. Note their head position and if they hold their head to one side or the other. Watch their movements. Do they have fluid, coordinated movements? Or do they appear stiff, slow, or uncontrolled?

The spine has several landmarks that can assist in palpation, including the mastoid process, individual spinous processes (C7 is usually the most prominent), and individual facet joints, which lie approximately 1 inch lateral to each spinous process. These joints are not always palpable. Soft-tissue palpation should include paraspinal musculature, the sternocleidomastoid muscle, and the trapezius muscle. Tenderness over the midline of the cervical spine when palpating the spinal processes could be indicative of a spinous process fracture.

Cervical range of motion includes flexion, extension, lateral rotation to the left and right, and lateral bending to the left and right. The majority of flexion/extension occurs between the occiput and C1, with the majority of rotation occurring between C1 and C2. Normal values for the cervical spine range of motion are:

- Flexion: 45 degrees (**Figure 15.14A**)
- Extension: 55 degrees (**Figure 15.14B**)
- Lateral bending: 40 degrees (**Figure 15.14C**)
- Lateral rotation: 70 degrees (**Figure 15.14D**)

Do not test for passive range of motion if unstable spine injury is suspected.

A proper cervical spine examination would also include dermatome and myotome examinations of the upper extremities, along with reflex testing of the biceps (C5), brachioradialis (C6), and triceps (C7; **Table 15.2**).

Special Tests of the Cervical Spine

Spurling test—This test looks to identify if a nerve root is being compressed because of intervertebral disc pathology. Passively extend and rotate the patient's neck to the affected side. Slowly start applying axial pressure by pressing down on the top of the patient's head (**Figure 15.15**). Radicular pain extending down the arm on the same side as the test is considered a positive test. Current evidence indicates that this test is highly specific but has only mild-to-moderate sensitivity (Jones & Miller, 2019). Be sure to rule out cervical instability, vertebral artery injury, and vertebral fracture before performing. It should not be performed in an acute trauma setting.

Extension–rotation test—This test is best used to eliminate facet joint etiology. Start by moving the patient into cervical extension, then laterally flex and rotate to the same side. Repeat with the contralateral side. The test is considered positive if the maneuver increases pain or causes numbness/tingling on the side of the neck being tested.

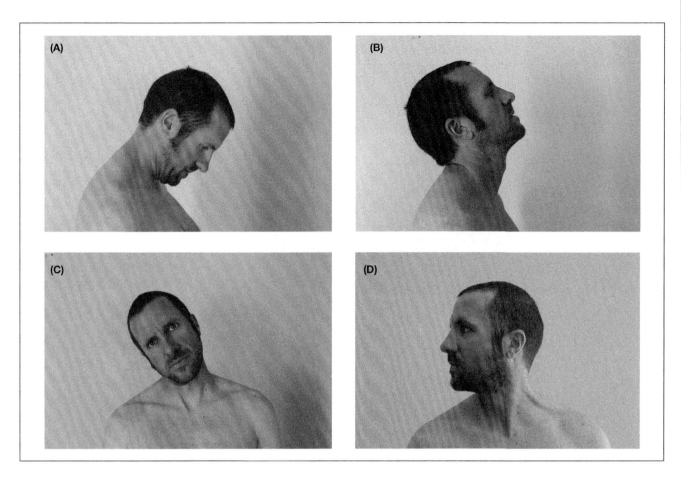

FIGURE 15.14 Range of motion of the cervical spine. (A) Flexion: 45 degrees. (B) Extension: 55 degrees. (C) Lateral bending: 40 degrees. (D) Lateral rotation: 70 degrees.

TABLE 15.2 Tomes of the Upper Extremity

Nerve	Dermatome	Myotome	Reflex
C5	Lateral upper arm	Deltoid	Biceps
C6	Radial side of forearm to thumb and index finger	Biceps, wrist extensors	Brachioradialis
C7	Middle finger	Triceps, wrist flexors, finger extensors	Triceps
C8	Ulnar forearm to fourth and fifth digits	Finger flexors and interossei muscles	None
T1	Ulnar side of elbow	Interossei muscles	None

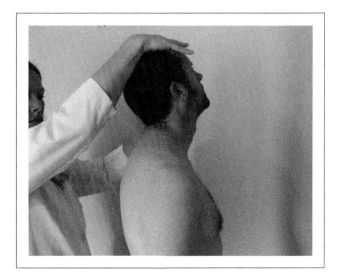

FIGURE 15.15 Spurling test.

THORACIC/LUMBAR SPINE

Low back pain is among the most common musculo-skeletal concerns. The lumbar spine supports the entire upper body, allowing humans to walk upright. Having a precise history and physical examination can significantly increase the efficiency with which patients can be correctly diagnosed and treated. A proper history and examination can be used to differentiate between hip, knee, and lumbar spine etiologies. Be sure to ask about the timing of symptoms. Often lumbar extension will stress facet injuries, as indicated with the extension–rotation test, while flexion movements will exacerbate central stenosis issues. Worsening of back pain symptoms with bowel movements can also be indicative of lumbar or thoracic pathologies because the Valsalva maneuver increases the pressure in the central nervous system. Burning or electrical/zinging type pain is indicative of nerve etiology rather than a musculoskeletal etiology.

Inspect the spine, looking for increased lumbar lordosis, kyphosis, and side curvature of the spine (scoliosis; **Figure 15.16**). Spinal curvature is best examined by having the patient flex forward while observing the spinous processes. The spinal processes should form a straight line. There are two natural lordoses and when viewed from the side, the spine should form an "S-"shaped curve. The skin should be inspected for any abnormalities, including hairy patches, café-au-lait spots, or doughy lipomata. These findings could be indicative of underlying neurological pathology. Observe the iliac crests, gluteal folds, posterior superior iliac spines (PSIS), and the anterior superior iliac spines (ASIS) while the patient is standing. Note any differences in height between the left and right sides. While the patient is supine, measure from the ASIS to the medial malleolus to check for true leg length discrepancies. This can then be compared to apparent leg length discrepancies as measured from the umbilicus to the medial malleolus to evaluate for possible pelvic obliquity. Any significant findings should be confirmed with radiography.

Palpation of the lumbar and thoracic spines, as shown in **Figure 15.17**, should include individual spinous processes, the iliac crests (approximately at L4–L5 interspace), bilateral ASIS, greater trochanters, ischial tuberosities, and bilateral PSIS. The umbilicus often lies near the L3–L4 interspace. When palpating the spinous processes, be sure to look for any step-off deformities from one process to the next. A significant drop between one spinous process and the next is considered a step-off deformity. The transition from one spinous process to the neighboring ones should be smooth, with a slight divot between each.

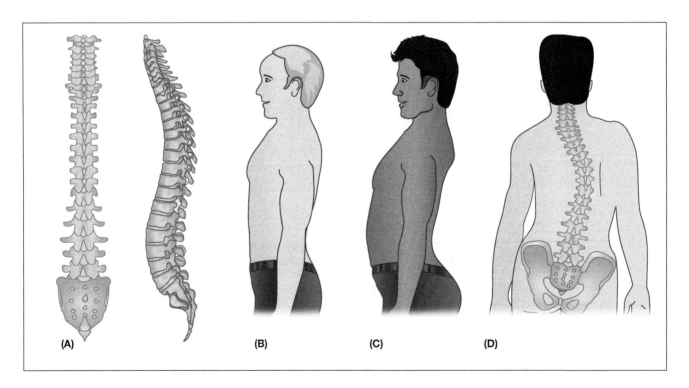

FIGURE 15.16 Spine curvatures. (A) Normal spinal curvature. (B) Lordosis. (C) Kyphosis. (D) Scoliosis.

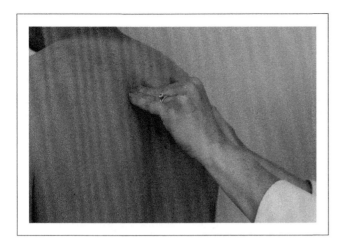

FIGURE 15.17 Palpation of spinal processes.

Normal values for the lumbar spine range of motion are:

- Flexion: 40 to 60 degrees (**Figure 15.18A**)
- Extension: 20 to 35 degrees (**Figure 15.18B**)
- Lateral bending: 15 to 20 degrees (**Figure 15.18C**)
- Lateral rotation: 5 to 20 degrees (**Figure 15.18D**)

Table 15.3 includes a listing of dermatomes originating from the spine that affect the lower extremities.

SPECIAL TESTS OF THE LUMBAR SPINE

Straight leg raise—This test looks to identify lumbar radiculopathy. Have the patient lie supine. Lift one leg at a time to 90 degrees or as far as the patient can tolerate. Place your other hand on the knee to ensure full knee extension (**Figure 15.19**). The test is considered positive if there is pain between 30 and 70 degrees of hip flexion that radiates below the knee. To further confirm neurologic etiology, slightly lower the leg and dorsiflex the foot; this will often also reproduce the radicular symptoms.

Valsalva maneuver—This test looks to identify if pain is coming from the spinal canal. With the patient sitting, have them take a deep breath and bear down as if trying to have a bowel movement. Localized or radicular pain is considered a positive test. Be careful as this maneuver can lead to lightheadedness/dizziness.

UPPER EXTREMITIES

Shoulder

As mentioned before, the shoulder is a ball-and-socket joint that typically sacrifices mobility for stability. When inspecting the shoulder, evaluate the patient's arm swing. Does it appear equal or does the motion seem limited in one side? Movements should be smooth and coordinated. As with all extremity examinations, use the contralateral side for comparison, not just during inspection, but also when testing range of motion, strength, and special tests. Look for any muscle atrophy (indicative of a nerve palsy or extreme deconditioning), deformity (fracture or dislocation), winging scapula, discoloration, or scars. When the proximal biceps tears, the tension on the muscle is altered. This results in the belly of the muscle bulging distally, giving a Popeye deformity (**Figure 15.20**). A Popeye deformity is indicative of a proximal biceps tear. Of note, the cephalic vein typically lies in the groove between the pectoralis and the deltoid. The spine of the scapula lies on the level of T3 and the entire scapula typically covers ribs 2 through 7.

Precise palpation of the shoulder can offer many clues about the underlying etiology of a shoulder-related concern. Being methodical when approaching the exam is the easiest way to ensure no areas or points of tenderness are missed during the examination. The following bony landmarks should be included: the scapula (including the coracoid process, acromion process, spine of scapula, superior and inferior angles of the scapula, and the medial and lateral borders of the scapula), clavicle (including sternal end, acromial end, and entire shaft), and humerus (including the deltoid tuberosity, the greater tuberosity [lateral], the bicipital groove, and the lesser tuberosity [medial]). The following joints and ligaments should be palpated: the sternoclavicular joint, AC joint, sternoclavicular ligament, and the AC ligament. The following areas of soft tissue should be palpated: the insertion point of the rotator cuff muscles at greater tuberosity; the axilla borders; the serratus anterior muscles; the pectoralis major muscles; the upper, middle, and lower trapezius; the deltoid (anterior, middle, and posterior bellies); the sternocleidomastoid; the biceps insertion and belly; and the latissimus dorsi muscles. When palpating the musculature, feel for tenderness and tone, and compare the muscles to the contralateral side.

There are a number of ways to actively test the range of motion (**Figure 15.21**). To perform the Apley's scratch test (**Figure 15.21A**), ask the patient to abduct and externally rotate their arms, then reach behind their back and touch the contralateral scapula. Next, have the patient abduct and internally rotate their arm, then ask the patient to reach behind their back as if tucking in their shirt and reach as far up their back as possible. Remember to compare the range of motion bilaterally. To test active horizontal adduction, have the patient abduct their arms to 90 degrees, flex the elbow to 90 degrees, then reach across the front of their body and touch the contralateral AC joint. To test for full abduction range of motion, be sure the patient externally rotates their arm to allow the humeral head to clear under the acromion.

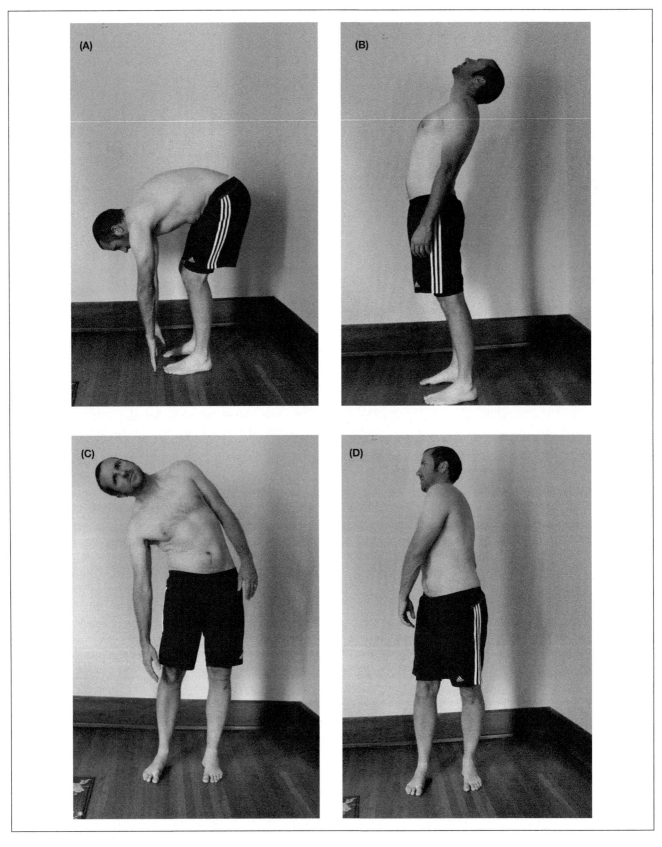

FIGURE 15.18 Range of motion of the spinal column. (A) Flexion: 40–60 degrees. (B) Extension: 20–35 degrees. (C) Lateral bending: 15–20 degrees. (D) Lateral rotation: 5–20 degrees.

TABLE 15.3 Tomes of the Lower Extremity

Nerve	Dermatome	Myotome	Reflex
L4	Medial leg and medial foot	Anterior tibialis	Patella tendon
L5	Lateral leg and dorsum of foot	Extensor hallucis longus	None
S1	Lateral foot	Peroneus longus and brevis	Achilles tendon

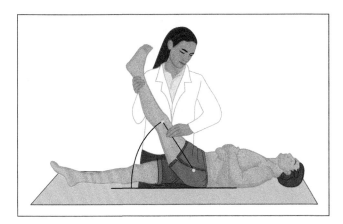

FIGURE 15.19 Straight leg raise.

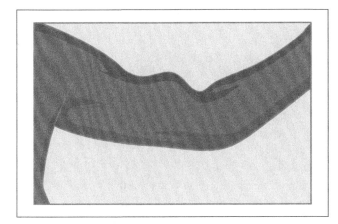

FIGURE 15.20 Popeye deformity.

Passive Range of Motion Normal Values
- Abduction: 180 degrees (approximately two-thirds of motion comes from glenohumeral joint and one-third from scapulothoracic joint; **Figure 15.21B**)
- Adduction: 45 degrees (**Figure 15.21C**)
- External rotation: 90 degrees (**Figure 15.21D**)
- Internal rotation: 90 degrees
- Forward flexion: 180 degrees

- Extension: 50 degrees
- Horizontal adduction: 45 degrees

It is important to know what muscles are activated with which movements. Test all nine shoulder movements and compare bilaterally. See **Table 15.4** for associated muscle involvement with various movements.

Special Tests of the Shoulder
A meta-analysis and systematic review by Lange et al. (2017) demonstrated that there is moderate-to-substantial inter-rater reliability for the Hawkins–Kennedy test, Neer test, empty can test, and the painful arc test. There was considerable heterogeneity among currently available research studies, and all shoulder tests lack proven validity because of insufficient methodological quality of studies. Shoulder tests should be completed in clusters, in contrast to completing a single test, to improve the reliability of results (Hegedus et al., 2015; Lange et al., 2017).

Hawkins–Kennedy test—This test helps to identify shoulder impingement, particularly of the supraspinatus. While holding the patient's elbow at 90 degrees with one hand and their wrist with the other hand, flex the shoulder to 90 degrees, then internally rotate (**Figure 15.22**). Pain and apprehension are considered positive tests.

Neer test—This test also looks to identify supraspinatus impingement. While stabilizing the patient's scapula, passively forward flex the arm while the arm is in the pronated position (**Figure 15.23**). Pain and apprehension are considered positive tests.

Empty can test—This test helps to identify supraspinatus weakness because of a tear, impingement, or a nerve injury. Have the patient abduct both of their arms to 90 degrees in the scapular plane (approximately 30 degrees of horizontal adduction). Next have them internally rotate the shoulder so their thumbs are pointing to the ground (**Figure 15.24**). Then, have the patient try to actively resist adduction. A positive test is an inability to hold the arm in the testing position.

Painful arc test—Ask the patient to forward flex the arm in 30 degrees of horizontal adduction. Ask them to slowly move their arms overhead to 180 degrees (**Figure 15.25**). Pain in the 60 to 120 degrees of flexion range is considered positive. Pain will often be worse with internal rotation and somewhat relieved with external rotation. A positive test is indicative of subacromial impingement.

External rotation resistance test—This test is used to identify rotator cuff pathology, particularly of the infraspinatus and teres minor. Have the patient flex their elbow to 90 degrees, then have them try to externally rotate the shoulder while providing resistance (**Figure 15.26**). Pain or weakness is considered

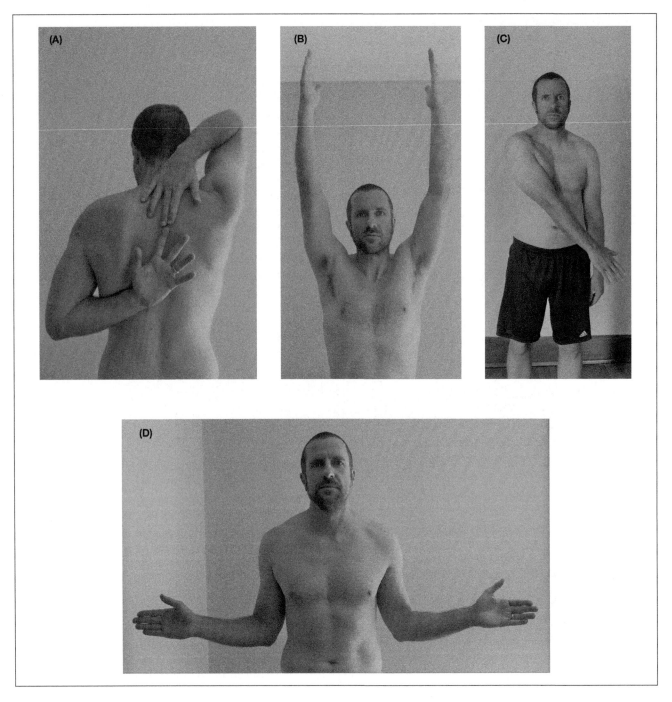

FIGURE 15.21 Shoulder range of motion. (A) Apley's scratch test. (B). Abduction: 180 degrees. (C) Adduction: 45 degrees. (D) External rotation: 90 degrees.

a positive result. The test can be repeated with the arm abducted to 90 degrees.

Lag test—This test also looks to identify rotator cuff pathology. With the patient seated, have them flex their elbow to 90 degrees, then abduct to 90 degrees. Move them 5 degrees less of full external rotation, then ask them hold the position. An inability to hold

the position when support is removed is considered a positive test.

Elbow

When inspecting the elbow, it is important to examine it in both flexion and extension. Identify the carrying angle with the elbow in extension. A normal carrying

TABLE 15.4 Shoulder Movements With Associated Muscle Involvement

Motion	Muscles (Secondary)
Flexion	Anterior deltoid, coracobrachialis (pectoralis major, biceps)
Extension	Latissimus dorsi, teres major, posterior deltoid (teres minor, triceps)
Abduction	Middle deltoid, supraspinatus (anterior/posterior deltoid, serratus anterior)
Adduction	Pectoralis major, latissimus dorsi (teres major, anterior deltoid)
External rotation	Infraspinatus, teres minor (posterior deltoid)
Internal rotation	Subscapularis, pectoralis major, latissimus dorsi, teres major (anterior deltoid)
Scapular elevation	Trapezius, levator scapulae (rhomboid major, rhomboid minor)
Scapular retraction	Rhomboid major, rhomboid minor (trapezius)
Scapular protraction	Serratus anterior

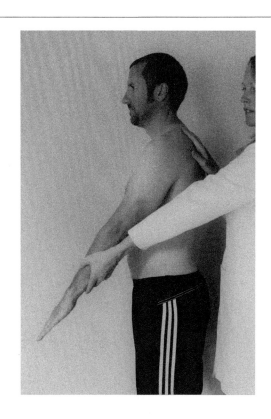

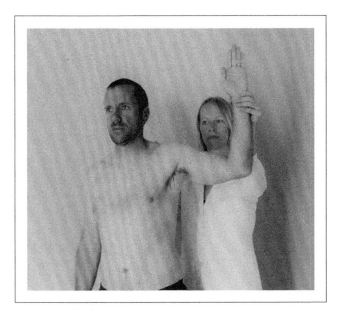

FIGURE 15.22 Hawkins–Kennedy test.

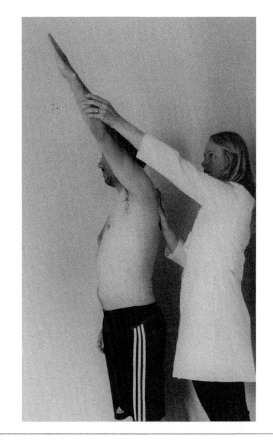

FIGURE 15.23 Neer test.

angle is considered to be between 5 and 15 degrees valgus. An increase in the angle is known as cubitus valgus. Cubitus varus is a decrease in that angle, also known as gunstock deformity; in children, this can be a

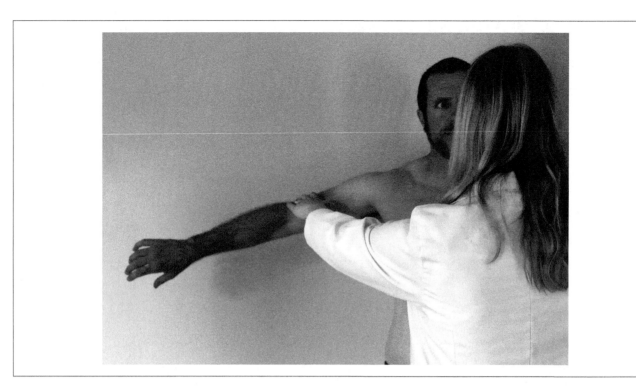

FIGURE 15.24 Empty can test.

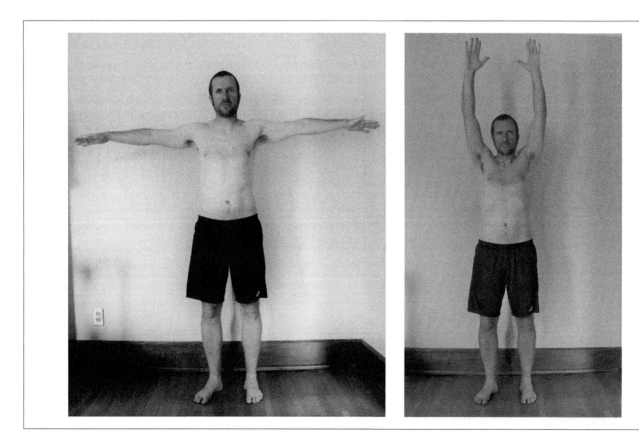

FIGURE 15.25 Painful arc test.

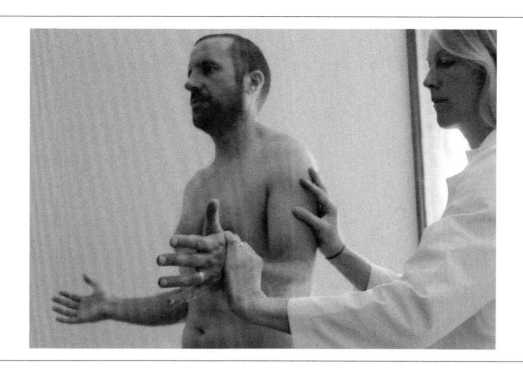

FIGURE 15.26 External rotation resistance test.

sign of a fracture affecting the rotation of the distal end of the humerus. Also, look for edema at the tip of the elbow over the olecranon fossa, as olecranon bursitis is a common complication of falling onto the tip of the elbow. Be sure to keep in mind proper anatomic position when referring to anatomic landmarks on the elbow. The ulnar side is medial and the radial side is lateral. Anatomic landmarks are often interchanged, with the ulnar collateral ligament often being called the medial collateral ligament of the elbow.

Important bony landmarks of the elbow to note during palpation include the medial and lateral epicondyles, origins for the wrist flexors and extensor bundles, the medial and lateral supracondylar lines of the humerus, the olecranon, the olecranon fossa, the ulnar border, and the radial head. The radial head is felt about an inch distal to the lateral epicondyle during pronation and supination.

When examining soft tissue, palpate the medial side of the elbow, feeling for the origin of the flexor bundle (pronator teres, flexor carpi radialis, palmaris longus, and flexor carpi ulnaris), and the ulnar nerve. Palpate for any tenderness over the ulnar collateral ligament. On the lateral side, palpate the extensor bundle (brachioradialis, extensor carpi radialis longus, and the extensor carpi radialis brevis) and feel for any tenderness over the radial collateral and the annular ligaments. The hand should be moved anteriorly to find the insertion of the biceps tendon and the brachial artery, which lies just medial to the biceps insertion point. The median nerve is found medial to the brachial artery.

See **Table 15.5** for associated muscle involvement with various movements.

Passive Range of Motion Normal Values
- Flexion: 135 degrees (**Figure 15.27A**)
- Extension: 0 to 5 degrees hyperextension (**Figure 15.27B**)
- Supination: 90 degrees (**Figure 15.27C**)
- Pronation: 90 degrees (**Figure 15.27D**)

TABLE 15.5 Elbow Movements With Associated Muscle Involvement	
Motion	Muscles (Secondary)
Flexion	Brachialis (biceps, brachioradialis, supinator)
Extension	Triceps (anconeus)
Pronation	Pronator teres, pronator quadratus (flexor carpi radialis)
Supination	Biceps, supinator (brachioradialis)

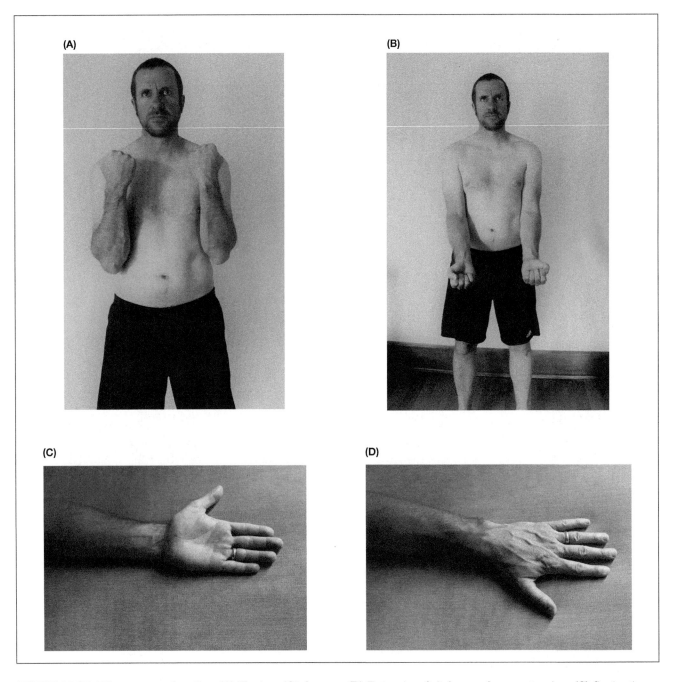

FIGURE 15.27 Elbow range of motion. (A) Flexion: 135 degrees. (B) Extension: 0–5 degrees hyperextension. (C) Supination: 90 degrees. (D) Pronation: 90 degrees.

Special Tests of the Elbow

Cozen test—This test looks to identify lateral epicondylitis, also known as tennis elbow. With the elbow stabilized and the hand pronated and in a fist, have the patient extend their wrist against resistance. Pain over the lateral epicondyle is considered a positive test.

Golfer elbow test—In contrast, this test looks to identify medial epicondylitis, or golfer's elbow. Again

with the elbow stabilized, have the patient supinate their hand and close their fist. Next, have the patient flex their wrist against resistance. Pain over the medial epicondyle is considered a positive test.

Varus stress test—This test looks to identify injury to the radial (lateral) collateral ligament of the elbow. With the wrist stabilized, apply a varus force to the medial side of the elbow while it is flexed to 20 or

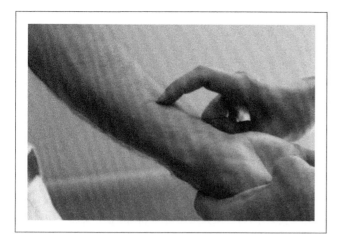

FIGURE 15.28 Tinel's sign.

30 degrees. Pain or excess motion compared to the contralateral side is considered a positive test.

Valgus stress test—This test seeks to identify injury to the ulnar (medial) collateral ligament of the elbow. With the elbow flexed to 20 or 30 degrees and the wrist stabilized, apply a valgus force to the lateral elbow. Pain or excess motion compared to the contralateral side is considered a positive test.

Tinel's sign—This test looks to identify compression of the ulnar nerve. With the elbow relaxed and the wrist supported, tap the ulnar nerve as it courses through the ulnar notch (**Figure 15.28**). Tingling or pain along the ulnar distribution is considered a positive test.

Wrist and Hand

When inspecting the wrist and hand, ensure all five fingers are present. Missing digits or parts of digits are not always noticeable at first glance. Observe the creases on the hands. Often times, the creases will be deeper and more prominent on the dominant hand as the musculature is more developed. Note the thenar eminence, the thick muscle belly at the base of the thumb, and the hypothenar eminence at the base of the little finger. In the middle of the palmar surface, there should be a slight depression, giving the palm a cup-like appearance. This is formed by the three main arches that give the hand its structural support. Damage to the intrinsic muscles of the hand will cause flattening of this arch.

Inspection of the fingers and nails is also essential for a thorough examination. With the fingers extended, look for rotation or crossing over of the fingers. This could be a sign of a phalange or metacarpal fracture. With a closed fist, the fingers should lay next to each other and, again, not cross one another. Bony nodules at the distal interphalangeal (IP) joint are known as

Heberden's nodes (**Figure 15.29**). The overgrowths at the proximal interphalangeal (PIP) joint are known as Bouchard's nodes (see **Figure 15.29**). Both Heberden's and Bouchard's nodes are a sign of osteoarthritis. Edema at the metacarpophalangeal (MCP) joints and ulnar deviation of the fingers are signs of possible RA.

Palpate the styloid processes of both the radius and the ulna. Then, move to the anatomical snuffbox, the depression on the radial side of the wrist bordered by the abductor pollicis longus and the extensor pollicis brevis tendons (**Figure 15.30**). Tenderness in this area is a sign of a possible scaphoid fracture. Feel for fullness and good muscle tone in the thenar and hypothenar eminences. Palpate the entire length of each metacarpal, again feeling for any tenderness or deformity. Finish the bony palpation at the fingers with each phalange and IP joint.

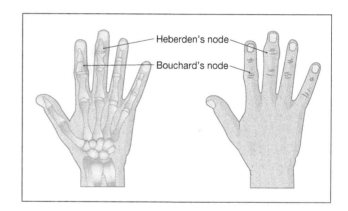

FIGURE 15.29 Heberden's and Bouchard's nodes.

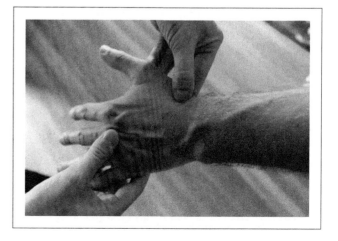

FIGURE 15.30 Area of snuffbox tenderness.

Passive Range of Motion Normal Values
- Wrist extension: 70 degrees
- Wrist flexion: 80 degrees
- Radial deviation: 20 degrees
- Ulnar deviation: 30 degrees
- MCP flexion: 80 to 90 degrees
- MCL extension: 30 to 45 degrees
- PIP flexion: 100 degrees
- PIP extension: 0 degrees
- DIP flexion: 90 degrees
- DIP extension: 20 degrees
- Finger abduction: 20 degrees
- Finger adduction: 0 degrees
- Thumb MCP flexion: 50 degrees
- Thumb MCP extension: 20 degrees
- Thumb abduction: 70 degrees
- Thumb adduction: 0 degrees

Special Tests for the Wrist and Hand

Finkelstein test—This test helps to identify tenosynovitis of the abductor pollicis longus and extensor pollicis brevis tendons, also known as De Quervain's syndrome. With the forearm stabilized, have the patient grasp their thumb in their fist, then perform ulnar deviation of the hand (**Figure 15.31**). Pain over the tendons is considered a positive test. Be sure to slowly deviate the hand, as this test, when positive, can be exquisitely painful.

Phalen's test—This test looks to identify median nerve pathology, particularly carpal tunnel syndrome. Have the patient sit with the dorsum of their hands touching, in maximal wrist flexion, applying force through the wrists, for 1 minute (**Figure 15.32**). Numbness or tingling in the median nerve distribution is considered a positive test.

Varus/valgus test—As with the elbow, the collateral ligaments in the fingers can be tested with a varus or valgus force applied while the joint is relaxed and supported. Pain or excess motion compared to the contralateral side is considered a positive test. This test is particularly useful at the MCP joint of the thumb to identify skier's thumb or a tear of the ulnar collateral ligament at the base of the thumb with increased motion or pain with a valgus force.

LOWER EXTREMITIES

Hip

When inspecting the hips, first assess gait patterns. Look for altered gait patterns as these can be a clue to a variety of lower extremity conditions. A Trendelenburg gait could be a sign of weak abductors. Shuffling of the feet or a wide base gait is important to note as these can be signs of Parkinson's or cerebellar disease. Bony landmarks, including the levels of the iliac crests, PSIS, ASIS, gluteal folds, and medial malleoli, should be examined and used to determine the symmetry of the lower limbs, leg length, or possible pelvic obliquity. Note the bony landmarks while the patient is standing and laying supine. A measurement from the ASIS to the medial malleolus is considered a true leg-length measurement and should be done bilaterally for comparison. A measurement from the umbilicus to the medial malleolus is considered an apparent leg-length measurement and can be compared to the true leg-length measurement to help identify possible soft tissue adaptations that can result in apparent leg-length differences even when true ones do not exist (Konin, Wiksten, Isear, & Brader, 2002).

When palpating, remember that true hip joint pathology typically presents as pain and tenderness in the groin. Pain on the lateral hip, over the greater

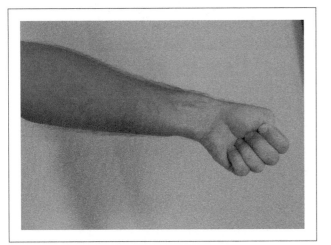

FIGURE 15.31 Finkelstein test.

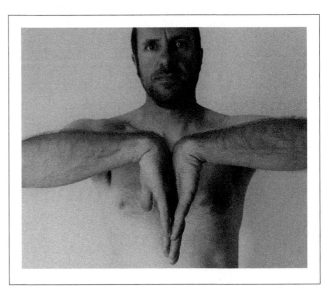

FIGURE 15.32 Phalen's test.

trochanter, is more commonly a trochanteric bursitis or abductor tendinitis, possibly related to a tight IT band or gluteal musculature. Palpate the ischial tuberosities deep in the gluteal folds as this is the origin of the hamstrings and a common area of injury.

See **Table 15.6** for associated muscle involvement with various movements.

TABLE 15.6 Hip Movements With Associated Muscle Involvement	
Motion	Muscles (Secondary)
Flexion	Iliopsoas, sartorius, rectus femoris
Extension	Gluteus maximus, hamstrings
Abduction	Gluteus medius (gluteus minimus)
Adduction	Adductor longus (adductor brevis, adductor magnus, pectineus, gracilis)
Internal rotation	Gluteus medius, gluteus minimus, adductor longus, adductor brevis
External rotation	Gluteus maximus, piriformis, quadratus femoris

Passive Range of Motion Normal Values
- Flexion: 120 degrees
- Extension: 20 to 30 degrees (**Figure 15.33A**)
- Abduction: 40 degrees (**Figure 15.33B**)
- Adduction: 20 degrees
- Internal rotation: 30 degrees
- External rotation: 60 degrees

Special Tests for the Hip

Thomas test—This test is used to identify hip flexor contracture and tightness. With the patient supine, have them bring one knee to their chest. When completing this maneuver, it is imperative for the clinician to control for lumbopelvic movement (i.e., pelvic tilt; Vigotsky, Lehman, Beardsley, Chung, & Feser, 2016). Passive flexion in the contralateral leg is considered a positive test on the contralateral side.

FABER test—This test identifies hip flexor, sacroiliac, or hip intra-articular pathology. FABER stands for **F**lexion, **AB**duction, and **E**xternal **R**otation. With the patient supine, have them flex, abduct, and externally rotate the hip until the ankle rests upon the contralateral knee. Then, apply downward pressure, moving the knee closer to the table (**Figure 15.34**). Pain or decreased range of motion is considered a positive test.

Log roll—This test identifies intra-articular pathology, particularly symptomatic arthritis. With the patient

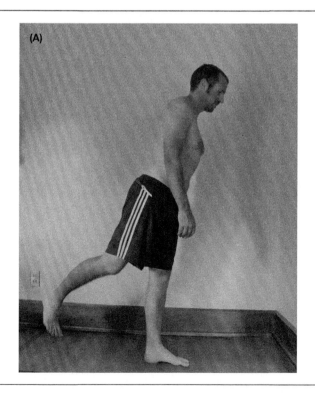
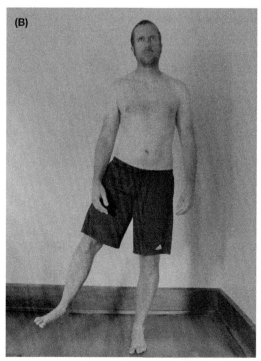

FIGURE 15.33 Hip range of motion. (A) Extension: 20–30 degrees. (B) Abduction: 40 degrees.

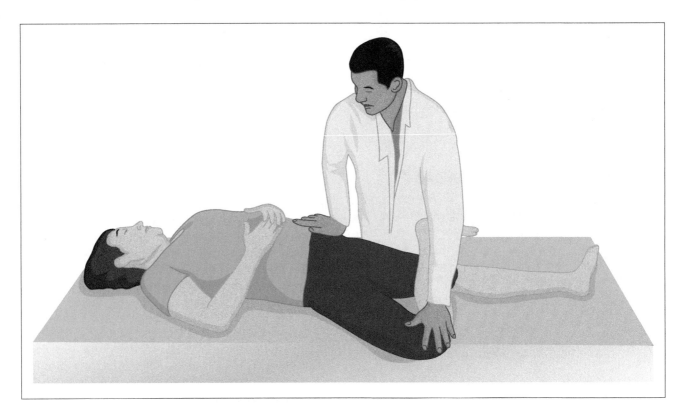

FIGURE 15.34 FABER test.

supine, hold the ankle or knee and passively internally and externally rotate the leg. Pain in the groin is considered a positive test.

Stinchfield's test—This test identifies intra-articular hip pathology. With the patient supine, have them flex the hip to 30 or 45 degrees. Apply a downward pressure on the ankle with the patient resisting. Pain in the groin is considered a positive test.

Trendelenburg's test—This test looks to identify weakness of the abductor musculature. Have the patient stand on one leg for 10 seconds, then switch legs (**Figure 15.35**). Weakness of the gluteus medius on the standing side will lead to a dip of the pelvis on the unsupported side. If this is seen, it is considered a positive test.

Knee

When inspecting the knee, look for any deformity, asymmetry, and/or edema. Evaluate for genu valgus (knock-knee) and genu varus (bow-legged; **Figure 15.36**). A prominent tibial tuberosity can be a sign of Osgood–Schlatter disease, which is common in adolescence.

Be systematic when completing palpation on the knee. The knee has a number of bony landmarks that can differentiate pathologies. On the lateral side of the knee, palpate the fibular head, lateral joint line, lateral femoral condyle, IT band and insertion on Gerdy's tubercle, biceps femoris insertion, and the lateral collateral ligament. On the medial side, palpate the medial joint line, MCL origin and insertion, pes anserine, and muscle bellies of the semitendinosus and semimembranosus. Feel anteriorly for the patella and its borders, the tibial tuberosity, and the patellar and quadriceps tendons. On the posterior side, feel in the popliteal fossa for a possible fluid collection, known as a Baker's cyst. This can be a sign of a meniscus tear. Often, meniscus tears will refer pain to the popliteal fossa.

See **Table 15.7** for associated muscle involvement with various movements.

Passive Range of Motion Normal Values
- Flexion: 130 to 140 degrees
- Extension: 0 to 5 degrees hyperextension

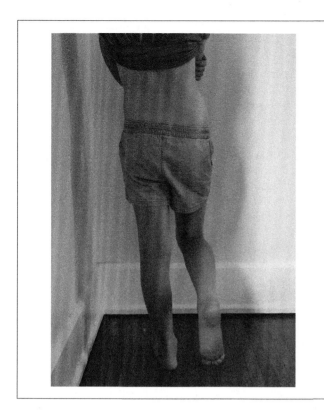

TABLE 15.7 Knee Movements With Associated Muscle Involvement	
Motion	Muscles (Secondary)
Flexion	Semimembranosus, semitendinosus, biceps femoris
Extension	Rectus femoris, vastus medialis, vastus lateralis, vastus intermedius

FIGURE 15.35 Negative trendelenburg test. No dip of the pelvis noted on the unsupported side.

Special Tests for the Knee

Valgus stress test—This test helps to identify injury to the medial collateral ligament. With the patient supine and relaxed, hold the ankle of the patient and apply a valgus stress to the lateral knee (**Figure 15.37**). Test in full extension and in 20 to 30 degrees of knee flexion. Pain or excessive laxity is considered a positive test.

Varus stress test—This test looks to identify injury to the lateral collateral ligament. With the patient supine and relaxed, hold the ankle of the patient and apply a varus stress to the medial knee (**Figure 15.38**). Test in full extension and in 20 to 30 degrees of knee flexion. Pain or excessive laxity is considered a positive test.

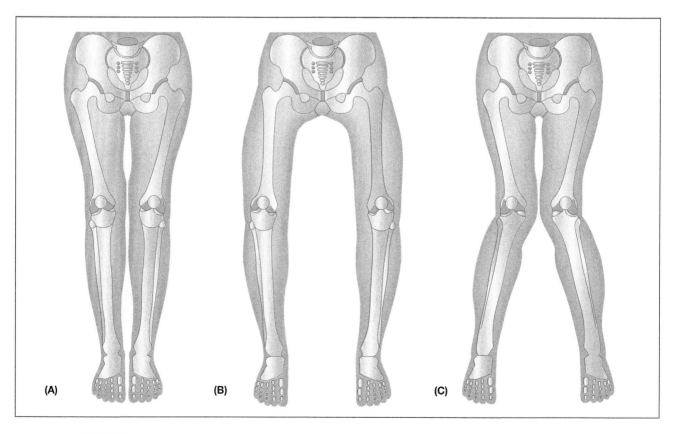

FIGURE 15.36 Knee deformity. (A) Normal. (B) Genu varus (bow-legged). (C) Valgus (knock-knee).

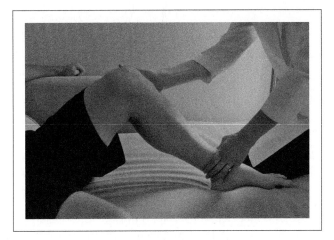

FIGURE 15.37 Valgus stress test.

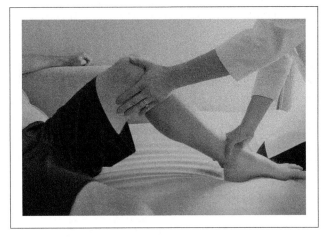

FIGURE 15.38 Varus stress test.

Anterior drawer test—This test helps to identify injury to the anterior cruciate ligament. With the patient supine, have them flex the hip to 45 degrees and flex the knee to 90 degrees, resting their foot on the table. Next, the clinician should sit on the patient's foot to stabilize the leg and place their hands behind the proximal tibia, resting the thumbs on the tibial tuberosity. Use the index fingers to ensure relaxation of the hamstring muscles. Apply an anterior force (**Figure 15.39A**). Increased anterior translation is indicative of an ACL tear.

Posterior drawer test—This test looks to identify injury to the posterior cruciate ligament. With the patient supine, have them flex their hip to 45 degrees and flex the knee to 90 degrees, resting their foot on the table. Next, sit on the patient's foot to stabilize the leg. Hands should be placed behind the proximal tibia, resting the thumbs on the tibial tuberosity. Use the index

fingers to ensure relaxation of the hamstring muscles. Apply a posterior force (**Figure 15.39B**). Increased posterior translation in indicative of a PCL tear.

Lachman test—This test is used to identify a tear to the ACL. With the patient supine and relaxed, place the outside or proximal hand over the distal thigh and inside hand, or distal hand, over the proximal tibia. Allowing the hip to externally rotate can help ensure the patient is relaxed. Next, apply anterior translation force on the tibia with the distal hand while stabilizing the thigh with the proximal hand (**Figure 15.40**). Excessive anterior tibial translation is indicative of an ACL tear. This test can be challenging if the patient is guarding.

McMurray's test—This test identifies meniscus pathology. With the patient supine, use one hand to grasp the patient's ankle, and the other hand to stabilize the patient's knee. With the knee flexed, externally rotate the tibia and apply a valgus force while extending the knee. Next, move the knee from flexion while internally rotating the tibia and applying a varus force (**Figure 15.41**). Pain or clicking over the medial or lateral joint lines is considered a positive test.

Apprehension test—This test looks to identify patellar laxity or subluxations/dislocations. With the patient supine and relaxed, place the knee in full extension. Next, apply a lateral force to the medial border of the patella (**Figure 15.42**). Pain or guarding is considered a positive test.

Ballottement test—This test looks for joint effusion in the knee. Joint effusion is most commonly caused by trauma to the knee. The patient should lay in the supine position with the legs extended. The clinician should place one hand superior to the patella and use the other hand to apply downward pressure in an anterior-to-posterior "milking" motion. If there is fluid present, the clinician will feel it against their lower hand. Then gently push down on the patella. If the patella can be depressed, it means that it was "floating" in fluid and signifies a positive test.

Bulge sign—This is another test commonly used to test for knee effusion. Gently press slightly medial to the patella. Then move the hand in an ascending motion and apply pressure firmly on the lateral aspect of the knee. A positive test would be if a "bulge" is seen on the medial aspect of the knee after the lateral pressure was applied. This would indicate that a moderate amount of fluid is present. A medial aspect that does not bulge but tensely reflects lateral pressure is consistent with a large amount of fluid.

Ankle and Foot

Observation and inspection of the feet should start with examination of the patient's footwear. Shoes can provide information on wear patterns and show where a person is putting pressure on their feet throughout

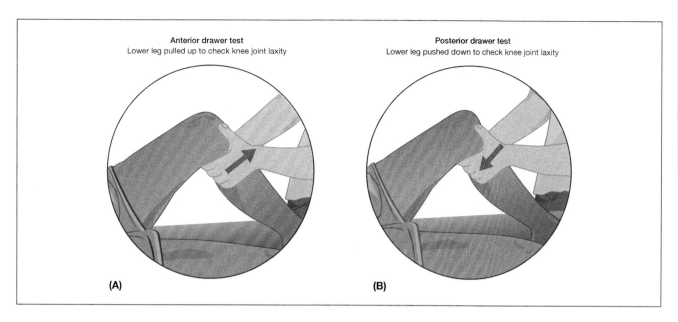

FIGURE 15.39 Drawer tests. (A) Anterior. (B) Posterior.

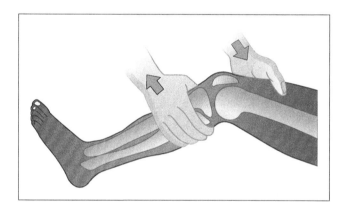

FIGURE 15.40 Lachman test.

their gait cycle. This can provide information about possible foot deformities or gait patterns. Observe the foot and ankle of the patient both in standing and sitting positions. Look for deformities and asymmetries as with any other joint. It is important to note any areas of calluses or corn formations. Calluses can indicate abnormal weight-bearing or improperly fitting shoes. The skin should be the thickest around the heel, at the lateral border, and over the metatarsal heads. Look at the arches in the patient's feet. The arches should be more pronounced when the patient is not bearing weight. Pes planus, known as flat feet, occurs when the arch does not become prominent when the patient is non–weight-bearing. If the patient does have pes planus, it is important to ensure the toes lay next to each other and are not overlapping. Overlapping toes can be a sign of pathology to the metatarsals and can lead to pressure sores between the toes or where the toes rub against

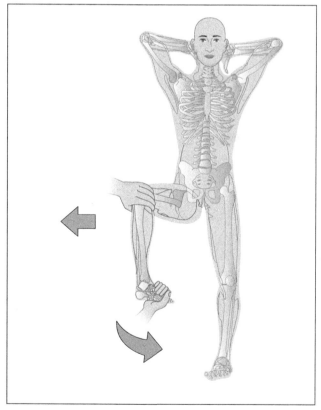

FIGURE 15.41 McMurray's test.

shoes. Pes cavus, or the high-arched foot, is seen when the arch remains high even when bearing weight. There are also a number of toe deformities, including claw toes, hammertoes, and mallet toes, that should be noted on inspection (**Figure 15.43**).

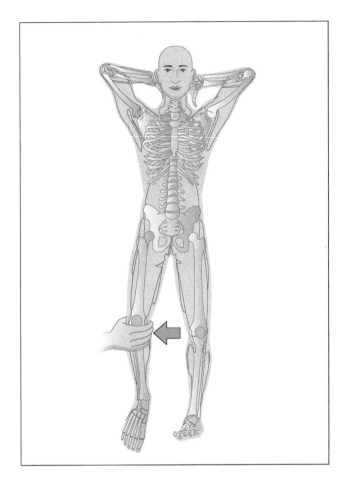

FIGURE 15.42 Apprehension test.

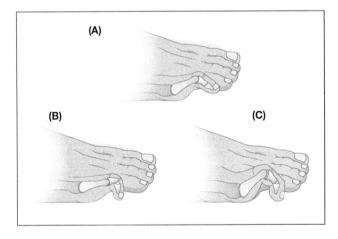

FIGURE 15.43 Toe deformities. (A) Hammer toe. (B) Mallet toe. (C) Claw toe.

On the medial side of the ankle and foot, palpate over the medial malleolus, then down the foot to the navicular bone (most prominent bone on the medial side). Palpate the medial head of the talus, which is just proximal to the navicular bone. Move down the foot to the first

TABLE 15.8 Ankle/Foot Movements With Associated Muscle Involvement	
Dorsiflexion	Tibialis anterior, extensor hallucis longus, extensor digitorum longus
Plantar flexion	Peroneus longus and brevis, gastrocnemius and soleus, flexor hallucis longus, flexor digitorum longus, tibialis posterior
Inversion	Tibialis anterior, extensor hallucis longus, tibialis posterior, flexor digitorum longus, flexor digitorum brevis
Eversion	Peroneus longus, peroneus brevis

metatarsal, then distally to the first phalange and the IP joint. On the lateral side, start palpation at the lateral malleolus, then move inferiorly to palpate the peroneus longus and brevis. Just distal to the lateral malleolus is the area of the anterior talofibular ligament. This is the most commonly sprained ligament with ankle injuries. Palpate down the foot and feel for the styloid process of the fifth metatarsal. This is a common area of avulsion or stress fractures. Lastly, palpate the shaft of the metatarsals and phalanges, feeling for the metatarsophalangeal (MTP) and IP joints.

On the posterior foot, palpate the Achilles tendon and its insertion site, feeling for any crepitus or nodularity. Then, move to the plantar surface and the calcaneus. Typically, plantar fasciitis will present as pain first thing in the morning at the distal end of the calcaneus that gradually eases with light activity. Continue moving distally and palpate the metatarsal shafts and heads, feeling for any tenderness.

Palpating for pedal pulses should also be included in an ankle/foot assessment. The posterior tibial artery can be palpated just posterior to the medial malleolus, and the dorsalis pedis artery can be palpated between the extensor hallucis longus and the extensor digitorum longus tendons. Absent or diminished pedal pulses can indicate peripheral vascular disease, compartment syndrome, or other pathology.

See **Table 15.8** for associated muscle involvement with various movements.

Passive Range of Motion Normal Values
- Dorsiflexion: 20 degrees
- Plantar flexion: 50 degrees
- Inversion: 30 degrees
- Eversion: 20 degrees
- Abduction: 10 degrees
- Adduction: 20 degrees
- First MTP flexion: 45 degrees
- First MTP extension: 70 degrees

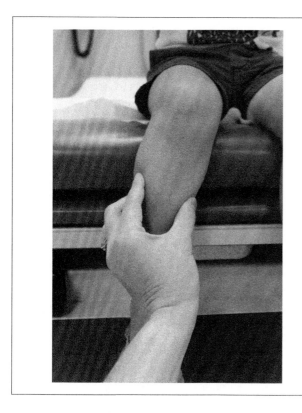

FIGURE 15.44 Squeeze test.

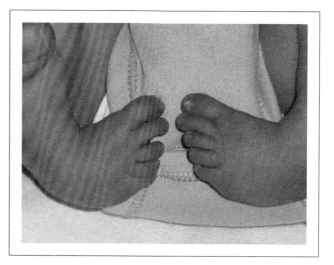

FIGURE 15.45 Clubfoot.
Source: Image courtesy of Brachet Youri.

Special Tests for the Ankle and Foot

Squeeze test—This test is used to identify syndes-motic (or high) ankle injuries or fractures. With the patient relaxed, squeeze the proximal tibia and fibula together (**Figure 15.44**). Pinpoint pain or pain distally is considered a positive test.

Talar tilt—This test identifies ankle ligamentous injury. With the patient relaxed and the foot in a neu-tral position, passively move the foot into an adducted position; pain or increased motion is considered posi-tive and a sign of damage to the lateral ankle ligaments. Next, passively move the foot into an abducted position. Pain or increased motion is considered a positive test.

Thompson test—This test is used to evaluate the in-tegrity of the Achilles tendon complex. With the patient prone or seated with the foot unsupported, squeeze the belly of the gastrocnemius. With an intact complex, the foot should passively plantar flex when the calf is squeezed. No plantar flexion of the foot is considered a positive test.

LIFE-SPAN CONSIDERATIONS FOR PHYSICAL EXAMINATION

Pediatric Considerations

Clubfoot

Clubfoot, or talipes equinovarus, is a congenital condi-tion where the forefoot is adducted, while the heel is in varus (**Figure 15.45**). Early treatment will include casting and bracing, with surgery becoming an op-tion around month 3 or 4, though it can be delayed if necessary.

Developmental Dysplasia of the Hip

Dysplasia of the hip encompasses a range of hip issues in infants, from dysplasia with no instability to dislo-cated hips. All infants should be evaluated for the sym-metry of the gluteal, inguinal, and thigh skin folds. The Barlow–Ortolani maneuvers are designed to test for hip dislocations and subluxations in 0- to 1-year-olds. With the infant supine, flex the hips and knees to 90 degrees. The clinician's thumbs should rest on the medial side of the knees, fingers resting on the greater trochanters. Adduct the thighs and put gentle pressure through the femurs, trying to shift them out of the acetabulums. A clunk is considered positive. For the next step, slowly abduct the thighs and use the fingers to put pressure on the trochanters to guide the femoral head back into po-sition. Again, a clunk is considered a positive test and could be a sign of hip subluxation or dislocation. If dys-plasia is suspected within the first 6 months of life, an ultrasound evaluation is preferred to x-ray. If any tests are abnormal, refer to a pediatric orthopedic clinician for intervention(s) and/or treatment options.

Scoliosis

Scoliosis is an abnormal curvature of the spine (**Figure 15.46**). In normal alignment, the spine should have four major curvatures: a cervical lordosis, thoracic kyphosis, lumbar lordosis, and sacral kyphosis, all in the sagittal plane. Although preventive screening for scoliosis is not recommended by the U.S. Preventive

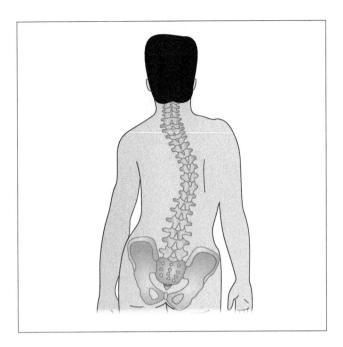

FIGURE 15.46 Scoliosis.

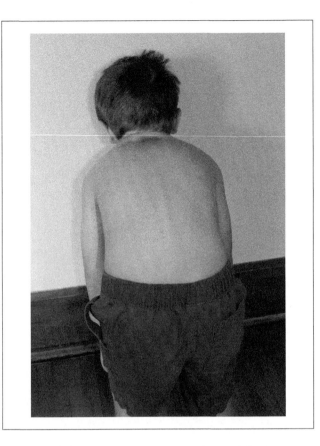

FIGURE 15.47 Normal spine in forward flexion.

Services Task Force ([USPSTF] 2018), clinicians need to be aware how to identify it. First, have the patient stand and observe them from the front. Note the symmetry of the patient's shoulders. The shoulders should be even. Uneven shoulder height can be a clue to scoliosis. Then, ask the patient to turn around and bend at the waist (**Figure 15.47**). The clinician should stand behind the patient and observe the patient from the rear. The spine should be straight without curvature and centered over the sacrum. Angles of less than 10 degrees can often be followed with periodic radiographs. Angles of up to 30 degrees typically show no lasting effects into adulthood. Angles over 50 will lead to complications later in life. In more severe cases of scoliosis, a unilateral rib hump may be present. Appropriate intervention early in the process helps to avoid possible complications later in life, including restrictive pulmonary disease and severe low back pain. Treatment aims to prevent the progression of the curvature through bracing or surgery if necessary.

Legg-Calve-Perthes Disease
Legg-Calve-Perthes disease typically affects boys aged 4 to 10 years. This condition occurs when the blood supply to the femoral head is temporarily severed, then eventually restored. Bone weakening and breakdown occurs, causing the round, ball-like femoral head to lose its shape. Patients will often present with groin, hip, thigh, or anterior knee pain; stiffness and limited range of motion in the hip joint; and a limp. Upon further imaging, the femoral head will appear mottled and sclerosed. Treatment can vary depending on the

patient's age and the progression of the disease. Treatments can range from bracing and observation to femoral osteotomy.

Slipped Capital Femoral Epiphysis
Slipped capital femoral epiphysis (SCFE) occurs typically in patients aged 8 to 14 years. They often present with hip, thigh, or knee pain, and will normally have a limp. The most common patient will be male and overweight. Radiographs will have the appearance of ice cream falling off a cone. Treatment is surgical unless the disease is significantly progressed and the growth plates are closed. Referral to orthopedics is necessary.

Muscular Dystrophy
MD is a rare group of diseases that cause muscle weakening. These diseases are due to genetic defects and can run in families. There are over 30 different types of MD, but there are nine major types. Each type has different characteristics. Age of onset, muscle group affected, severity, and genetic defects are all different depending on the subtype. Duchenne MD is the most well-known. It is typically seen in males and starts in early childhood (before age 5; Centers for Disease Control and Prevention, n.d.). Muscle weakness and degeneration are progressive with the average life expectancy in the early

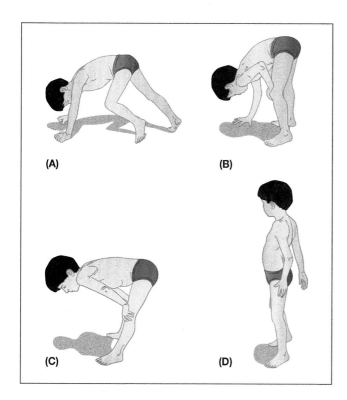

(A)

(B)

(C)

(D)

FIGURE 15.48 Gower's sign. In a positive test, the child will move from hands and knees (A) to hands and feet (B), then move hands to knees (C) to help push themselves to a standing position (D).

30s. Gower's sign is a sign of muscle weakness in the proximal hip muscles and is commonly associated with MD. See **Figure 15.48** for the typical pattern seen with Gower's sign. Gower's sign is witnessed when the child moves from sitting on the floor to standing. In a positive test, the child will move from hands and knees to hands and feet, then move hands to knees to help push themselves to a standing position.

IMAGING CONSIDERATIONS FOR THE MUSCULOSKELETAL SYSTEM

X-RAY

With musculoskeletal concerns, the majority of information will be derived from x-rays. Plain films provide a quick, inexpensive evaluation of the general health of a joint. X-rays can identify numerous abnormalities, including fractures, disruption in the cortex of the bones, osteoarthritis, bony tumors, or punch-out lesions as seen in multiple myeloma. Often, unless an acute injury is known or there are red flags, imaging can be deferred until after the patient has trialed a course of formal physical therapy. There are many evidence-based clinical decision rules available with high sensitivity and specificity that can be used to determine the need for

radiographs. For instance, the Ottawa ankle and knee rules indicate that x-rays are only needed with certain physical findings (Beutel, Trehan, Shalvoy, & Mello, 2012; Jenkin, Sitler, & Kelly, 2010). See **Box 15.2** for the Ottawa knee and ankle rules. There are similar clinical decision-making tools for acute back pain.

Interpreting x-rays in children presents its own unique challenges as growth plates are still open and can easily be confused for a fracture if the clinician is not mindful. **Table 15.9** shows the classification for growth plate fractures, known as the Salter–Harris classification. Also, of note in children, advanced imaging studies (computed tomography [CT] and/or magnetic resonance imaging [MRI]) should not be ordered on children until all appropriate clinical, laboratory, and plain films have been completed (American Academy

---

BOX 15.2
OTTAWA KNEE AND ANKLE RULES

Indications for Knee Radiographs*:

- ≥55 years old
- Inability to bear weight (for four steps, regardless of limp) immediately after trauma and in the emergency department (ED)
- Isolated patellar tenderness
- Fibular head tenderness
- Inability to flex the knee to 90 degrees

Indications for Ankle Radiographs:

- Pain in the malleolar zone and any of the following:
  ○ Bony tenderness on the posterior edge of the lateral malleolus
  ○ Bony tenderness on the posterior edge of the medial malleolus
  ○ Inability to bear weight both immediately and in the ED
- Pain in the mid-foot zone and any of the following:
  ○ Bony tenderness at the base of the fifth metatarsal
  ○ Bony tenderness at the navicular bone
  ○ Inability to bear weight both immediately and in the ED

*At least one of the criteria must be present.
Sources: Jenkin, M., Sitler, M. R., & Kelly, J. D. (2010). Clinical usefulness of the Ottawa Ankle Rules for detecting fractures of the ankle and mid-foot. *Journal of Athletic Training, 45*(5), 480–482. doi:10.4085/1062-6050-45.5.480; Stiell, I. G., Greenberg, G. H., Wells, G. A., McDowell, I., Cwinn, A. A., Smith, N. A., . . . & Sivilotti, M. L. (1996). Prospective validation of a decision rule for the use of radiography in acute knee injuries. *The Journal of the American Medical Association, 275*(8), 611–615. doi:10.1001/jama.1996.03530320035031

TABLE 15.9 Salter–Harris Classification System

Classification	Description
I	Transverse fracture through physeal plate
II	Transverse fracture extending into metaphysis
III	Transverse fracture extending into epiphysis
IV	Fracture extending into both metaphysis and epiphysis
V	Comminution of physeal plate

of Pediatrics-Section on Orthopaedics & Pediatric Orthopaedic Society of North America, 2018).

MAGNETIC RESONANCE IMAGING

MRI is a better tool to evaluate soft tissue injury, including sprained or torn ligaments, strained muscles or tendons, meniscal tears, and labral pathology in the hip and shoulder. MRIs involve the use of magnets so patients with artificial joints might not have the ideal picture quality, and some patients might be contraindicated if they have other metal implants or certain types of pacemakers. MRI or bone scans can also be utilized to evaluate for bony injuries not present on plain x-rays, including stress fractures or reactions. A reaction is an early bone irritation that can lead to a stress fracture.

ULTRASOUND

Ultrasound has many advantages as an imaging modality for musculoskeletal conditions. It is relatively inexpensive, quick, noninvasive, and does not cause exposure to radiation. It is also portable and can provide onsite, real-time evaluation when necessary. It does have limitations, including difficulty in visualization of deeper structures, restricted access to certain joints, and reliance on the ability and training of the operator, which can jeopardize its reliability. RA, psoriatic arthritis, osteoarthritis, lateral/medial epicondylitis, carpel tunnel syndrome, and sports injuries are just some conditions where ultrasound can be useful when imaging is required (Patil & Dasgupta, 2012).

DUAL-ENERGY X-RAY ABSORPTIOMETRY SCAN

Dual-energy x-ray absorptiometry (DEXA/DXA) is an enhanced x-ray that is used to measure bony mineral density. For women aged 65 years and older and for women who are postmenopausal but younger than 65 years and at an increased risk for osteoporosis, the USPSTF (2018) recommends screening for osteoporosis

> **BOX 15.3**
> **SIMPLE CALCULATED OSTEOPOROSIS RISK ESTIMATION (SCORE) CLINICAL RISK ASSESSMENT TOOL**
>
> **Components:**
> - Race
> - Rheumatoid arthritis diagnosis
> - Fracture history
> - Age
> - Estrogen use
> - Weight
>
> **Calculation Formula:**
>
> SCORE = Race + RheumArth + FractureHx + Estrogen + $(3 \times Age/10) - (Weight/10)$
>
> Online calculator available at: https://reference.medscape.com/calculator/osteoporosis-risk-score
>
> *Source:* Geusens, P., Hochberg, M. C., van der Voort, D. J., Pols, H., van der Klift, M., Siris, E., ... Ross, P. (2002). Performance of risk indices for identifying low bone density in postmenopausal women. *Mayo Clinic Proceedings*, 77(7), 629–637. doi:10.4065/77.7.629

to prevent osteoporotic fractures (Grade B). Evidence-based clinical risk assessment tools for osteoporosis include the Simple Calculated Osteoporosis Risk Estimation (SCORE, Merck), Osteoporosis Risk Assessment Instrument (ORAI), Osteoporosis Index of Risk (OSIRIS), and the Osteoporosis Self-Assessment Tool (OST). **Box 15.3** shows the criteria for the SCORE clinical assessment risk tool. Each of these tools have demonstrated moderate accuracy at predicting osteoporosis. Central DXA is the recommended test in lieu of peripheral DXA and quantitative ultrasound. DXA scans should not be repeated more often than once every 2 years (American College of Rheumatology, 2013). There is currently insufficient evidence to screen men of any age for osteoporosis (Grade I).

EVIDENCE-BASED PRACTICE CONSIDERATIONS

The Choosing Wisely Initiative® has multiple recommendations for imaging and treatment considerations for musculoskeletal conditions. The American Medical Society for Sports Medicine (AMSSM), the American College of Rheumatology (ACR), the American Academy of Pediatrics' Orthopaedics (AAP-SOOr) and the Pediatric Orthopaedic Society of North America

(PONSA), the North American Spine Society (NASS), and the American Orthopaedic Foot & Ankle Society (AOFAS) are just some of the organizations that have contributed to the initiative with their recommendations and suggestions for providing better care. These organizations also provide screening, diagnosis, and treatment/intervention guidelines on a variety of conditions. Clinicians should review and become familiar with these guidelines and recommendations statements to ensure they are integrating evidence-based practice into their patient care.

ABNORMAL FINDINGS OF THE MUSCULOSKELETAL SYSTEM

CARPAL TUNNEL SYNDROME

Carpal tunnel syndrome is inflammation and compression of the median nerve as it moves through the carpal tunnel of the wrist. It is common in patients who do repetitive wrist motions such as typing.

Key History and Physical Findings

- Numbness and tingling over the median nerve distribution into the hand (thumb and index, middle or ring fingers; **Figure 15.49**)
- History of repetitive activity such as writing or typing
- Pain with gripping objects
- Decreased grip strength
- Atrophy of thenar eminence (later stages)
- Positive Phalen's and Tinel's tests
- Weakness of thumb strength and opposition

NURSEMAID'S ELBOW (RADIAL HEAD SUBLUXATION)

Nursemaid's elbow is a subluxation of the radial head. It is most often seen in young children, typically occurring after a jerking motion of the arm. It can also be seen if a child falls while holding onto an object, such as monkey bars, leading to the distraction force at the elbow.

Key History and Physical Findings

- Seen in young children, aged 1 to 4
- History of arm jerking motion
- Pain at the elbow or wrist
- Child will not want to move the arm
- Child is holding arm in a flexed and pronated position

DUPUYTREN'S CONTRACTURE

Dupuytren's contracture is a progressive nodularity and flexion contracture of the palmar fascia and digital flexors in the hand (**Figure 15.50**). It happens slowly over years and is usually seen in people over the age of 50. Tobacco, alcohol, and diabetes are all risk factors. Eventually, it can lead to flexion contractures of the MCP and PIP joints.

Key History and Physical Findings

- Commonly seen in fourth and fifth digits
- Inability to completely straighten affected finger(s)
- Nodules on flexor tendons on palmar side of hand
- Without intervention, it can progress to skin puckering and flexion contracture

ROTATOR CUFF TEAR

The rotator cuff is prone to injury owing to the inherent mobility of the shoulder. Tears in the rotator cuff muscles, the supraspinatus, infraspinatus, subscapularis, and teres minor can lead to decreased shoulder movement and strength. It can cause significant deficits when it comes to ADLs. The risk of injury increases with age.

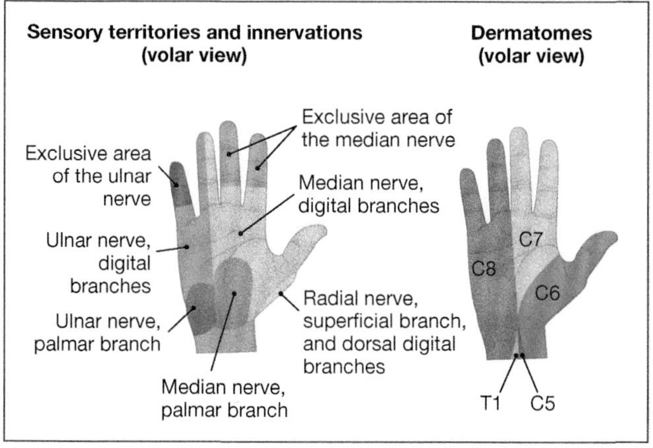

FIGURE 15.49 Median and ulnar nerve distribution (volar view).

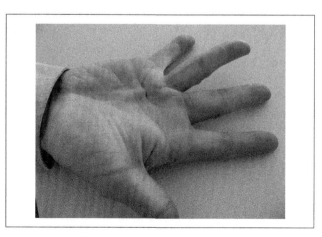

FIGURE 15.50 Dupuytren's contracture.
Source: Image courtesy of Frank C. Müller.

Key History and Physical Findings

- History of traumatic injury or repetitive movements
- Degenerative tears can be exacerbated insidiously
- Pain and weakness with overhead activities
- Dominant arm
- Described pain as a dull ache
- Decreased range of motion, including forward flexion and internal and/or external rotation
- Positive empty can test, external rotation resistance test, and/or the lag test
- Often negative x-rays or with subtle changes
- MRI shows partial or full thickness tear

LATERAL EPICONDYLITIS

Lateral epicondylitis, commonly called tennis elbow, is an inflammation and eventual chronic degeneration of the common extensor bundle on the lateral elbow. It is thought to be an overuse injury, seen in individuals who do activities causing repetitive wrist extension.

Key History and Physical Findings

- Pain over lateral epicondyle of humerus with activation of wrist extensors
- Pain may radiate from the lateral side of the elbow into the forearm and wrist.
- Pain is worse when shaking hands or squeezing objects.
- Pain is worse when holding the wrist stiff or moving the wrist with force.
- Decreased grip strength
- Positive Cozen's test

OSGOOD–SCHLATTER DISEASE

Osgood–Schlatter disease is common in adolescents. When the growth plates are still open, excess force can be generated through the tibial tuberosity, leading to an apophysitis injury. Similar injuries can be seen at the inferior pole of the patella (Sinding-Larsen–Johansson disease) and at the calcaneus (Sever's disease).

Key History and Physical Findings

- Anterior knee pain, centered over tibial tubercle or distal patellar tendon
- Common in adolescents during puberty
- Often worsens during activity and resolves with rest
- Typically unilateral
- Painful, bony bump on the tibia just below the knee

OSTEOARTHRITIS

Wearing of the articular cartilage at the end of the long bones is known as osteoarthritis. A wearing of the cartilage can then lead to increased force seen at the bone, leading to joint space narrowing, osteophyte formation, and sclerosis of the bones. It is often age-related or related to previous trauma.

Key History and Physical Findings

- History of previous trauma or injury
- Pain isolated to single joint
- Pain will often improve with mild-to-moderate activity.
- Pain worsens in the morning and improves throughout the day.
- Worsens with prolonged activity
- Pain typically with active and passive range of motion
- Often decreased range of motion
- Tenderness to palpation over joint line (if applicable)
- Positive x-ray showing joint cartilage degeneration

OSTEOPOROSIS/OSTEOPENIA

Osteoporosis is a condition that causes bones to weaken. This bone condition occurs when the body loses too much bone, does not make enough bone, or both of these issues. As bone density declines, the bones become porous and brittle, and fracture risk increases (**Figure 15.51**). Risk factors include smoking, having a diet low in calcium and/or vitamin D, being a female, certain medications, and lack of weight-bearing exercise. Early stages of bone loss are considered as osteopenia. As the disease progresses, osteoporosis can develop.

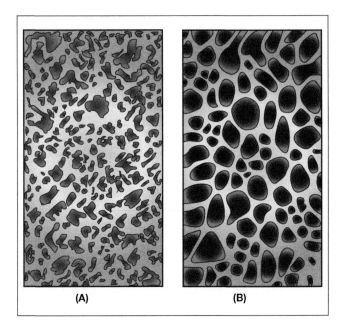

FIGURE 15.51 (A) Normal bone matrix. (B) Osteoporotic bone matrix.

- Typically asymptomatic in the beginning
- Loss of height over time
- Bone fracture, often with no associated trauma
- A t-score <–2.5 indicates osteoporosis; between –1.0 and –2.5 indicates osteopenia

RHEUMATOID ARTHRITIS

RA is a chronic autoimmune inflammatory disease affecting the joints. It is more common in women and can lead to debilitating pain and deformity, most commonly of the MCP and PIP joints in the hands (**Figure 15.52**). The deformity occurs through the stretching of tendons and ligaments and the destruction of joints through the erosion of cartilage and bone. According to the 2010 ACR/European League Against Rheumatism (EULAR) classification criteria for RA, five criteria must be present for diagnosis: inflammatory arthritis involving three or more joints; positive rheumatoid factor (RF) and/or anti-citrullinated peptide/protein antibody (such as anti-cyclic citrullinated peptide [anti-CCP]) testing; elevated levels of C-reactive protein (CRP) or the erythrocyte sedimentation rate (ESR); diseases with similar clinical features have been excluded; and the duration of symptoms is greater than 6 weeks.

Key History and Physical Findings

- More common in women
- Onset typically in middle age
- History of smoking
- Positive family history of RA
- Pain in multiple joints (smaller joints are typically affected first)

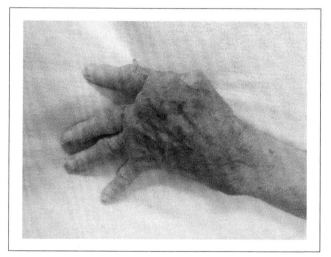

FIGURE 15.52 Ulnar deviation of fingers due to rheumatoid arthritis.
Source: Image courtesy of James Heilman, MD.

- Tender, warm, edematous joints
- Morning stiffness typically lasting more than 1 to 2 hours
- Anorexia
- Fatigue
- Commonly affects PIP and MCP joints first
- Firm lumps (rheumatoid nodules) under the skin that form close to joints
- Ulnar deviation of the fingers
- Positive RF
- Positive antinuclear antibody (ANA)
- Positive anti-CCP serum levels
- Possible short-term elevation of CRP
- Possible long-term elevation of ESR

GOUT

Gout is typically related to hyperuricemia with an excessive amount of uric acid production. The uric acid crystalizes, leading to uric acid crystals being deposited into the synovial fluid. This deposition leads to exquisitely, painful joints. It is most commonly seen in middle-aged men.

Key History and Physical Findings

- History of alcohol use
- Diets high in purines
- Red, inflamed, exquisitely tender joint, most often the thumb, great toe, or knee
- Acute onset with no known injury
- Joint discomfort that lasts several weeks
- Limited range of motion in the affected joint
- Joint aspiration analysis is positive for monosodium urate crystals
- Serum ESR and CRP may be elevated during acute attack

DE QUERVAIN'S SYNDROME

De Quervain's syndrome is a tenosynovitis of the abductor pollicis longus and extensor pollicis brevis tendons. It is often seen in patients with repetitive thumb movements and is an inflammation between the tendon and tendon sheath.

Key History and Physical Findings

- Tenosynovitis of the abductor pollicis longus and extensor pollicis brevis
- A "sticking" sensation in the thumb when moving it
- Pain and edema over radial styloid
- Pain that is exacerbated with active wrist ulnar deviation
- Difficulty moving the thumb and wrist when performing activities that involve grasping or pinching
- Positive Finkelstein's test

CASE STUDY: Knee Pain, Swelling, and Instability

A 22-year-old intramural soccer player presents to clinic complaining of pain, swelling, and instability of her left knee. She states the night before she went to turn and felt a pop in her knee. She did not have immediate pain and tried to continue playing. She was unable to continue due to her knee giving out.

Most Likely Diagnosis

The patient is presenting with classic ACL tear symptoms. It is not uncommon to lack pain in the acute phase of a tear, but instability is the hallmark sign of an ACL tear.

Special Tests

The Lachman test is the gold standard to check for ACL tears. An anterior drawer test also helps to determine ACL laxity. It would also be prudent to check a McMurray's test to evaluate the meniscus as well.

Imaging Considerations

Obtaining an x-ray would be important to ensure there is not a fracture. In adolescents, it is common to have a tibial spine avulsion rather than an ACL tear. An MRI is the definitive imaging for an ACL evaluation, as it allows visualization of the soft tissues of the knee.

Definitive Treatment

ACL reconstruction is the definitive treatment in a young, athletic patient.

Unique Population Considerations

Some patients can do well without having a surgical ACL reconstruction. Typically, these people are not as active, and slightly older. They can trial a course of physical therapy to see how they recover and move to surgical intervention if they are not pleased with conservative measures.

CASE STUDY: Insidious Knee Pain and Limp

A 12-year-old boy presents with insidious knee pain and with a noticeable limp. He denies known injury to the knee. He is mildly overweight. On examination, he has limited range of motion of his hip and knee due to spasm. His Lachman test, anterior drawer test, posterior drawer test, valgus stretch test, varus stretch test, and McMurray's tests were all negative.

Possible Diagnoses

This is the classic presentation of a slipped capital femoral epiphysis (SCFE). Often clinicians can be confused because, though the problem is at the hip,

patients can present with no hip symptoms at all. If only knee x-rays are obtained, the entire diagnosis can be missed.

Imaging Considerations

If the clinician is concerned about a possible SCFE, evaluate the hip joint with x-ray. On x-ray, the head of the femur will have the classic, "scoop of ice cream falling off the cone" appearance.

Definitive Treatment

Once the diagnosis is made, referral should be made to orthopedics for surgical intervention.

Clinical Pearls

- Ask the patient where their musculoskeletal pain is located and have them specifically point to the location with one finger.
- Most clavicular fractures will be mid-shaft.
- It can be helpful to passively extend the shoulder when feeling for the insertion point of the rotator cuff muscles.
- The rhomboids can be palpated with the patient pushing off with their arm internally rotated behind their back (same position for internal rotation lag sign).

Key Takeaways

- History questions for the individual who presents with chronic musculoskeletal problems include assessing for fever, weakness, inability to bear weight, stiffness, and/or swelling.
- History questions for the individual who presents with acute musculoskeletal injury include asking about the mechanism of injury and subsequent limitation in movement.
- To be both systematic and thorough when completing a physical examination related to injury or pain in a joint, remember to begin with inspection, then palpate and assess strength; proceed to assess range of motion and use special tests to note joint stability if there are no obvious deformities or point tenderness.

REFERENCES

American Academy of Pediatrics-Section on Orthopaedics & Pediatric Orthopaedic Society of North America. (2018). *Five things patients and physicians should question.* Retrieved from http://www.choosingwisely .org/societies/american-academy-of-pediatrics-section-on -orthopaedics-and-the-pediatric-orthopaedic-society -of-north-america

American College of Rheumatology. (2013). *Five things patients and physicians should question.* Retrieved from http://www.choosingwisely.org/societies/american-college -of-rheumatology

Betts, J. G., Young, K. A., Wise, J. A., Johnson, E., Poe, B., Kruse, D. H., . . . DeSaix, P. (2013). *Anatomy and physiology.* Houston, TX: OpenStax. Retrieved from http://cnx.org/ contents/14fb4ad7-39a1-4eee-ab6e-3ef2482e3e22@8.24

Beutel, B. G., Trehan, S. K., Shalvoy, R. M., & Mello, M. J. (2012). The Ottawa knee rule: Examining use in an academic emergency department. *The Western Journal of Emergency Medicine, 13*(4), 366–372. doi:10.5811/ westjem.2012.2.6892

Biga, L. M., Dawson, S., Harwell, A., Hopkins, R., Kaufmann, J., LeMaster, M., . . . Runyeon, J. (Eds.). (2019). *Anatomy & physiology.* Corvallis: Open Oregon State. Retrieved from http://library.open.oregonstate.edu/aandp

Centers for Disease Control and Prevention. (n.d.). *What is muscular dystrophy?* Retrieved from https://www.cdc .gov/ncbddd/musculardystrophy/facts.html

Geusens, P., Hochberg, M. C., van der Voort, D. J., Pols, H., van der Klift, M., Siris, E., . . . Ross, P. (2002). Performance of risk indices for identifying low bone density in postmenopausal women. *Mayo Clinic Proceedings, 77*(7), 629–637. doi:10.4065/77.7.629

Hegedus, E. J., Cook, C., Lewis, J., Wright, A., & Park, J. Y. (2015). Combining orthopedic special tests to improve diagnosis of shoulder pathology. *Physical Therapy in Sport, 16,* 87–92. doi:10.1016/j.ptsp.2014.08.001

Jenkin, M., Sitler, M. R., & Kelly, J. D. (2010). Clinical usefulness of the Ottawa ankle rules for detecting fractures of the ankle and midfoot. *Journal of Athletic Training, 45*(5), 480–482. doi:10.4085/1062-6050-45.5.480

Jones, S. J., & Miller, J.-M. (2019). Spurling test. In *StatPearls* [Internet]. Treasure Island, FL: StatPearls Publishing. Retrieved from https://www.ncbi.nlm.nih.gov/books/ NBK493152

Konin, J. G., Wiksten, D. L., Isear, J. A., Jr., & Brader, H. (2002). *Special tests for orthopedic examination* (2nd ed.). Thorofare, NJ. Slack Incorporated.

Lange, T., Matthijs, O., Jain, N. B., Schmitt, J., Lützner, J., & Kopkow, C. (2017). Reliability of specific physical examination tests for the diagnosis of shoulder pathologies: A systematic review and meta-analysis. *British Journal of Sports Medicine, 51,* 511–518. doi:10.1136/ bjsports-2016-096558

Patil, P., & Dasgupta, B. (2012). Role of diagnostic ultrasound in the assessment of musculoskeletal diseases. *Therapeutic Advances in Musculoskeletal Disease, 4*(5), 341–355. doi:10.1177/1759720X12442112

Stiell, I. G., Greenberg, G. H., Wells, G. A., McDowell, I., Cwinn, A. A., Smith, N. A., . . . & Sivilotti, M. L. (1996). Prospective validation of a decision rule for the use of radiography in acute knee injuries. *Journal of the American Medical Association, 275*(8), 611–615. doi:10.1001/ jama.1996.03530320035031

U.S. Department of Health and Human Services, National Institute of Arthritis and Musculoskeletal and Skin Diseases. (2018). *What is bone?* (NIH Publication No.18-7876). Retrieved from https://www.bones.nih.gov/health-info/bone/ bone-health/what-is-bone

U.S. National Library of Medicine. (n.d.). *Aging changes in the bones - muscles - joints.* Retrieved from https://medlineplus .gov/ency/article/004015.htm

U.S. Preventive Services Task Force. (2018). Final recommendation statement: Osteoporosis to prevent fractures: Screening. Retrieved from https://www .uspreventiveservicestaskforce.org/Page/Document/ RecommendationStatementFinal/osteoporosis-screening1

Vigotsky, A. D., Lehman, G. J., Beardsley, C., Chung, B., & Feser, E. H. (2016). The modified Thomas test is not a valid measure of hip extension unless pelvic tilt is controlled. *PeerJ, 4,* e2325. doi:10.7717/peerj.2325

Wieckiewicz, M., Boening, K., Wiland, P., Shiau, Y., & Paradowska-Stolarz, A. (2015). Reported concepts of the treatment modalities and pain management of temporomandibular disorders. *The Journal of Headache and Pain, 16,* 106. doi:10.1186/s10194-015-0586-5

16

Evidence-Based Assessment of the Abdominal, Gastrointestinal, and Urological Systems

Leigh Small, Tammy Spencer, Rosario Medina, Kerry Z. Reed, Sandy Dudley, and Kate Gawlik

"Develop a passion for learning. If you do, you will never cease to grow."

—ANTHONY J. D'ANGELO

 VIDEO

- Patient Case: Young Adult With Abdominal Pain (Appendicitis)

LEARNING OBJECTIVES

- Describe the structure and function of the gastrointestinal system.
- Describe the structure and function of the urological system.
- Understand the components of a comprehensive, evidence-based history and physical exam of the gastrointestinal and urological systems.
- Distinguish between normal and abnormal findings in the gastrointestinal and urological systems.

Visit https://connect.springerpub.com/content/book/978-0-8261 -6454-4/chapter/ch00 to access the videos.

ANATOMY AND PHYSIOLOGY

LANDMARKS, MUSCULATURE, AND CONTENTS OF THE ABDOMEN

Assessment of the **abdomen** requires an understanding of the bony and muscular architecture of the abdomen and the organs, muscles, and structures contained within it (**Figure 16.1**). The abdominal contents lie inferior to the diaphragm and superior to the pelvic floor. The abdominal cavity is framed by the costal margins of the 7th, 8th, 9th, 10th, and 11th ribs and their distal cartilaginous extensions/ends. The bony landmarks that outline the inferior aspect of the abdomen include the right and left iliac crests and the pubic tubercle (**Figure 16.2**). When the patient is lying in the prone position and the posterior aspect of the abdomen is visible, the bony structure overlying the abdomen begins at the T10 spinal vertebrae and the articulating ribs. The inferior aspect of the abdomen in the prone position is formed by the bilateral iliac crests.

The musculature overlying the abdominal cavity serves to protect the inner organs and structures. There are two main muscular layers. The innermost muscle layer comprises the internal obliques and the transverse abdominis muscles. The external muscular layer comprises the external obliques and the rectus abdominis.

443

Therefore, light and deep palpation techniques should be implemented with these muscular layers in mind so that the clinician can approximate what is being palpated and the origin of the pain/discomfort the patient is experiencing. As this muscular structure is designed to protect the organs of the abdomen, it is important to encourage the patient to relax for the examination, which can be facilitated by several distraction strategies discussed in the Physical Examination section of this chapter.

The contents of the abdomen include the gastrointestinal (GI) tract, organs that aid digestion but are not part of the GI tract, and abdominal structures of other systems (accessory digestive organs). In this chapter,

the focus will be the GI tract and the organs that aid digestion (**Figure 16.3**).

Any discomfort to the mid region of the anterior torso is described as **abdominal pain** and is one of the most common reasons for seeking care. Despite the commonality of the symptom, determining the cause of abdominal pain is challenging due to the nonspecific neuro receptors found in the visceral cavity that are only sensitive to stretch and chemical irritation (Hogan-Quigley, Palm, & Bickley, 2012). There are also multiple organs in the viscera, each of which can result in abdominal pain when inflamed or dysfunctional. The most common diagnoses related to abdominal discomfort are "nonspecific" (43% of patients), acute appendicitis (4%–20% of patients), acute cholecystitis (3%–9% of patients), and small bowel obstruction represented by 4% of patients (McGee, 2017). Other common causes of abdominal pain include gastroenteritis, gastritis, peptic ulcer disease (PUD), reflux esophagitis (gastroesophageal reflux disease [GERD]), irritable bowel syndrome (IBS), and diverticulitis (Seller & Symons, 2018).

It is imperative to consider referred pain from different areas of the abdomen or different body systems when assessing for the origin of abdominal pain. The abdomen is commonly divided into either four or nine quadrants in order to describe the location of symptoms and pain (**Figure 16.4**).

The complexity of determining the cause of abdominal pain is related to the structure and function of the abdomen and abdominal contents and requires a comprehensive health history to direct and focus physical assessment and achieve diagnostic accuracy. Abdominal discomfort can be considered functional or organic in cause, and acute or chronic in nature. Acute

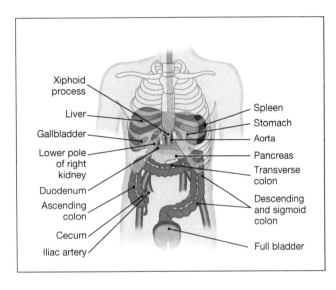

FIGURE 16.1 Abdominal cavity.

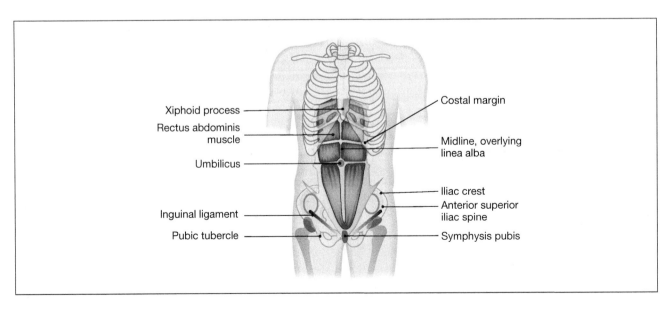

FIGURE 16.2 Abdominal landmarks.

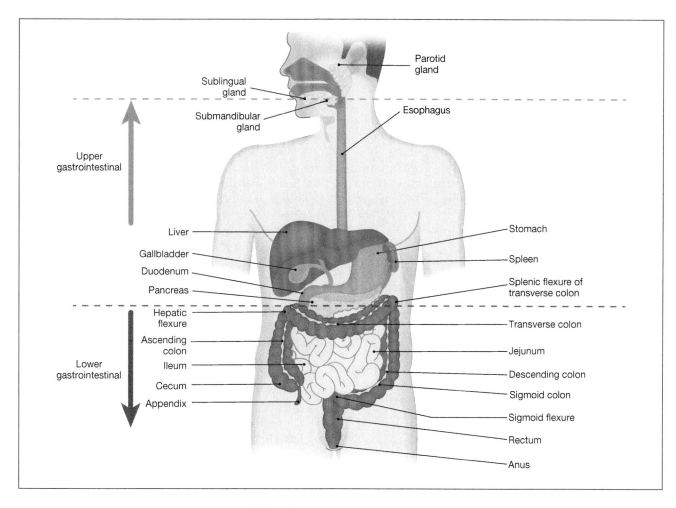

FIGURE 16.3 Gastrointestinal tract.

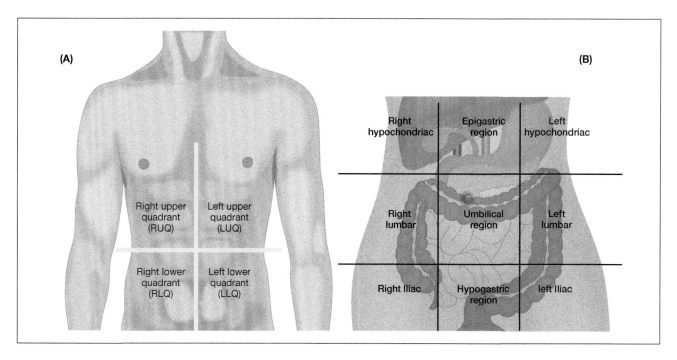

FIGURE 16.4 Quadrants of the abdomen to describe the location and symptoms of pain. (A) Four quadrants. (B) Nine quadrants.

abdominal pain is considered to be any abdominal pain with a sudden onset (Goolsby & Grubbs, 2015) and may indicate a life-threatening situation that requires immediate medical attention (Seller & Symons, 2018). It is more difficult to determine an accurate description of pain from young children because of language and cognitive limitations and an older adult who presents with multiple preexisting conditions (Seller & Symons, 2018). It is imperative for the clinician to be familiar with the underlying structures and organs found in the abdomen. Knowing this anatomy greatly assists the clinician in determining the correct diagnosis.

GASTROINTESTINAL TRACT

The GI tract includes the alimentary canal and the accessory organs. Each component plays an integral role in the digestive system. The alimentary canal is a hollow muscular tube that extends from the oral cavity (mouth) to the anus, much of which lies in the abdominal cavity. The accessory organs that are attached to the alimentary canal include the liver, gallbladder, and pancreas. The vermiform appendix, while it does not aid in digestion, is an appendage stemming from the cecum and should be noted because it can play a role in the assessment of the abdomen and consideration of diagnoses.

The mouth and esophagus mark the beginning of the alimentary canal. After the physical breakdown of food by chewing (mastication), the food passes down the pharynx to the stomach through the esophagus (D'Amico & Barbarito, 2016). Although not in the abdominal cavity, damage or dysfunction of the esophagus can result in significant pain or symptoms, which require assessment and diagnosis. Through the coordinated muscular action of peristalsis, food is propelled into the stomach. At the lower end of the esophagus is the lower esophageal sphincter (LES), sometimes referred to as the cardiac sphincter. This is a critical juncture that separates the esophagus (usually at a normal pH) from the stomach and stomach acid (a low pH). Low or poor LES pressures fail to keep the stomach contents from entering the esophagus and result in acid reflux or GERD.

The stomach extends from the LES to the pyloric sphincter that marks the beginning of the duodenum. The stomach is located in the left upper abdomen just beneath the xiphoid process and inferior to the diaphragm. It is a sac-like structure, and its purpose is to facilitate the physical and chemical digestion of food by mixing it with digestive juices and acid. At this point, the food is now referred to as *chyme*.

Chyme leaves the stomach through the pyloric sphincter into the small intestine. The primary purpose of the small intestine is to facilitate further digestion and absorption. The three segments of the small intestine are the duodenum, jejunum, and ileum. The most striking aspect of the small intestine is its length at 18 to 21 feet. Within the lumen of the small intestine are villi that further increase the digestive surface of the intestine. Through coordinated neuromuscular innervation, the peristaltic waves propel chyme through the small intestine. Bile and digestive enzymes are secreted in the duodenum, promoting the digestion of fats and starches. Chyme flows from the duodenum to the jejunum. In the jejunum, absorption of nutrients in the form of minerals, electrolytes, carbohydrates, proteins, and fats occurs. The primary digestive actions that occur in the ileum are the absorption of vitamin B12 and bile salts. The end of the ileum is marked by the terminal ileum and ileocecal valve or sphincter. This valve controls the flow of chyme into the large intestine. Inflammation of the terminal ileum is called terminal ileitis. **Crohn's disease** is an **inflammatory bowel disease** (IBD) that frequently affects the ileum and terminal ileum.

The last portion of the alimentary canal is the large intestine, or large bowel. The large intestine is approximately 5 to 6 feet in length and is composed of seven segments: the cecum, ascending colon, transverse colon, descending colon, sigmoid colon, rectum, and anus (**Figure 16.5**). The vermiform appendix is attached to the proximal portion of the cecum and does not contribute to digestion; however, it can become inflamed and lead to a number of health problems. The large intestine, as the name implies, is wider and shorter than the small intestine and its main functions are to absorb water and electrolytes from the chyme and facilitate the elimination of the residual, undigested food as feces. The ileocecal valve is a sphincter muscle that prevents the backflow of chyme from the cecum back to the ileum. The cecum is very short and marks the beginning

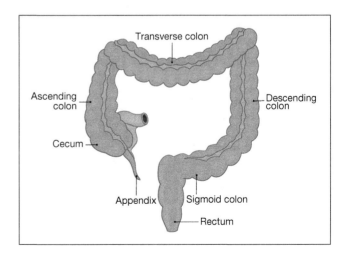

FIGURE 16.5 Anatomy of the large intestine.

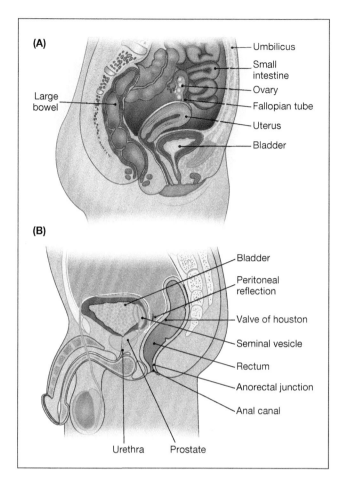

FIGURE 16.6 Anus and rectum (sagittal view). (A) Female. (B) Male.

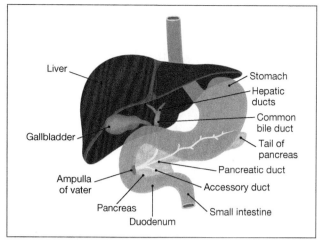

FIGURE 16.7 Accessory digestive organs.

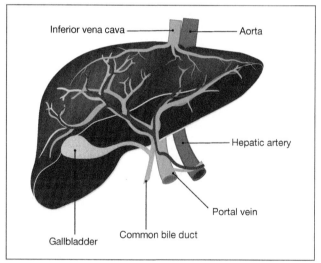

FIGURE 16.8 Anatomy of the liver.

of the ascending colon that lies on the right side of the abdomen. The ascending colon ends just beneath the liver and gallbladder at a bend known as the hepatic flexure. Thirty percent of cancerous tumors are found in the ascending colon. The transverse colon lies inferior to the stomach and it crosses the abdominal cavity where it becomes the descending colon (down the left side of the abdomen). The descending colon ends in the sigmoid colon, rectum, and anus (**Figure 16.6**).

ACCESSORY DIGESTIVE ORGANS

Other organs of the abdomen contribute to the function of the GI system and the digestion of food. These accessory digestive organs include the liver, gallbladder, and pancreas (**Figure 16.7**).

The liver is located in the right upper quadrant (RUQ) of the abdomen. It is a triangular- or wedge-shaped organ and is in charge of over 500 vital functions for the body (**Figure 16.8**). The liver is composed of two lobes. Within each lobe, there are many smaller lobes called lobules. These lobules are made up of hepatocytes. Hepatocytes are the main functional cells of the

liver and perform metabolic, endocrine, and secretory functions for the body. All blood that leaves the stomach and intestine passes through and is processed by the liver. Some of the key functions of the liver include metabolizing nutrients to produce energy for the body; producing bile, immune factors, cholesterol, and multiple types of essential proteins; breaking down harmful substances including bacteria and poisonous substances; converting ammonia to urea; removing bilirubin; regulating blood clotting; processing hemoglobin to extract its iron; and regulating blood levels of amino acids (Siddiqui, 2018).

The liver is protected by the lower right portion of the rib cage (ribs 6–10) and it extends across the abdomen and over the stomach. It can range in its span from 2 to 6 inches (6–15 cm); however, it is usually 4

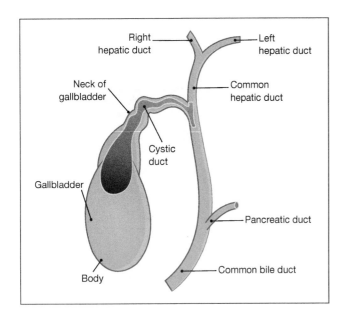

FIGURE 16.9 Anatomy of the gallbladder.

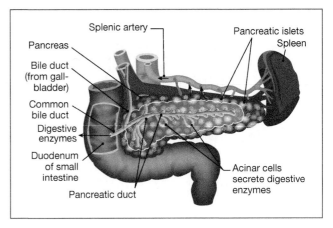

FIGURE 16.10 Anatomy of the pancreas.

to 5 inches (11–12 cm). The anatomical location of the liver below the ribs and its rubbery texture make palpation difficult, resulting in clinicians' underestimating the liver edge and span as compared with ultrasound (Pinsky & Wipf, n.d.).

Bile is transported out of the liver via a network of ducts. The common bile duct is formed by the junction of the common hepatic and cystic ducts. The majority (about 75%) of the bile secreted from the liver passes from the common hepatic duct into the gallbladder via the cystic duct. The rest of the bile drains directly into the common bile duct and into the duodenum. Blockage, stasis, inflammation, and infection of the ducts can cause significant pathology (Siddiqui, 2018).

The gallbladder stores bile in a thin-walled, pear-shaped sac, and it is located on the inferior, ventral surface of the liver, at the right mid-clavicular line (**Figure 16.9**). The digestive purpose of the gallbladder is to release bile stores into the duodenum via the common bile duct when stimulated. The bile promotes emulsification of fats.

The pancreas is a 6-inch long, thin gland that is located just below the stomach (**Figure 16.10**). There are two primary purposes of the pancreas. Digestive enzymes are produced and secreted into the duodenum through the pancreatic duct; this action makes the pancreas an exocrine gland. The other role of the pancreas is the production and release of insulin into the bloodstream; this action makes the pancreas an endocrine gland. Both the common bile duct and the pancreatic duct join together and release their digestive products into the duodenum through the ampulla of vater as controlled by the sphincter of Oddi. Advanced medical technology and endoscopic techniques now allow

noninvasive intervention in this small system of ducts and glands that cause multiple health problems.

URINARY SYSTEM

The urinary system also lies within the abdomen and includes the kidneys, ureters, urinary bladder, urethra, and the renal circulatory system (arteries and veins; **Figure 16.11**). The primary function of the urological system is to filter wastes, toxins, and foreign matter from the bloodstream. This is a sterile system. In addition to this, the kidneys prevent the accumulation of nitrogenous wastes, help to balance fluids and electrolytes, assist in the maintenance of blood pressure, and play a role in erythropoiesis. A discussion of each structure is outlined in the text that follows.

The kidneys are bean-shaped structures found in the retroperitoneal space (posterior to the abdominal peritoneum), protected by the 11th and 12th ribs at the costovertebral angle between T12 and L3 of the vertebral column (**Figure 16.12**). The left kidney is positioned slightly higher than the right. An adrenal gland lies on top of each kidney. Each kidney is composed of approximately one million nephrons, which are the functional units within the kidney. Nephrons contain glomeruli to filter the blood and tubules to excrete waste products and return filtered blood into the circulatory system. As a result of the needed proximity of the circulatory system to the kidney, each kidney has a renal artery that perfuses the kidney and a renal vein for the filtered blood to return to the circulatory system. Blood is supplied to the kidneys via the renal arteries that branch off the descending aorta and the renal veins return blood to the inferior vena cava.

After the blood is filtered, waste products, excess water, and electrolytes are excreted by the nephrons as urine and are eliminated from the kidney via a ureter. The urine flows through the ureters, aided by peristalsis, to the bladder which acts as a reservoir and holds

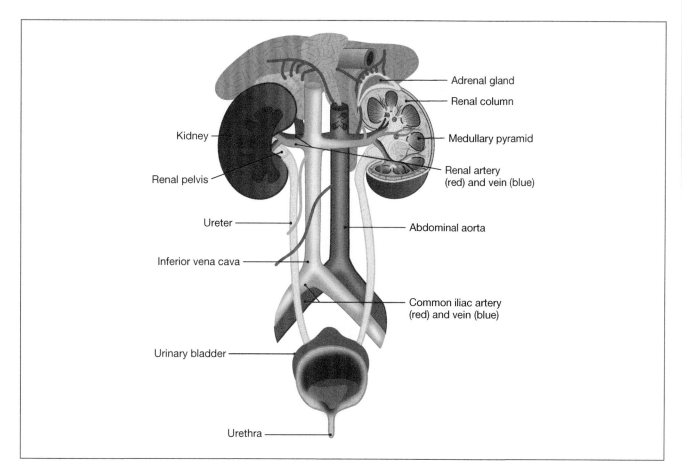

FIGURE 16.11 The renal system.

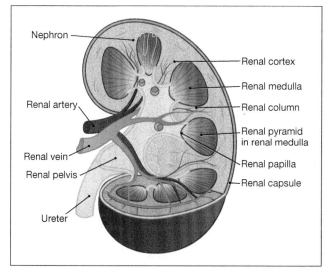

FIGURE 16.12 Anatomy of the kidney.

above the symphysis pubis. There are two parts of the bladder: (a) the rounded muscular sac composed of the detrusor muscle and (b) the urethra. The detrusor muscle allows urine to collect in the bladder and then contracts to empty the urine from the bladder into the urethra. This process is micturition (urination). When empty, the bladder lies low in the pelvis behind the symphysis pubis; however, when the bladder is full, the bladder fundus becomes palpable. In males, the neck of the bladder is encircled by the prostate. In females, the bladder lies anterior to the vagina and uterus.

The urethra is a single tube-like structure that is mucous lined (**Figure 16.13**). The length of the urethra is approximately 1.5 inches in females and approximately 20 inches in males. The urethra ends with the urethral opening, which is close to the anus in females. The short length of the urethra and proximity to the anus in females allow it to become contaminated with bacteria much more easily compared with the male urethra.

SPLEEN

The spleen is an organ of the immune system that is found in the left mid-axillary line when assessing the

the urine before micturition. Each ureter is approximately 10 to 12 inches (25–30 cm) in length.

The bladder is a hollow, muscular organ that lies on the pelvic floor of the retroperitoneal space located just

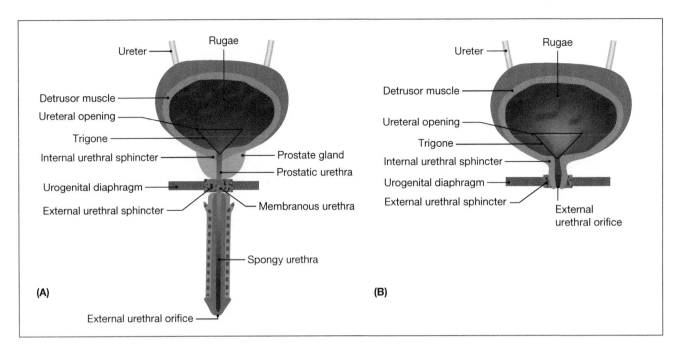

FIGURE 16.13 The urinary system. (A) Male. (B) Female.

abdomen. This small organ varies in size but is commonly fist-shaped and approximately 4 inches long. The spleen filters the blood, removing old or damaged red blood cells (RBCs) and old platelets; stores breakdown products of red blood cells and lymphocytes; returns the RBC breakdown products to the bone marrow; and fights infections. The spleen also stores blood that can be released in the case of significant blood loss. For additional information about the spleen's role in the immune system, refer to Chapter 10, Evidence-Based Assessment of the Lymphatic System.

LIFE-SPAN DIFFERENCES AND CONSIDERATIONS IN ANATOMY AND PHYSIOLOGY

The organs within the abdomen grow in size and function/dysfunction over the life course. For example, the size and location of the stomach changes from a horizontal position to a more vertical position as an infant grows. This change in the pitch of the stomach changes the food bolus to the distal portion of the stomach and increases the LES pressure. This results in a significant reduction of reflux of gastric contents over time. At age 4 months, approximately 50% of infants have GERD; however, by 12 months of age, only 5% to 10% have GERD (Esposito et al., 2015). Children often swallow more air compared with adults as they learn to coordinate eating, sucking, and swallowing. Therefore, the abdomen of a young child is more tympanic than that of adults.

The appearance of the abdomen changes during the life course, too. Infants have less abdominal muscle tone than do older children and have a protuberant abdomen. Interestingly, the older adult begins to lose muscle tone and often gains abdominal adiposity leading to a protuberant abdomen. Infants, as well as older adults, experience changes in dietary intake, the coordination of peristalsis (i.e., delayed gastric emptying time), and changes in the secretion of digestive enzymes or water reabsorption leading to indigestion, constipation, increased flatulence, and/or diarrhea.

Growth and maturation also change the organ functioning as well as structure. Infants have a significant change in blood flow and glomerular filtration compared with fetal functioning. This continues to increase until the first or second year of life. Fluid balance in young children is fragile because they are more prone to fluid loss due to thinner skin, proportionately greater skin surface, and susceptibility to illnesses that may cause significant and rapid imbalances in fluids and electrolytes and metabolic acidosis (e.g., GI illness).

Pregnancy presents a unique situation to women in terms of urinary functioning. During pregnancy, a growing uterus places pressure on the bladder, causing changes in urinary frequency which is most evident in the first and third trimester. This is accentuated by the increased production of urine in pregnancy. There is a tendency for some pregnant women to test positive for glucose in their urine (glycosuria), which may cause increased frequency and/or urgency of urination. Following childbirth, some women find that they have stress incontinence. In these situations, the weakened or damaged urethral sphincter or pelvic floor muscles are unable to stop urination (incontinence) to various degrees when there is stress on the bladder such as laughing, sneezing, jumping, or exercising (Bardsley, 2016).

Aging affects kidney size and functioning. The weight of the kidneys may drop by up to 30% and perfusion gradually decreases. Thirty to fifty percent of glomeruli degenerate due to fibrosis, hyalinization, and fat deposition leading to loss of the filtration surface area by age 75. Other age-related challenges to the urological system include hydration, urine concentrating ability, decreasing effectiveness of antidiuretic hormone, and reduced capacity to produce ammonia. The combination of these issues and the increase in urinary retention that comes with age makes the older adult prone to increased **urinary tract infection** (UTI), frequency, urgency, and urinary incontinence.

KEY HISTORY QUESTIONS AND CONSIDERATIONS

HISTORY OF PRESENT ILLNESS

Common reasons for seeking care include abdominal pain, nausea and vomiting, diarrhea, constipation, and urinary incontinence. Key history related to both GI and genitourinary (GU) disorders and systems are listed to guide decision-making regarding differential diagnoses. As an individual's history related to their presenting illness or reason for seeking care is reviewed, clinicians should be aware of red flags that indicate serious illness; these are listed in **Box 16.1**.

Example: Abdominal Pain

- Onset: Recent, chronic, reoccurring
- Location: Suprasternal, epigastric, left/right of the epigastric region, radiating to the back, periumbilical, diffuse, lower abdomen, right/left upper or lower quadrant
- Pain quality: Sharp, crampy, burning, dull, achy, squeezing
- Pain intensity: Severe, moderate, mild (intensity is easier to assess in acute pain. Indirect questions may help assess chronic pain such as if pain interferes with sleep or daily function.)
- Duration: Constant, intermittent or reoccurring—lasting minutes, hours, days
- Associated symptoms: Fever, nausea/vomiting, diarrhea/constipation, arthritis/arthralgias, rashes, headaches, anorexia, weight loss, jaundice, dysuria, urgency and/or frequency of urination, hematuria

---

BOX 16.1
RED FLAGS: CONCERNING SIGNS AND SYMPTOMS OF GI/GU SYSTEMS

- Arthritis
- Bilious emesis
- Deceleration of linear growth
- Delayed onset of puberty
- Dysphagia
- Family history of IBD, Lynch's syndrome, celiac disease, PUD, Barrett's esophagus, or hepatobiliary disease
- Hematuria
- Hematemesis
- Hepatosplenomegaly
- Nighttime pain or diarrhea
- Oral ulcers
- Perianal skin tags/fissures
- Persistent RUQ or RLQ pain
- Persistent vomiting or diarrhea
- Recurrent unexplained fever
- Rectal bleeding or melena
- Severe flank pain
- Severe groin pain
- Unexplained anemia
- Unintentional weight loss

GI, gastrointestinal; GU, genitourinary; IBD, inflammatory bowel disease; PUD, peptic ulcer disease; RLQ, right lower quadrant; RUQ, right upper quadrant.

- Aggravating/alleviating factors: Food ingestion, certain positions, passage of flatus or stool
- Treatment tried: Pharmacological treatments including acid-suppressives, laxatives, over-the-counter (OTC) pain relief

Differential Diagnoses

Functional GI disorder (IBS, abdominal migraine, functional abdominal pain syndrome, constipation), celiac disease, IBD, cholelithiasis, pancreatitis, esophagitis/gastritis, PUD, eosinophilic esophagitis, UTI, **pyelonephritis**, **appendicitis**, small bowel obstruction, gastroenteritis, hepatitis, abdominal aortic aneurysm (AAA), GERD, ectopic pregnancy, ovarian cyst, diverticulitis (Cosford, Leng, & Thomas, 2007)

Example: Nausea and Vomiting

- Onset: Acute (1–2 days), chronic (lasting >1 week)
- Triggers: Meal ingestion; delayed, early morning, unknown

- Character of vomiting: Undigested food, partial digested food, bile, blood, volume
- Frequency: Daily, intermittent
- Associated symptoms: Pain, diarrhea/constipation, fever, early satiety, heartburn, bloating, myalgia, weight loss, headaches, visual changes, altered mentation, neck stiffness, dizziness, palpitations
- Aggravating/alleviating factors: Food ingestion, sleep
- Treatment tried: Acid-suppressive medication

Differential Diagnoses

Functional GI disorder causing vomiting (functional regurgitation, rumination syndrome, cyclic vomiting syndrome), infection, celiac disease, GERD, peptic ulcers, *Helicobacter pylori*, gastric outlet obstruction, gastroparesis, chronic intestinal pseudo-obstruction, recurrent pancreatitis, cholecystitis, cholelithiasis, acute hepatitis, appendicitis, gastroenteritis, adverse medication reaction, alcohol induced, neurological cause, pregnancy

Example: Diarrhea

- Onset: Acute (<3 weeks), abrupt, gradual
- Character of diarrhea: Volume, consistency (watery, soft/unformed), greasy/bulky/foul-smelling, bloody
- Triggers: Dairy products, meals, certain foods, contaminated foods, uncertain
- Frequency: Daily, intermittent, number of stools per day, nocturnal stools
- Other pertinent questions for acute diarrhea: Travel, sexual practices, exposure to well water or poorly cooked food, exposure to high risk persons in day care, hospitals or nursing homes, change in diet
- Associated symptoms: Abdominal pain, pain with stooling, incontinence, fever, weight loss, nausea/vomiting
- Relieving factors and treatment tried: OTC medications, dietary changes, fluid intake

Differential Diagnoses

Functional GI disorder (chronic nonspecific diarrhea, IBS, overflow encopresis), infection, drugs, ingestion of osmotic substance, celiac disease, IBD, food allergy, gastroenteritis, postenteritis syndrome, inborn errors of electrolyte transport, carbohydrate intolerance, pancreatic disease (cystic fibrosis, Schwachman–Diamond)

Example: Constipation

- Onset: Birth/life long, recent change in bowel habits, recurrent periods of constipation
- Questions for the pediatric population: Meconium passage, onset of constipation (transition to formula/spoon feeds, toilet training, beginning school), overflow soiling, retentive posturing during stooling
- Frequency of stools: Daily, weekly
- Character of stool: Large/bulky, hard, presence of blood
- Associated symptoms: Pain, straining, bloating, sense of incomplete evacuation, urine infection, urinary incontinence, nausea/vomiting, heartburn, early satiety, weight loss/gain, intermittent episodes of diarrhea
- Aggravating and alleviating factors: Dietary choices, fluids, activity level
- Treatment tried: Review current and past use of medications to relieve symptoms

Differential Diagnoses

Functional GI disorder causing constipation (constipation, fecal retention, IBS), Hirschsprung's disease, celiac disease, mechanical obstruction (colorectal neoplasm, strictures from diverticulitis, anal narrowing), hypothyroidism, tethered cord, dairy/food intolerance

Example: Urinary Incontinence

- Onset: May be a rapid, strong urge to urinate, little to no urge to urinate, or inability of the individual to reach the restroom in time to urinate
- Character: Mild leaking to total loss of bladder control
- Aggravating factors or triggers: Sneezing; coughing; laughing; jumping; exercising; UTI; certain drinks, foods, and medications; pregnancy; menopause; prostate hypertrophy; urinary tract obstruction; and overweight/obesity
- Frequency and duration: Daily, occasion, rare
- Alleviating factors and treatment tried: Avoidance of exercise or activity, medications

Differential Diagnoses

Stress incontinence, urge incontinence, overflow incontinence, functional incontinence, mixed-type incontinence

MEDICAL HISTORY FOR GASTROINTESTINAL CONCERNS

- Chronic diseases (cancers, congenital disorders, autoimmune disorders)
- Food allergies
- Birth history, meconium passage
- History of abdominal surgeries
- Development and growth
- Recent illness, trauma
- Cardiovascular disease (history of myocardial infarction)

- Mental health conditions
- History of *H. pylori*

FAMILY HISTORY FOR GASTROINTESTINAL CONCERNS

- Family history of GI disease (celiac disease, IBD, GERD, eosinophilic esophagitis [EoE], liver disease, IBS)
- Cancer (esophageal, gallbladder, liver, pancreatic, gastric, small intestine, colon, rectal)
- Autoimmune disorders (thyroid disease, diabetes mellitus type 1, IBD)
- Polyposis syndromes (including Lynch's syndrome)
- Cystic fibrosis
- Migraines
- Mental health disorders (mild, moderate, or severe anxiety; depression; mental illness)

SOCIAL HISTORY FOR GASTROINTESTINAL CONCERNS

- Impact on daily living (missing school/work)
- Family dynamics/environment
- Socioeconomic factors
- Life event stress
- Emotional/behavioral symptoms
- Recent travel out of the country
- Exposure to lakes/streams
- Animal or food contact
- Smoking history/history of tobacco use
- Substance use including alcohol

MEDICAL HISTORY FOR URINARY CONCERNS

- History of UTI and/or pyelonephritis (any untreated UTIs)
- Incontinence: Current, acute, chronic
- Recent or previous vaginal childbirth
- Overweight/obesity
- Pelvic prolapse
- Neurological disease or disorders including neurogenic bladder
- Dementia and/or confusion
- Diabetes and/or hypertension
- Benign prostatic hypertrophy
- Disability related to mobility; arthritis
- Medications including diuretics, antibiotics, anticholinergics, hypertensive medications
- Hematuria

FAMILY HISTORY FOR URINARY CONCERNS

- Chronic diseases: Hypertension, diabetes, arthritis
- Overweight/obesity
- Renal or bladder carcinoma
- Diabetes

SOCIAL HISTORY FOR URINARY CONCERNS

- Caffeine intake
- Sexual activity
- Water/fluid intake
- Impact on daily living (missing school/work)
- Family dynamics/environment
- Socioeconomic factors
- Stressors
- Smoking history/history of tobacco use
- Substance use including alcohol

REVIEW OF SYSTEMS FOR GASTROINTESTINAL/ GENITOURINARY SYSTEMS

- General: Fever, fatigue, malaise, anorexia, weight loss, weight gain
- Cardiovascular/respiratory: Chest pain, ankle edema, dyspnea
- GI: Abdominal pain, nausea, vomiting, constipation, diarrhea, heartburn, increased abdominal girth, irritable bowel symptoms, and/or dysphagia
- GU: Dysuria, urinary frequency and/or urgency, suprapubic pain, lower back pain (flank pain), hematuria, turbid or cloudy urine, foul-smelling urine, concentrated or dilute urine
- Reproductive: Vaginal or urethral discharge, recent or current pregnancy
- Neurological: Memory loss, confusion, disorientation, mental/physical disability
- Musculoskeletal: Back pain, muscle aches, arthritic joints, arthritis pain
- Psychiatric: Mild, moderate, or severe anxiety, depression, or mental illness

PREVENTIVE CARE CONSIDERATIONS RELATED TO THE GASTROINTESTINAL SYSTEM

- Health lifestyle behaviors including diet and exercise
- Proper food handling and cooking
- Colonoscopy

LIFE-SPAN CONSIDERATIONS FOR HISTORY

Developmental changes related to cognition are likely to cause significant complexities when noting historical information. For example, young children may have difficulty identifying where their pain is located and how to describe their discomfort. Somewhat similarly, the older adult with cognitive declines in memory, dementia, or Alzheimer's disease may not be able to articulate discomfort or location of the discomfort. Because historical questions related to the abdomen are often based on the understanding of a series of events (i.e., proximity to eating, consequences after eating certain foods) and because infants/toddlers and older adults may not always be in the care of the primary historian, clinicians may have incomplete or inaccurate information.

UNIQUE POPULATION CONSIDERATION FOR HISTORY

A reported history of recent increased abdominal girth, weight gain, ankle edema, and/or a history of hepatitis are suggestive of liver disease; recognizing health disparities on the basis of race and ethnicity especially for liver disease is essential for early diagnosis. Hepatitis C (HCV), for example, occurs more commonly in Asian and African Americans. This may be the result of the global prevalence rates. The infection rates are estimated to be high (>3.5%) in Central and East Asia, North Africa, and the Middle East; as intermediate (1.5%–3.5%) in South and Southeast Asia, sub-Saharan Africa, Central and Southern Latin America, Caribbean, Oceania, Australia, and Central, Eastern, and Western Europe; and low (<1.5%) in Asia-Pacific, Tropical Latin America, and North America (Mohd Hanafiah, Groeger, Flaxman, & Wiersma, 2013). While hepatitis C rates are higher in the countries noted, chronic hepatitis C in the United States is now estimated at 4 million, with 50% to 75% of those infected being unaware; the Centers for Disease Control and Prevention (CDC, n.d.) recommends screening individuals born between 1945 and 1965.

GI disorders overall occur disproportionately in certain ethnic groups. Gallstones and gallbladder cancer have an increased prevalence in Mexican Americans and Native Americans. Gastric or stomach cancer is more common in individuals from Japan, China, Southern and Eastern Europe, and South and Central America. The prevalence of substance use disorders, including alcoholism and addiction, impacts the prevalence of liver disease for at-risk populations, including Native Americans and African Americans.

PHYSICAL EXAMINATION

PREPARATION FOR THE EXAMINATION

Assessment of other body systems proceeds as follows: inspection, palpation, percussion, and auscultation. In the abdominal exam, the sequence is inspection, auscultation, percussion, and palpation. Palpation should occur last because there is the possibility that pain can be elicited during this aspect of the exam and can alter the clinical findings that occur following the occurrence of pain.

To prepare for the exam, ensure adequate lighting and a patient who is relaxed. This allows for a thorough examination of the abdomen and underlying abdominal organs and structures. Make sure the patient has been adequately draped with the abdomen exposed while maintaining privacy of the genitalia and breasts. Several techniques, such as deep breathing and having the patient empty their bladder before the exam, can be helpful to relax the abdominal musculature, maintain patient comfort, and assist in all elements of the abdominal exam, especially palpation. The patient should be placed in the supine position with the arms at the side and knees bent. Positioning the patient with their arms above the head can cause the abdominal muscles to have tension, making the abdominal exam difficult. A warm room and stethoscope can also help to relax tense abdominal muscles. Any painful areas should be examined last to prevent muscle guarding and decrease patient anxiety due to fear of pain.

INSPECTION

Inspection of the abdomen is similar to inspection of any other body system. It requires a keen sense of observation and yields a surprising amount of information. While performing inspection of the abdomen, think about the underlying organs. This will be important when thinking about differential diagnoses and symptom management. Use tangential lighting while seated next to the patient in order to highlight skin characteristics and color as well as the contour of the abdomen and any underlying organs or masses. Inspect the abdomen from the side as well as while looking down at the abdomen for symmetry and contour. The contour of the abdomen—described as flat, scaphoid, rounded, or protuberant—equates to the nutritional status of the patient, and may also be associated with gas, enlarged organs, or fluid (**Figure 16.14**). Inspect the skin for bruises, discoloration, and lesions (Williams & Simel, 1992).

Note any scars as they may give clues about previous surgical interventions related to the abdomen. The umbilicus should be in the midline position without obvious venous patterns, hernias, or nodules. Visible pulsations of the aorta and peristalsis may be seen in the epigastric area in thin patients.

Ask the patient to take a deep breath and hold it; this helps to lower the diaphragm and move the abdominal organs downward to better assess bulges or masses that may not have been previously noted. When performing this maneuver, the abdominal contour should remain symmetric and smooth. Following this maneuver, ask the patient to raise their head off the exam table. This allows the abdominal muscles to contract, and again allows the clinician to assess for previously undetected masses, bulges, or nodules.

Ecchymosis is an ominous finding on the abdominal visual inspection as this can be an indicator of abdominal trauma and/or hemorrhage. Specifically, Grey Turner's sign (flank ecchymosis; **Figure 16.15**) and Cullen's

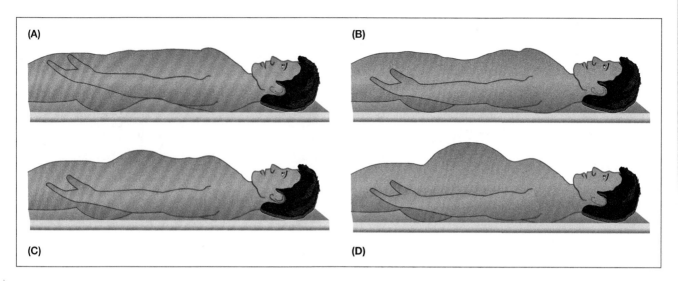

FIGURE 16.14 Inspection of the abdomen: abdominal contour. (A) Flat. (B) Scaphoid. (C) Rounded. (D) Protuberant.

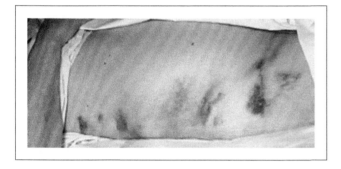

FIGURE 16.15 Grey Turner's sign.
Source: Image courtesy of Herbert L. Fred, MD and Hendrik A. van Dijk.

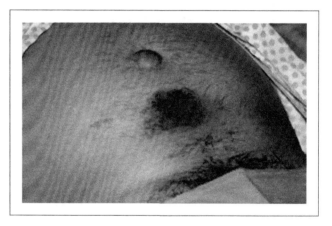

FIGURE 16.16 Cullen's sign.
Source: Image courtesy of Herbert L. Fred, MD and Hendrik A. van Dijk.

sign (umbilical ecchymosis; **Figure 16.16**) are rare findings that have been thought to be important clues to abdominal hemorrhage, acute pancreatitis, or ectopic pregnancy; however, controversy exists about whether these signs are sensitive or specific for these conditions (Wright, 2016). Note that abdominal visual findings are important but do not seem to be specifically related to ectopic pregnancy or acute pancreatitis; more evidence is needed to identify whether and how abdominal ecchymosis indicates internal hemorrhage.

Another visual abdominal finding is a Sister Mary Joseph nodule. This umbilical nodule can either be an initial sign of malignancy or a sign of a metastatic cancer (**Figure 16.17**). Individuals with this finding often succumb to cancer quickly. Inspection of the abdomen for obvious swelling, deformities, and skin changes is essential for individuals who present with weight loss, fatigue, loss of appetite, and/or abdominal distention.

Jaundice is another important visual finding that should be noted as well as abdominal venous patterns.

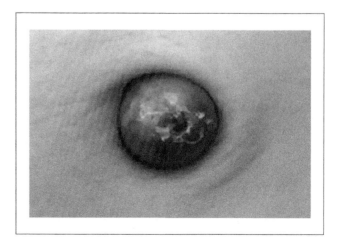

FIGURE 16.17 Sister Mary Joseph nodule.

These visual findings may suggest liver involvement of various etiologies. Evidence suggests that the probability of hepatocellular disease in patients with jaundice increases with various assessment findings; with a palpable spleen (+LR [likelihood ratio], 2.9), with abdominal ascites (+LR, 4.4), with spider angiomas (+LR, 4.7), with palmar erythema (+LR, 9.8), and with dilated abdominal veins (+LR, 17.5; McGee, 2017).

AUSCULTATION

Historically, clinicians have listened for abdominal bowels sounds; however, the auscultation of bowel sounds has limited value in the clinical setting in terms of being an accurate diagnostic tool. The lack of usefulness of auscultation of bowel sounds as a diagnostic tool is heavily reported in the literature (Durup-Dickenson, Christensen, & Gade, 2013; Felder, Margel, Murrell, & Fleshner, 2014; Massey, 2012). Although a few small studies point to auscultation of bowel sounds as being a useful diagnostic tool (Gade, Kruse, Anderson, Pedersen, & Boesby, 1998; Gu, Lim, & Moser, 2010), the majority of available evidence does not exist to recommend auscultating bowel sounds (Zuin, Rigatelli, Andreotti, Fogato, & Roncon, 2017).

Listen for vascular sounds or bruits, which may indicate turbulent blood flow associated with vascular disease. Auscultate for bruits over the aorta (**Figure 16.18**), iliac, renal (**Figure 16.19**), and femoral arteries. Normally, no bruits are auscultated. Abdominal bruits (during systole) heard in the epigastric region of the abdomen are likely a normal finding in a healthy person; however, continuous bruits (across systole and diastole) or a bruit heard away from the midline are more concerning and deserve a more focused assessment. Friction rubs may also be heard over the liver and spleen due to inflammation of the peritoneal surface of these organs from a mass or tumor.

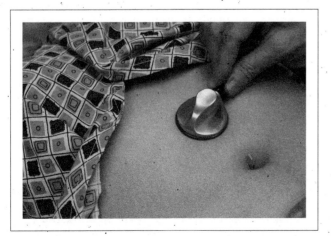

FIGURE 16.18 Auscultation of abdominal aorta.

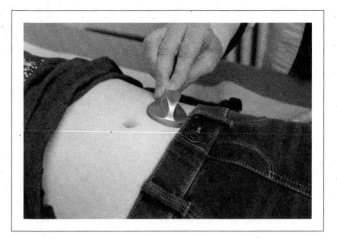

FIGURE 16.19 Auscultation of renal arteries.

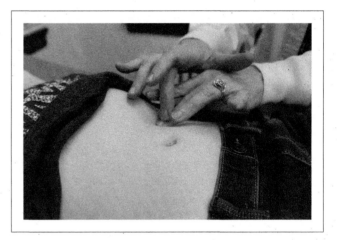

FIGURE 16.20 Abdominal percussion technique.

PERCUSSION

Percussion helps to assess the size, density, and location of abdominal organs and structures. In addition, percussion can help to detect fluid or air in the abdomen. To percuss, place the distal joint and tip of the middle finger of the nondominant hand firmly on the abdomen, avoiding the ribs (**Figure 16.20**). Do not place any other portion of the hand on the abdomen as doing this will dampen the percussion notes. Use the middle finger of the dominant hand to strike the distal interphalangeal joint of the stationary finger on the abdomen. Use short, quick motions while listening for the percussion tone produced from vibration of underlying organs and structures.

To begin, percuss lightly in all four quadrants of the abdomen. Generalized tympany can be found over the majority of the abdomen due to gas. Dullness occurs over fluid, organs, masses, or a distended bladder.

Percussion of the Liver

Percussion can be used to estimate liver size; however, this technique is a general estimation of the size of the liver, or the liver span. It is often inaccurate due to the difficulty of the technique, especially for females owing to the presence of breast tissue. Enlargement of the liver associated with hepatitis or ascites may be easier to detect than the normal liver size. While percussion of the liver may be useful in determining the location of the lower border of the liver, the findings of percussion should be interpreted with caution.

Dullness is typically heard over the liver when percussed. To estimate the size or span of the liver, percussion should be used to determine both the lower and upper borders. Start percussion at the right mid-clavicular line over an area of lung resonance. Percuss at the interspaces between the ribs and move down the right mid-clavicular line, listening for a change in percussion tones from resonance to dullness. Mark this change in tone associated with the upper border of the liver, typically at the fifth intercostal space, with tape or an appropriate writing device. Next, start percussion at an area of tympany in the abdomen at the right mid-clavicular line. Percuss upward along the mid-clavicular line, noting the change from tympany to dullness and mark this spot associated with the lower border of the liver. Measure the distance between the two marks; the normal liver span at the right mid-clavicular line is 6 to 12 cm (2–5 inches) at the right mid-clavicular line.

Liver tenderness may be elicited by using indirect fist percussion. Using this technique, place the left hand on the lower right rib cage and then gently strike the left hand with the ulnar surface of the right fist. Tenderness should not be produced in the normal healthy liver using this technique. The sensitivity of indirect fist percussion of the liver for diagnosing hepatobiliary infection is 60% and specificity is 85% (Ueda & Ishida, 2015).

Percussion of the Spleen

The spleen is also difficult to percuss because of the other organs such as the stomach and intestine, which lie in the abdominal cavity. Listen for the dullness of the spleen while percussing just posterior to the left mid-axillary line. Splenic dullness may be heard from the sixth to tenth rib. Dullness at Traube's space—the area in the left lower chest area between lung resonance and the costal margin (**Figure 16.21**)—has been shown to have moderate sensitivity and specificity in association with splenomegaly; however, this finding is less accurate with overweight/obese patients. There is limited evidence for the use of spleen percussion techniques to rule out splenomegaly (specificity 32.6%–87%; sensitivity 22%–85.7%; Stewart, Derck, Long, Learman, & Cook, 2013).

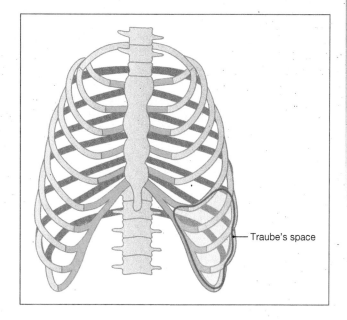

FIGURE 16.21 Traube's space. Surface markings: left sixth rib, left mid-axillary line, left costal margin.

The spleen can also be assessed by percussing the lowest intercostal space in the left anterior axillary line before and after the patient takes a deep breath. Using this method, the area should remain tympanic with the patient's breathing. If the spleen is enlarged, tympany changes to dullness as the spleen moves forward and down with inspiration.

Percussion of the Kidneys

Percuss the right and left costovertebral angle to assess for tenderness or pain, indicating kidney inflammation or musculoskeletal problems. Direct fist percussion can be used. This is when the clinician directly strikes the costovertebral angle using the ulnar surface of the fist (**Figure 16.22**). Conversely, indirect fist percussion may be used by placing the palm of the right hand on the back and striking this hand with the ulnar surface of the fist of the left hand.

PALPATION

Similar to percussion, palpation can be used to assess for masses, tenderness, and fluid in the abdomen. In addition, abdominal organs can be evaluated for size, shape, mobility, and consistency using palpation techniques (**Figure 16.23**). Remember to review techniques that allow the patient to relax, especially during the palpation portion of the exam. Pressing too firmly, having cold hands, and/or having used a cold stethoscope may cause the abdominal muscles to tense or cause voluntary guarding to occur, which may interfere with deep palpation. Palpate the painful areas last as

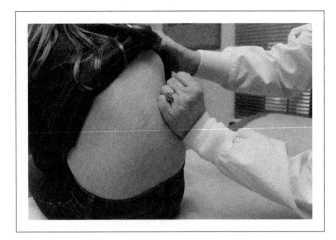

FIGURE 16.22 Percussion of the costovertebral angle to assess for tenderness.

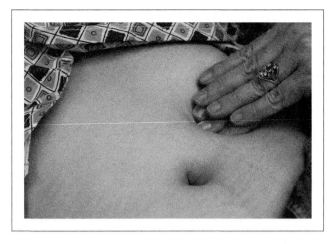

FIGURE 16.24 Abdominal palpation.

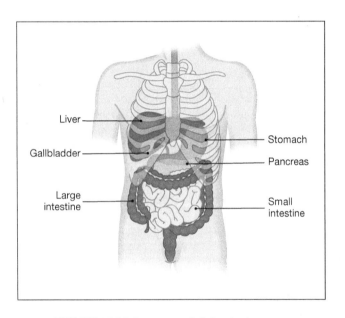

FIGURE 16.23 Location of abdominal organs.

examining these areas will cause pain and muscle tension that skew palpation findings.

Light Palpation

Start with light palpation of the abdomen, moving in a systematic way through all four quadrants (see **Figure 16.4**). Place the palmar surface of the hand lightly on the abdomen with fingers outstretched and close together. Press down on the abdominal wall no more than 1 cm with light palpation. Keep the hands low and parallel to the abdomen; keeping the hands high and pointing downward increases the likelihood of the patient tensing the abdomen. Use a light and circular motion, avoiding disjointed, jabbing, or hurried

motions. Pick up the hand when moving to the next area of the abdomen; do not drag the fingers. The abdomen should normally feel soft and smooth.

Deep Palpation

Deep palpation requires the clinician to depress the abdomen 5 to 8 cm (**Figure 16.24**). Similar to light palpation, move in a systematic way throughout all four quadrants of the abdomen. Deep palpation is useful in helping to determine abdominal organs and masses that may not be large enough to detect with light palpation. In addition, deep palpation may reveal tenderness not evident with light palpation. When performing deep palpation, note any masses, tenderness, and pulsations. Exam findings of guarding, rigidity, rebound tenderness, percussion tenderness, and pain with coughing nearly double the likelihood of peritonitis. Review the Special Tests for the Abdomen section later in this chapter for information on how to elicit rebound tenderness. Rigidity alone makes the diagnosis of peritonitis almost four times as likely.

Liver Palpation

Because the rib cage covers most of the liver, it is difficult to palpate. To palpate the liver, the clinician should place their left hand under the patient at the 11th and 12th ribs while pressing up in order to elevate the liver toward the abdominal wall. The right hand should be placed on the abdomen, fingers parallel to the midline. Using the right hand, push deeply under the right costal margin. Ask the patient to take a deep breath while trying to feel the edge of the liver as the diaphragm brings it down to the fingertips of the clinician's hand. Normally, the liver is not palpable, although it may be palpated in thin patients without any underlying disease and in children. If the liver edge is palpated, it should feel smooth, nontender, and without nodules.

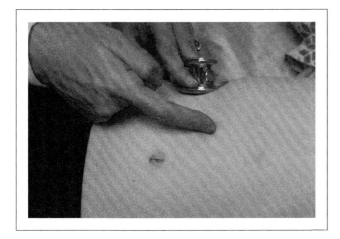

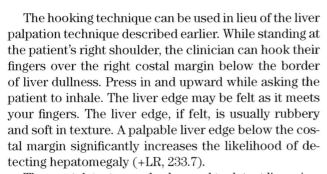

FIGURE 16.25 Scratch test.

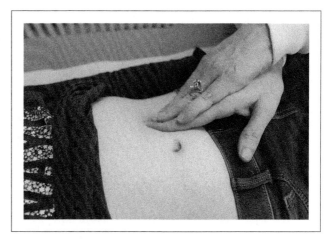

FIGURE 16.26 Palpation of the spleen.

The hooking technique can be used in lieu of the liver palpation technique described earlier. While standing at the patient's right shoulder, the clinician can hook their fingers over the right costal margin below the border of liver dullness. Press in and upward while asking the patient to inhale. The liver edge may be felt as it meets your fingers. The liver edge, if felt, is usually rubbery and soft in texture. A palpable liver edge below the costal margin significantly increases the likelihood of detecting hepatomegaly (+LR, 233.7).

The scratch test may also be used to detect liver size. To perform this technique, place a stethoscope on the xiphoid process while using the finger to scratch the abdominal surface (**Figure 16.25**). Note the differences in sound transmission over solid and hollow organs; when the liver is reached, the sound of the finger scratching the abdominal surface becomes louder. The scratch test has shown high reproducibility and moderate agreement between the scratch test findings and ultrasound; nevertheless, obesity can jeopardize these results (Gupta., Dhawan, Abel, Talley, & Attia, 2013).

Palpation of the Spleen

There is moderate evidence for the use of spleen palpation tests for confirming an enlarged spleen (specificity 82%–93%; sensitivity 31%–85.6%; Stewart et al., 2013). To palpate the spleen, place the left hand across and behind the patient's left side at the costovertebral angle, lifting up the spleen. Place the right hand on the patient's abdomen below the left costal margin, pressing the fingers toward the spleen. Ask the patient to take a deep breath while attempting to feel the spleen as it moves toward the fingers (**Figure 16.26**). Another equivalent method is the hook technique previously discussed for liver edge palpation; only when assessing the spleen, use the fingers to "hook" over the left costal boarder. Normally, the spleen is not palpable, although approximately 3% of the population have a palpable

TABLE 16.1 Hackett's Grading System for Palpable Splenomegaly

Grade 0	Normal impalpable spleen
Grade 1	Spleen palpable only on deep inspiration
Grade 2	Spleen palpable on mid-clavicular line, halfway between umbilicus and costal margin
Grade 3	The spleen expands toward the umbilicus
Grade 4	The spleen goes past the umbilicus
Grade 5	The spleen expands toward the pubis symphysis

Note: Modest correlation (r ≤0.62, p <.001).

spleen tip. In case of a palpable spleen, the exam is considered abnormal if it is greater than 2 cm below the costal margin (Chapman & Azevedo, 2019). A palpable spleen increases the likelihood of detecting splenomegaly (+LR, 8.5). The spleen must be enlarged three times before it is palpable. See **Table 16.1** for Hackett's Grading System for a palpable spleen.

Palpation of the Kidneys

To palpate the right kidney, stand at the right side of the patient and place one hand on the patient's right flank and the other hand at the right costal margin (**Figure 16.27A**). Press the two hands together and ask the patient to take a deep breath. The kidney edge may be felt between the fingers, or not palpated at all—both finds are normal. To palpate the left kidney, reach across the patient and behind the left flank with the left hand (**Figure 16.27B**). Press the right hand into the

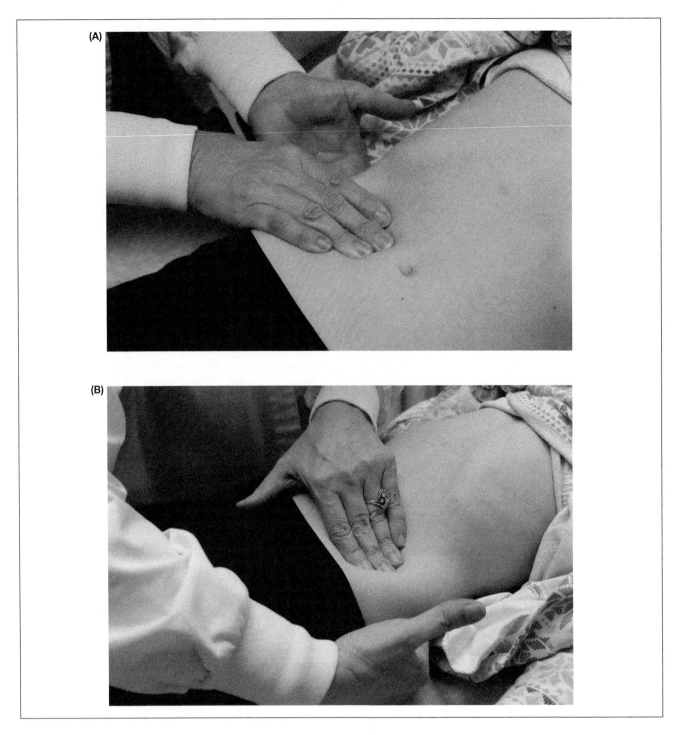

FIGURE 16.27 Palpation of the (A) right kidney and (B) left kidney.

abdomen while asking the patient to inhale. Press firmly between the two hands; there should be no change with inhalation.

Palpation of the Aorta

Palpate the aorta with the opposing thumb and fingers slightly left of the midline in the upper abdomen (**Figure 16.28**). Alternatively, assess the width of the aorta by pressing on either side of the aorta in the upper abdomen with one hand on each side of the aorta. The ability to palpate the aorta is related to the size of the aneurysm, but the inability to palpate the aorta is not efficient at ruling out an aneurysm in obese patients or in those who cannot relax their abdomen to facilitate the examination. The normal aorta is 2.5 to 4.0 cm wide in the adult.

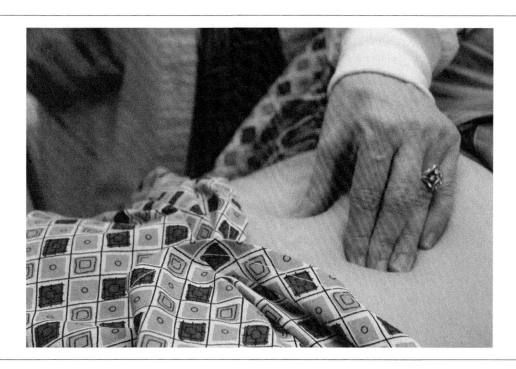

FIGURE 16.28 Palpation of the aorta.

Palpation of the Gallbladder

If a gallbladder is palpable during an abdominal exam, this is an abnormal finding. A palpable and tender gallbladder suggests acute cholecystitis and has a positive likelihood of detecting obstruction of the bile ducts (+LR, 26.0). If enlarged, a gallbladder can be felt behind the smooth liver border in the tight upper quadrant of the abdomen. Compared with the smooth liver, an enlarged gallbladder feels like a firm mass. If palpable, an inflamed gallbladder is exquisitely tender, making palpation difficult due to abdominal muscle guarding.

Special Tests for the Abdomen

The following tests are typically considered positive when pain is associated with the maneuver. Therefore, these specialized tests need to be completed last because the pain response may cause peritoneal irritation and could jeopardize any future exam findings. Similar to other clinical exam tests, combinations of findings from the clinical examination are more powerful than any single finding.

McBurney's Point

Pain with palpation of the right lower quadrant (RLQ) of the abdomen indicates a positive McBurney's point (sometimes called McBurney's sign). A positive test can be associated with the diagnosis of appendicitis.

Rebound Tenderness or Blumberg's Sign

Palpate the abdomen by applying slow and steady pressure to the suspected area followed by abrupt removal of the pressure. The test is considered positive if pain is worsened upon release of the hands (verses application of the pressure) when the underlying structure(s) shift back into place. A positive sign indicates peritoneal irritation. The odds of appendicitis triple in children who exhibit rebound tenderness (LR, 3.0; 95% CI [confidence interval], 2.3–3.9) and reduce the likelihood of its occurrence if rebound tenderness is absent (summary LR, 0.28; 95% CI, 0.14–0.55; Bundy et al., 2007). The results do not appear as favorable for adults (LR+, 1.59; 95% CI, 1.22–2.06; LR−, 0.65; 95% CI, 0.54–0.61; Ahn et al., 2016).

Rovsing's Sign

Deeply palpate the left iliac fossa. If pain is felt in the right iliac fossa, this is considered a positive Rovsing's sign (Figure 16.29). Historically, a positive Rovsing's sign has been associated with acute appendicitis. Rovsing's sign has a sensitivity of 30.1% and specificity of 84.4% (Kharbanda, Taylor, Fishman, & Bachur, 2005).

Psoas Test

With the patient in the supine position, place one hand just above the patient's right knee. Ask the patient to raise the leg while applying downward pressure on the leg (Figure 16.30). Pain can indicate irritation of the psoas muscle due to inflammation of the appendix. According to some sources, a positive test can indicate a retrocecal (behind the cecum) appendicitis presentation due to retroperitoneal inflammation

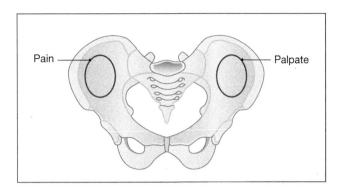

FIGURE 16.29 Rovsing's sign. Location of the iliac fossa and eliciting the Rovsing's sign.

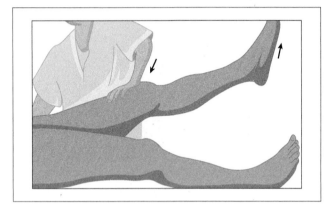

FIGURE 16.30 Psoas test.

(LR+, 2.38; 95% CI, 1.21–4.57; LR–, 0.90; 95% CI, 0.83–0.86).

Obturator Test

The obturator sign is commonly discussed in assessment texts and literature; however, there is little to no research regarding its clinical effectiveness in diagnosing appendicitis. Due to this fact, other tests are encouraged in lieu of the obturator test.

Heel Drop Test (Also Called the Markle's Test or Heel Jar Test)

Have the patient stand on their toes. Then ask the patient to abruptly release back onto the heels, creating a jarring sensation to the body. If there is pain in the RLQ, this is a positive test and contributes further information toward a possible diagnosis of appendicitis (LR+, 1.95; 95% CI, 1.51–2.52; LR–, 0.48; 95% CI, 0.38–0.61).

Digital Rectal Examination

Digital rectal exams (DREs) are sometimes warranted when a patient has a GI or urinary concern. Chapter 19, Evidence-Based Assessment of Male Genitalia, Prostate, Rectum, and Anus, reviews how to complete a DRE.

Murphy's Sign

Place one hand at the costal margin in the RUQ and ask the patient to breathe in deeply (**Figure 16.31**). If the gallbladder is inflamed, the patient will experience pain in the RUQ upon palpation and will have abrupt cessation of the breath (i.e., catch the breath) due to pain

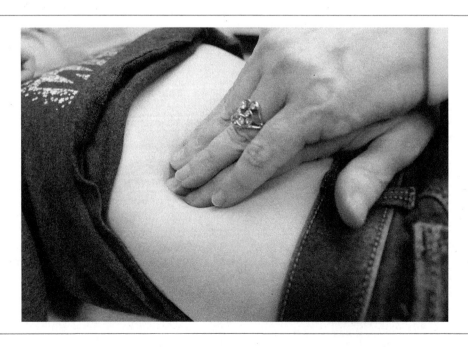

FIGURE 16.31 Murphy's sign.

as the gallbladder descends and contacts the palpating hand. Murphy's sign (LR+, 2.8; 95% CI, 0.8–8.6) is considered positive when the patient experiences pain in the RUQ with palpation. Sensitivity is 80% for diagnosis of cholecystitis (Ueda & Ishida, 2015).

Life-Span Considerations for Physical Examination

In the infant, the contour of the abdomen is protuberant because of the undeveloped abdominal musculature. The abdomen should be symmetric. In addition, inspection of the abdomen may reveal respiratory movement and peristalsis. Auscultation and percussion techniques do not differ for the infant and child. No vascular sounds are audible in the abdomen of the infant; however, these are common in thin children. Percussion findings include tympany over the stomach and dullness over the liver. Similar to the adult, tympany is associated with gas, and dullness can reflect fluid or a mass. The spleen is not percussed in the infant. The liver predominates in the RUQ, and the liver edge may be palpated at the right costal margin or slightly below. The spleen, kidneys, and bladder may be palpated in the infant. In children 4 years and older, the liver is still palpable as is the spleen. The liver span is 3.5 cm at age 2, 5 cm at age 5, and 6 to 7 cm during adolescence. The right and left kidneys may also be palpated. Abdominal exam findings for the school-aged child are the same as for the adult. Modifications in how the abdominal exam is performed may be necessary in young children (**Figure 16.32**).

Palpation of the abdominal organs may be easier in the older adult because of thinning of the abdominal wall and weakness of the abdominal musculature. The liver is easier to palpate and may be found 1 to 2 cm below the costal margin with inhalation. Decreased motility occurs with aging, which in turn means symptoms of gas and distention, as well as tympany upon percussion.

LABORATORY CONSIDERATIONS

GI and urological conditions often require laboratory testing, which can aid the clinician in ruling in or out certain conditions as well as assist the clinician in determining the correct diagnosis. The following labs should be considered on the basis of the presenting concern and possible differential diagnoses.

CELIAC DISEASE

- Celiac disease antibody tests that include tissue transglutaminase antibody; deaminated gliadin peptide antibodies; anti-endomysial antibodies; anti-reticulin antibodies; and quantitative immunoglobulin A
- The gold standard testing is endoscopy that shows shortened or flattened intestinal villi.

INFLAMMATORY BOWEL DISEASE

- Complete blood count (CBC) with differential that has a high white blood cell (WBC) count (low predictive validity)
- Electrolyte panel may show low levels of sodium, potassium, chloride, and carbon dioxide with chronic diarrhea.

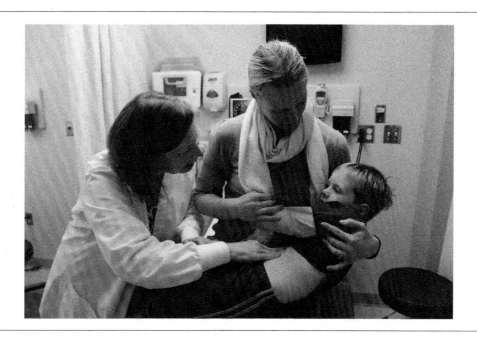

FIGURE 16.32 Abdominal examination in a young child.

- Liver function tests (LFT) may show low albumin and prealbumin levels but otherwise normal unless there is concomitant liver damage or poor liver functioning.
- Positive hemoccult stool test
- Elevated erythrocyte sedimental rate (ESR) and C-reactive protein (CRP) levels
- The gold standard testing is endoscopy with biopsy that shows crypt abscesses.

HEPATITIS

- An acute viral hepatitis panel detects hepatitis infection. **Table 16.2** reviews how to interpret the test results of a hepatitis panel.
- A comprehensive metabolic panel (CMP) should also be obtained and includes the following tests that assess liver health/function: alanine ami-notransferase (ALT), aspartate aminotransferase (AST), alkaline phosphatase (ALP), bilirubin, albumin, total protein, prothrombin, and gamma-glutamyl transpeptidase (GGT).
- These would often be elevated in acute hepatitis.

PANCREATITIS

- Amylase and/or lipase (digestive enzymes of the pancreas) rise following hepatic injury; levels two to four times normal are considered diagnostic for pancreatitis.
- Trypsinogen and elastase have no significant advantage over amylase or lipase.
- If lipase and/or amylase are not elevated and the diagnosis is uncertain, abdominal imaging, such as a computed tomography (CT) scan, might be indicated.

URINARY TRACT INFECTION OR PYELONEPHRITIS

Urinalysis (UA) findings (sensitivity 74.02% for UTI)—positive nitrites, pyuria, and hematuria (Mambatta et al., 2015):

- "Do not initiate a workup for hematuria or proteinuria before repeating an abnormal urine dipstick analysis (UA)" (American Academy of Pediatrics [AAP] & American Society of Pediatric Nephrology [ASPN], 2018, #2).

Urine culture (>10,000 colony-forming units of a uropathogen/mL):

- Positive urine cultures provide definitive evidence of a urinary infection that requires treatment.
- "Avoid ordering follow-up urine cultures after treatment for an uncomplicated urinary tract infection (UTI) in patients that show evidence of clinical resolution of infection" (AAP & ASPN, 2018, #3).

White blood cell casts on microscopy with signs and symptoms of a UTI:

- Indicates acute pyelonephritis and differentiates this condition from a UTI.

IMAGING CONSIDERATIONS

CHOLECYSTITIS

Ultrasonography used to detect acute cholecystitis has an adjusted sensitivity of 88% and specificity of 80%. The hepatobiliary (HIDA) scan is a nuclear medicine scan that tracks the flow of the nuclear tracer from

TABLE 16.2 Interpretation of Hepatitis Panel				
Anti-Hepatitis A, IgM	Hepatitis B Surface Antigen	Anti-Hepatitis B Core, IgM	Anti-Hepatitis C	Interpretation of Results
Positive	Negative	Negative	Negative	Acute hepatitis A
Negative	Positive	Positive	Negative	Acute hepatitis B
Negative	Positive	Negative	Negative	Chronic hepatitis B infection
Negative	Negative	Positive	Negative	Acute hepatitis B; quantity of hepatitis B surface antigen is too low to detect
Negative	Negative	Negative	Positive	Acute or chronic hepatitis C; additional tests are required to make the determination

the liver into the gallbladder and small intestine. This is used to confirm a clinical diagnosis of cholecystitis (Simel, Rennie & Keitz, 2009).

GASTROESOPHAGEAL REFLUX DISEASE

Upper endoscopy and biopsy shows inflammation of the esophagus. Esophageal pH monitoring shows prolonged episodes of low pH in the esophagus independent of following meals or supine positioning. Esophageal manometry measures the pressure in the LES, which may be low and associated with other findings of esophageal acidity and/or inflammation (Rosen et al., 2018).

APPENDICITIS

Once acute appendicitis is suspected, no single history, physical examination, laboratory finding, or clinical score attained can eliminate the need for imaging studies, especially in the pediatric population (Benabbas, Hanna, Shah, & Sinert, 2017). A graded compression ultrasound is often used to detect acute appendicitis (sensitivity 86%, specificity 81%) and is superior to an x-ray or barium enema. An ultrasound should be the first imaging test completed for a case of suspected acute appendicitis, especially in children (American College of Radiology, 2017). While the sensitivity and specificity is less for ultrasound compared with magnetic resonance imaging (MRI) or CT, it is more cost-efficient and does not use ionizing radiation. This should be used in conjunction with a thorough physical exam that employs a scoring system like the Alvarado or Samuel scoring system (Mostbeck et al., 2016).

HEPATOMEGALY

The ultrasound is a fairly accurate radiological test for detecting hepatomegaly, but CT and MRI are the most reliable methods for determining vertical liver span and overall dimensions (Childs, Esterman, Thoirs, & Turner, 2016).

SPLENOMEGALY

Ultrasound or scintigraphy should be used to confirm the diagnosis of splenomegaly or both should be used if the diagnosis is an important clinical concern (Barkun & Grover, 2009).

OTHER TESTING CONSIDERATIONS

- "For a patient with functional abdominal pain syndrome (as per ROME IV criteria), computed tomography (CT) scans should not be repeated unless there is a major change in clinical findings or symptoms" (American Gastroenterology Association, 2012, #5).

- "Do not repeat colonoscopy for at least five years for patients who have one or two small (<1 cm) adenomatous polyps, without high-grade dysplasia or villous histology, completely removed via a high-quality colonoscopy" (American Gastroenterology Association, 2012, #3).
- "[Do not] routinely use computed tomography (CT) to screen pediatric patients with suspected nephrolithiasis" (American Urological Association [AUA], 2019, #15).
- "[Do not] diagnose microhematuria solely on the results of a urine dipstick (macroscopic urinalysis)" (AUA, 2019, #10).
- "[Do not] order routine screening urine analyses (UA) in healthy, asymptomatic pediatric patients as part of routine well child care" (AAP & ASPN, 2018, #1).
- "Avoid ordering CT of the abdomen and pelvis in young, otherwise healthy . . . patients (age <50) with known histories of kidney stones, or ureterolithiasis, presenting with symptoms consistent with uncomplicated renal colic" (American College of Emergency Physicians, Choosing Wisely, 2018, #10).

EVIDENCE-BASED PREVENTIVE PRACTICE CONSIDERATIONS

The U.S. Preventive Services Task Force (USPSTF; 2016) recommends all persons aged 50 to 75 get a colorectal screening (Grade A). Colonoscopy is considered the gold standard for detection of colorectal cancer but fecal occult blood testing and/or sigmoidoscopy may be better options for certain individuals. For adults 76 to 85 years old, the USPSTF states the decision to screen should be individualized with previous screening history and overall health taken into consideration (Grade C).

ABNORMAL FINDINGS OF THE GASTROINTESTINAL SYSTEM

CONSTIPATION

Constipation is the result of abnormal transport mechanisms of the GI tract where there is slow motility in the intestinal lumen. Most often, the decreased motility is noted in the large intestines. It is a common GI symptom. The most common causes of constipation are diets with high refined carbohydrates and low fiber intake, prolonged laxative use, drug usage (i.e., opiates), and decreased physical activity (Seller & Symons, 2018). It is more appropriately defined by the existence of having more than 25% of the following and at least a 3-month duration of symptoms: straining with bowel movements, hard stools, incomplete evacuation, and fewer than three bowel movements a week (Goolsby & Grubbs, 2015).

Key History and Physical Findings

- Dried, hard, small stools
- Infrequent bowel movements
- Straining with bowel movements
- Incomplete evacuation of stool

DIARRHEA

Diarrhea is the result of abnormal and rapid transport of chyme in the GI tract. This is marked by increased intestinal motility and changes in the osmotic mechanism that result in abnormal absorption (Goolsby & Grubbs, 2015). The rapid transport can be triggered by numerous causes that include bacterial, viral, organic, or functional. Most frequently, the episodes are self-limited and resolve within a few days without intervention. When the diarrhea is accompanied by high fever and intractable vomiting, dehydration can occur. This complication occurs particularly frequently in children and older adults and can require hospitalization (Goolsby & Grubbs, 2015). Increased intestinal motility can be visually apparent at times. Tenderness is often reported on palpation of the affected area. Viral gastroenteritis is the most common cause of diarrhea (Seller & Symons, 2018).

Key History and Physical Findings

- Loose, watery stools
- Frequent bowel movements
- Cramping due to inflammation
- Increased intestinal motility of the GI tract
- Gas formation
- Diffuse abdominal pain
- Dehydration

NAUSEA/VOMITING

Nausea and vomiting are frequent concerns associated with GI infections, functional GI obstruction, central nervous system disorders including those psychiatric in nature, pregnancy, and metabolic disorders; they also occur as side effects of drug intake or use (Goolsby & Grubbs, 2015). When vomiting is found in newborns or neonates, the cause may be due to esophageal atresia or a congenital anomaly (Seller & Symons, 2018), although clinicians should be cautioned to differentiate between vomiting and "spitting up." In adults, the most common causes of nausea and vomiting include gastritis (drug or alcohol induced), viral gastroenteritis, psychogenic conditions, and occasionally labyrinthine disorders (Seller & Symons, 2018). A careful history and good symptom analysis is likely to identify triggering events. Questions to ascertain important information include

the time at which meals are eaten and type of food ingested, associated motion or offensive odors, and the type, timing, and duration of pain. The report of vomiting may be associated with various symptoms such as accompanying queasiness/nausea, rapid onset of vomiting, and/or retching. The amount, consistency, color of vomitus, and presence of bile are important historical elements when trying to decipher the etiology of the vomiting episodes (Goolsby & Grubbs, 2015).

Key History and Physical Findings

- A queasy sensation including an urge to vomit
- Vomitus

ABNORMAL FINDINGS BASED ON LOCATION OF ABDOMINAL PAIN (Figure 16.33)

RIGHT UPPER QUADRANT PAIN: DUODENUM, LIVER, GALLBLADDER, LIVER, PANCREAS

The RUQ of the abdomen has several underlying organs, whose dysfunction can cause pain and pathology. RUQ pain encompasses a variety of diagnostic possibilities. Most common etiologies are diseases of the liver, gallbladder, or pancreas. A careful history and physical exam can help the clinician differentiate the etiology of the pain but all underlying structures need to be considered.

Acute Pancreatitis

Pancreatitis is an inflammation of the pancreas. It can be acute or chronic with symptoms ranging from mild to severe. It can be the result of a variety of disorders including gallstones, biliary disease, alcohol abuse, cystic fibrosis, autoimmune diseases, or certain heredity diseases or can occur as a side effect of medication administration. Pancreatitis occurs when digestive enzymes start digesting the pancreas itself.

Key History and Physical Findings

- RUQ or epigastric abdominal pain that is characterized as piercing/penetrating
- Pain radiating to the back
- Nausea and vomiting (Goolsby & Grubbs, 2015)
- Fever
- Tachycardia
- Shallow respirations
- Postural hypertension
- Diaphoresis (Seller & Symons, 2018)

Cholecystitis/Cholelithiasis

Gallbladder disease is usually due to an occlusion of the bile duct. This can be due to either infection or stones. The term *cystitis* implies infection as a result of bacteria while *lithiasis* refers to any obstruction as a result

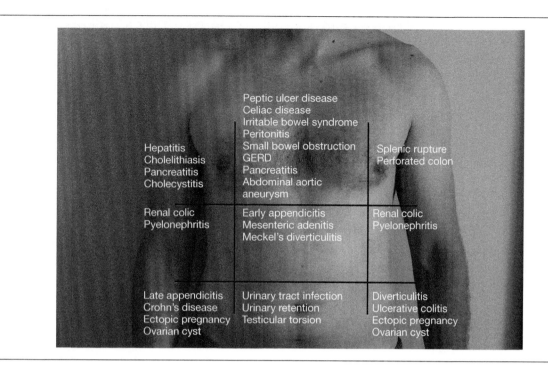

FIGURE 16.33 Differential diagnoses according to localization of abdominal pain.
GERD, gastroesophageal reflux disease.

of stones. A frequently used mnemonic to describe the most common incidence of gallbladder disease is the four Fs: female, fat, forty, and fertile (Goolsby & Grubbs, 2015).

Key History and Physical Findings
- Acute, colicky RUQ pain with radiation to back or right shoulder
- Anorexia
- Nausea
- Vomiting
- Low-grade fever
- Increased neutrophilic leukocyte counts (Seller & Symons, 2018)
- Jaundice can occur if obstruction is present.

Hepatitis/Hepatomegaly/Cirrhosis

Liver disease can be caused by a viral infection (hepatitis A, B, C, D, E), structural changes such as liver enlargement (hepatomegaly), or cirrhosis, which is most commonly found due to alcohol-related causes. Hepatocellular injury in the liver caused by an accumulation of fat not associated with alcohol is also increasingly common; nonalcoholic fatty liver disease (NFLD) is associated with obesity, type 2 diabetes, and dyslipidemia. Infiltrative liver disease, irrespective of the cause, increases the firmness of liver tissue and, if enlarged, can result in a palpable liver edge or increased liver girth. Ultrasonic studies are used to confirm liver structural

changes (Seller & Symons, 2018); lab studies confirm cellular changes or damage. Note that the incubation, infectivity, and transmission of viral hepatitis vary depending on the type. See **Table 16.3** for more information on incubation, infectivity, and transmission.

Key History and Physical Findings
- Abnormal liver function test (ALT, AST, and alkaline phosphatase elevations)
- Thrombocytopenia
- Jaundice
- Hepatomegaly on ultrasound
- Portal hypertension
- Ascites
- Eventually encephalopathy (Goolsby & Grubbs, 2015)

RIGHT LOWER QUADRANT PAIN: APPENDIX, ASCENDING COLON

Important to consider in the evaluation of RLQ pain is the potential for radiated pain or referred pain from a different site or to another part of the body (Goolsby & Grubbs, 2015). Pain referred to the back is a commonly referred pain associated with RLQ pain. Always consider a female GU etiology when a female patient presents with left lower quadrant (LLQ) pain. For more information on female GU etiologies, refer to Chapter 20, Evidence-Based Assessment of the Female Genitourinary System.

TABLE 16.3 Incubation, Infectivity, and Transmission of Hepatitis Subtypes

Type	Incubation	Infectivity	Transmission
HAV	Above 30 days	Few weeks prior through 1 week after	Fecal–oral
HBV	60–90 days	Weeks to years	Blood, secretions, saliva, body fluid
HCV	50 days	Weeks to years	Blood, sexual contact, IV drugs
HDV	4–7 weeks	Coinfection HBV; usually short lived	Rare in the U.S., intimate contact
HEV	About 40 days	While symptomatic	Fecal–oral

HAV, hepatitis A virus; HBV, hepatitis B virus; HCV, hepatitis C virus; HDV, hepatitis D virus; HEV, hepatitis E virus; IV, intravenous.
Source: Centers for Disease Control and Prevention. (n.d.). Hepatitis C questions and answers for the public. Retrieved from https://www .cdc.gov/hepatitis/hcv/cfaq.htm

TABLE 16.4 Alvarado Scoring Model for Acute Appendicitis in Adults (MANTRELs Score)

Signs	Score No (0)	Score Yes (1)
RLQ tenderness	0	+2
Elevated temperature (37.3°C or 99.1°F)	0	+1
Rebound tenderness in RLQ	0	+1
Symptoms		
Migration of pain to the RLQ	0	+1
Anorexia	0	+1
Nausea or vomiting	0	+1
Laboratory Values		
Leukocytosis >10,000	0	+2
Leukocyte left shift	0	+1
Total Score		

RLQ, right lower quadrant.
Note: Total score >7 = Sensitivity 66%, specificity 81%, positive predictive value 96%, negative predictive value 29%.

Appendicitis

Inflammation of the appendix is the most common cause of acute abdominal pain between the ages of 10 and 30 years (Seller & Symons, 2018). Inflammation of the appendix can result from a variety of elements that can obstruct the appendix lumen and cause subsequent bacterial growth. Appendicitis is a surgical emergency and can cause significant morbidity and mortality if not identified early. Perforation, gangrene, and peritonitis can result within the first 36 hours (Goolsby & Grubbs, 2015). See **Table 16.4** for the Alvarado Scoring Model for acute appendicitis in adults. There are several other scoring systems available including the MESH criteria and the Pediatric Appendicitis Score (PAS) for children.

Key History and Physical Findings
- Pain is initially vague and around umbilicus but migrates within hours to RLQ (LR+, 4.81; 95% CI, 3.59–6.44)
- Low-grade fever* (LR+, 3.4; 95% CI, 2.4–4.8)
- Elevated WBC count
- Feeling of constipation
- Nausea
- Vomiting
- Positive McBurney's point tenderness
- Cough/hop pain (LR+, 7.64; 95% CI, 5.94–9.83)
- Rovsing's sign tenderness (LR+, 3.52; 95% CI, 2.65–4.68)
- Rectal tenderness
- Positive psoas sign

*Applicable for children only

Strangulated Hernia

A strangulated hernia occurs when part of the intestine protrudes through a weak spot in the abdominal muscles and becomes trapped, resulting in decreased circulation to the lumen and eventual necrosis. There is usually a history of straining, heavy lifting, or previous abdominal surgery (Goolsby & Grubbs, 2015). Most commonly found are inguinal or groin hernias where a mass may be palpable in the left or right groin area. An abdominal ultrasound can be used to confirm the condition (Mayo Clinic, 2018).

- Often initiated with coughing, bending over, or lifting heavy objects
- Nausea and vomiting
- Palpable mass on the abdomen that turns red, purple, or dark in color
- Acute pain
- Fever

Regional Ileitis/Crohn's Disease

Regional ileitis is a disease of the terminal ileum, affecting mainly young adults. It is characterized by a subacute or chronic necrotizing inflammation. Crohn's disease is an autoimmune, inflammatory bowel disease associated with intermittent exacerbations of mucosal inflammation and ulceration. It can affect any part of the GI tract and can affect all layers of the bowel wall. Severity can range from mild to severe. **Table 16.5** provides an evidence-based clinical scoring tool called the

TABLE 16.5 Harvey-Bradshaw Index–Pro (HBI–PRO) Score to Assess Endoscopic Disease Activity in Crohn's Disease

Item	Score	Score and Meaning
General well-being (for the previous day)		0 = very well 1 = slightly below 2 = poor 3 = very poor 4 = terrible
Abdominal pain (for the previous day)		0 = none 1 = mild 2 = moderate 3 = severe
Number of stools/day (for previous day)		Indicate the number of stools as the score
Abdominal mass		0 = none 1 = dubious 2 = definite 3 = definite and tender
Complications (score 1 per item)		Arthralgia, uveitis, erythema nodosum, aphthous ulcers, pyoderma gangrenosum, anal fissure, new fistula, abscess
Total HBI score		Clinical remission <5 = 0 Mild disease 5–7 = 1 Moderate disease 8–16 = 2 Severe disease >16 = 3
PROp (patient-reported outcome: Is your CD active/ inactive [remission] in the last 2 weeks previously to the colonoscopy?)		0 = inactive 1 = active
PROc (provider-reported outcome: If you had to scope your patient today, do you think your patient would have had…?)		0 = inactive disease 1 = mild active disease 2 = moderately active disease 3 = severely active disease
Optional—CRP		
Total HBI-PRO score		0 = clinical remission (+CRP 0–0.47 = inactive) 1 = mild disease (+CRP 0.47–1.01 = mild) 2 = moderate disease (+CRP 1.01–3.75 = moderate) 3 = severe disease (+CRP >3.75 = severe)

CD, Crohn's disease; CRP, C-reactive protein.

Note: Improved sensitivity and specificity is noted in this combined model rather than HBI or PROp or PROc alone. The addition of CRP significantly improved the accuracy of this model.

Harvey-Bradshaw Index–Pro (HBI–PRO) that is used to access current clinical disease severity.

Key History and Physical Findings

- Intermittent, cramping abdominal pain
- Severe diarrhea usually with blood, pus, and mucus
- Fatigue and malaise
- Fever
- Weight loss
- Arthralgias
- Decreased hemoglobin and hematocrit
- ESR is usually high during exacerbations
- Skip lesions on colonoscopy
- Other body systems can be affected.

LEFT UPPER QUADRANT: SPLEEN, STOMACH, CARDIAC

Pain in the left upper quadrant (LUQ) can be associated with splenic, gastric, or cardiac diseases. Always rule out a cardiac etiology when a patient presents with LUQ pain. For more information on cardiovascular etiologies, refer to Chapter 6, Evidence-Based Assessment of the Heart and Circulatory System.

Splenomegaly/Ruptured Spleen

Enlargement of the spleen can be due to infections, inflammatory diseases, or neoplasms such as hepatitis, endocarditis, malaria, mononucleosis, lupus, or leukemia (Goolsby & Grubbs, 2015). Splenic rupture occurs due to blunt trauma or injury. Motor vehicle accidents, sports injuries, and fighting are common causes of splenic rupture. Splenic rupture is a medical emergency that causes life-threatening internal bleeding.

Key History and Physical Findings
Splenomegaly
- Asymptomatic in some
- Pain and/or fullness in LUQ that can radiate to the left shoulder
- Fatigue
- Frequent infections
- Anemia

Splenic Rupture
- Sudden onset abdominal pain
- Splenomegaly and/or tenderness in LUQ on abdominal exam
- Hemodynamic instability
- Confusion
- Lightheadedness
- Dizziness

Perforated Colon

Perforated colon is an opening that occurs anywhere in the intestinal tract resulting in stool contents leaking into the viscera or peritoneal cavity (Seller & Symons, 2018). This can occur due to trauma or during an abdominal surgery. It can also occur as a complication from various disease states such as diverticulitis, IBD, PUD, strangulated hernia, or toxic megacolon. It can also occur due to swallowing a foreign object and should always be a consideration in young children. A perforated colon is a surgical emergency.

Key History and Physical Findings
- Gradual onset, but worsening, abdominal pain
- Board-like abdomen distention
- Fever
- Nausea/vomiting
- Elevated WBC

LEFT LOWER QUADRANT PAIN: DESCENDING COLON

LLQ pain is usually associated with diseases originating in the descending colon or sigmoid colon region.

Sigmoid Diverticulosis/Diverticulitis

Diverticulosis is the herniation or out-pouching of the walls of the colon. This herniation creates small pouches. When these pouches fill with food particles, or feces, it causes inflammation and/or the bacteria count to increase, causing infection. This results in diverticulitis (Goolsby & Grubbs, 2015).

Key History and Physical Findings
- Abdominal pain in LLQ
- Occasionally abdominal pain can be in RLQ
- History of chronic constipation or, less commonly, diarrhea
- Fever
- Nausea/vomiting
- Tenderness to LLQ palpation
- Leukocytosis

Ulcerative Colitis

Ulcerative colitis is an autoimmune disorder that can affect any area of the large colon. It is characterized by intermittent inflammation and ulceration of the colon mucosal lining. It is characterized by bloody and mucous stools (Goolsby & Grubbs, 2015). There are periods of exacerbations and remissions. Common diagnostics used range from CBC, stool samples, barium x-rays, and colonoscopy. Colonoscopy can assist in diagnosis by verifying the cobblestone, ulcerative appearance of the mucosal wall. A commonly used scoring system used to determine disease severity is the *Mayo Score: Disease Activity Index for Ulcerative Colitis*. Refer to **Table 16.6** for the criteria.

TABLE 16.6 Mayo Score: Disease Activity Index for Ulcerative Colitis

Symptom	+1	+2	+3
Stool frequency	1–2 stools/day more than usual	3–4 more stools/day more than usual	>4 stools/day more than usual
Rectal bleeding	Visible blood with stool <half the time	Visible blood with stool half the time or more	≥50% of stools with visible blood AND ≥1 stool with blood alone
Mucosal appearance at endoscopy	Mild disease (erythema, decreased vascular pattern, mild friability)	Moderate disease (marked erythema, absent vascular pattern, friability, erosions)	Severe disease (spontaneous bleeding, ulceration)
Health provider rating of disease activity (normal = 0)	Mild	Moderate	Severe
Total Score =			

Note: Sensitivity 88%, specificity 80%.

Key History and Physical Findings
- Abdominal pain, often in the LLQ
- Diarrhea with blood or pus
- Rectal pain and bleeding
- Weight loss
- Other systems can be affected.
- In severe cases, signs of systemic toxicity include fever, tachycardia, anemia, elevated ESR, and rapid weight loss.
- Anemia
- Stool cultures have WBCs.
- Colonoscopy shows cobblestoning.

PERIUMBILICAL/EPIGASTRIC PAIN: STOMACH, TRANSVERSE COLON, AORTA

Epigastric or periumbilical pain is a very common complaint of discomfort stemming from digestive structures but cardiac differentials should always be considered.

Abdominal Aortic Aneurysm

Abdominal aortic aneurysm should be considered and ruled out when abdominal pain is in the epigastric area as it can be a life-threatening condition. Chapter 6, Evidence-Based Assessment of the Heart and Circulatory System, provides an overview of AAA including associated signs and symptoms.

Celiac Disease

Celiac disease is an autoimmune disorder with strong genetic predisposition where the ingestion of gluten leads to damage of the small intestinal wall. Over time, the immune reaction to eating gluten creates inflammation that damages the small intestine's lining, leading to malabsorption of all nutrients (Goolsby & Grubbs, 2015).

Key History and Physical Findings
- Diarrhea
- Bloating
- Flatulence
- Fatigue
- Weight loss
- Iron-deficiency anemia
- Constipation
- Depression

Peptic Ulcer Disease

Peptic ulcer disease is an inflammation and ultimate ulceration of the stomach or duodenal lining. It is commonly associated with *H. pylori* and/or chronic use of nonsteroidal anti-inflammatory medications (NSAIDs). Disease characteristics are variable and depend on the location of the ulcer(s). Most patients present with dyspepsia and/or other GI symptoms. Other patients may initially present only with complications like GI bleeding. In rare cases, PUD can be due to Zollinger–Ellison syndrome (Goolsby & Grubbs, 2015).

Key History and Physical Findings
- Asymptomatic in some
- Abdominal pain, often in epigastric region, but can be in the LUQ or RUQ of the abdomen
- Pain is described as gnawing or burning.
- Pain can radiate to back.
- Pain worsens with immediate food intake (gastric) or 2 to 5 hours after food intake (duodenal).
- Heartburn
- Belching
- Bloating
- Nausea
- Positive guaiac test
- Positive *H. pylori* testing
- Gastroduodenal lesions found on endoscopy
- Complications include bleeding, gastric outlet obstruction, fistulas, and perforation

Gastroesophageal Reflux Disease/Dyspepsia

GERD is the most common cause of epigastric discomfort. It is often called heartburn, ingestion, reflux, or sour stomach. It can be associated with other diseases, food intake, or medication side effects. Common medication causes include theophylline, dopamine, diazepam, and calcium channel blockers. Food and other causes include caffeine, alcohol, chocolate, fatty foods, tobacco use, pregnancy, or hiatal hernia (Goolsby & Grubbs, 2015; North American Society for Pediatric Gastroenterology, Hepatology and Nutrition).

Key History and Physical Findings
- A burning sensation in the chest (heartburn), usually after eating
- Symptoms are worse at night with laying supine.
- Chest pain
- Difficulty swallowing
- Abdominal bloating
- Regurgitation of food or sour liquid
- Globus sensation
- Worse with certain foods and medications
- Worse after meals
- Relieved with antacids
- Cough
- Hoarseness
- Pain with palpation of epigastric area
- Negative *H. pylori* test

Irritable Bowel Syndrome

Irritable bowel syndrome is considered a functional bowel (motility) disorder. There are several types of functional bowel disorder. The Rome IV Classification system is used to classify these diseases and separate them into esophageal, gastroduodenal, and bowel disorders. See **Table 16.7** for further classification.

IBS is characterized by intermittent, mild-to-severe abdominal pain with a change in bowel habits. The cause is unknown but can be associated with other conditions, such as celiac disease, parasitic infection, or IBDs (Goolsby & Grubbs, 2015). The Rome IV criteria is the most widely used diagnostic criteria. There are different subtypes of IBS including IBS with predominant constipation, IBS with predominant diarrhea, IBS with mixed bowel habits, and IBS unspecified (Lacy et al., 2016).

Key History and Physical Findings
- Recurrent abdominal pain, at least 1 day/week in the last 3 months, with an altered bowel pattern
- Diarrhea
- Constipation
- Alternating diarrhea and constipation

TABLE 16.7 Rome IV Classification of the Functional Gastrointestinal Disorders—Disorders of Gut–Brain Interaction

A. Esophageal Disorders

A1. Functional chest pain	A4. Globus
A2. Functional heartburn	A5. Functional dysphagia
A3. Reflux hypersensitivity	

B. Gastroduodenal Disorders

B1. Functional dyspepsia	B3. Nausea and vomiting disorders
B1a. Postprandial distress syndrome	B3a. Chronic nausea vomiting syndrome
B1b. Epigastric pain syndrome	B3b. Cyclic vomiting syndrome
B2. Belching disorders	B3c. Cannabinoid hyperemesis syndrome
B2a. Excessive supragastric belching	B4. Rumination syndrome
B2b. Excessive gastric belching	

C. Bowel disorders

C1. Irritable bowel syndrome	C2. Functional constipation
IBS with predominant constipation	C3. Functional diarrhea
IBS with predominant diarrhea	C4. Functional abdominal bloating/distension
IBS with mixed bowel habits	C5. Unspecified functional bowel disorder
IBS unclassified	C6. Opioid-induced constipation

Source: Schmulson, M. J., & Drossman, D. A. (2017). What is new in Rome IV. *Journal of Neurogastroenterological Motility*, *23*(2), 151–163. doi:10.5056/jnm16214 (evidence-based information is available).

- Bowel movements generally occur during waking hours, most often in the morning or after meals.
- Abdominal bloating
- Increased gas production (belching and/or flatulence)
- Exacerbated with emotional stress and/or eating
- Abdominal pain is relieved with defecation.
- Periods of exacerbations and remissions

Small Bowel Obstruction

Bowel obstruction occurs when the normal flow of intraluminal contents is interrupted, causing partial or complete blockage of GI contents. The obstruction can be due to abnormal intestinal physiology or due to a mechanical obstruction. The most common causes of mechanical small bowel obstruction are postoperative adhesions and hernias. Obstruction or blockage to the intestinal lumen is associated with pain, nausea, or vomiting (Seller & Symons, 2018).

Key History and Physical Findings
- History of previous abdominal surgery
- Stools that have decreased in diameter and frequency
- Abrupt onset of periumbilical abdominal pain
- Paroxysmal, cramping abdominal pain
- Nausea
- Vomiting
- Abdominal distention
- Obstipation
- Dehydration, causing tachycardia, orthostatic hypotension, and reduced urine output
- Abdominal/inguinal hernias on exam

Peritonitis

Peritonitis is an inflammation to the peritoneal lining of the abdomen as a result of bacterial infection from a perforation in the bowel or as a result of surgical contamination (Goolsby & Grubbs, 2015). Spontaneous bacterial peritonitis primarily occurs in patients with advanced cirrhosis. It usually manifests with severe abdominal pain and is considered a medical emergency, requiring immediate intervention (McGee, 2017). If it is not found early in the course of infection, shock ensues, rapidly followed by multisystem organ failure.

Key History and Physical Findings
- History of advanced cirrhosis
- Fever
- Guarding
- Diffuse abdominal pain
- Rigidity and distention of abdomen
- Rebound tenderness
- Altered mental state
- Leukocytosis

ABNORMAL FINDINGS OF THE URINARY SYSTEM

LOWER URINARY TRACT INFECTION

The urinary tract is a sterile environment. Bacteria are typically introduced into the urinary tract through the urethra, making lower UTIs more common than upper UTIs (see later in this chapter for more information). Lower UTIs involve the bladder (cystitis) and urethra (urethritis). Different anatomical features and mechanisms can make certain individuals more susceptible to the introduction of bacteria into this sterile environment. Women are more susceptible to UTIs because their urethras are shorter and in closer proximity to the

TABLE 16.8 Clinical Decision Rule for Urinary Tract Infection in Women Without Signs of Complicated Disease

Clinical Score		Dipstick Score	
Symptom	Points	Dipstick Results	Points
Urine cloudiness	1.0	Nitrites	2.0
Burning dysuria	1.0	Leukocyte esterase	1.5
Any nocturia	1.0	Blood	1.0
Total		**Total**	
0 points: LR = 0.23, prevalence = 19%		0 points: LR = 0.16, prevalence = 14%	
1–2 points: LR = 0.82, prevalence = 46%		1–2.5 points: LR = 1.1, prevalence = 53%	
3 points: LR = 2.25, prevalence = 70%		≥3 points: LR = 5.4, prevalence = 85%	

LR, likelihood ratio.

anus and vagina. Incomplete bladder emptying due to a variety of possible mechanisms of obstruction (e.g., enlarged prostate, prolapsed bladder or uterus, kidney stones, pregnancy) provides bacteria an opportunity to proliferate, making UTIs more likely in these individuals. When other protective mechanisms of the urinary tract, such as immunological and mucosal barriers, are jeopardized because of disease, age, or procedures (i.e., urinary catheters), this can also make certain individuals more susceptible to this condition. Gram-negative organisms are most commonly the causative agent in UTIs with strains of *E. coli* accounting for the majority of cases (Hertz et al., 2015). See **Table 16.8** for the Clinical Decision Rule for UTI in Women Without Signs of

Complicated Disease and **Box 16.2** for clinical pearls related to UTIs.

Key History and Physical Findings

- Dysuria
- Urinary frequency
- Urinary urgency
- Suprapubic pain
- Lower back pain
- Gross hematuria
- Appearance of turbid urine
- Low-grade fever
- Urethral discharge (primarily in men)
- Positive nitrites, pyuria, and hematuria on urinalysis (sensitivity of 74.02%; Mambatta et al., 2015)
- Positive urine culture result

PYELONEPHRITIS

Pyelonephritis is an inflammation and infection of the upper urinary tract involving the renal pelvis and kidney. An infection of the upper urinary tract is more severe and can have more serious implications than an infection of the lower urinary tract. Pyelonephritis occurs when bacteria ascend into the kidney, typically from an untreated lower UTI. For this reason, risk factors for pyelonephritis are similar to the risk factors for lower UTIs (see earlier section on lower UTIs). *E. coli* accounts for 90% of pyelonephritis cases in healthy young women (Johnson & Russo, 2018). Pyelonephritis can lead to sepsis if left untreated. Genitourinary causes account for 10.3% of sepsis cases in males and 18.0% of sepsis cases in females (Mayr, Yende, & Angus, 2013).

Key History and Physical Findings

- History of untreated lower UTI
- Sudden onset of systemic symptoms (fever, chills, malaise)
- Urinary frequency
- Urinary urgency

BOX 16.2
CLINICAL PEARLS: URINARY TRACT INFECTIONS

- Cloudy and/or foul-smelling urine should not be used to diagnose a UTI.
- Positive leukocyte esterase may signal pyuria and UTI.
- Positive WBCs in the urine do not diagnose UTI.
- Positive nitrite testing of a urine sample is highly specific for gram-negative bacteria (such as *E. coli*). Negative urine nitrates do not rule out UTI because of the bladder dwell time necessary for positive testing.
- Positive squamous cells do not necessarily indicate contamination of a urine specimen.
- Urine culture should be utilized to confirm a UTI.
- Bacteriuria but no pyuria = colonization/bacteriuria
- Pyuria alone but no bacteria = inflammation
- Pyuria + bacteriuria + nitrites = infection

UTI, urinary tract infection; WBCs, white blood cells.

- Dysuria
- Unilateral flank pain
- Abdominal pain
- Nausea/vomiting
- Gross hematuria
- Unilateral costovertebral angle tenderness
- Enlarged kidney (palpable on exam)
- Urinalysis showing pyuria, bacteriuria, and nitrites
- White blood cell casts on microscopy
- Urine culture (>10,000 colony-forming units of a uropathogen/mL)
- Acute pyelonephritis will classically present as a triad of fever, unilateral flank pain, and nausea or vomiting, but not all symptoms have to be present.

RENAL COLIC (UROLITHIASIS, URETEROLITHIASIS)

Renal colic is severe abdominal/flank pain from an obstructing calculus (renal/kidney stone) within the urinary system. Renal calculi can affect any part of the urinary tract. Depending on the location and size of the calculus, location of pain and presentation can vary. The pain from renal colic is caused by dilation, stretching, and spasm of the ureters. Most kidney stones are formed from calcium oxalate. Kidney stones are treated in different ways depending on the location and size of the stones (Leveridge et al., 2016).

Key History and Physical Findings

- Sudden-onset, unilateral, severe pain in the flank
- Intermittent, colicky pain (comes in waves and fluctuates in intensity)
- Pain can radiate to the lower abdomen, groin, or genitals.
- Nausea/vomiting
- Dysuria
- Urinary frequency
- Urinary urgency
- Low voided volumes (distal ureteric stones)
- Positive CVA tenderness
- Pink, red, or brown urine
- Tachycardia
- Patient often paces and has constant movement due to pain.

- Microscopic hematuria
- Calculus on imaging

URINARY INCONTINENCE

Urinary incontinence is the involuntary leakage of urine. Urinary incontinence can range from mild leaking to total loss of bladder control. There are different etiologies of urinary incontinence. The four main types are stress incontinence, urge incontinence, overflow incontinence, and functional incontinence (Bardsley, 2016). There can be overlap of two or more of these conditions called mixed incontinence. Stress incontinence occurs because of a weakened or damaged urethral sphincter or pelvic floor muscles (or both). When individuals have this condition, any type of activity that increases abdominal pressure, which then causes pressure on the bladder, can lead to urinary leakage or stress incontinence (Bardsley, 2016). Urge incontinence (i.e., overactive bladder) can be the result of another physical injury or chronic condition such as a brain injury, spinal injury, various neurological diseases, or diabetes. In other cases, there is no identifiable cause. Urge incontinence causes the patient to feel a strong urge to urinate even when the bladder is not full, immediately followed by the loss of urine before reaching the bathroom (Bardsley, 2016). Overflow incontinence occurs because of an obstruction in the urinary tract that prohibits urine from flowing normally out of the bladder. This causes the bladder muscle to weaken, which causes the individual to lose the urge to urinate. This, in turn, causes the bladder to overflow, allowing urine to leak. Some examples of types of obstruction include an enlarged prostate, a tumor, and urinary stones (Bardsley, 2016). Functional incontinence is when the patient's urinary tract is functioning properly, but the patient has a physical or mental comorbidity or disability that prohibits them from effectively reaching or using the bathroom. Examples include dementia/cognitive impairment, diuretic medications, impaired mobility that makes it difficult to get to the toilet in a timely manner, and arthritis that causes difficulty getting clothing removed (Bardsley, 2016). See **Table 16.9** for the Historical Symptom Assessment tool.

TABLE 16.9 Urinary Incontinence: Historical Symptom Assessment				
Symptom	Stress Incontinence	Urge Incontinence	Mixed Incontinence	Overflow Incontinence
Leak with cough, sneeze, exercise	+	−	+	−
Leak with urgency	−	+	+	−
Frequent urination	−	+	+	−
Continuous leakage	−	−	−	+

Key History and Physical Findings

- Stress incontinence: History of vaginal childbirth; being overweight or obese; history of pelvic prolapse; pregnancy; loss of urine when sneezing, laughing, coughing, jumping, exercising, or increasing abdominal pressure
- Urge incontinence: History of neurological disease or injury; history of diabetes; urinary frequency; intense urinary urgency immediately followed by the involuntary loss of urine

- Overflow incontinence: History of benign prostatic hypertrophy, neurogenic bladder, diabetes, or any other condition that can damage the nerves or bladder; constant or frequent dribbling of urine
- Functional incontinence: Dementia; disabilities related to mobility; history of arthritis; diuretic medications; any physical or mental impairment that causes difficulty in effectively getting to the bathroom

CASE STUDY: Epigastic Abdominal Pain

History

A 40-year-old obese male presents with intermittent epigastric abdominal pain for the past 2 years. The pain feels like burning. The pain worsens after eating "Flaming Hot Cheetos," soda, orange juice, and salsa. He has occasional nausea and rare episodes of vomiting. He passes bowel movements one to two times a day. The stools are soft without blood or mucus. He takes antacids as needed, which is typically two to three times a day with little relief. He reports no associated fevers, weight loss, blood in the stools, or melena.

Physical Examination

- Height: 5′8″, weight: 200 lb; HR: 80, RR: 18, BP: 132/84
- General appearance: Well-appearing
- HEENT: Head is normocephalic, atraumatic. Pupils are equal, round, and reactive to light. Conjunctiva are pink; sclera are not icteric. Nares clear without exudate or flaring. Posterior pharynx is pink with 2+ tonsils, tongue is midline, and he has normal dentition.

- Neck: Neck is supple without thyromegaly, adenopathy, or decreased range of motion.
- Chest: Lungs are clear to auscultation bilaterally with unlabored respiratory effort. Regular rate and rhythm without murmur. No jugular venous distention.
- Abdomen: Abdomen is soft, obese, and nondistended without hepatosplenomegaly or masses. There is tenderness to deep palpation in the epigastric area.
- Anorectal: Deferred
- Skin: Pink, warm, well perfused, no jaundice, no rashes

Differential Diagnosis

GERD, nonerosive reflux disease (NERD), functional dyspepsia, rumination syndrome, eosinophilic esophagitis, *H. pylori* gastritis, hiatal hernia, celiac disease, achalasia, Barrett's esophagus, pancreatitis

Final Diagnosis

GERD

CASE STUDY: Periumbilical Abdominal Pain

History

A 12-year-old girl presents for abdominal pain intermittently for the past year. The pain is periumbilical and she has difficulty describing its characteristics, indicating that the pain "comes and goes." She may have pain daily for a week, and then have no pain for 1 to 2 weeks. The pain does

not wake her at night. Eating sometimes makes the pain better but can also make it worse. There are no particular food triggers. She denies stress, but the mother feels stress may worsen the pain. She has occasional nausea but no vomiting. Stooling sometimes makes the pain better but can also make it worse. She is having bowel movements one to two

(continued)

CASE STUDY: Periumbilical Abdominal Pain (*continued*)

times a day with soft-formed stools without blood or mucus. She has tried Tums and Pepcid without improvement. She has no recurrent fevers, weight loss, dysuria, arthralgias, or diarrhea. She has missed over 10 days of school this year due to the pain.

Physical Examination
- Height: 155 cm, weight: 36 kg, HR: 92, RR: 14, BP: 114/66
- General appearance: Well-appearing
- HEENT: Head is normocephalic, atraumatic. Conjunctiva are pink; sclera are not icteric. Nares clear without exudate or flaring. Throat is not injected, with tongue midline and normal dentition.
- Neck: Neck is supple without thyromegaly, adenopathy, or decreased range of motion.
- Chest: Lungs are clear to auscultation bilaterally with unlabored respiratory effort. Regular rate and rhythm without murmur. No jugular venous distention.

- Abdomen: Abdomen is soft and nondistended without hepatosplenomegaly or masses. There is tenderness in all four quadrants. There is no guarding or rebound tenderness.
- Anorectal: No skin tags or fissures. Normal anal tone, nondilated rectum, small soft stool within rectal vault.
- Stool analysis: Hemoccult negative
- Skin: Pink, warm, well perfused, no jaundice, no rashes

Differential Diagnosis
Functional abdominal pain, IBS, abdominal migraines, constipation, GERD, peptic ulcers, celiac disease, food allergy or intolerance, hepatobiliary disease, pancreatitis, IBD, renal stones, gynecological disorders

Final Diagnosis
Functional abdominal pain

Clinical Pearls

- Abdominal pain is COMMON, and most individuals with abdominal pain have a benign or self-limiting condition. The initial goal of assessment is to identify those individuals with a serious etiology.
- Functional abdominal pain disorders (FAP) account for 50% of GI consults. Indicators of functional pain disorders include absence of red flags, onset after apparent GI infection, worse on weekdays and/or during school year, history of anxiety/depression in child or parent, family history of IBS or chronic pain disorder, "excruciating" pain during visit, missing school or work.
- Rome IV criteria (see criteria in **Table 16.9**) has been established for disorders of gut–brain interaction (DGBI) to help in the diagnosis of DGBIs and differentiate between different clinical entities. More information can be found at www.theromefoundation.org.
- Although children with chronic abdominal pain and their parents are more often anxious or depressed than are children without chronic pain, the presence of anxiety, depression, behavior

problems, or recent negative life events does not appear to be useful in distinguishing between FAP and organic disease (Di Lorenzo et al., 2005).
- Lactose intolerance may be found in teenagers and adults, but is less common in infants and children. Dairy protein intolerance is often associated with atopic disease (allergies, asthma, and eczema).
- Dairy and gluten are common foods reported to cause GI symptoms; however, true food allergies, without other atopic disease, is much lower than what is self-reported in patients with IBS or chronic pain.
- GI allergic diseases occur more often in children than in adults.
- Constipation is a common problem in children and adults. Most patients have no underlying medical disease responsible for symptoms.
- Red flags in constipation include onset <1 month of age, passage of meconium >48 hours, family history of Hirschsprung's disease, ribbon stools, blood in stool, failure to thrive, unexplained weight loss, fever, bilious vomiting, severe abdominal distention, absent anal or cremasteric reflex, tuft of hair on spine,

abnormal thyroid, abnormal anal position, anal scars, and extreme fear during anal inspection.

- Obesity does not exclude celiac disease.
- Diagnostic testing for celiac must take place when a patient is consuming gluten.
- Most infants with reflux are "happy spitters" and do not require extensive testing.
- Most cases of pancreatitis in children are mild and self-limiting. Early oral feeding is recommended rather than NPO (nil per os) in managing acute pancreatitis (Crockett, Wani, Gardner, Falck-Ytter, & Barkun, 2018).
- The first 2 years of life are critical for linear growth. Severe nutritional deficits can have long-term effects on growth.
- Eating disorders should be considered when there is dramatic weight loss, nonspecific GI concerns, extreme concern about body size and weight, frequent dieting, or excessive exercise.

Key Takeaways

Assessment of the abdomen requires an understanding of the bony and muscular architecture of the abdomen and the organs, muscles, and structures contained within it.

Abdominal pain is one of the most common subjective chief concerns.

Abdominal pain can be challenging to diagnosis due to the nonspecific neuroreceptors found in the visceral cavity.

Abdominal pain can be referred pain from outside the GI/GU system so other systems should always be considered and ruled out.

REFERENCES

Ahn, S., Lee, H., Choi, W., Ahn, R., Hong, J. S., Sohn, C. H., . . . Kim, W. Y. (2016). Clinical importance of the heel drop test and a new clinical score for adult appendicitis. *PLoS One*, *11*(10), e0164574. doi:10.1371/journal.pone.0164574

American Academy of Pediatrics & American Society of Pediatric Nephrology. (2018). Five things physicians and patients should question. Retrieved from http://www.choosingwisely.org/societies/american-academy-of-pediatrics-section-on-nephrology-and-the-american-society-of-pediatric-nephrology

American College of Emergency Physicians. (2018). *Ten things physicians and patients should question.*
Retrieved from https://www.choosingwisely.org/societies/american-college-of-emergency-physicians

American College of Radiology. (2017). *Ten things physicians and patients should question.* Retrieved from https://www.choosingwisely.org/societies/american-college-of-radiology

American Gastroenterology Association. (2012). *Five things physicians and patients should question.* Retrieved from https://www.choosingwisely.org/societies/american-gastroenterological-association

American Urological Association. (2019). *Fifteen things physicians and patients should question.* Retrieved from http://www.choosingwisely.org/societies/american-urological-association

Bardsley, A. (2016). An overview of urinary incontinence. *British Journal of Nursing, 25*(18), S14–S21. doi:10.12968/bjon.2016.25.18.S14

Barkun, A., & Grover, S. A. (2009). Splenomegaly. In D. L. Simel & D. Rennie (Eds.), *The rational clinical examination: Evidence-based clinical diagnosis.* New York, NY: Mc-Graw-Hill. Retrieved from http://jamaevidence.mhmedical.com/content.aspx?bookid=845&sectionid=61357591

Benabbas, R., Hanna, M., Shah, J., & Sinert, R. (2017). Diagnostic accuracy of history, physical examination, laboratory tests, and point-of-care ultrasound for pediatric acute appendicitis in the emergency department: A systematic review and meta-analysis. *Academy of Emergency Medicine, 24*(5), 523–551. doi:10.1111/acem.13181

Bundy, D. G., Byerley, J. S., Liles, E. A., Perrin, E. M., Katznelson, J., & Rice, H. E. (2007). Does this child have appendicitis? *Journal of the American Medical Association, 298*(4), 438–451. doi:10.1001/jama.298.4.438

Centers for Disease Control and Prevention. (n.d.). Hepatitis C questions and answers for the public. Retrieved from https://www.cdc.gov/hepatitis/hcv/cfaq.htm

Chapman, J., & Azevedo, A. M. (2019, January). Splenomegaly. In *StatPearls* [Internet]. Treasure Island, FL: StatPearls Publishing. Retrieved from https://www.ncbi.nlm.nih.gov/books/NBK430907/

Childs, J. T., Esterman, A. J., Thoirs, K. A., & Turner, R. C. (2016). Ultrasound in the assessment of hepatomegaly: A simple technique to determine an enlarged liver using reliable and valid measurements. *Sonography, 3*(2), 47–52. doi:10.1002/sono.12051

Cosford, P. A., Leng, G. C., & Thomas, J. (2007). Screening for abdominal aortic aneurysm. *Cochrane Database of Systematic Reviews,* (2), CD002945. doi:10.1002/14651858.CD002945.pub2

Crockett, S. D., Wani, S., Gardner, T. B., Falck-Ytter, Y., & Barkun, A. N. (2018). American Gastroenterological Association Institute guideline on initial management of acute pancreatitis. *Gastroenterology, 154,* 1096–1101. Retrieved from https://www.gastrojournal.org/article/S0016-5085(18)30076-3/pdf

D'Amico, D., & Barbarito, C. (2016). *Health and physical assessment in nursing* (3rd ed.). New York, NY: Pearson Education.

Di Lorenzo, C., Colletti, R., Lehmann, H., Boyle, J., Gerson, W., Hyams, J., . . . Kanda, P. (2005). Chronic abdominal pain in children: A technical report of the American Academy of Pediatrics and the North American Society for Pediatric

Gastroenterology, Hepatology and Nutrition. *Journal of Pediatric Gastroenterology and Nutrition, 40*, 249–261. doi:10.1097/01.mpg.0000154661.39488.ac

Durup-Dickenson, M., Christensen, M. K., & Gade, J. (2013). Abdominal auscultation does not provide clear clinical diagnosis. *Danish Medical Journal, 60*, 1–5. Retrieved from http://ugeskriftet.dk/dmj/abdominal-auscultation-does-not-provide-clear-clinical-diagnoses

Esposito, C., Roberti, A., Turrà, F., Escolino, M., Cerulo, M., Settimi, C., . . . Di Mezza, A. (2015). Management of gastroesophageal reflux disease in pediatric patients: A literature review. *Pediatric Health Medical Therapy, 6*, 1–8. doi:10.2147/PHMT.S46250

Felder, S., Margel, D., Murrell, Z., & Fleshner, P. (2014). Usefulness of bowel sound auscultation: A prospective evaluation. *Journal of Surgical Education, 71*, 768–773. doi:10.1016/j.jsurg.2014.02.003

Gade, J., Kruse, P., Anderson, O. T., Pedersen, S. B., & Boesby, S. (1998). Physicians' abdominal auscultation. A multi-rater agreement study. *Scandinavian Journal of Gastroenterology, 33*, 773–777. doi:10.1080/00365529850171756

Goolsby, M. J. and Grubbs, L. (Eds.). (2015). *Advanced assessment interpretation of findings and formulating differential diagnoses* (3rd ed.). Philadelphia, PA: F. A. Davis.

Gu, Y., Lim, H. J., & Moser, A. A. J. (2010). How useful are bowel sounds in assessing the abdomen? *Digestive Surgery, 27*, 422–426. doi:10.1159/000319372

Gupta, K., Dhawan, A., Abel, C., Talley, N., & Attia, J. (2013). A re-evaluation of the scratch test for locating the liver edge. *BMC Gastroenterology, 13*, 35. doi:10.1186/1471-230X-13-35

Hertz, F., Schønning, K., Rasmussen, S., Littauer, P., Knudsen, J., Løbner-Olesen, A., & Frimodt-Møller, N. (2015). Epidemiological factors associated with ESBL- and non ESBL-producing *E. coli* causing urinary tract infection in general practice. *Infectious Diseases, 48*(3), 241–245. doi:10.3109/23744235.2015.1103895

Hogan-Quigley, B., Palm, M. L., & Bickley, L. (2012). *Bates' nursing guide to physical assessment and history taking.* Philadelphia, PA: Wolters Kluwer/ Lippincott Williams & Wilkins.

Johnson, J., & Russo, T. (2018). Acute pyelonephritis in adults. *New England Journal of Medicine, 378*(1), 48–59. doi:10.1056/NEJMcp1702758

Kharbanda, A. B., Taylor, G. A., Fishman, S. J., & Bachur, R. G. (2005). A clinical decision rule to identify children at low risk for appendicitis. *Pediatrics, 116*(3), 709–716. doi:10.1542/peds.2005-0094

Lacy, B. E., Mearin, F., Chang, L., Chey, W. D., Lembo, A. J., Simren, M., & Spiller, R. (2016). Bowel disorders. *Gastroenterology, 150*(6), 1393–1407. doi:10.1053/j.gastro.2016.02.031

Leveridge, M., D'Arcy, F. T., O'Kane, D., Ischia, J., Webb, D., Bolton, D. M., & Lawrentschuk, N. (2016). Renal colic: Current protocols for emergency presentations. *European Journal of Emergency Medicine, 23*(1), 2–7. doi:10.1097/MEJ.0000000000000324

Mambatta, A. K., Jayarajan, J., Rashme, V. L., Harini, S., Menon, S., & Kuppusamy, J. (2015). Reliability of dipstick assay in predicting urinary tract infection. *Journal of Family Medicine and Primary Care, 4*(2), 265–268. doi:10.4103/2249-4863.154672

Massey, R. L. (2012). Return of bowel sounds indicating an end of postoperative ileus: Is it time to cease this long-standing nursing tradition? *Medical Surgical Nursing, 21*, 146–150. Retrieved from https://www.ncbi.nlm.nih.gov/pubmed/22866434

Mayo Clinic. (2018). Patient care and health information: Inguinal hernia: Diagnosis and treatment. Retrieved from https://www.mayoclinic.org/diseases-conditions/inguinal-hernia/diagnosis-treatment/drc-20351553

Mayr, F. B., Yende, S., & Angus, D. C. (2013). Epidemiology of severe sepsis. *Virulence, 5*(1), 4–11. doi:10.4161/viru.27372

McGee, S. (2017). *Evidence based physical diagnosis* (4th ed.). St. Louis, MO: Elsevier.

Mohd Hanafiah, K., Groeger, J., Flaxman, A., & Wiersma, S. (2013). Global epidemiology of hepatitis C virus infection: New estimates of age-specific antibody to HCV seroprevalence. *Hepatology, 57*, 1333–1342. doi:10.1002/hep.26141

Mostbeck, G., Adam, E. J., Nielsen, M. B., Claudon, M., Clevert, D., Nicolau, C., . . . Owens, C. M. (2016). How to diagnose acute appendicitis: Ultrasound first. *Insights Imaging, 7*(2), 255–263. doi:10.1007/s13244-016-0469-6.

North American Society for Pediatric Gastroenterology, Hepatology and Nutrition. *Guidelines on GERD, constipation, celiac, eosinophilic esophagitis, chronic abdominal pain, in addition to many other GI resources.* Retrieved from https://www.naspghan.org/

Pinsky, L. E., & Wipf, J. E. (n.d.). *Advanced physical diagnosis learning and teaching at the bedside.* Seattle: University of Washington Department of Medicine. Retrieved from https://depts.washington.edu/physdx/liver/evid2.html

Rosen, R., Vandenplas, Y., Singendonk, M., Cabana, M., DiLorenzo, C., Gottrand, F., . . . Tabbers, M. (2018). Pediatric gastroesophageal reflux clinical practice guidelines: Joint recommendations of the North American Society for Pediatric Gastroenterology, Hepatology and Nutrition and the European Society for Pediatric Gastroenterology, Hepatology and Nutrition. *Journal of Pediatric Gastroenterology and Nutrition, 66*(3), 516–554. doi:10.1097/MPG.0000000000001889

Schmulson, M. J., & Drossman, D. A. (2017). What is new in Rome IV. *Journal of Neurogastroenterological Motility, 23*(2), 151–163. doi:10.5056/jnm16214

Seller, R. H., & Symons, A. B. (2018). *Differential diagnosis of common complaints* (7th ed.). St. Louis, MO: Elsevier.

Siddiqui (2018). Overview of biliary function. In R. S. Porter (Ed.), *MSD manual: Professional version.* Retrieved from https://www.msdmanuals.com/professional/hepatic-and-biliary-disorders/gallbladder-and-bile-duct-disorders/overview-of-biliary-function

Simel, D.L., Rennie, D., & Keitz, S. (Eds.). (2009). *The rational clinical examination: Evidence-based clinical diagnosis.* New York, NY: McGraw-Hill.

Stewart, K. R., Derck, A. M., Long, K. L., Learman, K., & Cook, C. (2013). Diagnostic accuracy of clinical tests for the detection of splenomegaly. *Physical Therapy Reviews, 18*(3), 173–184. doi:10.1179/1743288X13Y.0000000081

Ueda, T., & Ishida, E. (2015). Indirect fist percussion of the liver is a more sensitive technique for detecting hepatobiliary infections than Murphy's sign. *Current Gerontology and Geriatrics Research, 2015*, 6. doi:10.1155/2015/431638

U.S. Preventive Services Task Force. (2016). Final update summary: Colorectal cancer: Screening. Retrieved from https://www.uspreventiveservicestaskforce.org/Page/Document/UpdateSummaryFinal/colorectal-cancer-screening

Williams, J. W., & Simel, D. L. (1992). Does this patient have ascites? How to divine fluid in the abdomen. *Journal of the American Medical Association, 267,* 2645–2648. doi:10.1001/jama.1992.03480190087038

Wright, W. (2016). Cullen sign and Grey Turner sign revisited. *The Journal of the American Osteopathic Association, 116,* 398–401. doi:10.7556/jaoa.2016.081

Zuin, M., Rigatelli, G., Andreotti, A. N., Fogato, L., & Roncon, L. (2017). Is abdominal assessment still a relevant part of the physical examination? *European Journal of Internal Medicine, 43,* e24–e25. doi:10.1016/j.ejim.2017.04.013

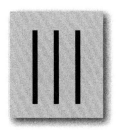

III

EVIDENCE-BASED PHYSICAL EXAMINATION AND ASSESSMENT OF SEXUAL AND REPRODUCTIVE HEALTH

17

Evidence-Based Assessment of the Breasts and Axillae

Brenda M. Gilmore and Brittany B. Hay

"We know what we are but know not what we may be."

—WILLIAM SHAKESPEARE

LEARNING OBJECTIVES

- Review the prominent anatomic and physiologic features of the breast and the axillae.
- Identify key components of a comprehensive health history and evidence-based physical examination of the breast and axillae.
- Identify common assessment tools for screening and diagnoses for the breast and axillae.
- Delineate common abnormal findings of the breast and the axillae.

ANATOMY AND PHYSIOLOGY OF THE BREASTS AND AXILLAE

At birth and throughout childhood, the structure and function of male and female breasts are similar. The prepubertal breast consists of rudimentary breast components, including estrogen and androgen receptors, and several lobes, or small divisions in breast tissue, located under the areola and nipple. With the onset of puberty, and in response to the influence of sex hormones, dramatic structural and functional changes occur. Maturation of the ductal and glandular system results in the specialized lobules required for **lactation**, or the production and secretion of milk. The mature female breast contains the mammary gland, the milk-producing gland, and the lobules and ducts required to secrete and eject human milk, part of the process of lactation.

The adult female breast is a dome-like structure that lies vertically between the second and the sixth ribs and horizontally between the sternal edge and the mid-axillary line. The breast also extends into the axilla; this area of breast tissue is known as the tail of Spence. Two fascial layers envelop the breast and secure its position. The superficial pectoral fascia covers the breast, and the deep pectoral fascia, at the undersurface of the breast, covers the pectoralis major and anterior serratus muscles. Cooper suspensory ligaments are fibrous bands that connect the two fascial layers and offer structural support for the breast (Obsorne, 2014).

The breast is approximately 10 to 12 cm in diameter, with an average thickness of 5 to 7 cm centrally. The nipple, located over the fourth intercostal space and surrounded by the areola, contains abundant sensory nerve endings and 15 to 20 lactiferous ducts (Ellis & Mahadevan, 2013). The areola is circular and pigmented and contains visible sebaceous glands, known as the glands of Montgomery, and apocrine sweat glands. The breast is composed of skin, breast tissue, and subcutaneous tissue. The skin of the breast is thin and contains hair follicles, sebaceous glands, and eccrine sweat glands. Most of the breast tissue is localized in the upper outer quadrant of the breast and is composed of both parenchyma and stroma. The functional or glandular breast tissue, known as the parenchyma, is divided into 15 to 20 lobes that come together at the nipple in a radial configuration. Within each of the lobes are 20 to 40 lobules, and each of these lobules consists

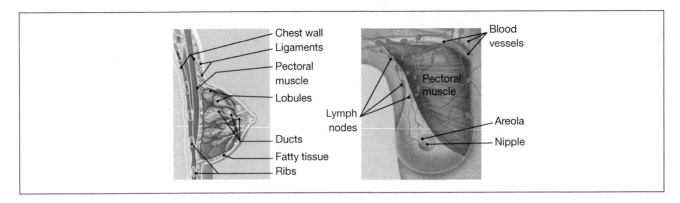

FIGURE 17.1 Breast anatomy, front (right) and lateral (left) views. The breast is composed of skin, breast tissue, and subcutaneous tissue. The functional or glandular breast tissue, known as the parenchyma, is divided into 15 to 20 lobes that come together at the nipple in a radial configuration.

of milk-producing alveoli or secretory units. These units are unremarkable in nonlactating women. Each lobe is connected at the nipple by lactiferous ducts that drain milk onto the nipple surface during lactation. The stroma and subcutaneous tissues of the breast contain fat, connective tissue, blood vessels, nerves, and lymphatics (Obsorne, 2014). See **Figure 17.1** for overall breast anatomy (front and lateral views).

The complex vascular supply and lymphatic drainage networks of the breast can be best understood by considering each region of the breast, as medial and lateral regions have unique structures to support breast function. The primary blood supply for the breast arises from the internal thoracic artery, which supplies the majority of the breast medially and centrally. This region of the breast is drained by the internal thoracic vein and the adjacent parasternal lymph nodes exiting the medial side of the breast. The upper outer or lateral side of the breast is supplied by the lateral thoracic artery, a branch of the axillary artery, and lateral branches of the intercostal arteries. This region of the breast is drained by the lateral thoracic and intercostal veins with lymphatic vessels that lead mainly to the pectoral group of lymph nodes. Ultimately, lymph from the right breast drains into the right lymphatic duct, and that from the left breast drains into the thoracic lymphatic duct (Morton, Foreman, & Albertine, 2011; **Figure 17.2**).

Cyclic hormonal changes during the menstrual cycle profoundly influence breast tissue morphology. Under the premenstrual influence of increasing estrogen and progesterone levels, the breasts are full related to the increasing interlobular edema and enhanced ductular–acinar proliferation. With the onset of menstruation, after a rapid decline in the circulating estrogen and progesterone levels, secretory activity within the epithelial tissue regresses. After menstruation, the tissue edema continues to abate, and the regression of the epithelium ends as a new menstrual cycle begins. The lowest breast volume is observed 5 to 7 days after menstruation (Obsorne, 2014).

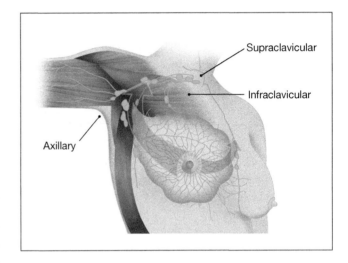

FIGURE 17.2 Blood supply and lymphatic drainage. The breasts contain a highly complex network of vasculature and lymphatic drainage.

LIFE-SPAN DIFFERENCES AND CONSIDERATIONS IN ANATOMY AND PHYSIOLOGY OF THE BREASTS AND AXILLAE

Adolescence/Tanner Staging

Puberty begins in females by the ages of 10 to 12 years, and breast development is one of the first signs. Rising hormonal levels and ovarian function induce changes to the rudimentary breast tissue. The synergistic effects of estrogen and progesterone are responsible for ductular–lobular–alveolar maturation of mammary tissues (Ellis & Mahadevan, 2013). Breast evolution from childhood to maturity is differentiated by external morphologic changes delineated by the five Tanner stages. **Table 17.1** identifies the physical findings associated with the five phases of breast development. Menstruation in the majority of females occurs by the third or fourth Tanner stage of development (Obsorne, 2014). While breast development occurs through identifiable

TABLE 17.1 Tanner Staging: Phases of Breast Development

Estimated Age (Years)	Phase	Physical Findings
≤10	1	Preadolescent elevation of the nipple with no palpable glandular tissue or areolar pigmentation
10–12	2	Presence of glandular tissue in the subareolar region; nipple and breast project as a single mound from the chest wall
11–13	3	Increase in the amount of readily palpable glandular tissue with enlargement of the breast and increased diameter and pigmentation of the areola; contour of the breast and nipple remains in a single plane
12–14	4	Enlargement of the areola and increased areolar pigmentation; nipple and areola form a secondary mound above the level of the breast
13–17	5	Final adolescent development of a smooth contour with no projection of the areola and nipple

phases, breast growth is unique to each individual, varies in timing, and can be asymmetrical.

Pregnancy/Lactation

During pregnancy, owing to estrogen, progesterone, and placental hormonal secretion, significant ductular, lobular, and alveolar growth occurs in the breast (Obsorne, 2014). There are two specific hormones that induce lactation in pregnancy. Prolactin, excreted by the anterior pituitary gland, is progressively released during pregnancy; prolactin release begins slowly during the first half of pregnancy and then rises three to five times higher than normal during the second and third trimesters (Ellis & Mahadevan, 2013; Obsorne, 2014). Human placental lactogen, produced by the placenta, peaks during the third trimester and prepares the breast for the production of human milk. While prolactin and placental lactogen prepare the breast during pregnancy for lactation, elevated estrogen and progesterone levels inhibit milk production. Soon after birth, an immediate cessation of placental lactogen and a marked drop in estrogen and progesterone levels occurs (Ellis & Mahadevan, 2013). Within the first 4 to 5 days postpartum, the breasts enlarge as a result of the accumulation of secretions in the

alveoli and ducts. Oxytocin, a lactogenic hormone produced in the hypothalamus and stored in the posterior pituitary gland, mediates prolactin secretion with neonatal sucking. The initial postbirth mammary secretion is **colostrum**, a thin, serous fluid that is, at first, sticky and yellow. After colostrum secretion, transitional milk and then mature milk are produced (Ellis & Mahadevan, 2013; Obsorne, 2014). During well-established lactation, a liter of human milk can be produced per day (Ellis & Mahadevan, 2013).

Menopausal Changes

Owing to diminishing ovarian function, the menopausal transition is associated with a natural and marked decline in the production of estrogen and progesterone. The diminution of hormonal stimulus leads to an overall decline in epithelial and stromal structures. There is significant reduction in the number of ducts, lobules, and lymphatic channels. This culminates in a progressive attenuation or reduction in glandular breast tissue and a concurrent proliferation in fatty tissue. Consequently, these menopausal changes reduce breast density, which affords better breast cancer detection by mammography than in premenopausal women (Ellis & Mahadevan, 2013; Obsorne, 2014). **Breast cancer** is the uncontrolled growth of breast cells that can spread and invade surrounding tissues (Centers for Disease Control and Prevention [CDC], n.d.-c).

KEY HISTORY QUESTIONS AND CONSIDERATIONS FOR THE BREASTS AND AXILLAE

HISTORY OF PRESENT ILLNESS

Symptoms of breast pathology are diverse, ranging from painful lumps of variable onset to minor abnormalities, which may be dismissed by patients and their partners. Therefore, it is important for any clinician to be well versed with obtaining a comprehensive health history and associated physical examination. The careful history and exam drives development of appropriate differential diagnoses to support evidence-based diagnostic evaluation and management strategies. With breast concerns, the following should be addressed:

- Onset of symptoms: Sudden or gradual
- Location: Area of the breast with primary concern and presence of any radiation to other areas of the breast or axilla; unilateral or bilateral presentation
- Duration: Intermittent or persistent; lasting hours, days, weeks, months, or years
- Character: Burning or stinging; sharp/lancinating; dull; feeling of heaviness, throbbing, or pulling/drawing

- Aggravating factors: Hormonal influences, use of bras or binders
- Associated signs or symptoms: Change in appearance of the breast(s), including dimpling, peau d'orange, pain, nipple discharge (include amount, color, and consistency), or localized skin changes (erythema or other discoloration, increased warmth, flaking, crusting), presence of skin lesions or open areas, dilated blood vessels
- Relieving factors: Medications, change in position, application of heat or cold
- Timing: Relationship to menstrual cycle or a traumatic event
- Severity: Mild, moderate, or severe intensity (American Cancer Society [ACS], 2019; CDC, n.d.-b; National Cancer Institute [NCI], n.d.-a, n.d.-b).

PAST MEDICAL HISTORY

Pertinent medical history, including any regarding past breast health concerns that may inform the current clinical encounter and differential diagnoses, should also be obtained (ACS, 2019; CDC, n.d.-a; NCI, 2019). Assessment of past medical history includes the following:

- Previous breast conditions, including dense breasts, previous biopsies, past malignancy (including treatment and follow-up plan), past nonmalignant conditions
- History of radiation (as a teen or young adult)
- Trauma to the chest or breast
- Presence of breast implants, including length of time, type, and complications
- Genetic disorders
- Hepatic disorders
- Hormonal disorders
- Testicular cancer in men
- Medications: Hormonal therapies (including hormonal contraception and treatment for infertility), antipsychotics, antidepressants, spironolactone, chemotherapeutic agents, cimetidine, omeprazole, antiadrenergic therapies, exposure to diethylstilbestrol (DES)
- Early menarche (before the age of 12) or late menopause (after the age of 55)
- Pregnancy, childbirth, and breastfeeding history
- Other malignancies (e.g., ovarian, colon)

FAMILY HISTORY

Information regarding family history can be instrumental in determining the presence of any genetic basis for breast cancer risk in both male and female patients (ACS, 2019; CDC, n.d.-a; NCI, 2019). The family health history related to breast disorders that should be explored includes the following:

- Breast cancer history (female: mother, sister, or daughter; male), especially in a first-degree relative, including age of diagnosis and type of breast cancer if known
- Family history of premalignant lesions of the breast (hyperplasia or atypical hyperplasia)
- First-degree relative with ovarian or peritoneal cancer
- First-degree relative with pancreatic cancer
- Family history of testicular or high-grade (Gleason score >7) prostate cancers
- Known *BRCA1* and *BRCA2* genetic mutations

SOCIAL HISTORY

Lifestyle behaviors have been shown to impact an individual's breast cancer risk (ACS, 2019; CDC, n.d.-a; NCI, 2019). Unlike family history, these risk factors can be changed and include the following:

- Smoking/history of tobacco or marijuana use
- Alcohol

PREVENTIVE CARE CONSIDERATIONS

Factors for preventive care for the breast and the axillae include healthy lifestyle behaviors. These encompass healthy diet, routine exercise, and breast self-awareness (ACS, 2019; CDC, n.d.-a; Hoffman & Pearson, 2016; NCI, 2019).

LIFE-SPAN AND UNIQUE POPULATION CONSIDERATION FOR HISTORY

Overall, breast cancer risk increases with age following menopause (e.g., age over 55 years). However, certain races/ethnicities carry a significant risk of breast malignancy. Caucasian women, in general, are more likely to develop breast cancer. Yet African American women are more likely to be diagnosed at a younger age and with more advanced disease, negatively impacting overall survival rates. Comparatively, women of Asian, Hispanic, and Native American ethnicities have a lower risk of developing breast cancer and exhibit higher survival rates (Baquet, Mishra, Commiskey, Ellison, & DeShields, 2008). It is also important to note that the *BRCA* genetic mutations known to significantly increase breast cancer risk are more prevalent in Jewish people of Ashkenazi descent. A careful history with attention to the three-generation pedigree will help to alert clinicians to these associated risks (ACS, 2019; NCI, 2019).

BREAST CANCER RISK ASSESSMENT TOOLS

There are many risk assessment models employed to determine a patient's risk for breast cancer. One of the most common is the NIH Breast Cancer Risk Assessment Tool (BCRAT) based on the Gail Model (available on the NCI website: https://bcrisktool.cancer.gov). This tool rates a woman's risk of developing of breast cancer on the basis of age, age at menarche and at first live birth, family history of breast cancer, and personal history of breast abnormalities. This model has been shown to accurately predict the incidence of breast cancer in American and European women (Wang et al., 2018). There are several risk assessment tools recommended by the U.S. Preventive Services Task Force (USPSTF; Moyer, 2014). Himes, Root, Gammon, and Luthy (2016) offer one of several software-based lifetime breast cancer risk calculator options.

PHYSICAL EXAMINATION OF THE BREASTS AND AXILLAE

The **clinical breast examination (CBE)** is a key component of a well-woman exam, although its use as a screening tool is controversial. At one time widely accepted as both a screening and a diagnostic assessment, research studies have not found that CBE has a significant correlation with findings of breast cancer. As a result, the value of CBE is being questioned. (See Evidence-Based Practice Considerations for the Breasts and Axillae section later in this chapter.) Even though there is controversy regarding the actual benefit of the CBE for population-health screening, CBE may identify a small proportion of breast malignancies not detected with mammography, may be requested by an individual as a component of their exam, and can be used to document the presence of palpable masses and cysts in young women who are not typical candidates for mammography. The CBE includes visual inspection and palpation of the breast and **axillae** (or underarm; Hoffman & Pearson, 2016). If the patient has concerns about a possible breast lump, or a possible mass is detected on exam, more extensive evaluation is required.

INSPECTION OF THE BREASTS

CBE begins with inspection of the breasts, with the patient in a sitting position facing the clinician (**Figure 17.3A**). With the patient sitting and disrobed to the waist, note breast size, shape, and contour. Note the patient's natural breast asymmetry, nipple placement, and nipple configuration (Morton et al., 2011). Look for bulging or flattening of the breast contour, nipple displacement or retraction, skin dimpling, dilated superficial veins, or edema of the skin, also known as peau d'orange skin changes (Hoffman & Pearson, 2016). Inspect the nipples for fissures, scaling, excoriation, retraction, or deformity of the nipple; recent deformities suggest acquired disease. Observe the anterior trunk for the presence of any supernumerary nipples. Have the patient raise her arms overhead, and observe for a

shift in nipple position, as well as any unusual dimpling or bulging (Morton et al., 2011). Next, the breasts are viewed as a woman sits on the table's edge with her hands pressed together and with the pectoralis muscles flexed (**Figure 17.3B**) or her hands placed at the hips (**Figure 17.3C**). These positions can accentuate any dimpling by increasing tension on the breast ligaments arising from the pectoralis major fascia. When the breasts are large and pendulous, have the patient lean forward in a sitting position. This way the breasts are suspended away from the chest wall. This may facilitate the inspection process by rendering skin abnormalities and making them more easily visible (Hoffman & Pearson, 2016; Morton et al., 2011).

PALPATION OF THE BREASTS AND AXILLAE
Palpation of the Axillae

Following breast inspection, axillary, supraclavicular, and infraclavicular lymph nodes are palpated most easily with a woman seated and her arm supported by the clinician. The axilla is surrounded by the pectoralis major muscle ventrally and the latissimus dorsi muscle dorsally. Lymph nodes are detected as the clinician's fingers glide superiorly to inferiorly in the axilla and momentarily compress nodes against the lateral chest wall (**Figure 17.4**). In a thin patient, one or more normal, mobile lymph nodes less than 1 cm in diameter may be palpated. The first lymph node to become involved with breast cancer metastasis (the sentinel node) is nearly always located just behind the midportion of the pectoralis major muscle (Hoffman & Pearson, 2016).

Palpation of the Breast

Palpation of the breast is done with a woman in the supine position with one hand above her head. The entire breast is examined from the second to sixth ribs and from the left sternal border to the midaxillary line (Hoffman & Pearson, 2016). The majority of breast masses identified during the CBE are found during palpation. The supine position facilitates palpation of the breast tissue against the chest wall, as this position minimizes the normal stromal density and allows for abnormalities to be more evident on exam (**Figure 17.5**).

For a thorough assessment and documentation of the breast exam findings, imagine the breast divided into four quadrants with vertical and horizontal lines intersecting at the nipple. These quadrants are known as the upper inner, upper outer, lower inner, and lower outer (**Figure 17.6**). The upper outer quadrant encompasses the axillary tail of breast tissue that extends into the axilla. Palpate in all four quadrants of both breasts by compressing breast tissue between the pads of the three middle fingers and the chest wall (Morton et al., 2011).

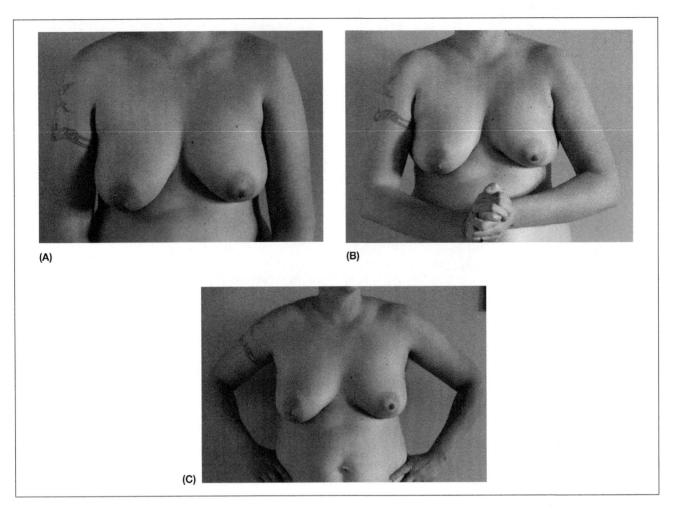

FIGURE 17.3 Positioning during breast inspection. (A) Inspection of breasts in the sitting position at front and lateral sides. (B) Inspection of breasts with hands pressed together. (C) Inspection of breasts with hands pressed on hips.

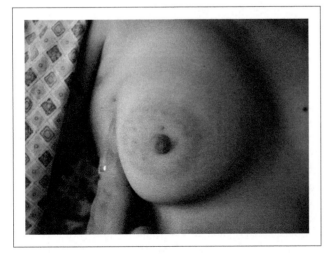

FIGURE 17.4 Palpation of upper outer quadrant while patient is seated.

Proper breast palpation technique encompasses the use of the three middle finger pads in a continuous rolling, gliding circular motion in the vertical strip, circular, or wedge pattern (**Figure 17.7**). The pressure of the fingers should be varied from light to medium to deep palpation. The areola and the nipple are included inherently in the palpation of the breast. However, nipple expression to assess for the presence of nipple discharge is not recommended unless the patient describes spontaneous discharge that requires evaluation (Hoffman & Pearson, 2016). During palpation, the breast tissue is carefully appraised for the presence of increased heat, tenderness, or masses. If abnormal breast findings are noted, they are described by their location in the right or left breast, clock position, distance from the areola, and size. The mobility and consistency of the abnormality should also be established (Klein, 2005; Morton et al., 2011). The physical characteristics of palpable

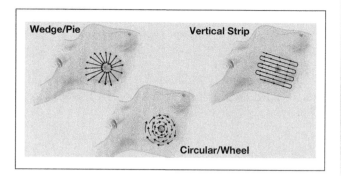

FIGURE 17.7 Breast palpation methods. Breast palpation should be completed in one of these three ways (clockwise, left to right): wedge/pie, vertical strip, or circular/wheel. These examination techniques provide a systematic way to ensure the clinician palpates the entire breast.

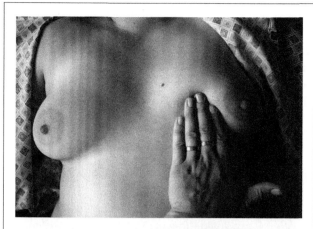

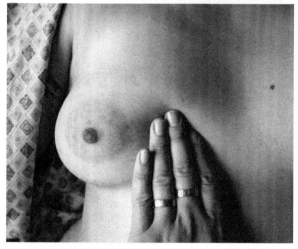

FIGURE 17.5 Breast palpation in the supine position.

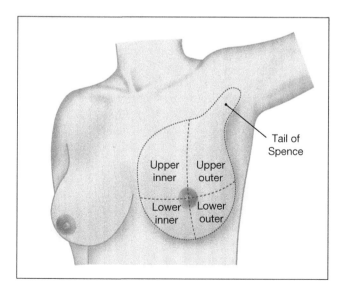

FIGURE 17.6 Breast quadrants. This figure shows the four quadrants of the breast. This anatomic system is commonly used to describe exam findings in breast conditions.

breast masses correlated with benign and malignant findings are listed in **Table 17.2**.

LIFE-SPAN CONSIDERATIONS FOR PHYSICAL EXAMINATION OF THE BREASTS AND AXILLAE

The breasts may be engorged and tender the week prior to menses and during pregnancy. This can render the breast examination more uncomfortable for the patient and less accurate. The breast exam during pregnancy should be reserved for women with specific breast-related concerns. For premenopausal women who have a low risk of breast cancer, 1 week after onset of menses is the time frame least likely to cause pain and most likely to allow for exam accuracy (Morton et al., 2011).

UNIQUE POPULATION CONSIDERATIONS FOR PHYSICAL EXAMINATION OF THE BREASTS AND AXILLAE

Men

CBEs are not recommended as a routine screening or diagnostic tool for men. However, breast tissue in men, primarily located behind and concentric to the nipple-areola complex, can develop enlargement and/or suspicious lumps that do require assessment. Enlargement of the breast tissue, gynecomastia, is typically described as disk or plate-like, and can present as a central breast mass. Gynecomastia can be a normal finding during puberty; common causes of gynecomastia beyond puberty include certain pharmacotherapies and hepatic dysfunction. Medications such as H_2 blockers, phenytoin, and marijuana have been associated with gynecomastia. Hepatic dysfunction can impair testosterone clearance, increase peripheral conversion of testosterone to estradiol and estrone, and result in breast tissue stimulation and hypertrophy. Important to note

TABLE 17.2 Physical Characteristics of Benign Versus Malignant Breast Masses

Benign	Malignant
Well-defined, distinct shape and size	Indistinct, irregular borders
Smooth, soft, or rubbery consistency	Hard, asymmetrical texture
Mobile and nonfixed to surrounding tissues	Immobile and fixed to adjacent structures
No skin changes	Dimpling, edema, nipple retraction
Scattered symmetrical tissue thickening in upper outer quadrants of both breasts	Unilateral localized thickening of the breast tissue surrounding the mass site

Source: Klein, S. (2005, May 1). Evaluation of palpable breast masses. *American Family Physician, 71*(9), 1731–1738. Retrieved from https://www.aafp.org/afp/2005/0501/p1731.html

during inspection of the male breast is whether there is distortion of the nipple and areola, as puckering of the skin, discoloration of the nipple, and/or displacement of the areola can indicate an underlying cyst or lump. Despite the smaller amount of breast tissue, the assessment, documentation, and diagnostic decision-making related to male breast exam findings are similar to female breast assessment and diagnoses (Bleicher, 2014).

Sexual and Gender Minorities

Sexual and gender minorities are populations or groups whose sexual orientation, gender identity, gender expression, and/or sexual practices differ from majority groups. Chapter 19, Evidence-Based Assessment of Sexual Orientation, Gender Identity, and Health, discusses the assessment of individuals who identify as a part of sexual and/or gender minority groups, including preventive care considerations. Sexual and gender minority populations are known to have less access to care and experience poorer health outcomes. For example, lesbian women, or women who are romantically interested in other women, are 10 times more likely to forgo breast cancer screening despite being at increased risk for breast cancer–related mortality than their heterosexual counterparts. A trans-man, whose gender identity is male but who was assigned female at birth, who is undergoing androgen hormonal treatment may be at significant risk for breast cancer if he has the *BRCA1* or *BRCA2* genetic mutation; this increased risk is because testosterone is partially metabolized into an estrogen that can stimulate any remaining breast tissue.

Complicating increased risk of breast cancer in sexual and gender minority populations is their increased likelihood to experience health disparities, gender dysphoria, and implicit or explicit bias. When combined with physical changes associated with hormonal influences and/or surgical interventions, elements of a clinical examination may be traumatic. Such perceptions and experiences hold the potential to negatively impact patient engagement in recommended screening and health promotion behaviors. Clinicians should be cognizant that discussing sexual history, partners, or practices may be difficult for individuals who identify as belonging to a sexual and gender minority. During clinical encounters, it is imperative for clinicians to ensure confidentiality, make no assumptions regarding sexual orientation, and establish a respectful, trusting clinician–patient relationship (Gillespie & Capriotti, 2016).

LABORATORY CONSIDERATIONS FOR THE BREASTS AND AXILLAE

GENETIC TESTING FOR *BRCA* AND OTHER GENE MUTATIONS

Evaluating a patient's risk of hereditary breast cancer should include a detailed personal medical history and family history. Genetic testing is recommended when the results of a detailed risk assessment suggest the potential for an inherited cancer syndrome (American College of Obstetricians and Gynecologists [ACOG], 2017b). The USPSTF recommends that women who have a family history of breast, ovarian, tubal, or peritoneal cancer and are at increased risk for having hereditary gene mutations such as *BRCA1* or *BRCA2* be offered genetic testing (Moyer, 2014). The hereditary gene mutations, *BRCA1* and *BRCA2*, account for the majority of cases of hereditary breast and ovarian cancer syndrome. The estimated risk of breast cancer in individuals with these gene mutations is 45% to 85% by age 70 years. Owing to new technologies, there are other genes being discovered that impart varying risks of breast cancer, ovarian cancer, and other types of cancer as well. Although not as highly correlated as the *BRCA1* and *BRCA2*, the gene mutations *ATM, CDH1, CHEK2, PALB2, PTEN, STK11,* and *TP53* have also shown a correlation with an increased risk of breast cancer. Currently, the main genetic testing options for hereditary breast cancer syndromes include both *BRCA* and multigene panel testing.

Technologic advances have resulted in multigene testing that is done rapidly and is more cost effective than in the past. Offering genetic testing for hereditary cancers in the clinical setting allows more precise identification of women who are at an increased risk for inherited breast cancer. The goal of the genetic testing is to find significant mutations that lead to effective changes in medical management, including rigorous screening and preventive strategies, that can reduce the risks for the patient when specific genes are identified (ACOG, 2017b).

PROLACTIN LEVELS

Measurement of a serum prolactin level is indicated for the individual who is not pregnant nor breastfeeding, yet has breast or nipple discharge (galactorrhea). Breast discharge not associated with pregnancy or lactation, especially large amounts of milky or white discharge, whether unilateral or bilateral, can be indicative of a pituitary tumor (Galea, 2015). The normal serum prolactin level, outside of pregnancy and lactation, is less than 30 mcg/L. Prolactin-secreting pituitary adenomas or prolactinomas are the most common cause of prolactin levels greater than 200 mcg/L regardless of gender. Less pronounced prolactin elevation can be induced by other pathology such as pituitary stalk compression, hypothyroidism, and renal failure (Melmed & Jameson, 2018). Certain pharmacologic agents or breast overstimulation can cause incremental prolactin level elevations. In any case, if the prolactin is notably elevated, then a referral to an endocrinologist for consideration of brain magnetic resonance imaging (MRI) is indicated (Galea, 2015).

IMAGING CONSIDERATIONS FOR THE BREASTS AND AXILLAE

MAMMOGRAPHY

Greater than 90% of the imaging centers in the United States use the digital mammogram, which is a low-dose x-ray converted into a digital picture. The digital mammogram can be used for diagnostic evaluation of breast lumps or palpable abnormalities and is considered the gold standard for breast cancer screening. The USPSTF found sufficient data to support the use of mammography for screening in reducing breast cancer mortality in women aged 40 to 74 years. Since the risk of breast cancer increases with age, women aged 40 to 49 years benefit the least from screening (C recommendation), and women aged 60 to 69 years benefit the most (B recommendation). However, limitations to mammography exist. The numbers of women aged 70 to 75 were low, so a recommendation was difficult to make in this age group. Furthermore, there is minimal evidence regarding the benefits of screening mammography in women aged 75 years or older (I recommendation). Lastly, women who have dense

breasts (more breast parenchyma and less adipose tissue) have a higher risk of undetected breast cancer on mammography. Patients with dense breast tissue may inquire about repeat mammographic images and adjuvant screening tests. Unfortunately, there are no studies that show adjuvant testing contributes to earlier detection of breast cancer or improved prognosis (Nelson et al., 2016; USPSTF, 2016).

DIGITAL BREAST TOMOSYNTHESIS

Digital Breast Tomosynthesis (DBT) is a three-dimensional (3D) mammogram. The 3D image is made up of multiple mammographic images of the breast that are captured from different angles and then reconstructed into a 3D image set similar to the image "slices" of computed tomography (CT). DBT images tend to be clearer and could potentially improve the accuracy of evaluating the size, shape, and location of breast abnormalities. In preliminary studies, DBT seemed to reduce recall rates and increase cancer detection rates compared with conventional digital mammography alone. DBT has shown earlier detection of smaller hidden breast cancers, which may be promising for women with dense breast tissue; however, recent study designs could not determine whether the discovery of these additional small breast cancers would have become clinically significant, suggesting possible overdiagnosis. It is also unclear whether there is any quantifiable benefit to detecting these cancers earlier than occurs with conventional digital mammography. Additionally, studies to date do not provide a comparison of clinical outcomes, such as breast cancer morbidity or mortality or quality of life with the use of the 3D mammogram versus the conventional mammogram (Skaane et al., 2018). Currently, the USPSTF reports that evidence regarding the benefits and harms of DBT is inadequate to recommend it as a principal screening method for breast cancer or as adjuvant screening for women with dense breasts (Nelson et al., 2016; USPSTF, 2016).

ULTRASOUND

This noninvasive mode of testing employs sound waves to produce images of the breast. Diagnostic ultrasound is employed in differentiating the composition of a breast mass, for example, solid versus fluid-filled, and is frequently used for guidance during interventional breast procedures such as core biopsy or cyst aspiration. Owing to high false-positive and false-negative result rates, breast ultrasound is not appropriate for first-line screening for breast cancer. Whole breast ultrasound was recently approved by the U.S. Food and Drug Administration (FDA) as an adjuvant screening for women with dense breasts. Unfortunately, there are no studies showing a survival benefit for adjuvant screening in this population. Given the lack of evidence on the benefits of ultrasound and the effect on the rates of breast cancer incidence, mortality, and overdiagnosis, the USPSTF does not recommend this adjuvant therapy in women with dense breast and normal mammography (Nelson et al., 2016).

MAGNETIC RESONANCE IMAGING

MRI uses magnetic fields to create breast images. There is no radiation exposure as with the mammogram, but the MRI is not an appropriate initial breast cancer screening tool for women of average risk because of its expense and high rate of false-positive results. The USPSTF also does not recommend the MRI as adjuvant therapy for women with dense breasts. However, the MRI has been shown to perform well as a screening measure for women at elevated risk for breast cancer,

including women with a strong family history or a genetic predisposition to breast cancer as with a *BRCA1* or *BRCA2* mutation (Nelson et al., 2016).

See **Table 17.3** for a summary of the American College of Radiology (ACR) recommendations for evaluation of a palpable breast mass.

EVIDENCE-BASED PRACTICE CONSIDERATIONS FOR THE BREASTS AND AXILLAE

CURRENT RECOMMENDATIONS FOR BREAST CANCER SCREENING

Self-Breast Examination

Although a sizable number of malignant breast masses are self-detected, the personal act of inspecting the breasts on a regular, repetitive basis for breast cancer screening and detection, known as **self-breast examination** or SBE, is no longer recommended for a woman at average risk for breast cancer. When compared with no screening and incidental discovery of abnormalities, the SBE does not reduce breast cancer mortality (Nelson et al., 2016; Oeffinger et al., 2015). In fact, there is notable evidence that the SBE can lead to more harm due to false-positive test results, increased invasive diagnostics such as breast biopsies, and increased findings of benign breast conditions (ACS, 2019; NCI, 2019). Breast self-awareness, unlike SBE, focuses more on the overall personal awareness of the normal feel and appearance of the breasts. Education should be provided to increase breast familiarity and be cognizant of any deviations or potential concerns of the breasts. The signs and symptoms of breast cancer such as pain, a palpable mass, new onset of nipple discharge, or redness in their breasts should be discussed, and these changes should be reported to the clinician (ACOG, 2017a).

Clinical Breast Examination

There are also differing recommendations in regard to the performance of the CBE during the well-woman visit by the healthcare clinician. The USPSTF, the ACS, and the NCI concluded that there is insufficient evidence to recommend the CBE for average risk, asymptomatic women regardless of age (NCI, 2019; Nelson et al., 2016; Oeffinger et al., 2015). The consensus is that the time with the patient may be better spent by evaluating for pertinent risk factors, counseling women on being cognizant of breast changes, and recommending appropriate breast cancer screening such as mammography (Oeffinger et al., 2015). The

TABLE 17.3 Summary of American College of Radiology Recommendations for Evaluation of a Palpable Breast Mass

	Mammogram/ DBT	Ultrasound	Biopsy
Women aged <30		✓	
Women aged 30–39	✓		
Women aged >40	✓		
Highly suspicious mass noted on imaging (regardless of CBE findings)			✓
Highly suspicious mass noted on CBE (regardless of imaging findings)			✓

CBE, clinical breast examination; DBT, digital breast tomosynthesis.
Source: Moy, L., Heller, S. L., Bailey, L., D'Orsi, C., DiFlorio, R. M., Green, E. D., . . . Newell, M. S. (2017). ACR appropriateness criteria palpable breast masses. *Journal of the American College of Radiology, 14*, S203–S224. doi:10.1016/j.jacr.2017.02.033

ACOG (2017a) acknowledges the limitations and the potential for false-positive detection rates with CBE. It proposes offering the CBE to women who have an average risk of breast cancer by endorsing clinician- and patient-shared decision-making and by fully disclosing the risk and the ambiguity of the benefits of the CBE for breast cancer screening. If the CBE is performed for screening, the recommended intervals are every 1 to 3 years for women aged 25 to 39 years and annually for women 40 years and older. The evidence suggests that CBE alone is not adequate screening for breast cancer and should be used in conjunction with evidence-based breast cancer screening methods. The CBE continues to be the standard initial physical evaluation tool for high-risk and symptomatic women. For mammogram screening recommendations, see the Imaging Considerations for the Breasts and Axillae section.

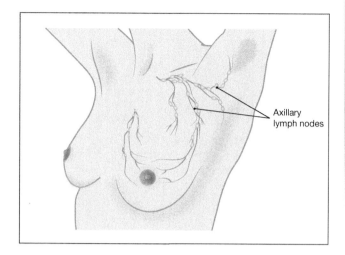

FIGURE 17.8 Axillary lymph nodes.

ABNORMAL FINDINGS OF THE BREAST AND AXILLAE

Common symptoms of breast conditions requiring further evaluation include the presence of a breast or axillary lump/mass (painless or painful), breast pain or discomfort, and/or nipple abnormalities, including changes in appearance (scaling, redness, thickening), discharge, or retraction. Other symptoms of breast cancer include swelling of the breast or skin changes (peau d'orange, irritation, or dimpling/retraction).

LYMPHADENOPATHY

Some masses, discovered by SBE or CBE, may be difficult to assess if located in the axillae or in the tail of the breast; associated axillary lymph node enlargement, or lymphadenopathy, can indicate that further evaluation is required to determine the nature of the mass. Lymph node assessment is a key to recognizing the urgent need for additional breast evaluation. Specific and detailed attention should be given to the number of palpable nodes, fixation, laterality, and size (Bleicher, 2014).

Key History and Physical Findings

- Normal axillary lymph nodes tend to be discrete oblong nodules that are not usually palpable; however, small lymph nodes may be detected, especially in thin individuals. (**Figure 17.8**)
- Lymph nodes vary greatly in size:
  - Normal axillary lymph nodes tend to be small (a few to several millimeters in size) and mobile.
  - Abnormal axillary lymph nodes can be several centimeters in size when enlarged and may be fixed to each other and/or the chest wall.

ACCESSORY BREAST TISSUE

Accessory breast tissue and/or nipples; that is, additional mammary tissue remote from the primary breast tissue, can occur along "milk lines" anywhere from the axilla to the groin. Accessory breast tissue is benign; this finding is common, although it can be a source of embarrassment or concern (Galea, 2015).

Key History and Physical Findings

- The accessory tissue is so small it is mistaken for a freckle or mole.
- Accessory tissue can be present without an observable accessory nipple. The tissue presents as a soft subcutaneous lump near or in the axillae (**Figure 17.9**).
- The area of the accessory breast tissue can be tender and enlarged in response to the hormonal fluctuations of the normal menstrual cycle.
- The accessory tissue can also become full and active with pregnancy and lactation.

BREAST MASS

The self-detection of a breast mass or lump is the most common reason for women presenting for clinical breast evaluation in reproductive healthcare practices, accounting for more than half of the reasons for seeking care. The presence of a breast mass causes considerable anxiety and concern for the potential of having breast cancer. Fortunately, in most cases, the findings are benign. However, the goal in evaluating any breast abnormality or patient concern is to exclude the presence of a malignancy and to find the most efficient path to an accurate diagnosis and management. Regardless of age, gender, or positive/negative family history of cancer, the presence of a breast mass should never be

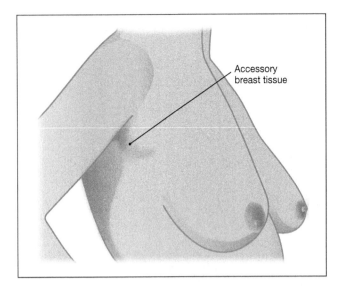

FIGURE 17.9 Accessory breast tissue.

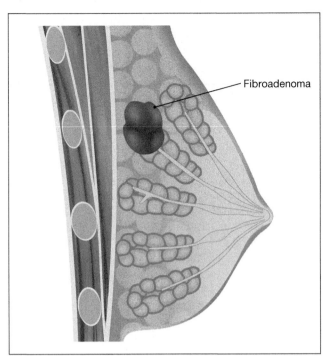

FIGURE 17.10 Fibroadenoma.

dismissed. Although the delayed diagnosis for breast cancer may need to be 8 months or longer to be detrimental, delayed diagnosis of cancer continues to be a common cause of litigation (Bleicher, 2014).

Benign Breast Mass

Benign breast disorders encompass a large group of heterogeneous nonmalignant conditions that originate from one of the three main components of the breast: fat, supportive parenchyma, and the ductal–alveolar epithelium. Most of these conditions are not pathologic and stem from exaggerated physiology of normal breast development and involution. As a result, many benign disorders are age related (Galea, 2015). The two most common benign breast masses are fibroadenomas and breast cysts (Collins & Schnitt, 2014; Galea, 2015).

Fibroadenoma

Fibroadenomas are composed mainly of parenchymal/stromal tissue and they typically present in women under 25 (**Figure 17.10**). Fibroadenomas are proliferative lesions, and they have the propensity to change over time, potentially increasing breast cancer risk. In many cases, removal of the lesion is recommended (Galea, 2015).

Key History and Physical Findings
* A single well-defined mobile ovoid and discrete lump is palpable on exam.
* The palpable mass may be tender to touch.
* Multiple fibroadenomas can be present.

Breast Cyst

Breast cysts are fluid-filled, round-to-ovoid structures and are the most common cause of discrete breast lumps in women in their forties. The breast cyst is considered a nonproliferative lesion with a minimal breast cancer risk, and, in the majority of cases, does not require intervention (Collins & Schnitt, 2014).

Key History and Physical Findings
* Breast cyst formation can be related to hormonal changes induced by natural reproductive cyclic variations, oral contraceptives, and hormone replacement therapy (Galea, 2015).
* Palpable cysts vary greatly in size, present as single or multiple entities, and can be unilateral or bilateral (Collins & Schnitt, 2014; **Figure 17.11**).
* Upon palpation, they are often tender and, unlike a malignant mass, usually round and mobile.

MALIGNANT MASS

Breast cancer is the most common female cancer and the second leading cause of cancer death in women in the United States. A woman presenting with a new palpable breast mass should have a thorough clinical breast evaluation since, frequently, the breast mass is a common presenting sign of breast cancer. Additionally, since many breast masses may not exhibit unique physical findings typical of malignancy, imaging evaluation is necessary in almost all cases to characterize the palpable lesion (Moy et al., 2017). Invasive breast cancers constitute a heterogeneous group of lesions that differ with regard to their clinical, radiographic,

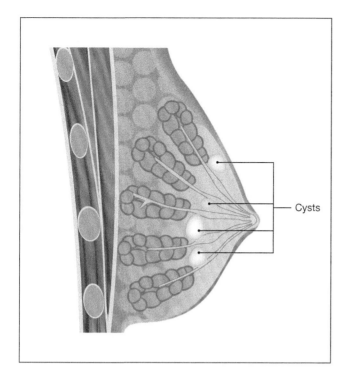
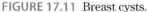
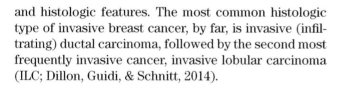

FIGURE 17.11 Breast cysts.

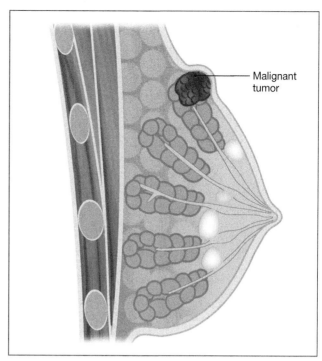

FIGURE 17.12 Malignant breast mass.

and histologic features. The most common histologic type of invasive breast cancer, by far, is invasive (infiltrating) ductal carcinoma, followed by the second most frequently invasive cancer, invasive lobular carcinoma (ILC; Dillon, Guidi, & Schnitt, 2014).

Invasive Ductal Carcinomas

Key History and Physical Findings

- Often presents as a discrete firm mass on palpation
- An abnormality such as speculated mass on a mammogram
- There are no clinical or mammographic characteristics that are specific to invasive ductal carcinomas (IDCs) and apart from other histologic types of invasive cancer.
- Prognosis varies and depends on tumor size, histologic grade, hormonal receptor expression, lymph node status, and whether lymphovascular invasion has occurred; still, favorable-prognoses, specialized tumor types, have been identified within this group (Dillon et al., 2014).

Invasive Lobular Carcinomas

Key History and Physical Findings

- They may present as a palpable mass or a mammographic abnormality similar to those of IDC, but the findings may be subtle and substantially underestimated.
- On exam, there may be only an area of thickening or induration, without distinct margins (**Figure 17.12**).

- The mammogram may show no more than a poorly defined area of asymmetric density with architectural distortion, even in the presence of a palpable mass.
- Prognosis with ILC is similar and reliant on the same factors as with IDC. There are many clinical follow-up studies that indicate that patients with ILC can be effectively managed with conservative surgery and radiation therapy following complete gross excision of the tumor, with similar recurrence rates seen in patients with IDC (Dillon et al., 2014).

BREAST PAIN (MASTALGIA)

Breast pain or mastalgia is extremely common. The majority of all women experience this symptom during their reproductive years. Unfortunately, many women mistakenly think that breast pain alone is associated with early breast cancer. There are no data to support any strong relationship with breast pain and malignancy (Mansel, 2014). If the mastalgia is the primary concern and no breast mass is present, then the pain is categorized as cyclical or noncyclical. Although it can be difficult to determine and varies with the individual, this distinction is instrumental in delineating the underlying cause of the discomfort (Galea, 2015).

Cyclical Pain

If the breast pain is cyclical, it is more likely to be related to hormonal fluctuations. There is a wide continuum of cyclical pain intensity among women that is not fully understood. There are several etiologic theories that include the presence of elevated estradiol levels, insufficient progesterone, and enhanced receptor sensitivity to otherwise normal circulating hormones that, so far, have limited supporting evidence.

Key History and Physical Findings

- The pain is bilateral and has some association with the menstrual cycle.
- The pain is often generalized and described as heaviness and tenderness.
- In younger women, nodularity can be associated with cyclic mastalgia, and this is considered normal (Galea, 2015; Mansel, 2014).

Noncyclical Pain

Noncyclical pain is more likely to be musculoskeletal in origin, especially if upon CBE there are no palpable abnormalities and appropriate imaging is normal. The pain may originate from the breast or the chest wall since the pectoral muscle lies beneath the breast. Inquiry regarding recent sport activities, history of trauma, and previous musculoskeletal disorders should be considered, and a focused exam on the pectoral muscle or the costochondral junctions should be considered to identify the trigger activity in inducing the pain (Galea, 2015; Mansel, 2014).

Key History and Physical Findings

- The pain is more likely to be unilateral.
- The pain severity is typically related to a specific area of the breast and/or the chest.
- Pectoral tendinitis or fasciitis can cause lateral chest wall tenderness and discomfort behind the nipple.

NIPPLE CHANGES

Nipple Discharge

Discharge from the nipple of a woman is a relatively common occurrence and may represent either benign or pathologic conditions. According to the American Society of Breast Surgeons Foundation (n.d.-a), physiologic (normal) nipple discharge is often characterized as occurring with breast manipulation (not spontaneous), from more than one duct, and associated with pregnancy or breastfeeding, thyroid disease, or medications. Nipple discharge is suspicious for an underlying malignancy if it is unilateral, occurs spontaneously, persists, appears to be coming from one duct, or is clear/colorless, bloody, or serous. Milky nipple discharge in a nonlactating woman is likely associated with certain pharmacologic agents or pituitary/hypothalamic

disease, warranting further evaluation. Any nipple discharge in males is considered abnormal and requires prompt evaluation.

Key History and Physical Findings

- Milky, serous, bloody, or purulent discharge from one or both breasts
- Presence or absence of a breast mass
- Relation to menses or menopausal status
- Medications—hormonal therapies, opiates, antipsychotics, select antidepressants, or phenothiazines
- History of endocrine disorders or tumors, pituitary or hypothalamic disease

Paget's Disease of the Breast

Paget's disease of the breast is a rare type of breast cancer affecting the skin, nipple, and areola. It can occur in men or women from adolescence to the late 80s and represents 1% to 4% of breast cancers (NCI, n.d.-b). Owing to the benign appearance, it is often initially mistaken for dermatitis or eczema.

Key History and Physical Findings

- Itching, tingling, or erythema of the nipple and/or areola
- Thickening, flaking, or crusting of the skin on/around the nipple (**Figure 17.13**)
- Flat nipple

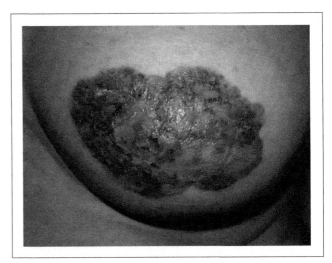

FIGURE 17.13 Paget's disease of the breast.

Source: From Muttarak, M., Siriya, B., Kongmebhol, P., Chaiwun, B., & Sukhamwang, N. (2011). Paget's disease of the breast: Clinical, imaging, and pathologic findings: A review of 16 patients. *Biomedical Imaging and Intervention Journal, 7*(2), e16. Retrieved from https://www.ncbi.nlm.nih.gov/pmc/articles/PMC3265154

- Yellowish or bloody nipple discharge
- Breast lump(s) in the same breast

CONDITIONS ASSOCIATED WITH SKIN CHANGES OF THE BREAST

Mastitis

Mastitis is an infection in the breast (**Figure 17.14**). It occurs in up to 10% of women who are lactating and 1% to 2% who are not (American Society of Breast Surgeons Foundation, n.d.-b; Kasales et al., 2014). Note that mastitis is not common in women who are not breast-feeding and not pregnant; breast tissue that appears infected or inflamed in nonlactating women should be evaluated for conditions other than mastitis.

Key History and Physical Findings

- Trauma/chafing to the nipple
- Breast engorgement that is prolonged
- Smoking
- Nipple piercings
- A warm, tender, erythematous, firm area of the breast; possibly complicated with a palpable abscess
- Fever (over 100°F)
- Fatigue, chills, arthralgias, myalgias, malaise, and/or poor appetite
- Unilateral presentation most likely
- Abrupt onset of symptoms

Inflammatory Breast Cancer

Inflammatory breast cancer is a rare, highly aggressive malignant breast condition occurring in women or men, accounting for 1% to 5% of all breast cancers (NCI, n.d.-a).

Key History and Physical Findings (Figure 17.15)

- Hispanic women with youngest average age of onset (50.5 years), African American women (55.2 years), Caucasian women (58.1 years; van Uden, van Laarhoven, Westenberg, de Wilt, & Blanken-Peeters, 2015)
- More common in young African American women than Caucasian women
- Younger age at menarche and first live birth
- Obesity
- Unilateral presentation of an erythematous or purplish, edematous, or inflamed appearing breast involving one third or more of the breast area
- Peau d'orange skin changes of the affected breast
- Rapid change in breast size (<3 months)
- Sensation of fullness/heaviness, burning, or tenderness
- Inverted nipple
- Axillary or supraclavicular lymphadenopathy; metastatic disease present in one third of patients at diagnosis
- Presence or absence of breast mass

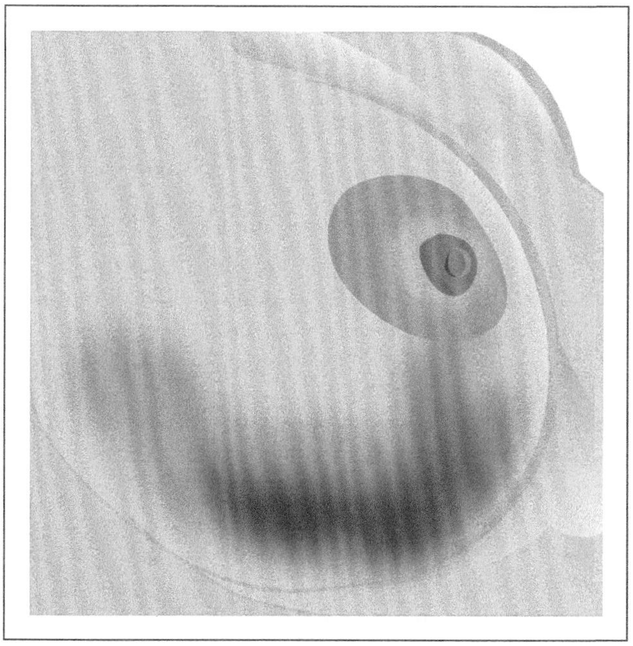

FIGURE 17.14 Mastitis.

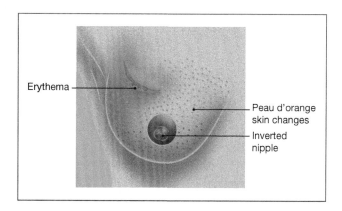

FIGURE 17.15 Inflammatory breast cancer.

CASE STUDY: Bilateral Breast Pain

History

A healthy 29-year-old female comes to the office with a concern of bilateral breast pain. She describes the pain as achy and tender, especially around the nipple and on the lateral aspect of both breasts near the axillary border. She denies noting any distinct masses during self-examination. However, she has difficulty determining what is significant during self-examination since her breasts "always feel lumpy." Her symptoms started 3 months ago. The discomfort is intermittent but persistent. She denies the risk of pregnancy. She is currently on oral combination contraceptives. She is in an intimate relationship with one male partner. She denies any family history of breast cancer. She is a nonsmoker and denies alcohol use. She does not have any chronic medical conditions. Her only surgical history is an appendectomy when she was 10 years old. She has no drug allergies. She is a high school teacher and currently coaches the cross-country ski team.

Physical Examination

On inspection, in the sitting position, both breasts are found to be symmetrical, with no skin changes or dimpling. The nipples are everted and directionally symmetrical. The axillae are palpated in the sitting position, and no adenopathy is present. The patient denies tenderness during palpation of the axillae.

The patient is placed in the supine position for palpation. During the breast exam, diffuse, nonspecific nodularity is noted; however, no distinct masses were palpated. Tenderness was noted during palpation of the nipple, areola, and lateral breast tissue near the axillary line bilaterally.

Differential Diagnoses

Cyclic mastalgia; noncyclic mastalgia

Laboratory and Imaging

With the patient's age, negative family history, and no palpable masses on exam, concern for breast abnormalities or malignancy is low. There is no indication for diagnostic testing (Galea, 2015; Mansel, 2014).

Final Diagnosis

On further discussion, the patient had started her oral contraceptives about 4 months ago, and her current symptoms started soon after. The final diagnosis was cyclic mastalgia related to the initiation of oral contraceptive use.

CASE STUDY: Well-Woman Exam

History

A 60-year-old female comes to the office for a well-woman exam. She has been without insurance and healthcare for about 5 years. She recently started a job that provides health insurance coverage. She has scheduled the appointment to get established and caught up with her healthcare. Her main concern is that she has a firm lump near the nipple on her left breast. She states that it has been there for "quite some time now." She denies any pain or tenderness related to the lump. She denies any nipple discharge. She just kept thinking the lump would go away, but it has actually become more prominent over the past year. She has a maternal grandmother who was diagnosed with breast cancer at the age of 70. She has a 20-pack-year smoking history. She quit smoking 5 years ago. She denies alcohol use. Her medical history includes asthma and hypertension. Her surgical history includes a partial hysterectomy (i.e., both ovaries remain intact) at age 40 for fibroids. Medications include lisinopril 10 mg daily and a rescue inhaler that she uses just before exercise. She has no drug allergies. She denies fatigue; weight loss; or any respiratory, cardiac, or gastrointestinal symptoms.

Physical Examination

On inspection, in the sitting position, the breasts are asymmetrical. There is dimpling and significant nipple retraction and distortion on the left breast. The axillae are palpated in the sitting position. No adenopathy is palpable on the right,

(continued)

CASE STUDY: Well-Woman Exam (*continued*)

but significant adenopathy is present on the left. The patient denies tenderness during palpation of the axillae.

The patient is placed in the supine position for palpation. The right breast is negative for palpable masses, skin changes, or tenderness. On the left breast, there is a mass noted just under the surface of the areola at approximately the 3 o'clock position. The mass is palpated at 2 to 3 cm in diameter. It is flat, irregular, and fixed. It extends from the nipple to the edge of the areola. There is no tenderness noted during palpation bilaterally.

Differential Diagnoses

Malignant breast mass or nonmalignant mass. Owing to the clinical presentation and history, there is a

very high suspicion of malignancy unless diagnostic testing indicates otherwise.

Laboratory and Imaging

Considering this patient's age, positive family history, and suspicious exam findings, a diagnostic mammogram with DBT and/or compression views is ordered. A surgical referral is also merited in case mammographic findings are suspicious or indicate malignancy, which is then an indication for an ultrasound-guided biopsy (Moy et al., 2017).

Final Diagnosis

The mammographic findings showed a suspicious subareolar lesion in the left breast. IDC was confirmed by an ultrasound-guided biopsy.

Clinical Pearls

- Breast tissue is denser in young patients.
- Mammograms can be done on men.
- All breast masses require imaging for full evaluation.
- Unilateral, spontaneous, bloody nipple discharge, originating from one breast duct with or without a breast mass, is highly suspicious for malignancy.
- Eczematous appearing skin changes at or near the nipple should be biopsied.
- Always carefully and fully listen when individuals share concerns about breast lumps or masses, even when the clinical level of suspicion is low.

Key Takeaways

- The adult female breast is a dome-like structure that lies vertically between the second and the sixth ribs and horizontally between the sternal edge and the midaxillary line. The breast also extends into the axilla; this area of breast tissue is known as the tail of Spence.
- While breast development occurs through identifiable phases, breast growth is unique to each individual, varies in timing, and can be asymmetrical.

- Multiple changes occur in the breasts during adolescence, pregnancy, lactation, and menopause.
- Self- and clinical breast exams are not currently recommended for asymptomatic women at average risk for breast cancer.
- The primary screening imaging modality for breast cancer is mammography. Other imaging should be considered on the basis of current evidence available, patient presentation, and breast specialist recommendation.
- Breast and axillae examination should include inspection and palpation of the breast/axillae, the surrounding lymph nodes (axillary, supraclavicular, and infraclavicular), and the tail of Spence.
- Regardless of age, gender, or positive/negative family history of cancer, the presence of a breast mass should never be dismissed.

REFERENCES

American Cancer Society. (2019, September 18). Breast cancer signs and symptoms. Retrieved from https://www .cancer.org/cancer/breast-cancer/about/breast-cancer -signs-and-symptoms.html

American College of Obstetricians and Gynecologists. (2017a, July). Practice Bulletin Number 179: Breast cancer risk assessment and screening in average-risk women.

Obstetrics and Gynecology, 130(1), e1–e16. doi:10.1097/AOG.0000000000002158

American College of Obstetricians and Gynecologists. (2017b, September 3). Practice Bulletin No 182: Hereditary breast and ovarian cancer syndrome. *Obstetrics & Gynecology, 130*(3), e110–e126. doi:10.1097/AOG.0000000000002296

American Society of Breast Surgeons Foundation. (n.d.-a). Nipple discharge. Retrieved from https://breast360.org/topics/2017/01/01/nipple-discharge

American Society of Breast Surgeons Foundation. (n.d.-b). *Topics: Infection.* Retrieved from https://breast360.org/topics/category/infection

Baquet, C. M., Mishra, S. I., Commiskey, P., Ellison, G. L., & DeShields, M. (2008). Breast cancer epidemiology of blacks and whites: Disparities in incidence, mortality, survival rates, and histology. *Journal of the National Medical Association, 100*(5), 480–488. doi:10.1016/s0027-9684(15)31294-3

Bleicher, R. J. (2014). Management of the palpable breast mass. In J. R. Harris, M. E. Lippman, M. Morrow, & C. K. Osborne (Eds.), *Diseases of the breast* (5th ed., pp. 29–37). Philadelphia, PA: Wolters Kluwer.

Centers for Disease Control and Prevention. (n.d.-a). What are the risk factors for breast cancer? Retrieved from https://www.cdc.gov/cancer/breast/basic_info/risk_factors.htm

Centers for Disease Control and Prevention. (n.d.-b). What are the symptoms of breast cancer? Retrieved from https://www.cdc.gov/cancer/breast/basic_info/symptoms.htm

Centers for Disease Control and Prevention. (n.d.-c). What is breast cancer? Retrieved from https://www.cdc.gov/cancer/breast/basic_info/what-is-breast-cancer.htm

Collins, L. C., & Schnitt, S. J. (2014). Pathology of benign breast disorders. In J. R. Harris, M. E. Lippman, M. Morrow, & C. K. Osborne (Eds.), *Diseases of the breast* (5th ed., pp. 71–88). Philadelphia, PA: Wolters Kluwer.

Dillon, D., Guidi, A. J., & Schnitt, S. J. (2014). Pathology of invasive breast cancer. In J. R. Harris, M. E. Lippman, M. Morrow, & C. K. Osborne (Eds.), *Diseases of the breast* (5th ed., pp. 381–410). Philadelphia, PA: Wolters Kluwer.

Ellis, H., & Mahadevan, V. (2013). Anatomy and physiology of the breast. *Surgery, 31*(1), 11–14. doi:10.1016/j.mpsur.2012.10.018

Galea, M. (2015). Benign breast disorders. *Surgery, 34*(1), 19–24. doi:10.1016/j.mpsur.2015.10.006

Gillespie, A., & Capriotti, T. (2016, July 14). Healthcare issues of the LGBT community: What the primary care clinician should know. *Clinical Advisor.* Retrieved from https://www.clinicaladvisor.com/practice-management-information-center/healthcare-issues-of-the-lgbt-community-what-the-primary-care-clinician-should-know/article/509329

Himes, D. O., Root, A. E., Gammon, A., & Luthy, K. (2016, October). Breast cancer risk assessment: Calculating lifetime risk using the Tyrer-Cuzick model. *The Journal for Nurse Practitioners, 12*(9), 581–591. doi:10.1016/j.nurpra.2016.07.027

Hoffman, B. L., & Pearson, M. J. (2016). Well woman care. In B. L. Hoffman, J. O. Schorge, K. D. Bradshaw, L. M. Halvorson, J. I. Schaffer, & M. M. Corton (Eds.), *Williams gynecology* (3rd ed., pp. 2–21). New York, NY: McGraw-Hill.

Kasales, C. J., Han, B., Smith, J. S., Jr., Chetlen, A. L., Kaneda, H. J., & Shereef, S. (2014). Nonpuerperal mastitis and subareolar abscess of the breast. *American Journal of Roentgenology, 202*(2), 133–139. doi:10.2214/AJR.13.10551

Klein, S. (2005, May 1). Evaluation of palpable breast masses. *American Family Physician, 71*(9), 1731–1738. Retrieved from https://www.aafp.org/afp/2005/0501/p1731.html

Mansel, R. E. (2014). Management of breast pain. In J. R. Harris, M. E. Lippman, M. Morrow, & C. K. Osborne (Eds.), *Diseases of the breast* (5th ed., pp. 51–57). Philadelphia, PA: Wolters Kluwer.

Melmed, S., & Jameson, J. (2018). Pituitary tumor syndromes. In J. Jameson, A. S. Fauci, D. L. Kasper, S. L. Hauser, D. L. Longo, & J. Loscalzo (Eds.), *Harrison's principles of internal medicine* (20th ed., Chapter 168). New York, NY: McGraw-Hill.

Morton, D. A., Foreman, K. B., & Albertine, K. H. (2011). *The big picture: Gross anatomy* (pp. 25–40). New York, NY: McGraw-Hill.

Moy, L., Heller, S. L., Bailey, L., D'Orsi, C., DoFlorio, R. M., Green, E. D., . . . Newell, M. S. (2017). ACR Appropriateness Criteria® palpable breast masses. *Journal of the American College of Radiology, 14*(5, Suppl.), S203–S224. doi:10.1016/j.jacr.2017.02.033

Moyer, V. A. (2014, February 10). Risk assessment, genetic counseling, and genetic testing for BRCA-related cancer in women: U.S. Preventive Task Force recommendation statement. *Annals of Internal Medicine, 160*(4), 271–281. doi:10.7326/M13-2747

Muttarak, M., Siriya, B., Kongmebhol, P., Chaiwun, B., & Sukhamwang, N. (2011). Paget's disease of the breast: Clinical, imaging, and pathologic findings: A review of 16 patients. *Biomedical Imaging and Intervention Journal, 7*(2), e16. Retrieved from https://www.ncbi.nlm.nih.gov/pmc/articles/PMC3265154

National Cancer Institute. (n.d.-a). Inflammatory breast cancer. Retrieved from https://www.cancer.gov/types/breast/ibc-fact-sheet

National Cancer Institute. (n.d.-b). Paget disease of the breast. Retrieved from https://www.cancer.gov/types/breast/paget-breast-fact-sheet

National Cancer Institute. (2019, October 30). *Breast cancer screening (PDQ)—Health professional version.* Retrieved from https://www.cancer.gov/types/breast/hp/breast-screening-pdq#link/_15_toc

Nelson, H. D., Cantor, A., Humpfrey, L., Fu, R., Pappas, M., Daegas, M., & Griffin, J. (2016). *Screening for breast cancer: A systematic review to update the 2009 U.S. Preventive Services Task Force recommendation.* Rockville, MD: Agency for Healthcare Research and Quality.

Osborne, M. (2014). Breast anatomy and development. In J. R. Harris, M. E. Lippman, M. Morrow, & C. K. Osborne (Eds.), *Diseases of the breast* (5th ed., pp. 3–14). Philadelphia, PA: Wolters Kluwer.

Oeffinger, K. C., Fontham, E. T., Etzioni, R., Herzig, A., Michaelson, J. S., Shih, Y.-C. T., . . . Wender, R.; American Cancer Society. (2015, October 20). Breast cancer screening for women at average risk: 2015 guideline update from the American Cancer Society. *Journal of the American Medical Association, 314*(15), 1599–1614. doi:10.1001/jama.2015.12783

Skaane, P., Sebuodegard, S., Bandos, A. I., Gur, D., Osteras, B. H., Gullen, R., & Hofvind, S. (2018). Performance of breast cancer screening using digital breast tomosynthesis: Results for the prospective population-based Oslo tomosynthesis screening trial. *Breast Cancer Research and Treatment, 169,* 489–496. doi:10.1007/s10549-018-4705-2

U.S. Preventive Services Task Force. (2016, November). Final recommendation statement—Breast cancer: Screening. Retrieved from https://www.uspreventiveservicestaskforce .org/Page/Document/RecommendationStatementFinal/ breast-cancer-screening1

van Uden, D. J., van Laarhoven, H. W., Westenberg, A. H., de Wilt, J. H., & Blanken-Peeters, C. F. (2015). Inflammatory breast cancer: An overview. *Critical Reviews in Oncology/Hematology, 93*(2), 116–126. doi:10.1016/j .critrevonc.2014.09.003

Wang, X., Huang, Y., Li, L., Dai, H., Song, F., & Chen, K. (2018). Assessment of performance of the Gail model for predicting breast cancer risk: A systematic review and meta-analysis with trial sequential analysis. *Breast Cancer Research, 20*(1), 18. doi:10.1186/s13058-018-0947-5

18

Evidence-Based Assessment of Sexual Orientation, Gender Identity, and Health

Kathryn Tierney and Britta Shute

"If you do not know how to ask the right question, you discover nothing."

—W. Edward Deming

✓

LEARNING OBJECTIVES

- Describe key questions needed to ascertain a patient's sexual orientation and gender identity.
- List common physical changes associated with gender transition.
- Recognize health conditions that are more common in the LGBTQ+ population.

ANATOMY AND PHYSIOLOGY

Sexual orientation and gender identity are central to every person's sense of self and well-being. Determining how each person identifies himself or herself and the kind of behaviors each individual engages in based on those identities is critical to providing quality, patient-centered healthcare. Patients who identify as **lesbian, gay, bisexual, transgender, queer, and more (LGBTQ+)** are part of a minority group that experience health disparities at a rate higher than that of the general population and have unique healthcare needs (Lunn et al., 2017). On average, only 5 hours of training on information specific to the LGBTQ+ population is included in medical school curricula (Obedin-Maliver et al., 2011); while this measure may vary, many clinicians are unprepared to address the specific health needs of this population. A survey of transgender individuals found that 50% had experienced situations in

healthcare where they had to teach their clinician how to take care of them, and 19% reported being refused healthcare outright (James et al., 2016). Being able to competently and confidently assess each person's sexual orientation and gender identity at every clinician visit is crucial to reducing barriers to care and improving the health of this marginalized population.

To clarify terms, **sexual orientation** is a label assigned by one's culture that refers to a person's romantic or intimate preferences. The label of one's sexual orientation as heterosexual, bisexual, asexual, or homosexual is determined by the gender identities of the people involved in the romantic or intimate relationship. **Gender identity** refers to each individual's internal sense of self and their own understanding of their gender within a cultural context, rather than on their physical body. Typically, in American culture, gender identity is either male or female; gender identity can also be **nonbinary**, that is, both male and female or neither male nor female.

It is essential to understand that sexual orientation and gender identity are related to each other but are not the same. The two labels are often conflated. Knowing the difference will help clinicians avoid mislabeling or misgendering patients. Sexual orientation is a description of the type of romantic relationship a person is in as it relates to the genders of people involved, while gender identity refers to each individual's internal sense of self. Although gender identity is not related to their romantic interests, changes in gender may alter the cultural label applied to a relationship despite romantic interests being unchanged. For example, if both a romantic partner and an individual identify as female, they are labeled as homosexual within the American culture. If one of the individuals transitions to male and they maintain the same relationship as romantic partners, the culture changes their label to heterosexual.

SEXUAL ORIENTATION

Sexual orientation must be assessed in order for a clinician to determine what preventive care should be recommended and/or what specific health risks an individual may have. Sexual orientation is based on each individual person's romantic and intimate relationships and attractions, and, in general, the label is determined by culture and applied to individuals on the basis of their relationships. There are many ways to categorize sexual orientation (**Table 18.1**). Patients may identify with one or more of these labels, or they may not identify with any of them, and identity can change over time. It is important to note that sexual orientation does not always predict what kind of sexual behaviors the person is engaging in. For example, a person who identifies as male and heterosexual may be engaging in sexual behaviors with other men. Relying on his sexual orientation or identity alone hinders the clinician's

ability to accurately assess the patient's healthcare needs. Targeted questions regarding behavior, asked without judgment, will help the clinician elicit important information.

GENDER IDENTITY

Gender identity is based on an internal sense of self and how a person best fits into cultural expectations of male and female. It can be determined only by the person and not by genitals or DNA. A person's **sex assigned at birth** is determined by visually assessing genitalia. For most people, sex assigned at birth and gender identity are the same thing (i.e., a person who has female genitalia most often also has a female gender identity, and a person who has male genitalia most often has a male gender identity). This is not true for everyone, however. There are approximately 1.4 million people in the United States for whom their assigned sex at birth does not match their gender identity (Flores, Herman, Gates, & Brown, 2016). *Transgender* is the umbrella term used to describe someone whose gender identity is different than the sex assigned at birth. For example, someone who was assigned female at birth and identifies their gender as male is a transgender man. The term *nonbinary* refers to people who do not identify as only male or only female. They may identify as both male and female, as neither, androgynous, or a hybrid of characteristics typically associated with male or female. See **Table 18.2** for other terms related to gender identity.

Culture plays a significant role in how gender identity is developed and expressed. In general, the American culture views gender as binary, meaning that individuals are expected to be either male or female. In addition, there are specific expectations for expressing that gender in terms of appearance and role in society. The expectations of how male and female gender are expressed change over time and are also dependent on geographical location. Gender roles and expectations are different now than they were 100 years ago, for example. **Gender nonconforming** is a term used when someone is not adhering to cultural expectations in terms of gender presentation and role. It is important to note that nearly everyone makes choices not to conform to gender norms, whether it be choices in clothes, hair, activities, or toys. For example, some people who identify as male have long hair, and some people who identify as female have short hair. These are gender nonconforming, but it does not necessarily make the person transgender.

Correct gender pronouns and the name that the patient chooses to use must be utilized during all encounters with each patient. Gender identity can be determined only by the individual; therefore, it is imperative that patients be given the opportunity to provide their preferred name and gender pronouns. This is easily assessed by

TABLE 18.1 Sexual Orientation Vocabulary	
Term	**Definition**
Heterosexual or straight	Relationship between two people of the opposite sex or gender
Homosexual or gay	Relationship between two people of the same sex or gender
Lesbian	Relationship between two people who identity as female
Bisexual	Romantic interest in both male- and female-identified people regardless of person's own gender identity
Asexual	A person with reduced or lack of sexual interest or desire
Aromantic	A person who has no interest in or desire for romantic relationships
Polyamorous	A person with interest in romantic or sexual relationships with more than one person

Note: These definitions are not all encompassing. Ask the patient with which label, if any, they identify.

TABLE 18.2 Gender Identity Vocabulary

Term	Definition
Sex or sex assigned at birth	Male or female based on chromosomal makeup or physical presentation of genitalia
Transgender	Umbrella term encompassing any person whose internal sense of gender identity differs from their sex assigned at birth. Also known as *gender incongruence*
Cisgender	Person whose sex assigned at birth and gender identity are the same
Gender dysphoria	Discomfort or distress that a person experiences when their gender identity and sex assigned at birth are not in alignment. Not all transgender individuals experience dysphoria
Transman	Person whose gender identity is male but who was assigned female at birth
Transwoman	Person whose gender identity is female but who was assigned male at birth
Nonbinary, gender nonconforming, or genderqueer	Person whose gender identity is neither female nor male or is both female and male
Two spirit	Native American term for people of a third, nonbinary gender

Note: These definitions are not all encompassing. Ask the patient with which label, if any, they identify.

simply asking the individual what they prefer. A sample conversation is provided later in this chapter to demonstrate how to elicit this information. Careful attention to these details, including vocabulary, can reduce barriers to healthcare and improve experience among transgender patients accessing health systems.

LIFE-SPAN DIFFERENCES AND CONSIDERATIONS IN ANATOMY AND PHYSIOLOGY

Sexual orientation and gender identity are expressed in different ways at all stages of life. Both are deeply rooted in the culture and the belief system of the person, as

well as their family, community, and support systems. Experiences of family rejection, homelessness, discrimination in the workplace, and financial instability lead to disparities that are further compounded by lack of access to appropriate and affirming healthcare. Geographical differences in the likelihood of being accepted by family and community, as well as religious, financial, and safety considerations, can affect whether and when a person can outwardly identify or present as their preferred sexual orientation or gender at any given time.

Sexual Orientation

Mental health assessment and support are priorities for LGBTQ+ youth. While awareness and acceptance of LGBTQ+ people are increasing, multiple studies detail how youth deal with stressors related to having a stigmatized identity or orientation (Rosario, Schrimshaw, & Hunter, 2012). LGBTQ+ youth may be exposed to negative experiences, including bullying, social rejection and isolation, diminished peer support, discrimination, verbal abuse, and violence at a disproportionate rate when compared with cisgender, heterosexual peers. Youth who identify as LGBTQ+ are two to three times more likely to attempt suicide (Garofalo, Wolf, Wissow, Woods, & Goodman, 1999).

LGBTQ+ older adults face additional barriers due to isolation, lack of social services, and culturally incompetent clinician. LGBTQ+ older adults are more likely to be single or living alone and less likely to have children to care for them; studies find resilient older adults rely on chosen families, community organizations, and affirmative religious groups for care and support (Choi & Meyer, 2016). Lifetime disparities in earnings, employment, and opportunities to build savings, as well as discriminatory access to legal and social programs, including housing, put LGBTQ+ older adults at greater financial risk (Choi & Meyer, 2016).

Gender Identity

Gender identity is often solidified by 3 years of age. Elementary school–aged children will explore their gender prior to puberty as a way to determine how they best fit into the culture. This may include experimenting with clothes or toys that are typically assigned to the opposite gender; this experimentation is a normal developmental activity.

Adolescents who are transgender may experience a significant worsening of gender dysphoria as they start puberty, as the development of secondary sex characteristics can precipitate significant anxiety and/or depression. A teenager assigned male at birth who identifies as female and starts developing male secondary sex characteristics—such as deepening of the voice or facial hair—can have a feeling of powerlessness over their body and outward appearance. Similarly, a teenager assigned female at birth who identifies as male and starts developing female secondary sex characteristics, such as breast development or menstrual bleeding, can have acutely worsening depression and anxiety. Assessing gender identity and providing support through this process has the potential to significantly decrease negative mental health outcomes (Olson, Durwood, DeMeules, & McLaughlin, 2016).

The process of developing gender identity can continue through adulthood as well. Because of situations beyond the person's control, including financial instability or lack of family support, some people do not start their gender transition until much later in life. The medical treatment of that transition will change depending on the patient's age and other health risks, but assessing for gender identity and supporting the patient with use of their preferred name and pronoun is an intervention that is effective and safe at all stages of life.

Safety concerns are significant for transgender individuals. The year 2017 was the deadliest on record for transgender people in the United States, with 29 deaths, some of which were hate crimes perpetrated by acquaintances or strangers, and some by intimate partners (Human Rights Campaign [HRC] Foundation, 2018). In 2018, there were 26 transgender deaths, 82% of which were women of color, 64% under the age of 35, and 55% lived in the south; these numbers are likely widely underreported (HRC Foundation, 2018).

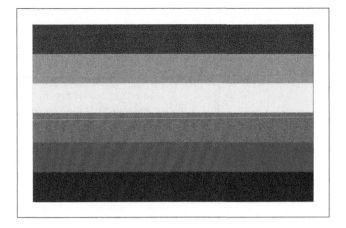

FIGURE 18.1 LGBT Pride Flag. The LGBT Pride Flag is internationally recognized as a symbol of the gay rights movement, unity, and acceptance of this population.

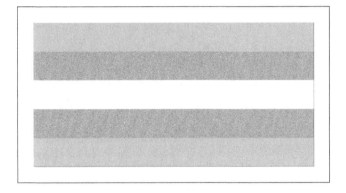

FIGURE 18.2 Transgender Pride Flag, created by Monica Helmes. The design features the colors light blue and pink, which are traditionally associated with baby boys and girls, and white, which represents those who are intersex, training, or have a neutral or undefined gender.

KEY HISTORY QUESTIONS AND CONSIDERATIONS

Sensitive history taking encompasses much more than just the interview with the clinician. The environment of the healthcare facility, intake forms, and the vocabulary used by staff and clinicians contribute to the comfort of the patient and willingness to communicate information about their identity. Creating a welcoming environment for LGBTQ+ persons can be accomplished by hanging posters that reflect many different races and gender expressions. Posting gay and transgender pride flags in a highly visible area signifies commitment to nondiscriminatory care (**Figures 18.1** and **18.2**). Gender-neutral bathrooms should be available for all patients. Forms should account for diverse sexual orientations and gender identities by providing multiple checkbox options and a space for patients to write in their identity if the options do not accurately reflect their internal sense of self. This can sometimes be challenging as electronic medical record (EMR) systems are often

not flexible to free text, nor do they always include an "other" option. Each individual practice should plan for how identities not listed in the EMR can be included in the patient's chart to avoid misidentification. It is critical that every member of the healthcare team address the patient with the name and gender pronoun indicated by the patient at all times and that documentation in the chart reflect these preferences. Keep in mind that both name and pronoun can change over time and must be reassessed periodically. Many people will change their name and gender pronoun legally, but this is not always possible depending on financial, employment, and legal issues in some states.

Consider how the environment and verbal and nonverbal cues impact the individual during history taking. For example, be intentional about how the exam room is configured for a patient visit. Face the patient and allow the computer screen to be visible to them; this simple move of transparency fosters trust. Ask routine open-ended questions the same way to every patient, every time. If the clinician assumes someone is cisgender or heterosexual and that is not how they identify, the clinician will likely miss an opportunity to adequately assess that patient's specific health needs. Explain the rationale for asking questions that may seem intrusive; make it transparent that the questions will augment the patient's care and that they are not being asked out of curiosity. Before asking a question, consider and assess whether the information gleaned from the response will help to make clinical decisions in regard to the individual's care. Respond to patients with empathy and understanding, and reassure them of confidentiality. Some patients may share identities with a clinician that they have never shared with anyone else, including family. Clinicians who establish trust, remain open-minded, and are careful about using unassuming language find that patients willingly share the information needed to provide evidence-based, sensitive, high-quality care that supports their health and well-being.

Key health and well-being assessments pertinent to sexual orientation and gender identity, including past medical history, family, and social history, are included with rationale in **Exhibit 18.1**.

PREVENTIVE CARE CONSIDERATIONS

Assessments of health and well-being allow the clinician to consider and individualize preventive care services. Health disparities, including disparities in sexual health, affect sexual and gender minorities at higher rates. Key history and physical exam considerations are intended to assess risks to health and well-being and need for preventive care. Risks include the following:

- Gay men and men who have sex with men are at higher risk for human immunodeficiency virus (HIV) and other sexually transmitted infections (STIs), particularly men of color.
- Lesbians are less likely to get preventive services for cancer.
- LGBTQ+ groups have high rates of tobacco, alcohol, and other drug use.
- Lesbians and bisexual females are more likely to be overweight or obese.
- Transgender individuals have the highest rate of attempted suicide of any population group.

Sexual Orientation, Sexual Health, and Sexually Transmitted Infections

Ask all patients about sexual orientation and sexual practices to ensure adequate STI screening. Asking

---

EXHIBIT 18.1 Script for Health History Assessment: Clinician Questions With Rationale and Considerations

Hello, my name is _____. How do you like to be addressed? *All individuals should have the opportunity to state their name and preferred pronouns.*

Tell me about your health history. Have you ever been diagnosed with a chronic condition? Have you had surgery? Any hospitalizations? Do you take any prescribed medications? Over-the-counter medications? *Assessing past medical and surgical history should be conducted in a similar way for all patients, regardless of sexual orientation and/or gender identity.*

Where do you live? Does anyone live in the home with you? Is your housing safe and stable? *Assessing social determinants of health is imperative, especially for individuals who identify with vulnerable minority groups.*

To understand if you have any inherited health risks, could you tell me about your biological parents' health? Any cancer, heart disease, diabetes . . . ? *It may be important to ask specifically about genetic relationships as many LGBTQ+ people have chosen families that are not genetically related.*

How is your relationship with your family of origin? Are they supportive of you? Who are your best supports? *Assessing family and social support systems is a key component of health assessment.*

Do you now or have you ever smoked tobacco? Do you drink alcohol? Any past or present drug use? *Screening all patients for tobacco, alcohol, and drug use is an evidence-based priority.*

Tell me about your gender identity. *It is important to allow the person the space to explain their identity to you, but you may need to ask specifically if the person identifies as female, male, nonbinary, or some other description.*

Tell me about your gender journey. When did you first realize your identity differed from your sex assigned at birth? What steps have you taken to affirm your gender identity? *Allow the individual to share their history. Options include, but are not limited to, using a different name and/or gender pronoun, changes in physical appearance, medical treatment, and/or surgical treatment; include dates of initiation of medical treatments such as puberty suppressors and hormones.*

(continued)

EXHIBIT 18.1 Script for Health History Assessment: Clinician Questions With Rationale and Considerations (*continued*)

What organs were present at birth? *An organ inventory should be done to determine what organs the person has or had, including breast tissue, cervix, uterus, ovaries, penis, testes, prostate, and so forth. It should be performed for all patients, as cisgender people may also have had surgeries that alter their reproductive organs.*

What organs are present currently? *Assess for surgical removal of the cervix, uterus, ovaries, breast tissue, penis, and testes.*
  * **Organs enhanced with hormones?** *Clitoral tissue, breast tissue*
  * **Organs enhanced with surgery?** *Breast augmentation, vaginoplasty, facial feminization, metoidioplasty, phalloplasty, testicular implants*

Have you shared your identity with friends? Family? Partners? School? Work? *Responses to these questions provide information related to social, family, community, and professional support and/or concerns.*

Do you have safe access to bathroom facilities? *Urinary stasis from holding the bladder for extended periods of time is a risk factor for urinary tract infections (UTIs). Also assess safety in environment.*

Do you tuck? *Tucking is the process of moving the penis and testes between the legs to conceal the organs; this may be accomplished by wearing tight clothing or using some type of binder or strap. Sometimes, the testes are pressed up into the inguinal canal, risking incarceration/strangulation. Escherichia coli UTIs are more common in individuals who tuck.*

Do you bind? *Binding is the process of flattening breast tissue so that the chest appears more masculine. This is typically achieved with medical-grade binders and can cause fungal infections and skin breakdown.*

Do you need help changing legal documents to align with your identity? *Know where to refer patients, such as www .lambdalegal.org*

Are you sexually active? Do you have a regular partner? *Sexual health screening is a key assessment for all individuals.*

How do you identify sexually? *If the person does not understand, provide options such as, "Do you identify as straight, gay, lesbian, bisexual, or something else?"*

In order to know which screenings would benefit you, can you tell me with whom you have sex? What parts of your body do you use when having sex? How do your partners identify their gender and sexual orientation? *If the person does not understand, provide options such as, "Do you have sex with women, men, both? Are your partners cisgendered? Do you participate in oral sex (receptive/insertive), oral–vaginal contact, oral–anal contact, anal sex (receptive/insertive), vaginal sex (receptive/insertive)? Do you use shared sex toys or have any type of genital-to-genital contact?" Note: For individuals who identify as transgender, it may be important to first ask about "triggering" labels for body parts; for example, an individual who identifies as transgender male may prefer to use the term* frontal canal *instead of vagina, and may find that the term* vagina *triggers feelings of gender dysphoria. Reflecting preferred labels or terms within sexual health history questions is most appropriate.*

Are you in a relationship? *Not all people who are sexually active, even with regular partners, are in a relationship, and a relationship is not always exclusively between two people.*

Is your relationship open or closed? *Some relationships have consensual agreements that partners have other sexual partners outside of the relationship. Some relationships are between multiple people, rather than two.*

Are you satisfied with your sexual function? *Key assessment for all individuals.*

How do you protect yourself from STIs? *If using barrier protection such as condoms ask, "Do you wear protection 100% of the time? Are barriers used for oral–genital contact?"*

When was the last time you had STI screening? *Key assessment related to sexual health for all individuals.*

Do you use drugs or alcohol when having sex? Do you exchange sex for money, drugs, or a place to stay? *These questions are intended to identify behaviors and situations that increase risks to health and well-being.*

Do you desire to have biological children? Do you desire pregnancy? *For transgender patients, also ask if they desire to have preserved fertility, such as cryopreservation of sperm and eggs, prior to starting hormonal or surgical transition. This issue is especially complicated in individuals on puberty blockers as they are never exposed to natal hormones necessary for gamete development.*

Have you felt isolated, trapped, or like you are walking on eggshells in an intimate relationship? Has someone pressured or forced you to do something sexual that you didn't want to do? Has someone hit, kicked, punched, or otherwise hurt you? *Screen for intimate partner violence, as well as past and/or current history of physical, sexual, emotional, economic, or verbal abuse.*

about sexual practices can more accurately direct targeted testing for specific STIs. For example, patients practicing oral or anal sex may require testing at sites other than just urethral or vaginal/cervical samples. Gonorrhea can flourish in the pharynx and rectum, and chlamydia can cause asymptomatic rectal infection, which if untreated may progress to lymphogranuloma venereum (LGV) and, subsequently, rectal fistulas and strictures.

Anyone who practices anilingus, or anal–oral stimulation, can become infected with fecal oral route infections such as hepatitis A, *Giardia lamblia*, *Entamoeba histolytica*, ectoparasites, *Shigella*, and *Campylobacter* (Centers for Disease Control and Prevention [CDC], n.d.).

Hepatitis A, B, and C can be transmitted through anal intercourse. Routine screening and vaccination for hepatitis A and B are recommended for all men who have sex with men (MSM). Screening for hepatitis C is recommended if engaging in unprotected intercourse with multiple partners, injecting drugs, or being sexually active with intravenous drug users (CDC, n.d.).

Any patient who is HIV-positive and practices anal receptive intercourse may require an anal pap smear as anal HPV can progress to cancer similarly to cervical HPV. Evidence for use of anal pap smears in people who are not HIV-positive and practicing anal receptive sex is limited (CDC, n.d.). However, clinicians may consider anal pap if the patient is practicing anal receptive sex and has anal warts or has undiagnosed gastrointestinal or rectal symptoms, such as local pain, itching, bleeding, discharge, irritation, or tenesmus. Consider anal screening for any person with high-grade cervical dysplasia (Aberg et al., 2014).

Women who have sex with women are at risk for vaginal infections and STIs as well. STIs like human papillomavirus (HPV), gonorrhea, chlamydia, pubic lice, genital herpes, and trichomoniasis can spread easily between women. HIV transmission between two cisgender females is thought to be low, but it is theoretically possible through vaginal secretions or menstrual blood (CDC, n.d.). Women who have sex with women have increased risk of bacterial vaginosis (BV). Oral sex and manual stimulation of the clitoris, vagina, or rectum can also spread infections. This risk is increased with shared penetrative sex toys, genital-to-genital contact, and transmission of bodily fluids on hands.

Individuals at risk for HIV infection can further protect themselves with pre-exposure prophylaxis (PrEP) by taking a daily medication to prevent HIV. High-risk individuals include those with an HIV-positive sexual partner, recent STI diagnosis, multiple partners, inconsistent condom use, commercial sex work, region with high prevalence of HIV, intravenous drug use, or sexual partner who uses intravenous drugs (CDC, 2019).

Sexual Orientation, Sexual Health, and Cervical Cancer Screening

Any individual with a cervix should follow the recommendations by the United States Preventive Services Task Force (USPSTF) for cervical cancer screening (Curry et al., 2018). Abnormal pap testing results should be managed in compliance with American Society for Colposcopy and Cervical Pathology (ASCCP) guidelines (Saslow et al., 2012). Refer to Chapter 3, Approach to Implementing and Documenting Patient-Centered, Culturally Sensitive Evidence-Based Assessment, and Chapter 20, Evidence-Based Assessment of the Female Genitourinary System, for more information on these guidelines.

Transmasculine patients, or patients whose sex assigned at birth is female but whose identified gender is male, may be less likely to present for cervical cancer screening because of multiple factors, including fear of presenting male in a gynecology office, fear of the procedure, or lack of understanding of the need for screening. It is important to keep in mind that 47% of transgender people have been sexually assaulted at some point in their lives (James et al., 2016). Clinicians must explain the process and rationale for cervical cancer screening, including risk of HPV documented in women who have sex with women, regardless of vaginal penetration. Clinicians must also ensure a safe space and environment, as well as individualized considerations for the exam, including chaperone, family member support, practice inserting speculum at home privately, insertion of the speculum personally in the office, or use of a short-acting benzodiazepine 20 to 30 minutes prior to exam. In a harm-reduction model and after counseling related to limited adequacy of surveillance, it is appropriate to offer any patient with a cervix who declines a pap test a self-administered vaginal HPV screening with polyester swab and ThinPrep vial. It must be made clear on the requisition that the specimen is a cervical sample; note that the patient is amenorrheic and whether the person is using testosterone, especially if the chart gender marker is not female. It is common to receive an insufficient cervical sample even with careful collection, and it is important to discuss this possibility with patients at the time of pap testing in the event of a need to repeat the test. Using a short course of topical estrogen in the vaginal or frontal canal for 1 to 2 weeks prior to collection of pap test specimens can improve comfort in masculine-identified patients with atrophy and can improve chances of adequate collection. Reassure patients that topical estrogens used short term are unlikely to be absorbed systemically.

Sexual Orientation, Sexual Health, and Fertility

It is important to review fertility and pregnancy prevention with each patient. While women who have sexual intercourse exclusively with women or with individuals who do not produce sperm are not at risk for unintended pregnancy, they may desire pregnancy at some point in their lives. It is also important to assess whether the person's partner is capable of producing sperm and offering pregnancy prevention information if necessary. It is not appropriate to assume that all women of childbearing age require or desire birth-control options.

Some transmasculine patients may desire the experience of pregnancy or see it as a means to have biological children. For others, thinking of using reproductive organs may cause triggering of gender dysphoria. There are limited data to guide discussions around the effect of hormones on fertility, and certainly some gender reassignment surgeries are sterilizing with available technologies today. There are multiple case reports of transmasculine people discontinuing testosterone after years of use and having healthy pregnancies, deliveries, and children.

Sexual Orientation, Sexual Health, and Intimate Partner Violence

Intimate partner violence (IPV) is violence incurred by a current or former intimate partner. IPV can take many shapes, including physical, verbal, emotional, economic, and sexual abuse. LGBTQ+ individuals experience different barriers to seeking help for IPV as the partner experiencing abuse may not be believed as there is a "common knowledge" myth that IPV exists only between heterosexual couples and affects mostly women. Furthermore, the National Coalition of Anti-Violence Programs (NCAVP, 2009) reports that police are 15 times more likely to arrest both partners in cases of homosexual IPV cases and that judges are more likely to place restraining orders on both partners. This does not allow justice for the victim and can be further traumatizing. In healthcare settings, the person who is abusive might introduce themselves as a friend and be allowed to stay with the abused person during the visit, depriving the abuser of an opportunity to seek help (Basham, Presley, & Potter, 2015). From the NCAVP (2012):

- Of all LGBTQ+ victims of IPV, 50.5% identified as female, 38.7% as gay, and 31.3% as lesbian; 66.8% were people of color.
- More than half, 63.2%, of the LGBTQ+ homicide victims of IPV identified as male.
- LGBTQ+ youth, young adults, and gay people are more likely to experience injuries as a result of IPV.
- LGBTQ+ individuals who experience abuse may have difficulty finding a safe shelter. A study of LGBTQ+ domestic violence survivors found 61.6% of survivors who sought shelter were denied access.

Transwomen/Feminine Preventive Care Considerations

- Estrogen is not a reliable form of birth control, and a barrier method should be used as needed.
- Patients may need to be instructed to wipe front to back after vaginoplasty.
- Patients will need to adhere to a dilation schedule long term to maintain vaginal depth.
- The prostate is not removed during vaginoplasty, and infectious prostatitis must be considered for at-risk women.
- Screening mammograms should be started at age 50 if there is a history of 5 to 10 years of feminizing hormones, and it is recommended to be repeated every 2 years.

Transmen/Masculine Preventive Care Considerations

- Pelvic inflammatory disease should be considered for all at-risk men with a uterus and fallopian tubes.
- Testosterone is not a reliable form of birth control, and testosterone is teratogenic. Some form of birth control should be considered as needed, including progesterone-only emergency contraception, Depo Provera, or a long-acting contraceptive or an implanted or intrauterine device.
- Some men retain vaginas with or without reproductive organs after metoidioplasty, but not all are safe to penetrate. Consult with the patient's surgeon.
- There is less concern for endometrial hyperplasia and cancer on chronic testosterone than previously thought, but any vaginal bleeding after cessation of menses should be evaluated as such.
- Not all breast tissue is removed in male chest reconstruction, and breast cancer risk should be assessed. Imaging is limited, but would most likely involve ultrasound.

PHYSICAL EXAMINATION

Every physical exam should be targeted to the specific health concerns of an individual at the time of the encounter, regardless of gender identity or sexual orientation. Questions about gender identity or transition-related physical changes should be asked only if pertinent to the current problem. For example, if the person has a sprained ankle, questions about or exam of physical changes related to their hormones or the person's genitalia are likely not appropriate. The reverse also holds true; if the person has a concern that is in some way related to or affected by gender-related hormonal or surgical procedures or sexual practices, clinicians must ask further questions and do the appropriate exam. It is important to think critically about

TABLE 18.3 Transmen/Transmasculine Considerations for Physical Examination	
Consideration	Rationale
Chest surgery	Transmen commonly have chest surgery to remove breast tissue; approximately 20%–30% of natal tissue remains after surgery for contouring
Binding	Transmen often bind breast tissue to be able to present as male with a flattened chest
Vaginal atrophy	Testosterone therapy can cause vaginal atrophy similar to that seen in menopause
Clitoral enlargement	Testosterone therapy causes clitoral enlargement
Metoidioplasty	Genital surgery that creates a microphallus with or without a neo-urethra; vaginectomy may or may not be done at the time of the surgery
Phalloplasty	Genital surgery that creates a phallus using skin grafts from other sites and contains a neo-urethra; vaginectomy is done at the time of the surgery

TABLE 18.4 Transwomen/Transfeminine Considerations for Physical Examination	
Consideration	Rationale
Breast growth and breast augmentation	Breast tissue develops with use of estrogen therapy; if insufficient growth over time, the patient may opt to have breast augmentation performed.
Silicone pumping	As a result of lack of access to feminizing procedures, patients may inject nonmedical grade-free silicone, sometimes upward of 1–2 L, in an attempt to augment breasts, cheeks, or buttocks. This is sometimes done in groups, raising concern for infectious diseases from needle sharing, bacterial skin infections, silicone calcification, local tissue necrosis, migration of silicone, and potential for pulmonary embolism.
Vaginoplasty	Surgical construction of a vaginal canal, usually penile inversion procedure; the anatomy of the neovagina is a blind cuff and may have a more downward sloping presentation. In the first 3–6 months after vaginoplasty, it is imperative to receive clearance from the surgeon prior to internal exam, and an anoscope should be used rather than a speculum.
Prostate	The prostate will be small and withdrawn in patients on feminizing hormone therapy. For patients who have undergone vaginoplasty, it may be reasonable to assess the prostate digitally through the neovagina as access from the rectum may be obscured by the vaginal wall.

each situation to avoid over- or underexamining the patient.

Each chapter of this text identifies key physical exam techniques and findings. Additional surgical procedures, physical changes, and hormonal adaptations that might require supplementary considerations for physical exam are listed for transmen/transmasculine individuals in **Table 18.3** and for transwomen/transfeminine individuals in **Table 18.4**.

LABORATORY CONSIDERATIONS

CONSIDERATIONS RELATED TO SEXUAL ORIENTATION

Clinicians should check with individual laboratories, as policies and recommendations for which collection device is used for various screenings will vary, especially for rectal samples. For a gonorrhea and chlamydia screening rectal sample, labs will often approve the use of the same collection kit as used for urethral or cervical samples. Anal pap tests are typically done by using the same swabs, collection procedure, and preservative solutions as cervical pap testing. Note to clinicians: Always be sure to label anal specimens as such, especially as the patient exam and screenings may involve the use of swabs from several different sites. Knowing the source of samples is imperative for pathologists to interpret cytology findings.

TABLE 18.5 Changes in Laboratory Values Related to Hormone Therapy

Laboratory Test	Transmasculine on Testosterone	Transfeminine on Estrogen
HCT	↑	↓
RBC	↑	Unchanged
Creatinine	↑	↓
PSA	NA	↓

HCT, hematocrit; NA, not applicable; PSA, prostate surface antigen; RBC, red blood cells.

CONSIDERATIONS RELATED TO GENDER IDENTITY

The most common laboratory tests have normal ranges based on gender, which presents a unique challenge when a transgender patient has lab work completed. Both feminizing and masculinizing hormone therapy can alter some results. The most common of these changes are listed in **Table 18.5.**

Consideration must be given to the labeling of the laboratory sample within the EMR. How the individual's gender is documented in the EMR will communicate to the lab how to handle the specimen and which set of normal values, male or female, to use to determine abnormalities. Some EMR systems use sex assigned at birth, and some use legal gender. Keep in mind that not all transgender patients will have the ability to change their name and/or gender marker because of financial issues, family expectations, work situation, or local and state laws. Computerized flags for normal and abnormal lab results may not be applicable; critical thinking must be used in interpreting all lab results.

One additional, specific consideration for transfeminine-identified patients after vaginoplasty: It is not known whether a urethral sample for gonorrhea and chlamydia is sufficient screening; therefore, an additional neovaginal swab should be completed for at-risk individuals and can be done with or without the anoscope (Deutsch, 2016).

IMAGING CONSIDERATIONS

CONSIDERATIONS RELATED TO GENDER IDENTITY

Communication among members of the healthcare team is important to ensure that information about the patient's gender identity is relayed so as to avoid putting the patient through the process of exposing it to every person. Telling the radiologist or radiology technician that a patient is transgender can prevent potentially uncomfortable or damaging interactions. An organ

inventory should be completed prior to imaging to determine necessary pretest screening and protection. Transmasculine patients should be screened for pregnancy with the same guidelines as cisgender women. Consider the invasiveness of transvaginal ultrasound, and ensure that the patient feels safe and that the ultrasound technician is sensitive to the situation. Patients may be more comfortable if afforded the opportunity to insert their own probe and should be asked if they prefer that the clinician gently place it. Considerations may include offering a short-acting benzodiazepine and offering a chaperone, including the patient's own support person.

EVIDENCE-BASED PRACTICE CONSIDERATIONS

LGBTQ+ medicine presents a particular challenge for the development of evidence-based guidelines due to limitations in the available body of evidence, as well as the exclusion of gender and sexual identities in many existing mechanisms for collecting population-based data (Cahill & Makadon, 2013; Deutsch & Bucholz, 2015; Hembree et al., 2017; Lambda Legal, 2014; Reisner et al., 2016). This is further compounded by the stigma and bias that can decrease the likelihood of LGBTQ+ and transgender individuals to self-identify. Existing studies often have small sample sizes, are based on collective expert experience, or use data collected outside of the United States. While research findings are limited, guidelines that have been established for the primary care of LGBTQ+ individuals include the following:

- American Psychological Association Practice Guidelines (2019)
- Gay and Lesbian Medical Association Guidelines for Care of LGBT Patients (2014)

Although based mostly on expert opinions, current guidelines for transgender health are available through the following organizations:

- The World Professional Association for Transgender Health Standards of Care (Coleman et al., 2012)
- University of California San Francisco (UCSF) Guidelines for the Primary and Gender-Affirming Care of Transgender and Gender Non-Binary People (Deutsch, 2016)
- Endocrine Society Clinical Practice Guidelines (Hembree et al., 2017)

At this time, there are no transgender medicine–specific certifying boards or fellowships available for research or for training primary care clinicians, endocrinology specialists, or surgeons. The guidelines listed provide the most current evidence-based assessment and practice considerations and aim to address disparities by equipping clinicians with the tools and knowledge to meet the healthcare needs of LGBTQ+ and transgender and gender nonconforming individuals.

CASE STUDY: Rectal Pain

Reason for Seeking Care
A healthy 36-year-old male with no history of chronic medical conditions or past surgical history presents to clinic with 4 weeks of rectal pain. He is a nonsmoker, has infrequent use of alcohol, and denies use of illicit substances. He is married to his husband of 5 years, and they have an open relationship. He has engaged in unprotected anal receptive intercourse; his last encounter was 2 weeks ago. He denies oral or insertive intercourse. Over the past month, he complains of progressive rectal pain, which is constant, but exacerbates with bowel movements, which have had a normal consistency.

Further History and Review of Systems
- Fever, chills, weight loss, flu-like symptoms?
- Pharyngitis?
- Lymphadenopathy?
- Rash, lesions?
- Bleeding or discharge from anus?

Physical Examination
- General appearance
- Skin exam
- If individual has flu-like symptoms, examine HEENT
- Lymphatic assessment for lymphadenopathy
- Rectal exam—inspect for lesions, condylomata, fissures, hemorrhoids
- Digital rectal exam for masses, internal condylomata, prostatic tenderness
- Guaiac for blood

Differential Diagnoses
- Hemorrhoids or fissure secondary to rectal trauma, rectal gonorrhea, chlamydia, or LGV given chronicity of symptoms
- If he had abdominal pain/diarrhea, differential would include fecal oral pathogens as well.
- Consider acute retroviral syndrome (HIV) if associated symptoms of fever, pharyngitis, rash, and flu-like symptoms

Next Steps
- Given history of unprotected rectal intercourse, it may be reasonable to treat empirically for gonorrhea and chlamydia. STI screening, including hepatitis A and B (including immunity); consider HCV if additional risk factors; HIV (antibody and antigen—given that his last encounter was 2 weeks ago, it is prudent to repeat HIV testing again in 4 weeks if initial testing is negative); rapid plasma reagin (RPR); rectal swab for gonorrhea and chlamydia (consider urine for urethral site and oral gonorrhea swab if indicated).
- If not immune to hepatitis A or B, vaccinate
- Consider PrEP
- Educate in a nonjudgmental manner about benefits of barrier methods of preventing STIs; provide access to condoms

Clinical Pearls

- Healthcare clinicians must be experts in compassion. Giving all patients the space to be who they are can dramatically improve patient encounters and improve health outcomes.
- Maintain a neutral line of questioning with all patients to ensure that the patient is not misidentified, thereby limiting the quality of the history. If a mistake is made, apologize, correct the mistake, and move on to the next question.

Key Takeaways

- Sexual orientation must be assessed to determine what preventive care should be recommended and/or what specific health risks an individual may have.
- Gender identity can be determined only by the individual; therefore, it is imperative that individuals be given the opportunity to provide their preferred name and gender pronouns. Correct gender pronouns and the name that the patient chooses to use must be used during all encounters with each patient.

REFERENCES

Aberg, J. A., Gallant, J. E., Ghanem, K. G., Emmanuel, P., Zingman, B. S., & Horberg, M. A. (2014). Primary care guidelines for the management of persons infected with HIV: 2013 update by the HIV Medicine Association of the Infectious Diseases Society of America. *Clinical Infectious Diseases, 58,* e1–e34. doi:10.1093/cid/cit665

American Psychological Association. (2019). *Practice guidelines for LGB clients.* Retrieved from https://www.apa.org/pi/lgbt/resources/guidelines

Basham, C., Presley, C., & Potter, J. (2015). *Implementing routine intimate partner violence screening in a primary care setting* [PowerPoint slides]. Retrieved from https://www.lgbthealtheducation.org/webinar/lgbt-ipv-screening

Cahill, S., & Makadon, H. (2013). Sexual orientation and gender identity data collection in clinical settings and in electronic health records: A key to ending LGBT health disparities. *LGBT Health, 1*(1), 34–41. doi:10.1089/lgbt.2013.0001

Centers for Disease Control and Prevention. (n.d.). *Sexually transmitted disease treatment guidelines.* Retrieved from https://www.cdc.gov/std/tg2015/default.htm

Centers for Disease Control and Prevention. (2019). *Pre exposure prophylaxis (PrEP).* Retrieved from https://www.cdc.gov/hiv/risk/prep/index.html

Choi, S. K., & Meyer, I. H. (2016). *LGBT aging: A review of research findings, needs, and policy implications.* Retrieved from https://williamsinstitute.law.ucla.edu/research/lgbt-older-adults-highlighting-isolation-discrimination/

Coleman, E., Bockting, W., Botzer, M., Cohen-Kettenis, P., DeCuypere, G., Feldman, J., . . . Zucker, K. (2012). *Standards of care for the health of transsexual, transgender, and gender nonconforming people* (7th version). Minneapolis, MN: World Professional Association for Transgender Health. Retrieved from https://www.wpath.org/publications/soc

Curry, S. J., Krist, A. H., Owens, D. K., Barry, M J., Caughey, A. B., Davidson, K. W., . . . Wong, J. B. (2018). Screening for cervical cancer: U.S. Preventive Services Task Force recommendation. *Journal of the American Medical Association, 320*(7), 674–686. doi:10.1001/jama.2018.10897

Deutsch, M. B. (Ed.). (2016). *Guidelines for the primary and gender-affirming care of transgender and gender nonbinary people* (2nd ed.). San Francisco, CA: Center of Excellence for Transgender Health. Retrieved from http://transhealth.ucsf.edu/trans?page=guidelines-home

Deutsch, M. B., & Bucholz, D. (2015). Electronic health records and transgender patients—Practical recommendations for the collection of gender identity data. *Journal of General Internal Medicine, 30*(6), 843–847. doi:10.1007/s11606-014-3148-7

Flores, A. R., Herman, J. L., Gates, G. J., & Brown, T. N. T. (2016). How many adults identify as transgender in the United States? Retrieved from https://williamsinstitute.law.ucla.edu/research/how-many-adults-identify-as-transgender-in-the-united-states

Garofalo, R., Wolf, R. C., Wissow, L. S., Woods, E. R., & Goodman, E. (1999). Sexual orientation and risk of suicide attempts among a representative sample of youth. *Archives of Pediatrics and Adolescent Medicine, 153*(5), 487–493. doi:10.1001/archpedi.153.5.487

Gay and Lesbian Medical Association. (2014). *Guidelines for care of lesbian, gay, bisexual, and transgender patients.* Retrieved from https://npin.cdc.gov/publication/guidelines-care-lesbian-gay-bisexual-and-transgender-patients

Hembree, W. C., Cohen-Kettenis, P. T., Gooren, L., Hannema, S. E., Meyer, W. J., Murad, M. H., . . . T'Sjoen, G. G. (2017). Endocrine treatment of gender-dysphoric/gender-incongruent persons: An Endocrine Society clinical practice guideline. *The Journal of Clinical Endocrinology & Metabolism, 102*(11), 3869–3903. doi:10.1210/jc.2017-01658

Human Rights Campaign Foundation. (2018). *A national epidemic: Fatal anti-transgender violence in America in 2018.* Retrieved from https://www.hrc.org/resources/a-national-epidemic-fatal-anti-transgender-violence-in-america-in-2018

James, S. E., Herman, J. L., Rankin, S., Keisling, M., Mottet, L., & Anafi, M. (2016). *The report of the 2015 U.S. transgender survey.* Washington, DC: National Center for Transgender Equality. Retrieved from https://transequality.org/sites/default/files/docs/usts/USTS-Full-Report-Dec17.pdf

Lambda Legal. (2014). *When health care isn't caring: Lambda Legal's survey on discrimination against LGBT people and people living with HIV.* Retrieved from https://www.lambdalegal.org/health-care-report

Lunn, M. R., Cui, W., Zack, M. M., Thompson, W. W., Blank, M. B., & Yehia, B. R. (2017). Sociodemographic characteristics and health outcomes among lesbian, gay, and bisexual U.S. adults using *Healthy People 2020* leading health indicators. *LGBT Health, 4*(4), 203–294. doi:10.1089/lgbt.2016.0087

National Coalition of Anti-Violence Programs. (2009). *Lesbian, gay, bisexual, transgender and queer domestic/intimate partner violence in the United States in 2009.* Retrieved from https://avp.org/wp-content/uploads/2017/04/2009_NCAVP_IPV_Report.pdf

National Coalition of Anti-Violence Programs. (2012). *Lesbian, gay, bisexual, transgender, queer, and HIV-affected intimate partner violence: 2011.* New York: New York

City Gay & Lesbian Anti-Violence Project. Retrieved from https://avp.org/wp-content/uploads/2017/04/2011_NCAVP _IPV_Report.pdf

Obedin-Maliver, J., Goldsmith, E. S., Stewart, L., White, W., Tran, E., Brenman, S., . . . Lunn, M. R. (2011). Lesbian, gay, bisexual, and transgender-related content in undergraduate medical education. *The Journal of the American Medical Association, 306,* 971–977. doi:10.1001/jama.2011.1255

Olson, K. R., Durwood, L., DeMeules, M., & McLaughlin, K. A. (2016). Mental health of transgender children who are supported in their identities. *Pediatrics, 137*(3), 1–8. doi:10.1542/peds.2015-3223

Reisner, S. L., Deutsch, M. B., Bhasin, S., Bockting, W., Brown, G. R., Feldman, J., . . . Goodman, M. (2016). Advancing methods for US transgender health research. *Current Opinion in Endocrinology, Diabetes and Obesity, 12*(2), 198–207. doi:10.1097/MED.0000000000000229

Rosario, M., Schrimshaw, E. W., & Hunter, J. (2012). Different patterns of sexual identity development over time: Implications for psychological adjustment of lesbian, gay, and bisexual youths. *The Journal of Sex Research, 48*(1), 3–15. doi:10.1080/00224490903331067

Saslow, D., Solomon, D., Lawson, H. W., Killackey, M., Kulasingam, S. L., Cain, J., . . . Myers, E. R. (2012). American Cancer Society, American Society for Colposcopy and Cervical Pathology, and American Society for Clinical Pathology screening guidelines for the prevention and early detection of cervical cancer. *Journal of Lower Genital Tract Disease, 16*(3), 175–204. doi:10.1097/ LGT.0b013e31824ca9d5

Tillery, B., Ray, A., Cruz, E., & Waters, E. (2018). *Lesbian, gay, bisexual, transgender, queer, and HIV-affected intimate partner violence in 2017.* Retrieved from http://avp.org/ wp-content/uploads/2019/01/NCAVP-HV-IPV-2017-report.pdf

19

Evidence-Based Assessment of Male Genitalia, Prostate, Rectum, and Anus

Rosie Zeno and Alice M. Teall

"Never let the fear of striking out keep you from playing the game."

—BABE RUTH

VIDEO

- Well Exam: Male Sexual History and Genitourinary Exam

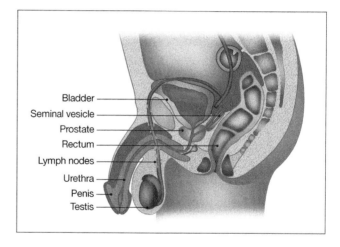

FIGURE 19.1 Male pelvic organs.

LEARNING OBJECTIVES

- Review the anatomy and physiology of the male genitalia, including prostate.
- Determine key assessments for evaluating the structure and function of the male genitalia, prostate, rectum, and anus.
- Identify assessment findings, signs, and symptoms indicating abnormalities, problems, and/or disorders affecting the male genitalurinary system, prostate, rectum, and anus.

ANATOMY AND PHYSIOLOGY OF MALE GENITALIA

MALE PELVIC ORGANS AND REPRODUCTIVE SYSTEM

Male genitalia includes external, internal, and glandular accessory structures that function to produce and

Visit https://connect.springerpub.com/content/book/978-0-8261-6454-4/chapter/ch00 to access the videos.

transport viable sperm for reproduction (**Figures 19.1 and 19.2**).

External Organs: Penis and Scrotum

The shaft of the **penis** is composed of three columns of erectile tissue, the two corpora cavernosa on the dorsal side and the corpus spongiosum ventrally, and the enveloping layers of fascia, nerves, lymphatics, and blood vessels. Two suspensory ligaments, composed primarily of elastic fibers, support the penis at its base. The corpus spongiosum extends into the rounded cone of erectile tissue, the glans; the expanded base or border of the glans is the corona. The urethra, surrounded and supported by the corpus spongiosum, opens as a slit-like vertical opening, the urinary meatus, approximately

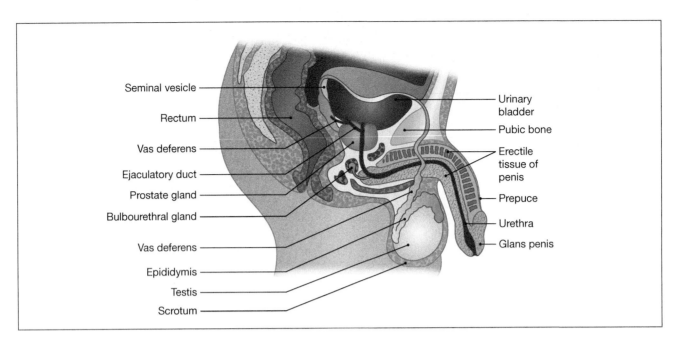

FIGURE 19.2 Male reproductive system.

2 mm ventral to the tip of the glans (Dyer, 2016). The darker-pigmented skin of the penis is continuous with that of the lower abdominal wall proximally, and confluent with the smooth, hairless skin covering the glans distally. At the corona, it is folded on itself to form the prepuce (foreskin), which overlies the glans. Unless the foreskin has been surgically removed through **circumcision**, the prepuce covers the glans.

The **scrotum** is a fibromuscular pouch, continuous with the abdominal wall and perineal skin, and divided medially by a septum that forms two compartments, each of which contains a testis and accessory structures. The lymphatics of the penis and scrotal surface drain into the inguinal lymph nodes. The layers of the scrotum consist of skin, dartos and cremaster muscles, and external and internal fascia. One function of the scrotum is to maintain the temperature necessary for sperm production by locating the testes outside of the body cavity. Temperature receptors are located in the scrotum. When the temperature is too low, the dartos muscle contracts, causing the scrotal skin to wrinkle, minimizing surface area for heat loss. Cold temperatures also cause the cremaster muscle to contract, which raises the testes to bring them closer to the warmer groin region. When the scrotal temperature rises, these muscles relax, the surface area of the scrotum increases, and the scrotum descends.

Internal and Accessory Structures of the Male Reproductive System

The **testes** are paired reproductive glands suspended in the scrotum by the dartos muscle and spermatic cord. The left testis often is lower than the right. Each testis is covered by the tunica vaginalis, a double-layered membrane that separates it from the scrotal wall; testes are normally 1.5 to 2 cm in length before puberty, and 3.5 to 5 cm after puberty (Dyer, 2016). A normal variation found within the upper portion of the testis is the appendix testis, a small appendage of normal tissue, 1 to 3 mm in length. Primarily responsible for testosterone and sperm production, the testes are composed mainly of seminiferous tubules. Leydig cells surrounding the seminiferous tubules produce and secrete testosterone and other androgens important for sexual development, libido, spermatogenesis, and erectile function. The seminiferous tubules are lined with germ cells that produce sperm and nutrient fluid. These tubules empty their contents into a network of ducts, which ultimately flow into the epididymis.

The comma-shaped, elongated epididymis is a duct formed from a single tubular structure estimated to be up to 20 feet in length, highly convoluted, and compressed to the point of appearing solid (Dyer, 2016). Owing to its length, the epididymal duct allows space for storage and maturation of sperm. Progressively tapering in width, the narrow, lower part of the epididymis is continuous with a muscular duct, the vas deferens.

The vas deferens approximates with arteries, veins, lymphatics, muscle fibers, and nerves to form the spermatic cord. The spermatic cord ascends along the posterior border of the testes, and into the pelvic cavity through the inguinal canal. The vas deferens then loops anteriorly over and behind the bladder to the prostate, where it merges with seminal vesicles to form the ejaculatory duct, which traverses the prostate and empties into the urethra.

Secretions from the ducts of the vas deferens, seminal vesicles, prostate, and bulbourethral glands, located adjacent to the urethra just below the prostate gland, are essential to fertility. Although the seminal vesicles secrete a significant portion of the fluid that ultimately becomes semen, sperms are rarely in contact with thick seminal fluid from seminal vesicles, and the exact role of seminal fluid is unclear. Fluid from the prostate carries the sperm in the ejaculate. During sexual arousal, preejaculate, viscous fluid produced by the bulbourethral glands, lubricates the urethra and neutralizes acidity associated with residual urine.

Erectile function involves complex hemodynamic, neurologic, endocrine, and psychogenic signaling and mechanisms (Gratzke et al., 2010). Sexual stimulation triggers release of neurotransmitters and responses in hormonal and neural pathways that result in vasodilation and engorgement of the penis, causing erection. The relationship between erection and arousal is not an absolute direct correlation. Older adults may not have an erection when sexually aroused, and male erection can occur during sleep (nocturnal penile tumescence). During sexual arousal, blood flow to the male genitalia increases, and the muscles of the pelvic floor, the seminal vesicles, and the prostrate contract, resulting in the onset of orgasm and sperm ejaculation. Dysfunction in the hypothalamic-pituitary axis, impaired circulation from atherosclerotic or arterial occlusive disease, pathologic neurogenic processes, and/or generalized or situational inhibition of arousal can impair erectile function (Dean & Lue, 2005; Gratzke et al., 2010).

ANATOMY OF THE RECTUM AND ANUS

The rectum and anus or **anal canal** constitute the terminal end of the large intestine. Chapter 16, Evidence-Based Assessment of the Abdomen, Gastrointestinal, and Urologic Systems, reviewed the anatomy and physiology of the colon, which included an illustration of the sagittal view of the rectum in both men and women (see **Figure 16.6**). The anal canal is the most terminal part of the lower large intestine, which lies between the rectum and the anal verge or orifice in the perineum (**Figure 19.3**).

There are three primary components of the anal canal:

- *Transitional zone:* In the upper portion of the anal canal is the transitional zone, where the columnar or glandular epithelial cells of the rectum transition to the squamous cells of the anus.
- *Dentate line:* Within the anal canal, the mucosal lining folds and merges with muscle sphincters, valves, and sinuses; this occurs at the dentate or pectinate line. Below the dentate line, further changes in arterial and venous circulation, nerve innervation, and

lymphatic drainage cause the mucosa/skin to be similar to the external perianal area.
- *Anal verge:* The anal verge is the opening or orifice to the external perineum, defined by the external anal sphincter. The perianal skin of the buttocks around the anal verge is composed of keratinized epithelial cells, in addition to hair, sweat glands, and sebaceous glands.

STRUCTURE AND FUNCTION OF THE PROSTATE GLAND

The **prostate** is a male exocrine accessory gland located inferior to the bladder (**Figure 19.4**). A thin layer of connective tissue separates the prostate and seminal vesicles from the rectum posteriorly. The prostate contains two main types of tissue: exocrine glandular tissue and fibromuscular tissue. Exocrine glandular tissue in the prostate is epithelial tissue specialized

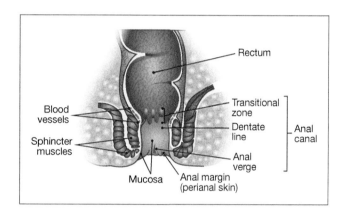

FIGURE 19.3 Anatomy of the anus and rectum.

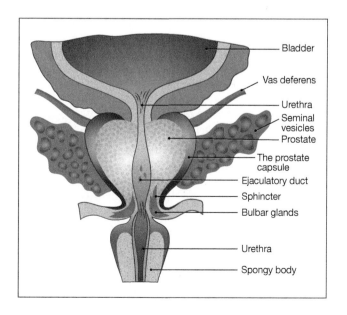

FIGURE 19.4 Anatomy of the prostate.

for the secretion of the components of semen. Most of the prostate is made of exocrine glandular tissue, as the prostate's primary function is the secretion of fluid that facilitates sperm motility and survival. Fibromuscular tissue is a mixture of smooth muscle tissue and dense connective tissue. The collagen fibers of the connective tissue provide strength, while the smooth muscle permits the tissue to contract to expel fluids. Fibromuscular tissue forms the outermost layer of the prostate, the prostate capsule, and the tissue surrounding the urethra. Under normal conditions, urine in the urethra passes through the prostate without flow being impeded.

Distinct lateral, anterior, median, and posterior lobes form the structure of the prostate. The lateral lobes, which are rounded and shaped like orange slices when viewed in a transverse section, are the largest lobes and meet at the midline of the prostate. The median lobe, which lies between the anterior and posterior lobes, contains the ejaculatory ducts of the prostate.

As the understanding of prostatic diseases has evolved, so has the understanding of the structure and function of the prostate. Consequently, the relevance of zones of the prostate has taken on more significance than lobes (Fine & Reuter, 2012). There are three distinct zones found in the prostate gland, and each is associated differently with neoplastic processes (Fine & Reuter, 2012). These are as follows:

- *Peripheral zone:* Approximately 70% of the volume of the prostate is in this zone, which is the most common location for carcinoma.
- *Central zone:* Approximately 25% of the volume of the prostate gland is in this area, which is cone-shaped, located at the base of the prostate adjacent to the seminal vesicles, and contains approximately one-third of the ducts that secrete prostate fluid. Less than 10% of prostate cancers originate in this zone.
- *Transition zone:* This zone contains 5% volume of the gland, surrounds the urethra, and is the site where benign prostatic hyperplasia (BPH) originates.

LIFE-SPAN DIFFERENCES AND CONSIDERATIONS

Anatomic and physiologic differences exist across the life span, beginning with fetal development. During fetal development, the male sex organs are formed under the influence of testosterone secreted from the fetal testes; the differentiation of male and female external genitalia occurs by 12 weeks of gestation. During the third trimester of pregnancy, the testes descend through the retroperitoneal space through the inguinal canal to the scrotum. At full-term, one or both of the testes may not have fully descended and may be in the inguinal canal until early in the postnatal period. Also at birth, the separation of the prepuce from the glans may

be incomplete and may remain so until 3 or 4 years of age in uncircumcised males.

Reproductive maturity begins with the onset of puberty. Testicular growth is the first sign of puberty; normal onset is between the ages of 9 and 14 years. As discussed in Chapter 4, Evidence-Based Assessment of Children and Adolescents, *Tanner staging* is the staging of sexual development by inspection. Male sexual development is staged according to genitalia size and the distribution of pubic hair.

Sexual function wanes during older adulthood, and erectile dysfunction becomes increasingly common. Pubic hair thins, the scrotum becomes more pendulous, and orgasms may develop more slowly. Testosterone levels decline, primarily due to the decline in Leydig cell mass. The prostate enlarges slowly throughout a man's lifetime, potentially leading to the restriction or blockage of urine flow through the urethra.

KEY HISTORY QUESTIONS AND CONSIDERATIONS FOR MALE GENITALIA, PROSTATE, RECTUM, AND ANUS

HISTORY OF PRESENT ILLNESS

As part of a well visit, the clinician assesses for normal functioning of male genitourinary (GU) and reproductive systems, health maintenance, and health promotion needs. During an episodic visit, the clinician focuses on specific concerns. A sensitive, patient-centered, detailed history will inform the components of the physical examination. The elements of the history listed are intended to be used in conjunction with the assessments discussed in Chapter 16, Evidence-Based Assessment of the Abdomen, Gastrointestinal, and Urological Systems, and Chapter 18, Evidence-Based Assessment of Sexual Orientation, Gender Identity, and Health.

Common Presenting Symptoms

Common concerns include penile discharge or lesions; scrotal pain, swelling, or lesions; inguinal or groin swelling; pubic area rash/itching; reproductive health; and/or sexual health concerns, including exposure to sexually transmitted infections (STIs). Often the presenting symptoms are general or nonspecific, as noted in the examples.

Example: Possible Hernia
- Onset: Manner in which symptoms began (i.e., acutely or gradually over time)
- Location: Specific location (i.e., right or left inguinal area, scrotum, abdomen)
- Duration: Persistent or intermittent
- Character: Painful or painless; tenderness, swelling, erythema, or bruising at site

- Associated symptoms: None or fever, nausea, vomiting; dysuria or discharge
- Relieving symptoms: Pressure at/on site of the hernia causes it to be relieved (reduced)
- Timing or temporal factors: Worse with exercise, activity, movement, straining
- Red Flag symptoms indicating need for emergency evaluation: Scrotal pain, irreducible
- Differential diagnoses: Direct inguinal hernia; indirect inguinal hernia; femoral hernia; lymphadenopathy associated with urethritis

Example: Discharge
- Onset: Recent, intermittent, and/or chronic
- Location: Penis/urethra or surrounding lesions
- Duration: Persistent symptoms; increasing amount of discharge or worsening associated symptoms versus lingering, improving, or intermittent symptoms
- Character: Odor (none, or foul odor), color (gray, yellow, green, white), consistency (frothy, thin), amount (minimal or copious)
- Associated symptoms—local: Pruritus (internal, external, or both), painful skin lesions, dysuria, frequent urination, abdominal pain.
- Associated symptoms—systemic: Fever, nausea, vomiting
- Relieving symptoms: Over-the-counter antifungal cream, cool compresses, showering
- Timing or temporal factors: Recent antibiotics; symptoms after use of latex condoms; recent sexual activity, new partner, or history of infection in current partner
- Red Flag symptoms indicating need for emergency evaluation: Testicular or scrotal pain
- Differential diagnoses: STI (chlamydia, gonorrhea, trichomonas, herpes simplex, scabies, trichomoniasis); nongonococcal urethritis, complicated urethritis, prostatitis, epididymitis, orchitis, balanitis

PAST MEDICAL HISTORY
- Chronic diseases (cancers, congenital disorders, autoimmune disorders)
- History of rectal surgeries, hemorrhoids, rectal polyps, rectal bleeding
- History of urinary tract infection (UTI), pyelonephritis, incontinence, weak urinary stream, hematuria
- History of inguinal, femoral, or abdominal hernias, including surgery
- History of prostate enlargement, prostate surgery
- Reproductive health, fertility/infertility, condom use, vasectomy
- Sexual function/dysfunction; concerns regarding sexual response, libido
- History of STIs, treatment, recurrence
- Recent illness, trauma, accidents, injuries, environmental or occupational exposures

- Allergies
- Medications

FAMILY HISTORY
- Family history of colon or rectal cancers, breast or ovarian cancers
- Family history of renal or bladder cancers, prostate cancer
- Family history of hypertension, diabetes, heart disease

SOCIAL HISTORY
- Use of tobacco, smoking history
- Substance use, including alcohol
- Family dynamics, relationships, friends
- Sexual relationships with men, women, or both
- Type of intercourse (oral, vaginal, or anal)
- Safety of home and work environments
- Social determinants of health; socioeconomic factors impacting health
- Victim of violence or assault; adverse childhood events
- Behaviors involving risk-taking

REVIEW OF SYSTEMS
- General/dermatologic: Recent illness, weight loss, lesions or rashes, fever, chills
- Head, Eyes, Ears, Nose, Throat (HEENT): Oral lesions, eye drainage or redness, pharyngitis
- Lymphatic: Lymphadenopathy, tender lymph nodes in groin area
- Cardiovascular/respiratory: Chest pain, edema, dyspnea, cough
- Gastrointestinal (GI): Localized pain, change in bowel habits, blood in the stool, pain with defecation, dyschezia
- GU: Urinary frequency, dysuria, weak urinary stream, "dribbling," urinary frequency, nocturia, hematuria, rectal bleeding, rectal pain, anal itching
- Musculoskeletal: Back pain, myalgias
- Neurologic/psychiatric: Worry; sadness, helplessness, hopelessness; fatigue or insomnia; change in mood, stress, coping; healthy lifestyle behaviors

PREVENTIVE CARE CONSIDERATIONS
- Healthy lifestyle behaviors, including diet and exercise
- Condom use, STI prevention; fertility, infertility, or pregnancy prevention concerns
- Management of stress, coping with stressors
- Concerns or worries about health/wellness, reluctance to share
- Recent/needed health screenings

LIFE-SPAN AND POPULATION CONSIDERATIONS FOR HISTORY

Owing to the personal nature of discussions about sexual and reproductive health, there are populations who are vulnerable to disparities in care related to implicit or unconscious bias and/or related to reluctance to share information for fear of bias. Care should be taken to provide sensitive assessment and counseling for individuals with respect for gender identity and sexual orientation; please review the Script for Health History Assessment: Clinician Questions with Rationale and Considerations (**Exhibit 18.1**) in Chapter 18, Evidence-Based Assessment of Sexual Orientation, Gender Identity, and Health.

In addition, gender and ethnic disparities are significant related to men's health. Men have shorter life expectancy than women, despite having relative social and economic advantages; across the globe, women outlive men by an average of almost 6 years (Baker et al., 2014). According to the World Health Organization (WHO), this gender disparity reflects numerous factors, including greater levels of occupational exposure to physical and chemical hazards, behaviors associated with male norms of risk-taking, health behavior paradigms related to masculinity, and the detail that men are less likely to visit a clinician when they are ill, and when they do they are less likely to report symptoms of disease or illness (Baker et al., 2014). In addition, the health disparities experienced by African American men contribute to the overall decreased life expectancy of all men in the United States. Specifically, African American men have significantly higher morbidity and/or mortality rates associated with heart disease, diabetes, stroke, injuries, liver disease, mental and behavioral illnesses, and cancers, including prostate cancer (Noonan, Velasco-Mondragon, & Wagner, 2016).

When assessing personal and family health history, the evidence suggests that clinicians prioritize health and wellness screening related to environmental exposures, risk-taking, and concerns that men may be reluctant to discuss. Health promotion and disease prevention strategies to address social determinants of health are a priority.

PHYSICAL EXAMINATION OF MALE GENITALIA, PROSTATE, RECTUM, AND ANUS

Clinical examination of the adult male genitalia is not typically performed as part of routine male wellness examinations. However, a thorough examination should be performed for any individual presenting with a GU concern. Male GU conditions may be inflammatory, infectious, neoplastic, or traumatic in nature.

The clinician should maintain patient modesty by only exposing the male's groin and anogenital region as required. It is important to maintain a professional tone and avoid any joking, sarcasm, or inappropriate comments. The genital examination can be performed with the patient supine or sitting but the ideal approach is to have the patient stand with the clinician in a sitting position to best assess for hernia or testicular abnormalities. The anorectal examination can be performed with the male in a side-lying position with hips and knees flexed.

INSPECTION

The clinician should begin the examination by inspecting the inguinal area, pubic region, penis, and scrotum for lice/nits, and any signs of infection or disease, including ulcers, papules, pustules, vesicles, abnormal soft tissue growths, condylomata, discoloration, or swelling. Note whether the penis is circumcised or uncircumcised. Retract the prepuce (foreskin) of the uncircumcised penis to inspect the glans and urethral meatus. **Figure 19.5** depicts the prepuce and glans. Gently compress the glans penis between the thumb and first finger to inspect for patency, inflammation, or urethral discharge. Following the genital examination, the clinician should inspect the anus for skin tags, fissures, hemorrhoids, or other skin lesions.

PALPATION

Palpate the shaft of the penis for nodules, plaques, or other soft tissue masses. The index or middle finger of the clinician's hand should be placed posteriorly while the thumb of the same hand is placed anteriorly. The testis should be gently palpated for nodules, hard masses, or abnormal shape. A normal testis should feel smooth, ovoid, and nontender. Continue by palpating

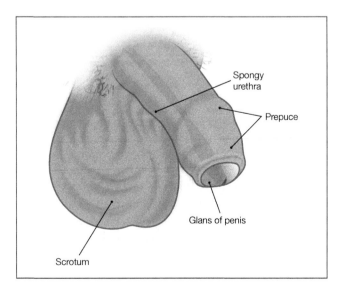

FIGURE 19.5 Prepuce and glans.

the epididymis along the posterior aspect of the testis and up along the spermatic cord (**Figure 19.6**). Clinicians should also note any swelling or soft tissue masses within the scrotal sac, epididymis, or spermatic cord. It is important to additionally palpate the inguinal nodes for enlargement and/or tenderness, especially when evaluating for concern of infection or malignancy of the genitalia.

Cremasteric Reflex

The clinician can attempt to elicit the cremasteric reflex when evaluating for certain testicular concerns that cause scrotal pain. Stroking the inner thigh with the index and middle finger should trigger the reflex. An intact reflex will cause the ipsilateral cremaster muscle to contract, thereby raising the testis. In some conditions, like testicular torsion, the cremasteric reflex will be negative because the cremaster muscles surrounding the spermatic cord are twisted and unable to contract. The absence of the cremasteric reflex for individuals presenting with scrotal pain is a useful sign. Ultrasound is recommended to confirm diagnosis of testicular torsion; further information is included in the Imaging Considerations for Male Genitalia, Prostate, Rectum, and Anus and Common Abnormalities of the Male Genitalia, Prostate, Rectum, and Anus sections of this chapter.

Transillumination

Transillumination is a technique for evaluating the scrotal sac for certain concerns such as scrotal swelling.

Perform the procedure by dimming the lights of the exam room and shining a bright light (e.g., penlight, otoscope, flashlight) through the wall of the scrotum. Fluid will illuminate; soft tissue masses will not.

Assessment of Hernias

A **hernia** is a protrusion of a body organ through the wall of the cavity that contains it. Abdominal hernias develop as a result of a weakening or defect in the abdominal wall allowing for an abnormal protrusion of a peritoneal-lined sac of abdominal contents (usually bowel). Abdominal wall hernias are classified by location (**Figure 19.7**):

- Ventral hernias: Epigastric, umbilical, spigelian (through fascia and musculature)
- Groin hernias: Obturator, femoral (direct inguinal), inguinal (indirect inguinal)

Abdominal wall hernias occur in approximately 2% of people. Inguinal hernias account for 75% of abdominal wall hernias requiring surgery with a lifetime risk of 27% in men (Kingsnorth & LeBlanc, 2003).

A patient history of pain, swelling, and/or presence of a mass in the groin area should raise concern for inguinal hernia. Symptoms worsen with increased abdominal pressure (coughing, sneezing, straining). In infants, the only symptom may be a caregiver concern of intermittent swelling or bulging in the groin with crying or straining. An inguinal hernia occurs when there is a

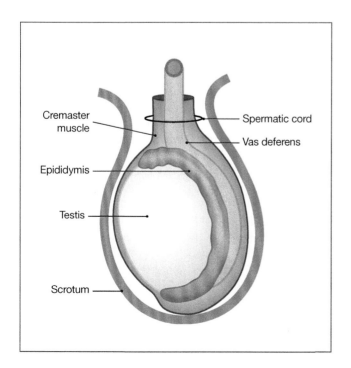

FIGURE 19.6 Scrotal anatomy.

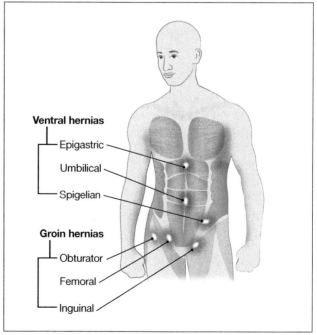

FIGURE 19.7 Location of abdominal wall hernias.

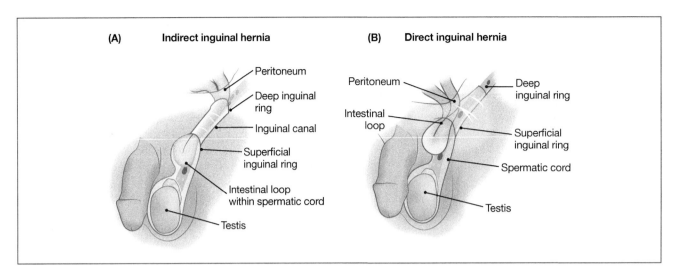

FIGURE 19.8 Inguinal hernias. (A) Indirect. (B) Direct.

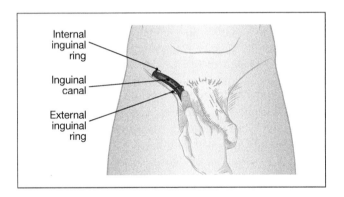

FIGURE 19.9 Technique for assessing inguinal hernias.

fascial defect in the inguinal canal that allows bowel to protrude through the deep inguinal ring and sometimes through the superficial inguinal ring into the scrotum (**Figure 19.8**). When bowel protrudes through the deep inguinal ring and becomes entrapped, it is considered an "incarcerated inguinal hernia." If the bowel cannot be reduced (pushed back into the abdominal cavity), emergent surgery is required to preserve viability of the bowel. A femoral hernia, or direct inguinal hernia, enters the inguinal canal via a defect inferior to the deep inguinal ring.

The examination for inguinal hernia should be performed with the patient in a standing position and the clinician in a seated position facing the patient. With a gloved index or middle finger, gather loose skin from the scrotum and invaginate the scrotal sac with the finger upward along the inguinal canal until the external ring is reached (**Figure 19.9**). Ask the patient to cough or bear down as when making a bowel movement. If a hernia is present, a bulging sensation can be palpated or felt at the tip of the finger. While the patient bears

down, also observe the inguinal area for bulging over the femoral canal that can indicate a femoral hernia.

Digital Rectal Examination

A **digital rectal examination** (DRE) can be performed to evaluate the lower rectum and prostate. A DRE is typically performed for presenting concerns of unexplained blood in the stool, an abnormal mass in the anus or rectum, a significant change in bowel or bladder habits, change in urinary stream, and/or urethral discharge or bleeding. Otherwise, DRE is not performed as a routine element of male wellness examinations.

For this examination, the individual should be unclothed from the waist down and in a gown and/or covered with a drape. Ideal positioning for the examination is either with the male standing with a forward bend at the waist or side-lying with knees to chest. Separate the buttocks and inspect for fissures, hemorrhoids, bleeding, skin tags, and rashes. Lubricate the index or middle finger of a gloved hand. The clinician should inform the patient that a finger will be inserted into the rectum. Ask the patient to take a deep breath, and relax and breathe out while gently inserting the examining finger into the anal canal. Palpate the prostate anteriorly, noting size, symmetry, and texture. A normal prostate is walnut-sized, symmetrical, and smooth with a cartilaginous texture (similar to the tip of the nose). The prostate has a midline groove (sulcus) that should be palpable. The proximity of the prostate to the rectum during a DRE is depicted in **Figure 19.10**.

Rotate the finger 360° to palpate the span of the rectal wall for masses or irregularities. Stool may be palpated in the rectal vault. Note the consistency (hard or soft). Assess anal tone by asking the patient to tighten their anal sphincter on the finger. Once the patient relaxes, withdraw the finger and inspect for blood, stool, or mucus. Redrape the patient, provide tissues or cleansing

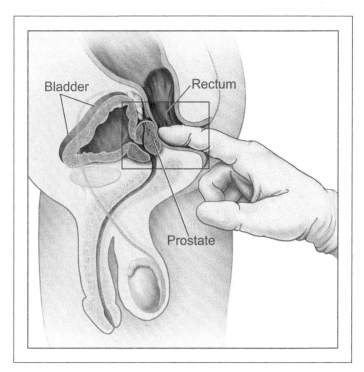

FIGURE 19.10 Digital rectal examination, including examination of the prostate.

Source: U.S. Department of Health and Human Services, National Institutes of Health, and the National Cancer Institute.

cloths, and allow privacy so the patient can clean up and get dressed.

PEDIATRIC AND ADOLESCENT CONSIDERATIONS FOR PHYSICAL EXAMINATION

The anogenital examination of the infant or child should be performed with a caregiver present. If the caregiver is unable to be present, a chaperone should be present. Ideally, the chaperone should be another healthcare clinician. The American Academy of Pediatrics (AAP) asserts that if an adolescent patient requires a physical examination of the genitalia, the use of a chaperone is recommended; however, this should be a shared decision between the clinician and the adolescent (Curry et al., 2011). Some states have mandatory chaperone laws so it is important for clinicians to be aware of their respective state laws. A chaperone can be a caregiver or another healthcare clinician, but this should be the adolescent's choice.

Routine GU examinations should be performed during all infant and child wellness examinations. Inspect the skin of the groin, pubis, penis, scrotum, and perineum for rashes, lesions, discoloration, or swelling (**Figure 19.11**). The clinician should gently retract the foreskin to visualize the urethral meatus. The foreskin of uncircumcised newborns and young infants may be tightly adhered to the glans penis and should never be forcefully retracted. The newborn examination, in particular, should include inspection for congenital malformations, ambiguous genitalia, and placement and patency of the anus.

The clinician should palpate the scrotal sac for soft tissue masses and to ensure that both testes have descended and can be brought down into the lower third of the scrotal sac. If the testis cannot be palpated in the scrotum, the clinician should palpate the inguinal canal and upper scrotal sac for the testis. Some testes are "retractile," meaning they can move between the inguinal canal and scrotum. A retractile testis can be located and brought down into the lower third of the scrotum. Retractile testes should resolve by puberty.

For adolescents, the genital examination can produce anxiety. Adolescence is the transition from childhood to adulthood. Growth and development is rapid. Adolescents can be unsure whether their developing bodies are "normal" and they have a greater need for modesty and privacy during sensitive examinations. It is important to reassure the adolescent male when physical examination findings are normal. Assessment of the adolescent genitalia is similar to the adult, except the clinician should assess for sexual maturity, or Tanner staging, while inspecting the genitalia.

The sexual maturity rating for preadolescent and adolescent males uses a scale from 1 (prepubertal) to 5 (adult-like), based on changes in pubic hair distribution and growth of the penis and testes. The Tanner stages are as follows:

1. Testes are more than 2.5 cm, no change in penis size, no pubic hair
2. Enlargement of testes, pigmentation of scrotal sac; no change in penis size; pubic hair is long, downy, and variable in pattern

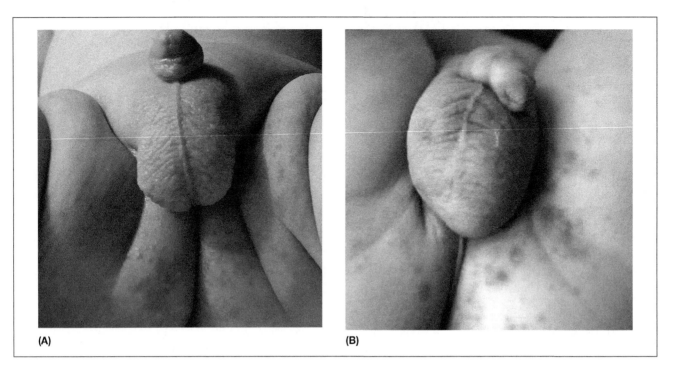

(A) **(B)**

FIGURE 19.11 Infant genitalia examination. (A) Circumcised penis. (B) Uncircumcised penis.

3. Further enlargement of testes; significant enlargement of penis, especially in diameter; increase in amount and curling of pubic hair
4. Further enlargement of testes and penis, pubic hair is adult in type but not distribution, development of axillary and facial hair begins
5. Testes and penis are adult in size, pubic hair is adult in distribution, body hair continues to grow; overall growth (height/weight/muscle) velocity peaks

LABORATORY CONSIDERATIONS FOR MALE GENITALIA, PROSTATE, RECTUM, AND ANUS

SCREENING FOR SEXUALLY TRANSMITTED INFECTIONS

- HIV screening can be performed as a rapid, point-of-care test with a cheek swab or finger prick for blood. Ideally, diagnostic testing is conducted via a venous blood draw for a combination antigen/antibody immunoassay.
- The following STIs require a venous blood draw for testing: (a) syphilis: nontreponemal testing (rapid plasma reagin [RPR], venereal disease research laboratory [VDRL]) is first line for testing and is reported as a titer. Treponemal testing (antibody testing) is complex, expensive, and typically performed as a confirmatory test when the nontreponemal test is reactive; (b) hepatitis B virus (HBV): laboratory test

includes surface antigen (HBsAg), surface antibody (HBsAb), and core antibody (HBcAb); and (c) hepatitis C virus testing is available for hepatitis C virus antibody.
- Nucleic acid amplification testing (NAAT) can be performed on urine for gonorrhea (*Neisseria gonorrhea*) and chlamydia (*Chlamydia trachomatis*). NAAT can also be performed on self- or clinician-collected rectal swabs (gonorrhea and chlamydia) or pharyngeal swabs (gonorrhea) if infection is possible based on sexual history. Urine NAAT for gonorrhea and chlamydia is less expensive, more time effective, highly sensitive and specific, and preferable to a urethral swab for most men. However, a swab for microbiologic culture remains an important diagnostic clinical approach when antibiotic resistance is a concern. Specimen collection is depicted in **Figure 19.12**.
- Herpes simplex virus (HSV) and human papillomavirus (HPV) condylomata lesions can typically be diagnosed clinically following the history and physical examination. If the diagnosis is not clear or confirmation is needed, the clinician can evaluate for HSV by culture or polymer chain reaction (PCR) testing. To obtain a viral swab, remove the top of a vesicular lesion and swab the vesicular fluid. If no vesicles are present, the clinician can swab an ulcerative lesion, but this will be more painful.
- There are insufficient data regarding the evolution of anal dysplasia from HPV. In addition, there is a lack of evidence regarding the efficacy of anal Pap smears

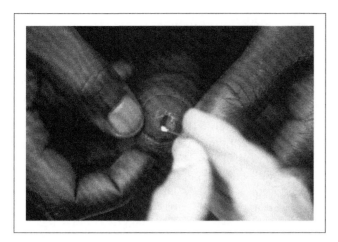

FIGURE 19.12 Collection of specimen for sexually transmitted infection testing.

Source: Centers of Disease Control and Prevention/Susan Lindsley.

and subsequent interventions for the prevention of anal cancer. These data would be needed to provide recommendations for the use of anal Pap screening in individuals (men who have sex with men [MSM] and women who have engaged in anal sex). It is not known whether treating the high-grade disease prevents anal cancer (Centers for Disease Control and Prevention, n.d.).

TESTING FOR PROSTATE-SPECIFIC ANTIGEN

Prostate-specific antigen (PSA) is a protein produced by the prostate gland. PSA is typically found in the semen, with minimal levels in blood or systemic circulation. PSA testing is primarily performed to screen for prostate cancer. Malignancy of the prostate gland can cause elevated PSA levels. However, other conditions can also elevate prostate levels like BPH (enlarged prostate) or prostatitis (inflamed prostate). PSA levels also normally increase with age. Elevated PSA levels often lead to prostate biopsy, which has associated risks.

Of every 1,000 men offered PSA screening, 1 to 2 men will avoid death due to prostate cancer, while 60 men will experience serious complications as a result of the screening, such as urinary incontinence and erectile dysfunction (U.S. Preventive Services Task Force [USPSTF], 2019). A substantial number of men who opt for PSA screening receive false-positive results leading to biopsy, while some men with prostate cancer actually have normal PSA levels. An estimated 20% to 40% of men who received prostate cancer treatment following PSA testing did not in fact have the type of tumors that would have caused symptoms in their lifetime. For these reasons, PSA screening for

prostate cancer should only be performed if an individual expresses interest in testing following a discussion regarding individualized risks and benefits with a knowledgeable clinician. Treatment decisions involve repeated PSA testing to determine if PSA levels are persistently elevated.

IMAGING CONSIDERATIONS FOR MALE GENITALIA, PROSTATE, RECTUM, AND ANUS

ULTRASOUND

Scrotal ultrasound is the initial imaging study of choice for evaluating acute, urgent testicular concerns. While male GU emergencies are uncommon, emergent diagnosis is needed to preserve the structure and function of the male genitalia. Presenting signs and symptoms that necessitate an emergent scrotal ultrasound include acute testicular pain and swelling. Emergent conditions may be infectious, traumatic, or vascular in nature.

Testicular torsion is the primary condition that should prompt a time-sensitive ultrasound. Clinicians should refer to the emergency department, if necessary. If testicular torsion is suspected but scrotal ultrasound is unavailable, surgical exploration is advised. Torsion of the testis can result in testicular ischemia and death within 6 to 12 hours.

Other testicular diagnoses that may prompt concern include torsion of the testicular appendix, hydrocele, epididymitis, orchitis, and testicular cancer. These conditions may result in loss of blood flow and subsequent tissue necrosis, or become at risk for abscess and gangrene. Urgent or emergent scrotal ultrasound is indicated, especially if there is any doubt in the diagnosis.

EVIDENCE-BASED PRACTICE CONSIDERATIONS FOR MALE GENITALIA, PROSTATE, RECTUM, AND ANUS

- Evidence-based practice considerations that address colorectal health are covered in Chapter 16, Evidence-Based Assessment of the Abdomen, Gastrointestinal, and Urologic Systems.
- Recommendations for prevention and immunization for HPV, STI prevention and screening, HIV screening, and pregnancy prevention are covered in Chapter 20, Evidence-Based Assessment of the Female Genitourinary System; these evidence-based guidelines are applicable for men and women.

TESTICULAR CANCER SCREENING

- The USPSTF (2016) does not recommend routine clinician or self-testicular examinations for testicular cancer screening in asymptomatic males of any age. Screening by a clinician or a self-examination is not likely to yield significant health benefits given the low incidence (5.4 cases per 100,000 males) and high cure rate even in cases of advanced disease. There is insufficient evidence that these examinations reduce mortality or improve outcomes. While periodic clinician or self-testicular examination may lead to detection of malignancy before it causes noticeable symptoms, there are no studies on the sensitivity or specificity of these examinations, so the benefit is unknown.
- The American Cancer Society (ACS, 2018) advises men to consider doing a monthly self-testicular examination if certain risk factors are present, such as a history of cryptorchidism or personal or family history of testicular cancer.

PROSTATE CANCER SCREENING

- The USPSTF (2019) recommends against screening for prostate cancer in men aged 70 and older.
- For men aged 55 to 69 years, the decision to screen for prostate cancer should be an individual one (USPSTF, 2019). While there is a small potential benefit in reducing mortality from prostate cancer in some men, the potential harms of routine screening include false-positive results that result in further testing, possible prostate biopsy, and overdiagnosis and treatment which can lead to complications like urinary and erectile dysfunction. Following a discussion of individualized risks and benefits, PSA-based screening should only be performed for men who express a desire in screening.
- The ACS (2016) advises men to make an informed decision whether to undergo PSA-based screening for prostate cancer following a conversation with the healthcare clinician about their individual risks and benefits. The conversation should occur at age 50 for men who are at average risk; at age 45 for men at higher risk, including African Americans, and men with a first-degree relative with a history of prostate cancer at a young age (<65 years old); and at age 40 for men with more than one first-degree relative with a history of early prostate cancer. In addition to PSA-based screening, a DRE may also be performed. If no prostate cancer is found as a result of screening, the time between future screenings depends on the results of the PSA blood test:
  - Men who choose to be tested, who have a PSA of less than 2.5 ng/mL, may only need to be retested every 2 years.
  - Screening should be done yearly for men whose PSA level is 2.5 ng/mL or higher.

COMMON ABNORMALITIES OF THE MALE GENITALIA, PROSTATE, RECTUM, AND ANUS

CONGENITAL OR DEVELOPMENTAL ABNORMALITIES

Epispadias and Hypospadias

Hypospadias is a congenital malformation of the male GU tract in which the urethral opening is abnormally located on the ventral aspect of the penis (**Figure 19.13**). The condition varies in severity, as the urethral meatus may be located on the glans, penile shaft, scrotum, or perineum. Similarly, but less commonly, epispadias is an abnormal dorsal placement of the urethral meatus (**Figure 19.14**). These conditions require surgical correction.

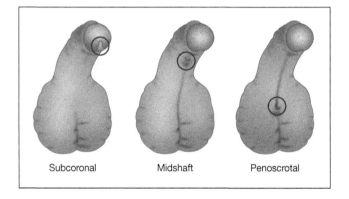

Subcoronal   Midshaft   Penoscrotal

FIGURE 19.13 Hypospadias.

Source: Centers for Disease Control and Prevention, National Center for Birth Defects and Developmental Disabilities.

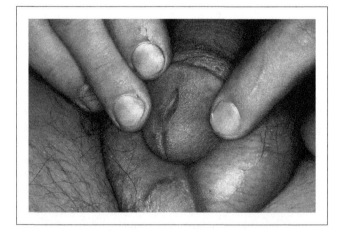

FIGURE 19.14 Epispadias.

Source: Centers for Disease Control and Prevention/Gavin Hart, MD.

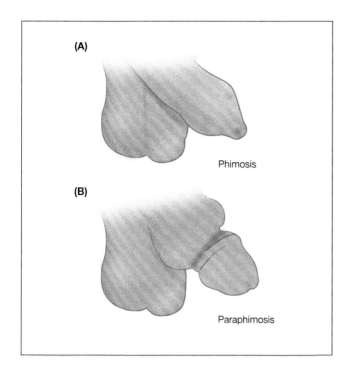

FIGURE 19.15 Phimosis (A) and paraphimosis (B).

Phimosis and Paraphimosis

Phimosis is a condition in which the foreskin of an un-circumcised penis cannot be retracted over the glans. This condition can be physiologic or pathologic. Physiologic phimosis occurs in almost all newborn males due to naturally occurring adhesions between the foreskin and glans penis during fetal development. The adhesions spontaneously resolve over time with intermittent erections and foreskin retraction. Physiologic phimosis is expected to resolve prior to puberty, but usually by age 3. Key findings of physiologic phimosis can vary from an inability to retract the foreskin far enough to view the urethral meatus to an inability to retract the foreskin fully past the corona of the glans penis (**Figure 19.15A**).

Pathological phimosis is acquired as a result of distal scarring of the prepuce due to infection or inflammation. The key finding is a contracted fibrous ring around the opening of the distal prepuce with an inability to retract the foreskin. Pathological phimosis requires medical treatment.

Paraphimosis is a condition that results from forcefully retracting tight foreskin back over the glans penis. The foreskin becomes entrapped behind the corona of the glans. Key signs and symptoms include painful swelling of the distal glans penis with a constricted band of tissue proximal to the corona (**Figure 19.15B**). Paraphimosis is a medical emergency because it will eventually result in tissue ischemia and necrosis.

Undescended Testes

An undescended testis fails to descend into the lower third of the scrotum by 4 months of age. The testis may be located in the intra-abdominal space (cryptorchidism), the inguinal canal, or the upper third of the scrotum (**Figure 19.16**). There is no advantage to clinical observation of an undescended testis longer than 12 months of age. Surgical correction is required prior to puberty to preserve fertility and decrease the risk of testicular cancer.

Hydrocele

A communicating **hydrocele** is a collection of peritoneal fluid in the scrotal sac that results from a fascial defect in the inguinal canal (**Figure 19.17**). All males have this defect at some point during gestation, but when it persists, it allows peritoneal fluid to travel back and forth. This can be normal up to age 1 to 2 years.

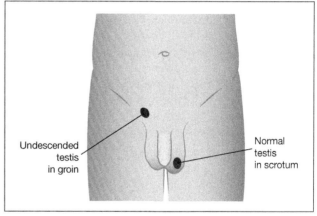

FIGURE 19.16 Undescended testicle and normal testicle.

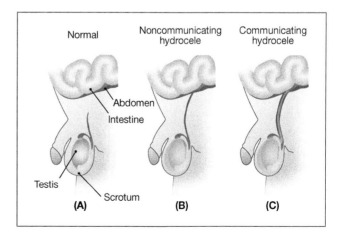

FIGURE 19.17 Hydrocele. (A) Normal scrotum. (B) Noncommunicating hydrocele. (C) Communicating hydrocele.

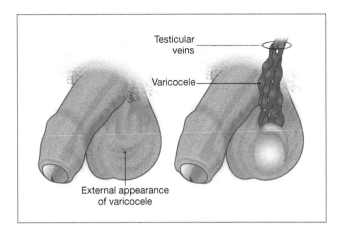

FIGURE 19.18 Varicocele.

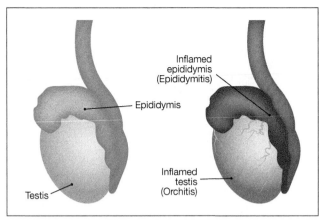

FIGURE 19.19 Epididymitis and orchitis.

When the defect is large enough to admit bowel tissue, an inguinal hernia can result. Key signs and symptoms of a hydrocele include painless scrotal swelling (unilateral or bilateral) that may fluctuate in size. Transillumination of the scrotum can be helpful for diagnosis. Peritoneal fluid will illuminate in the scrotal sac, while bowel tissue will not. Communicating hydroceles that persist beyond age 1 to 2 years require surgical correction. In older children and adults, a noncommunicating hydrocele can be idiopathic or develop secondary to infection, inflammation, trauma, or malignancy. Primary causes must be ruled out.

Varicocele

A **varicocele** is a collection of dilated twisted veins surrounding the spermatic cord that typically occurs in the left hemiscrotum. Key signs and symptoms include a soft mass with a "bag of worms" texture and appearance that worsens with increased venous pressure as with standing or performing the Valsalva maneuver (**Figure 19.18**). Most cases are asymptomatic, but some will present with a dull ache in the left scrotum. A varicocele usually does not require intervention unless there is atrophy of the testicle, which can lead to infertility.

Epididymitis, Orchitis, and Scrotal Cellulitis

Acute epididymitis is a clinical syndrome involving pain, swelling, and inflammation of the epididymis that can last up to 6 weeks. When the testis is also affected, it is referred to as epididymo-orchitis (**Figure 19.19**). Epididymitis typically occurs secondary to infection but can also be a result of trauma or autoimmune disease. Infectious etiology is most likely a result of UTI in children or an STI in adolescents and adults.

Cellulitis of the scrotum is an infection of the dermis of the scrotal tissue, which occurs from bacterial

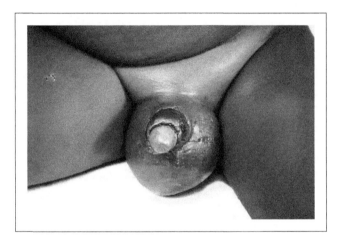

FIGURE 19.20 Scrotal cellulitis.
Source: Centers for Disease Control and Prevention/Robert S. Craig.

entry via a break in the integrity of the epidermal barrier. Scrotal cellulitis presents with scrotal pain, swelling, and inflammation (**Figure 19.20**). Urgent medical treatment is required to prevent an abscess or gangrene.

Testicular Torsion

Testicular torsion can result from a failure of the testis/epididymis to affix posteriorly inside the scrotum, allowing the testis to twist on the spermatic cord (**Figure 19.21**). Torsion of the testis can result in testicular ischemia and death within 6 to 12 hours. Emergency surgery is required to preserve the viability of the testicle. Key signs and symptoms include acute onset of testicular pain and swelling, a transverse testicular lie, and a negative cremasteric reflex. Testicular ultrasound with a perfusion scan can be critical for timely diagnosis.

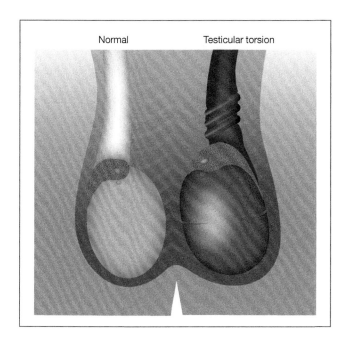

FIGURE 19.21 Testicular torsion.

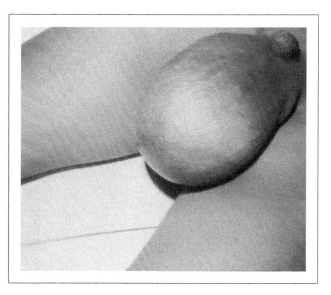

FIGURE 19.22 Testicular tumor.
Source: Centers for Disease Control and Prevention/Mr. Gust.

The appendix testis is a small embryologic remnant found on the anterosuperior aspect of the testis that is approximately 3 mm in length. Torsion of the testicular appendix can present with acute onset of mild-to-severe testicular pain. Other key signs and symptoms include localized tenderness to the superior or inferior pole of the testis, reactive hydrocele, normal vertical testicular lie, and intact cremasteric reflex. Blood flow to the testis is normal and management is supportive.

Testicular Tumor/Malignancy

A normal testis is smooth, ovoid, and freely mobile. Any solid, firm mass, or fixed area within the testis should be evaluated for malignancy (**Figure 19.22**). A scrotal ultrasound is indicated for any suspicious testicular mass. Males with a history of cryptorchidism are particularly at an increased risk for testicular cancer; the average age at time of diagnosis is 33 years (ACS, 2018). Testicular cancer is not uncommon; 1 in approximately 250 males will develop a testicular malignancy in their lifetime; however, testicular cancer can be treated successfully (ACS, 2018).

Anorectal Agenesis/Imperforate Anus

Anorectal agenesis, or imperforate anus, is a congenital anorectal malformation in which there is an absence of or abnormal location of the anal opening (**Figure 19.23**). An imperforate anus is not always readily evident on examination. The key finding is failure of the newborn to pass meconium within the first 24 to 48 hours following birth. Imperforate anus can be a

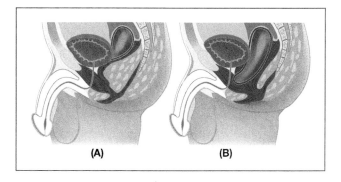

FIGURE 19.23 Anorectal agenesis/imperforate anus.
(A) Imperforate anus with rectovesical fistula.
(B) Imperforate anus without fistula.

solitary finding or part of a cluster of findings of a more complex congenital syndrome. Surgical correction is required.

INFECTION OR INFLAMMATORY DISORDERS
Balanitis and Balanoposthitis

Balanitis describes an inflammation of the glans penis, while balanoposthitis describes an inflammation of the glans penis and foreskin in uncircumcised males (**Figure 19.24**). Key signs and symptoms can include genital itching, pain, dysuria, exudate, erythema, swelling of glans or the foreskin, foul odor, and phimosis. Causes include poor hygiene and infectious agents like STIs and other bacterial, fungal, and viral organisms.

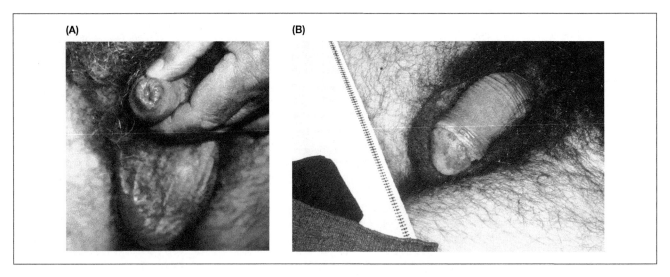

FIGURE 19.24 Balanoposthitis. (A) Diabetic balanoposthitis. (B) Hemorrhagic balanoposthitis.
Source: (A) Centers for Disease Control and Prevention/Brian Hill. (B) Centers for Disease Control and Prevention/NJ Fiumara, MD.

Male Genital Candidiasis

Candidiasis is a fungal infection caused by yeast. Key signs and symptoms include a painful, itchy, erythematous, and potentially fissured rash (**Figure 19.25**). A white, curd-like exudate is possible, especially in uncircumcised males. Candida infections can affect the glans, foreskin, scrotum, thighs, gluteal folds, and buttocks. This condition is more common among men with diabetes, uncircumcised males, and males with female sex partners with recurrent vaginal yeast infections.

Nonspecific Urethritis

Urethritis describes an inflammation of the urethra. Urethritis can be caused by a UTI or chemical irritants, but is often a common indicator of STIs among males. In particular, urethritis with purulent penile discharge is often associated with chlamydia and/or gonorrhea. Key signs and symptoms include dysuria, itching, burning, and/or discharge at the urethral meatus (**Figure 19.26**). Infectious organisms should be investigated first.

Sexually Transmitted Infections

Gonorrhea and chlamydia are the most common STIs in male adolescents and adults. Though these infections can be asymptomatic, the most common signs and symptoms include urethritis and/or urethral discharge. Other common STIs in men can present with dermatologic findings, including scabies (inflamed, erosive papules; **Figure 19.27**), HPV (condyloma; **Figure 19.28**), genital herpes (vesicles/ulcers; **Figure 19.29**), syphilis (chancre; **Figure 19.30**), and chancroid (**Figure 19.31**).

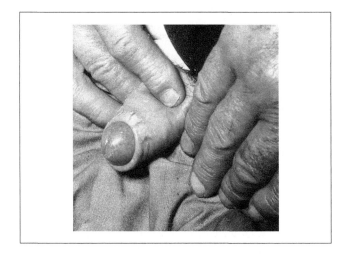

FIGURE 19.25 Male genital candidiasis.
Source: Centers for Disease Control and Prevention/Brian Hill.

OTHER ABNORMALITIES OF MALE GENITALIA

Manifestations of Systemic Conditions

Systemic conditions can cause dermatologic symptoms in the male genitalia. In particular, reactive arthritis can manifest in part as vesicles and crusted plaques on the penis (**Figure 19.32**). Chronic, generalized pruritus and dermatologic changes can signify an underlying systemic disease; disorders such as connective tissue disease, lichen planus, seborrheic dermatitis, lichen sclerosus, atopic dermatitis, and psoriasis cause cutaneous findings.

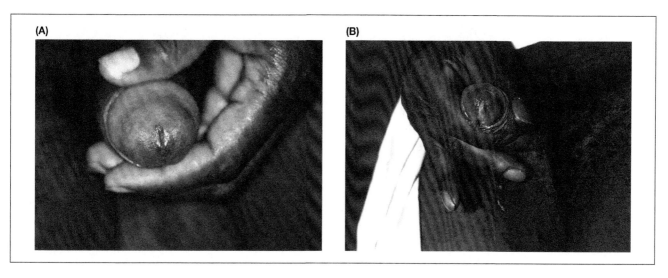

FIGURE 19.26 Nonspecific urethritis. (A) Urethritis with mucoid discharge. (B) Urethritis with purulent discharge.

Source: (A) Centers for Disease Control and Prevention/Jim Pledger. (B) Centers for Disease Control and Prevention/Renelle Woodall.

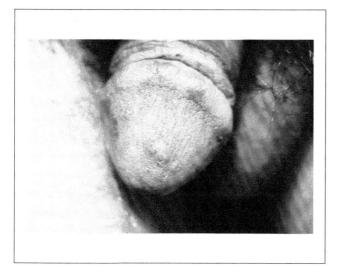

FIGURE 19.27 Scabies. Note the presence of erosive, inflamed lesions on the glans penis and preputial skin.

Source: Centers for Disease Control and Prevention/Gavin Hart, MD.

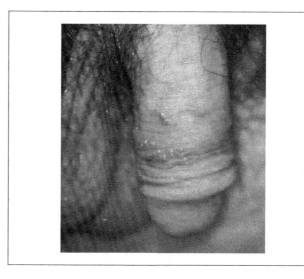

FIGURE 19.28 Condyloma. Note the presence of soft, wart-like growths about the penile shaft, known as condylomata acuminate or anogenital warts.

Source: Centers for Disease Control and Prevention/MF Rein, MD.

Peyronie's Disease

Peyronie's disease is an acquired condition resulting in penile deformity, mass, pain, and possible erectile dysfunction. The etiology is unknown but likely multifactorial. The primary finding is dorsal fibrous plaques that alter penile anatomy and can impair function (**Figure 19.33**). It is thought to be a result of the postinflammatory healing process. Risk factors include genital injuries, urethral instrumentation, and prostatectomy. Key signs and symptoms include penile pain, nodules, penile curvature, or deformity along with erectile penile shortening and sexual dysfunction.

Skin Cancer

The first sign of penile cancer is often a change in the skin of the foreskin, glans penis, or penile shaft. Key signs and symptoms may include thickening of skin, changes in skin color, ulcers, or well-defined, velvety red plaques (**Figure 19.34**). Initial assessment and evaluation should be guided on the likelihood of whether

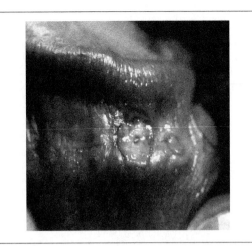

FIGURE 19.29 Genital herpes. Note the presence of vesicular lesions on the underside of the penile shaft, just proximal to the corona of the glans.

Source: Centers for Disease Control and Prevention/Susan Lindsley.

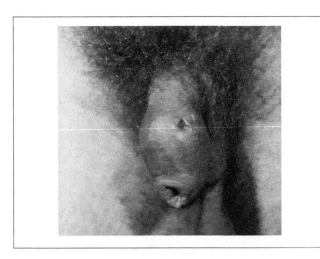

FIGURE 19.30 Syphilis. Note the presence of a penile chancre due to a primary syphilitic infection. The chancre is usually firm, round, small, and painless.

Source: Centers for Disease Control and Prevention/Susan Lindsley.

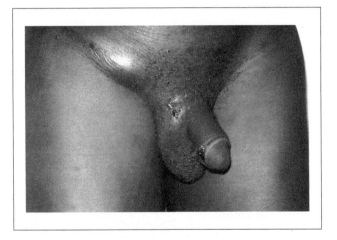

FIGURE 19.31 Chancroid. Note the presence of erosive, bleeding lesions on the distal penis and penile base caused by the Gram-negative bacterium *Haemophilus ducreyi*. Note that a lymph node in the right inguinal region had become swollen, as it drained the infected, ipsilateral region.

Source: Centers for Disease Control and Prevention/J. Pledger.

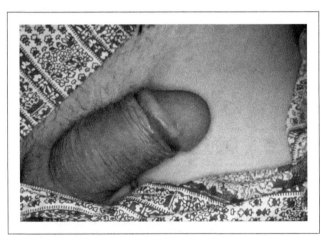

FIGURE 19.32 Manifestations of systemic conditions. Note the presence of a painless sore on the corona of the glans penis known as balanitis circinata, a form of keratoderma blennorrhagicum, due to reactive arthritis.

Source: Centers for Disease Control and Prevention/Susan Lindsley.

an infection or malignancy is more likely. While penile cancer is rare, 95% are squamous cell carcinomas.

ABNORMALITIES OF THE ANUS, RECTUM, AND PROSTATE

Anal Fissures

An anal fissure is a small tear in the mucosal lining of the anus. A fissure can be a result of constipation and straining during bowel movements or anal penetration

during sexual intercourse. Key signs and symptoms can include bleeding or pain with bowel movements and/or visible cracks in the skin around the anus (**Figure 19.35**).

External and Internal Hemorrhoids

Hemorrhoids are enlarged, bulging veins of the distal rectum and anus. Risk factors include family history of hemorrhoids, obesity, pregnancy, chronic constipation, and straining with bowel movements.

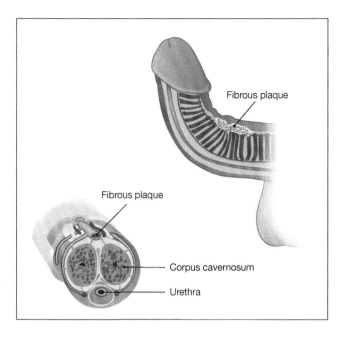

FIGURE 19.33 Peyronie's disease.

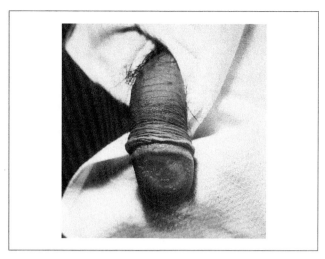

FIGURE 19.34 Skin cancer. The erythematous patch on this patient's glans penis was diagnosed as a case of Bowen's disease, or squamous cell carcinoma in situ.

Source: Centers for Disease Control and Prevention/Susan Lindsley.

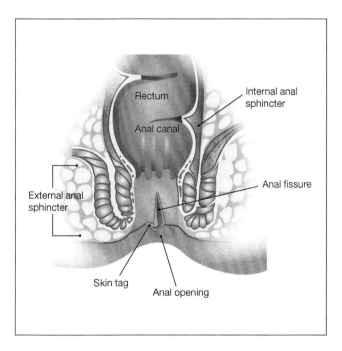

FIGURE 19.35 Anal fissures.

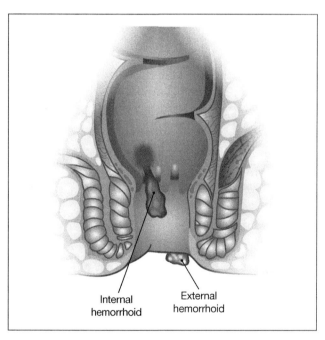

FIGURE 19.36 External and internal hemorrhoids.

Internal hemorrhoids are located in the distal rectum. External hemorrhoids are located within the anus (**Figure 19.36**). Key signs and symptoms include painless, bright red bleeding with bowel movements, anal itching, acute onset of perianal pain (thrombosed hemorrhoid), and/or fecal soiling. Hemorrhoids may prolapse outside the anal sphincter.

Benign Prostatic Hyperplasia

BPH is an enlargement of the prostate gland (**Figure 19.37**). This condition becomes more common as men age. Key signs and symptoms include uncomfortable urinary symptoms: urinary frequency, impaired flow, weak urine stream, nocturia, and/or urinary dribbling posturination.

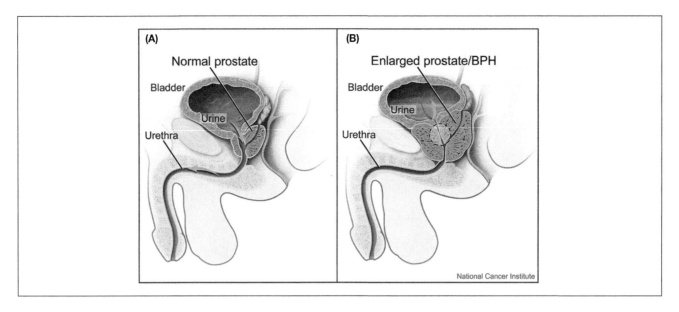

FIGURE 19.37 Benign prostatic hyperplasia (BPH). Flow of urine with a normal prostate (A) and with an enlarged prostate/BPH (B).

Source: National Cancer Institute.

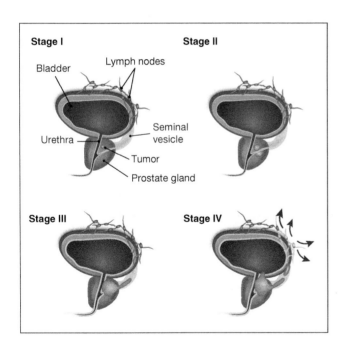

FIGURE 19.38 Stages of prostate cancer.

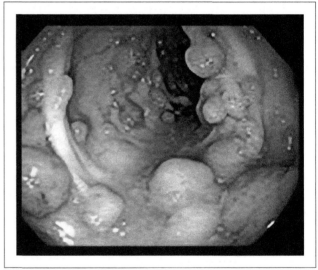

FIGURE 19.39 Rectal polyps.

Source: National Cancer Institute/Miguel Rodriguez-Bigas, MD.

Prostate Cancer

Cancer of the prostate gland is typically detected at an asymptomatic stage (**Figure 19.38**). Key signs of prostate cancer include abnormal finding of the prostate on DRE, that is, nodules or asymmetry, and/or elevated PSA levels. PSA is not specific for prostate cancer, however, and can be elevated in other conditions.

Abnormal DRE or urinary/rectal symptoms warrant further investigation.

Rectal Polyps and Rectal Cancer

Rectal polyps refer to a protrusion of the rectal mucosa into the lumen of the rectum (**Figure 19.39**). Polyps are usually asymptomatic but may ulcerate and bleed if they become enlarged and obstruct the colon. Polyps can be benign, inflammatory lesions or neoplastic lesions. Inflammatory polyps are an endoscopic physical finding of inflammatory bowel disease like Crohn's disease or ulcerative colitis. Neoplastic polyps are an endoscopic physical finding of rectal cancer.

CASE STUDY: Scrotal Pain

History

Luca is a 16-year-old male who presents to the emergency department with concerns of left-sided scrotal pain for the past 3 hours. The pain is constant and does not change with position. There is no history of recent trauma. He denies dysuria, fever, chills, nausea, or vomiting. He is sexually active with one female partner. He reports consistent condom use.

Physical Examination

On examination, Luca appears in moderate distress secondary to left scrotal pain. His heart rate is 110 beats/minute. He is afebrile and his blood pressure is 120/80 mmHg. The left hemiscrotum is edematous and erythematous. The left testis exhibits a transverse lie with marked tenderness to light palpation. Left cremasteric reflex is absent. Right hemiscrotum and testis are normal. Normal circumcised penis with no urethral discharge.

Differential Diagnoses

Differential diagnoses include testicular torsion, torsion of the testicular appendix, epididymitis/orchitis, hernia and/or hydrocele, and varicocele.

Laboratory and Imaging

Testicular ultrasound and perfusion scan demonstrate absence of blood flow to the left testis and epididymis. Normal blood flow to the right testis is present. No testicular masses were noted. Complete blood count (CBC) and urinalysis (UA) were normal. Urine NAAT is negative for gonorrhea and chlamydia.

Final Diagnosis

Testicular torsion requiring emergent surgical intervention

Clinical Pearls

- As part of a well visit, the clinician assesses for normal functioning of male GU and reproductive systems, health maintenance, and health promotion needs.
- During an episodic visit, the clinician focuses on specific concerns. A thorough examination is done for any individual presenting with a GU concern.
- Clinical examination of the adult male genitalia is not typically done as part of routine wellness examinations. However, GU examinations should be performed during *all* infant and child wellness examinations.
- The anogenital examination of the infant or child should be performed with a caregiver present.

Key Takeaways

- Male GU and anogenital conditions may be inflammatory, infectious, neoplastic, or traumatic in nature.
- Sudden onset of severe testicular pain must be considered testicular torsion until proven otherwise.
- Evidence-based recommendations for prostate cancer screening indicate the need for patient-centered, shared decision-making.

REFERENCES

American Cancer Society. (2016). American Cancer Society recommendations for prostate cancer early detection. Retrieved from https://www.cancer.org/cancer/prostate -cancer/early-detection/acs-recommendations.html

American Cancer Society. (2018). Can testicular cancer be found early? Retrieved from https://www.cancer.org/cancer/ testicular-cancer/detection-diagnosis-staging/detection .html

Baker, P., Dworkin, S. L., Tong, S., Banks, I., Shand, T., & Yamey, G. (2014). The men's health gap: Men must be included in the global health equity agenda. *Bulletin of the World Health Organization, 92*(8), 618–620. doi:10.2471/ BLT.13.132795

Centers for Disease Control and Prevention. (n.d.). *Screening/questions and answers/2015 STD treatment guidelines.* Retrieved from https://www.cdc.gov/std/tg2015/qa/ screening-qa.htm

Curry, E., Hammer, L., Brown, O., Laughlin, J., Lessin, H., Simon, G., & Rodger, C. (2011). Policy statement: Use of chaperones during the physical examination of the pediatric patient. *Pediatrics, 127*(5), 991–993. doi:10.1542/ peds.2011-0322

Dean, R. C., & Lue, T. F. (2005). Physiology of penile erection and pathophysiology of erectile dysfunction. *Urologic Clinics of North America, 32*(4), 379–395. doi:10.1016/j. ucl.2005.08.007

Dyer, R. (2016). The male genital tract. In R. J. Zagoria, R. Dyer, & C. Brady (Eds.) *Genitourinary imaging: The requisites* (3rd ed., pp. 304–336). Philadelphia, PA: Elsevier. FIGURE 19.1 Male pelvic organs.

Fine, S. W., & Reuter, V. E. (2012). Anatomy of the prostate revisited: Implications for prostate biopsy and zonal origins of prostate cancer. *Histopathology, 60*(1), 142–152. doi: 10.1111/j.1365-2559.2011.04004.x

Gratzke, C., Angulo, J., Chitaley, K., Dai, Y., Kim, N. N., Paick, J.-S., . . . Stief, C. G. (2010). Anatomy, physiology, and pathophysiology of erectile dysfunction. *Journal of Sexual Medicine, 7*(1 Pt. 2), 445–475. doi:10.1111/j.1743-6109.2009.01624.x

Kingsnorth, A., & LeBlanc, K. (2003). Hernias: Inguinal and incisional. *Lancet, 362*(9395), 1561–1571. doi:10.1016/ S0140-6736(03)14746-0

Noonan, A. S., Velasco-Mondragon, H. E., & Wagner, F. A. (2016). Improving the health of African Americans in the USA: An overdue opportunity for social justice. *Public Health Reviews, 37*, 12. doi:10.1186/s40985-016-0025-4

U.S. Preventive Services Task Force. (2016). Final recommendation statement: Testicular cancer: Screening. Retrieved from https://www.uspreventiveservicestaskforce.org/ Page/Document/RecommendationStatementFinal/ testicular-cancer-screening

U.S. Preventive Services Task Force. (2019). Final summary: Prostate cancer: Screening. Retrieved from https:// www.uspreventiveservicestaskforce.org/Page/Document/ UpdateSummaryFinal/prostate-cancer-screening1

20

Evidence-Based Assessment of the Female Genitourinary System

Sherry Bumpus and Amber Carriveau

"I am not afraid. … I was born to do this."

—JOAN OF ARC

 VIDEO

- Well Exam: Women's Health History and Gynecological Exam

LEARNING OBJECTIVES

- Describe the structures and functions of the female genitourinary (GU) system.
- Explain the relationship between the organs of the female GU system and the endocrine system.
- Discuss the menstrual cycle.
- Understand the key components of a comprehensive, evidence-based history and physical examination of the female GU system.
- Distinguish between normal and abnormal findings in the female GU system.

ANATOMY AND PHYSIOLOGY OF THE FEMALE GENITOURINARY SYSTEM

Knowledge of pelvic anatomy is the first step of the female GU examination. Normal and abnormal findings

Visit https://connect.springerpub.com/content/book/978-0-8261 -6454-4/chapter/ch00 to access the videos.

are easier to identify with a solid knowledge base of anatomy, which includes recognition of key landmarks and an understanding of the structure and function of the female GU system.

THE BONY PELVIS

The bony pelvis serves many functions. Bones of the pelvis provide a supportive cradle for pelvic structures, anchor connective tissue and muscle attachments, and form a bridge between the trunk and the lower extremities. The pelvis is the connection and point of articulation for the lower extremities. In females, the bony pelvis serves to accommodate the passage of the fetus during childbirth (King & Brucker, 2019).

Four bones make up the structure of the pelvis: the two hip bones (known as the innominate bones), the sacrum, and the coccyx. The innominate bones are composed of three parts: the ilium, the ischium, and the pubis. These three bones are joined at the acetabulum initially by cartilage, but by approximately 16 to 18 years of age they fuse together to form a single bony structure (Drake, Vogl, & Mitchell, 2015). **Figure 20.1** depicts the bony structures of the female pelvis from the anterior and lateral views.

The ilium forms the uppermost posterior portion of the pelvis. The uppermost ridge is called the iliac crest. It provides an attachment site for many muscular structures of the abdomen, back, and lower limbs (Drake et al., 2015). The ischium is located inferior to the ilium in the posterior pelvis. The ischial spine is a prominent bony structure arising from the posterior margin of the ischium (Drake et al., 2015). The ischial

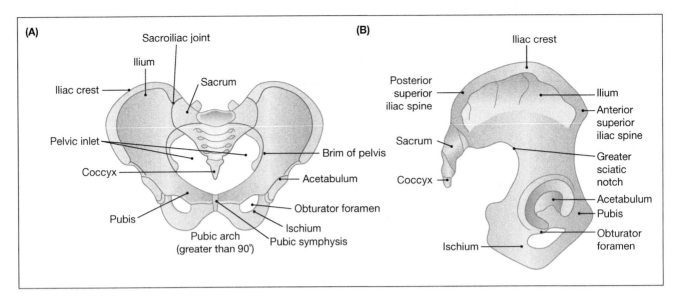

FIGURE 20.1 Female bony pelvis. (A) Anterior view. (B) Posterior view.

spines are a commonly used landmark to monitor fetal descent during childbirth (Hays & Clarks, 2017). The ischial tuberosity is the most prominent landmark and is located on the inferior aspect of the ischium. The ischial tuberosities serve as attachment sites for muscles of the lower extremities, as well as a support structure when sitting (Drake et al., 2015). The pubis is the most anterior portion of the bony pelvic structure. The pubic bones are joined by a fibrous cartilage and further supported by pubic ligaments (Drake et al., 2015). The pubic arch forms another pelvic landmark, which is bordered by the inferior portion of the pubic symphysis and the inferior pubic rami.

The posterior portion of the pelvis is shaped by the sacrum and coccyx. The concave shape of the sacrum is derived from the fusion of five sacral vertebrae. The sacral promontory is an important landmark and represents the anterior edge of the most superior vertebral body. The coccyx serves as a pelvic landmark and consists of four fused coccygeal vertebrae. It is located just inferior to the sacrum and is joined by the sacrococcygeal symphysis (Drake et al., 2015).

The *true pelvis* refers to the opening in the pelvis the fetus passes through during childbirth. It is composed of the pelvic inlet, the pelvic wall, and the pelvic outlet. The pelvic inlet is the opening from the abdomen into the pelvis. The pelvic wall consists of the sacrum and coccyx, along with the muscular and ligamentous structures supporting the lateral walls of the pelvis. The pelvic outlet describes the inferior portion of the bony pelvis and is composed of the inferior portion of the bony pelvic bones, along with the supporting ligaments.

Caldwell and Moloy (1933) developed a classification system to describe the four basic female pelvic shapes: gynecoid, android, anthropoid, and platypelloid. The features of the posterior portion of the pelvic inlet determine the pelvic shape. Further research has suggested that most female pelvic shapes do not adhere to one of the four Caldwell and Moloy classifications but are composed of a combination of them instead (Kolesova & Vetra, 2012).

The bony pelvis contains four joints: two sacroiliac (SI) joints, the pubic symphysis, and the sacrococcygeal symphysis. The SI joints are synovial joints that connect the ilium and the sacrum and redistribute forces from the lower limbs to the vertebral column. They are designed to allow only minimal movement and are supported by several ligaments. The pubic symphysis is a fibrocartilaginous joint connecting the anterior pubic bones and is supported by the superior and inferior pubic ligaments. The sacrococcygeal symphysis is a hinge joint that connects the distal portion of the sacrum to the coccyx, allowing for flexion and extension of the coccyx (King & Brucker, 2019).

PELVIC SUPPORT

Pelvic support is reliant on many ligaments, muscles, and connective tissues. These structures provide the framework for the pelvic floor and vaginal walls, support the organs of the abdomen and pelvis, assist with elimination and urination, preserve continence, and aid in the delivery of a fetus (King & Brucker, 2019).

The many muscles supporting the bony pelvis can be divided into two main groups: those that attach to the pelvis outside the pelvic cavity and those that attach inside the pelvis (Madadevan, 2018). The muscles located inside the pelvic cavity are found bilaterally and include the piriformis, obturator internus, coccygeus, and levator ani. The piriformis and the obturator internus originate in the pelvic cavity and form the lateral

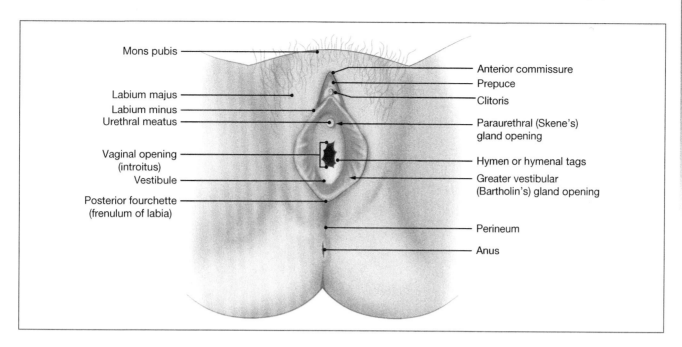

FIGURE 20.2 External female genitalia (vulva).

walls of the pelvis. Both exit the pelvic cavity to attach to the greater trochanter of the femur (Drake et al., 2015). The levator ani and coccygeus muscles provide support for the pelvic floor. Muscles that attach outside the bony pelvis support many other structures. They include the perineal muscles, the iliacus muscle, and muscles of the anterior abdominal wall and lower limbs (Madadevan, 2018).

EXTERNAL GENITALIA

Also known as the vulva, the female external genitalia include the mons pubis, labia majora and minora, clitoris, vaginal introitus, hymen, vestibule, urethral meatus, and the posterior fourchette (**Figure 20.2**). The *mons pubis* refers to the mound of fatty tissue overlying the pubic symphysis. Pubic hair develops here during puberty. The labia majora are the external folds of fatty tissue and supportive connective tissue that begin at the mons and extend inferiorly, where they end at the posterior commissure, a depression formed between the inferior edges of the labia majora. The labia majora have many sebaceous and sweat glands and the external surface is covered with hair follicles (R. P. Smith, 2018). The labia majora serve to protect the sensitive vulvar tissues, aid in keeping the introitus closed, and prevent infection (Hays & Clarks, 2017). Inside the folds of the labia majora lie the labia minora, which consist of thin folds of skin. Similar to the labia majora, the tissue of the labia minora contains many sebaceous glands (R. P. Smith, 2018). Superiorly, the lateral folds of the labia minora join to form the prepuce, or clitoral

hood, and the medial folds form the frenulum. The labia minora extend inferiorly and unite to form a small fold, the posterior fourchette. The area enclosed by the labia minora is referred to as the vestibule. The clitoris is located just inferior to the prepuce. The vaginal introitus marks the opening of the **vagina**; just inside the introitus is the ringlike fold of tissue referred to as the hymen. The hymen has marked variation in normal size and shape. The urethral meatus is located inside the vestibule, inferior to the frenulum of the labia minora.

Glandular openings found at the entrance of the urethra and vagina are also considered part of the external genitalia, although not externally visible. The Bartholin and Skene glands are found under the soft tissue of the vestibule (see **Figure 20.2**). The Bartholin gland ducts open in the fold of the vaginal introitus and hymenal remnants at the 4 o'clock and 8 o'clock positions. The Skene or paraurethral gland ducts are found along the lateral margins of the urethra. The Bartholin and Skene glands function to secrete mucus during sexual arousal. Blockage of either of the ducts can result in inflammation, cyst formation, or abscess.

INTERNAL STRUCTURES OF THE FEMALE GENITOURINARY SYSTEM AND REPRODUCTIVE SYSTEMS

The internal structures of the female GU system are depicted in **Figure 20.3**. The internal structures of the female *reproductive system* are shown in **Figure 20.4** and include the vagina, cervix, uterus, fallopian tubes, and ovaries.

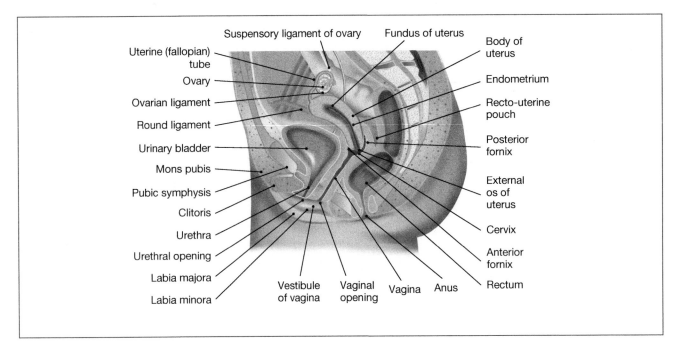

FIGURE 20.3 Female genitourinary system.

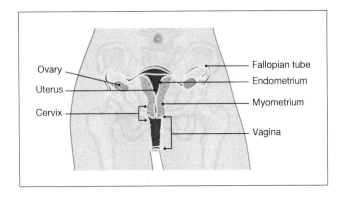

FIGURE 20.4 Female reproductive system.

Vagina

In the sagittal plane, the vagina lies inferior to the bladder, separated by the vesicovaginal septum. It is superior to the rectum and is separated by the rectovaginal septum in the lower segment; the upper segment is separated by the cul-de-sac of Douglas.

The thin muscular walls of the vagina are normally flattened and consist of a potential space, which stretches to become tubelike during sexual activity or childbirth. The vagina begins at the introitus and extends internally ending at the cervix. The length of the vagina varies and increases to some extent based on the height and weight of the woman. The vaginal walls are defined based on their anatomic position: anterior, posterior, and (two) lateral walls. Transverse folds, known as rugae, line the vaginal walls of women

of reproductive age and are composed of squamous epithelial cells. They are most prominent in the lower one-third of the vagina and assist with vaginal distensibility (Valea, 2017). The cervix extends down into the upper portion of the vaginal vault, creating a pocket of vaginal tissue referred to as the fornices. The four fornices are the anterior, posterior, and (two) lateral fornices. The anterior fornix is shorter than the posterior fornix, with the anterior vaginal length approximately 6 to 9 cm and posterior length approximately 8 to 12 cm (Valea, 2017).

Cervix

The cervix is the lower, narrow portion of the uterus and is made up of fibrous tissue. The cervix may be cylindrical or conical in shape; the cervical canal is tapered at both ends, opening into the vagina via the external cervical os and connecting to the uterus via the internal cervical os. The shape of the external cervical os is small and round in a nulliparous woman, with a variety of other shapes noted after vaginal delivery. **Figure 20.5** identifies normal variations of the cervical os.

The external surface of the cervix, referred to as the ectocervix, is covered with squamous epithelial cells. The endocervix, the cervical canal, is lined with columnar epithelial cells. The transformation zone is an important anatomical landmark, as it is the area where the squamous epithelial cells and the columnar epithelial cells meet. The transformation zone, also referred to as the squamocolumnar junction, is the

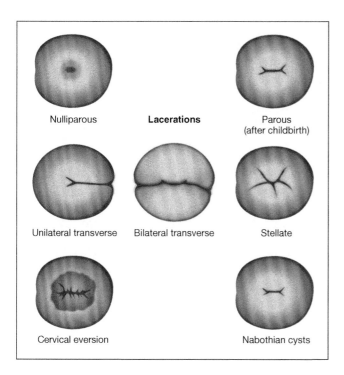

FIGURE 20.5 Normal variations of the cervical os.

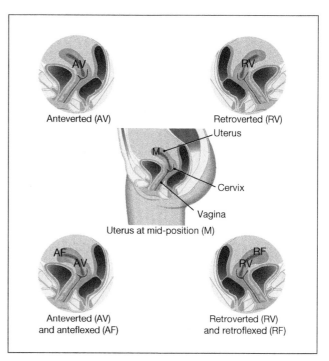

FIGURE 20.6 Normal variations in the position of the uterus.

location from which Papanicolaou (Pap) sampling is performed and which is the origin of most cervical cancers. The location of the transformation zone on the cervix is dependent on several factors, including age, pregnancy status, and use of contraceptive hormones (King & Brucker, 2019). Eversion of the transformation zone onto the surface of the cervix is a normal finding and is referred to as cervical ectropion, eversion, or ectopy.

Uterus

The uterus lies centrally in the pelvis, posterior to the bladder and anterior to the rectum, and is supported laterally by the broad ligaments. It is a pear-shaped organ with thick, muscular walls. The superior portion of the uterus is referred to as the fundus, the middle portion is the body of the uterus, and the lower portion of the uterus enters the vagina at the cervix. The size and weight of the uterus change depending on the hormonal status and pregnancy history. The average uterus is approximately 8 cm long, 5 cm wide, and weighs about 40 to 50 g (Valea, 2017). The position of the uterus in the pelvis is variable. **Figure 20.6** depicts normal variations in the position of the uterus, which include midline, anteverted, anteflexed, retroverted, and retroflexed.

The uterus consists of three layers: the endometrium, the myometrium, and the serosa. The endometrium is the innermost lining of the uterus. The stratum functionalis layer of the endometrium is responsible for

the changes that occur in the endometrial tissue during the proliferative and menstrual phase of the menstrual cycle (see "The Menstrual Cycle" section for more information). The majority of the uterus is composed of the myometrium, which is the muscular layer. The outermost layer is the serosa, which arises from the peritoneum.

Fallopian Tubes

The fallopian tubes are located at the upper lateral edges of the body of the uterus, called the cornua. They are approximately 10 to 14 cm in length, and are thin, muscular tubes (Valea, 2017). The fallopian tubes laterally extend out from the cornua and open into the peritoneal cavity near the ovaries. Fertilization often takes place in the fallopian tubes as they serve as the passageway for the ovum from the **ovary** to the uterus.

Ovaries

The ovaries sit adjacent to the fimbriae of the fallopian tube and are held in place by the broad ligaments. The ovaries are approximately 4 cm in length during reproductive years and are similar in size to an almond (Valea, 2017). The ovaries are responsible for oogenesis and are considered part of the endocrine system for their role in the hormone production of estrogen and progesterone. The term *adnexa* refers to the physical area, including the ovary, fallopian tube, and surrounding ligamentous structures.

THE MENSTRUAL CYCLE

The reproductive cycle requires a complex coordinated effort involving the endocrine system and the female reproductive system. The hypothalamic–pituitary–ovarian axis controls the flux of gonadotropin hormones by secreting releasing factors and inhibiting factors, which regulate the menstrual cycle. These hormones affect both the endometrium of the uterus and the ovaries. The subsequent discussion of the menstrual cycle includes the endometrial cycle and the ovarian cycle as depicted in **Figure 20.7**.

The Ovarian Cycle

Gonadotropin-releasing hormone (GnRH) is released by the hypothalamus and provides stimulus for the release of gonadotropin from the pituitary gland. The pulsed release of GnRH is required for proper follicle development, subsequent ovulation, and the corpus luteum development. The anterior pituitary gland releases the gonadotropins luteinizing hormone (LH) and follicle-stimulating hormone (FSH). Two other hormones are required for the reproductive cycle: estradiol and progesterone. These are produced by the ovaries and are controlled by the levels of FSH and LH. The three phases of the ovarian cycle are follicular, ovulatory, and luteal, and are described next.

Follicular Phase

The follicular phase of the ovarian cycle begins on day 1 of the menstrual cycle and lasts through approximately day 14. A primary ovarian follicle develops as a result of the release of FSH from the anterior pituitary gland. During the course of maturation, this developing follicle releases estradiol. In response to increasing levels of estradiol secretion, the anterior pituitary decreases secretion of FSH. When estradiol levels have reached a threshold, the anterior pituitary gland is signaled through the positive feedback loop to release a surge of LH.

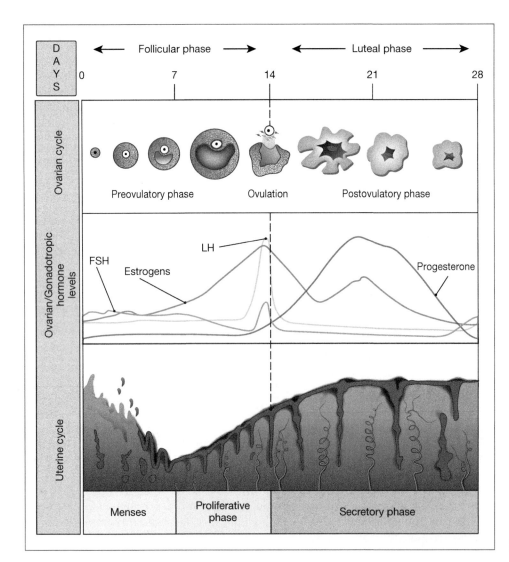

FIGURE 20.7 Menstrual cycle.

Ovulatory Phase

The ovulatory phase begins with a surge in LH and FSH levels. The surge in LH stimulates the release of an egg (ovulation) within 16 to 32 hours after the surge begins. The estrogen level decreases during the surge and the progesterone level starts to increase.

Luteal Phase

The luteal phase begins with the surge of LH at approximately day 14 of the cycle and ends with the first day of menses. This rapid rise in LH stimulates the production of progesterone and the production of these hormones ultimately results in ovulation, which describes the release of the mature ovum from the follicle. If fertilization fails to occur, hormone production dwindles and the decreasing levels of estradiol and progesterone result in a rise in FSH, starting the cycle over again.

The Endometrial Cycle

The endometrial cycle consists of three phases: the menstrual phase, the proliferative phase, and the secretory phase. The changes in the endometrial tissue are a result of its response to cyclic changes in estradiol and progesterone levels that normally occur during the reproductive cycle.

The Menstrual Phase

The menstrual phase begins on the first day of menses, referred to as day 1 of the menstrual cycle, and lasts approximately 3 to 5 days, although this is variable, and bleeding for 2 to 7 days is considered to be normal. During this phase, the endometrial glands disintegrate and the stratum functionalis desquamates, causing the vaginal bleeding characteristic of the menstrual cycle. The average volume of menstrual blood loss is approximately 35 mL, with the normal range being 10 to 80 mL (Douglas & Lobo, 2017).

The Proliferative Phase

The proliferative phase begins on approximately the fourth or fifth day of the menstrual cycle and lasts for about 10 days. During this time, the endometrial tissue undergoes significant growth, tripling in size (Douglas & Lobo, 2017). This growth is triggered by rising levels of estradiol. The proliferative phase begins the preparation of the endometrium for implantation of a fertilized ovum.

The Secretory Phase

The secretory phase begins on approximately day 15 of the menstrual cycle or about 1 day after ovulation occurs. Progesterone levels rise after ovulation, which stimulates the glands of the endometrium to increase secretion. The increased secretions provide a thick, nutrient-rich environment for implantation. If fertilization and subsequent implantation fail to occur, falling progesterone and estradiol levels trigger the initiation of endometrial regression, ending in the menstrual phase.

LIFE-SPAN DIFFERENCES AND CONSIDERATIONS IN ANATOMY AND PHYSIOLOGY

There are several life-span considerations worth mentioning as knowledge of them will improve the clinician's ability to differentiate normal findings associated with age or developmental stage from abnormal findings requiring further evaluation.

Infancy and Childhood

Oocytes, the precursors to the ovum, develop in the fetus while in utero. The maximum number of oocytes are present by about the 20th week of gestation; they initially number in the millions but decrease to hundreds of thousands by puberty because of a process called atresia (Hsueh, Eisenhauer, Chun, Hsu, & Billig, 1996). It can be said that when a woman is pregnant with a female child, she is carrying both her child and her future grandchildren.

Sexual Maturity Rating

Assessment of the sexual maturity of the female child is important in clinical practice as it confirms expected sexual development and identifies potential alterations in expected development. It also offers an opportunity for anticipatory guidance for the child and parents. The most commonly used sexual maturity rating tool is Tanner staging, which is shown for female pubertal development in **Table 20.1**. The American Academy of Pediatrics (AAP) recommends visual inspection of the female breast and genitalia begin at age 7 through 17 for assessment of sexual maturity rating (AAP, 2017a, 2017b).

Differences in Female Versus Male Anatomy

Males and females share similarities in the pelvic structure until puberty, at which time the female pelvic dimensions change, which is an adaptation to allow for childbearing. This pelvic accommodation appears to regress around 40 years of age, when the pelvic structure again narrows and becomes more similar to that of the male (Huseynov et al., 2016).

In order to potentially accommodate the delivery of a fetus, there are some specific differences between the fully developed female and male pelvis. The female pelvis has a more circular pelvic inlet when compared with the heart-shaped inlet seen in the male pelvis. The angle formed at the pubic arch is another area of difference. This angle in the female pelvis is approximately 80° to 85° in women, which is much wider when compared with 50° to 60° of the male pelvis. And finally, the medial

TABLE 20.1 Tanner Stages of Female Development

	Breast		Pubic Hair	
Stage 1	Small nipples. No breast.		No pubic hair.	
Stage 2	Breast and nipples have just started to grow. The areola has become larger. Breast tissue bud feels firm behind the nipple.		Initial growth of long pubic hairs. These are straight, without curls, and of light colors.	
Stage 3	Breast and nipples have grown additionally. The areola has become darker. The breast tissue bud is larger.		The pubic hair is more widespread. The hair is darker and curls may have appeared.	
Stage 4	Nipples and areolas are elevated and form an edge toward the breast. The breast has also grown a little larger.		More dense hair growth with curls and dark hair. Still not entirely as an adult woman.	
Stage 5	Fully developed breast. Nipples are protruding and the edge between areola and breast has disappeared.		Adult hair growth. Dense, curly hair extending toward the inner thighs.	

projection of the ischial spines into the pelvic cavity is much less prominent in the females compared with their male counterparts (Drake et al., 2015).

Pregnancy

The significant anatomic and physiologic changes that occur in women during pregnancy and postpartum are reviewed in Chapter 21, Evidence-Based Obstetric Assessment.

Menopause

Whereas there are no reliable methods to predict the exact time when a woman's reproductive ability ceases, the average age of menopause is 52 years; natural menopause may occur in women at any time between the ages of 40 and 58 years (The North American Menopause Society [NAMS], 2014). Menopause is defined as the cessation of menstrual bleeding for 12 consecutive months in a woman with a uterus. Menopause that occurs prior to age 40 is considered premature and warrants further investigation (Lobo, 2017). In addition to

naturally occurring menopause that results from decreasing gonadal hormone levels, menopause may be induced by surgery, chemotherapy, or radiation therapy to the pelvis. Perimenopause is defined as the phase prior to the cessation of menses that is characterized by fluctuating estrogen levels and postmenopause is defined as the time frame that begins after 12 months of amenorrhea. See **Figure 20.8** that outlines the stages of a woman's reproductive life span.

Anatomic changes to the external and internal female genitalia occur during the menopausal transition as a direct result of declining levels of estrogen (Bradshaw, 2016). The epithelium of the urogenital tract thins, collagen levels and elasticity decrease, and the concentration of blood vessels diminishes (Portman & Gass, 2014). These changes result in the thinning of the labia majora and retraction of the introitus (Portman & Gass, 2014). The overall length of the vagina and size and weight of the uterus diminish with the menopausal transition (Valea, 2017).

					Final Menstrual Period (FMP)		
Stages:	-5	-4	-3	-2	-1	0	+1	+2
Terminology	Reproductive			Menopausal Transition		Postmenopause		
	Early	Peak	Late	Early	Late*	Early*		Late
				Perimenopause				
Duration of stage:	Variable	Variable		Variable		(a) 1 yr	(b) 4 yrs	Until demise
Menstrual cycles:	Variable to regular	Regular		Variable cycle length (>7 days different from normal)	≥2 skipped cycles and an interval of amenorrhea (≥60 days)	Amen x 12 mos	None	
Endocrine:	Normal FSH		↑FSH	↑FSH		↑FSH		

*Stages most likely characterized by vasomotor symptoms   ↑ = elevated

FIGURE 20.8 Female reproductive life span.
FSH, follicle-stimulating hormone.
Source: Adapted from Harlow, S.D., Gass, M., Hall, J.E., Lobo, R., Maki, P., Rebar, R.W., … de Villiers, T.J. (2012). Executive summary of the Stages of Reproductive Aging Workshop + 10: addressing the unfinished agenda of staging reproductive aging. *The Journal of Clinical Endocrinology & Metabolism, 97*(4), 1159–1168.

Physiologic changes attributable to the menopausal transition also occur. These include rising FSH levels and decreasing levels of estrogen and androgens. Women experience a wide range of symptoms as a result, which include vasomotor instability, commonly called "hot flashes," insomnia, mood changes, fatigue, and menstrual irregularities. These symptoms are most commonly attributed to declining estrogen levels. Postmenopausal women have an increased risk for declining health and wellness and should therefore be screened for heart disease, osteoporosis, urinary problems, and cancers. Details regarding recommended screenings are discussed later in this chapter.

KEY HISTORY QUESTIONS AND CONSIDERATIONS FOR THE FEMALE GENITOURINARY SYSTEM

There are two main reasons to conduct a history and physical examination related specifically to the GU system: wellness and illness. As part of a well visit, the clinician must assess for normal functioning, health maintenance, and health promotion needs. During an acute or episodic visit, the clinician focuses on specific concerns. A sensitive, patient-centered, detailed history will inform what physical examination needs to be done; more specifically, when breast and pelvic examinations, or cervical inspection, are warranted. Patients should be asked about their menstrual, obstetric, and sexual history (American College of Obstetricians and Gynecologists [ACOG], 2018a). The elements of the history pertinent to the well-woman examination are included in **Table 20.2**.

Clinicians should begin the **women's health** history only when the environment has been satisfactorily prepared for privacy and a rapport has been established with the patient. Note in **Table 20.2** there are four supplementary subject areas essential for a complete women's health history in addition to the traditional elements: menstrual, **gynecologic**, obstetric, and sexual histories. Although generally considered as part of the past medical history, little consensus exists on where these elements should be documented. It is not uncommon for the gynecologic history to be embedded in the past medical history or in the review of systems. Most commonly, the menstrual, obstetric, and sexual histories are documented as their own sections either before or after the past medical history.

HISTORY OF PRESENT ILLNESS

The history of present illness (HPI) aides the clinician in appropriately addressing the individual's reason for seeking care and health concerns. Presenting symptoms related to the female GU system vary greatly depending on the organs or structures involved. For example, vaginal discharge is a common condition because of vaginitis (although more aggressive infections can arise from organs deeper in the pelvis), chronic pelvic

TABLE 20.2 Elements of History Pertinent to the Well-Woman Examination

History Component	Description of Assessment
Chief concern (CC) or reason for seeking care	The patient's chief concern (This can also be written as reason for visit.)
History of present illness (HPI)	Describes the major characteristics of the chief concern (onset, location, duration, character, associated symptoms, aggravating factors, relieving symptoms, temporal factors)
Menstrual history	Describes the patient's menstrual cycle, flow, and present status (adrenarche through menopause)
Gynecologic history	Describes the patient's self-care behaviors, health promotion or risk behaviors, and past medical history pertaining to breast and gynecologic health (including Pap smears and pelvic examinations)
Obstetric history	Provides a detailed account of each pregnancy, outcome, and complication; summarized using the GTPAL system
Sexual history	Describes the patient's current and past sexual experiences and the patient's physical, emotional, and mental responses and well-being; includes partners, practices, protection, past history of sexually transmitted infections, pregnancy prevention, trauma/violence screening
Past medical history	Includes the traditional elements of the past medical history such as allergies, medications, and immunizations, as well as a thorough review of all other current acute or chronic conditions that may influence one's gynecologic or sexual health
Family history	Serves as a risk assessment; provides a list of illnesses occurring in first-degree relatives
Social history	Includes current lifestyle, social, and behavioral activities that may have an impact on a woman's overall health (marital status, employment, social support, habits—smoking, alcohol, illicit drugs, gun exposure, etc.)

GTPAL, gravida, term births, preterm births, abortions, living children.

pain is typically related to pelvic organs or muscular/supportive structures, and menstrual irregularities including amenorrhea may have underlying endocrine or pregnancy causes. Therefore, to better understand questions pertaining to the HPI for the female GU system, three examples of common presenting symptoms are provided:

- Vaginal discharge
- Pelvic pain
- Amenorrhea

Example: Vaginal Discharge

- Onset: Recent, intermittent, or chronic
- Location: Vulvovaginal
- Duration: Persistent symptoms, increasing amount of discharge or worsening associated symptoms versus lingering, improving, or intermittent symptoms
- Character: Odor (none, fishy [amine], putrid), color (gray, yellow, green, white), consistency (frothy, thin, clumped), amount
- Associated symptoms—local: Pruritus (internal, external, or both), painful skin lesions, dyspareunia, dysuria, frequent urination
- Associated symptoms—systemic: Fever, nausea, vomiting; any prior history of similar symptoms

- Aggravating factors: Intercourse, urination, antibiotics, douching, soaking in a bathtub or hot tub
- Relieving symptoms: Over-the-counter (OTC) antifungal cream, cool compresses, sitz bath, or other treatments
- Temporal factors: Timing in relation to menstrual cycle, recent antibiotics, symptoms after presence of foreign objects, or latex in vagina; recent sexual activity, new partner, or history of infection in current partner.
- Differential diagnoses: Local infections (candida, bacterial vaginosis [BV], trichomoniasis, gonorrhea, chlamydia, herpes simplex); systemic ions (pelvic inflammatory disease [PID], toxic shock syndrome [TSS]); atrophic vaginitis; dermatitis; irritant or allergic vaginitis; physiologic leukorrhea; malignancy; retained foreign body; fistula

Example: Pelvic Pain

- Onset: Recent, intermittent, or chronic
- Location: Vaginal, superpubic or suprapubic, lower abdomen, adnexal, umbilical; highly localized (patient can point to one place) versus a more generalized discomfort or pain that moves around
- Duration: Persistent symptoms; constant, recurrent, cyclical

- Character: Sharp, dull, burning, achy, crampy, colicky
- Associated symptoms: Vaginal discharge, menstruation, urination, defecation, fever, nausea, vomiting, violence
- Aggravating factors: Intercourse, urination, defecation, movement, tampon use
- Relieving symptoms: Rest, warm compresses, pain relievers, end of menses, repositioning, exercise
- Temporal factors: Last menstrual period (LMP), timing in relation to menstrual cycle (premenstrual, during menstruation, postmenstrual, postmenopausal); recent sexual activity, new partner, or history of infection in current partner
- Differential diagnoses: Uterine (leiomyoma, malignancy, endometriosis); ovarian (cyst, torsion, malignancy); structural (musculoskeletal, ligamentous); menstrual-related (premenstrual syndrome, Mittelschmerz); pregnancy (normal pregnancy, spontaneous abortion, ectopic pregnancy); systemic (PID, TSS); urinary (urinary tract infection, renal calculi); gastrointestinal

Example: Amenorrhea

- Onset: Number of missed cycles or no menses by age 16.
- Location: Not applicable
- Duration: Menses never started, pattern of missed cycles
- Character: Bleeding pattern (e.g., no menses, spotting, irregularity); character of flow (scant, moderate, heavy); number of days and duration between
- Associated symptoms—local: Vaginal discharge, vaginal dryness, pain, unprotected intercourse, new sexual partner(s), last sexually transmitted infection (STI) testing
- Associated symptoms—systemic: Nausea, vomiting, weight change, stress, mood changes, breast tenderness, hot flashes, night sweats, acne, facial hair, headaches, fatigue
- Aggravating factors: Recently gave birth, other chronic illness, chronic medications (including contraception), breastfeeding (frequency, duration), radiation exposure
- Relieving symptoms: Not applicable
- Temporal factors: Age, sexual activity, current contraception, LMP
- Differential diagnoses: Primary amenorrhea—pregnancy, constitutional delay, pituitary tumors, obstructed outflow tract, stress, or certain genetic (androgen insensitivity, congenital adrenal hyperplasia) or chromosome (Turner syndrome) abnormalities; secondary amenorrhea—pregnancy, breastfeeding, ovarian disease (polycystic ovarian syndrome, premature ovarian failure), hypothalamic dysfunction, pituitary disease, Asherman's syndrome, hormonal contraception

MENSTRUAL HISTORY

Menstrual history is often the first supplemental section of the health history addressed in a women's health examination. Understanding where a woman is in her overall menstrual cycle (from adrenarche to menopause) as well as the characteristics of each cycle result from these assessments.

- Age of menarche (first episode of menstruation)
- Duration of flow
- Cycle length (from the first day of one to the first day of the next)
- Regularity of cycle
- Describe any irregularities (e.g., spotting between cycles)
- Symptoms that accompany menstruation
- Age at last menstrual cycle

GYNECOLOGIC HISTORY

In this section, the clinician should specifically address the following:

- Breast history
  - History of breast disease
  - Breastfeeding
  - Self-breast examination
  - Last mammogram
- Gynecologic history
  - Last pelvic examination
  - Last Pap test
  - History of STIs: note when and how treated
  - History of abnormal Pap testing
  - Abnormal Pap results and/or treatments
  - Last human papillomavirus (HPV) testing and result
  - Gynecologic surgery
  - Fertility
  - Exposure to diethylstilbestrol (DES)

OBSTETRIC HISTORY

The obstetric history tells the story of every pregnancy that a woman has had. Common terms used to describe the number of pregnancies and the disposition of each pregnancy are listed in **Table 20.3**. The clinician should document the year of each pregnancy, the duration of each pregnancy (in weeks), and the method of delivery, as well as any complications during or after the pregnancy for the mother and infant. It is also important to obtain details about each child born, such as gender, weight, and the current condition of each child today. The GTPAL (gravida, term births, preterm births, abortions, living children) system (**Table 20.4**) is used to summarize these assessment findings. This five-digit system may be documented in table format, as a series of numbers with

TABLE 20.3 Common Terminology of Gravidity and Parity	
Term	Definition
Gravida	A pregnant woman; the number of pregnancies, regardless of outcome
Primigravida	A woman in her first pregnancy or who has been pregnant only once
Multigravida	A woman who is or has been pregnant more than once
Nulligravida	A woman who has never been pregnant
Primipara	A woman who has carried one pregnancy beyond 20 weeks
Multipara	A woman who has carried a pregnancy beyond 20 weeks two or more times
Nullipara	A woman who has never carried a pregnancy or never carried one beyond 20 weeks

TABLE 20.4 GTPAL System		
	Term	Definition
G	Gravida	Number of pregnancies
T	Term	Number of full-term births (≥37 weeks' gestation)
P	Preterm births	Number of preterm births (≥20 weeks, <37 weeks' gestation)
A	Abortions	Number of abortions (spontaneous, elective, ectopic) <20 weeks' gestation
L	Living children	Number of living children

dashes between them, and as an acronym with values as superscript. How the clinician was trained, their area of specialty, or the standard of practice in the current environment determines GTPAL documentation.

SEXUAL HISTORY

The sexual health history provides an opportunity for the clinician to acknowledge the importance of sexuality, relationships, and sexual behavior to one's overall health. Therefore, this part of the examination should not be limited to a disease-oriented perspective, but should provide an opportunity to further the patient–clinician relationship and support behaviors that encourage sexual health across the life span (ACOG, 2017). **Box 20.1** provides a list of possible questions covering the five Ps listed by the ACOG: **P**artners, **P**ractices, **P**rotection from STIs, **P**ast history of STIs, and **P**regnancy **P**revention, and lists a sixth, **P**lus additional questions, to remind clinicians to be sure to assess each individual's concerns and questions regarding sexual health. Sexual health history questions should be asked with an understanding that sexual orientation and gender identity are central to every person's sense of self and well-being. Sensitive history taking allows an opportunity for the

patient to discuss their satisfaction or dissatisfaction with their own or their partner's sexual function and to speak frankly about issues related to orgasm and desire.

PAST MEDICAL HISTORY

In the past medical history, the clinician should include subsections to document allergies, medications, immunizations, and any other current, chronic, or other medical conditions during her lifetime. This would include hospitalizations, surgeries, and potentially specific questions about diabetes, cancer, and cardiovascular disease. The clinician should review and discuss these conditions as they pertain to the patient's overall health as well as her gynecologic health.

FAMILY HISTORY

A thorough family history, specifically of first-degree relatives (parents, siblings, and children), is a critical element in assessing health risks in women. The clinician should note ages, cause of death, and any serious illnesses such as diabetes, cardiovascular disease, hematologic or coagulation disorders, mental illness, and cancer. The clinician should also inquire about

BOX 20.1
SIX Ps OF SEXUAL HEALTH HISTORY

1. Partners
- Are you currently sexually active? (Are you having sex?)
  - If no, have you ever been sexually active?
- In recent months, how many sex partners have you had?
- In the past 12 months, how many sex partners have you had?
- Are your sex partners men, women, or both?
  - If the answer is "both," repeat first two questions for each specific gender.

2. Practices
- I am going to be more explicit here about the kind of sex you have had over the past 12 months to better understand if you are at risk of sexually transmitted infections (STIs).
- What kind of sexual contact do you have or have you had?
  - Genital (penis in the vagina)?
  - Anal (penis in the anus)?
  - Oral (mouth on penis, vagina, or anus)?

3. Protection from Sexually Transmitted Infections
- Do you and your partner(s) use any protection against STIs?
  - If not, could you tell me the reason?
  - Are you comfortable asking your partner to use condoms? (If appropriate)
  - If so, what kind of protection do you use?
  - How often do you use this protection?
  - If "sometimes," in what situations or with whom do you use protection?
- Do you have any other questions, or are there other forms of protection from STIs that you would like to discuss today?

4. Past History of Sexually Transmitted Infections
- Have you ever been diagnosed with an STI?
  - When? How were you treated?
  - Have you had any recurring symptoms or diagnoses?
- Have you ever been tested for HIV or other STIs?
  - Would you like to be tested?
- Has your current partner (or former partners) been diagnosed or treated for an STI?
  - Were you tested for the same STI(s)?
  - If yes, when were you tested? What was the diagnosis? How was it treated?

5. Prevention of Pregnancy
- Are you currently trying to become pregnant?
- Are you concerned about getting pregnant?
- Are you using contraception or practicing any form of birth control?
- Is your partner supportive of you using birth control?
- Do you need any information on birth control?

6. Plus Additional Questions to Complete the History
- What other things about your sexual health and sexual practices should we discuss to help ensure your good health?
- What other concerns or questions regarding your sexual health or sexual practices would you like to discuss?

Source: Adapted from the American College of Obstetricians and Gynecologists. (2017). Committee Opinion No 706. *Obstetrics & Gynecology, 130*(1), e42–e47. doi:10.1097/aog.0000000000002161

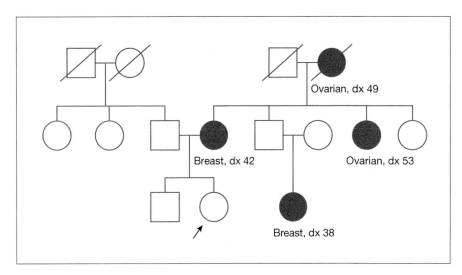

FIGURE 20.9 Classic *BRCA1* pedigree.

Source: National Cancer Institute.

congenital malformations or genetic conditions, and recurrent pregnancy losses, as these may have an impact on an individual's reproductive life plan.

As a clinician, a family pedigree is a useful aide to addressing genetic risk. Clinicians can encourage individuals to create and regularly update their family history using the Surgeon General's "My Family Health Portrait" available through the Centers for Disease Control and Prevention (CDC; https://phgkb.cdc.gov/FHH/html/index.html). **Figure 20.9** provides an illustration of how a family pedigree can be useful when considering the penetrance of gynecologic malignancies. This figure specifically highlights the *BRCA1* gene, which is associated with breast and ovarian cancer.

SOCIAL HISTORY

A women's health visit is a prime opportunity to inquire about an individual's health, wellness, and lifestyle behaviors. Whereas there are overlaps in assessing HPI, sexual history, family history, and social history, be sure to learn about the environment that a client lives and works in, their social support systems, and their personal habits and safety practices that may support wellness or increase risk of illness.

Social history questions may be assessed along with discussion of an individual's plan for pregnancy. The CDC recommends that all individuals who are of reproductive age be asked about their reproductive life plan (Gavin et al., 2014). Knowing whether an individual desires or does not desire pregnancy and has or does not have a plan is a priority for addressing reproductive and sexual health in context with wellness, risk factors, and behavioral health.

Social

What is their marital status? Who lives in the home with them? Does she live in a safe community? Inquire about

relationships with family and friends and ask about her social support network.

Occupational

What is the patient's employment status? Do they have a vocation? Where does the patient work? How are things going at work?

Substance Use

Patients who engage in or have a history of high-risk behavior are at increased risk for STIs, including HIV and hepatitis C (Feaster et al., 2016; National Institute on Drug Abuse, National Institutes of Health, & U.S. Department of Health and Human Services, 2019). Be sure to address high-risk behaviors such as alcohol use, tobacco use, or illicit drugs (e.g., marijuana, cocaine, opiates). Asking these questions can be difficult. Use open-ended questions and be more specific when needed. How much and how often does the patient drink? What do they drink? Document smoking in pack years (number of packs smoked per day × the number of years smoked). Note the number of years smoke-free as well.

PREVENTIVE CARE CONSIDERATIONS

The women's health visit may be the only routine well visit that a woman has during her reproductive years, which means that assessment and discussion of health, wellness, and lifestyle behaviors are imperative. Numerous organizations, such as the ACOG, the U.S. Preventive Services Task Force (USPSTF), and the American Academy of Family Physicians (AAFP), have published key recommendations for the well-woman examination. The Women's Preventive Services Initiative is a collaborative effort, led by the ACOG and in agreement with the Department of Health and Human Services, charged to review and update recommendations for women's preventive healthcare. The recommendations

are updated annually and are available at www
.womenspreventivehealth.org. To partner with individuals to meet these guidelines, inquire about personal
habits and safety issues when addressing preventive
care. As the primary point of contact for health promotion, clinicians should be prepared to listen without
being judgmental and to provide evidence-based recommendations. Two specific areas to assess are personal
habits related to healthy lifestyle behaviors and safety.

Personal Habits

How active is the patient? What type of exercise do they
do and how much? How much sleep do they get at night?
Do they awaken feeling rested? Ask the patient to describe their diet or do a 24-hour recall of the foods they
ate. Does the patient use sunscreen? Do they use feminine
hygiene products such as scented sprays or douches?

Safety

Safety covers a broad range of behaviors from wearing a seatbelt in a car to appropriately storing firearms
in the home. Be sure to privately screen for intimate
partner violence to identify concerns. Ask whether the
individual feels safe in their current relationships.

LIFE-SPAN CONSIDERATIONS FOR HISTORY

The types of questions that need to be addressed during
a gynecologic history vary greatly by age and development. It is worth noting, however, that this is not necessarily an additional area that needs to be covered during
the history, as most concerns relevant to the patient's developmental stage were likely addressed through the HPI,
menstrual, gynecologic, obstetric, sexual, past medical,
family, and social history components. A few additional
considerations are discussed in the text that follows.

Gender-specific examinations are appropriate for all
age groups—from infancy through older adult. As children grow, the clinicians must adjust how they approach
advance assessment and what components of the
health history are prioritized. During infancy and childhood, the parent should be asked pertinent questions
about the child, and also about the mother's pregnancy
and medications taken during the pregnancy. In early
adolescence, secondary sexual characteristics may
begin to develop (breast budding, pubic hair growth,
and fat deposition). Adolescents at this stage are often
uncomfortable discussing these changes. Care should
be taken when inquiring about these changes. Note
that parents often stop seeing their children unclothed
at this point and may be unaware that these changes
are taking place. Adolescence is often a time of questioning and experimentation. The clinician should be
comfortable answering questions about sexuality and
be cautious not to encroach on cultural or religious beliefs and practices. As adults, much of the well-woman

health history is centered around health maintenance
and health promotion. As women approach menopause,
more care should be taken to inquire about physiologic,
cognitive, and emotional changes resulting from perimenopause. Sensitivity should be used to discuss issues related to intimacy and intercourse.

UNIQUE POPULATION CONSIDERATIONS FOR HISTORY

Owing to the intimate nature of the gynecologic examination, there are a few populations who are vulnerable
to disparities in care. Care should be taken to provide
culturally sensitive counseling and education to patients and families who identify as LGBTQ+, are sexual
assault survivors, or are victims of female genital mutilation (formerly female circumcision). Each of these
groups has experienced trauma, isolation, insensitivity, and often lack of access to care. Further, clinicians
are often ill-prepared to care for these individuals. One
study concluded that fewer than half of certified obstetricians and gynecologists reported that they had training in LGBTQ health (Mehta, 2018). There is a known
national shortage in trained sexual assault forensic examiners (SAFEs; Clowers, 2018), and evidence suggests
an overall lack of knowledge and training in how to diagnose and care for victims of female genital mutilation
(Abdulcadir, Say, & Pallitto, 2017; Lane, Johnson-Agbakwu, Warren, Budhathoki, & Cole, 2018; Zurynski,
Sureshkumar, Phu, & Elliott, 2015). *Note: Please review
the HPI script provided in Chapter 18, Evidence-Based
Assessment of Sexual Orientation, Gender Identity,
and Health, to develop sensitivity regarding assessment of gender identity and sexual orientation.*

PHYSICAL EXAMINATION OF THE FEMALE GENITOURINARY SYSTEM

Whereas this chapter is focused specifically on the female GU anatomy and related concerns, it is important to remember that for a well-woman examination,
a thorough head-to-toe examination is recommended.
Components of the well-woman examination include
examination of the mouth and throat; thyroid examination (when indicated); examination of the cardiac,
respiratory, and integumentary systems; and abdominal, pelvic, and breast examinations (when indicated).
Recommendations regarding the frequency and specific breast and pelvic examination components are
discussed later in the chapter.

The presence of a chaperone during the physical examination should be offered to all women, regardless of
the clinician's sex (ACOG, 2007; E. S. Curry et al., 2011).
This is especially important when performing a breast
or anogenital examination.

PERFORMING THE PELVIC EXAMINATION

The pelvic examination is often a source of anxiety and stress for women. The clinician's approach should be respectful, open, and caring. Providing education about the examination and answering any questions is an important part of establishing a trusting patient–clinician relationship. This step is especially important for women who have never experienced a pelvic examination.

The female genital examination is most commonly performed with the patient in the lithotomy position, a supine position with the legs separated, flexion at the hips and knees, and feet resting in foot rests. A supine position, as opposed to a semi-Fowler's position, allows for relaxation of the abdominal rectus muscle. Consider semi-Fowler's position for patients with mobility limitations or those with difficulty lying supine. Other optional positioning for a pelvic examination includes the V, M, diamond, or lateral positions. See **Table 20.5** for position options for pelvic examinations. Use of optional positioning may be helpful in patients with mobility limitations. Regardless of the chosen positioning, attention should be paid to appropriate draping of the patient during the examination. Care should be taken to adequately cover the patient to preserve modesty and warmth. Ideally, the clinician should drape the patient to ensure eye contact with the patient throughout the examination.

INSPECTION AND PALPATION OF EXTERNAL GENITALIA

The pelvic examination begins with a thorough examination of the external genitalia. Beginning with the mons pubis, evaluation should include a description of the pattern and quality of hair distribution on both the mons and the labia majora. For adolescent patients, assess their Tanner stage of sexual maturity (see **Table 20.1**). Inspect for signs of infestation with pediculosis. Proceed to inspection of the skin of the mons and perineum. The skin inspection should evaluate for discoloration or hypopigmentation, erythema, and excoriation. Note any visible ulcerations, pustules, vesicles, growths, lesions, nevi, varicosities, or scars.

The size and shape of the clitoris should be documented. Normal clitoral length is approximately 1 to 1.5 cm (Mendiratta & Lentz, 2017). Evaluate labia for development or atrophy. Inspect the introitus, noting its shape—closed or gaping—in the lithotomy position. The Bartholin and Skene glands should be inspected for swelling and purulent exudates. The perineal body should then be assessed. This area begins with the posterior aspect of the labia and extends to the anus. Similar to the inspection of the skin of the mons pubis and labia majora, the inspection of the perineal body should include the items previously described. Finally, the perianal area should be examined. Inspect for injury, lesions, warts, hemorrhoids, or other abnormalities. Evidence of trauma found on the external genitalia examination should prompt further investigation into its origin. Care should be taken to approach questions in a sensitive and caring manner.

INTERNAL INSPECTION: SPECULUM EXAMINATION

Performing a speculum examination allows for direct visualization of the cervix and the surrounding vaginal walls. A speculum examination for the sole purpose of screening for STIs is not necessary, as other methods for sample collection are available (see Laboratory Considerations for the Genitourinary System section).

Choice of speculum: The appropriately sized speculum should be chosen prior to starting the examination. Speculum choices typically include metal or plastic. See **Table 20.6** for a listing of the considerations for choosing metal or plastic specula and images of speculum. The most commonly used metal specula are the Grave and Pederson. The Grave speculum is wider and more appropriate for parous or obese women. The Pederson blades are narrower, and thus may be more appropriate for a virginal, thin, or postmenopausal woman. It may also be beneficial for women with dyspareunia or vaginal/pelvic pain. Both the Grave and Pederson specula are available in several different lengths. In more recent years, the use of plastic, disposable specula have become more common. Typically, plastic specula are found in three sizes. Pediatric specula are also available in both metal and plastic.

Traditionally, the choice of speculum type has been left to the clinician preference, with limited data on patient preference for the use of metal versus plastic specula. Unpublished data from a randomized controlled trial suggested that use of plastic specula may reduce perceived discomfort by the patient during a pelvic examination (Rempe et al., 2018). Given that the data is sparse at best, no specific recommendations can be made. The appropriately sized speculum should be chosen taking into consideration the woman's size, history, and anatomical findings. This can, at times, present a clinical challenge, and in such circumstances, evaluation with a bimanual examination may be performed first to assess for vaginal length, laxity, and anatomical variants. Bear in mind that the use of a wider speculum increases the potential for patient discomfort with the examination and a narrower speculum may impair visualization (Bates, Carroll, & Potter, 2011).

Insertion of the Speculum

By convention, the speculum examination is performed first, followed by the bimanual examination. This order of examination was initially adopted to avoid contamination of the cervix with lubricant that was thought to impede the interpretation of cytologic samples, HPV, or

TABLE 20.5 Positioning for the Pelvic Examination		
Position	Description	Illustration
Lithotomy	Most commonly used for the pelvic examination. Can elevate the head of the bed (semi-Fowler's position) if the woman cannot tolerate lying supine. Stirrups can be lowered for comfort.	
V position	Supine, hips abducted, and knees extended	
M position	Supine, hips abducted, knees flexed, feet at edges of the table	
Diamond position	Supine, hips abducted, knees flexed, soles of feet touching	
Lateral position	Side lying with hips and knees flexed	

common vaginal bacterial pathogens. Multiple studies have refuted this long-held belief (Amies, Miller, Lee, & Koutsky, 2002; Griffith, Stuart, Gluck, & Heartwell, 2005; Harer, Valenzuela, & Lebo, 2002; Pergialiotis et al., 2015). Use of a small amount of water-soluble lubrication does not interfere with the interpretation of cytology, and, in fact, has been shown to decrease discomfort in postmenopausal women during speculum

TABLE 20.6 Speculum Types and Considerations			
Type	Positives (Pros)	Negatives (Cons)	Illustration
Metal	• More variability in size and shape • Less waste • More adjustability, may improve visibility	• Requires clean up and access to autoclave • More knobs for adjustment, more places to check before use • Requires accessory light source • Accessory light source can be difficult to position for optimal visualization	
Plastic	• Disposable • Clear plastic bills increase visibility of vaginal walls • Light source attaches directly to speculum for ease of use. • Some brands available with cordless light source	• Less durable, may crack or break under stress • Cordless light source is sometimes accidentally discarded and is costly to replace. • Fewer choices in size/shape	

insertion (Uygur et al., 2012). Current recommendations suggest that a small amount (dime-sized) be applied to the introitus and bills of the speculum for ease of insertion (Bates et al., 2011).

The speculum should be warmed using either warm water or a warming device. If a metal speculum is used, touch it to the patient's leg to ensure the temperature is acceptable to her prior to insertion. Lubrication should be applied after warming and prior to insertion.

Begin by separating the labia with the thumb and first finger of the nondominant hand for visualization of the introitus. The traditional approach to insertion of the speculum recommends holding the speculum with the bills completely closed facing the lateral aspects of the vagina. With the speculum angled slightly downward, apply gentle pressure toward the coccyx and direct the speculum inward. Avoid a severe angle downward as this will cause the base of the speculum to compress the sensitive structures of the upper genitalia. Upon full insertion of the speculum, rotate the handle of the speculum downward so the bills are in the inferior/superior position and open the speculum for visualization of the cervix. Open the speculum only as wide as needed for visualization. It is not necessary to open it completely. The evidence to support this method of insertion is lacking. Furthermore, in the supine position, the vaginal walls are flattened and form an H-shape, which should be taken into consideration when inserting the speculum (Valea, 2017). Therefore, an alternative method for insertion can also

be considered, which involves inserting the speculum directly into the vagina with the bills in the inferior/superior position (Royal College of Nursing, 2016). Application of a gentle downward pressure on the vaginal wall aids in the insertion of the speculum. The evidence in support of this method of insertion is also lacking, so no recommendations can be made at this time in support of one method over another. Further research in this area is needed.

No matter the method of speculum insertion, care should be taken to avoid the involution of the labia majora tissue. Apply gentle traction to the labial tissue should this occur. Also, be mindful to avoid pinching the vaginal or labial tissue in the bills of the speculum, or pulling on pubic hair. If the clinician has difficulty-finding the cervix or determining the appropriately sized speculum to use, consideration should be given to performing a bimanual examination first for assessment of anatomy and position of the cervix.

Evaluation of the Vagina

The vaginal tissue should be inspected during both insertion and removal of the speculum. If using a plastic speculum, the bills are clear, which can aid in visualization. Use of a metal speculum will require tilting the position of the bills, so visualization of the entirety of the vaginal vault can be performed. The vagina should be inspected for color, tissue appearance, moisture, discharge, moles, or lesions, and any unusual odors should be noted.

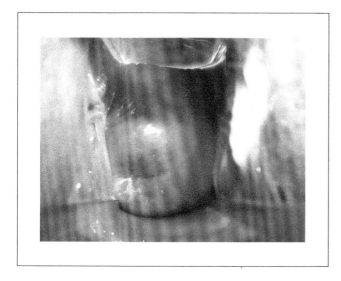

FIGURE 20.10 Cervix as viewed using a speculum.

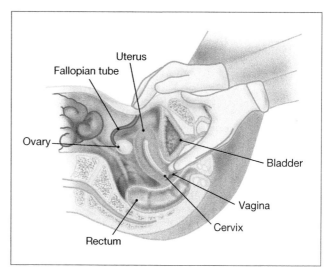

FIGURE 20.11 Bimanual examination.

Evaluation of the Cervix

The speculum should be positioned to allow for visualization of the entire surface of the cervix. A visual inspection of the cervix should be performed and include the size and shape of the os, color, bleeding or discharge, the evaluation of the squamocolumnar junction, and assessment for any lesions or growths (**Figure 20.10**). Collection of any necessary specimens can be completed at this time. A detailed description of common specimens collected during a speculum examination is discussed in the Laboratory Considerations for the Genitourinary System section.

Removal of the Speculum

Upon completion of the inspection of the cervix and collection of necessary specimens, the speculum lock should be released, and the speculum should be opened slightly while simultaneously drawing upward with the handle of the speculum, following the same plane used with insertion. This allows the bills of the speculum to release the cervix. A final inspection of the vaginal walls should be performed if needed. The bills of the speculum should be allowed to fall closed naturally, which avoids pinching the vaginal tissue and labia in the bills. Gently remove the speculum from the vagina.

PALPATION: BIMANUAL EXAMINATION

Uterus and Adnexa

The bimanual examination is performed to assess the uterus and adnexa. The index and middle finger of the dominant hand are lubricated with a water-soluble lubricant and inserted into the vagina until the cervix is palpable, moving fingers to the posterior fornix, located below the cervix. Take care to tuck the thumb out of the way to avoid compressing the sensitive structures of the pubic symphysis, mons pubis, and clitoris. The clinician should place the same leg as the dominant hand on the step of the examination table, leaning forward slightly so weight is shifted forward a bit. The nondominant hand is placed on the lower abdomen, above the pubic symphysis. Using the flat surface of the fingers, a sweeping downward motion toward the internal fingers is used to isolate the uterus. The internal fingers direct the uterus up to the fingers, gently compressing the uterus. This procedure allows for palpation of the uterine size and position in the pelvis. In nonpregnant women, the uterus is approximately 6 × 4 cm, although may be larger in multiparous women (Mendiratta & Lentz, 2017). The size, shape, and symmetry of the uterus should be documented, as well as the position and consistency of the uterus. In normal circumstances, palpation of the uterus is not painful, and any discomfort should be noted and may warrant further evaluation. See **Figure 20.11** for a cross-sectional view of a bimanual examination.

Palpation of the adnexa serves to assess the ovaries and fallopian tubes. To assess the right adnexa, the clinician shifts the internal fingers to the patient's right side, moving the fingers to the right vaginal fornix. The flat surface of the fingers of the nondominant hand are placed just medial to the right anterior superior iliac spine and directed downward to meet the internal fingers. The goal is to capture the adnexa between the internal and external fingers for palpation. The ovary is approximately 3 × 2 cm and is often compared with the size of a walnut (Mendiratta & Lentz, 2017). This maneuver is repeated on the left side for assessment of the left adnexa. Documentation should include a description of the size and mobility of the adnexa, as well as consistency. Palpation of the ovaries in postmenopausal women is not considered a normal finding; if this should be identified on examination, it requires further evaluation.

Regarding the assessment of women who may have a cystocele or rectocele, consider using just one bill of the speculum. Specifically, when performing a speculum examination on a woman where cystocele is a concern, consider removing the upper bill of the speculum and inserting the speculum in the upright direction with only the lower bill. Application of gentle downward pressure will allow for an unobstructed view of the upper vaginal wall for assessment of the pelvic organ prolapse (POP). Having the patient bear down during this time will determine the extent of the prolapse, if it is not readily apparent at rest. Similarly, one can perform a single-billed speculum examination to evaluate for rectocele. In this circumstance, the speculum should be inserted with the single bill supporting the anterior vaginal wall to allow unobstructed evaluation of the posterior vaginal wall. Asking the patient to bear down can reveal the presence of a rectocele that is not visible at rest.

Assessment of Cervical Motion Tenderness

Cervical motion tenderness (CMT) is found in several pathologic conditions, including PID, appendicitis, and ectopic pregnancy (Piepert et al., 2001). It is performed by placing the index and middle finger on either side of the cervix and gently pulling the cervix first to one side, then the other. Positive CMT is noted when the patient experiences pain with traction on the adnexa. Inter-rater reliability for CMT is low, but there is still evidence that suggests its clinical significance in assisting with diagnosis of pelvic inflammatory disorder (Farrukh, Sivitz, Onogul, Patel, & Tejani, 2018; Simms, Warburton, & Westrom, 2003).

Rectovaginal Examination

The rectovaginal examination (RVE) can be used for additional evaluation, if needed, and is typically performed after bimanual examination is completed. It is used to further assess the uterus, uterosacral ligaments, and the rectovaginal septum. Clean gloves should be donned prior to completing the RVE. The first finger of the dominant hand is placed into the vagina and the middle finger of the same hand is placed into the rectum. Gentle upward pressure of the middle finger allows for the assessment of the rectovaginal septum. The uterosacral ligaments can be palpated by locating them along the posterior wall of the cervix, lateral to the sacrum. A retroverted uterus can also be examined using this method. Examination should evaluate for any abnormalities, including tenderness, nodules, or apparent thickening or thinning. Abnormalities

found on this examination will require further evaluation. See the Evidence-Based Practice Considerations section for the Female Genitourinary System for more information on appropriate use of this assessment technique.

LIFE-SPAN CONSIDERATIONS FOR PHYSICAL EXAMINATION

Infancy

The physical examination for the infant should include an evaluation of the genitalia to assess for any abnormal findings (AAP, 2017b). This is best performed with the infant in the supine position with hips flexed and abducted. Inspection should include evaluation of the labia, clitoris, vaginal introitus, and urethral meatus. Any abnormal findings of the genitalia will require further evaluation.

Atypical/Ambiguous Genitalia

Atypical/ambiguous genital is a term used to describe an infant with visible atypical appearing genitalia. Further evaluation is indicated for all infants presenting with atypical genitalia.

Imperforate Hymen

An *imperforate hymen* refers to hymenal tissue that is completely fused together, forming an obstruction to the vaginal opening. This is a relatively uncommon finding and can be identified with a thorough genital examination of an infant. Failure to diagnose this problem early can result in fertility issues, endometriosis, and renal issues (Lee et al., 2019).

Precocious Puberty

Precocious puberty refers to pubertal development at an age of 2 to 2.5 standard deviations earlier than population norms. It should be suspected in a child with early development of secondary sexual characteristics. Precocious puberty may reflect a normal variant of puberty or, less commonly, a pathologic condition with associated morbidity and mortality. Historically, puberty is considered precocious if it starts before age 8 in females. Several studies have identified that in addition to age, the child's body mass index (BMI) and racial/ethnic background need to be taken into consideration. Black and Hispanic girls, as well as overweight girls, have been noted to undergo earlier pubertal development (Biro et al., 2010; Rosenfield, Lipton, & Drum, 2009). Although the majority of cases of precocious puberty, particularly in girls, are a normal variant of pubertal development, close monitoring and further evaluation may be necessary to rule out the underlying pathology (Kaplowitz & Bloch, 2016).

Middle Childhood

The AAP (2017c) identifies physical growth and development as priorities in the middle-aged child. An assessment for sexual maturity should be performed at each well-child visit.

Adolescence

The AAP (2017a) suggests that beginning in early adolescence, the clinician should arrange to spend part of the visit alone with the adolescent. This avenue allows for the adolescent to develop a personal relationship with their healthcare clinician (AAP, 2017a). A personal relationship can encourage full disclosure of health information and support developing self-confidence and self-management (AAP, 2017a). Priorities during this time include risk reduction—including pregnancy and STIs (AAP, 2017a). The developing adolescent female often has concerns about her changing body. The well examination is an opportunity to discuss these changes in a safe environment and to provide accurate messages regarding body image, menstrual cycle, and developmental changes.

Genital examination in this age group should include an assessment of the hymen. Bulging in the hymenal area, amenorrhea with cyclic lower abdominal pain, or urinary retention should prompt further evaluation as they are signs of an imperforate hymen. Diagnosis of imperforate hymen can be overlooked in infancy and childhood (Lee et al., 2019).

Postmenopausal Considerations

The decrease in estrogen levels during the menopause transition results in thinning of the vaginal tissue. This thinning causes decreased elasticity of the tissue, a paler appearance, and more fragile tissue (Lobo, 2017). This can result in vaginal dryness and petechiae (Lobo, 2017). These changes can range from asymptomatic to moderate-to-severe dyspareunia, vaginal discomfort, and irritation (Bachman, Lobo, Gut, Nachtigall, & Notelovitz, 2008). As a result of these changes, speculum examination may be uncomfortable for the postmenopausal patient. Consider use of water-based lubrication, as previously discussed, and a smaller size speculum.

SPECIAL POPULATION CONSIDERATIONS FOR PHYSICAL EXAMINATION

Victims of Sexual Violence and Trauma

A victim of sexual violence is defined as having experienced one or more of the following: "rape, being made to penetrate someone else, sexual coercion, and unwanted sexual contact" (S. G. Smith et al., 2018, p. 1). It is a common occurrence among females, affecting approximately 43.6% of women in the United States (S. G. Smith et al., 2018). According to the U.S. Agency for Healthcare Research and Quality (AHRQ, 2015), "one out of every 6 American women has been the victim of an attempted or completed rape in her lifetime" (para. 2).

Sexual violence is only one form of trauma a woman can experience. Currently in the United States, "nearly one in three adult women experience at least one physical assault by a partner during adulthood" (AHRQ, 2015, para. 1). Equally concerning is that "by the age of 13 . . . one out of every five girls are sexually abused" (AHRQ, 2015, para. 3). Given the significance of this problem, clinicians caring for women of all ages should be aware of the potential for a history of violence or other trauma. Trauma-informed care provides a framework for assisting patients with this unfortunate history. Chapter 24, Evidence-Based Assessment and Screening for Traumatic Experiences: Abuse, Neglect, and Intimate Partner Violence, provides more information on this topic.

Trauma-Informed Care

Trauma-informed care provides a framework for engaging with individuals who have had a history of trauma. There are four basic principles that direct trauma-informed care: an awareness of the prevalence of traumatic events, an ability to recognize the signs and symptoms of trauma, development of policies and practices that integrate knowledge regarding trauma, and avoiding retraumatization of the individual during the history and patient examination (AHRQ, 2015).

The pelvic examination can be an anxiety-inducing experience for a woman and is often more problematic for women who have experienced sexual violence. It is important to have an open dialogue with the patient during all portions of the examination. Obtain permission to perform each part of the examination, explaining what the examination entails and the purpose for doing it. And finally, give her permission to stop the examination at any time should she wish to end it or take a break. Review the suggestions regarding preparing the patient as these are applicable for the woman who has been a victim of violence. Identification of trauma-affected women and a sensitive approach to their individual concerns and needs will strengthen the clinician–patient relationship and allow for appropriate referrals for further assessment, support, and treatment.

LGBTQ+ Populations

See Chapter 18, Evidence-Based Assessment of Sexual Orientation, Gender Identity, and Health.

Women With Disabilities

Disability, as defined by the World Health Organization (WHO, n.d.-a), is "an umbrella term, covering impairments, activity limitations, and participation restrictions" (para. 1). Approximately 12.8% of all Americans report having a disability (Kaiser Family Foundation [KFF], 2019). Individuals with disabilities are at increased risk for social and health-related disparities (Havercamp & Scott, 2015).

Women with disabilities are still in need of the same screening and preventive care offered to those without disabilities. Clinicians must be sure to use a sensitive approach and avoid making assumptions about a woman's abilities based on appearances. The examination approach may need to be modified to accommodate the patient's disability.

Female Genital Cutting

Female genital cutting has also been referred to as female circumcision or genital mutilation. It is a cultural practice, predominantly in Asia and Africa, defined as "all procedures involving partial or total removal of the external female genitalia or other injury to the female genital organs for non-medical reasons" (WHO, n.d.-b, "Overview"). Female genital cutting affects approximately 200 million girls and women worldwide (United Nations Children's Fund, 2019). Female genital cutting has no health benefits and causes short- and long-term complications. Immediate complications include severe pain, fever, swelling, bleeding, and urinary problems. These procedures have associated morbidity and mortality. Long-term complications include chronic infection, menstrual disorders, dyspareunia, sexual dysfunction, and an increased risk of childbirth complications for the mother and baby. The WHO has been involved in international, regional, and local efforts to eliminate the practice of female genital cutting and to provide care for those who have experienced this practice.

LABORATORY CONSIDERATIONS FOR THE GENITOURINARY SYSTEM

CERVICAL CYTOLOGY

Cervical cytology testing is most commonly obtained for routine screening for cervical cancer. There are two types of cervical cytology samples: the conventional Pap smear and the liquid-based thin-layer preparation, which is the most commonly used preparation for cervical cytology testing. Use of the liquid-based thin-layer preparation has improved the quality of cytology samples collected (Sigurdsson, 2013). See the Evidence-Based Practice Considerations for the Female Genitourinary System section for a discussion on the guidelines for cervical cytology collection.

There are several collection tools available. Most commonly a broomlike tool or cervix-brush is used, although using both a cytobrush and plastic spatula is also appropriate. These collection tools are shown in **Figure 20.12**. Wooden spatulas should be avoided for Pap testing as cellular material has been found to stick to the spatula. It is best practice to use the sampling devices provided by the supplier of the liquid-based thin-layer testing kit.

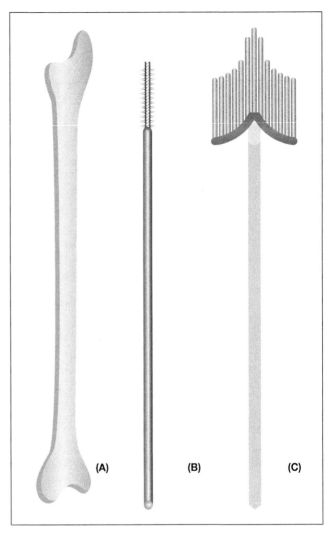

FIGURE 20.12 Collection tools for Pap testing. (A) Spatula. (B) Cytobrush. (C) Cervix-brush.

Ideally, women should avoid use of douching, intravaginal medications, intercourse, or tampon use 48 hours prior to Pap smear collection, and sampling should be avoided, if possible, during heavy menstrual cycle bleeding, all of which can prevent collection of adequate cells for evaluation. Use a cotton swab to remove excessive mucus, discharge, or menstrual blood if it is obscuring the os.

Carefully completing the collection of endocervical and cervical cells by meticulously following the technique recommended is required if an adequate specimen is to be evaluated for cellular changes. These techniques vary depending on the collection tools used. For example, using the cervix-brush requires rotating this broomlike device when placed in the cervical os for specimen collection. **Figure 20.13** depicts the collection of a cervical specimen using the broomlike tool. With the two-device technique, the spatula is placed on the surface of the cervix for collection of endocervical

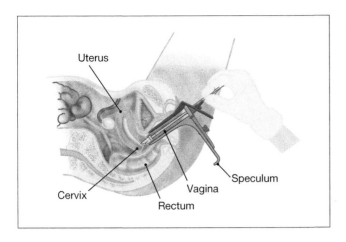

FIGURE 20.13 Collection of cervical specimen for Pap testing.

cells and rotated 360°; next, the cytobrush is inserted into the cervical os, completing no more than a 180° rotation, using care not to overrotate (Hologic, 2017). Care should also be taken to note how the cells should be transferred from the tools into the collection vial. The following link provides video instructions on proper liquid-based cytology collection protocol: https://cytologystuff.com/watch/specimen-collection-video.

WET MOUNT

A vaginal wet mount or wet prep is a laboratory test that involves evaluating a sample of vaginal discharge under a microscope. A wet mount is performed for evaluation of vaginal symptoms, including odor, discharge, irritation, itching, or discomfort. The microscopy may be done in office or may be sent to a laboratory; the sample is collected by using a cotton-tipped swab to collect discharge from the vaginal walls. The sample of vaginal secretions is typically placed into a collection vial with normal saline. Infections commonly diagnosed by using a wet mount include candidiasis, trichomoniasis, and BV. In lieu of saline, potassium hydroxide (KOH) can also be used to diagnosis vulvovaginal candidiasis (VVC). Visualization of blastospores and pseudohyphae (commonly called buds and hyphae) would indicate that a fungal infection is present.

Traditionally, the sample for evaluation with wet or KOH mount has been collected by the clinician during a speculum examination. Recent evidence suggests that patient self-collected samples in uncomplicated cases of vaginal concerns provide adequate sensitivity and specificity when compared with clinician-collected samples, with sensitivity of 70% to 100% and specificity of 97% to 100%, respectively (Kashyap, Singh, Bhalla, Arora, & Aggarwal, 2008; Morgan et al., 1996; Nelson, Bellamy, Gray, & Nachamkin, 2003; Strauss, Eucker, Savitz, & Thorp, 2005; Tanksale et al., 2003). To obtain

a sufficient self-collected sample, the patient should be instructed to insert the cotton-tipped swab into the vagina at least 1 inch (Paladine & Desai, 2018).

TESTING FOR SEXUALLY TRANSMITTED INFECTIONS

Nucleic acid amplification tests are used to screen for gonorrhea and chlamydia. These DNA tests can be performed from specimens collected from a variety of sites including urine, clinician-collected endocervical samples, and clinician or patient-collected vaginal specimens (USPSTF, 2014). See the Evidence-Based Practice Considerations for the Female Genitourinary System section for a discussion on the guidelines for testing for STI.

HUMAN PAPILLOMAVIRUS TESTING

HPV is a double-stranded DNA virus known to infect epithelial cells (J. K. Wolf & Ramirez, 2001) and is spread by sexual contact during oral, vaginal, or anal sex (CDC, n.d.-e). There are over 200 different types of HPV, classified as high-risk HPV (oncogenic, or cancer-causing) and low-risk HPV (wart-causing; National Cancer Institute, 2019a). More than 90% of cervical cancers are caused by infection with high-risk HPV (Bosch, Lorincz, Munoz, Meijer, & Shah, 2002). Of the multiple high-risk types of HPV, types 16 and 18 are most commonly associated with cervical cancer, which account for approximately 70% of all cervical cancers (Braaten & Laufer, 2008; Lowy & Schiller, 2012).

Testing for HPV can be performed as a stand-alone test or in conjunction with collection of cervical cytology. There are several types of HPV tests approved by the U.S. Food and Drug Administration (FDA) and all of them test for the 13 most common types of high-risk HPV. There is no role for screening for low-risk HPV types (American Society for Colposcopy and Cervical Pathology, 2017). See the Evidence-Based Practice Considerations for the Female Genitourinary System section for HPV testing guidelines.

IMAGING CONSIDERATIONS FOR THE FEMALE GENITOURINARY SYSTEM

TRANSVAGINAL AND TRANSABDOMINAL PELVIC ULTRASOUND

Ultrasound is the radiologic modality of choice to evaluate the pelvic structures in women, as good visualization of the pelvic anatomy is possible without the risk of radiation exposure. A transvaginal ultrasound (TVUS) is the most commonly performed ultrasound and involves introducing an ultrasound probe into the vagina to evaluate uterine and ovarian structures. A TVUS is performed with the ultrasound probe on the abdomen and is frequently done in conjunction with a TVUS to complement the TVUS images. Occasionally, when a woman cannot tolerate the vaginal ultrasound probe (e.g., in a virginal patient), transabdominal images are performed without the TVUS. Fetal evaluation is also performed using the transabdominal approach. Common indications for ultrasound imaging include abnormal vaginal bleeding, pelvic pain, and evaluation for ectopic pregnancy (American College of Radiology, 2014).

EVIDENCE-BASED PRACTICE CONSIDERATIONS FOR THE FEMALE GENITOURINARY SYSTEM

THE WELL-WOMAN EXAMINATION

Until recently, it was a common practice for women to have a gynecologic examination annually. In fact, most insurance companies allowed female patients to have two primary care clinicians: one for their reproductive needs and one for their general health needs. In practice, some women did see both a general practitioner and a clinician focused on women's health, whereas some would choose to only see a women's health clinician for all their needs and some a family practice clinician for all their needs.

Historically, during an annual women's health examination in a nonpregnant female, practitioners would conduct a history focused primarily on reproductive issues and perform a gynecologic-focused physical examination. This examination usually consisted of a breast examination, a speculum examination, bimanual pelvic examination, and a Pap test. Whereas many women's health clinicians also examined other organ systems (thyroid, heart, lungs, abdomen), the annual reproductive-focused gynecologic examination and Pap testing became the norm in this setting.

Today, the ACOG (2018a) continues to promote the benefits of a periodic well-woman examination. They acknowledge the benefit of a comprehensive health history and support the visit as an opportunity for health promotion and counseling, as well as engaging patients in shared decision-making as outlined in the **Exhibit 20.1**.

PELVIC EXAMINATIONS FOR ASYMPTOMATIC AND NONPREGNANT ADULT WOMEN

Recent changes to recommendations for cervical cancer screening and prevention have brought into question not only how frequently women's health

examinations are warranted, but also what type of examination *should* be done. Because of the extensive evidence correlating cervical cancer and high-risk strains of HPV, in addition to improved technology for screening of high-risk HPV, current guidelines no longer recommend the annual Pap test (Practice Bulletin No. 168, ACOG, 2016a). Instead, the focus has shifted to prevention through vaccination.

However, whereas yearly Pap testing is no longer recommended, Bibbins-Domingo et al. (2017) concluded that there was no direct evidence to support or discourage periodic pelvic examinations (apart from the annual "Pap smear"). In fact, the USPSTF notes that no trials have evaluated the screening pelvic examination in relation to mortality, cancer reduction, disease-specific morbidity, or quality of life (Bibbins-Domingo et al., 2017). Few studies evaluated the screening accuracy of a pelvic examination for identifying ovarian cancer, BV, trichomoniasis, or genital herpes. Studies examining infectious disease were frequently conducted in high-prevalence populations, and, despite high specificity, largely demonstrated low specificity and negative predictive value (Guirguis-Blake, Henderson, & Perdue, 2017). Conversely, ovarian cancer, because of its low prevalence, was found to have a wide range of sensitivity (0%–100%) and low positive predictive value. Consequently, the USPSTF found insufficient evidence to make a recommendation on the screening pelvic examination (grade I; Bibbins-Domingo et al., 2017).

CERVICAL CANCER SCREENING AND HUMAN PAPILLOMAVIRUS TESTING

Screening recommendations for the detection of cervical cancer are complex. As previously noted, infection from high-risk strains of HPV is the most common cause of cervical cancer. The current evidence-based guidelines from the USPSTF (2018a) for women aged 21 to 65 years are considered grade A recommendations and for women older than 65 years or younger than 21 years are considered grade D recommendations. See **Table 20.7** for a summary of current USPSTF recommendations regarding the use of cytology or Pap testing and screening for HPV.

HUMAN PAPILLOMAVIRUS VACCINATION

HPV is the most common sexually transmitted infection. A total of 79 million Americans currently have HPV, and 14 million more become infected each year; while some types of HPV resolve without causing health problems, other types cause genital warts, and cancers of the cervix, vulva, penis, or anus (CDC, n.d.-e). Every year in the United States, more than 19,000 women and 12,000

EXHIBIT 20.1 Education Handout: Why You Should Have a Well-Woman Exam!

Family Planning

Birth control	Discuss birth control options, which can be using pills, patch, intrauterine device, condom, or implant, and choose a method that is best for you.
Prepregnancy counseling	If you are planning to become pregnant, schedule a time to talk about your reproductive and family history. Discuss diet, exercise, and activities that can lead to a healthier pregnancy and a healthier you!

Preventive Care

Vaccinations	Discuss risks and benefits of protecting yourself from diseases such as flu, human papillomavirus (HPV), rubella, and more. Take action to stay healthy.
Weight control	Learn about healthy weight, your ideal body mass index (BMI), and risks of obesity. Your healthcare clinician can help you with diet, exercise, and weight-related problems.

Disease Screenings

Cancer screening	Schedule time for your healthcare clinician to inform you about recommended screening for breast cancer, cervical cancer, colon cancer, and others based on your age, gender, race, and risk factors. Early detection leads to better outcomes.
Depression screening	Depression is both common and a serious health issue. Depression can range from mild to severe. Your healthcare clinician can discuss your symptoms and concerns and help identify ways to help.
Screening for STIs	STIs such as genital herpes, gonorrhea, chlamydia, HIV, and some forms of hepatitis can all be transmitted through sexual contact. Talk to your healthcare clinician about your risk.
Disease screening	Your annual well-woman examination is a great time to check your blood pressure, screen you for diabetes, and assess your risk for osteoporosis and heart disease.

Concerns

Concerns about sex/sexuality	A well-woman examination is the ideal time to address concerns related to intimacy, sexual orientation, sexual expression, and gender identification. These common, sensitive issues can be discussed during a well examination.
Menstrual issues	Premenstrual syndrome, heavy bleeding, weight gain, painful cramping, and irregular cycles are some of the concerns that you may want to discuss.
Other reasons	Other concerns related to female organs or to general women's health can be addressed at your well-woman examination.

STIs, sexually transmitted infections.
Source: Adapted from The American College of Obstetricians and Gynecologists. (2015). Annual well-woman exam infographic. Retrieved from https://www.acog.org/About-ACOG/ACOG-Departments/Annual-Womens-Health-Care/Annual-Well-Woman-Exam-Infographic?IsMobileSet=false

men are diagnosed with a cancer caused by HPV infection; subsequently, more than 4,000 women die every year from cervical cancer (CDC, n.d.-e).

The CDC recommends routine HPV vaccination for adolescents at age 11 or 12 years; this is a grade A evidence-based recommendation according to the Advisory Committee on Immunization Practices (ACIP; CDC, n.d.-a; Markowitz et al., 2014; Meites, Kempe, & Markowitz, 2016). The vaccine may be started as early as 9 years of age and is also recommended for females aged 13 to 26 years and males aged 13 to 21 years who

are not previously vaccinated. The safety and efficacy of the HPV vaccine is well-researched and documented.

ASSESSMENT AND SCREENING FOR BREAST, OVARIAN, AND ENDOMETRIAL CANCERS

The most common malignancies related specifically to women's health are breast, ovarian, and endometrial cancers (ACOG, 2015). Routine assessments should be completed to determine each individual's personal risk for developing malignancies. Because

TABLE 20.7 USPSTF Cervical Cancer Screening Recommendations

Population	Women aged 21–29 years	Women aged 30–65 years	Women aged <21 years, women aged >65 years with adequate prior screening, and women posthysterectomy
Recommendation	Screen for cervical cancer every 3 years with cytology alone	Screen for cervical cancer every 3 years with cytology alone, every 5 years with high-risk HPV testing alone, or every 5 years with co-testing.	Do not screen for cervical cancer
Risk assessment	All women aged 21–65 years are at risk for cervical cancer because of potential exposure to high-risk HPV types through sexual intercourse and should be screened. Certain risk factors further increase risk for cervical cancer, including HIV infection, a compromised immune system, in-utero exposure to diethylstilbestrol (DES), and previous treatment of a high-grade precancerous lesion or cervical cancer. Women with these risk factors should receive individualized follow-up.		
Screening tests	Screening with cervical cytology alone, primary testing for high-risk HPV alone, or both at the same time (co-testing) can detect high-grade precancerous cervical lesions and cervical cancer. Clinicians should focus on ensuring that women receive adequate screening, appropriate evaluation of abnormal results, and indicated treatment, regardless of which screening strategy is used.		

HPV, human papillomavirus; USPSTF, U.S. Preventative Services Task Force.
Source: From U.S. Preventive Services Task Force. (2018a, August). Clinical summary: Cervical cancer: Screening. Retrieved from https://www.uspreventiveservicestaskforce.org/Page/Document/ClinicalSummaryFinal/cervical-cancer-screening2

cancer risk is determined by a complex interaction between genetics and the environment, no single set of personal characteristics or behaviors, history questions, family history, or genetic tests can independently predict the likelihood of developing a malignancy. It is for this reason that routine history and physical examination continue to play an important role in primary, secondary, and tertiary prevention. Women should be routinely advised of modifiable behaviors, for example, smoking, and exposures that place them at higher risk for a malignancy. In addition to screening for risks of these cancers, the American Society of Clinical Oncology (ASCO) recommends that patients *with* cancer have a more detailed family history completed at diagnosis and periodically thereafter (Lu et al., 2014). Minimum recommended elements for adequate cancer family history include both maternal and paternal cancer diagnoses, age of cancer diagnoses in family member, type of cancers in both first- and second-degree relatives, and results of any genetic testing.

It should be noted that the presence or absence of hereditary breast or ovarian cancer (HBOC) genetic markers does not make or exclude a diagnosis of malignancy. There are a number of secondary prevention measures commonly recommended for women. Refer to Chapter 17, Evidence-Based Assessment of the Breasts and Axillae, for specific screening recommendations

for breast cancer screening, and Chapter 15, Evidence-Based Assessment of the Musculoskeletal System, for colon cancer screening recommendations. The USPSTF (2018b) currently recommends against (grade D) screening for ovarian cancer in asymptomatic women.

The current USPSTF (2019) recommendation for BRCA screening is grade B for a woman who has a family history of breast, ovarian, tubal, or peritoneal cancer; for women without a family history, recommending BRCA screening is grade D. Identification of risks can be done with any number of validated risk assessment tools. The USPSTF evaluated specifically the Ontario Family History Assessment Tool, Manchester Scoring System, Referral Screening Tool, Pedigree Assessment Tool, and Family History Screen 7 (FHS-7) in developing these recommendations (Moyer et al., 2014). Women who are screened positive should be referred for genetic counseling. Only after genetic counseling should a decision be made regarding genetic testing.

HIV SCREENING

Both the CDC and the USPSTF recommend that all pregnant women should be screened for HIV as part of a prenatal assessment (Branson et al., 2006; Moyer et al., 2013). Additionally, screening recommendations from the CDC encourage the screening of all individuals 13 to 64 years of age at least once and persons at higher risk annually (CDC, 2015). An update to the USPSTF HIV screening recommendations is currently underway; refer to Chapter 10, Evidence-Based Assessment of the Lymphatic System, for more information on the pathophysiology, assessment, and diagnosis of HIV.

SEXUALLY TRANSMITTED INFECTION SCREENING

Gonorrhea

Screening recommendations from the USPSTF (2014) and the CDC (2015) encourage annual screening for gonorrhea for all sexually active women aged 24 years and younger and older women who are at increased risk.

Chlamydia

Screening recommendations from the USPSTF (2014) and the CDC (2015) encourage annual screening for chlamydia for all sexually active women aged 24 years and younger and older women who are at increased risk.

Trichomonas

The CDC does not have a formal recommendation for screening for trichomonas. Consideration should be given for screening women at high risk for infection and those receiving care in high-prevalence settings, such as correctional institutions or STI clinics (CDC, 2015). Women infected with HIV should be screened initially when care is established, and then annually (CDC, Health Resources and Services Administration, National Institutes of Health, HIV Medicine Association of the Infectious Diseases Society of America, HIV Prevention in Clinical Care Working Group, 2004).

Syphilis

Screening recommendations from the USPSTF (2016) encourage screening of all asymptomatic, nonpregnant adults and adolescents at increased risk. Those at increased risk include women living with HIV, individuals who have been incarcerated, and those who participate in commercial sex work. Clinicians should also consider the incidence and prevalence of syphilis in their community and patient population.

Genital Warts

Genital warts are most commonly caused by HPV types 6 and 11, which are considered low-risk for cervical cancer. Neither the USPSTF nor the CDC recommend screening for genital warts. Cervical screening cannot detect whether an individual has genital warts.

Diagnosis of genital warts can only be made with direct visualization. However, there is insufficient evidence based on this alone to recommend annual pelvic examinations.

Genital Herpes

The USPSTF (2016) recommends against routine serologic screening for genital herpes simplex virus (HSV) infection in asymptomatic adolescents and adults, including pregnant women. This is supported by the American Academy of Family Physicians (AAFP, 2018). The CDC (2015) suggests that consideration be given for HSV serologic testing for women that request an STI evaluation, particularly if they have multiple sexual partners.

FAMILY PLANNING

Family planning is one of the major reasons that women seek gynecologic care. Although much of this chapter has focused on health promotion, disease prevention, and illness diagnosis, the importance of family planning should be underscored. After all, the need for well-woman care stems from the need to provide care for a woman's reproductive needs. According to *Healthy People 2020* (Office of Disease Prevention and Health Promotion, n.d.), family planning is one of the top 10 public health achievements of the 20th century. Access to family planning allows women to plan for birth spacing and family size, which contributes to improved health outcomes.

Providing Quality Family Planning (QFP) is a joint initiative by the CDC and the Office of Population Affairs of the Department of Health and Human Services. In recognizing the challenges that the United States faces, including high rates of unintended pregnancy, adolescent pregnancy, preterm births, and infant mortality, these agencies developed recommendations for providing family planning services to address these issues (Gavin et al., 2014). They identified and provided recommendations in six key areas: contraception, pregnancy testing and counseling, achieving pregnancy, basic infertility services, preconception health, and STI diagnosis and treatment (Gavin et al., 2014). The Oregon Health Authority proposed the One Key Question (Allen, Hunter, Wood, & Beeson, 2017) "Would you like to become pregnant in the next year?" as a simple way to begin the conversation about family planning.

It is beyond the scope of this physical assessment text to review the guidelines for family planning, as most relate to management and shared decision-making of care. However, it is worth noting that the Joint Committee of the American College of Obstetricians and Gynecologists and the American

Society of Reproductive Medicine (2019) recommend that any patient encounter with a nonpregnant women or male with reproductive capacity be used as an opportunity for promoting wellness counseling toward improving reproductive and obstetric outcomes and support the use of "Would you like to become pregnant in the next year?" The QFP further recommends contraceptive services to all who wish to prevent pregnancy (Gavin et al., 2014). Together, these two recommendations have the potential to promote discussions and shared decisions between patients and clinicians that can help reach the *Healthy People 2020* Family Planning goals (Office of Disease Prevention and Health Promotion, n.d.).

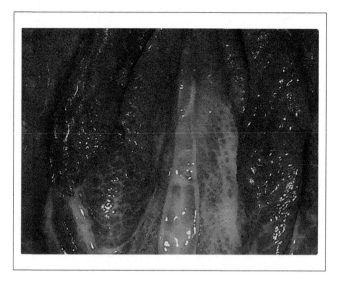

FIGURE 20.14 Cervical discharge caused by gonococcal infection.

ABNORMAL FINDINGS OF THE FEMALE GENITOURINARY SYSTEM

SEXUALLY TRANSMITTED INFECTIONS

Gonorrhea

Gonorrhea is an STI caused by the bacterium *Neisseria gonorrhoeae*, which most commonly infects the cervix, uterus, fallopian tubes, and urethra. Gonorrhea is transmitted by sexual contact via the mouth, penis, vagina, or anus of an infected partner and is the second most commonly reported STI (CDC, n.d.-g).

Key History and Physical Findings
- Asymptomatic in majority of women
- Mid-cycle vaginal bleeding
- Vaginal discharge (**Figure 20.14**)
- Dysuria
- In severe or untreated cases, PID may develop

Chlamydia

Chlamydia is the most commonly reported bacterial STI, and women aged 15 to 24 years account for 44% of cases (CDC, 2019). It is caused by an infection with the bacterium *Chlamydia trachomatis* and is transmitted through sexual contact, similar to gonorrheal infections (**Figure 20.15**). It is a common cause of cervicitis in women, although most women with chlamydia are not symptomatic (CDC, n.d.-d).

Key History and Physical Findings
- Asymptomatic in majority of women (only 5%–30% develop symptoms)
- Abnormal vaginal discharge
- Easily induced endocervical bleeding
- Dysuria
- Pyuria
- Urinary frequency

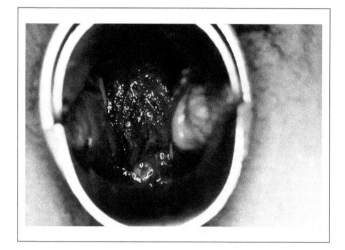

FIGURE 20.15 *Chlamydia trachomatis* infection. Colposcopic view of a female patient's cervix, which manifested signs of erosion and erythema because of infection.

Source: Centers for Disease Control and Prevention; Lourdes Fraw, MD; and Jim Pledger.

- Severe or untreated infections can result in PID, infertility, increased risk for ectopic pregnancy, and chronic pelvic pain (CDC, n.d.-d). See the Pelvic Inflammatory Disease section for details of this problem
- If the infection is in the rectum, it may cause rectal pain, rectal bleeding, and/or rectal discharge (CDC, n.d.-d).

Trichomonas

Trichomoniasis is an STI that is caused by an infection with the protozoal parasite *Trichomonas vaginalis*. It is the most common nonviral STI in the world (Kissinger, 2015). The majority of infected women are asymptomatic (CDC, n.d.-j). Historically, trichomonas has been thought of as just a bothersome STI; however, it is now recognized for its role in increasing infection with and transmission of HIV (Guenthner, Secor, & Dezzutti, 2005).

Key History and Physical Findings
- Asymptomatic in majority of women
- Greenish-yellow, frothy, and malodorous vaginal discharge
- Dysuria
- Irritation and itching of the vulva (n.d.-j)
- Erythematous vulvar tissue and vaginal mucosa
- Trichomonas noted on microscopy
- "Strawberry cervix" is a rare but pathognomonic finding that results from punctate hemorrhages on the cervix and vaginal tissue (**Figure 20.16**)

Syphilis

Syphilis is an STI caused by the bacterium *Treponema pallidum*. An infection with syphilis can present in a variety of ways depending on the stage of infection. It is referred to as "The Great Pretender," as its symptoms are similar to many other diseases (CDC, n.d.-i). Syphilis infections are on the rise and have increased by 34% in women from 2017 to 2018 (CDC, 2019). Syphilis is

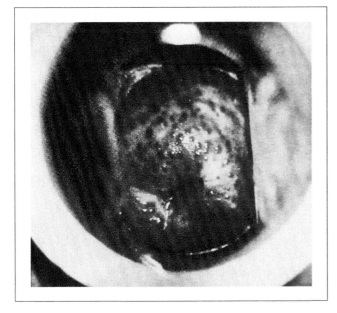

FIGURE 20.16 *Trichomonas vaginalis* infection.
Colposcopic view of a female patient's cervix, revealing what is referred to as a strawberry cervix.

Source: Centers for Disease Control and Prevention.

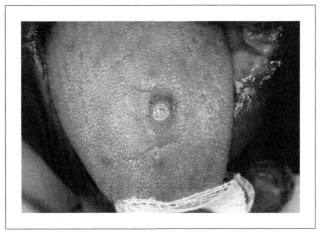

FIGURE 20.17 Primary syphilitic chancre of the tongue.
Source: Centers for Disease Control and Prevention/Robert E. Sumpter.

spread by direct contact with a painless sore, known as a chancre. Chancres are typically found on the genitals, mouth/throat, anus, or vagina (**Figure 20.17**). Syphilis can also spread from a pregnant woman to her fetus, which is referred to as congenital syphilis. Congenital syphilis can lead to stillbirth, developmental delay, seizures, and death (CDC, n.d.-i). Syphilis is progressive if not treated and is classified by stage (primary, secondary, latent, or tertiary).

Key History and Physical Findings
Primary stage
- Chancre (raised lesion, with an indurated margin, approximately 1–2 cm in size)
- Typically occurs 21 days after exposure
- Positive nontreponemal test (i.e., Venereal Disease Research Laboratory [VDRL] or rapid plasma reagin [RPR]) *and* a positive treponemal test (i.e., fluorescent treponemal antibody absorbed [FTA-ABS] tests, the *T. pallidum* passive particle agglutination [TP-PA] assay, various enzyme immunoassays [EIAs], chemiluminescence immunoassays, immunoblots, or rapid treponemal assays; CDC, n.d.-i)

Secondary stage
- Palmar rash on the hands and bottoms of the feet (typically appears rough and red and does not usually cause itching; **Figure 20.18**)
- Fatigue
- Fevers
- Lymphadenopathy
- Hair loss
- Weight loss
- Myalgias
- The symptoms will eventually resolve even if no treatment is provided (CDC, n.d.-i).

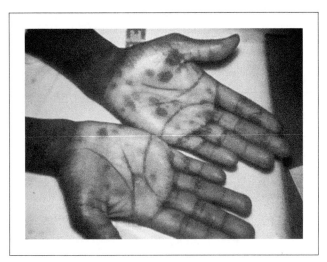

FIGURE 20.18 Palmar rash on palms of hands because of secondary syphilis.
Source: Centers for Disease Control and Prevention.

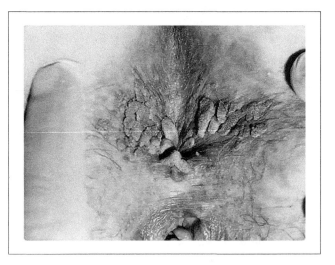

FIGURE 20.19 Genital warts found on perineum.
Source: Image courtesy of SOA-AIDS Amsterdam.

Latent stage
- Time when no symptoms are present
- Can last for years
- Continue to be contagious (CDC, n.d.-i)

Tertiary stage
- Typically occurs 10 to 30 years after initial infection
- Can be fatal
- Symptoms of tertiary syphilis depend on the organ system affected and can cause infection in the nervous system, eyes, vascular and cardiac system, liver, bones, and joints (CDC, n.d.-i).

Genital Warts (Condyloma acuminata)

HPV types 6 and 11 are the most common cause of genital warts. In the United States, approximately 1 in 100 sexually active adults has genital warts (CDC, n.d.-e). Vaccination with the HPV vaccine provides protection against HPV types 6 and 11, which is most commonly associated with genital warts (CDC, n.d.-d).

Key History and Physical Findings
- Flat, papular, or pedunculated growths on the genital mucosa and surrounding skin of the perineal area, including the groin, suprapubic or perianal region, and vulva (**Figure 20.19**)
- Can also develop on the cervix, urethra, and in the anal canal
- Can appear as single lesions or grouped together in a cauliflower-shaped growth
- Can present in a variety of colors and include flesh tones, white, pink, or red
- Rarely painful or pruritic

Genital Herpes

Genital herpes is a viral STI that is caused by the herpes simplex virus type 1 (HSV-1) or type 2 (HSV-2). The prevalence of HSV-2 infections among people 14 to 49 years of age was 11.9% (McQuillan, Kruszon-Moran, Flagg, & Paulose-Ram, 2018). Females have a higher prevalence of both HSV-1 and HSV-2 infections than their male counterparts (McQuillan et al., 2018). Although there is no cure for a viral herpes infection, there are treatment options available to help manage outbreaks (CDC, n.d.-f).

Historically, HSV-1 infection typically occurred during childhood and was transferred nonsexually, whereas HSV-2 was almost always sexually transmitted (Bradley, Markowitz, Gibson, & McQuillan, 2014). More recently, genital herpes infections with HSV-1 have been increasing and are now more common than genital herpes infection with HSV-2 in young women (Bernstein et al., 2013). HSV infections can be transmitted via contact with infected herpes lesions, genital and oral secretions, or mucosa. The virus can be shed from normal appearing skin/tissues, and many people are not aware they are infected and have no symptoms (Wald et al., 2000). A primary herpes infection occurs when a patient without antibodies to HSV develops an infection (Garland, Eundem, & Steben, 2014). Only 10% to 25% of people develop clinically evident lesions with a primary herpes infection (Garland et al., 2014). Recurrent outbreaks usually have a shorter duration and less severe symptoms.

Key History and Physical Findings
- One or more vesicular lesions that rupture and become ulcerated (**Figure 20.20**)
- Lesions are usually located around the mouth or genital area, including the rectum.

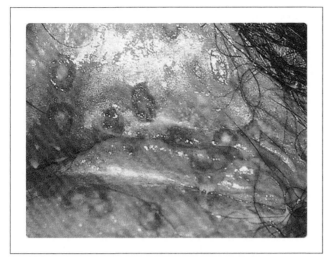

FIGURE 20.20 Ulcerated lesions of genital herpes infection.
Source: Image courtesy of SOA-AIDS Amsterdam.

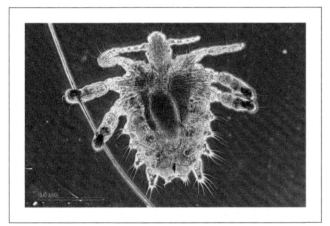

FIGURE 20.21 Optical microscopic image of a pubic (crab) louse.
Source: Image courtesy of Josef Reischig, CSc.

- Lesions are very painful and remain so until they have healed.
- In a primary infection, individual can experience flu-like symptoms, including body aches, fever/chills, headache, and lymphadenopathy (Kimberlin & Rouse, 2004).

Pubic Lice (Pediculosis Pubis)

Pubic lice are translucent parasites that are usually spread through sexual contact (**Figure 20.21**). They feed on the blood of their human host (CDC, n.d.-c). Transmission through fomites (e.g., towels, clothing, or linens) is possible, but much less likely (Leone, 2007). Condoms do not provide protection against pubic lice infestation (Leone, 2007).

Key History and Physical Findings
- Itching in the pubic area because of irritation from the feeding lice (Leone, 2007)
- Visible live lice and/or nits in the pubic hair

Pelvic Inflammatory Disease

PID involves infection and inflammation of the upper genital tract organs, including the uterus and/or fallopian tubes. PID can arise from a variety of infections; gonorrheal and chlamydial infections account for almost one-half of all cases of PID. BV, mycoplasma genitalium, and other endogenous microorganisms have also been known to cause PID (Haggerty et al., 2016). PID can lead to infertility resulting from damage to the upper genital tract organs (CDC, n.d.-h). The symptoms of PID range from mild to severe.

Key History and Physical Findings
- Asymptomatic
- Lower abdominal/pelvic pain
- Vaginal discharge
- Fever
- Pain with intercourse
- Frequent urination
- Tenderness on bimanual examination, including CMT (CDC, n.d.-h)
- Positive STI culture (gonorrhea, chlamydia, trichomonas, and/or BV)

VAGINITIS/VAGINOSIS

Bacterial Vaginosis

BV is a vaginal infection caused by an imbalance in the vaginal flora and is the most common vaginal infection in women aged 15 to 44 years (CDC, n.d.-b). Infection with BV is associated with preterm labor and infection and transmission of HIV (Hillier et al., 1995). The cause of BV or how it is spread is not known; however, it is more common in sexually active women. Known risk factors for BV include having a new sexual partner or multiple sexual partners and douching (CDC, n.d.-b). Women identified as having a BV infection should be evaluated for signs and symptoms of PID, as BV is known to be a causative agent of PID in some women (Haggerty et al., 2016).

Key History and Physical Findings
- Often asymptomatic
- Vaginal itching or irritation
- White or gray vaginal discharge
- Strong fishy odor that is particularly noticeable after intercourse (CDC, n.d.-b)
- Positive whiff test
- Clue cells (more than 20%) on microscopy

Candidiasis

VVC is an inflammation of the vulvar and vaginal tissues owing to an infection with *Candida* yeast. Approximately 50% of women will experience a yeast infection at least once in their lifetime (Welsh, Howard, & Cook, 2004). There are several different species of *Candida* that cause VVC; however, *Candida albicans* is by far the most common (Welsh, Howard, & Cook, 2004). Risk factors for VVC include sexual debut, pregnancy, uncontrolled diabetes mellitus (DM), and an immunosuppressed state (Lopez, 2015).

Key History and Physical Findings
- Vulvar itching/irritation
- Dysuria
- Dyspareunia
- Symptoms frequently worsening in the week prior to the start of the menstrual cycle (Lopez, 2015)
- Curd-like discharge that is adherent to the vaginal walls (**Figure 20.22**)
- Erythematous vagina and vulvar tissue (see **Figure 20.22**)
- Blastospores and pseudohyphae on microscopy

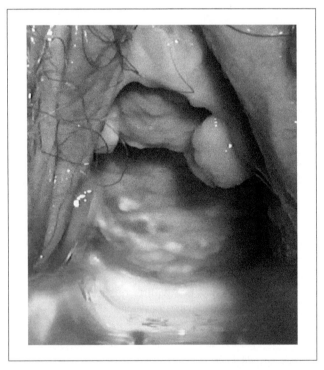

FIGURE 20.22 Vulvovaginal candidiasis. Speculum examination showing thick, curd-like plaque on vaginal wall. A slightly erythematous base is visible close to the center of the image, where some of the plaque was scraped off.

Source: Image courtesy of Mikael Haggstrom.

Genitourinary Syndrome of Menopause (Formerly Atrophic Vaginitis)

Genitourinary syndrome of menopause (GSM) refers to symptoms because of changes that occur in the vulvovaginal and urethra areas during the menopause transition. The decreased levels of estrogen result in a thinning of the epithelial tissue of the vagina, with a subsequent decrease in elasticity and vascularity (Portman & Gass, 2014). Care should be taken to use water-soluble lubrication when performing a speculum examination on women suspected to have this condition, as insertion of the speculum can be painful. Early recognition and treatment of this condition improve symptoms and quality of life.

Key History and Physical Findings
- Vaginal dryness, burning, and irritation
- Dyspareunia
- Vaginal spotting or bleeding (NAMS, 2014)
- Dysuria
- Urinary urgency
- Frequent or recurring urinary tract infections

VULVAR/VAGINAL/URETHRAL LESIONS

Lichen Planus

Vulvar lichen planus (LP) is a chronic autoimmune condition of unknown etiology that affects the skin and mucous membranes, including the vulva and vagina. There are several different types of vulvar LP, with erosive LP being the most common presentation (Schlosser & Mirowski, 2015). LP typically affects women in their 50s to 60s; however, younger women can also be affected (Schlosser & Mirowski, 2015). It is uncertain if there is a correlation between LP and vulvar malignancy (Cooper & Wojnarowska, 2006; Simpson & Murphy, 2012). Suspicion for this diagnosis should prompt referral for further evaluation and treatment.

Key History and Physical Findings
- Dysuria
- Dyspareunia
- Vulvar itching
- Postcoital bleeding
- Irritation of vulvar area
- Erosion and scarring can occur in erosive LP (Schlosser & Mirowski, 2015).

Lichen Sclerosus

Lichen sclerosus (LS) is one of the most common vulvar dermatoses. Similar to LP, it is an autoimmune-mediated, chronic inflammatory disease, with an unknown etiology (Schlosser & Mirowski, 2015). Although it shares some similarities with LP, there are some important

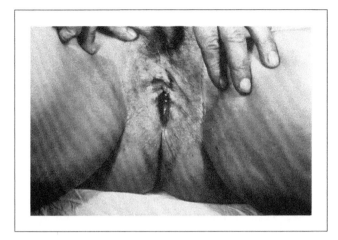

FIGURE 20.23 Waxy, wrinkled patches/skin erosions associated with lichen sclerosus.

Source: Centers for Disease Control and Prevention/Susan Lindsley.

differences that should be known. Similar to LP, postmenopausal women are most affected, although with LS there is a bimodal distribution of presentation, with peaks of onset in both prepubertal and postmenopausal women (Wallace, 1971). Another distinguishing feature is that vulvar LP involves the vaginal tissue, whereas in LS, vaginal involvement almost never occurs (Cooper & Wojnarowska, 2006). The mucous membranes are most commonly affected and include the medial labia, clitoris, posterior fourchette, and perianal skin (Schlosser & Mirowski, 2015). A figure-eight appearance may be noted, with involvement of genital structures and perianal structures (Schlosser & Mirowski, 2015). It is important to note that women with LS are at 200 to 300 times increased risk of developing squamous cell carcinoma of the vulva (Carli et al., 1995). Women suspected of this condition should be referred for further evaluation and treatment.

Key History and Physical Findings
- Vulvar itching, typically worse at night
- Dysuria
- Pain
- Urine/stool retention
- Plaques and patches that are ivory in color with a waxy or wrinkled appearance (**Figure 20.23**)
- Fissures, ulcerations, lichenification, scarring, and destruction of normal tissue structures may also be present

Intertrigo

Intertrigo affects the superficial layers of the skin and is an inflammatory condition that occurs in places where two skin surfaces rub together. This is compounded

by the subsequent development of moisture, which together with the friction of the skin results in irritation, redness, and maceration of the skin surfaces, which are the symptoms commonly described by affected patients (Shinkai & Fox, 2019). Intertrigo is susceptible to secondary infections (R. Wolf, Oumeish, & Parish, 2011). Factors increasing risk for development include hot and humid conditions, obesity, diabetes, incontinence, malnutrition, and poor hygiene (R. Wolf et al., 2011).

Key History and Physical Findings
- Irritation, erythema, and itching in the skin folds
- Typically occurs in areas such as the axilla, groin folds, inner thighs, and breast and abdominal folds

Vulvar Cancers and Vulvar Intraepithelial Neoplasia

Vulvar cancers are relatively rare and affect at a rate of 2.6 per 100,000 women (U.S. Cancer Statistics Working Group, 2019). Most vulvar cancers are squamous cell carcinomas (Faber et al., 2017). HPV infection is associated with about 40% of vulvar malignancy cases (Faber et al., 2017). Vulvar intraepithelial neoplasia (VIN) is a premalignant condition of the vulva (Reyes & Cooper, 2014). There are two common categories of VIN, usual and differentiated (Faber et al., 2017). Usual VIN develops as a result of HPV infection and is responsible for 40% of vulvar squamous cell carcinoma cases (Faber et al., 2017). Differentiated VIN results from skin conditions such as LS, and is associated with approximately 60% of vulvar squamous cell carcinoma cases (Bigby, Eva, Fong, & Jones, 2016). Squamous cell carcinomas of the vulva associated with HPV infections are found more commonly in younger women, whereas those associated with differentiated VIN are typically found in older women. Risk factors associated with vulvar cancer include HPV infection, cervical cancer history, smoking, and chronic vulvar skin conditions, such as LS (Division of Cancer Prevention and Control & CDC, n.d.). Early identification and referral for treatment is important in patients with suspected VIN.

Key History and Physical Findings
- Chronic vulvar itching
- Dyspareunia
- Burning, tingling, or soreness in the vulvar region
- Change in appearance of the affected skin including areas of redness or white, discolored skin
- Slightly raised skin lesions; some may appear darkened like a mole or freckle

Urethral Caruncle

A urethral caruncle is a benign lesion of the urethra most commonly found in postmenopausal women and premenarchal girls and suspected to be a result of decreased levels of estrogen (Dolan, Hill, & Valea, 2017).

It is a benign polypoid mass of the posterior urethral meatus.

Key History and Physical Findings
- Asymptomatic
- Dyspareunia
- Dysuria
- Hematuria
- Vaginal bleeding
- Bright red, vascular lesion located on the posterior lip of the urinary meatus

Bartholin Gland Cyst

Bartholin gland cysts develop when the Bartholin gland becomes blocked—a common gynecologic problem (Dolan et al., 2017). These cysts are most common in reproductive-aged women (Maldonado, 2014). The blockage of the duct causes a collection of secretions to develop that leads to swelling (Pundir & Auld, 2008). An uninfected cyst is typically painless and presents as a palpable, nontender lump or swelling (Pundir & Auld, 2008). Bartholin cysts can become infected, and when that occurs, women typically report significant pain (Pundir & Auld, 2008). Visible erythema and acute tenderness are suggestive of an inflamed cyst and possible abscess (**Figure 20.24**).

Key History and Physical Findings
- If uninfected, the cyst will be painless.
- If infected, the cyst will be significantly painful.
- Discomfort while walking or sitting
- Dyspareunia
- Fever
- Unilateral swelling or lump at the introitus in the 5 o'clock or 7 o'clock position
- Can develop into an abscess

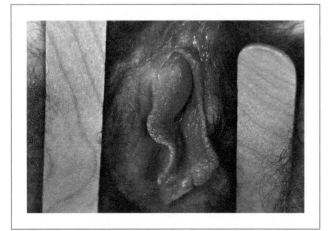

FIGURE 20.24 Infected Bartholin cyst.
Source: Centers for Disease Control and Prevention/Susan Lindsley.

PELVIC SUPPORT ISSUES
Pelvic Organ Prolapse

POP describes a condition in which there is failure of the anatomic supportive structures to adequately support the organs of the pelvis. It is a common and most often asymptomatic problem that does not require intervention for most women (Dolan et al., 2017). Symptoms vary depending on the severity of the defects in the supportive structures (Haylen et al., 2010). Risk factors for development of POP include pregnancy, vaginal delivery and delivery-related injury, family history/genetic component, obesity, and connective tissue diseases (Cartwright et al., 2015; Fornell, Wingren, & Kjolhede, 2004; Handa et al., 2011). Women identified as having POP should be referred for a formal assessment and quantification of prolapse (Aguilar, White, & Rogers, 2017). See **Table 20.8** for descriptions and depictions of the most common types of POP, including cystocele, rectocele, and uterine prolapse.

Key History and Physical Findings
- Low-back discomfort
- Pelvic pressure
- Vaginal bleeding or discharge
- Bulging in the vulvar area
- A need to displace the prolapse in order to urinate or defecate

GENITAL LESIONS/MASSES: MALIGNANT AND NONMALIGNANT
Cervical Intraepithelial Neoplasia and Cervical Malignancy

Cervical intraepithelial neoplasia (CIN) is a premalignant condition of the squamous epithelial cell of the cervix. Infection with HPV is the most common cause of CIN lesions (Kaufman et al., 1997; Schiffman et al., 1993). There are two common types of CIN: low-grade squamous intraepithelial lesion (LSIL) and high-grade squamous intraepithelial lesion (HSIL). Low-risk types of HPV infection are associated with LSIL, which have a low risk for oncogenic potential. High-risk types of HPV infection are associated with HSIL, which have a much higher risk of oncogenic potential. Several risk factors have been identified in the development of HSIL and cervical cancer, including the subtype of HPV infection, the persistence of the HPV infection, cigarette smoking, and immunosuppressed state (Appleby et al., 2006; Louie et al., 2011). **Figure 20.25** depicts the differences between low- and high-grade lesions, and cervical cancer. Cervical cancer is the third most common gynecologic cancer (U.S. Cancer Statistics Working Group, 2019). The majority of cervical cancers are squamous cell carcinomas, with adenocarcinomas accounting for 15% to 20% of cases (Jhingran & Meyer, 2017). Most cervical cancers are a result of HPV infection. It

TABLE 20.8 Types and Descriptions of Pelvic Organ Prolapse

Type	Description	Illustration
Cystocele	Loss of pelvic support in the anterior vaginal wall causes the bladder to prolapse into the vaginal canal. This can vary in severity from minimal, which may only be seen on examination when the patient is bearing down, or severe, in which the bladder has prolapsed and everted outside the genital tract. Common symptoms associated with a cystocele include urinary urgency, slow urine stream, and/or feeling of incomplete emptying; women may also report feeling a bulge or soft mass in the vagina or at the introitus (Dolan et al., 2017).	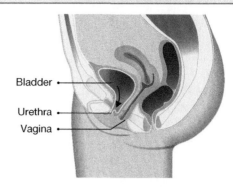
Rectocele	Loss of pelvic support in the posterior vaginal wall allows the small bowel and/or rectum to prolapse. Similar to a cystocele, women can be asymptomatic. Symptomatic women report feeling a vaginal bulge, pelvic pressure or pulling, difficulty with defecation, or sexual dysfunction (Ellerkmann et al., 2001; Handa, Cundiff, Chang, & Helzlsouer, 2008).	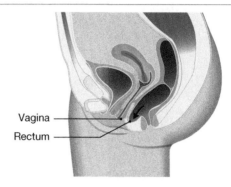
Uterine prolapse	Loss of pelvic support allows the uterus and cervix to prolapse through the vaginal canal. It is often associated with a concurrent cystocele and rectocele. Common symptoms in uterine prolapse include pelvic fullness, pressure, heaviness, and a bulge or visible tissue at the introitus of the vagina; irritation, pain, and bleeding may occur if the cervix is at or beyond the introitus (Dolan et al., 2017).	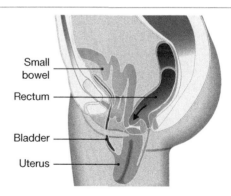

takes several years for a HSIL to develop into cervical cancer (ACOG, 2018b). Cervical cancer rates in the United States have been declining over the last 40 years because of increased screening, detection, immunization, and treatment (U.S. Cancer Statistics Working Group, 2019).

Key History and Physical Findings
- History of HSIL
- Watery, bloody vaginal discharge that may be heavy and malodorous
- Unusual vaginal bleeding (specifically after intercourse, between periods, or after menopause)
- Pelvic pain
- Dyspareunia
- Cervix appearance on examination shows gross erosion, ulcer, or mass

ADNEXAL MASSES
Adnexal masses have many etiologies, most of which are benign. Most masses are detected incidentally on physical examination or pelvic imaging (ACOG, 2016b). Appropriate evaluation and monitoring of women with an adnexal mass is important to differentiate between a benign versus a malignant mass (ACOG, 2016b). It is important to obtain a thorough medical history, as the woman's age, family history, and menstrual history,

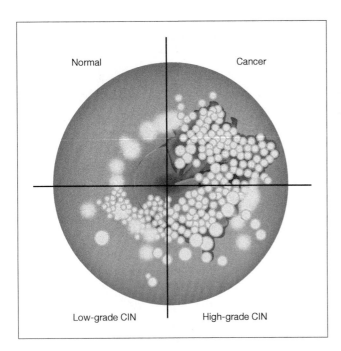

FIGURE 20.25 Cervical intraepithelial neoplasia (CIN) and cervical cancer.

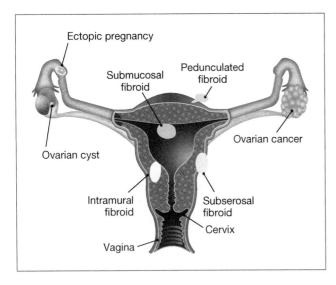

FIGURE 20.26 Adnexal masses including ovarian cysts, ectopic pregnancy, ovarian cancer, and uterine fibroids.

along with her presenting symptoms, will determine the differential diagnosis and appropriate work up. TVUS is recommended as first-line imaging for evaluation of adnexal masses. (ACOG, 2016b). **Figure 20.26** depicts adnexal masses, including ovarian cysts, ectopic pregnancy, ovarian cancer, and uterine fibroids.

Ovarian Cyst

Ovarian cysts are a common ultrasound finding and are more common in premenopausal women than in

postmenopausal women (Pavlik et al., 2013). Ovarian cysts have various etiologies. They are fluid-filled sacs that form in or on a woman's ovaries. Most ovarian abnormalities resolve without intervention (Pavlik et al., 2013). Occasionally, a cyst may require surgical intervention.

Key History and Physical Findings
- Often asymptomatic
- Unilateral, sometimes acute, pelvic pain
- Irregular menstrual periods
- Bloating
- Ovarian cysts may be palpable during the bimanual physical examination.

Ectopic Pregnancy

Ectopic or tubal pregnancy is a potential life-threatening emergency that results from the implantation of a fertilized egg outside of the uterus, most commonly in the fallopian tube (Bouyer, Coste, Fernandez, Pouly, & Job-Spira, 2002). Ectopic pregnancy accounts for 2% of all pregnancies and for approximately 4% to 10% of pregnancy-related deaths (Marion & Meeks, 2012). Failure to diagnose an ectopic pregnancy in a timely fashion can result in rupture of the fallopian tube, leading to hemorrhage and possible death.

Key History and Physical Findings
- Vaginal bleeding
- Increasing unilateral pelvic pain
- Altered menstrual cycle
- Positive pregnancy test
- Palpable adnexal mass on bimanual examination
- CMT

Ovarian Cancer

Ovarian cancer is the second most common gynecologic cancer, although overall it is rare (National Cancer Institute, 2019b; U.S. Cancer Statistics Working Group, 2019). The death rates of ovarian cancer have been falling over the last 10 years, and 5-year survival rates are 47.6% (National Cancer Institute, 2019b). Ovarian cancer is most commonly diagnosed in women aged 55 to 64 years (National Cancer Institute, 2019b).

Key History and Physical Findings
- Symptoms often nonspecific and present late in the disease process
- Abdominal pain
- Abdominal bloating
- Increased abdominal size (girth)
- Urinary symptoms
- Constipation
- Early satiety or difficulty eating

Uterine Fibroids

Uterine fibroids, also known as uterine leiomyomas, are benign growths arising from the smooth muscle (myometrium) of the uterus (Cramer & Patel, 1990). They occur in about 77% of women, making them the most common pelvic growth (Baird, Dunson, Hill, Cousins, & Schectman, 2003; Cramer & Patel, 1990). Uterine fibroids develop after menarche and usually regress with the menopausal transition (Segars et al., 2014).

Key History and Physical Findings
- Can be asymptomatic
- Heavy menstrual bleeding
- Pelvic pain
- Dyspareunia
- Bladder dysfunction
- Lump or mass on abdominal examination
- Enlarged uterus in a nonpregnant woman on bimanual examination
- Irregular contour of the uterus on bimanual examination

MENSTRUAL IRREGULARITIES

Polycystic Ovarian Syndrome

Polycystic ovarian syndrome (PCOS) is a complex endocrine disorder of unknown etiology. It is thought to be genetically linked (Vink, Sadrzadeh, Lambalk, & Boomsma, 2006). It is a common cause of menstrual irregularity and infertility (Hull, 1987). Women with PCOS are at increased risk for metabolic syndrome, type 2 diabetes, dyslipidemia, and cardiovascular disease (Celik, Tasdemir, Abali, Bastu, & Yilmaz, 2014; Phelan et al., 2010; Schmidt, Landin-Wilhelmsen, Brannstrom,

& Dahlgren, 2011). Women suspected of having PCOS require a thorough evaluation for diagnosis as well as risk assessment for associated conditions.

Key History and Physical Findings
- Presentation is variable.
- Can be asymptomatic
- Irregular menstrual cycles
- Infertility
- Signs of hyperandrogenism (e.g., acne, hirsutism, acanthosis nigricans)
- Polycystic ovaries on ultrasound

Vasomotor Symptoms (Hot Flashes)

Vasomotor symptoms (VMS) is a term used to describe the constellation of symptoms frequently and commonly referred to as hot flashes or night sweats. VMS are a common perimenopause symptom and are described as "recurrent, transient episodes of flushing accompanied by a sensation of warmth to intense heat on the upper body and face" (NAMS, 2014, p. 55). VMS have been associated with diminished quality of life for some women (Burleson, Todd, & Trevathan, 2010). Women identified as suffering from moderate-to-severe VMS that are interfering with quality of life should be referred for further evaluation and treatment.

Key History and Physical Findings
- Hot flashes
- Night sweats
- Severe sweating
- Flushing
- Chills

CASE STUDY: Abdominal Pain and Discharge

History

A healthy 24-year-old female presents to the clinic with concerns of lower abdominal pain and "liquid coming out of her vagina." She is Muslim and speaks very little English. She is accompanied by her spouse who is translating for her. Symptoms began 8 months ago. Her spouse translates that once a month she has bad lower abdominal pain lasting 5 to 7 days. The pain radiates into her back. She also has similar pain intermittently that lasts about 10 minutes and resolves spontaneously. The pain is described as cramping and is improved with a heating pad and ibuprofen. She reports that in association with the pain that lasts 5 to 7 days, she sometimes has dark

brown liquid come out of her vagina, not the usual bright red. At other times, when she has the cramps for only a few minutes, she has clear sticky liquid; when she wipes, it is thin and does not have any odor. She notices that the short episodes of pain are always right after intercourse. She reports that she has been healthy, walks daily, eats a variety of foods including fruits and vegetables, and has not had any changes in her weight. She has not had any fever or chills, no nausea or vomiting, and no breast tenderness.

Menstrual history: Her last menstrual period was 1 month ago that lasted 7 days. Before that, her cycle was 2 months ago that lasted about 5 days. She does

(continued)

CASE STUDY: Abdominal Pain and Discharge (*continued*)

not use tampons, but goes through about five pads per day. She started her menses at age 13. For much of her life, her period has been somewhat irregular—sometimes every 28 to 30 days and sometimes 1 week or 2 weeks late. She does not track it regularly, but states that it should come on the 10th of every month.

Gynecologic history: Client has never had a well-woman examination. She was seen once in urgent care for the pain and clear discharge and was motivated to be seen by the fear that the pain and discharge might prevent her from being able to have children. She had an examination at that time only. She also reports that she douches with plain water after her cycle and intercourse.

Obstetric history: gravida 0, term 0, para 0, abortion 0, living children 0.

Sexual history: Client was recently married (8 months ago). Her first sexual encounter was 8 months ago. She has had one lifetime partner. They are hoping to have children and are not currently using any form of birth control. She denies ever being a victim of violence.

Past medical history: She denies any chronic health problems or surgeries. She currently takes a multivitamin, and is on no other medications.

Family history: She denies any first-degree relatives with breast or ovarian cancer.

Social history: She is a lifelong nonsmoker and denies any illicit drug use.

Physical Examination

- General: Normotensive, in no acute distress
- Chest: Lungs clear to auscultation bilaterally, anteriorly, and posteriorly
- Heart: Regular, rate and rhythm, no murmurs
- Abdomen: Soft, nontender, no masses

- Pelvis:
  - External genitalia: Pubic hair present; labia are intact and without lesions or excoriations; Bartholin and Skene glands nonpalpable
  - Vagina: Walls are pink, supple with rugae; small amount of clear mucus noted
  - Cervix: Nulliparous, pink, smooth, without lesion or discharge, freely mobile without tenderness
  - Uterus: Retroverted; normal size and mobility, without tenderness on palpation
  - Adnexa: No masses palpated, no tenderness

Differential Diagnoses

Diagnoses specific to pain and vaginal discharge, as well as diagnoses that overlap: Menstrual cramping, postcoital uterine cramping, endometriosis, sexually transmitted infection, vaginal infection, urinary tract infection, uterine fibroids, pregnancy

Laboratory and Imaging

As with all sexually active women of childbearing age, a pregnancy test is typically the first test to be done. Her pregnancy test was negative. A urine dipstick was also negative for RBC, WBC, and nitrites. An in-office wet mount revealed no yeast or clue cells and no amine odor. Cytology and HPV typing were also completed and there were no abnormal cells or HPV strains found. Gonorrhea and chlamydia testing was negative.

Final Diagnosis

Menstrual cramping and postcoital cramping with normal intercycle leukorrhea. Note: The dark brown blood occasionally reported with regular menses is not usually an abnormal finding.

CASE STUDY: Abdominal Pain and Bleeding

History

A healthy 48-year-old female presents to the OB/GYN office with concerns of lower abdominal pain and heavy menstrual bleeding. Symptoms began yesterday. The pain is in her lower abdomen and in her buttocks. The pain is described as severe cramping; that is, "it feels like labor pain and nothing has helped it." Patient reports taking 600 mg of ibuprofen every 6 hours, drinking plenty of fluids and resting with her feet up. She is using a tampon and a nighttime pad and has to change them about every 2 to 3 hours. She had a similar episode about 4

(continued)

CASE STUDY: Abdominal Pain and Bleeding (*continued*)

months ago. She reports that she does not exercise as often as she should and that she is not following any specific diet. She drinks one or two glasses of wine (4 ounces) daily. She has not had fever, chills, nausea, vomiting, breast tenderness, constipation, or diarrhea.

Menstrual history: Her last menstrual period was 4 months ago and was similar to her current episode. Over the last 4 months, she has occasionally had some spotting, but "not a period." She uses tampons and pads as previously described. She started her menses at age 11. She reports that her cycle has always been very regular. She took birth control pills from age 18 to 29. She stopped taking birth control pills to have children. Over the last few years, her periods had been getting heavier, but also more irregular.

Gynecologic history: Last well-woman examination was 2 years ago. Her cytology was normal and additional HPV typing was negative. She denies ever having abnormal Pap test results. She does not douche.

Obstetric history: Gravida 3, term 3, para 0, abortion 0, living children 3. All pregnancies were vaginal deliveries without complications.

Sexual history: Client reports having five lifetime partners; one for 22 years. All male. She was on birth control pills for pregnancy prevention and used condoms with partners before she was married and after her divorce. She had chlamydia once about 5 years ago. That is how she found out her spouse had an affair. He is now living with his same-sex partner. She has not been sexually active for the last 6 months. She tested negative for all STIs at that time. She denies any unwanted sexual experiences or having ever been a victim of mental or physical abuse.

Past medical history: Client has a history of hypothyroidism and elevated cholesterol. She had repair of a torn rotator cuff 10 years ago and tonsillectomy as a child.

Family history: Her parents are alive and well. Her mother also has hypothyroidism. Her father has high blood pressure. She denies any first-degree relatives with cancer, psychiatric, or neurologic conditions.

Social history: She smoked for 5 years in her 20s (one pack per day) but nothing since. She drinks wine as previously noted, but denies any other substances. She enjoys recreational shooting and has three guns at home. She reports that she keeps the guns in a locked cabinet, unloaded and separate from the ammunition.

Physical Examination

- General: Pleasant female, in no acute distress. BMI 28.5, T 98.8°F, HR 88, RR 12, BP 118/68
- Chest: Lungs clear to auscultation bilaterally, anteriorly, and posteriorly
- Heart: regular, rate and rhythm, no murmurs
- Abdomen: soft, nontender, no masses
- Pelvis:
   ○ External genitalia: Shaved pubic hair; labia large, thin, and without lesions
   ○ Vagina: Bartholin and Skene glands nonpalpable; visible vaginal walls are pale pink, smooth; large amount of blood noted obscuring examination
   ○ Cervix: Multiparous, pale pink, granular transformation zone where visualized, no lesions, minimal tenderness during examination but freely mobile
   ○ Uterus: Anteverted; larger than normal and tender on palpation
   ○ Adnexa: No masses palpated

Differential Diagnoses

Spontaneous abortion, abnormal uterine bleeding, uterine fibroid, malignancy, endometriosis, perimenopause

Laboratory and Imaging

In-office pregnancy test was negative. Additional labs included a complete blood count (CBC) and erythrocyte sedimentation rate (ESR). Her hemoglobin was slightly low at 11.8 g/dL and her ESR was 28 mm/hr.

Subsequent pelvic ultrasound revealed an anteverted uterus with two fibroids. The first was in the anterior wall measuring 16 mm and the other at the posterior wall measuring 32 mm. Endometrial thickness measures 5 mm.

Final Diagnosis

Abnormal uterine bleeding secondary to uterine fibroids. The patient is also likely perimenopausal.

Clinical Pearls

- Be sure the space where the examination takes place is private. Many women feel uncomfortable speaking about their "private parts." If the clinical space is noisy or if the patient can hear the patient in the next room or the medical assistant in the hall, they are less likely to share personal health history.
- Ideally, patients should have an opportunity to speak with a clinician privately, without anyone else in the room . . . even if a patient says "it's okay, they can stay." Sometimes practices have a policy to meet with a patient alone. Clinicians can be more creative and ask for a urine specimen and then meet the patient at the restroom to inquire if there is anything they need to discuss privately.
- Try to conduct the health history while the patient's clothes are on. Sitting naked on an examination table under a flimsy gown increases the likelihood the patient may feel vulnerable. They may be less inclined to provide any detailed responses. Additionally, the more tense a patient is, the more challenging the physical examination can be.
- Consider having a patient view their genitalia while the examination is being conducted by holding a mirror. This demystifies the examination and can be empowering for the patient.
- A thorough evaluation of the external genitalia can sometimes be challenging because of overlying skin folds. Visualization can be improved by holding the labia majora between the thumb and first finger and lifting gently.
- Concerns related to sexual health or sexual activity identified during the history may be further explored during the pelvic examination. Women may be more inclined to share personal information when they do not have to look the clinician in the eye.
- If a patient's body habitus is limiting visualization of the cervix, have the patient rotate their hips forward by placing their hands under their buttocks. Additional assistance may be needed to mobilize the pannus out of the way for better visualization.
- For women with very little vaginal tone, try cutting the fingers off of a large glove or the end off of a condom and covering the bills of the speculum. This will prevent vaginal tissue from rolling inside the speculum and obscuring the visual field. A large cotton-tipped swab can also be used to manipulate the vaginal wall or hold it to the side to aid in better visualization.

Key Takeaways

- When a woman presents for a well-woman examination, advanced assessment includes a comprehensive, thorough, evidence-based history and physical examination.
- Testing to consider in addition to the physical examination for a well-woman visit includes Pap testing, HPV testing, STI screening, Wet Prep, and breast, ovarian, endometrial, cervical, and colon cancer screening.
- Understanding the anatomy and physiology of the female GU system, female reproductive system, menstrual cycle, and reproductive life span is the key to providing family planning and reproductive health guidance.

REFERENCES

Abdulcadir, J., Say, L., & Pallitto, C. (2017). What do we know about assessing healthcare students and professionals' knowledge, attitude and practice regarding female genital mutilation? A systematic review. *Reproductive Health*, *14*(1), 64–77. doi:10.1186/s12978-017-0318-1

Agency for Healthcare Research and Quality. (2015). Trauma-informed care. Retrieved from https://www.ahrq.gov/professionals/prevention-chronic-care/healthier-pregnancy/preventive/trauma.html

Aguilar, V. C., White, A. B., & Rogers, R. G. (2017). Updates on the diagnostic tools for evaluation of pelvic floor disorders. *Current Opinion in Obstetrics and Gynecology*, *29*(6), 458–464. doi:10.1097/GCO.0000000000000415

Allen, D., Hunter, M. S., Wood, S., & Beeson, T. (2017). One Key Question®: First things first in reproductive health. *Maternal and Child Health Journal*, *21*(3), 387–392. doi:10.1007/s10995-017-2283-2

American Academy of Family Physicians. (2018). *Twenty things physicians and patients should question*. Retrieved from http://www.choosingwisely.org/clinician-lists/aafp-genital-herpes-screening-in-asymptomatic-adults

American Academy of Pediatrics. (2017a). *Bright futures: Adolescence visits: 11 through 21 years*. Retrieved from https://brightfutures.aap.org/Bright%20Futures%20Documents/BF4_AdolescenceVisits.pdf

American Academy of Pediatrics. (2017b). *Bright futures: Infancy visits: Prenatal through 11 months*. Retrieved from https://brightfutures.aap.org/Bright%20Futures%20Documents/BF4_InfancyVisits.pdf

American Academy of Pediatrics. (2017c). *Bright futures: Middle childhood visits: 5 through 10 years*. Retrieved from https://brightfutures.aap.org/Bright%20Futures%20Documents/BF4_MiddleChildhoodVisits.pdf

American College of Obstetricians and Gynecologists. (2007). *Committee Opinion Number 373: Sexual misconduct* [Reaffirmed 2016]. Retrieved from https://www.acog.org/

Clinical-Guidance-and-Publications/Committee-Opinions/Committee-on-Ethics/Sexual-Misconduct

American College of Obstetricians and Gynecologists. (2015). Committee Opinion No. 634: Hereditary cancer syndromes and risk assessment. *Obstetrics & Gynecology, 125*(6), 1538–1543. doi:10.1097/01.aog.0000466373.71146.51

American College of Obstetricians and Gynecologists. (2016a). Practice Bulletin No. 168: Cervical cancer screening and prevention. *Obstetrics & Gynecology, 128*(4), e111–e130. doi:10.1097/aog.0000000000001708

American College of Obstetricians and Gynecologists. (2016b). Practice Bulletin No. 174: Evaluation and management of adnexal masses. *Obstetrics & Gynecology, 128*(5), e210–e226. doi:10.1097/AOG.0000000000001768

American College of Obstetricians and Gynecologists. (2017). Committee Opinion No. 706: Sexual health. *Obstetrics & Gynecology, 130*(1), e42–e47. doi:10.1097/aog.0000000000002161

American College of Obstetricians and Gynecologists. (2018a). ACOG Committee Opinion No. 755: Well-woman visit. *Obstetrics & Gynecology, 132*(4), e181–e186. doi:10.1097/AOG.0000000000002897

American College of Obstetricians and Gynecologists. (2018b). *Frequently asked questions: Gynecologic problems.* Retrieved from https://www.acog.org/Patients/FAQs/Cervical-Cancer

American College of Obstetricians and Gynecologists, & American Society for Reproductive Medicine. (2019). ACOG Committee Opinion No. 762: Prepregnancy counseling. *Obstetrics & Gynecology, 133*(1), e78–e89. doi:10.1097/AOG.0000000000003013

American College of Radiology. (2014). *ACR appropriateness criteria.* Retrieved from https://acsearch.acr.org/docs/69458/Narrative

American Society for Colposcopy and Cervical Pathology. (2017). *Five things physicians and patients should question.* Retrieved from http://www.choosingwisely.org/clinician-lists/asccp-screening-tests-for-low-risk-hpv-types

Amies, A. M. E., Miller, L., Lee, S. K., & Koutsky, L. (2002). The effect of vaginal speculum lubrication on the rate of unsatisfactory cervical cytology diagnosis. *Obstetrics & Gynecology, 100*(5), 889–892. doi:10.1016/S0029-7844(02)02348-7

Appleby, P., Beral, V., Berrington de González, A., Colin, D., Franceschi, S., Goodill, A., . . . Sweetland, S. (2006). Carcinoma of the cervix and tobacco smoking: Collaborative reanalysis of individual data on 13,541 women with carcinoma of the cervix and 23,017 women without carcinoma of the cervix from 23 epidemiological studies. *International Journal of Cancer, 118*(6), 1481–1495. doi:10.1002/ijc.21493

Bachman, G., Lobo, R. A., Gut, R., Nachtigall, L., & Notelovitz, M. (2008). Efficacy of low-dose estradiol vaginal tablets in the treatment of atrophic vaginitis: A randomized controlled trial. *Obstetrics & Gynecology, 111*(1), 67–76. doi:10.1097/01.AOG.0000296714.12226.0f

Baird, D. D., Dunson, D. B., Hill, M. C., Cousins, D., & Schectman, M. (2003). High cumulative incidence of uterine leiomyoma in black and white women: Ultrasound evidence. *American Journal of Obstetrics and Gynecology, 188*(1), 100–107. doi:10.1067/mob.2003.99

Bates, C. K., Carroll, N., & Potter, J. (2011). The challenging pelvic exam. *Journal of General Internal Medicine, 26*(6), 651–657. doi:10.1007/s11606-010-1610-8

Bernstein, D. I., Bellamy, A. R., HookIII, E. W., Levin, M. J., Wald, A., Ewell, M. G., . . . Belshe, R. B. (2013). Epidemiology, clinical presentation, and antibody response to primary infection with herpes simplex virus type 1 and type 2 in young women. *Clinical Infectious Disease, 56,* 344–351. doi:10.1093/cid/cis891

Bibbins-Domingo, K., Grossman, D. C., Curry, S. J., Barry, M. J., Davidson, K. W., Doubeni, C. A., . . . Tseng, C. W. (2017, March 7). Screening for gynecologic conditions with pelvic examination: U.S. Preventive Services Task Force recommendation statement. *Journal of the American Medical Association, 317*(9), 947–953. doi:10.1001/jama.2017.0807

Bigby, S. M., Eva, L. J., Fong, K. L., & Jones, R. W. (2016). The natural history of vulvar intraepithelial neoplasia, differentiated type: Evidence for progression and diagnostic challenges. *International Journal of Gynecological Pathology, 35*(6), 574–584. doi:10.1097/PGP.0000000000000280

Biro, F. M., Galvez, M. P., Greenspan, L. C., Succop, P. A., Vangeepuram, N., Pinney, S. M., . . . Wolff, M. S. (2010). Pubertal assessment method and baseline characteristics in a mixed longitudinal study of girls. *Pediatrics, 126*(3), e582–e590. doi:10.1542/peds.2009-3079

Bosch, F. X., Lorincz, A., Munoz, N., Meijer, C. J., & Shah, K. V. (2002). The causal relation between human papillomavirus and cervical cancer. *Journal of Clinical Pathology, 55*(4), 244–265. doi:10.1136/jcp.55.4.244

Bouyer, J., Coste, J., Fernandez, H., Pouly, J. L., & Job-Spira, N. (2002). Sites of ectopic pregnancy: A 10-year population-based study of 1800 cases. *Human Reproduction, 17*(12), 3224. doi:10.1093/humrep/17.12.3224

Braaten, K. P., & Laufer, M. R. (2008). Human papillomavirus (HPV), HPV-related disease, and the HPV vaccine. *Reviews in Obstetrics and Gynecology, 1*(1), 2–10. Retrieved from http://medreviews.com/journal/reviews-in-obstetrics-gynecology/vol/1/no/1/human-papillomavirus-hpv-hpv-related-disease-and-hpv-vaccine

Bradley, H., Markowitz, L. E., Gibson, T., & McQuillan, G. M. (2014). Seroprevalence of herpes simplex virus types 1 and 2—United States, 1999–2010. *Journal of Infectious Diseases, 209*(3), 325–333. doi:10.1093/infdis/jit458

Bradshaw, K. D. (2016). Menopausal transition. In B. L. Hoffman, J. O. Schorge, K. D. Bradshaw, L. M. Halvorson, J. I. Schaffer, & M. M. Corton (Eds.), *Williams gynecology* (3rd ed., pp. 471–491). New York, NY: McGraw-Hill.

Branson, B. M., Handsfield, H. H., Lampe, M. A., Janssen, R. S., Taylor, A. W., Lyss, S. B., Clark, J. E. (2006). Revised recommendations for HIV testing of adults, adolescents, and pregnant women in health-care settings. *Morbidity and Mortality Weekly Report. Recommendations and Reports, 55*(RR-14), 1–17. Retrieved from https://www.cdc.gov/mmwr/preview/mmwrhtml/rr5514a1.htm

Burleson, M. H., Todd, M., & Trevathan, W. R. (2010). Daily vasomotor symptoms, sleep problems, and mood: Using daily data to evaluate the domino hypothesis in middle-aged women. *Menopause, 17*(1), 87–95. doi:0.1097/gme.0b013e3181b20b2d

Caldwell, W. E., & Moloy, H. C. (1933). Anatomical variations in the female pelvis and their effect in labor with a suggested classification. *American Journal of Obstetrics and Gynecology*, 26, 479–505. doi:10.1016/S0002-9378(33)90194-5

Carli, P., Cattaneo, A., De Magnis, A., Biggeri, A., Taddei, G., & Giannotti, B. (1995). Squamous cell carcinoma arising in vulval lichen sclerosus: A longitudinal cohort study. *European Journal of Cancer Prevention*, *4*(6), 491–495. doi:10.1097/00008469-199512000-00008

Cartwright, R., Kirby, A. C., Tikkinen, K. A. O., Mangera, A., Thiagamoorthy, G., Rajan, P., . . . Khullar, V. (2015). Systematic review and metaanalysis of genetic association studies of urinary symptoms and prolapse in women. *American Journal of Obstetrics & Gynecology*, *212*(2), 199.e1–199.e24. doi:10.1016/j.ajog.2014.08.005

Celik, C., Tasdemir, N., Abali, R., Bastu, E., & Yilmaz, M. (2014). Progression to impaired glucose tolerance or type 2 diabetes mellitus in polycystic ovary syndrome: A controlled follow-up study. *Fertility and Sterility*, *101*(4), 1123–1128. doi:10.1016/j.fertnstert.2013.12.050

Centers for Disease Control and Prevention. (n.d.-a). About HPV vaccines. Retrieved from https://www.cdc.gov/vaccines/vpd/hpv/hcp/vaccines.html

Centers for Disease Control and Prevention. (n.d.-b). Bacterial vaginosis—CDC fact sheet. Retrieved from https://www.cdc.gov/std/bv/stdfact-bacterial-vaginosis.htm

Centers for Disease Control and Prevention. (n.d.-c). Biology. Retrieved from https://www.cdc.gov/parasites/lice/pubic/biology.html

Centers for Disease Control and Prevention. (n.d.-d). Chlamydia—CDC fact sheet (detailed). Retrieved from https://www.cdc.gov/std/chlamydia/stdfact-chlamydia-detailed.htm

Centers for Disease Control and Prevention. (n.d.-e). Genital HPV infection—Fact sheet. Retrieved from https://www.cdc.gov/std/hpv/stdfact-hpv.htm

Centers for Disease Control and Prevention. (n.d.-f). Genital HSV infections. Retrieved from https://www.cdc.gov/std/tg2015/herpes.htm

Centers for Disease Control and Prevention. (n.d.-g). Gonorrhea—CDC fact sheet (detailed version). Retrieved from https://www.cdc.gov/std/gonorrhea/stdfact-gonorrhea-detailed.htm

Centers for Disease Control and Prevention. (n.d.-h). Pelvic inflammatory disease (PID)—CDC fact sheet. Retrieved from https://www.cdc.gov/std/pid/stdfact-pid-detailed.htm#ref1

Centers for Disease Control and Prevention. (n.d.-i). Syphilis—CDC fact sheet (detailed). Retrieved from https://www.cdc.gov/std/syphilis/stdfact-syphilis-detailed.htm

Centers for Disease Control and Prevention. (n.d.-j). Trichomoniasis—CDC fact sheet. Retrieved from https://www.cdc.gov/std/trichomonas/stdfact-trichomoniasis.htm

Centers for Disease Control and Prevention. (2015). 2015 sexually transmitted diseases treatment guidelines. Retrieved from https://www.cdc.gov/std/tg2015/screening-recommendations.htm

Centers for Disease Control and Prevention. (2019). *CDC fact sheet: Reported STDs in the United States, 2018*. Retrieved from https://www.cdc.gov/nchhstp/newsroom/docs/factsheets/STD-Trends-508.pdf

Centers for Disease Control and Prevention, Health Resources and Services Administration, National Institutes of Health, HIV Medicine Association of the Infectious Diseases Society of America, & HIV Prevention in Clinical Care Working Group. (2004). Recommendations for incorporating human immunodeficiency virus (HIV) prevention into the medical care of persons living with HIV. *Clinical Infectious Diseases*, *38*(1), 104–121. doi:10.1086/380131

Clowers, A. N. (2018, December 12). *GAO: Sexual assault information on the availability of forensic examiners (GAO-19-259T)*. Retrieved from https://www.gao.gov/assets/700/695914.pdf

Cooper, S. M., & Wojnarowska, F. (2006). Influence of treatment of erosive lichen planus of the vulva on its prognosis. *Archives Dermatology*, *142*(3), 289–294. doi:10.1001/archderm.142.3.289

Cramer, S. F., & Patel, A. (1990). The frequency of uterine leiomyomas. *American Journal of Clinical Pathology*, *94*(4), 435–438. doi:10.1093/ajcp/94.4.435

Curry, E. S., Hammer, L. D., Brown, O. W., Laughlin, J. J., Lessin, H. R., Simon, G. R., & Rodgers, C. T. (2011). Policy statement: Use of chaperones during the physical examination of the pediatric patient. *Pediatrics*, *127*(5), 991–993. doi:10.1542/peds.2011-0322

Division of Cancer Prevention and Control, Centers for Disease Control and Prevention. (n.d.). Basic information about vaginal and vulvar cancers. Retrieved from https://www.cdc.gov/cancer/vagvulv/basic_info

Dolan, M. S., Hill, C., & Valea, F. A. (2017). Benign gynecologic lesions: Vulva, vagina, cervix, uterus, oviduct, ovary, ultrasound imaging of pelvic structures. In R. A. Lobo, D. M. Gershenson, G. M. Lentz, & F. A. Valea (Eds.), *Comprehensive gynecology* (7th ed., pp. 370–422). Philadelphia, PA: Elsevier.

Douglas, N. C., & Lobo, R. A. (2017). Reproductive endocrinology: Neuroendocrinology, gonadotropins, sex steroids, prostaglandins, ovulation, menstruation, hormone assay. In R. A. Lobo, D. M. Gershenson, G. M. Lentz, & F. A. Valea (Eds.), *Comprehensive gynecology* (7th ed., pp. 77–107). Philadelphia, PA: Elsevier.

Drake, R. L., Vogl, A. W., & Mitchell, A. W. M. (2015). *Gray's anatomy for students* (3rd ed., pp. 421–532). Philadelphia, PA: Churchill Livingstone Elsevier.

Ellerkmann, R. M., Cundiff, G. W., Melick, C. F., Nihira, M. A., Leffler, K., & Bent, A. E. (2001). Correlation of symptoms with location and severity of pelvic organ prolapse. *American Journal Obstetrics Gynecology*, *185*(6), 1332–1337. doi:10.1067/mob.2001.119078

Faber, M. T., Sand, F. L., Albieri, V., Norrild, B., Kjaer, S. K., & Verdoodt, F. (2017). Prevalence and type distribution of human papillomavirus in squamous cell carcinoma and intraepithelial neoplasia of the vulva. *International Journal of Cancer*, *141*, 1161–1169. doi:10.1002/ijc.30821

Farrukh, S., Sivitz, A., Onogul, B., Patel, K., & Tejani, C. (2018). The additive value of pelvic examinations to history in predicting sexually transmitted infections for young female patients with suspected cervicitis or pelvic inflammatory disease. *Annals of Emergency Medicine*, *72*(6), 703–712. doi:10.1016/j.annemergmed.2018.05.004

Feaster, D. J., Parish, C. L., Gooden, L., Matheson, T., Castellon, P. C., Duan, R., . . . Metsch, L. R. (2016). Substance use and STI acquisition: Secondary analysis from the AWARE study. *Drug and Alcohol Dependence, 169,* 171–179. doi:10.1016/j.drugalcdep.2016.10.027

Fornell, E. U., Wingren, G., & Kjolhede, P. (2004). Factors associated with pelvic floor dysfunction and emphasis on urinary and fecal incontinence and genital prolapse: An epidemiological study. *Acta Obstetricia et Gynecologica Scandinavica, 83*(4), 383–389. doi:10.1080/j.0001-6349.2004.00367.x

Garland, S. M., Eundem, A., & Steben, M. (2014). Genital herpes. *Best Practice & Research: Clinical Obstetrics & Gynaecology, 28*(7), 1098–1110. doi:10.1016/j.bpobgyn.2014.07.015

Gavin, L., Moskosky, S., Carter, M., Curtis, K., Glass, E., Godfrey, E., . . . Zapata, L. (2014). Providing quality family planning services: Recommendations of CDC and the U.S. Office of Population Affairs. *Morbidity and Mortality Weekly Report. Recommendations and Reports, 63*(RR-4), 1–54. Retrieved from https://www.cdc.gov/mmwr/pdf/rr/rr6304.pdf

Griffith, W. F., Stuart, G. S., Gluck, K. L., & Heartwell, S. F. (2005). Vaginal speculum lubrication and its effects on cervical cytology and microbiology. *Contraception, 72,* 60–64. doi:10.1016/j.contraception.2005.01.004

Guenthner, P. C., Secor, W. E., & Dezzutti, C. S. (2005). Trichomonas vaginalis-induced epithelial monolayer disruption and human immunodeficiency virus type 1 (HIV-1) replication: Implications for the sexual transmission of HIV-1. *Infection and Immunity, 73,* 4155–4160. doi:10.1128/IAI.73.7.4155-4160.2005

Guirguis-Blake, J. M., Henderson, J. T., & Perdue, L. A. (2017). Periodic screening pelvic examination: Evidence report and systematic review for the U.S. Preventive Services Task Force. *Journal of the American Medical Association, 317*(9), 954–966. doi:10.1001/jama.2016.12819

Haggerty, C. L., Totten, P. A., Tang, G., Astete, S. B., Ferris, M. J., Norori, J., . . . Ness, R. B. (2016). Identification of novel microbes associated with pelvic inflammatory disease and infertility. *Sexually Transmitted Infections, 92*(6), 441–446. doi:10.1136/sextrans-2015-052285

Handa, V. L., Blomquist, J. L., Knoepp, L. R., Hoskey, K. A., McDermott, K. C., & Munoz, A. (2011). Pelvic floor disorders 5-10 years after vaginal or cesarean childbirth. *Obstetrics & Gynecology, 118*(4), 777–784. doi:10.1097/AOG.0b013e3182267f2f

Handa, V. L., Cundiff, G., Chang, H. H., & Helzlsouer, K. J. (2008). Female sexual function and pelvic floor disorders. *Obstetrics & Gynecology, 111*(5), 1045–1052. doi:10.1097/AOG.0b013e31816bbe85

Harer, W. B., Jr., Valenzuela, G., & Lebo, D. (2002). Lubrication of the vaginal introitus and speculum does not affect Papanicolaou smears. *Obstetrics & Gynecology, 100*(5 Pt. 1), 887–888. doi:10.1016/S0029-7844(02)02168-3

Harlow, S.D., Gass, M., Hall, J.E., Lobo, R., Maki, P., Rebar, R.W., . . . de Villiers, T.J. (2012). Executive summary of the Stages of Reproductive Aging Workshop + 10: addressing the unfinished agenda of staging reproductive aging. *The Journal of Clinical Endocrinology & Metabolism, 97*(4), 1159–1168. doi:10.1210/jc.2011-3362

Havercamp, S. M., & Scott, H. M. (2015). National health surveillance of adults with disabilities, adults with intellectual and developmental disabilities, and adults with no disabilities. *Disability and Health Journal, 8*(2), 165–172. doi:10.1016/j.dhjo.2014.11.002

Haylen, B. T., de Ridder, D., Freeman, R. M., Swift, S. E., Berghmans, B., Lee, J., . . . Schaer, G. N. (2010). An International Urogynecological Association (IUGA)/International Continence Society (ICS) joint report on the terminology for female pelvic floor dysfunction. *Neurourology and Urodynamics, 29*(1), 4–20. doi:10.1002/nau.20798

Hays, D., & Clarks, N. R. (2017). Gynecologic anatomy and physiology. In K. D. L. Schuiling & F. E. Likis (Eds.), *Women's gynecologic health* (3rd ed., pp. 77–93). Burlington, MA: Jones & Bartlett.

Hillier, S. L., Nugent, R. P., Eschenbach, D. A., Krohn, M. A., Gibbs, R. S., & Martin, D. H. (1995). Vaginal Infections and Prematurity Study Group. Association between bacterial vaginosis and preterm delivery of a low-birth-weight infant. *New England Journal of Medicine, 333*(26), 1737–1742. doi:10.1056/NEJM199512283332604

Hologic. (2017). *Liquid based cytology collection: Quick reference guide.* Retrieved from http://www.thinprep.com.au/assets/MED-00247-AUS-ENRev001_ThinPrep%20AU_Sample_collection_protocols_updated.pdf

Hsueh, A. J. W., Eisenhauer, K., Chun, S. Y., Hsu, S. Y., & Billig, H. (1996). Gonadal cell apoptosis. *Recent Progress in Hormone Research, 51,* 433–456. Retrieved from https://www.sciencedirect.com/book/9780125711487/recent-progress-in-hormone-research

Hull, M. G. (1987). Epidemiology of infertility and polycystic ovarian disease: Endocrinological and demographic studies. *Gynecological Endocrinology, 1*(3), 235–245. doi:10.3109/09513598709023610

Huseynov, A., Zollikofer, C. P. E., Coudyzer, W., Gascho, D., Kellenberger, C., Hinzpeter, R., & Ponce de Leon, M. S. (2016). Developmental evidence for obstetric adaptation of the human female pelvis. *Proceedings of the National Academy of Sciences of the United States of America, 113*(19), 5227–5232. doi:10.1073/pnas.1517085113

Jhingran, A., & Meyer, L. A. (2017). Malignant diseases of the cervix: Microinvasive and invasive carcinoma: Diagnosis and management. In R. A. Lobo, D. M. Gershenson, G. M. Lentz, & F. A. Valea (Eds.), *Comprehensive Gynecology* (7th ed., pp. 666–684). Philadelphia, PA: Elsevier.

Kaiser Family Foundation. (2019). *Percentage of non-institutionalized population who reported a disability.* Retrieved from https://www.kff.org/other/state-indicator/disability-prevalence/?currentTimeframe=0&sortModel=%7B%22colId%22:%22Location%22,%22sort%22:%22asc%22%7D

Kaplowitz, P., & Bloch, C. (2016). Evaluation and referral of children with signs of early puberty. *Pediatrics, 137*(1), e20153732. doi:10.1542/peds.2015-3732

Kashyap, B., Singh, R., Bhalla, P., Arora, R., & Aggarwal, A. (2008). Reliability of self-collected versus provider-collected vaginal swabs for the diagnosis of bacterial vaginosis. *International Journal of STD & AIDS, 19,* 510–513. doi:10.1258/ijsa.2007.007235

Kaufman, R. H., Adam, E., Icenogle, J., Lawson, H., Lee, N., Reeves, K. O., . . . Reeves, W. C. (1997). Relevance of human papillomavirus screening in management of cervical intraepithelial neoplasia. *American*

Journal of Obstetrics and Gynecology, 176(1, Pt. 1), 87–92. doi:10.1016/S0002-9378(97)80017-8

Kimberlin, D. W., & Rouse, D. J. (2004). Genital herpes. *New England Journal of Medicine, 350*(19), 1970–1977. doi:10.1056/NEJMcp023065

King, T. L., & Brucker, M. C. (2019). Anatomy and physiology of the female reproductive system. In T. L. King, M. C. Brucker, K. Osborne, & C. M. Jevitt (Eds.), *Varney's midwifery* (6th ed., pp. 327–356). Burlington, MA: Jones & Bartlett.

Kissinger, P. (2015). Epidemiology and treatment of trichomoniasis. *Current Infectious Disease Reports, 17*(6), 31. doi:10.1007/s11908-015-0484-7

Kolesova, O., & Vetra, J. (2012). Female pelvic types and age differences in their distribution. *Papers on Anthropology, 21*, 147–154. doi:10.12697/poa.2012.21.11

Lane, J. L., Johnson-Agbakwu, C. E., Warren, N., Budhathoki, C., & Cole, E. C. (2018). Female genital cutting: Clinical knowledge, attitudes, and practices from a provider survey in the US. *Journal of Immigrant and Minority Health, 21*(5), 954–964. doi:10.1007/s10903-018-0833-3

Lee, K. H., Hong, J. S., Jung, H. J., Jeong, H. K., Moon, J. S., Park, W. H., . . . Shin, J. I. (2019). Imperforate hymen: A comprehensive systematic review. *Journal of Clinical Medicine, 8*(56), 1–14. doi:10.3390/jcm8010056

Leone, P. A. (2007). Scabies and pediculosis pubis: An update of treatment regimens and general review. *Clinical Infectious Diseases, 44*(Suppl. 3), S153–S159. doi:10.1086/511428

Lobo, R. A. (2017). Menopause and care of the mature woman: Endocrinology, consequences of estrogen deficiency, effects of hormone therapy, and other treatment options. In R. A. Lobo, D. M. Gershenson, G. M. Lentz, & F. A. Valea (Eds.), *Comprehensive gynecology* (7th ed., pp. 48–76). Philadelphia, PA: Elsevier.

Lopez, J. E. M. (2015, March 16). Candidiasis (vulvovaginal). *BMJ Clinical Evidence, 2015*, 815. Retrieved from https://www.ncbi.nlm.nih.gov/pmc/articles/PMC4360556/pdf/2015-0815.pdf

Louie, K. S., Castellsague, X., de Sanjose, S., Herrero, R., Meijer, C. J., Shah, K., . . . Bosch, F. X. (2011). Smoking and passive smoking in cervical cancer risk: Pooled analysis of couples from the IARC multicentric case-control studies. *Cancer Epidemiology, Biomarkers & Prevention, 20*(7), 1379–1390. doi:10.1158/1055-9965.EPI-11-0284

Lowy, D. R., & Schiller, J. T. (2012). Reducing HPV-associated cancer globally. *Cancer Prevention Research, 5*(1), 18–23. doi:10.1158/1940-6207

Lu, K. H., Wood, M. E., Daniels, M., Burke, C., Ford, J., Kauff, N. D., . . . Hughes, K. S. (2014, March 10). American Society of Clinical Oncology expert statement: Collection and use of a cancer family history for oncology providers. *Journal of Clinical Oncology, 32*(8), 833–840. doi:10.1200/JCO.2013.50.9257

Madadevan, V. (2018). Anatomy of the pelvis. *Surgery (Oxford), 36*(7), 333–338. doi:10.1016/j.mpsur.2018.04.005

Maldonado, V. A. (2014). Benign vulvar tumors. *Best Practice & Research Clinical Obstetrics and Gynaecology, 28*(7), 1088–1097. doi:10.1016/j.bpobgyn.2014.07.014

Marion, L. L., & Meeks, G. R. (2012). Ectopic pregnancy: History, incidence, epidemiology, and risk factors. *Clinical Obstetrics and Gynecology, 55*(2), 376–386. doi:10.1097/GRF.0b013e3182516d7b

Markowitz, L. E., Dunne, E. F., Saraiya, M., Chesson, H. W., Curtis, C. R., Gee, J., . . . Unger, E. R. (2014). Human papillomavirus vaccination: Recommendations of the Advisory Committee on Immunization Practices (ACIP). *Morbidity and Mortality Weekly Report, 63*(RR-05), 1–30. Retrieved from https://www.cdc.gov/mmwr/preview/mmwrhtml/rr6305a1.htm

McQuillan, G., Kruszon-Moran, D., Flagg, E. W., & Paulose-Ram, R. (2018, February). *Prevalence of herpes simplex virus type 1 and type 2 in persons aged 14–49: United States, 2015-2016* (NCHS Data Brief No. 304). Retrieved from https://www.cdc.gov/nchs/products/databriefs/db304.htm

Mehta, P. K., Easter, S. R., Potter, J., Castleberry, N., Schulkin, J., & Robinson, J. N. (2018). Lesbian, gay, bisexual, and transgender health: Obstetrician-gynecologists' training, attitudes, knowledge, and practice. *Journal of Women's Health, 27*(12), 1459–1465. doi:10.1089/jwh.2017.6912

Meites, E., Kempe, A., & Markowitz, L. E. (2016). Use of a 2-dose schedule for human papillomavirus vaccination—Updated recommendations of the Advisory Committee on Immunization Practices. *Morbidity and Mortality Weekly Report, 65*, 1405–1408. doi:10.15585/mmwr.mm6549a5

Mendiratta, V., & Lentz, G. M. (2017). History, physical examination, and preventive health care. In R. A. Lobo, D. M. Gershenson, G. M. Lentz, & F. A. Valea (Eds.), *Comprehensive gynecology* (7th ed., pp. 48–76). Philadelphia, PA: Elsevier.

Morgan, D. J., Aboud, C. J., McCaffrey, I. M. B., Bhide, S. A., Lamont, R. F., & Taylor-Robinson, D. (1996). Comparison of gram-stained smears prepared from blind vaginal swabs with those obtained at speculum examination for the assessment of vaginal flora. *British Journal of Obstetrics and Gynaecology, 103*, 1105–1108. doi:10.1111/j.1471-0528.1996.tb09591.x

Moyer, V. A., LeFevre, M. L., Siu, A. L., Baumann, L. C., Bibbins-Domingo, K., Curry, S. J., . . . Pignone, M. P. (2013). Screening for HIV: U.S. Preventive Services Task Force recommendation statement. *Annals of Internal Medicine, 159*(1), 51–60. doi:10.7326/0003-4819-159-1-201307020-00645

Moyer, V. A., LeFevre, M. L., Siu, A. L., Baumann, L. C., Bibbins-Domingo, K., Curry, S. J., . . . Pignone, M. P. (2014). Risk assessment, genetic counseling, and genetic testing for BRCA-related cancer in women: U.S. Preventive Services Task Force recommendation statement. *Annals of Internal Medicine, 160*(4), 271–281. doi:10.7326/m13-2747

National Cancer Institute. (2019a). *HPV and cancer*. Retrieved from https://www.cancer.gov/about-cancer/causes-prevention/risk/infectious-agents/hpv-fact-sheet#r1

National Cancer Institute. (2019b). *SEER cancer stat facts: Ovarian cancer*. Retrieved from https://seer.cancer.gov/statfacts/html/ovary.html

National Institute on Drug Abuse, National Institutes of Health, & U.S. Department of Health and Human Services. (2019, July). Drug use and viral infections (HIV, Hepatitis). Retrieved from https://www.drugabuse.gov/publications/drugfacts/drug-use-viral-infections-hiv-hepatitis

Nelson, D. B., Bellamy, S., Gray, T. S., & Nachamkin, I. (2003). Self-collected versus provider-collected vaginal swabs for the diagnosis of bacterial vaginosis: An assessment of validity and reliability. *Journal of Clinical Epidemiology, 56*, 862–866. doi:1016/S0895-4356(03)00073-8

The North American Menopause Society. (2014 *Menopause practice: A clinician's guide* (pp. 21–43, 45–105). Mayfield Heights, OH: Author.

Office of Disease Prevention and Health Promotion. (n.d.). *Family planning.* Retrieved from https://www.healthy people.gov/2020/topics-objectives/topic/family-planning

Paladine, H. L., & Desai, U. A. (2018). Vaginitis: Diagnosis and treatment. *American Family Physician, 97*(5), 321–329. Retrieved from https://www.aafp.org/afp/2018/0301/p321 .html

Pavlik, E. J., Ueland, F. R., Miller, R. W., Ubellacker, J. M., DeSimone, C. P., Elder, J., . . . van Nagell, J. R., Jr. (2013). Frequency and disposition of ovarian abnormalities followed with serial transvaginal ultrasonography. *Obstetrics & Gynecology, 122*(2, Pt. 1), 210–217. doi:10.1097/AOG.0b013e318298def5

Pergialiotis, V., Vlachos, D. G., Rodolakis, A., Thomakos, N., Christakis, D., & Vlachos, G. D. (2015). The effect of vaginal lubrication on unsatisfactory results of cervical smears. *Journal of Lower Genital Tract Disease, 19*(1), 55–61. doi:10.1097/LGT.0000000000000037

Phelan, N., O'Connor, A., Kyaw-Tun, T., Correia, N., Boran, G., Roche, H. M., & Gibney, J. (2010). Lipoprotein subclass patterns in women with polycystic ovarian syndrome (PCOS) compared with equally insulin-resistant women without PCOS. *The Journal of Clinical Endocrinology & Metabolism, 95*(8), 3933–3939. doi:10.1210/jc.2009-2444

Piepert, J. F., Ness, R. B., Blume, J., Soper, D. E., Holley, R., Randall, H., . . . Bass, D. C. (2001). Clinical predictors of endometriosis in women with symptoms and signs of pelvic inflammatory disease. *American Journal of Obstetrics and Gynecology, 184*, 856–864. doi:10.1067/mob.2001.113847

Portman, D. J., & Gass, M. L. S. (2014). Genitourinary syndrome of menopause: New terminology for vulvovaginal atrophy from the International Society for the Study of Women's Sexual Health and The North American Menopause Society. *Menopause, 21*(10), 1063–1068. doi:10.1097/gme.0000000000000329

Pundir, J., & Auld, B. J. (2008). A review of the management of diseases of the Bartholin's gland. *Journal of Obstetrics and Gynaecology, 28*(2), 161–165. doi:10.1080/01443610801912865

Rempe, J. R., Paladino, P., Mazey, M., Gilbert-Ahee, L., Colman, R., & Shaw, M. (2018). *Metal versus plastic speculums.* Manuscript in preparation.

Reyes, M. C., & Cooper, K. (2014). An update on vulvar intraepithelial neoplasia: Terminology and a practical approach to diagnosis. *Journal of Clinical Pathology, 67*, 290–294. doi:10.1136/jclinpath-2013-202117

Rosenfield, R. L., Lipton, R. B., & Drum, M. L. (2009). Thelarche, pubarche, and menarche attainment in children with normal and elevated body mass index. *Pediatrics, 123*(1), 84–88. doi:10.1542/peds.2008-0146

Royal College of Nursing. (2016, March 14). *Genital examination in women: A resource for skills development and assessment.* London, United Kingdom: Author. Retrieved from https://www.rcn.org.uk/professional-development/publications/pub-005480

Schiffman, M. H., Bauer, H. M., Hoover, R. N., Glass, A. G., Cadell, D. M., Rush, B. B., . . . Wacholder, S. (1993). Epidemiologic evidence showing that human papillomavirus infection causes most cervical intraepithelial neoplasia. *Journal of the National Cancer Institute, 85*(12), 958–964. doi:10.1093/jnci/85.12.958

Schlosser, B. J., & Mirowski, G. W. (2015). Lichen sclerosus and lichen planus in women and girls. *Clinical Obstetrics and Gynecology, 58*(1), 125–142. doi:10.1097/GRF.0000000000000090

Schmidt, J., Landin-Wilhelmsen, K., Brannstrom, M., & Dahlgren, E. (2011). Cardiovascular disease and risk factors in PCOS women of postmenopausal age: A 21-year controlled follow-up study. *The Journal of Clinical Endocrinology & Metabolism, 96*(12), 3794–3803. doi:10.1210/jc.2011-1677

Segars, J. H., Parrott, E. C., Nagel, J. D., Guo, X. C., Gao, X., Birnbaum, L. S., . . . Dixon, D. (2014). Proceedings from the Third National Institutes of Health International Congress on Advances in Uterine Leiomyoma Research: Comprehensive review, conference summary, and future recommendations. *Human Reproduction Update, 20*(3), 309–333. doi:10.1093/humupd/dmt058

Shinkai, K., & Fox, L. P. (2019). Dermatologic disorders. In M. A. Papadakis, S. J. McPhee, & M. W. Rabow (Eds.), *Current medical diagnosis & treatment 2019* (58th ed., pp. 103–173). New York, NY: McGraw-Hill.

Sigurdsson, K. (2013). Is a liquid-based cytology more sensitive than a conventional Pap smear? *Cytopathology, 24*(4), 254–263. doi:10.1111/cyt.12037

Simms, I., Warburton, F., & Westrom, L. (2003). Diagnosis of pelvic inflammatory disease: Time for a rethink. *Sexually Transmitted Infections, 79*, 491–494. doi:10.1136/sti.79.6.491

Simpson, R. C., & Murphy, R. (2012). Is vulval erosive lichen planus a premalignant condition? *Archives of Dermatological, 148*(11), 1314–1316. doi:10.1001/2013.jamadermatol.84

Smith, R. P. (2018). *Netter's obstetrics & gynecology* (3rd ed., pp. 11–12). Philadelphia, PA: Elsevier.

Smith, S. G., Zhang, X., Basile, K. C., Merrick, M. T., Wang, J., Kresnow, M., & Chen, J. (2018, November). *The national intimate partner and sexual violence survey: 2015 data brief—Updated release.* Atlanta, GA: National Center for Injury Prevention and Control, Centers for Disease Control and Prevention. Retrieved from https://www.cdc.gov/violenceprevention/pdf/2015data-brief508.pdf

Strauss, R. A., Eucker, B., Savitz, D. A., & Thorp, J. M., Jr. (2005, March). Diagnosis of bacterial vaginosis from self-obtained vaginal swabs. *Infectious Diseases in Obstetrics and Gynecology, 13*(1), 31–35. doi:10.1080/10647440400025611

Tanksale, V. S., Sahasrabhojanee, M., Patel, V., Nevrekar, P., Menezes, S., & Mabey, D. (2003). The reliability of a structured examination protocol and self administered vaginal swabs: A pilot study of gynaecological outpatients in Goa, India. *Sexually Transmitted Infections, 79*, 251–253. doi:10.1136/sti.79.3.251

United Nations Children's Fund. (2019, October). *Female genital mutilation.* Retrieved from https://data.unicef.org/topic/child-protection/female-genital-mutilation

U.S. Cancer Statistics Working Group. (2019). *U.S. Cancer Statistics Data Visualizations Tool, based on November*

2018 submission data (1999-2016). Retrieved from https://gis.cdc.gov/Cancer/USCS/DataViz.html

U.S. Preventive Services Task Force. (2014, September). Clinical summary: Chlamydia and gonorrhea: Screening. Retrieved from https://www.uspreventiveservicestaskforce .org/Page/Document/ClinicalSummaryFinal/chlamydia -and-gonorrhea-screening

U.S. Preventive Services Task Force. (2016, November). Genital herpes infection: Serologic screening. Retrieved from https://www.uspreventiveservicestaskforce.org/ Page/Document/UpdateSummaryFinal/genital-herpes -screening1?ds=1&s=genital%20herpes

U.S. Preventive Services Task Force. (2018a, August). Clinical summary: Cervical cancer: Screening. Retrieved from https://www.uspreventiveservicestaskforce.org/Page /Document/ClinicalSummaryFinal/cervical-cancer -screening2

U.S. Preventive Services Task Force. (2018b, February). Final recommendation statement: Ovarian cancer: Screening. Retrieved from https://www.uspreventiveservicestaskforce .org/Page/Document/RecommendationStatementFinal/ ovarian-cancer-screening1

U.S. Preventive Services Task Force. (2019, August). BRCA-related cancer: Risk assessment, genetic counseling, and genetic testing. Retrieved from https://www .uspreventiveservicestaskforce.org/Page/Document/ UpdateSummaryFinal/brca-related-cancer-risk-assessment -genetic-counseling-and-genetic-testing1

Uygur, D., Guler, T., Yayci, E., Atacag, T., Comunoglu, C., & Kuzey, G. M. (2012). Association of speculum lubrication with pain and Papanicolaou test accuracy. *American Board of Family Medicine, 25*(6), 798–804. doi:10.3122/ jabfm.2012.06.120021

Valea, F. A. (2017). Reproductive anatomy: Gross and microscopic, clinical correlations. In R. A. Lobo, D. M. Gershenson, G. M. Lentz, & F. A. Valea (Eds.), *Comprehensive gynecology* (7th ed., pp. 48–76). Philadelphia, PA: Elsevier.

Vink, J. M., Sadrzadeh, S., Lambalk, C. B., & Boomsma, D. I. (2006). Heritability of polycystic ovary syndrome in a Dutch twin-family study. *The Journal of Clinical Endocrinology & Metabolism, 91*(6), 2100–2104. doi:10.1210/ jc.2005-1494

Wald, A., Zeh, J., Selke, S., Warren, T., Ryncarz, A. J., Ashley, R., . . . Corey, L. (2000). Reactivation of genital herpes simplex virus type 2 infection in asymptomatic seropositive persons. *New England Journal of Medicine, 342*(12), 844–850. doi:10.1056/NEJM200003233421203

Wallace, H. J. (1971). Lichen sclerosus et atrophicus. *Transactions of the St. John's Hospital Dermatological Society, 57*, 9–30.

Welsh, B., Howard, A., & Cook, K. (2004). Vulval itch. *Australian Family Physician, 33*(7), 505–510. Retrieved from https://www.racgp.org.au/afpbackissues/2004/200407/ 20040703welsh.pdf

Wolf, J. K., & Ramirez, P. T. (2001). The molecular biology of cervical cancer. *Cancer Investigation, 19*(6), 621–629. doi:10.1081/CNV-100104290

Wolf, R., Oumeish, O. Y., & Parish, L. C. (2011). Intertriginous eruption. *Clinics in Dermatology, 29*, 173–179. doi:10.1016/j.clindermatol.2010.09.009

World Health Organization. (n.d.-a). *Disabilities*. Retrieved from https://www.who.int/topics/disabilities/en

World Health Organization. (n.d.-b). *Female genital mutilation*. Retrieved from https://afro.who.int/health-topics/ female-genital-mutilation

Zurynski, Y., Sureshkumar, P., Phu, A., & Elliott, E. (2015). Female genital mutilation and cutting: A systematic literature review of health professionals' knowledge, attitudes and clinical practice. *BMC International Health and Human Rights, 15*, 32–50. doi:10.1186/s12914-015-0070-y

21

Evidence-Based Obstetric Assessment

Emily Neiman

"To be pregnant is to be vitally alive, thoroughly woman, and distressingly inhabited. Soul and spirit are stretched—along with body—making pregnancy a time of transition, growth, and profound beginnings."

—ANNE CHRISTIAN BUCHANAN

 VIDEO

- Well Exam: Prenatal Exam

LEARNING OBJECTIVES

- Describe the normal physiologic changes associated with pregnancy and why these occur.
- Understand the key components of a comprehensive evidence-based history and physical exam of a pregnant patient.
- Recognize abnormal findings in a pregnant patient, and initiate appropriate testing and treatment.
- Diagnose common pregnancy complications and initiate appropriate testing and treatment.

ANATOMY AND PHYSIOLOGY

The potential childbearing period takes up a majority of a woman's life—theoretically from menarche to menopause. Conception, pregnancy, labor, and birth are major life events and affect women and families both physically and emotionally. This section will focus specifically on anatomic and physiologic changes during

Visit https://connect.springerpub.com/content/book/978-0-8261 -6454-4/chapter/ch00 to access the videos.

pregnancy. The approximate length of a full-term **pregnancy** is 38 weeks from ovulation, or 40 weeks from the first day of the last menstrual period (LMP). Over this time, the reproductive organs and almost every other body system adapt to support the developing fetus and prepare to support an infant. These changes are outlined in the text that follows.

BREASTS

There are two phases of change to the **breasts** during pregnancy: mammogenesis and lactogenesis I. Mammogenesis starts in early pregnancy and is responsible for breast enlargement due to cellular hyperplasia (cellular proliferation). The breast lobules increase in size, and alveoli proliferate at the end of the breast lobules. The areola become darker and bigger, and the breasts may become tender during this phase (**Figure 21.1**). Mid-pregnancy, the lactogenesis I phase begins, and the alveoli epithelial cells become secretory epithelium. The alveoli produce colostrum, but this process is mostly suppressed during pregnancy because of increased progesterone (King, Brucker, Osborne, & Jevitt, 2019).

UTERUS

The **uterus** undergoes multiple changes during pregnancy (**Figure 21.2**). The size of the uterus changes, driven by hormonal effects on smooth muscle cells (causing hyperplasia) and increased ability for both contractility and elasticity.

The three layers of the uterus (endometrium, myometrium, and perimetrium) become clearly defined during pregnancy. The endometrial layer of the uterus becomes

585

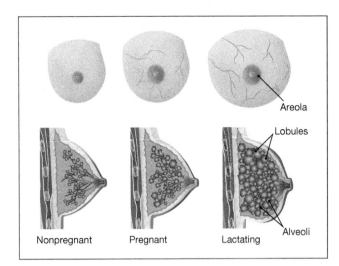

FIGURE 21.1 Breast changes during pregnancy. Breast lobules increase in size, alveoli proliferate at the end of the breast lobules, and the areola become darker and bigger.

the decidua during pregnancy, facilitating implantation and remodeling the extracellular matrix. Once the blastocyte is present at the implantation site, the stromal cells become decidual cells, which are stronger and larger. These cells have a membrane to which the trophoblast can attach, which triggers a chemical process causing remodeling of the spiral arteries. The endothelial and smooth muscle portion of the arteries are destroyed, which makes them unable to contract or expand in response to vasoactive agents. This remodeling of the spiral arteries is critical for the development of a healthy placenta and a healthy pregnancy—if the remodeling does not happen as it should, maternal and fetal morbidity can result, such as fetal growth restriction, reduced placental oxygenation, or preeclampsia. The decidual tissue that is formed during pregnancy will be shed after the birth. The innervation of the uterus also changes during pregnancy—there is less innervation at the fundus (top) of the uterus and more nerve fibers remain near the cervix.

CERVIX

The **cervix** softens as early as 2 weeks after conception (Goodell's sign) owing to increased estrogen production. Additionally, cervical vascularization increases, which may lead to spotting during pregnancy, particularly after intercourse. The increased vascularization may also contribute to a cyanotic appearance to the cervix in early pregnancy (Chadwick's sign), first seen at 6 to 8 weeks' gestation. Mucus production from glandular tissue is increased, which serves to prevent ascending bacteria or pathogens during pregnancy. There are four distinct phases of cervical change during pregnancy, labor, birth, and postpartum. The first stage is softening, or "remodeling." The second stage occurs toward the end of pregnancy and is called "ripening," or extreme

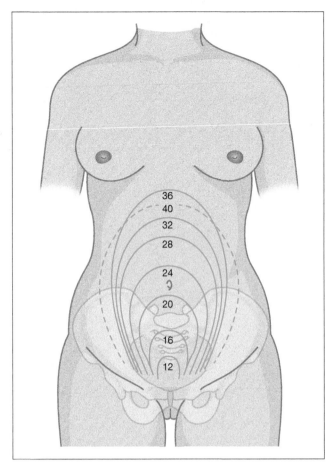

FIGURE 21.2 Changes in fundal height. Changes in fundal height during pregnancy: At 12 weeks' gestation, the fundus of the uterus is palpable just superior to the symphysis pubis. At 16 weeks' gestation, the fundus is palpable midway between the symphysis pubis and the umbilicus. At 20 weeks' gestation, the fundus is in line with the umbilicus. At approximately 28 weeks' gestation, the fundus is palpable midway between the umbilicus and the xyphoid process; the clinician should be able to determine fetal presentation. At 34 weeks' gestation, the fundus is palpable just below the xyphoid process. It should be noted that sometimes fundal height will decrease at term, as the fetal head engages in the maternal pelvis.

softening. "Dilation" is the third stage, which happens just prior to and during labor. During the postpartum period, the fourth stage, "repair," occurs (King et al., 2019).

Cervical ripening begins in the weeks prior to labor. This ripening is thought to be due to interactions of hormonal and mechanical factors: progesterone levels decrease, estrogen levels increase, the water content and vascularization of the cervix increase, and the strength of collagen bundles in the cervix decreases. Effacement and dilatation of the cervix may also start to occur in the weeks before labor begins and continue through labor. Uterine contractions stimulate cervical effacement, or the shortening of the length of the cervix. Dilation of the cervix occurs as labor progresses, opening

BOX 21.1
STAGES OF LABOR

- The first stage of labor begins when the woman starts having regular contractions, causing progressive changes in the cervix. The cervix softens, shortens, and thins (termed effacement). This stage is divided into three phases: early labor, active labor, and transition.
  - Early labor: Contractions begin. The cervix softens and begins to dilate (cervical dilation: 0–5 cm).
  - Active labor: Contractions intensify and are longer, stronger, and more frequent. The cervix dilates more rapidly (cervical dilation: 6–10 cm).
  - Transition: This is the most intense stage of labor. Contractions are strong and frequent and can last up to 90 seconds at a time.
- The second stage of labor begins when the cervix is fully dilated. This is commonly referred to as the "pushing stage." It ends with the birth of the baby.
- The third (and final) stage of labor begins right after the birth of the baby and ends on delivery of the placenta.

the internal os from its prepregnancy closed state to 10 cm (King et al., 2019). Ten centimeters' dilation marks the end of the first stage of labor and the start of the second stage of labor. See **Box 21.1** for the stages of labor and **Figure 21.3** for a depiction of the cervical changes that occur during labor.

ENDOCRINE SYSTEM

The placenta produces human chorionic gonadotropin (hCG) and human placental lactogen (hPL) and is an additional source of estrogen and progesterone production during pregnancy. Prior to implantation, hCG is secreted by the blastocyst and works to prevent degeneration of the corpus luteum after ovulation, which then continues to produce estrogen and progesterone. The free beta unit of hCG (beta-hCG) is often measured, either through urine or serum, in order to diagnose pregnancy (it is the basis for pregnancy tests) and to ensure that an early pregnancy seems to be progressing normally. The level of beta-hCG doubles approximately every 48 hours until it reaches a peak of approximately 100,000 mIU/mL around 8 to 11 weeks' gestation (King et al., 2019).

The fetus does not produce any detectable level of glucose during development and is dependent on the maternal supply. hPL alters maternal glucose metabolism

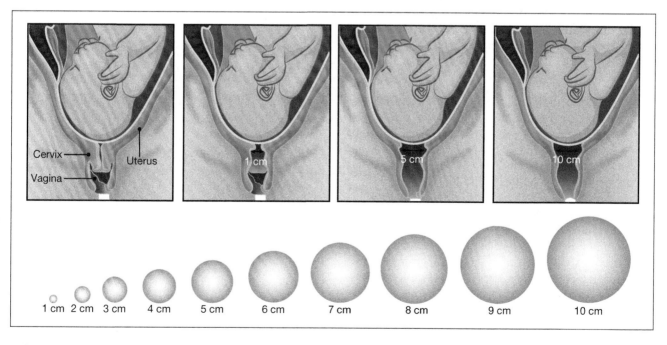

FIGURE 21.3 Cervical dilatation and effacement during labor. The cervix dilates from 0 (closed) to 10 cm throughout the first stage of labor. This progress is not linear and varies by individual. Effacement also occurs throughout the first stage of labor, thinning the cervix from 0% effaced to 100% effaced. Once the cervix is 10 cm dilated and 100% effaced, the second stage of labor begins.

in order to provide glucose for adequate fetal nutrition. The effect of this change in metabolism by hPL is a state of maternal insulin resistance during pregnancy and is most pronounced between 24 and 28 weeks' gestation.

Progesterone is initially produced by the corpus luteum; the placenta eventually takes over progesterone production. Progesterone is a steroid hormone that is responsible for maintenance of pregnancy—primarily through uterine quiescence or preventing contractions. Low levels of progesterone in early pregnancy may lead to an increased risk of miscarriage, and progesterone is sometimes given in early pregnancy to treat threatened miscarriage.

Estradiol (E3) is the primary type of estrogen produced during pregnancy. It is initially produced by the corpus luteum until the fetal adrenal glands and placenta work together to produce estradiol. Some functions of estrogen during pregnancy include increasing blood flow to the uterus, encouraging growth of mammary tissue, and stimulating uterine contractility/response to oxytocin.

CARDIOVASCULAR SYSTEM

Cardiovascular changes are also seen during pregnancy, with the aim of maximizing oxygenation to both the mother and the fetus. Blood volume increases by 40% to 50% over the course of pregnancy; this can often result in a physiologic anemia due to hemodilution. Cardiac output increases 30% to 50%, which may lead to systolic ejection murmurs. Heart rate increases by 10 bpm, while blood pressure (BP) decreases. Mainly as a result of the effects of progesterone, there is a decrease in overall vascular resistance, often causing dependent edema and varicosities (Gabbe et al., 2017; King et al., 2019).

HEMATOLOGIC STATE

Pregnant and postpartum women are at increased risk for venous thromboembolic events, owing to an increase in clotting factors, decreased fibrinolysis, and decreased anticoagulant activity. As discussed earlier, physiologic anemia is common during pregnancy owing to hemodilution, but fetal uptake of hemoglobin also decreases maternal iron stores and can lead to further (and symptomatic) anemia.

Pregnancy is a state of slight immunosuppression, resulting in a small increase in the risk of gram-negative organism infections and mycotic or fungal infections. The white blood cell count rises throughout pregnancy. There is increased morbidity among pregnant women who do contract gram-negative infections, influenza, and varicella. Additionally, pregnant women are at greater risk for becoming infected with herpes simplex virus (HSV), poliovirus, cytomegalovirus (CMV), malaria, and hepatitis. In terms of preexisting autoimmune conditions, some of these are improved by pregnancy and some are worsened (King et al., 2019).

RESPIRATORY SYSTEM

Lung capacity is affected during pregnancy. Physical adaptations drive some of these changes, including an increased thoracic diameter and rise in the diaphragm. Hyperventilation results from increased tidal volume and vital capacity, as well as the effects of progesterone. This leads to a state of respiratory alkalosis as well as frequent dyspnea.

GASTROINTESTINAL SYSTEM

Gastrointestinal (GI) structures are shifted by the growing uterus. Increased progesterone levels slow gastric motility and gastric emptying time. These factors, combined with the uterus' pressure on the descending colon, can contribute to constipation during pregnancy. Heartburn and reflux are extremely common during pregnancy, particularly during the second and third trimesters.

URINARY SYSTEM

Urinary frequency and nocturia are both common concerns during pregnancy. These are generally due to renal changes—an increase in renal blood flow and an increase in the glomerular filtration rate. Progesterone causes dilation of the ureters, urethra, and bladder, which causes pregnant women to be at increased risk for urinary tract infections (UTIs). This dilation can also make it more likely that UTIs progress to pyelonephritis. Stress incontinence is also often reported during pregnancy owing to both urinary stasis and the pressure of the uterus on the bladder and pelvic floor.

SKELETAL STRUCTURE AND FUNCTION

The bony skeleton undergoes changes during pregnancy. Lordosis (or increasing anterior convexity of the lumbar spine) is progressive throughout pregnancy. This adaptation aids a woman in keeping her center of gravity over her legs, but may often cause lower back pain. Additionally, the pubic symphysis widens during pregnancy (increases from 3–4 to 7.7–7.9 mm). The widening may also cause discomfort in the pregnant woman, and women often describe inner thigh pain or bony pelvic pain with walking or standing (Gabbe et al., 2017).

KEY HISTORY QUESTIONS AND CONSIDERATIONS

The initial prenatal visit is an opportunity to provide a wealth of information to women about the foregoing changes and what to expect throughout pregnancy. This visit is ideally performed by 10 weeks' gestation (Lockwood & Magriples, 2019). It typically includes education about nutrition during pregnancy, food

CULTURALLY APPROPRIATE TERMINOLOGY

Obstetric clinicians will care for pregnant people who identify as LGBTQ+. As such, it is important to be inclusive in the language that is used and familiar with current terminology. Terminology will change over time, but it benefits the patient–clinician relationship for the clinician to be knowledgeable about the distinction between sex and gender and to be comfortable with current terms such as "agender," "cisgender," "chestfeeding," "gender nonconfirming," and "transgender." See Chapter 18, Evidence-Based Assessment of Sexual Orientation, Gender Identity, and Health for more information about appropriate terminology.

Source: American College of Nurse-Midwives Gender and Equity Taskforce. (2017). *ACNM issue brief: Use of culturally-appropriate terminology for gender diverse populations.* Retrieved from http://www.midwife.org/ACNM/files/ACNMLibraryData/UPLOADFILENAME/000000000313/Issue-Brief-Use-of-Culturally-Appropriate-Terminology-for-Gender-Diverse-Populations-FEB-2018.pdf

METHODS OF DETERMINING ESTIMATED DUE DATE

- The first day of the LMP may be used if the LMP is certain, cycles are regular (ideally every 28–30 days), and the LMP was normal for that woman. The accuracy of this can be compromised by several factors: Some women may not know their LMP, some may ovulate later in their cycle than others, and some may have some early pregnancy bleeding that they mistake for a period. Naegele's rule is based on an LMP from a 28-day menstrual cycle. The formula for Naegele's rule is the first day of LMP + 7 days – 3 months = EDD. This is the basis for the calculations performed by most pregnancy wheels and apps. The variation in EDDs obtained by these methods is 1–7 days (King et al., 2019).
- If the pregnancy is conceived using ART such as IUI or IVF, the date of insemination or embryo transfer may be used as the LMP.
- Ultrasound may also be used to confirm an EDD. First trimester ultrasound (performed before 14 weeks and 0 days) is most accurate (within 5–7 days). Second trimester ultrasound is less accurate in terms of dating the pregnancy, with a variance of 7–14 days.

ART, artificial reproductive technologies; EDD, estimated due date; IUI, intrauterine insemination; IVF, in vitro fertilization; LMP, last menstrual period.

safety, exercise recommendations, safety of various over-the-counter medications, options for genetic screening during pregnancy, expected weight gain based on starting weight and current body mass index (BMI), common discomforts of pregnancy, and relief measures. Prenatal visits are usually scheduled every 4 weeks until week 28, then every 2 weeks until week 36, and then weekly until birth. It is important for the clinician to use culturally appropriate terminology during these visits (**Box 21.2**). The initial visit is also used to gather a complete history and often to perform a physical exam.

HISTORY OF PRESENT ILLNESS
- LMP date: Unknown, approximate, definite
  - There are multiple methods of calculating an estimated due date (EDD) for a pregnancy, and an accurate calculation is an extremely important part of prenatal care (**Box 21.3**). An accurate due date can aid the clinician in determining appropriate intervention for preterm labor, timing of screening, evaluating fetal growth, and timing of labor induction if needed. The accuracy of dating becomes less accurate as the pregnancy progresses, and the EDD should not be recalculated after the second trimester (King et al., 2019).
- Last normal menstrual period (LNMP) date (if different than LMP)
- Age at menarche
- Age at EDD

- Typical cycle length (28–30 days most reliable in terms of dating)
- Is this a planned pregnancy? Was any contraception used at the time of conception?
- Is this a desired pregnancy? If not, discussion of pregnancy options—continuing pregnancy and keeping child, continuing pregnancy and adoption, pregnancy termination.

PAST MEDICAL HISTORY
- Allergies
- Hypertension
- Diabetes mellitus (also relevant: polycystic ovary syndrome [PCOS] or insulin resistance)
- Asthma
- Autoimmune disorders
- Anxiety/depression/postpartum depression or other mental health disorders
- History of varicella (disease or vaccination? If vaccination, how many doses?)

- History of cytomegalovirus (CMV)
- History of clotting disorders

Obstetric History (If Relevant)

- GTPAL (Gravida [number of pregnancies], Term [number of full-term births], Preterm [number of preterm births, after 20 weeks' gestation], Abortions [number of elective terminations and/or miscarriages, including births prior to 20 weeks' gestation], Living [number of living children])
- Method of prior births: Vaginal—spontaneous, vacuum, or forceps; Cesarean section—type of incision, reason for cesarean
- Length of labor
- Complications during previous pregnancies and/or births: Gestational diabetes mellitus (GDM; diet-controlled, controlled with oral medication, controlled with insulin); essential hypertension; gestational hypertension; preeclampsia; eclampsia; hemolysis, elevated liver enzymes, and low platelet count (HELLP); postpartum hemorrhage; shoulder dystocia; retained placenta; third- or fourth-degree perineal laceration; issues with child's health
- History of elective termination or miscarriage: Any complications; required dilation and curettage (D&C)
- History of miscarriage(s): Age of fetus at time of miscarriage
- History of preterm labor or birth (20 weeks 0 days to 36 weeks 6 days)
- History of fetal/neonatal demise
- History of ectopic pregnancy

Note: *A poor outcome in previous pregnancy increases the risk for a poor outcome in the next pregnancy.*

Gynecologic History

- Date of last Pap test
- History of abnormal Pap tests
- History of loop electrosurgical excision procedure (LEEP) or cone biopsy; if yes, there is an increased risk of cervical incompetence/preterm labor/preterm birth.
- History of gynecologic surgery
- History of endometriosis

FAMILY HISTORY

- Genetic disorders: Known or suspected genetic disease, multiple malformations, multiple miscarriages, recurrence of the same or similar disorders, intellectual disability, autism spectrum disorders, and consanguinity (Lockwood & Magriples, 2019)
- Type 2 diabetes mellitus (DM)
- Preeclampsia

SOCIAL HISTORY

- Marital status: Married, single, divorced, widowed, or partnered
- Partner: Is partner involved? If not, who is support? Does partner have any other children?
- Living situation
- Housing situation; feelings of safety
- Tobacco use; if yes, assess readiness to quit.
- Alcohol use
- Illicit drug use (marijuana may or may not be legal, depending on state, but still need to warn of unknown effects during pregnancy)
- History of alcohol/drug use or addiction
- Occupation: Exposure to workplace hazards (e.g., chemicals/fumes, radiation, chemotherapeutic agents, patients with CMV)
- Intimate partner violence or history of reproductive or sexual coercion of:
  - Markers for interpersonal violence and reproduction and sexual coercion: Clinicians should note any nonverbal markers of intimate partner violence or reproductive and sexual coercion. These may include bruising, improbable injury, depression, late prenatal care (initiation of care in second or third trimester), missed prenatal visits, and/or appointments canceled on short notice (Lockwood & Magriples, 2019).

REVIEW OF SYSTEMS

- Constitutional: Fatigue, weight gain, weight loss, change in appetite
- Head, eyes, ears, nose, throat (HEENT): Visual changes (blurred vision, spots, or floaters), epistaxis, nasal drainage/congestion, bleeding gums, tooth pain
- Cardiovascular: Heart palpitations, leg swelling
- Respiratory: Shortness of breath, wheezing, snoring
- GI: Nausea, vomiting, food aversions, abdominal pain, constipation, diarrhea
- Genitourinary (GU): Pelvic pain, vaginal bleeding, vaginal discharge, frequent urination, hematuria, dysuria, urinary urgency, urinary incontinence, sexually transmitted infections (STIs) exposure
- Musculoskeletal: Muscle cramping, muscle pain, joint pain
- Skin: Itching, breast tenderness, breast lumps, nipple discharge
- Neurologic: Headache, seizure, dizziness, lightheadedness, syncope
- Psychiatric: Anxiety, depression, irritability, suicidality
- Endocrine: Heat or cold intolerance
- Hematologic: Easy bruising, excess bleeding
- Allergic: Hives, seasonal allergies

PREVENTIVE CARE CONSIDERATIONS

- Cervical cancer screening
- Mammography screening (if applicable)
- Influenza vaccine: Seasonal, recommended during pregnancy regardless of gestational age (American College of Nurse-Midwives [ACNM], 2017)
- Tetanus diphtheria and pertussis (Tdap) vaccine: Recommended between 27 and 36 weeks' gestation during each pregnancy (ACNM, 2017)
- Depression screening (U.S. Preventive Services Task Force [USPSTF], 2016a, Grade B recommendation)
- Intimate partner violence screening (USPSTF, 2018a, Grade B)
- Tobacco use counseling if patient uses tobacco (advise patient to stop smoking, and provide behavioral interventions for cessation; USPSTF, 2015c, Grade A)
- Screening for unhealthy alcohol use: Provide brief behavioral counseling interventions to reduce unhealthy alcohol use (USPSTF, 2018d, Grade B)
- Pets at home: Patients with cats must be counseled on the risk of toxoplasmosis and precautions; patients who own reptiles must be counseled on the risk of listeriosis and precautions.
- Recent travel for patient or partner to areas with Zika and timing of travel; if so, any mosquito bites or symptoms
- Current medications/vitamins/supplements (consider safety profile in pregnancy)
- Prepregnancy weight
- Preferred pronouns (he/him, she/her, they/their)

UNIQUE POPULATION CONSIDERATIONS FOR HISTORY

Advanced Maternal Age

Women who will be age 35 or older at their EDD are considered to be advanced maternal age (AMA). There are increased risks with AMA pregnancies, including an increased risk of chromosomal abnormalities, fetal growth restriction, gestational diabetes, gestational hypertension, preeclampsia, placental insufficiency, preterm birth, and stillbirth. Women who are AMA should be counseled thoroughly on their options for genetic testing. They will often have a detailed (or level two) anatomy ultrasound, which looks for "soft markers" of genetic abnormalities. Recommendations often include growth ultrasounds in the third trimester and increased fetal surveillance (nonstress tests [NST]) close to full term. Induction at term (39 weeks) is often recommended for these women to mitigate the increased risk for stillbirth. The risk of stillbirth at term is lower for multiparous women than for those who are nulliparous (Frederiksen et al., 2018).

Trauma-Informed Care

Many studies have been conducted over the past several years to assess the prevalence of childhood maltreatment and its effect on adult mental health. This research has shown that one in five girls aged 0 to 17 have experienced trauma stemming from childhood maltreatment. It is estimated that one third of these girls will go on to develop posttraumatic stress disorder (PTSD). Not all of the childhood maltreatment is sexual in nature, but in women who have experienced this type of trauma and resultant PTSD, a gynecologic or obstetric exam may trigger PTSD symptoms. Labor and birth are also often triggering events for women with a history of sexual violence. Even without a history of abuse or maltreatment, some women are finding themselves traumatized by their care prenatally, or in labor and delivery (Sperlich, Seng, Li, Taylor, & Bradbury-Jones, 2017).

Another finding of recent studies is that PTSD can contribute to adverse perinatal outcomes such as prematurity, low birth weight, postpartum depression, delayed/impaired bonding with the infant, and lower rates of breastfeeding. It is necessary that clinicians educate themselves on trauma-informed care, as well as how best to care for these women during pregnancy without retraumatizing them. Trauma-informed care such as universal screening, clinician comfort with adjusting routine exams and responding to possible reactions of those affected by prior trauma, and the availability of PTSD resources and referrals all play a role in helping to establish a good clinician–patient relationship and contribute to improved perinatal outcomes (Sperlich et al., 2017). For more information on trauma-informed care, refer to Chapter 24, Evidence-Based Assessment and Screening for Traumatic Experiences: Abuse, Neglect, and Intimate Partner Violence.

PHYSICAL EXAMINATION

INSPECTION

The clinician should start the physical exam by noting the patient's vital signs. Height, weight (current and prepregnancy), and BP should be obtained. Note whether the patient appears visibly pregnant (fundus above the symphysis pubis). During inspection of the breasts, note whether the breasts are symmetric and if the nipples are everted, flat, or inverted. Note any changes to the skin of the breasts, including dimpling, peau d'orange appearance, erythema, or edema. A complete visual inspection of the external genitals should be performed, noting any lesions, erythema, edema, or

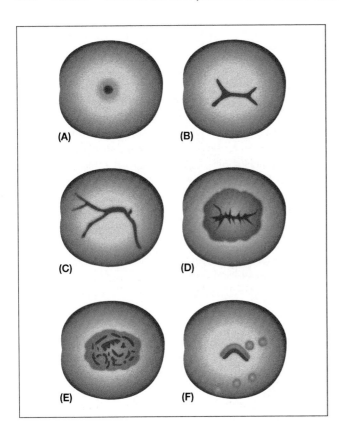

FIGURE 21.4 Appearance of normal cervix variations. (A) Nulliparous cervix. The os appears rounded. (B) Multiparous cervix. The os appears slit-like. (C) Multiparous cervix with scarring. (D) Everted cervix. The cells from the endocervical canal are present on the exterior of the cervix. (E) Eroded cervix. Also called cervical ectropion, this tissue is often friable. (F) Nabothian cysts. These are benign, mucus-filled cysts.

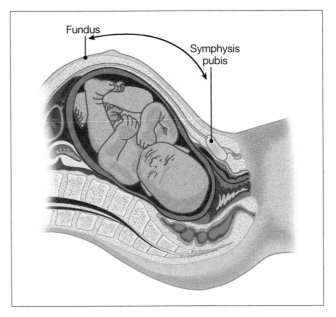

FIGURE 21.5 Measurement of fundal height. Measurement in centimeters from the top of the symphysis pubis to the fundus.

discharge. In early pregnancy, Chadwick's sign may be observed during a speculum exam— the cervix appears bluish-purplish in color or cyanotic (King et al., 2019). Note the presence of any lesions, erythema, edema, discharge, or bleeding inside the vaginal vault or at the cervix. The cervical os has a different appearance and feel in nulliparous women as compared with multiparous women (**Figure 21.4**). In the nulliparous woman, the cervical os is pinpoint in size and rounded. In the multiparous woman, the os has the appearance of a slit (King et al., 2019).

PALPATION

If greater than 12 weeks' gestation or if dates are unknown, an abdominal exam to assess whether the fundus is palpable in the abdomen is useful. At 12 weeks' gestation, the fundus should be palpable just caudally to the symphysis pubis. At 16 weeks' gestation, the fundus should be palpable midway between the symphysis pubis and the umbilicus. At 20 weeks' gestation, the fundus should be palpable at the umbilicus. As pregnancy

progresses past 20 weeks' gestation, the clinician will measure the fundal height at each visit. This is the measurement in centimeters from the top of the symphysis pubis to the fundus (**Figure 21.5**). The measurement approximately correlates with the current number of weeks' gestation. Clinicians will also assess the fetal presentation by utilizing Leopold's maneuvers after approximately 28 weeks' gestation (**Figure 21.6**).

Gestational age may be estimated by the size of the uterus, both abdominally and with a bimanual exam. In early pregnancy, the clinician may note Hegar's sign, in which the lower segment of the uterus becomes very soft and compressible in early pregnancy. The clinician may also note Goodell's sign, which is softening of the cervix in the first trimester (King et al., 2019). Clinical pelvimetry, or a measurement of the diameters of the pelvis, may be assessed by an experienced obstetric clinician, if indicated or desired. There is mixed evidence for the utility of measurements derived from pelvimetry, although this skill may be more useful during a labor in which cephalopelvic disproportion is suspected, or in low-resource countries, where a contracted pelvis may be more common (King et al., 2019).

When performing a speculum or bimanual pelvic exam, patient comfort, both physical and emotional, should be considered to be of the utmost importance. Many exams can be done without the need for stirrups, instead asking the patient to bend at the knee and come down toward the clinician on the exam table. Appropriate draping is important, as well as eye contact with the patient. It is helpful to ask the patient if they are ready to be touched before the clinician begins a pelvic exam

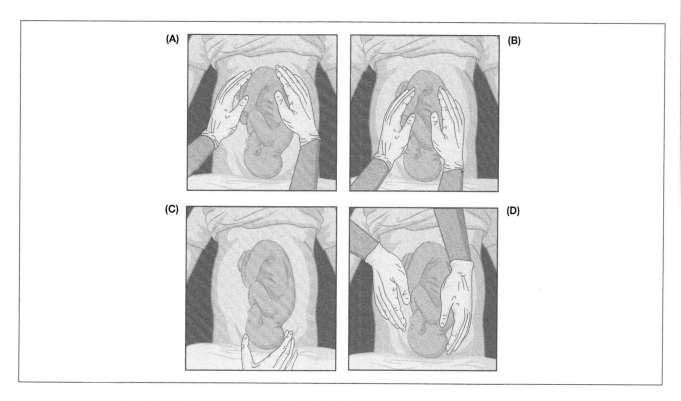

FIGURE 21.6 Performing Leopold's maneuvers. (A) Identify fetal part in uterine fundus. (B) Using the palmar surface of both hands, identify which side of the uterus contains the fetal back and which contains "small parts" such as hands and feet. (C) Use the thumb and third finger to identify fetal presenting part. (D) Use both hands to outline fetal presenting part.

and to initially touch on the inside of the thigh prior to touching the genitals.

In full-term pregnancy or for concerns prior to term, clinicians may again need to perform a cervical exam to evaluate for labor or preterm labor. There are five main findings from a cervical exam: dilation, effacement, fetal station (**Figure 21.7**), position of the cervix, and consistency of the cervix.

AUSCULTATION

The clinician may auscultate maternal heart and lungs during an initial physical exam. Fetal heart tones are auscultated at each visit, typically with a Doppler. Fetal heart tones can be heard with a Doppler after 10 to 12 weeks' gestation, depending on the strength of the Doppler. A fetoscope may also be used to auscultate fetal heart tones; however, this requires an experienced clinician, and the patient must typically be at least 24 weeks' gestation.

UNIQUE POPULATION CONSIDERATIONS FOR PHYSICAL EXAMINATION

If maternal BP is elevated at the initial prenatal visit, the clinician should attempt to find prepregnancy records to determine whether chronic hypertension

(cHTN) exists (Lockwood & Magriples, 2019). Maternal BMI should be calculated at the initial prenatal visit using the prepregnancy weight to guide weight gain recommendations during pregnancy as well as to assess for risk for comorbid conditions (**Table 21.1**; American College of Obstetricians and Gynecologists [ACOG], 2013).

Obesity

Obese pregnant patients should be counseled on their risks for the pregnancy, labor, and birth. Some of the effects of obesity on pregnancy include an increased risk of spontaneous abortion and recurrent miscarriage. Additional risks associated with obesity during pregnancy are increased findings of neural tube defects (NTDs); hydrocephaly; and cardiovascular, orofacial, and limb reduction anomalies. There is also an increased risk of cardiac dysfunction, proteinuria, sleep apnea, nonalcoholic fatty liver disease, GDM, and preeclampsia. The risk of stillbirth increases with class of obesity. Obese mothers also face an increased risk of cesarean birth, failed trial of labor, endometritis, wound rupture or dehiscence, and venous thrombosis. Long-term risks for mothers and children include increased risk of future metabolic dysfunction, postpartum weight retention, early termination of breastfeeding, postpartum anemia, and depression. The fetus of an obese mother is at greater risk for macrosomia and impaired growth during pregnancy. Long-term risks for offspring of mothers who were obese during pregnancy include an increase in metabolic syndrome and childhood obesity.

Women who have had bariatric surgery need to be evaluated for nutritional deficiencies during pregnancy.

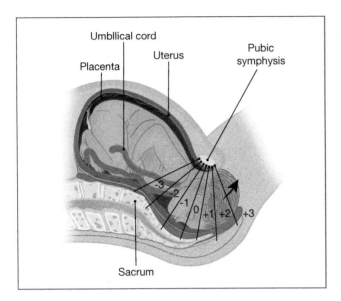

FIGURE 21.7 Fetal station. This is a measurement of the relationship of the presenting part to the ischial spines in the maternal pelvis and signifies the descent of the fetus in the pelvis. Negative numbers (e.g., –2, –1) indicate that the presenting part (typically, the bony aspect of the fetal vertex) is above the ischial spines by that many centimeters. Zero station indicates that the presenting part is in line with the ischial spines. Positive numbers (e.g., +1, +2) indicate that the presenting part is below the ischial spines by that many centimeters. The fetus descends as labor progresses. Most women will feel a spontaneous urge to push around 0 to +2 cm, particularly without an epidural.

Additionally, women with a history of certain types of bariatric surgery will not be able to complete a typical gestational diabetes screen during pregnancy, owing to the risk of dumping syndrome. Alternative screening for gestational diabetes must be considered for these women (ACOG, 2015b).

LABORATORY CONSIDERATIONS

INITIAL OBSTETRIC LAB WORK

Confirmation of pregnancy with urine pregnancy test or quantitative beta-hCG level.

Type and Screen

*   Rh (D) blood typing and antibody testing with repeated Rh (D) antibody testing for all unsensitized Rh (D)-negative women at 24 to 28 weeks' gestation, unless the biological father is known to be Rh (D) negative (USPSTF, 2015b). See **Box 21.4** for prevention of Rh (D) alloimmunization.
*   Syphilis (USPSTF, 2018c, Grade A recommendation)
*   Hepatitis B (USPSTF, 2019, Grade A recommendation)
*   HIV (USPSTF, 2018a, Grade A recommendation)
*   Complete blood count (CBC)
*   Rubella immunity
*   Urinalysis
*   Urine culture (USPSTF, 2015a, Grade A recommendation to screen for asymptomatic bacteriuria)
*   Gonorrhea/chlamydia

The following are frequently also ordered at the initial OB visit, dependent upon population, history, symptoms, and exposures:

*   Hepatitis C
*   Urine drug screen

TABLE 21.1 Institute of Medicine Weight Gain Recommendations for Pregnancy			
Prepregnancy Weight Category	Body Mass Index*	Recommended Range of Total Weight (lb)	Recommended Rates of Weight Gain† in the Second and Third Trimesters (lb; Mean Range [lb/week])
Underweight	<18.5	28–40	1 (1.0–1.3)
Normal weight	18.5–24.9	25–35	1 (0.8–1.0)
Overweight	25–29.9	15–25	0.6 (0.5–0.7)
Obese (includes all classes)	30 and greater	11–20	0.5 (0.4–0.6)

*Body mass index is calculated as weight in kilograms divided by height in meters squared, or as weight in pounds multiplied by 703, divided by height in inches.
†Calculations assume a 1.1–4.4 lb weight gain in the first trimester.
Source: Modified from Institute of Medicine. (2009). *Weight gain during pregnancy: Reexamining the guidelines.* Washington, DC. National Academies Press. © 2009 National Academy of Sciences.

BOX 21.4
PREVENTION OF RH (D) ALLOIMMUNIZATION

Approximately 15%–17% of women in the United States do not carry the Rhesus (Rh) D antigen in their blood. Women with these blood types are known as "Rh (D) negative." If a woman is carrying a fetus with the Rh (D) antigen and there is a mixing of maternal and fetal blood during pregnancy or birth, this can lead to Rh (D) alloimmunization. This mixing of the maternal and fetal blood may occur via many different mechanisms. Some common sensitizing events are threatened miscarriage or miscarriage, termination of pregnancy, antepartum hemorrhage, invasive genetic tests (chorionic villus sampling or amniocentesis), abdominal trauma, or birth. Administration of anti-D immune globulin (commonly known as Rhogam) is recommended within 72 hours of suspected mixing of fetal and maternal blood. Rhogam is given in the United States at 28 weeks' gestation for mothers who are Rh (D) negative to prevent alloimmunization at the time of birth. It is also given within 72 hours of birth once the baby has been typed and been shown to be Rh (D) positive.

Source: American College of Obstetricians and Gynecologists. (2017, reaffirmed 2019). ACOG Practice Bulletin No. 181: Prevention of Rh D alloimmunization. *Obstetrics & Gynecology*, 130(2), e57–e70. doi:10.1097/ AOG.0000000000002232

- Varicella immunity
- Toxoplasmosis
- CMV
- Vaginitis (yeast/bacterial vaginosis)
- Trichomonas
- Zika
- Lead level
- Cervical cancer screening, **if indicated**
- Thyroid function (**Box 21.5**)

GESTATIONAL DIABETES SCREENING

Early testing for undiagnosed type 2 diabetes is recommended in women with risk factors:

- BMI ≥25 (≥23 in Asian Americans) *plus* one or more of the following:
  - GDM in prior pregnancy
  - Hemoglobin A1C ≥5.7%, impaired glucose tolerance, or impaired fasting glucose on previous testing
  - First-degree relative with DM

BOX 21.5
THYROID DYSFUNCTION IN PREGNANCY

Thyroid function has physiologic variation during pregnancy. Primarily noteworthy is that thyroid-stimulating hormone (TSH) falls in the first trimester in response to increased levels of hCG, and free thyroxine (T4) has a corresponding increase. TSH typically returns to baseline levels after the first trimester and then gradually increases throughout the third trimester. The ACOG does not recommend universal thyroid function testing and states that this testing should be reserved for women who have a history of thyroid dysfunction or who are symptomatic. If women are found to be hypo- or hyperthyroid during pregnancy, they should be referred to their primary care clinician, an endocrinologist, or a perinatologist in order to regulate thyroid function. Recommendations for TSH ranges during pregnancy are: 0.1–2.5 mIU/L in the first trimester, 0.2–3.0 mIU/L in the second trimester, and 0.3–3.0 mIU/L in the third trimester.

Source: American College of Obstetricians and Gynecologists. (2015a, reaffirmed 2019). ACOG Practice Bulletin No. 148: Thyroid disease in pregnancy. *Obstetrics & Gynecology*, 125(4), 996–1005. doi:10.1097/01.AOG.0000462945.27539.93

- High-risk race/ethnicity (African American, Latino, Native American, Asian American, Pacific Islander)
- History of cardiovascular disease
- Previous birth of an infant weighing 4,000 g (8 lbs 13 oz) or more
- Hypertension or on therapy for hypertension
- High-density lipoprotein (HDL) <35 mg/dL and/or triglycerides >250 mg/dL
- PCOS
- Physical inactivity
- Other clinical condition associated with insulin resistance (BMI ≥40, acanthosis nigricans)

The diagnosis of pregestational diabetes is made by a plasma glucose level ≥126 mg/dL, an A1C ≥6.5%, or a random plasma glucose level ≥200 mg/dL. If no diagnosis of GDM or pregestational diabetes is made early in pregnancy, routine testing for gestational diabetes is performed between 24 and 28 weeks' gestation (ACOG, 2018b).

GENETIC TESTING

Labs for genetic screening are noninvasive and provide a risk specific to the current pregnancy as compared with the population risk for all women the same age/ethnicity/weight/gestational age as the patient. They are not diagnostic of any genetic condition. These tests include:

- First trimester screening, which is maternal serum screening of biochemical markers with ultrasound markers. This test may be referred to as the ultrascreen, the nuchal translucency screen, or the sequential screen. It is typically performed between 11 and 14 weeks' gestation and screens for Down syndrome (Trisomy 21), Trisomy 18, and Trisomy 13 (Gabbe et al., 2017; Lockwood & Magriples, 2019).
- The quadruple test, commonly called "quad screening," which is maternal serum screening of biochemical markers without ultrasound markers. This test measures levels of alpha-fetoprotein (AFP), unconjugated estriol (uE3), hCG, and inhibin A. It is typically performed between 15 and 22 weeks' gestation and screens for Down syndrome, Trisomy 18, and open NTDs such as spina bifida or anencephaly (Lockwood & Magriples, 2018).
- Cell-free DNA or noninvasive prenatal testing (NIPT) is an assessment of the fetal DNA in the maternal circulation to screen for Down syndrome, Trisomy 18, Trisomy 13, and sex chromosome aneuploidies. This test is performed after 9 to 10 weeks gestation, depending on the lab (Lockwood & Magriples, 2019). NIPT should not be offered to low-risk patients, and irreversible decisions should not be made on the basis of the results of this screening test in view of false-positive and negative results (Society for Maternal-Fetal Medicine, 2014).
- The single AFP test may be performed separately during the second trimester for women who opted for the first trimester screening or the cell-free DNA screening and who desire screening for open NTDs.

Chorionic villus sampling and amniocentesis are diagnostic tests for genetic abnormalities. These options are invasive and carry a risk of miscarriage; they are typically performed only if there is an indication. These tests are done by a perinatologist, often after counseling with a genetic counselor (ACOG, 2016a).

Testing may also be completed in early pregnancy to obtain genetic carrier status for diseases such as cystic fibrosis, spinal muscular atrophy, Fragile X, Tay–Sachs, sickle cell, or thalassemias. Appropriate testing options vary by ethnicity and country/area of descent. If a patient is found to be a carrier for one of these conditions, her reproductive partner should be offered testing, and a referral for genetic counseling may be considered (Lockwood & Magriples, 2019).

LABS AT 24–28 WEEKS' GESTATION

- Screening for gestational diabetes with oral glucose challenge
- CBC
- HIV 1/2
- Syphilis

LABS AT 35–37 WEEKS' GESTATION

- Group B streptococcus (GBS, with sensitivities if penicillin allergic)
- CBC, if indicated
- Gonorrhea/chlamydia, if indicated

IMAGING CONSIDERATIONS

Ultrasounds are frequently utilized during pregnancy for various indications. Prenatal ultrasounds may be performed by a sonographer, a radiologist, an obstetrician–gynecologist, a perinatologist, or a certified nurse-midwife, depending on the setting and the indication.

A dating ultrasound typically measures the embryonic or fetal crown–rump length in the first trimester. This ultrasound can be performed transvaginally or transabdominally and is typically used to confirm the EDD of the pregnancy. Prior to 14 weeks and 0 days, the gestational age based on crown–rump length is precise to 5 to 7 days. If less than 9 weeks' gestation and the EDD from crown–rump length versus from the LMP differs by more than 5 days, the EDD should be changed to correspond with the ultrasound dating. If between 9 weeks and 0 days and 13 weeks and 6 days, the EDD should be changed to correspond with the ultrasound dating if the difference is more than 7 days.

If ultrasound dating is not performed until the second trimester (14 weeks and 0 days or greater), the EDD is calculated using multiple biometric measurements instead of just the crown–rump length. Third trimester ultrasound measurements may vary by ±21 to 30 days. Discrepancies in the third trimester should typically *not* be used to change an EDD (ACOG, 2016b).

A dating ultrasound is most beneficial prior to 20 weeks, particularly with irregular menstrual cycles, an uncertain or unknown LMP, patients who conceive while on contraception, or when the uterine size by palpation does not correspond with dating from the LMP. Other structures that are typically seen and documented from a dating ultrasound are the ovaries, the yolk sac, a fetal pole, and fetal cardiac activity. The presence or absence of these findings is dependent on the gestational age as well as the viability of the pregnancy. A dating ultrasound may diagnose a fetal anomaly, but this is unlikely given the small size of the fetus. Dating ultrasounds may also detect some abnormal pregnancy findings: a missed abortion, a twin gestation, a subchorionic hemorrhage, ovarian cysts, uterine fibroids, or abnormal placentation.

Accurate pregnancy dating leads to significantly reduced frequency of labor induction for postterm pregnancy and significantly less use of tocolysis for suspected preterm labor. An accurate due date may also reduce planned cesarean delivery prior to 39 weeks (**Box 21.6**; Lockwood & Magriples, 2019).

An anatomy ultrasound is typically performed between 18 and 22 weeks' gestation. This ultrasound is performed transabdominally and assesses the number of fetuses, presentation of the fetus, fetal anatomic structures, fetal biometry, location of the placenta, cord insertion, and amniotic fluid volume. A cervical length ultrasound is sometimes performed with the anatomy ultrasound and is done transvaginally. This ultrasound is indicated for a history of preterm delivery or history of LEEP or cone biopsy. Some institutions now offer it to all pregnant women as a universal screening for risk of preterm labor. If the cervix is shortened at this time,

---

BOX 21.6
UTERINE SIZE GREATER THAN/ LESS THAN DATES

Uterine size greater than/less than date is when the fundal height or uterine size by palpation does not match the expected gestational age and is either larger or smaller than would be expected by the EDD. A diagnosis is typically confirmed by sonography.

- Differentials include:
  - In the first trimester:
    - Incorrect dating (unsure/unknown LMP or irregular menstrual cycles prior to conception)
    - Maternal obesity
    - Uterine fibroids
    - Uterine malposition (such as a retroverted uterus)
    - Multiple gestation
  - In the second or third trimester:
    - Maternal obesity
    - Fetus large for gestational age
    - Fetus small for gestational age
    - Malpositioned fetus (breech, transverse, oblique)
    - Polyhydramnios
    - Oligohydramnios
    - Uterine fibroids
    - Multiple gestation

EDD, estimated due date; LMP, last menstrual period.

Sources: Lockwood, C. J., & Magriples, U. (2018). Prenatal care: Second and third trimesters. In V. Berghella (Ed.), *UpToDate*. Retrieved from https://www.uptodate.com/ contents/prenatal-care-second-and-third-trimesters; Lockwood, C. J., & Magriples, U. (2019). Prenatal care: Initial assessment. In V. Berghella (Ed.), *UpToDate*. Retrieved from https://www.uptodate.com/contents/ prenatal-care-initial-assessment

---

recommendations include repeating an ultrasound, using progesterone injections or pills for supplementation, or placing a cervical cerclage.

Other ultrasounds that may be performed in pregnancy, depending on the indication, include a growth ultrasound, an amniotic fluid index, or a biophysical profile (BPP). However, prenatal ultrasounds for nonmedical purposes should not be performed (ACOG, 2016c).

EVIDENCE-BASED PRACTICE CONSIDERATIONS

FOLIC-ACID SUPPLEMENTATION

Most pregnant women in the United States take a daily prenatal vitamin that includes folic acid. Ideally, women begin taking a prenatal vitamin prior to conception in order to obtain additional folic acid. There is typically 0.8 mg of folic acid in an over-the-counter prenatal vitamin and 1 mg of folic acid in a prescription prenatal vitamin. The USPSTF (2017) currently recommends that all women who are planning or capable of pregnancy take 0.4 to 0.8 mg of folic acid. These levels are considered sufficient for most women. A woman with a history of a previous pregnancy affected by an NTD, spina bifida or anencephaly should take 4 mg of folic acid daily. A meta-analysis was performed by De-Rigil, Pena-Rosas, Fernandez-Gaxiola, and Rayco-Solon (2015) to evaluate the effect of folic acid supplementation on prevention of birth defects. Five trials were included with a total of 7,391 women. The meta-analysis concluded that folic acid, alone or in combination with other vitamins and minerals, prevents NTDs. The dose of folic acid varied between the trials and ranged from 0.36 to 4 mg daily. The effect on other birth defects such as cleft palate or cleft lip was unclear.

GESTATIONAL DIABETES SCREENING

The USPSTF (2016b) recommends screening for GDM in all asymptomatic pregnant women after 24 weeks of gestation. The test is typically performed between 24 and 28 weeks' gestation with an oral glucose challenge. It can be difficult to separate pregestational diabetes mellitus from GDM, particularly if no early pregnancy screening is performed. Between 6% and 7% of pregnant patients will have GDM. GDM that is well controlled with diet alone is called gestational diabetes type A1 (A1GDM), while GDM that requires medication for blood sugar control is called gestational diabetes type A2 (A2GDM). Patients with GDM have a greater risk of preeclampsia and cesarean delivery, as well as an increased risk of developing type 2 diabetes later in life. Infants born to mothers with GDM have an increased incidence of macrosomia, neonatal

TABLE 21.2 Diagnostic Criteria for the 3-Hour Glucose Tolerance

	Carpenter–Couston	National Diabetes Data Group
Fasting	95 mg/dL	105 mg/dL
1-hour	180 mg/dL	190 mg/dL
2-hours	155 mg/dL	165 mg/dL
3-hours	140 mg/dL	145 mg/dL

hypoglycemia, hyperbilirubinemia, shoulder dystocia, and birth trauma. There are two common testing protocols to screen for and diagnose GDM (ACOG, 2018b).

- Two-step test (most common method):
  - Initial screening: Nonfasting, consumption of 50-g glucose solution (Glucola), test blood sugar 1 hour later
  - If elevated (≥130–140 mg/dL depending on institution), perform diagnostic test
  - Diagnostic test: Fasting (overnight) blood sugar; consumption of 100-g glucose solution (Glucola); test blood sugar at 1, 2, and 3 hours after consumption
  - Typically, two or more elevated values on the diagnostic test are considered a diagnosis of gestational diabetes (ACOG, 2018b; Durnwald, 2019). Some clinicians are moving toward diagnosing GDM with just one elevated value on the 3-hour test. If this criterion is adopted nationally, the prevalence of GDM will increase (Durnwald, 2019).
  - There are two different diagnostic criteria for values on the 3-hour glucose tolerance test, depending on different organizations' guidelines (**Table 21.2**).
- One-step test:
  - Often used outside the United States
  - Fasting blood sugar, consumption of 75 g Glucola, test blood sugar at 1 and 2 hours after consumption
  - If one or more values are elevated, this is a diagnosis of gestational diabetes:
    - Fasting: 92 mg/dL
    - 1-hour: 180 mg/dL
    - 2-hours: 153 mg/dL (ACOG, 2018b; Durnwald, 2019)

INDUCTION OF LABOR

Ideal timing for delivery is a hotly contested topic among obstetric clinicians. The ARRIVE (A Randomized Trial of Induction Versus Expectant Management) trial was conducted with over 6,000 low-risk nulliparous

women at term. This trial found that induction of labor at 39 weeks, when compared with expectant management, did not show a difference of adverse perinatal outcomes, but did show a significantly lower rate of cesarean deliveries (Grobman et al., 2018). The implications of this finding have been the subject of much discussion since the study was published in 2018. While it is a goal of most clinicians and hospital systems to reduce the number of cesarean deliveries in nulliparous women, many have questioned whether induction of labor at 39 weeks is the best way to accomplish this. The ACNM, in response to the ARRIVE trial, pointed out that while the study was well-designed, the study population is not necessarily generalizable to the population at large. ACNM also noted that many women opted not to participate in the trial, highlighting the importance of collaborative decision-making between clinician and patient. It is unclear whether institutions or clinicians instituting a policy of 39-week inductions will follow the parameters of the trial. There are also multiple other interventions that have been shown to reduce the rate of cesarean delivery, many of which are low cost, low intervention, and do not require as much time in the hospital. These interventions include use of doulas for continuous labor support, use of intermittent auscultation rather than continuous monitoring for women in labor, and encouraging women to be upright and moving during labor rather than being in bed (ACNM, 2018).

FETAL SURVEILLANCE IN THIRD TRIMESTER

Women who need increased antepartum fetal surveillance in pregnancy are typically those with a higher risk of stillbirth. The aim of the surveillance is to prevent fetal death. Common pregnancy complications that are indications for antepartum fetal surveillance include:

- Advanced maternal age
- Decreased fetal movement
- Pregestational diabetes mellitus
- Gestational diabetes (typically reserved for medically treated)
- cHTN
- Gestational hypertension
- Preeclampsia
- Intrauterine growth restriction
- Systemic lupus erythematosus
- Hemoglobinopathies
- Oligohydramnios
- Prior fetal demise
- Postterm pregnancy

Fetal surveillance is composed of one or more of the following: maternal assessment (perception of fetal movement and performance of daily fetal kick counts), contraction stress tests (CST), NST, umbilical artery

Doppler velocimetry, BPP, and modified BPP. Identification of fetal compromise from these tests "provides the opportunity to intervene before progressive metabolic acidosis results in fetal death" (ACOG, 2014). When the testing is reassuring, it is unlikely that stillbirth will occur within 1 week of the normal test. Time of initiation of testing, frequency of testing, and mode of testing will vary by indication. Intervention for abnormal testing will also vary according to the complete clinical picture (ACOG, 2014).

MANAGEMENT OF WOMEN AT HIGH RISK FOR PRETERM BIRTH

The biggest risk factor for a preterm birth (<37 weeks' gestation) is having had a prior preterm birth. Other risk factors include a shortened cervix by ultrasound measurement, threatened preterm labor during the current pregnancy, multiple gestation, and history of cervical procedures such as a LEEP or cone biopsy. Infants born prior to 37 weeks' gestation (and particularly those born prior to 34 weeks' gestation) have an increased risk of complications, both at birth and during infancy. In recent years, studies have been performed to assess whether antepartum administration of progesterone (typically given either once weekly as an intramuscular injection or daily as a suppository) from weeks 16 through 36 weeks and 6 days is an effective strategy to prevent women who are at high risk for preterm birth. A meta-analysis performed by Dodd, Jones, Flenady, Cincotta, and Crowther (2013) that included 36 randomized controlled trials showed that progesterone was associated with beneficial effects for pregnancy length and neonatal morbidity and mortality. Progesterone is typically well tolerated by patients. The most common side effects are headache, breast tenderness, nausea, cough, and skin irritation (if administered intramuscularly).

HYPERTENSIVE DISORDERS

Hypertensive disorders of pregnancy are the leading cause of maternal and perinatal mortality worldwide. These disorders can be divided into several categories: cHTN, gestational hypertension, preeclampsia with and without severe features, HELLP, and eclampsia. In general, any type of hypertensive disorder during pregnancy is diagnosed using at least two elevated BP readings that are taken at least 4 hours apart. However, with severe hypertension, diagnosis may be made in a shorter interval for the purposes of BP treatment (ACOG, 2018d, 2018e). Current ACOG classifications for hypertension in pregnancy vary slightly from the 2018 guidelines from the American College of Cardiology (ACC) and the American Heart Association (AHA). Per ACOG, hypertension is diagnosed when there are two or more BP readings,

at least 4 hours apart, of a systolic BP of ≥140 mmHg or a diastolic BP of ≥90 mmHg (Whelton et al., 2018). Severe hypertension is defined as a systolic BP of ≥160 mmHg or a diastolic BP of ≥110 (ACOG, 2018e). This section will use the current ACOG classifications and will focus on the three most common presentations, diagnostic criteria, and treatment plans.

Low-dose aspirin (81 mg) therapy is now frequently recommended for women at high- and moderate risk for preeclampsia. High-risk factors include a previous pregnancy with preeclampsia, multiple gestation, renal disease, autoimmune disease, type 1 or type 2 diabetes mellitus, and cHTN. Moderate-risk factors include primiparous status, maternal age of 35 years or older, BMI greater than 30, and a family history of preeclampsia. Daily therapy with low-dose aspirin should be initiated between 12 and 28 weeks' gestation (ideally, prior to 16 weeks' gestation) and continued until delivery (ACOG, 2018d; USPSTF, 2016c).

ABNORMAL FINDINGS

ACUTE CYSTITIS URINARY TRACT INFECTION

Acute cystitis is an infection of the lower urinary tract. It is not uncommon in pregnant women owing to the effects of progesterone on the motility of the ureters. The urinary tract is typically sterile. UTIs occur when bacteria ascend into the urinary tract (Matuszkiewicz-Rowinska, Malyszko, & Wieliczko, 2015). The most common organism causing a UTI is *Escherichia coli*.

Key History and Physical Findings

- Dysuria
- Hematuria
- Increased urinary frequency
- Increased urinary urgency
- Incomplete emptying of bladder
- Flank and/or suprapubic pain
- Uterine contractions/cramping
- Fever
- Pyuria, positive nitrites, and hematuria on urinalysis

ASYMPTOMATIC BACTERIURIA

Asymptomatic bacteriuria is the presence of a high level of bacteria in the urine with no patient-reported symptoms (Hooton & Gupta, 2019). It is common in pregnancy and should be treated, as these infections have a higher likelihood of ascending to the kidneys. Pregnant women should be universally screened for asymptomatic bacteriuria at their initial prenatal visit. Asymptomatic bacteriuria may also cause preterm contractions, so it should be a consideration when preterm contractions or persistent cramping are concerns.

Key History and Physical Findings

- No signs or symptoms consistent with UTI
- High-level bacterial growth on urine culture ($\geq 10^5$ cfu/mL)
  - ○ If bacteriuria is due to GBS, treatment threshold is $\geq 10^4$, and women should be considered to be GBS positive for intrapartum care.

ANEMIA IN PREGNANCY

Iron deficiency is the most common cause of anemia in pregnancy because of increased maternal iron needs, fetal iron needs, and expanded maternal blood volume. Physiologic anemia is often seen during the second trimester of pregnancy owing to this increased blood volume. Iron-deficiency anemia is present when maternal iron stores begin to be depleted. Approximately 18% of pregnant women in the United States have iron deficiency, and the rates of iron deficiency increase with the trimester of pregnancy (from 6.9% to 14.3% to 28.4%; Cantor, Bougatsos, Dana, Blazina, & McDonagh, 2015; USPSTF, 2016d). Diagnosis and treatment are important as iron-deficiency anemia may contribute to preterm birth, intrauterine growth restriction, decrease in maternal blood reserves during birth and increase in need for transfusion after birth, and decreased milk production (Api, Breyman, Cetiner, Demir, & Ecder, 2015).

Key History and Physical Findings

- Fatigue
- Weakness
- Shortness of breath
- Leg cramps
- Cold intolerance
- Headaches
- Iron-deficient diet
- Pagophagia or pica
- GI issues affecting iron absorption
- History of closely spaced pregnancies
- Pallor
- Tachycardia
- Decreased hemoglobin and ferritin levels

CONSTIPATION IN PREGNANCY

Constipation is a common concern during all trimesters of pregnancy, although it is typically more prevalent during the first trimester. Elevated levels of progesterone are the main cause of constipation, as progesterone slows GI transit. Women may also experience more pressure on the GI tract from the uterus as it grows throughout pregnancy. Prenatal vitamins with iron or the addition of an iron supplement during pregnancy can also contribute to constipation (King et al., 2019). Constipation is a

frequent side effect of ondansetron, so the clinician will want to consider alternative medications for nausea and vomiting if the patient is extremely constipated.

Key History and Physical Findings

- Hard stools
- Difficult/painful bowel movements
- Straining with bowel movements
- Infrequent bowel movements (less than three times per week)
- Abdominal pain
- Low-fiber diet
- Decreased fluid intake
- Ignoring the urge to have a bowel movement
- Feeling bloated
- History of laxative or opioid use

FIRST-TRIMESTER BLEEDING

Vaginal bleeding in the first trimester of pregnancy occurs in approximately 20% to 40% of women. Understandably, this bleeding often causes a great deal of anxiety and worry for a pregnant woman and her family as they are concerned for the viability of the pregnancy. Between 15% and 20% of pregnancies will end in miscarriage, and about 80% of those losses will occur in the first trimester (ACOG, 2018c; Norwitz & Park, 2019). It is critical to exclude the possibility of an ectopic pregnancy in any patient with first trimester bleeding, as this can be a life-threatening complication.

First-Trimester Bleeding: Benign

This bleeding would include implantation bleeding, vaginitis, mistaken hematuria or rectal bleeding, or bleeding from a cervical polyp.

Key History and Physical Findings
- Light spotting/vaginal bleeding
- Recent intercourse
- Presence of fetal heart tones at 12 weeks' gestation or more with Doppler
- Presence of fetal cardiac activity/fetal movement on ultrasound
- Increasing levels of hCG

First-Trimester Bleeding: Cause for Increased Surveillance or Indicative of Miscarriage

This bleeding would include blighted ovum, subchorionic hemorrhage (carries increased likelihood of miscarriage), "disappearing" twin gestation, spontaneous abortion (either complete or incomplete), or missed abortion.

Key History and Physical Findings
- History of ectopic pregnancy or previous miscarriage, uterine anomaly, adnexal surgery, pelvic inflammatory disease, or endometriosis

- Presence of an intrauterine contraceptive device
- Varying amount of vaginal bleeding
- Passing tissue and/or large clots from vagina
- Abdominal cramping
- Back pain
- Lightheadedness
- Absence of fetal heart tones at 12 weeks' gestation or more with Doppler or fetal cardiac activity/fetal movement on ultrasound
- EDD by LMP inconsistent with crown–rump length on ultrasound or uterine size on bimanual exam
- Decreasing levels of hCG

HYPERTENSIVE DISORDERS

Chronic or Gestational Hypertension

Chronic hypertension (cHTN) is defined as "hypertension diagnosed or present before pregnancy or before 20 weeks of gestation" (ACOG, 2018e). Additionally, cHTN is hypertension diagnosed for the first time during pregnancy that does not resolve during the postpartum period. This type of hypertensive disorder is present in 0.9% to 1.5% of pregnant women. It should be noted, however, that clinicians may see an increase in women who are diagnosed with cHTN prior to pregnancy on the basis of newer (and more conservative) ACC/AHA guidelines (ACOG, 2018e).

Gestational hypertension (gHTN) is defined as a systolic BP of ≥140 mmHg or a diastolic BP of ≥90 mmHg on two separate occasions in a woman with previously normal BP. These measurements must be at least 4 hours apart and after 20 weeks' gestation. Gestational hypertension must be distinguished from preeclampsia by the absence of proteinuria or severe features. For a woman with gestational hypertension, BP readings return to normal in the postpartum period. A woman with gestational hypertension with severe range BP (a systolic BP of 160 mmHg or greater or a diastolic BP of 110 mmHg or greater) should be diagnosed instead as having preeclampsia with severe features (ACOG, 2018d). Up to 50% of women with gestational hypertension will eventually develop preeclampsia during their pregnancy.

Key History and Physical Findings

- History of kidney disease or diabetes
- Pregnant with multiples
- African-American descent
- Elevated BP
- May have no signs or symptoms (other than elevated BP)
- Headache
- Edema
- Nausea/Vomiting
- May progress to preeclampsia

Preeclampsia

Preeclampsia is traditionally defined as hypertension plus proteinuria during pregnancy, with an onset after 20 weeks' gestation. In women with gestational hypertension in the absence of proteinuria, preeclampsia may also be diagnosed with the new onset of any severe features (see the text that follows).

Key History and Physical Findings (in addition to symptoms listed earlier)

- Proteinuria
- Elevated BP
- Severe features (ACOG, 2018d):
  - ○ Thrombocytopenia (platelet count less than $100,00 \times 10^9/L$)
  - ○ Renal insufficiency (serum creatinine >1.1 mg/dL or a doubling of the serum creatinine)
  - ○ Impaired liver function (doubling of liver transaminases)
  - ○ New-onset headache unresponsive to medication and not accounted for by alternative diagnoses
  - ○ New-onset visual disturbances
  - ○ Severe persistent right upper quadrant or epigastric pain unresponsive to medication and not accounted for by alternative diagnoses
  - ○ Pulmonary edema

Eclampsia

When preeclampsia is left untreated, it can progress to the serious condition, eclampsia.

Key History and Physical Findings (in addition to symptoms listed earlier)

- Seizures
- Coma
- Expiry

THYROID DYSFUNCTION

Refer to Chapter 11, Evidence-Based Assessment of the Head and Neck, and **Box 21.5** for more information on thyroid dysfunction in pregnancy.

HYPEREMESIS GRAVIDARUM

Nausea and vomiting during pregnancy are among the most common concerns that clinicians will encounter when providing prenatal care. Nausea and vomiting of pregnancy is modulated by increased hCG and estrogen levels (ACOG, 2018a). Approximately 50% to 80% of pregnant women will report nausea, and 50% will experience both nausea and vomiting. "Normal" pregnancy-related nausea and vomiting should be differentiated from hyperemesis gravidarum (HG). Unfortunately, there is no widely accepted clinical distinction between the two. Often, women with HG will have more severe symptoms and often require inpatient management in the first and second trimesters.

Key History and Physical Findings

- Personal or family history of HG
- Severe nausea
- Having multiples
- Overweight
- Food aversions
- Dizziness/lightheadedness
- Headaches
- Persistent vomiting (>3–4 times daily)
- Large ketonuria
- Dehydration
- Weight loss (typically at least 5% of prepregnancy weight)
- Abnormalities with electrolytes, thyroid function, and liver function

PRURITIC URTICARIAL PAPULES AND PLAQUES OF PREGNANCY

Pruritic urticarial papules and plaques of pregnancy are typically seen in primiparous women toward the end of pregnancy (mean time of onset is 35 weeks' gestation). It is benign, self-limiting, and most often resolves within 7 to 10 days after delivery. It occurs in 0.3% to 0.6% of pregnancies and is more common with multiple gestation and male fetuses (Pomeranz, 2018).

Key History and Physical Findings

- Pruritic lesions (**Figure 21.8**)
- Lesions started in striae
- No lesions in periumbilical area
- Typically not on face, palms, or soles
- Scattered erythematous papules, most often found on abdomen with a clear area directly around the umbilicus
- Lesions may spread to the extremities, chest, and back.
- Lesions may combine to form plaques.
- In patients with fair skin, white halos may surround the papules.

GESTATIONAL THROMBOCYTOPENIA

Thrombocytopenia is defined as a platelet count of less than 150×10^9/L and occurs in 7% to 12% of pregnancies. A gradual decrease in platelets is expected as pregnancy progresses, but thrombocytopenia may result from both physiologic and pathologic conditions.

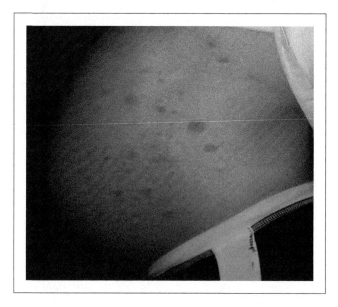

FIGURE 21.8 Pruritic urticarial papules and plaques of pregnancy rash.

Thrombocytopenia is often asymptomatic and may only be discovered on a routine CBC in pregnancy (ACOG, 2019).

Gestational thrombocytopenia is the most common cause of thrombocytopenia in pregnancy, affecting 5% to 11% of pregnant women. There is no significant maternal or fetal risk with gestational thrombocytopenia, and the diagnosis is one of exclusion. The clinician will want to assess for a history of any bleeding disorders or symptoms associated with platelet disorders, such as petechiae, ecchymosis, epistaxis, gingival bleeding, or a history of menometrorrhagia. It should be noted that most anesthesia clinicians will not place regional anesthesia (epidural or spinal anesthetic) with a platelet count of less than 70×10^9/L. For women with gestational thrombocytopenia, decisions about mode of delivery should be based on typical obstetric indications (ACOG, 2019).

Key History and Physical Findings

- Onset in the midsecond to third trimester
- Asymptomatic
- No history of bleeding or thrombocytopenia outside of pregnancy
- Thrombocytopenia resolves after pregnancy (1–2 months postpartum).

CASE STUDY: Routine Prenatal Visit

History

Maria is a 32-year-old G4P2012 at 25w2d gestation who presents to your office for a routine prenatal visit. During the visit, she states that her low back is "killing her." She reports having difficulty changing positions, standing for prolonged periods of time, and getting comfortable in bed, which contributes to difficulty sleeping. She has tried taking acetaminophen 650 mg every 4 to 6 hours, which she states has not improved her pain at all. She rates her pain currently at 5/10. She takes a prenatal vitamin daily, as well as a docosahexaenoic-acid (DHA) supplement. She reports preterm labor with her first pregnancy, stating that "they gave me medications to stop contractions" at 32 weeks' gestation. She went on to deliver at full term. She works full time as a preschool teacher and has a 4-year-old son and a 2-year-old daughter at home. She endorses normal, daily fetal movement and denies uterine contractions, vaginal bleeding, or leaking of fluid. She denies pelvic pressure, vaginal discharge, vaginal odor, or vaginal itching. She denies fever, dysuria, hematuria, urinary urgency, and urinary frequency. Her last instance of intercourse was 1 week ago. She denies any recent falls or injury to her back.

Physical Examination

She is well appearing and afebrile. Her weight increased 8 lb from her visit 4 weeks ago. On physical exam, she has no costovertebral angle (CVA) tenderness. A speculum exam shows normal external female genitalia. No vaginal discharge, erythema, or edema are visualized. Her cervix is closed, thick, and high.

Differential Diagnoses

Back pain in pregnancy, musculoskeletal strain or injury, preterm labor, vaginitis, urinary tract infection, and pyelonephritis

Laboratory and Imaging

A urinalysis was obtained in office and was not indicative of infection, so a urine culture was not sent. A vaginitis culture and fetal fibronectin were obtained during the speculum exam, but neither were sent as suspicion for either vaginitis or preterm labor was low.

Final Diagnosis

Back pain in pregnancy

CASE STUDY: Problem Obstetric Visit

History

Katie is a 25-year-old G1P0 at 11w1d gestation and presents to your office for a problem obstetric visit and reports that she is nauseated "all day long" and is vomiting at least five times per day. These symptoms have been persistent over the past week. She reports that she is unable to go to work because her nausea is so severe. She is keeping down bites of food and sips of water and ginger ale. She reports that she has tried ginger (in the form of ginger ale and ginger pops) to help with the nausea and vomiting. She reports feeling very fatigued, taking at least one 1-hour nap daily and sleeping approximately 9 to 10 hours per night. She has not yet felt any fetal movement. She denies cramping, vaginal bleeding, or leaking of fluid. She denies any sick contacts. She reports normal urine output. Her EDD has been set by a sure LMP and confirmed by a transvaginal ultrasound at 8 weeks. Her medical history is significant for Hashimoto's thyroiditis and anxiety. She reports taking her prenatal vitamin daily

but only when she feels that she can tolerate it, as well as daily sertraline (Zoloft) 50 mg.

Physical Examination

On exam, she appears fatigued. Her pulse is 101. She is afebrile, and her BP is 94/62. Fetal heart tones are obtained by handheld Doppler and are 155 bpm. Her weight is 181 lb, down 4 lb since her visit 3 weeks ago when she was still at her prepregnancy weight of 185 lb.

Differential Diagnoses

Nausea and vomiting of pregnancy, hyperemesis gravidarum, and gastroenteritis

Laboratory and Imaging

A urinalysis performed in the office is significant for trace ketones and trace protein.

Final Diagnosis

Nausea and vomiting of pregnancy

Clinical Pearls

- Women should be considered active participants in their care during pregnancy and encouraged to share decision-making with their clinician.
- Recognize that the childbearing year is a time of great growth, stress, and excitement for the entire family unit.
- Clinicians should perform universal screening for past or current violence, as well as have referrals to provide for a woman who is a victim of violence.
- The value of nutrition cannot be underestimated for a healthy pregnancy. Adequate time should be spent giving pregnant patients information about a well-balanced diet and food sources of various nutrients that are important for pregnancy.
- If a woman reports that her prenatal vitamin is contributing to her nausea, suggest a low-iron prenatal vitamin or a gummy prenatal vitamin (does not include iron) until her nausea subsides.

Key Takeaways

- The initial prenatal visit is an opportunity to provide a wealth of information to patients about their health and pregnancy, as well as an opportunity for the clinician to screen for problems that may arise in later pregnancy.
- The vast majority of women will have a healthy pregnancy.
- Prenatal care doubles as primary care for many women. This is a chance to educate women on preventive care, both during pregnancy and outside of pregnancy.
- The clinician should ask about fetal movement, contractions/cramping, vaginal bleeding, and loss of fluid at each visit.
- Collaboration with generalist obstetric clinicians or perinatologists is key for women with more complicated health histories.
- Many concerns in pregnancy are considered normal; the clinician's job is to determine when these concerns may actually be abnormal and to know how to assess for concerns.

REFERENCES

American College of Nurse-Midwives. (2017). *ACNM position statement: Immunization during pregnancy and the postpartum period*. Retrieved from http://midwife.org/ACNM/files/ACNMLibraryData/UPLOADFILENAME/000000000289/Immunization-in-Pregnancy-and-Postpartum-May-2014.pdf

American College of Nurse-Midwives. (2018). *ACNM responds to release of ARRIVE trial study results: Acknowledges quality of study but raises concerns about potential for misapplying results*. Retrieved from http://midwife.org/ACNM-Responds-to-Release-of-ARRIVE-Trial-Study-Results

American College of Nurse-Midwives Gender and Equity Taskforce. (2017). *ACNM issue brief: Use of culturally-appropriate terminology for gender diverse populations*. Retrieved from http://www.midwife.org/ACNM/files/ACNMLibraryData/UPLOADFILENAME/000000000313/Issue-Brief-Use-of-Culturally-Appropriate-Terminology-for-Gender-Diverse-Populations-FEB-2018.pdf

American College of Obstetricians and Gynecologists. (2013, reaffirmed 2018). ACOG Committee Opinion No. 548: Weight gain during pregnancy. *Obstetrics & Gynecology, 121*, 210–212. doi:10.1097/01.AOG.0000425668.87506.4c

American College of Obstetricians and Gynecologists. (2014, reaffirmed 2019). ACOG Practice Bulletin No. 145: Antepartum fetal surveillance. *Obstetrics & Gynecology, 124*(1), 182–192. doi:10.1097/01.AOG.0000451759.90082.7b

American College of Obstetricians and Gynecologists. (2015a, reaffirmed 2019). ACOG Practice Bulletin No. 148: Thyroid disease in pregnancy. *Obstetrics & Gynecology, 125*(4), 996–1005. doi:10.1097/01.AOG.0000462945.27539.93

American College of Obstetricians and Gynecologists. (2015b, reaffirmed 2018). ACOG Practice Bulletin No. 156: Obesity in pregnancy. *Obstetrics & Gynecology, 126*(3), e112–e126. doi:10.1097/AOG.0000000000001211

American College of Obstetricians and Gynecologists. (2016a, reaffirmed 2018). ACOG Practice Bulletin No. 162: Prenatal diagnostic testing for genetic disorders. *Obstetrics & Gynecology, 127*(5), e108–e122. doi:10.1097/AOG.0000000000001405

American College of Obstetricians and Gynecologists. (2016b, reaffirmed 2018). ACOG Practice Bulletin No. 175: Ultrasound in pregnancy. *Obstetrics & Gynecology, 128*(6), e241–e256. doi:10.1097/AOG.0000000000001815

American College of Obstetricians and Gynecologists. (2016c). Don't perform prenatal ultrasounds for non-medical purposes, for example, solely to create keepsake videos or photographs. Retrieved from http://www.choosingwisely.org/clinician-lists/american-college-obstetricians-gynecologists-prenatal-ultrasounds-for-non-medical-purposes

American College of Obstetricians and Gynecologists. (2017, reaffirmed 2019). ACOG Practice Bulletin No. 181: Prevention of Rh D alloimmunization. *Obstetrics & Gynecology, 130*(2), e57–e70. doi:10.1097/AOG.0000000000002232

American College of Obstetricians and Gynecologists. (2018a). ACOG Practice Bulletin No. 189: Nausea and vomiting of pregnancy. *Obstetrics & Gynecology, 131*(1), e15–e30. doi:10.1097/AOG.0000000000002456

American College of Obstetricians and Gynecologists. (2018b, reaffirmed 2019). ACOG Practice Bulletin No. 190: Gestational diabetes mellitus. *Obstetrics & Gynecology, 131*(2), e49–e64. doi:10.1097/AOG.0000000000002501

American College of Obstetricians and Gynecologists. (2018c). ACOG Practice Bulletin No. 200: Early pregnancy loss. *Obstetrics & Gynecology, 132*(5), e197–e207. doi:10.1097/AOG.0000000000002899

American College of Obstetricians and Gynecologists. (2018d). ACOG Practice Bulletin No. 202: Gestation hypertension and preeclampsia. *Obstetrics & Gynecology, 133*(1), e1–e25. doi:10.1097/AOG.0000000000003018

American College of Obstetricians and Gynecologists. (2018e). ACOG Practice Bulletin No. 203: Chronic hypertension in pregnancy. *Obstetrics & Gynecology, 133*(1), e26–e50. doi:10.1097/AOG.0000000000003020

American College of Obstetricians and Gynecologists. (2019). ACOG Practice Bulletin No. 207: Thrombocytopenia in pregnancy. *Obstetrics & Gynecology, 133*(3), e181–e193. doi:10.1097/AOG.0000000000003100

Api, O., Breyman, C., Cetiner, M., Demir, C., & Ecder, T. (2015). Diagnosis and treatment of iron deficiency anemia during pregnancy and the postpartum period: Iron deficiency anemia working group consensus report. *Turkish Journal of Obstetrics and Gynecology, 12*, 173–181. doi:10.4274/tjod.01700

Cantor, A.G., Bougatsos, C., Dana, T., Blazina, I., & McDonagh, M. (2015). Routine iron supplementation and screening for iron deficiency anemia in pregnancy: a systematic review for the U.S. Preventive Services Task Force. *Annals of Internal Medicine, 162*(8), 566–576. doi:10.7326/M14-2932

De-Rigil, L. M., Pena-Rosas, J. P., Fernandez-Gaxiola, A. C., & Rayco-Solon, P. (2015). Effects and safety of periconceptional oral folate supplementation for preventing birth defects. *Cochrane Database of Systematic Reviews*, (12), CD007950. doi:10.1002/14651858.CD007950.pub3

Dodd, J. M., Jones, L., Flenady, V., Cincotta, R., & Crowther, C. A. (2013). Prenatal administration of progesterone for preventing preterm birth in women considered to be at risk of preterm birth. *Cochrane Database of Systematic Reviews*, (7), CD004947. doi:10.1002/14651858.CD004947.pub3

Durnwald, C. (2019). Diabetes mellitus in pregnancy: Screening and diagnosis. In D. M. Nathan & E. F. Werner (Eds.), *UpToDate.* Retrieved from https://www.uptodate.com/contents/diabetes-mellitus-in-pregnancy-screening-and-diagnosis

Frederiksen, L.E., Ernst, A., Brix, N., Braskhøj Lauridsen, L.L., Roos, L., Ramlau-Hansen, C.H., & Ekelund, C.K. (2018). Risk of adverse pregnancy outcomes at advanced maternal age. *Obstetrics & Gynecology, 131*(3), 457–463. doi:10.1097/AOG.0000000000002504

Gabbe, S. G., Niebyl, J. R., Simpson, J. L., Landon, M. B., Galan, H. L., Jauniaux, E. R. M., . . . Grobman, W. A. (Eds.). (2017). *Obstetrics: Normal and problem pregnancies* (7th ed.). Philadelphia, PA: Elsevier.

Grobman, W. A., Rice, M. M., Reddy, U. M., Tita, A. T. N., Silver, R. M., Mallett, G., . . . Macones, G. A. (Eds.). (2018). Labor inductions versus expectant management in low-risk nulliparous women. *The New England Journal of Medicine, 379*(6), 513–523. doi:10.1056/NEJMoa1800566

Hooton, T. M., & Gupta, K. (2019). Urinary tract infections and asymptomatic bacteriuria in pregnancy. In S. B. Calderwood & C. J. Lockwood (Eds.), *UpToDate.* Retrieved from https://www.uptodate.com/contents/urinary-tract-infections-and-asymptomatic-bacteriuria-in-pregnancy

Institute of Medicine. (2009). *Weight gain during pregnancy: Reexamining the guidelines.* Washington, DC: National Academies Press.

King, T. L., Brucker, M. C., Osborne, K., & Jevitt, C. M. (Eds.). (2019). *Varney's midwifery* (6th ed.). Burlington, MA: Jones & Bartlett.

Lockwood, C. J., & Magriples, U. (2018). Prenatal care: Second and third trimesters. In V. Berghella (Ed.), *UpToDate.* Retrieved from https://www.uptodate.com/contents/prenatal-care-second-and-third-trimesters

Lockwood, C. J., & Magriples, U. (2019). Prenatal care: Initial assessment.In V. Berghella (Ed.), *UpToDate.* Retrieved from https://www.uptodate.com/contents/prenatal-care-initial-assessment

Matuszkiewicz-Rowinska, J., Malyszko, J., & Wieliczko, M. (2015). Urinary tract infections in pregnancy: Old and new unresolved diagnostic and therapeutic problems. *Archives of Medical Science, 11*(1), 67–77. doi:10.5114/aoms.2013.39202

Norwitz, E. R., & Park, J. S. (2019). Overview of the etiology and evaluation of vaginal bleeding in pregnant women. In C. J. Lockwood (Ed.), *UpToDate.* Retrieved from https://www.uptodate.com/contents/overview-of-the-etiology-and-evaluation-of-vaginal-bleeding-in-pregnant-women

Pomeranz, M. K. (2018). Dermatoses of pregnancy. In C. J. Lockwood & R. P. Dellavalle (Eds.), *UpToDate.* Retrieved from https://www.uptodate.com/contents/dermatoses-of-pregnancy

Society for Maternal-Fetal Medicine. (2014). *Ten things physicians and patients should question.* Retrieved from http://www.choosingwisely.org/societies/society-for-maternal-fetal-medicine/

Sperlich, M., Seng, J. S., Li, Y., Taylor, J., & Bradbury-Jones, C. (2017). Integrating trauma-informed care into maternity care practice: Conceptual and practical issues. *Journal of Midwifery & Women's Health, 62*, 661–672. doi:10.1111/jmwh.12674

U.S. Preventive Services Task Force. (2015a). Final update summary: Asymptomatic bacteriuria in adults: Screening. Retrieved from https://www.uspreventiveservicestaskforce.org/Page/Document/UpdateSummaryFinal/asymptomatic-bacteriuria-in-adults-screening

U.S. Preventive Services Task Force. (2015b). Final update summary: Rh(D) incompatibility: Screening. Retrieved from https://www.uspreventiveservicestaskforce.org/Page/Document/UpdateSummaryFinal/rh-d-incompatibility-screening

U.S. Preventive Services Task Force. (2015c). Final update summary: Tobacco smoking cessation in adults, including pregnant women: Behavioral and pharmacotherapy interventions. Retrieved from https://www

.uspreventiveservicestaskforce.org/Page/Document/ UpdateSummaryFinal/tobacco-use-in-adults-and -pregnant-women-counseling-and-interventions1

U.S. Preventive Services Task Force. (2016a). Final recommendation statement: Depression in adults: Screening. Retrieved from https://www.uspreventiveservicestaskforce .org/Page/Document/RecommendationStatementFinal/ depression-in-adults-screening1

U.S. Preventive Services Task Force. (2016b). Final update summary: Gestational diabetes mellitus, screening. Retrieved from https://www.uspreventiveservicestaskforce .org/Page/Document/UpdateSummaryFinal/gestational -diabetes-mellitus-screening

U.S. Preventive Services Task Force. (2016c). Final update summary: Low-dose aspirin use for the prevention of morbidity and mortality from preeclampsia: Preventive medication. Retrieved from https://www .uspreventiveservicestaskforce.org/Page/Document/ UpdateSummaryFinal/low-dose-aspirin-use-for-the -prevention-of-morbidity-and-mortality-from -preeclampsia-preventive-medication

U.S. Preventive Services Task Force. (2016d). Other supporting document for iron deficiency anemia in pregnancy women: Screening and supplementation. Retrieved from https://www.uspreventiveservicestaskforce.org/Page/ SupportingDoc/iron-deficiency-anemia-in-pregnant -women-screening-and-supplementation/evidence -summary22

U.S. Preventive Services Task Force. (2017). Final update summary: Folic acid for the prevention of neural tube defects: Preventive medication. Retrieved from https://www .uspreventiveservicestaskforce.org/Page/Document/ UpdateSummaryFinal/folic-acid-for-the-prevention -of-neural-tube-defects-preventive-medication?ds=1&s =folicacid

U.S. Preventive Services Task Force. (2018a). Final update summary: Human immunodeficiency virus (HIV)

infection: Screening. Retrieved from https://www .uspreventiveservicestaskforce.org/Page/Document/ UpdateSummaryFinal/human-immunodeficiency -virus-hiv-infection-screening

U.S. Preventive Services Task Force. (2018b). Final update summary: Intimate partner violence, elder abuse, and abuse of vulnerable adults: Screening. Retrieved from https://www.uspreventiveservicestaskforce.org/Page/ Document/UpdateSummaryFinal/intimate-partner -violence-and-abuse-of-elderly-and-vulnerable-adults -screening1

U.S. Preventive Services Task Force. (2018c). Final update summary: Syphilis infection in pregnant women: Screening. Retrieved from https://www.uspreventiveservicestaskforce .org/Page/Document/UpdateSummaryFinal/syphilis -infection-in-pregnancy-screening1?ds=1&s=syphilis

U.S. Preventive Services Task Force. (2018d). Final update summary: Unhealthy alcohol use in adolescents and adults: Screening and behavioral counseling interventions. Retrieved from https://www.uspreventiveservicestaskforce .org/Page/Document/UpdateSummaryFinal/unhealthy -alcohol-use-in-adolescents-and-adults-screening-and -behavioral-counseling-interventions

U.S. Preventive Services Task Force. (2019). Draft recommendation statement: Hepatitis B virus infection in pregnant women: Screening. Retrieved from https://www.uspreventiveservicestaskforce.org/Page/ Document/draft-recommendation-statement/ hepatitis-b-virus-infection-in-pregnant-women-screening

Whelton, P. K., Carey, R. M., Aronow, W. S., Casey, D. E., Jr., Collins, K. J., Dennison Himmelfarb, C., . . . Wright, J. T., Jr. (2018). 2017 ACC/AHA/AAPA/ABC/ACPM/AGS/APhA/ ASH/ASPC/NMA/PCNA guideline for the prevention, detection, evaluation, and management of high blood pressure in adults: Executive summary. *Journal of the American College of Cardiology, 71*(19), 2199–2269. doi:10.1016/j .jacc.2017.11.005

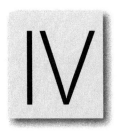

IV

EVIDENCE-BASED PHYSICAL EXAMINATION AND ASSESSMENT OF MENTAL HEALTH

22

Evidence-Based Assessment of Mental Health

Pamela Lusk and Bernadette Mazurek Melnyk

"You can't control everything. Sometimes you just need to relax and have faith that things will work out. Let go a little and just let life happen."

—KODY KIPLINGER

 VIDEO

- Patient History: Depression Symptoms

LEARNING OBJECTIVES

- Describe evidence-based screening instruments used to identify common mental health concerns.
- Delineate the key components of an evidence-based mental health history and interview, including how to document the encounter.
- Discuss the importance of including questions about the patient's strengths, experience of stress, and their usual coping strategies/supports.
- Identify skills and strategies that patients can follow to facilitate mental wellness.

ANATOMY AND PHYSIOLOGY

The mental health symptoms most often encountered when completing comprehensive patient assessments are related to anxiety and depression. Anxiety and

Visit https://connect.springerpub.com/content/book/978-0-8261 -6454-4/chapter/ch00 to access the videos.

depressive disorders are multidimensional and have been studied from physiological, neurobiological, cognitive, and behavioral perspectives (Tusaie & Fitzpatrick, 2017). Understanding the neurological system, as described in Chapter 14, Evidence-Based Assessment of the Nervous System, provides the foundation for appreciating the anatomic and physiological changes most associated with psychiatric/mental health conditions and symptoms, including anxiety and depression.

A study of the structure and function of the nervous system, or neuroanatomy, identifies the amygdala within the temporal lobe as the component of the brain and limbic system most associated with strong emotions, anxiety, and panic. The amygdala of the brain evolved to detect danger and mediate the fear response, that is, fight, flight, or freeze in response to a real or perceived threat. However, the evolution of the amygdala, the complexity of its interaction within the structures of the nervous system that modulate behavior, and how the amygdala is involved in forming memories are not clear; dysregulation of the amygdala is thought to have an impact on neurodevelopmental disorders, which results in impaired learning, mood, communication, and/or social interaction (Schumann, Bauman, & Amaral, 2011).

Clinical study of the complex structural and functional interactions among hormonal systems, the central nervous system, and behavior is known as psychoneuroendocrinology; the role of the hypothalamic–pituitary–adrenal (HPA) system has been central to this branch of science's research (Sadock, Sadock, & Ruiz, 2015). Knowledge of the HPA axis informs an appreciation of the underlying physical, hormonal, and environmental factors that impact the experience of stress, including the maintenance of homeostasis and adaptation to stress. **Figure 22.1** represents the feedback loop of the HPA axis, initiated when the hypothalamus responds to stress and cortisol levels by releasing corticotropin-releasing hormone (CRH). When CRH binds to receptors on the anterior pituitary gland, adrenocorticotropic hormone (ACTH) is released. ACTH then binds to receptors on the adrenal cortex and stimulates the release of cortisol. This hormonal response to stressors is affected by the characteristics of the stress itself and the individual's ability to cope with it. The HPA system affects and is affected by arousal, sensory processing, stimulus habituation, sleep, pain, and memory retrieval. To regain homeostasis after exposure to a stressor, the hypothalamus reduces CRH release. With repeated exposure to stressors, however, the brain and limbic system habituate to the stressor and sustain HPA axis activation.

The physiological basis for anxiety as a stress/resilience model was described by Hans Selye and is based on the HPA axis. "Resilient reactions to stress are associated with an ability to keep the hypothalamic–pituitary–adrenocortical system and noradrenergic activity within an optimal range during stress exposure and terminate the stress response once the stressor is no longer present…. Predictors of a resilient response to stress vary across developmental stages but generally include perceived social support (family and friends) as well as a sense of connectedness, optimism and cognitive flexibility" (Tusaie & Fitzpatrick, 2017, p. 153).

Complex interactions between the brain, nervous system, and endocrine system have an impact on cognition, behavior, and emotion. The function and processes of the brain to produce thought, movement, and sensation are a result of the transmission of information within and between neurons that are sensitive to an individual's physiological state. In Chapter 23, Evidence-Based Assessment of Substance Use Disorder, the impact of neurotransmitters on the brain and nervous system is reviewed in detail related to the diagnosis of substance use disorder. Specifically related to the diagnosis of depression, the *monoamine hypothesis* posits that depression is the result of deficiency in one or more of the three monoamines—serotonin, norepinephrine, and dopamine—and that this deficiency of neurotransmitters leads to upregulation of postsynaptic receptors in the brain and throughout the body. In simpler terms that can be used in discussion with patients, serotonin (5HT) is associated with mood, appetite, sleep, and anxiety. Norepinephrine (NE) is associated with an individual's energy, focus, initiative, and active adrenaline response (fight, flight, or freeze) to threat, and dopamine (DA) is most associated with pleasure, excitement, and movement. The monoamine hypothesis is central to the explanation for using current antidepressants such as selective serotonin reuptake inhibitors (SSRIs), selective norepinephrine reuptake inhibitors (SNRIs), and medications that act on the monoamines in different combinations. **Figure 22.2** includes a series of positron emission tomography (PET) scans of patients who are not depressed, who have depression, and following recovery; note that the entire brain, particularly the left prefrontal cortex, is more active when patients are well. Although PET scans are not used to diagnose depression, this type of imaging provides researchers with a better understanding of the neuroendocrine physiology that may impact recovery from mental health disorders.

In addition to understanding the structure and function of the nervous system in response to stress, hormones, and the uptake of neurotransmitters, a broader view of an individual's susceptibility is also key in addressing mental health disorders. For example, with bipolar disorder, there are strong genetic links. Disorders such as major depressive disorder (MDD), substance use disorder, and attention deficit hyperactivity disorder (ADHD) may have a component of family, genetic, and/or environmental tendencies that influence an individual's neuroanatomy.

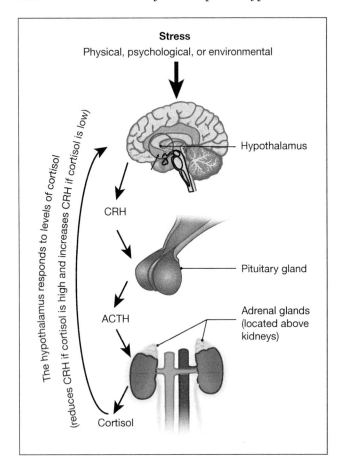

FIGURE 22.1 Hypothalamic–pituitary–adrenal (HPA) axis.

ACTH, adrenocorticotropic hormone; CRH, corticotropin-releasing hormone.

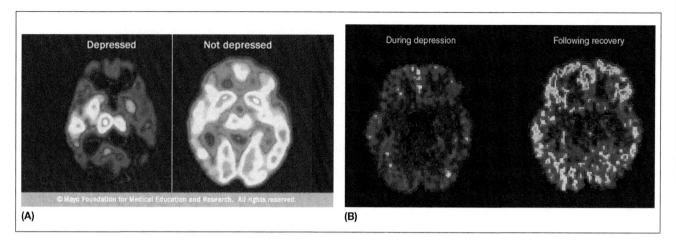

FIGURE 22.2 (A) PET scans (untreated depression and following treatment). (B) PET scans of a 45-year-old woman with recurrent depression. Note that her entire brain, particularly the left prefrontal cortex, is more active when she is well.

PET, positron emission tomography.

Part B courtesy of Mark George, MD, Biological Psychiatry Branch, National Institute of Mental Health.

Depression can occur as a result of depressogenic cognition, that is, a negative pattern of thinking (Beck, 2011; Melnyk, Kelly, & Lusk, 2014). The physiological and psychological impact of negative thinking increases vulnerability to depression, and this is the reason why cognitive-behavioral therapy (CBT) is the first-line recommended treatment for mild-to-moderate depressive symptoms (Lusk & Melnyk, 2013), physical health problems (e.g., hypothyroidism, anemia, chronic fatigue syndrome), environmental stressors, eating disorders, or substance abuse (Beck, 2011). Overcoming cognitive vulnerability has a powerful impact on an individual's health and well-being.

KEY HISTORY QUESTIONS AND CONSIDERATIONS

ASSESSMENT OF MENTAL STATUS

An assessment of an individual's mental status provides the basis for identifying signs and/or symptoms related to their overall mental health. As discussed in Chapter 5, Approach to the Physical Examination: General Survey and Assessment of Vital Signs, a mental status assessment gives the clinician an understanding of the patient's cognitive, emotional, personality, and psychological functioning. This assessment can be done in the course of an individual's routine history and physical examination. Reviewing the reason for seeking care, history of any recent symptoms or problems, as well as the medical and social history provides the clinician with valuable information about mental status and health.

Within the mental status assessment, the clinician can identify an individual's strengths and coping and note whether there are concerns that require more in-depth or formal assessment of mental health. A mental status assessment incorporates observational assessments which are components of the general survey as discussed in Chapter 5, Approach to the Physical Examination: General Survey and Assessment of Vital Signs, and neurological status as reviewed in Chapter 14, Evidence-Based Assessment of the Nervous System. The mental status assessment is performed within the context of the patient's age, developmental level, and cultural norms. Assessments of a person's affect, mood, attention, judgment, and memory can be remembered using the mnemonic "ABC" as listed in the following:

A: Appearance

- Affect: Appropriate for the situation, labile, pleasant, flat, nontoxic
- Posture: Lying, sitting, or standing; comfortable; obvious limitations or defects
- Hygiene and grooming: Appropriately dressed for the weather or situation, disheveled or neatly groomed
- Body habitus: Height, weight, waist circumference, and body mass index (BMI)

B: Behavior

- Verbal or nonverbal expressions of pain, anxiety, illness, anger, fear, frustration, contentment, or sadness
- Interactions: Cooperative, guarded, aggressive, withdrawn
- Activity level: Calm, active, flat, restless, previous/recent/current impulsivity
- Body movements and mobility: Coordinated, limited, assistive devices, abnormal movements or involuntary tics present, slowed or very quick movements

C: Cognition

- Oriented to time, person, and place; confused; disoriented; delirious
- Attention and concentration: Able to express coherent, organized thoughts, or rapidly shifting from one topic to next; any concerns with success in work, school, or at home
- Pattern and pace of speech: Appropriate, rushed, slow, loud or quiet, pressurized
- Judgment: Negative patterns of thinking (e.g., all-or-nothing thinking, catastrophizing, overgeneralization, blaming, emotional reasoning, or always being right), irrational fears, overwhelming worry
- Altered sensory perceptions: Hearing voices or hallucinations, able to control impulses, insight into personal strengths
- Memory: Able to repeat three unrelated words and remember and repeat these words again in 5 minutes; concerns about memory loss
- Mood: Feelings of sadness, guilt, worry, fear, helplessness, or hopelessness; recent insomnia, hypersomnia, loss of appetite, increased appetite, or difficulty feeling enjoyment; feelings of elation, grandiosity, or mood instability; previous or current suicidal and/or homicidal thoughts and/or plan

APPROACH TO ASSESSING MENTAL STATUS AND MENTAL HEALTH HISTORY

To begin the assessment of mental status and mental health, the clinician can use open-ended questions similar to beginning any episodic visit. These include:

- What brings you here to see me today?
- How were you hoping I might help you to feel better today?
- What do you expect from the visit?
- What do you think might be the best explanation for your symptoms?
- What do you feel will be the most helpful interventions/positive strategies to deal with the current concerns?

As the clinician talks with the patient, they can identify barriers to effective communication based on psychosocial, environmental, literacy, financial, and cultural considerations. If the reason for the visit includes psychiatric symptoms or concerns, it will be important to get a sense of the patient's understanding of their "anxiety," "depression," or other disorders. Many patients have learned what their symptoms/disorder/condition means (e.g., expected trajectory and best treatments) from information on the Internet or asking advice from friends/family. This is valuable information for the clinician. Validate or clarify observations from the history and physical examination.

As a reminder, assurance of confidentiality is the primary reason that patients hesitate to confide in or be truthful with their clinician. It is important for a clinician to first inform the patient that the information they share is confidential unless something is said about hurting self, harming others, or being harmed by others; that information will need to be shared with others for the safety of the self or others.

HISTORY OF PRESENT ILLNESS

The history of present illness (HPI) involves clarification of the patient's current symptoms of their mental health concern(s). It is important to gather detailed information on what symptoms are being experienced (e.g., depression, anxiety). Note that "**Are the symptoms currently interfering with functioning at work (school) and home?**" is a key question, as interference with functioning is often one important indicator of a mental health diagnosis. When are the symptoms worse or better? What tends to precipitate the symptoms? At what age do they first remember feeling their symptoms? When did they first receive counseling or other treatment as a child or adult? Has there been any past psychiatric hospitalizations and any substance use treatment/intervention/12-step program participation? What are the patient's associated symptoms (e.g., decreased appetite, headaches, difficulty sleeping)? What helps the symptoms? Is the patient currently on any medications? It is also important to ask about hopelessness/helplessness, as hopelessness is the #1 predictor of suicide.

FAMILY HISTORY

Within the mental health assessment, the family history is very important. Ask about who in the family has anxiety, depression, ADHD, bipolar disorder, schizophrenia, suicide/suicide attempts (SAs), neurological disorders, or substance use disorder. What have family members told the patient about their symptoms, onset, and treatment? What has been the trajectory of the illness? How has the patient been affected?

PAST MEDICAL HISTORY AND REVIEW OF SYSTEMS

It is important to conduct a thorough review of systems and past medical history because there can be physical conditions that are underlying the mental health issue. Symptoms related to mental health disorders, such as anxiety or panic disorder, can be a fast heart rate, sweating, and increased respiratory rate. The review of systems also provides an opportunity to review what interventions have been helpful in the past, for example, medications or integrative therapies, psychotherapy, or counseling.

SOCIAL HISTORY

A social history includes information about any recent changes in the patient's life/home and financial situation. Ask about friends, work or school, usual daily activities, relationships, joys, contributions to others, skills, strengths, interests, and goals. Ask the patient who they would talk to if a decision needed to be made or they wanted to talk about something; the answer to this question provides the clinician with a good sense of the individual's support systems. Asking about any pets and community activities can provide better information about their coping strategies.

STRENGTHS, GOALS, AND INTERESTS

Most electronic health records (EHRs) and charting systems have a "problem list." For patients of all ages, it is equally, if not more, important to also have a "strengths" list. Talk with the patient about the areas in which they excel. Find out the subjects and activities in which they have a great deal of interest. Explore their goals and aspirations. What are the patient's resources/supports, including religious beliefs, spiritual practices, and supportive family members (including pets)? Ask about the person's daily life to assess functioning, and get a sense of their wellness.

As the clinician identifies and builds the strengths list, they will gain a list of activities and goals that can be central to formulating intervention plans. If this assessment is part of a routine wellness check, the clinician can emphasize the individual's strengths and reinforce a commitment to healthy habits, lifelong learning, hobbies, contributions to others, and connectedness in their community.

PREVENTIVE CARE CONSIDERATIONS

Identify Skills and Strategies to Facilitate Mental Well-Being

Optimizing one's physical health with regular exercise, healthy eating, and adequate sleep (at least 7 hours a night for adults) also contributes to optimal mental health. Exercise is well known to be an evidence-based strategy to improve anxiety and depression symptoms. The evidence-based recommendation for adults is 150 minutes of moderate aerobic activity a week. Strategies that have strong evidence to support their use for managing stress and decreasing anxiety include (Lusk & Kahn-John, 2019):

- Removal of triggers (sources of stress, caffeine, nicotine)
- Deep breathing—just five deep abdominal breaths can reduce stress and lower blood pressure
- Movement therapies (yoga, tai chi) and physical activity
- Meditation

- Bibliotherapy—self-help books, workbooks, and psychoeducation
- Progressive muscle relaxation
- Mindfulness-based stress reduction
- CBT
- Acupuncture

UNIQUE POPULATION CONSIDERATIONS FOR HISTORY

Children and Adolescents

With children and adolescents, part of the assessment interview will be with parents or caregivers; if the young person can tolerate being separated from their parents, individual time spent with the child/teen is invaluable. In the individual time spent with the clinician (after confidentiality is made clear), the child/teen is often very forthcoming with their own concerns and experiences. The child/teen also can provide the clinician with best treatment options that fit with their values and preferences. Toys and props in the examination room allow the child/teen to keep their hands busy while talking, which is very helpful for their comfort with the interview.

For adolescents, the HEADSS assessment can be helpful in identifying mental health problems:

- **H**ome: Where is the teen living? Who lives in the home? How is the teen getting along with people in the home? Has the teen ever run away or been incarcerated?
- **E**ducation and/or **E**mployment: How is the teen functioning in school in terms of grades, performance in class, and teachers/peers? Any recent changes? Have there been any suspensions or missed school days? Any current or past employment? Any problems with work attendance?
- **A**ctivities: In which extracurricular and sports activities is the teen involved, if any? What do they do with their friends? What does the teen do for fun?
- **D**rugs: Which drugs, including alcohol, cigarettes, vaping, caffeine, stimulants, or pills, have been used by the teen, their family, and/or friends?
- **S**exuality: How does the teen express their gender identity? How does the teen identify their sexual orientation? Has the adolescent been sexually active? Are they currently in a relationship? Does the teen use contraception and/or condoms? How many partners have they had? What is the teen's past history of sexually transmitted infections (STIs), pregnancy, abortion, and sexual abuse? Has the adolescent been a victim of trauma?
- **S**uicide: Is there a history of isolation or being withdrawn, emotional outbursts, or impulsive behavior? Has the teen had depression symptoms, including suicidal ideation (SI) or a past history of SAs? If there has been SI, does the teen have a plan and access to the means to commit suicide?

In Chapter 25, Evidence-Based Therapeutic Communication and Motivational Interviewing in Health Assessment, the use of self to establish a therapeutic connection to facilitate open communication with the person is covered in more depth. How to ask sensitive questions and respond effectively to support positive health outcomes is a skill that requires empathy, openness, and authenticity; this is true for connecting with teens who are in distress. Being able to develop and sustain a person-centered relationship with a person in mental distress is central to effective mental healthcare. At the very least, this requires engagement with the adolescent's conceptualization of distress, strengths, and aspiration for the future.

RISK ASSESSMENT

A particularly sensitive part of the mental health assessment is a risk assessment for danger to self (DTS), danger to others (DTO), and ability to care for oneself (e.g., persistently or acutely disabled [PAD]). With vulnerable adults and children/teens, it is also important to assess for any danger they are in from others. Adding adverse childhood experiences (ACEs) screening (e.g., for violence, abuse, neglect) provides valuable information; the more ACEs a person has experienced, the higher is the likelihood for physical illnesses. Information about ACEs screening and trauma assessment is covered in Chapter 24, Evidence-Based Assessment and Screening for Traumatic Experiences: Abuse, Neglect, and Intimate Partner Violence.

Homicidal ideation (HI) is risk of DTO. If the patient acknowledges a desire to harm someone else, it is necessary to ask about their plan, intent, means, and availability of means. It is also important to ask about an identified target. If the patient identifies someone and has a plan, the intended victim must be informed according to the Tarasoff law/rule. The Tarasoff decision of 1976 states that the clinician has a responsibility to protect the potential victim; this generally involves informing the potential victim and law enforcement (Carlat, 2017).

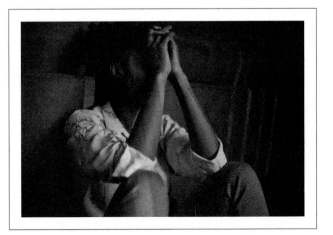

SI is risk of DTS. The majority of people who die by suicide visit a healthcare clinician within months before their death. This represents a tremendous opportunity to identify those at risk and connect them with mental health resources. Yet, most healthcare settings do not screen for suicide risk. In February 2016, The Joint Commission, the accrediting organization for healthcare programs in hospitals throughout the United States, issued a Sentinel Event Alert, recommending that all patients in all medical settings (e.g., inpatient hospital units, outpatient practices, emergency departments [EDs]) be screened for suicide risk. Using valid suicide risk screening tools that have been tested in the medical setting with adults and youth allows clinicians to accurately detect who is at risk and who needs further intervention. These screening tools (such as PHQ-9, PHQ-A for teens, Ask Suicide-Screening Questions [ASQ], and Columbia-Suicide Severity Rating Scale [C-SSRS]) are described in the "Evidence-Based Practice Considerations" section of this chapter. It is also important to obtain a history of self-injurious behavior, past SAs, hospitalizations for SI, or an SA. Of note, the period just following psychiatric hospital discharge is an extremely high-risk time for patients who struggle with SI (Olfson et al., 2016). Another major consideration is substance misuse or substance use disorder; asking about the use and availability of substances are critical questions when assessing suicide risk in primary care (Richards et al., 2019).

With risk assessment, it is important to identify protective factors. At the end of the risk assessment, evidence-based recommendations need to be put into place, including a safety plan with coping strategies that work for the patient, identified supports, and contact numbers for texting and calling when in crisis—especially suicidal crisis. It is also evidence-based to ensure a reduction of means to act on the SI and HI (e.g., remove bottles of medications, guns, and ropes from the environment). The *Stanley and Brown Patient Safety Plan* (template available at no cost at https://suicide preventionlifeline.org/wp-content/uploads/2016/08/Brown_StanleySafetyPlanTemplate.pdf) is an evidence-based format for actively writing down a plan (before leaving the office) and establishing with the patient that they will use the plan and contact identified support persons if they have SI.

LABORATORY CONSIDERATIONS

- Thyroid studies with the rationale that hypothyroidism presents like depression and hyperthyroidism presents like an anxiety disorder.
- Complete blood count (CBC) with differential with the rationale that anemia presents like depression. Underlying disease processes that can underlie

anemia include malignancies, viral illnesses (HIV, hepatitis C), impaired kidney function, and vitamin deficiencies (vitamin B12, folate).

- Testing may include assessing electrolytes, kidney function, urinalysis, and vitamin D levels, as well as tests for mono and lead levels, depending on age, signs, symptoms, and risks.

EVIDENCE-BASED PRACTICE CONSIDERATIONS

EVIDENCE-BASED DEPRESSION AND SUICIDALITY SCREENING

Assessing for depression, including the severity of symptoms, guides evidence-based interventions and treatment. The U.S. Preventive Services Task Force (USPSTF) recommendations related to depression assessment are listed in **Table 22.1**.

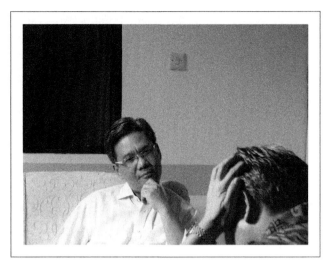

TABLE 22.1 USPSTF Recommendations for Depression Assessment

Age/Population	Recommendation
Adolescents aged 12–18 years	Screening for MDD in adolescents aged 12–18 years is recommended. Screening should be implemented with adequate systems in place to ensure accurate diagnosis, effective treatment, and appropriate follow-up.
Children aged 11 years or younger	Current evidence is insufficient to assess the balance of benefits and harms of screening for MDD in children aged 11 years or younger.
Adults, including pregnant and postpartum women	Screening for depression in the general adult population, including pregnant and postpartum women, is recommended. Screening should be implemented with adequate systems in place to ensure accurate diagnosis, effective treatment, and appropriate follow-up.

MDD, major depressive disorder; USPSTF, United States Preventive Services Task Force.
Sources: From Siu, A. L., Bibbins-Domingo, K., Grossman, D. C., Baumann, L. C., Davidson, K. W., Ebell, M., . . . Pignone, M. P. (2016). Screening for depression in adults: U.S. Preventive Services Task Force recommendation statement. *Journal of the American Medical Association, 315*(4), 380–387. doi:10.1001/jama.2015.18392; U.S. Preventive Services Task Force. (2016). Final update summary: Depression in children and adolescents: Screening. Retrieved from https://www.uspreventiveservicestaskforce.org/Page/Document/UpdateSummaryFinal/depression-in-children-and-adolescents-screening1

The depression screening instrument most often used in primary care, the nine-item Patient Health Questionnaire (PHQ-9), can be entirely self-administered by the patient; this tool includes an item that asks about how often one experiences thoughts of death/suicidal thoughts. The PHQ-9 has been adapted for teens (PHQ-A modified for adolescents). The PHQ is a valid and reliable instrument that is free and in the public domain, available at www.ncbi.nlm.nih.gov/pmc/articles/PMC1495268. The clinicians not only need to review the resultant scores from the screening, but they also need to follow up by **asking the patient directly** whether they have had SI or past SAs, and if they are currently struggling with these thoughts. Asking about suicide will not put that idea in a patient's mind. In fact, being asked is often a relief to patients who need to talk about their thoughts and fears. When the clinician explains that every individual is asked these questions, it gives a clear message that mental health is part of their total health and always can be discussed at their healthcare visits.

The USPSTF has not recommended specific screening for SI or suicide risk in all adolescents, adults, and older adults in primary care. The recommendations specific for suicide screening are listed in **Table 22.2**. However, screening for suicide risk in primary care is endorsed by the National Action Alliance for Suicide Prevention (Action Alliance: Transforming Health Systems Initiative Work Group, 2018) and supported by the NIMH Suicide Screening Toolkit (n.d.). The Action Alliance (2018) recommends a standard of care for people at high risk for suicide, including:

1. On intake and periodically, assess all patients for suicide risk using a standardized screening instrument or scale. If a person endorses suicidal thoughts, the recommendation is to enhance safety for the person by referring to specialized care and providing caring

TABLE 22.2 USPSTF Recommendations for Screening for Suicide Risk

Age/Population	Recommendation
Adolescents, adults, and older adults	Current evidence is insufficient to assess the balance of benefits and harms of screening for suicide risk in adolescents, adults, and older adults in primary care.

USPSTF, United States Preventive Services Task Force.
Source: From LeFevre, M. L., Siu, A. L., Bibbins-Domingo, K., Baumann, L. C., Curry, S. J., Davidson, K. W., . . . Pignone, M. P. (2014). Screening for suicide risk in adolescents, adults, and older adults in primary care: U.S. Preventive Services Task Force recommendation statement. *Annals of Internal Medicine, 160*(10), 719–726. doi:10.7326/M14-0589

contacts. (If acute risk is identified with plan, intent, and means, the clinician will "proceed with active referral for hospital or outpatient care as judged appropriate.")

2. Once referral for crisis is made for those at risk, the primary care clinician can begin safety planning.
3. Take action to reduce lethality. As part of the safety plan, discuss any lethal means considered by and available to the patient. This involves identifying possible means of self-harm that are available to the individual (especially ones they may have considered, such as use of a weapon or overdosing on medications) and reducing access by taking specific steps, such as self-storage. Reducing access to lethal means has repeatedly been shown effective in community-wide prevention and has been cited as a crucial factor in the success of suicide-prevention efforts. Arrange and confirm removal or reduction of lethal means as feasible.

Safety planning with means reduction has now been embedded in the suicide care protocols of hundreds of healthcare organizations. Safety planning is a brief intervention to help a patient develop a plan to recognize suicidal thoughts and manage them safely. Action steps may include calming activities, identifying supportive people to talk to, and providing contact information for crisis call or text lines. The *Stanley and Brown Safety Plan* in **Exhibit 22.1** is free, online, and easy to print, which allows this to be easily kept in the clinician's office or practice site. The tool is also available as a phone app *SAFETY NET* (NYS Office of Mental Health and Columbia University).

Safety planning includes assessing whether an individual is safe in their relationship(s), whether the individual feels afraid or threatened, and if they have a support system and safety plan if needed. A key USPSTF recommendation related to mental health assessment and exposure to violence is listed in **Table 22.3**.

For older adults, the Substance Abuse and Mental Health Services Administration (SAMHSA, 2011) has published *Treatment of Depression in Older Adults Evidence-Based Practices KIT*. This SAMHSA guide to evidence-based practices provides materials and information about assessing depression in older adults, including prevalence, risk factors, and symptoms. The evidence-based approach that is the foundation of the collected intervention strategies states, "Mental health services should have the goal of helping older adults achieve their health and personal recovery goals; develop resilience; and live, work, learn, and participate in the community" (SAMHSA, 2011, p. 3).

EVIDENCE-BASED MENTAL HEALTH SCREENING TOOLS

It is important for clinicians to understand that screenings are intended to identify concerning signs and/or symptoms that *may* indicate or raise red flags for mental health diagnoses; although these screenings are highly important for helping to identify mental health disorders, diagnoses must be confirmed with a careful diagnostic clinical evaluation, which goes beyond screening. Mental health disorders are diagnosed according to criteria in the *Diagnostic and Statistical Manual of Mental Disorders* (5th ed.; *DSM-5*; American Psychiatric Association [APA], 2013).

Patient Health Questionnaire (PHQ-9 and PHQ-2) Depression Scales

The PHQ-9, previously described, is a widely used valid and reliable nine-item tool used to diagnose and monitor the severity of depression. Question 9 of the tool screens for the presence and duration of SI. This screening tool and an instruction manual are available at no cost at www.phqscreeners.com. There is a valid and reliable adolescent version as well as an abbreviated screening, the PHQ-2, that is valid and reliable for teens (Richardson et al., 2010). The PHQ-2 screening contains the following two questions:

- Over the *past 2 weeks*, how often have you been bothered by the following problems?
  1. Little interest or pleasure in doing things
     - Not at all (0)
     - Several days (+1)
     - More than half the days (+2)
     - Nearly every day (+3)
  2. Feeling down, depressed, or hopeless
     - Not at all (0)
     - Several days (+1)
     - More than half the days (+2)
     - Nearly every day (+3)

The PHQ-2 score is obtained by adding the score for each question (total points) and interpreted based on the scoring:

EXHIBIT 22.1 Patient Safety Plan Template

Patient Safety Plan Template

Step 1: Warning signs (thought, images, mood, situation, behavior) that a crisis may be developing:

1. _____

2. _____

3. _____

Step 2: Internal coping strategies—things I can do to take my mind off my problems without contacting another person (relaxation technique, physical activity):

1. _____

2. _____

3. _____

Step 3: People and social settings that provide distraction:

1. Name _____ Phone _____

2. Name _____ Phone _____

3. Place _____ 4. Place _____

Step 4: People whom I can ask for help:

1. Name _____ Phone _____

2. Name _____ Phone _____

3. Name _____ Phone _____

Step 5: Professionals or agencies I can contact during a crisis:

1. Clinician Name _____ Phone _____

   Clinician Pager or Emergency Contact # _____

2. Clinician Name _____ Phone _____

   Clinician Pager or Emergency Contact # _____

3. Local Urgent Care Services _____

   Urgent Care Services Address _____

   Urgent Care Services Phone _____

4. Suicide Prevention Lifeline Phone: 1-800-273-TALK (8255)

Step 6: Making the environment safe:

1. _____

2. _____

Safety Plan Template ©2008 Barbara Stanley and Gregory K. Brown is reprinted with the express permission of the authors. No portion of the Safety Plan Template may be reproduced without their express permission. Completing and submitting the form on this web page www.suicidesafetlyplan.com/Page_8.html constitutes permission to use the template.

The one thing that is most important to me and worth living for is:

_____

TABLE 22.3 USPSTF Recommends Screening
for Intimate Partner Violence

Age/Population	Recommendation
Reproductive-aged women	The USPSTF recommends that clinicians screen for IPV in reproductive-aged women and provide or refer women who screen positive to ongoing support services.

IPV, intimate partner violence; USPSTF, United States Preventive Services Task Force.
Source: From Curry, S. J., Krist, A. H., Owens, D. K., Barry, M. J., Caughey, A. B., Davidson, K. W., . . . Wong, J. B. (2018). Screening for intimate partner violence, elder abuse, and abuse of vulnerable adults: U.S. Preventive Services Task Force final recommendation statement. *Journal of the American Medical Association, 320*(16), 1678–1687. doi:10.1001/jama.2018.14741

- A PHQ-2 score ranges from 0 to 6. The authors consider a score of 3 as the optimal cut point when using the PHQ-2 to screen for depression.
- If the score is 3 or greater, MDD is likely.
- Patients who screen positive should be further evaluated with the PHQ-9, other diagnostic instruments, and/or a direct interview to determine whether they meet criteria for a depressive disorder.

Columbia-Suicide Severity Rating Scale

The C-SSRS features questions that help determine whether an individual is at risk for suicide. There are brief versions of the C-SSRS often used as a screening tool (the first two questions) that, based on patient response, can lead to the administration of the longer C-SSRS to triage patients. The tool can be accessed at www.cssrs.columbia.edu.

Ask Suicide-Screening Questions

Ask Suicide-Screening Questions (ASQ) is a four-item suicide-screening tool designed to be used for people aged 10 to 24 years in EDs, inpatient units, and primary care facilities. The ASQ was developed by a team from the National Institute of Mental Health (NIMH) and is available at www.nimh.nih.gov/research/research-conducted-at-nimh/asq-toolkit-materials/asq-tool/screening-tool_155867.pdf

- Ask the patient:
  1. In the past few weeks, have you wished you were dead?
  2. In the past few weeks, have you felt that you or your family would be better off if you were dead?
  3. In the past week, have you been having thoughts about killing yourself?

4. Have you ever tried to kill yourself?
   - If yes, how? _____
   _____
- If the patient answers **Yes** to any of the previously mentioned questions, ask the following acuity question:
5. Are you having thoughts of killing yourself right now?
   - If yes, please describe: _____
- If the patient answers "yes" to #5, they require an immediate safety/full mental health evaluation. The patient cannot leave until evaluated for safety.
- If the patient answers "no" to question #5, they require a brief suicide safety assessment to determine whether a full mental health evaluation is needed. The patient cannot leave until evaluated for safety.
- Provide all patients who screen positively with the following resources:
  ○ 24/7 National Suicide Prevention Lifeline
    - In English: 1-800-273-TALK (8255); en Español: 1-888-628-9454
  ○ 24/7 Crisis Text Line: Text "HOME" to 741-741

In an NIMH study, a "yes" response to one or more of the four questions identified 97% of youth (aged 10–21 years) at risk for suicide. There is a free toolkit that can help to identify youth at risk at www.nimh.nih.gov/research/research-conducted-at-nimh/asq-toolkit-materials/index.shtml.

Outcome Questionnaire 45.2

The Outcome Questionnaire 45.2 (OQ-45.2®) helps mental health clinicians to assess symptom distress (depression and anxiety), interpersonal relationships (loneliness, conflicts with others, and marriage and family difficulties), and social roles (difficulties in the workplace, school, or home). It includes explicit questions about suicide and is for use with the adult population. There is a licensing fee for this instrument. See www.oqmeasures.com.

Mood Disorder Questionnaire

The Mood Disorder Questionnaire (MDQ) is a screening tool for bipolar disorder. The MDQ can be either administered by the clinician or self-administered by the patient; it consists of 15 questions and takes about 5 minutes to complete. The first 13 questions about possible symptoms are answered either "yes" or "no." The other two questions assess presentation of symptoms and disease severity.

7-Item Generalized Anxiety Disorder Scale

The 7-item Generalized Anxiety Disorder (GAD-7) is a screening tool most commonly used in primary care. Validated as a diagnostic tool and severity assessment scale, the GAD-7 is a three-point Likert-type self-report questionnaire with seven items. Scores greater than 10 indicate good diagnostic sensitivity and specificity for GAD. Higher scores correlate with more functional impairment. Download free at www.phqscreeners.com/sites/g/files/g10016261/f/201412/GAD-7_English.pdf.

Perceived Stress Scale 10

The 10-item Perceived Stress Scale (PSS-10) is a five-point Likert-type scale, with 10 items designed to determine the degree of stress associated with specific situations over the previous month. Total scores indicate how unpredictable, uncontrollable, and overloaded respondents perceive their life to be. There is also a four-item questionnaire called the PSS-4. This version has also been shown to have validity and reliability in the detection of stress. Download free at Mind Garden: www.mindgarden.com/documents/PerceivedStressScale.pdf.

Spielberger State-Trait Anxiety Inventory

One of the most widely used anxiety assessment instruments in research is the Spielberger State-Trait Anxiety Inventory. Note: There is a charge for this inventory. The inventory contains both state (how one feels at the present moment) and trait (how one generally feels) scales. State anxiety may be amenable to intervention, whereas trait anxiety is a personality trait that contributes to how an individual experiences and perceives anxiety. See Mind Garden: www.mindgarden.com.

Trauma and Substance Use Screenings

The likelihood of co-occurring exposure to trauma (see Chapter 24, Evidence-Based Assessment and Screening for Traumatic Experiences) and comorbid substance use disorder (see Chapter 23, Evidence-Based Assessment of Substance Use Disorder) can be assessed through screening instruments as well. See these chapters for further information about AUDIT-C for adult substance use screening, CRAFFT to assess adolescent risk for substance use disorder, and ACEs screening to assess for ACEs. The CRAFFT 2.1 includes vaping and edibles in their questions.

EVIDENCE-BASED SCREENING INSTRUMENTS SPECIFIC TO CHILDREN/TEENS

A full battery of screening tools for child and adolescent mental health/behavioral disorders is available from the American Academy of Pediatrics at www.aap.org/en-us/advocacy-and-policy/aap-health-initiatives/Mental-Health/Documents/MH_ScreeningChart.pdf. Three commonly used evidence-based instruments are listed as follows.

Pediatric Symptom Checklist

The Pediatric Symptom Checklist (PSC) is a valid and reliable 35-item questionnaire that lists a range of children's emotional and behavioral concerns as perceived by parents. There is also a youth self-reported form. It is used for children and youth who are 4 to 18 years of age. There is also a short form consisting of 17 items. The PSC has been adapted for young children, 18 to 60 months of age, and for children who are younger than 18 months. The scales are freely downloadable and available in multiple languages at www.massgeneral.org/psychiatry/services/treatmentprograms.aspx?id=2088.

The Screen for Child Anxiety-Related Disorders

The Screen for Child Anxiety-Related Disorders (SCARED) is a valid and reliable 41-item self-report questionnaire that measures anxiety-related disorders in 8- to 17-year-old children, teens, and their parents (Birmaher et al., 1999). The SCARED measures anxiety using four domains: panic/somatic, separation anxiety, generalized anxiety, and school phobia. It is free for download at www.midss.org/content/screen-child-anxiety-related-disorders-scared.

National Institute for Children's Health Quality Vanderbilt Assessment Scales

The National Institute for Children's Health Quality (NICHQ) offers a free download of the assessment scales used for children between the ages of 6 and 12 to identify signs and symptoms of ADHD; the tools are available at www.nichq.org/resource/nichq-vanderbilt-assessment-scales. Vanderbilt Assessment Scales include questionnaires for parents/guardians and teachers for initial and follow-up screenings; scales include symptoms assessments related to inattention, hyperactivity, and impulsiveness and screenings for other comorbidities including oppositional defiant disorder, conduct disorder, anxiety, and depression. These scales are not used alone to make a diagnosis, and information from multiple sources must be included. The American Academy of Pediatrics (AAP) recommends that healthcare clinicians ask parents, teachers, and other adults who care for the child about the child's behavior in different settings (e.g., home, school, or with peers).

FINDINGS IN COMMON MENTAL HEALTH DISORDERS

ANXIETY AND ANXIETY DISORDERS

Anxiety is multidimensional and has been studied from a variety of perspectives—physiological (neurobiological), cognitive, and behavioral. The etiology of anxiety-related disorders seems to be because of a combination of psychological traits, life stressors, and

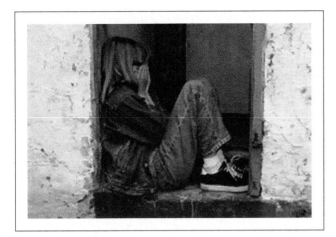

genetic vulnerability (Tusaie & Fitzpatrick, 2017). Often, the patient can identify another family member who also has had significant anxiety symptoms. When the patient identifies anxiety as a concern, the clinician will ask questions to determine whether the anxiety is within the range of normal or elevated as with panic attacks. The patient also may describe the symptoms of other anxiety disorders, such as social anxiety disorder, phobic disorder, and GAD (somatization, factitious).

To meet the *DSM-5* criteria for an anxiety disorder, there must be difficulty functioning owing to the anxiety symptoms at home, school, or in social situations (APA, 2013). The *DSM-5* criteria for diagnosis of mild, moderate, or severe anxiety or anxiety disorders are embedded in the GAD-2 and GAD-7 screenings. When screening for excessive worry, nervousness, and anxiousness, clinicians should recognize that this is a good time to also ask about the patient's usual coping strategies. It is also helpful to ask what strategies any affected relative(s) have found helpful for relieving anxiety. Many will describe deep breathing, yoga, therapy, strong family connections, friendships, or spending time alone in prayer or using guided imagery. All of these can be leveraged when engaged in a discussion of wellness and resilience strategies and coping.

TRAUMA AND STRESSOR-RELATED DISORDERS

In the previous *DSM*, posttraumatic stress disorder (PTSD) and acute stress disorders were listed in the Anxiety Disorders section. With the *DSM-5*, trauma and stressor-related disorders are discussed in a separate section. Trauma and stressor-related disorders have many of the same symptoms; however, they are diagnosed according to time from the experience. One thing is common to all the trauma and stressor-related disorders, in that they communicate clearly to clinicians that "something bad happened."

To meet criteria for a trauma or stressor-related disorder, there needs to have been:

1. Exposure to actual or threatened death, serious injury, or sexual violation in either:
   ○ Directly experiencing the traumatic event
   ○ Witnessing, in person, the event as it occurred to others
   ○ Learning that the event occurred to a close family member or close friend (violent or accidental)
   ○ Experiencing repeated or extreme exposure to aversive details of the traumatic event (e.g., first responders on site experiences, exposure to details of child abuse). (Does not apply to exposure through electronic media.)
2. Presence of the following symptoms:
   ○ Intrusive thoughts: Intrusive memories, flashbacks, recurrent nightmares
   ○ Negative mood: Inability to experience happiness, good emotions
   ○ Dissociation: Altered sense of reality, inability to remember aspects of the trauma
   ○ Avoidance symptoms: Efforts to avoid reminders, triggers of the event (isolation); efforts to avoid memories
   ○ Arousal symptoms: Hypervigilance, sleep disturbance, irritable, angry outbursts, exaggerated startle response, problems with concentration

With trauma and stressor-related disorders, it is important in teaching/psychoeducation that explanations are given to the patient clearly:

• "What you experienced was abnormal."
• "It was traumatic and of such severity that no person should ever have to experience that."
• "Your symptoms and your response are the normal human response to extreme trauma/stress. You are not abnormal. The event/experience was abnormal."

Note that the onset of the trauma, stressor-related symptoms, and emotional and behavioral reactions are the key to the diagnosis. Diagnoses include:

1. Adjustment disorders: Occur within 3 months of the onset of the stressor.
   ○ These include adjustment disorders with depressed mood; anxiety; mixed depressed mood and anxiety; disturbance of conduct, which might apply to children/ teens who have experienced trauma; and disturbance of emotions and conduct.
2. Acute stress disorder: Symptoms begin at time of event and last 3 days to 1 month.
3. PTSD: Symptoms or disturbance occur after 1 month.
   ○ There are criteria for PTSD for ages 6 to adulthood. In children under 6 years, there is a separate *DSM-5* criteria, and, generally, if it is determined at the time of the assessment that a child has experienced trauma or extreme ACEs, it is best to

document the examination/assessment and refer to a pediatric trauma specialist. Interestingly, young children respond very quickly to trauma-focused interventions, with much quicker response to treatment than adults.

DEPRESSION AND MOOD DISORDERS

Criteria for the diagnosis of depression (mild, moderate, and severe) are embedded in the evidence-based screenings reviewed. The acronym SIGECAPS is helpful to remember the signs and symptoms of depression:

- **S**leep: Increased (hypersomnia) or decreased (insomnia)
- **I**nterest: Decreased, loss of ability to enjoy activities that were once enjoyed
- **G**uilt: Feelings of worthlessness, hopelessness
- **E**nergy: Change in energy level, fatigued or restless
- **C**oncentration: Difficulty making decisions
- **A**ppetite changes, and/or weight increase or decrease
- **P**sychomotor activity: Increased (agitation) or decreased (slowed)
- **S**uicidal ideation: Recurrent thoughts of death, suicidal thoughts, plans for committing suicide

If the screening or history is positive for depression, obtain a sense of how long the depressive symptoms have been present. When was the first episode of depression? Persistent depressive disorder, or dysthymia, is a chronic form of depression. Depression can be related to medical illness, induced by substances including medication, and/or may be related to additional internal or external factors, such as premenstrual dysphoric disorder (PMDD) or seasonal affective disorder (SAD). The person with depression has a lack of energy, lack of interest, lack of initiative, and fewer interactions with others. Depression is more accurately a lack of vitality, not a disorder of "being sad" or having a "sad mood." Sadness is a normal emotion, often triggered by loss. Depression is a disorder characterized by self-diminishing negative patterns of thought.

Note that the SIGECAPS symptoms listed earlier are nonspecific; that is, they can be associated with other disorders. Clinicians are encouraged to use evidence-based screenings as symptoms warrant. If the PHQ-2 was used as a screening and it is positive, the PHQ-9 should then be administered. If only the PHQ-2 screening is used, the clinician should also ask about suicidal thoughts. SI is *not* one of the two questions on the PHQ-2.

It is imperative to conduct a suicide risk assessment. It is also important to assess for substance use because many individuals with depression will use substances to regulate their depressive symptoms. If the person endorses past SI, the clinician should ask whether there was an attempt or self-injurious behaviors. Then, ask

directly about current SI—clarify the plan, including how the patient plans to kill himself or herself, intent, and means (access to their plan, such as guns or drugs).

Signs and symptoms of mood disorder include periods of mood instability and changes in mood that can be daily or weekly. Screening for mania is key to identifying assessments that may indicate bipolar disorder; these include not needing sleep for days, excessive enthusiasm, and periods of great excitement and obsession. Key questions are as follows: (a) Do you have racing thoughts? (Those who do can describe those thoughts going so fast that they cannot keep track of them.) (b) Has your speech been so fast that it is hard to follow? Pressurized speech and flight of ideas are correlated with mania. (c) Have family or friends commented about your behavior or changes in behavior? If a family member or significant other is available, with the patient's permission, they can provide valuable input into the assessment of a mood disorder. With bipolar disorder, mania is sometimes not recognized by the person as insight is limited when bipolar symptoms are increased. DIGFAST is a mnemonic that can help the clinician to remember symptoms of mania:

- **D**istractibility: Difficulty blocking unimportant distractions
- **I**ndiscretion: Excessive involvement in pleasurable activities
- **G**randiosity: Feelings of invulnerability
- **F**light of ideas: Racing thoughts, rapid shifting of ideas
- **A**ctivity increase: Dramatic periods of excitement, enthusiasm
- **S**leep deficit: Decreased need for sleep
- **T**alkativeness: Pressured speech

Identifying symptoms of mania to differentiate unipolar and bipolar mood disorders significantly informs an individual's treatment plan. Antidepressants prescribed to persons with bipolar disorder can activate mania, often with negative outcomes for that person. Note that bipolar disorder can present first as a depressive disorder. The usual age of onset of serious mental disorders (bipolar disorder, thought disorders, and severe persistent mental health disorders) is generally in late adolescence and young adulthood, but can occur earlier or later.

THOUGHT DISORDERS

If the clinician has a difficult time following the patient's conversation while completing the history and physical examination, additional assessments may be needed for delusions, hallucinations, or thought disorder. Delirium and dementia, disorders that present as thought disorders, are reviewed in Chapter 14, Evidence-Based Assessment of the Nervous System. Assess thought processes, content, and perceptions.

The best way to assess and record these disordered thoughts is to write down what has been said—word for word. (It is very difficult to remember what the statement was because it does not follow usual logic.) The clinician might explore beliefs that they think are delusions, not based in common reality (e.g., "I am the king of this country."). It is not helpful to challenge delusions; delusions are strongly held false beliefs. Assess for auditory and/or visual hallucinations, and consider whether these occurred only with periods of substance use. Ask the patients whether they ever hear or see things that others do not. If they say this is occurring, ask them to describe the voices they hear or the things they see. It is more concerning if the voices are critical of the patient, and it is especially concerning if the voices are "commanding" the patient to do unsafe or harmful things (e.g., harming themselves or harming someone else, or engaging in risky behaviors like running on the highway).

These assessments help the clinician to identify red flags associated with severe, persistent mental illnesses (SPMIs), which are disorders defined by their level of severity and disability. The SPMI category includes the symptomatology of disordered thought processes that can be associated with severe MDD, schizoaffective bipolar disorders, schizophrenia, psychoses, and borderline personality disorder. SPMIs are characterized by marked difficulties in self-care, marked restriction of activities of daily living, frequent deficiencies of concentration, and significant difficulties in maintaining social functioning.

COMORBID MENTAL HEALTH CONDITIONS

When clinicians encounter individuals who are struggling with anxiety and/or depression, they should also consider that the patient may have other comorbidities, including physical and mental health disorders. These include:

- Eating disorders
- Sleep disorders
- Obsessive-compulsive disorder (OCD)
- Impulse control disorders
- ADHD
- Trauma/stress-related disorders, including PTSD
- Neurocognitive impairment, including delirium and dementia
- Substance misuse and substance use disorder

SPECIAL CONSIDERATIONS FOR CHILDREN AND ADOLESCENTS

ANXIETY

Anxiety and fear are a normal part of a child and adolescent's development, but they should not be excessive, interfere with functioning, or persist beyond what is appropriate for their developmental stage. Anxiety disorders are the most common mental health disorder in children and teens. Comorbidities are common, including depression, ADHD, and substance misuse (Melnyk & Jensen, 2013, p. 61).

Children with anxiety disorders often present with somatic symptoms, such as abdominal pain, headaches, or chest pain. They are often "worriers" and misdiagnosed with ADHD.

Key History/Assessment Questions for Children and Adolescents

- Is the anxiety appropriate for the age of the child/teen?
- Does the child/teen have symptoms in response to a specific trigger (e.g., social situations)?
- Has the child/teen experienced a traumatic event?
- Is there a history of recent stressful events, including marital transition?
- Does the anxiety interfere with functioning?
- What impact does anxiety have on the child's sleep, concentration, appetite, energy, and relationships?
- Are there associated signs of depression?
- What medications is the child taking? (Medications such as antihistamines, SSRIs, stimulants, antiasthmatics, hypoglycemia, marijuana, and nasal decongestants can cause anxiety.)
- Is the child or teen using substances to regulate anxiety symptoms?

It is important to rule out medical conditions, such as hyperthyroidism, lead intoxication, migraine headaches, and asthma.

Specific anxiety disorders include GAD, social anxiety disorder, panic disorder, and phobias. Somatic disorders are in their own separate category, as are OCDs. Anxiety is comorbid with many other mental disorders, including depression and ADHD.

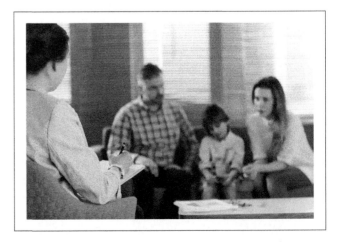

ATTENTION DEFICIT HYPERACTIVITY DISORDER

Clinicians use the *DSM-5* criteria to support an ADHD diagnosis; this standard is intended to help ensure that children, teens, young adults, and adults are diagnosed appropriately (APA, 2013). The diagnosis of ADHD involves assessment for a constellation of symptoms and is understood as one of a spectrum of neurological, developmental, cognitive, and genetic disorders. ADHD is often comorbid with other mental disorders and can present in adulthood. Individuals with ADHD show a persistent pattern of inattention and/or hyperactivity-impulsivity that interferes with function or development (APA, 2013). *DSM-5* criteria include (APA, 2013):

- Inattention: Six or more symptoms of inattention for children up to age 16, or five or more for adolescents 17 and older including adults; symptoms of inattention have been present for at least 6 months and are inappropriate for developmental level:
  - Often fails to give close attention to details or makes careless mistakes in schoolwork, at work, or with other activities.
  - Often has trouble holding attention on tasks or playing activities.
  - Often does not seem to listen when spoken to directly.
  - Often does not follow through on instructions and fails to finish schoolwork, chores, or duties in the workplace (e.g., loses focus, side-tracked).
  - Often has trouble organizing tasks and activities.
  - Often avoids, dislikes, or is reluctant to do tasks that require mental effort over a long period of time (such as schoolwork or homework).
  - Often loses things necessary for tasks and activities (e.g., school materials, pencils, books, tools, wallets, keys, paperwork, eyeglasses, mobile telephones).
  - Is often easily distracted.
  - Is often forgetful in daily activities.
- Hyperactivity and impulsivity: Six or more symptoms of hyperactivity-impulsivity for children up to age 16, or five or more for adolescents 17 and older including adults; symptoms of hyperactivity-impulsivity have been present for at least 6 months to an extent that is disruptive and inappropriate for the person's developmental level:
  - Often fidgets with or taps hands or feet, or squirms in seat.
  - Often leaves seat in situations when remaining seated is expected.
  - Often runs about or climbs in situations where it is not appropriate (adolescents or adults may be limited to feeling restless).
  - Often unable to play or take part in leisure activities quietly.
  - Is often "on the go," acting as if "driven by a motor."
  - Often talks excessively.
  - Often blurts out an answer before a question has been completed.
  - Often has trouble waiting for their turn.
  - Often interrupts or intrudes on others (e.g., butts into conversations or games).
- In addition, the following conditions must be met:
  - Several inattentive or hyperactive-impulsive symptoms were present before age 12 years.
  - Several symptoms are present in two or more settings (such as at home, school, or work; with guardians, friends, or relatives; in other activities).
  - There is clear evidence that the symptoms interfere with, or reduce the quality of, social, school, or work functioning.
  - The symptoms are not better explained by another mental disorder (such as a mood disorder, anxiety disorder, dissociative disorder, or a personality disorder). The symptoms do not happen only during the course of schizophrenia or another psychotic disorder.

Children, adolescents, and adults can have ADHD that predominantly presents as inattention, or hyperactivity-impulsivity, or both. Because symptoms can change over time, the presentation may change over time as well. ADHD often lasts into adulthood. To diagnose ADHD in adults and adolescents aged 17 years or older, only five symptoms are needed instead of six needed for younger children. Symptoms might look different at older ages. For example, in adults, hyperactivity may appear as extreme restlessness or wearing others out with their activity.

DEPRESSION

Important points to note regarding the assessment of depression in children and teens include:

- Young children less than 7 years of age with depression are often misdiagnosed with ADHD as they frequently present with inattention, impulsivity, and hyperactivity (Melnyk & Jensen, 2013).
- Anger is often a presenting symptom in adolescents.
- The mean age of onset for MDD is 14 years.
- Reoccurrence rate is as high as 60% to 70% and often reoccurs in adulthood; 40% to 70% of affected children/teens have comorbid mental health conditions, so it is critical to assess for other mental health disorders (e.g., anxiety, substance use, ADHD).

Specific Depression Assessment Questions for Children and Adolescents

- Mood: Have you been feeling sad, down, blue, or grouchy most of the days, more days than not? Do you find yourself crying a lot? Have you been getting into arguments more than usual?

- Anhedonia: Are you able to enjoy things you used to enjoy? Do you feel bored or tired a lot of the time?
- Negative self-concept: How do you feel about yourself on a scale of 0 (not good at all) to 10 (really good)?
- Guilt: Do you feel badly or guilty about what you have done?
- Relationships with friends: Do you have friends? Are you liked by your peers?
- Neurovegetative signs: Do you have trouble falling asleep or staying asleep? Do you have trouble concentrating? How is your appetite?
- Somatic symptoms: Do you have headaches and/or stomachaches?
- SIs: Do you ever wish you were dead? Do you think about death or hurting yourself? Have you ever hurt yourself?
- Current health and medications (e.g., benzodiazepines, beta-blockers, corticosteroids, accutane, oral contraceptives, etc.)
- Alcohol and drug use: What drugs are you taking? How often? How much alcohol do you drink? (Melnyk & Jensen, 2013, p. 102)

Always assess a depressed teen presenting with depressive symptoms for bipolar disorder, including elevated or irritable mood, inflated self-esteem, decreased sleep, more talkative, flight of ideas, distractibility, and excessive involvement in activities that have adverse consequences (e.g., buying sprees, drug use, promiscuity).

Physical diagnoses that should be ruled out include hypothyroidism (obtain thyroid-stimulating hormone [TSH], free T4 [FT4]), anemia (obtain CBC with differential), mononucleosis, eating disorders, substance use or withdrawal, premenstrual syndrome, diabetes, and lead intoxication (obtain lead level).

A supplementary handout that can be used as a resource for working with teens to assess physical, emotional, and behavioral symptoms (experiences) of stress can be accessed online (https://www.springerpub.com/ebpe).

THE WRITE-UP FOR A MENTAL HEALTH ASSESSMENT

Many of the symptoms discussed happen on a continuum from within normal limits in response to stress, to symptoms that impair functioning.

The purpose of the write-up or documentation of the mental health assessment is to build a narrative picture of the patient, including strengths and areas of concern, that will be informative to the clinician and to other colleagues, as well as provide a thorough assessment that will provide the data to support the clinician's diagnosis and treatment plan. Note that for the clinician using the EHR that there will be check boxes to complete, but using the free text fields will provide a description of the patient that will allow other readers to more deeply understand patient presentation and plan.

The identifying data are presented in a fairly long initial sentence that sets the stage for the entire assessment write-up. This sentence identifies the patient and includes age, sex, marital status, and source of referral. This information helps to provide context, providing a background of the patients within their social and cultural norms. This should include information about their occupation, living situation, family, and so on.

The chief concern is a verbatim quote from the patient regarding the reason they are being seen for assessment today. Using the patient's words signifies the main area of concern and also begins to tell their expectation for the visit.

The documentation should include a section specifically related to the individual's psychiatric and mental health history. This includes symptoms and diagnoses from their past, ideally beginning with the first significant symptoms. Document the psychiatric care received in the past (including outpatient, counseling services in schools and at work, inpatient hospitalizations and substance use disorder treatment, and recovery resources), the response to treatment, and what interventions were the most beneficial. Then, the clinician can review the onset, occurrence of the current symptoms, and/or additional concerns in detail to find out how they are being impacted now by symptoms.

Clinicians who work in pediatric settings will note that the initial mental health visits with children and teens are generally written up more descriptively. The pediatric case study that follows is an example. With children, there is less emphasis in assessment on their verbal accounts of distress; there is more notation about their behaviors and manner of relating to the parent(s) and clinician, as appropriate for their developmental level. Within the documentation, the clinician paints a picture of the child or teen's interactions and behaviors. As the child grows and develops, the written documentation of an initial assessment creates a baseline from which to monitor progress.

CASE STUDY: Adult Mental Health Assessment

Chart Review of Mental Health Assessment

MJ endorsed two previous periods of time where depressive symptoms required treatment with antidepressants, as treated by her primary care provider (PCP). She has a psychotherapist now that she has been seeing for 8 months. She denied any history of mania or hypomania. She has struggled with anxiety at times, but has never experienced panic or had obsessive thoughts and/or compulsive behaviors. There was no history of an eating disorder, attention deficit, or hyperactivity. She does not endorse past traumatic experiences or times when she was treated badly. She has never experienced impaired perceptions, no hallucinations, auditory or visual, no delusions or paranoia. There is no evidence of thought disorder. Her thoughts are organized and logical, and judgment and insight are good. No SI, no HI, no history of self-harm or SAs. She drinks alcohol occasionally, but has never experienced withdrawal symptoms or sought services for substance use disorder. She does not use other substances.

Assessment

MJ is a 44-year-old, married, white mother of three, and full-time nursing instructor who meets diagnostic criteria for MDD (recurrent; PHQ-9 today is 15) with current symptoms of low energy, decreased interest in activities she used to enjoy (such as going to the gym with friends), and hypersomnia. She also endorses anxiety, but this does not meet criteria for an anxiety disorder. She is still able to actively parent her three school-aged children, but makes negative statements, such as, "I used to be a better mother. They deserve a more involved mom now, and I'm just too tired and stressed to do as many activities with them." She does not endorse hopelessness and does not have SI. She is asking about restarting the SSRI that was so helpful to her in the past when she experienced episodes of depression. She still feels the sessions with her therapist are helpful, and she states the days she takes her dog for a 20-minute walk around the neighborhood increase her socialization with neighbors and increase her energy and sense of well-being.

Diagnosis and Follow-Up

Although the determination of management is beyond the focus of advanced assessment, it is useful to note that clinicians will be required to develop a treatment plan in partnership with patients who present similarly to MJ to manage MDD. The plan may include obtaining electrolytes, CBC with differential, and thyroid panel to rule out organic causes of symptoms. MJ has taken sertraline in the past with good therapeutic response for depression and anxiety and is interested in restarting this medication, which is reasonable. The prescribing clinician would review the expected response to SSRI, including that it takes about 4 to 6 weeks for optimal effects, and has possible adverse effects. Discussion of physical activity could incorporate MJ's willingness to walk her dog 3 to 4 days a week, continue with her therapist, and return to clinic in 3 weeks to assess her response to the treatment plan.

CASE STUDY: Pediatric Mental Health Assessment

Chart Review of Pediatric Mental Health Assessment

SCARED score: 29 (elevated, indicative of significant anxiety).

Zachary is a bright-eyed, thin 9-year-old boy with a buzz haircut who is wearing sports shorts and a T-shirt. He comes for this initial visit accompanied by his mother. When asked, Zachary says, "I'm here for stomachaches. I get stomachaches at school a lot." Mom agrees and says the school nurse and Zachary's teacher think Zachary's worries and stomachaches are getting in the way of his school performance now. Zachary is in fourth grade. Zachary's grades have dropped since the beginning of the winter term (4 months), and he is going to the school nurse three to four times a week for stomachaches. His teacher says he is very capable of doing fourth-grade work but gets visibly upset and shaky and appears on the verge of tears whenever she assigns a project or gives a test. He has difficulty concentrating. When he is at the nurse's office, he misses instruction. Zachary states that he likes his school and has been at the school since first grade. He has two

(continued)

CASE STUDY: Pediatric Mental Health Assessment (*continued*)

best friends, Alex and Tyrone. They mostly play tag or walk around before school and at recess.

He lives with his mom; dad; younger sister, Betty; and their black lab dog, Sport. He loves Legos and, at home, likes to play with Sport and spend time building things with his dad. Mom says Zachary is smart, responsible, kind, and really good at building with Legos. He has always been so advanced; he can build very complicated sets amazingly fast. He is a great helper at home, and he is very patient playing with his sister, even though she is 4 years younger.

He is happiest when all the family is together. If his dad is out of town or his mom is late picking him up, he worries and asks over and over when they will be back. He asks, "What if … ?" and lists the bad things that might happen. He is also very worried that a family member will get sick. Mom does think that Zachary's worry statements and stomachaches have increased since his dad's out-of-town work trips increased to two times every week. Mom is not aware of any traumatic events experienced by Zachary in the past. Zachary could not recall any extremely frightening experiences either.

During the visit, Zachary drew while his mother provided the history. Zachary had a normal birth, no complications, and met milestones at all the right times. He has never had counseling, but has always been a worrier. He has had times growing up when his parents have had to reassure him many times about the safety of his room and their home in order to address fears of monsters, robbers, or tornadoes. The only change in the home in the past 6 months is that his dad got a promotion at work and travels out of town a day or two each week.

Zachary has regular healthcare checkups and has been thoroughly worked up for gastrointestinal (GI) problems. His GI workup was normal. He is not on any medications. He has a fair appetite and eats foods from all food groups. He has no allergies/sensitivities. He sleeps well generally, and his growth has been steady for his height and weight. No head injuries/concussions. No surgeries or ED visits, except for having croup twice as a toddler.

Family history of anxiety/depression/mental/substance use disorders: Maternal history: Mom says she has always been anxious and mostly deals with anxiety by regular exercise, prayer, and self-talk that she learned in counseling when she was in her 20s. There have been a couple of times in her life when she took an SSRI and saw a counselor regularly—after

the birth of Zachary and when she was taking care of her ailing mother. She had trials of a couple of SSRIs, and sertraline has always worked best for her. Her mother was also anxious, and in her later years became so "nervous" that she could not go to church anymore. Paternal history: Only history is depression in two of his dad's brothers. Unsure what treatment they have had. No bipolar, no schizophrenia, no substance dependence on either side. No history of SI, SA, or death by suicide in family. No guns in home.

Throughout the visit, Zachary looked up and maintained eye contact when asked questions. He gave appropriate answers and exhibited logical, concrete thinking. Judgment is age appropriate. He smiled as he talked about his family and friends. There was an anxious quality to some of his responses, and he would look to his mom for the answer, before answering. He and his mom related warmly. He was most animated—explaining and gesturing about what he and his dad are going to build this summer out of their scrap wood. His affect was consistent with the content of his conversation. His three wishes are as follows: (a) He and his dad will build a go-cart; (b) his whole family will never be sick; and (c) *all* of the Lego sets will be made. Zachary has never had thoughts of wanting to hurt himself or thoughts of wanting to be dead. He has not heard things or seen things others did not hear or see. He has had nighttime dreams that were scary, and he went to his parents' room and told them. His mom says that has happened only a few times, and they do not watch certain movies now that were frightening to him. He has had times when he worried about school the next day and could not fall asleep easily.

He says if he needs to make a decision or talk with someone, he talks to his mom or dad. When he gets really stressed, he has learned to take deep breaths and he rubs his arms. He has not been teased or called names at school, but he fears that will happen. Sometimes he asks to go to the school nurse because he feels so bad, he thinks he might throw up in the classroom. The nurse lets him lay down and gives him crackers till he feels better.

Assessment

Zachary, a healthy-appearing, 9-year-old, fourth grader, presents with significant anxiety symptoms that are interfering with his functioning at school. History per mother who accompanies him: In the past 4 to 6 months, Zachary has had increased periods of difficulty concentrating, frequent stomachaches that

(*continued*)

CASE STUDY: Pediatric Mental Health Assessment (*continued*)

require visits to the school nurse, frequent expressed fears that something bad may happen to his family, and increased anxiety when his dad is working out of town. Anxiety symptoms increased when his dad was promoted to role of regional manager, which requires him to be out of town two to three times a week. Zachary has friends, many strengths including building abilities, and a close supportive family. A GI disorder has been ruled out by a pediatric practitioner/GI service. No evidence of thought disorder, no depressive/mood disorder, no SI, no history of trauma. Appetite and sleep OK. Has occasional bad dreams, worries that keep him awake. Grades are still B's and A's (previously all A's). Mood anxious, affect congruent with content of conversation. Good eye contact. Related warmly with his mom and conversed easily with interviewer. Speech normal rate/rhythm. Friendly and looking forward to summer building projects with his dad.

Diagnostic Impression

Generalized anxiety disorder

Plan

Cognitive-Behavioral Therapy: Reviewed the evidence (AAP handout) for CBT as the first-line treatment approach for children with significant anxiety. Mother and Zachary reviewed the seven-session Creating Opportunities for Personal Empowerment (COPE; Melnyk, 2003). CBT manual used in this practice for children with anxiety and depression. Both the mother and Zachary had good questions, and both agreed this will be a workable plan for their family. They want to do the seven weekly sessions this summer, to prepare Zachary for next school year.

Clinical Pearls

- If possible, the clinician should sit eye level with an individual as they listen.
- For a thorough clinical assessment, review the patient's history; level of functioning, including risk assessment; and review of systems. Be sure to allow time for the person to say what they want to say and to tell their story.
- The act of gathering information—the assessment of the patient—is the initial stage of developing a therapeutic relationship. Patients who feel their clinician is genuinely interested in them are more likely to follow agreed-upon treatment plans and health maintaining behaviors.
- Be observant for signs and symptoms that suggest a lack of vitality in individuals. Lack of energy and/or interest in activities that used to bring enjoyment are key signs of depression.
- Ask directly about past suicidal thoughts, self-harm, and SAs, as well as current SI. Clinicians should remind the patient that this is asked of every person seen. This is not going to give a patient the idea to kill themselves; this will give the patient the opportunity to discuss these thoughts.
- Optimizing one's physical health with regular exercise, healthy eating, and adequate sleep contributes to optimal mental health.

Key Takeaways

- Evidence-based screening tools can be used efficiently and effectively to assess for depression, anxiety, and suicidality in children and adults.
- When clinicians encounter individuals who are struggling with anxiety and/or depression, they should also consider that the patient may have other comorbidities, including physical and mental health disorders.
- Normalize discussion of mental health concerns as part of the assessment of health and well-being. Mental health assessment should be included as part of every health encounter.

REFERENCES

American Psychiatric Association. (2013). *Diagnostic and statistical manual of mental disorders* (5th ed.). Arlington, VA: American Psychiatric Publishing.

Beck, J. S. (2011). *Cognitive behavior therapy; Basics and beyond* (2nd ed.). New York, NY: Guilford Press.

Birmaher, B., Brent, D. A., Chiappetta, L., Bridge, J., Monga, S., & Baugher, M. (1999). Psychometric properties of the Screen for Child Anxiety Related Emotional Disorders (SCARED): A replication study. *Journal of the American Academy of Child and Adolescent Psychiatry, 38*(10), 1230–1236. doi:10.1097/00004583-199910000-00011

Carlat, D. J. (2017). *The psychiatric interview* (4th ed.). Baltimore, MD. Wolters Kluwer.

Curry, S. J., Krist, A. H., Owens, D. K., Barry, M. J., Caughey, A. B., Davidson, K. W., . . . Wong, J. B. (2018). Screening for intimate partner violence, elder abuse, and abuse of vulnerable adults: U.S. Preventive Services Task Force final recommendation statement. *Journal of the American Medical Association, 320*(16), 1678–1687. doi:10.1001/jama.2018.14741

Kroenke, K., Spitzer, R. L., & Williams, J. B. (2003). The Patient Health Questionnaire-2: Validity of a two-item depression screener. *Medical Care, 41*, 1284–1292. doi:10.1097/01.MLR.0000093487.78664.3C

LeFevre, M. L., Siu, A. L., Bibbins-Domingo, K., Baumann, L. C., Curry, S. J., Davidson, K. W., . . . Pignone, M. P. (2014). Screening for suicide risk in adolescents, adults, and older adults in primary care: U.S. Preventive Services Task Force recommendation statement. *Annals of Internal Medicine, 160*(10), 719–726. doi:10.7326/M14-0589

Lusk, P., & Kahn-John, M. (2019). Integrative nursing management of anxiety. In M. Kreitzer & M. Koithan (Eds.), *Integrative nursing* (2nd ed., pp. 221–239). New York, NY: Oxford Press.

Lusk, P., & Melnyk, B. M. (2013). Section 18: Brief evidence-based interventions for child and adolescent mental health disorders. In B. M. Melnyk & P. Jensen (Eds.), *Practical guide to child & adolescent mental health screening, early intervention, and health promotion* (2nd ed.). Cherry Hill, NJ: National Association of Pediatric Nurse Practitioners.

Melnyk, B. M. (2003). *COPE (Creating Opportunities for Personal Empowerment) for teens: A 7-session cognitive behavioral skills building program teen manual* (Teen Manual). Columbus, Ohio: COPE2Thrive.

Melnyk, B. M., & Jensen, P. (Eds.). (2013). *Practical guide to child & adolescent mental health screening, early intervention, and health promotion* (2nd ed.). Cherry Hill, NJ: National Association of Pediatric Nurse Practitioners.

Melnyk, B. M., Kelly, S., & Lusk, P. (2014). Outcomes and feasibility of a manualized cognitive-behavioral skills building intervention: Group COPE in school settings for depressed and anxious adolescents. *Journal of Child and Adolescent Psychiatric Nursing, 27*(1), 3–13. doi:10.1111/jcap.12058

National Action Alliance for Suicide Prevention: Transforming Health Systems Initiative Work Group. (2018). *Recommended standard care for people with suicide risk: Making health care suicide safe*. Washington, DC: Education Development Center. Retrieved from https://theactionalliance.org/sites/default/files/action_alliance_recommended_standard_care_final.pdf

National Institute of Mental Health Suicide Risk Screening Toolkit. (n.d.). Ask Suicide-Screening Questions (ASQ) toolkit. Retrieved from https://www.nimh.nih.gov/labs-at-nimh/asq-toolkit-materials/index.shtml

Olfson, M., Wall, M., Wang, S., Crystal, S., Liu, S. M., Gerhard, T., & Blanco, C. (2016). Short-term suicide risk after psychiatric hospital discharge. *JAMA Psychiatry, 73*(11), 1119–1126. doi:10.1001/jamapsychiatry.2016.2035

Richards, J., Whiteside, U., Ludman, E., Pabniak, C., Kirlin, B., Hidalgo, R., & Simon, G. (2019). Understanding why patients may not report suicidal ideation at a health care visit prior to a suicide attempt: A qualitative study. *Psychiatric Services, 70*(1), 40–45. doi:10.1176/appi.ps.201800342

Richardson, L. P., Rockhill, C., Russo, J. E., Grossman, D. C., Richards, J., McCarty, C., . . . Katon, W. (2010). Evaluation of the PHQ-2 as a brief screen for detecting major depression among adolescents. *Pediatrics, 125*, e1097–e1103. doi:10.1542/peds.2009-2712

Sadock, B. J., Sadock, V. A., & Ruiz, P. (2015). *Kaplan & Sadock's synopsis of psychiatry* (11th ed.). New York, NY: Wolters Kluwer.

Schumann, C. M., Bauman, M. D., & Amaral, D. G. (2011). Abnormal structure or function of the amygdala is a common component of neurodevelopmental disorders. *Neuropsychologia, 49*(4), 745–759. doi:10.1016/j.neuropsychologia.2010.09.028

Substance Abuse and Mental Health Services Administration. (2011). *Treatment of depression in older adults evidence-based practices kit*. Rockville, MD: Author. Retrieved from https://store.samhsa.gov/product/Treatment-of-Depression-in-Older-Adults-Evidence-Based-Practices-EBP-KIT/SMA11-4631CD-DVD

Siu, A. L., Bibbins-Domingo, K., Grossman, D. C., Baumann, L. C., Davidson, K. W., Ebell, M., . . . Pignone, M. P. (2016). Screening for depression in adults: U.S. Preventive Services Task Force recommendation statement. *Journal of the American Medical Association, 315*(4), 380–387. doi:10.1001/jama.2015.18392

Tusaie, K., & Fitzpatrick, J. (Eds.). (2017). *Advanced practice psychiatric nursing: Integrating psychotherapy, psychopharmacology, and complementary and alternative approaches across the life span* (2nd ed.). New York, NY: Springer Publishing Company.

United States Preventive Services Task Force. (2016). Final update summary: Depression in children and adolescents: Screening. Retrieved from https://www.uspreventiveservicestaskforce.org/Page/Document/UpdateSummaryFinal/depression-in-children-and-adolescents-screening1

23

Evidence-Based Assessment of Substance Use Disorder

Alice M. Teall and Kate Gawlik

"Empathy has no script. There is no right way or wrong way to do it. It's simply listening, holding space, withholding judgment, emotionally connecting, and communicating that incredibly healing message of 'You're not alone.'"

—Brené Brown

 VIDEO

- Patient History: Smoking and Smoking Cessation

LEARNING OBJECTIVES

- Evaluate the signs, symptoms, and risk factors associated with substance use disorder.
- Review the anatomic and physiological effects of substance use, including the areas of the brain and nervous system involved in substance use disorder and addiction.
- Recognize comorbidities of substance use disorder, including psychiatric and medical comorbidities.

OVERVIEW: DEFINING THE PROBLEM OF SUBSTANCE USE DISORDER

Substance misuse and **substance use disorders (SUDs)** are serious problems for adolescents and

Visit https://connect.springerpub.com/content/book/978-0-8261 -6454-4/chapter/ch00 to access the videos.

adults in the United States, affecting millions of Americans and imposing enormous costs.

The U.S. Surgeon General has identified the misuse of substances as one of the most pressing health crises of our time (U.S. Department of Health and Human Services [USDHHS], 2016). Staggering costs to individuals, families, and communities occur as a result of compromised physical and mental health; loss of productivity; reduced quality of life; and increased crime, violence, abuse, neglect, motor vehicle accidents, and healthcare costs. The most devastating consequences are experienced by tens of thousands each year who experience the death of a family member, friend, or colleague because of substance misuse (USDHHS, 2016).

Broadly defined, substances are psychoactive compounds with the potential to cause biological, psychological, and social disorders, including **addiction** (USDHHS, 2016). Substances with the potential to cause harm include alcohol, illicit drugs, and over-the-counter (OTC) substances, including tobacco. **Table 23.1** lists examples of substances included in each of these categories.

Although different in many aspects, these substances have three commonalities: (a) numerous individuals use and misuse them, (b) the substances can cause harm to the individual using them or others associated, and (c) prolonged and repeated misuse can change brain chemistry and function and lead to SUD.

TABLE 23.1 Types and Examples of Substances

Category	Examples
Alcohol	Beer, wine, distilled beverages (e.g., whiskey, gin, vodka, tequila)
Illicit drugs	Cocaine, crack cocaine, ecstasy, hallucinogens, heroin, ketamine, marijuana (as federally defined), methamphetamines (including crystal meth), synthetic drugs (e.g., K2, spice, bath salts); prescription medications used for nonmedical purposes: • Pain relievers, including opioids, fentanyl, codeine, oxycodone, hydrocodone, and tramadol • Tranquilizers, including benzodiazepines and muscle relaxants • Stimulants, including amphetamine, dextroamphetamine, phentermine, and methylphenidate • Sedatives, including any barbiturates
OTC drugs	Tobacco products, including cigarettes, smokeless tobacco, e-cigarettes, cigars, and pipe tobacco; cough and cold medicines; inhalants, including amyl nitrite, cleaning fluids, anesthetics, solvents, spray paint, and nitrous oxide

OTC, over-the-counter.

The prevalence of substance misuse is significant. For example, binge drinking at least once during the past month was self-reported by over 66 million individuals (Substance Abuse and Mental Health Services Administration [SAMHSA], 2019a). For a definition of binge drinking, and other terms related to substance misuse and SUD, including addiction and alcoholism, see **Box 23.1**.

BOX 23.1
DEFINITIONS OF TERMS RELATED TO SUBSTANCE MISUSE AND SUBSTANCE USE DISORDER

Substance Use: The use, even once, of any psychoactive compound or substance

Substance Misuse: The use of any substance in a manner, situation, amount, or frequency that can cause harm to users or to those around them

Substance Use Disorder (SUD): A medical illness caused by repeated misuse of a substance or substances. SUD is characterized by clinically significant impairments in health, social function, and impaired control over substance use and is diagnosed through assessing cognitive, behavioral, and psychological symptoms. SUDs range from mild to severe and from temporary to chronic. SUD typically develops gradually over time, leading to changes in brain chemistry and function. Multiple factors influence whether and how rapidly a person develops an SUD. These factors include the substance itself and the genetic vulnerability of the user.

○ **Tobacco Use Disorder** is the most common SUD, characterized by nicotine dependence and withdrawal symptoms with tobacco cessation attempts.

○ **Opioid Use Disorder** is characterized by the persistent use of opioids despite the adverse consequences of its use.

○ **Alcohol Use Disorder** can be mild, moderate, or severe repeated misuse of the consumption of alcohol. Alcoholism is the disease of addiction to alcohol, characterized by heavy drinking, dependence, tolerance, and use despite consequences.

Standard Drink: Based on the 2015–2020 Dietary Guidelines for Americans, a standard drink contains 14 g (0.6 ounce) of pure alcohol, which equates to one 12 ounce can of beer, one 5 ounce glass of wine, or one shot of 1.5 ounces of a distilled beverage.

Moderate Drinking: Up to 1 standard drink/day for women, and 2 drinks/day for men

Low-Risk Drinking: For women, low-risk drinking is defined as no more than 3 drinks on any single day and no more than 7 drinks/week. For men, it is defined as no more than 4 drinks on any single day and no more than 14 drinks/week.

Binge Drinking: Consuming an excessive amount of alcohol on a single occasion, or in about 2 hours. For men, this is defined as drinking 5 or more standard drinks, and for women, 4 or more standard drinks.

Heavy Drinking: Binge drinking on 5 days or more in the past month

Addiction: The most severe form of SUD, addiction, is a chronic brain disease characterized by compulsive or uncontrolled use of one or more substances. This disorder has the potential for **relapse** (recurrence after a significant time of abstinence), resistance to treatment, and recovery.

Recovery: A process of change through which individuals improve their health and wellness, live a self-directed life, and strive to reach their full potential. Being "in recovery" indicates that positive changes and values have become part of a voluntarily adopted lifestyle.

By definition, binge-drinking episodes have the potential for producing harm, and yet this type of substance misuse is often overlooked as socially appropriate, or misunderstood as developmentally acceptable, despite increasing an individual's risk of developing addiction.

The misuse of alcohol, tobacco, and illicit drugs, including prescription medications, affects the health and well-being of millions of Americans. SAMHSA (2019a) outlines the following health effects:

- Excessive alcohol consumption increases the risk of developing serious health problems, including type 2 diabetes, pancreatitis, cancers, cardiomyopathy, dementia, hepatitis, and cirrhosis, in addition to the short-term intoxication, disinhibition, stupor, and potential for coma and death.
- Tobacco use causes damage to nearly every organ in the body, often leading to lung cancer, heart disease, stroke, emphysema, and chronic bronchitis. Exposure to secondhand smoke also causes adverse health effects. Tobacco use is the single greatest cause of preventable death globally. **Figure 23.1** is a photo taken at the entryway of an office building in 2009; today, tobacco-free policies usually prohibit employees from smoking on work property.
- Marijuana has not only immediate effects like distorted perception, difficulty problem-solving, and

loss of motor coordination, but also effects with long-term use, including respiratory infections, impaired memory, and exposure to cancer-causing compounds.
- Opioids not only reduce the perception of pain, but also produce drowsiness, mental confusion, euphoria, nausea, constipation, and respiratory depression. Most overdose deaths from substance use are attributable to opioids.

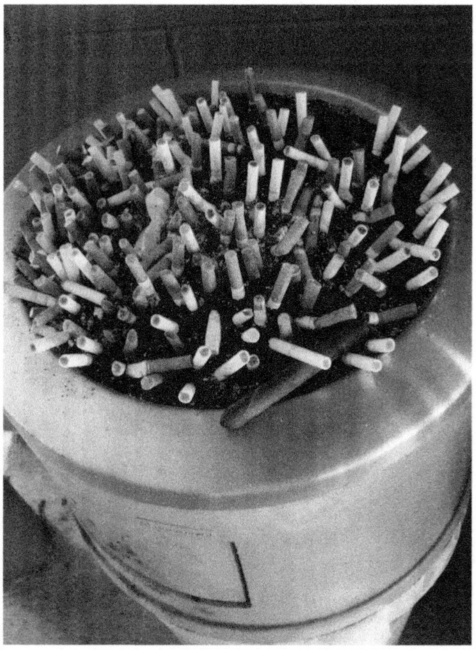

Although each substance can cause unique harm, the neurobiological changes that occur in the brain and nervous system with substance misuse can have damaging consequences. These changes are reviewed in the next section of this chapter. Like other chronic diseases, SUDs are influenced by genetic, biological, neurological, developmental, behavioral, social, and environmental factors. Often, substance use begins for one reason, and continues for another; the continuation of substance misuse despite consequences is correlated with changes in neurobiology.

ANATOMY AND PHYSIOLOGY OF THE BRAIN AND NERVOUS SYSTEM INVOLVED IN SUBSTANCE USE DISORDER

NEURONS, NEUROTRANSMITTERS, AND NERVOUS SYSTEM INVOLVEMENT

The brain is composed of billions of neurons, along with other cell types that help to support the function of the nervous system as reviewed in Chapter 14, Evidence-Based Assessment of the Nervous System. The function and processes of the brain to produce thought, emotion, movement, and sensation are a result of the transmission of information within and between neurons. To achieve this, neurons function unlike other cells. **Figure 23.2** identifies the

FIGURE 23.1 Ashtray in entryway of office building.

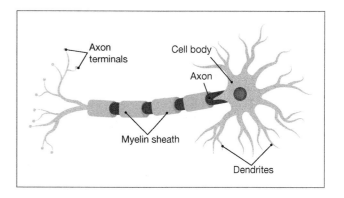

FIGURE 23.2 Neuronal structure.

components of a neuron. Each neuron consists of a cell body, dendrites, and an axon. Neurons use electrical signals to transmit information from the dendrite to the cell body and then down the axon to its terminals. The nerve terminal of an axon is in close proximity to the dendrites of another neuron; the space between neurons is the synapse, or synaptic gap. When an impulse travels down the axon to the terminals, it triggers release of chemical messengers, or **neurotransmitters**. The neurotransmitters diffuse across the synaptic gap and bind to receptors on the dendrites of postsynaptic cells. The binding of a neurotransmitter to its receptor is specific. Just as a key fits only a specific lock, a neurotransmitter binds only to a specified type of receptor.

Each neuron produces one or more dozens of neurotransmitters, including amino acids, acetylcholine, glutamine, glycine, dopamine, serotonin, and norepinephrine. Neurotransmitters and receptors can be excitatory, which causes a neuron to create another impulse, or inhibitory, causing an impulse to slow or stop. The effect of a neurotransmitter is dependent on location and distribution within the brain and nervous system; for example, dopamine is highly concentrated in the regions of the brain that regulate motivation and reward. The cycle within the nervous system of neurotransmitter release, receptor use, followed by breakdown and/or reuptake, maintains the amount of neurotransmitter in the synapse within certain limits. In most cases, the misuse of substances causes neurotransmission to increase or decrease dramatically beyond these limits (National Institute on Drug Abuse [NIDA], 2017).

All psychoactive substances act on the brain in some capacity. Some substances, such as opioids and cannabinoids, have specific receptors in the brain and act as nonconventional neurotransmitters. Other substances, such as cocaine and amphetamines, interact directly with receptors and transporters to produce a greater impact on neurons than occurs naturally. Because a neurotransmitter can excite or inhibit neurons that produce different neurotransmitters, substances that disrupt one neurotransmitter can have secondary impacts on others. For example, nicotine stimulates cells directly by activating receptors for acetylcholine and indirectly by inducing higher levels of glutamate, which accelerates neuron activity throughout the brain (NIDA, 2017). A key effect that all substances commonly cause is a dramatic increase in dopamine, which directly causes euphoria and indirectly creates desire to repeat the experience.

Long-term, permanent alterations in the brain can begin as adjustments to compensate for changes in neurotransmitter activity. For example, the brain responds to repeated, massive dopamine surges in part by reducing the number of dopamine receptors (NIDA, 2017). This alleviates the overstimulation of the dopamine system, but also contributes to dependence, as the reduction in dopamine receptors can cause an individual to have difficulty in experiencing feelings of normal enjoyment during withdrawal from the substance and during long-term recovery. The extent of recovery possible from the damage and disruption to neurons and neurotransmitters is related to the toxicity of substances and the cumulative effect of repeated exposures and is not well understood (NIDA, 2017). Researchers have identified that some changes in neurotransmission related to substance misuse, such as proliferation of new dendrites, can be epigenetic in nature (Anderson et al., 2018; NIDA, 2017).

Although the brain and nervous system are able to respond normally as substance levels decline during early or initial use, repeated use, misuse, and/or heavy use lead to long-lasting, permanent changes in neurobiology. These neuroadaptations compromise brain and nervous system function and lead to the development of SUD. Neuroadaptations may persist after an individual stops using a substance and can produce tolerance, withdrawal symptoms, and desire to use despite consequences and motivation to change (NIDA, 2017; USDHHS, 2016).

REGIONS OF THE BRAIN DISRUPTED WITH SUBSTANCE USE DISORDER

Three regions of the brain are involved in the neuroadaptations underlying the development and persistence of SUDs (NIDA, 2018; USDHHS, 2016). These three regions, the basal ganglia, extended amygdala, and prefrontal cortex, are shown in **Figure 23.3**.

The function of the basal ganglia structures located deep within the brain allows an individual to experience the pleasurable effects of behaviors. This region has an important role in generating motivation and reward to support the development of habits and routines. While the activation of dopamine and endogenous opioid receptors in response to sex, food, and human connection is vital to life, the basal ganglia are also activated during the bingeing of substances and intoxication. With continued use, substances overactivate this reward circuit, causing dysfunction in the brain's dopamine reward system and diminishing sensitivity to all pleasurable activities (NIDA, 2017, 2018; USDHHS, 2016).

The extended amygdala located beneath the basal ganglia regulates an individual's reaction to stress and negative emotions through interaction with the hypothalamus. Exposure to substances causes this region to become increasingly sensitive; heightened perception

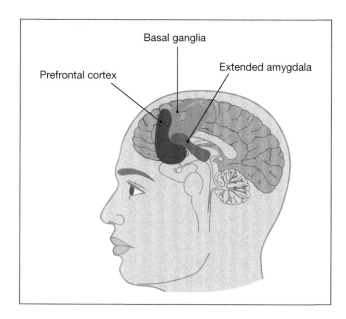

FIGURE 23.3 Primary regions of the brain altered with substance misuse.

of anxiety, irritability, and unease occur during withdrawal from substances, and creates motivation to use again for relief of increased discomfort. The negative feelings associated with substance withdrawal are thought to result from the diminished activity in the reward circuitry of the basal ganglia and activation of the brain's stress systems in the extended amygdala (NIDA, 2017, 2018; USDHHS, 2016).

The prefrontal cortex is responsible for complex cognitive processes, which include the ability to think, plan, organize, prioritize, problem-solve, express emotions, moderate social behavior, and exert control over impulses. This area of the brain is not fully mature until young adulthood. The developmental phase, complexity, and neuroplasticity of the prefrontal cortex are factors that result in increased vulnerability of adolescents to SUD. Neuroplasticity is the ability of the brain to form new connections, pathways, and circuitry; substance misuse takes advantage of neuroplasticity to "rewire" or delay maturity of the prefrontal cortex, using glutamate, an excitatory neurotransmitter, to trigger risk-taking and inhibit control. The shifting balance in neurotransmitters and changes in function of the prefrontal cortex, extended amygdala, and basal ganglia lead to alterations in brain chemistry, structure, and function that underlie compulsive substance use with reduced impulse control (NIDA, 2017, 2018; USDHHS, 2016).

Substance misuse or chronic use causes neurobiological changes in the basal ganglia, extended amygdala, and prefrontal cortex, which can help to explain the psychosocial manifestations of the disease of SUD, including the unmanageable use without regard to consequences. The cycle of addiction also maps to three areas: binge and intoxication to the basal ganglia; withdrawal and negative affect to the extended amygdala; and preoccupation and anticipation to the prefrontal cortex (USDHHS, 2016). The risk of these neurobiological changes occurring is heightened during adolescence, when the brain and nervous system are undergoing rapid change and growth.

LIFE-SPAN CONSIDERATIONS

The American Academy of Pediatrics (AAP) defines addiction as a developmental disorder and recommends screening for SUD as a routine part of adolescent care (AAP, 2015). The rationale for this position is based on the understanding of neurobiology and the neuroadaptations that result from substance use, which can be more dramatic and happen more quickly during adolescence. The AAP position statement (2015) notes:

- The adolescent brain is particularly vulnerable to the toxic effects of substances.
- The neuroplasticity of the adolescent brain increases their risk of SUD.
- Neuroadaptations can occur rapidly in the adolescent brain, leading to long-lasting changes in brain structure and function. Early identification is key. Most adults who develop SUD began use in adolescence.
- Trauma, social isolation, genetic factors, and comorbid physical and mental health disorders increase the likelihood of changes within the brain and nervous system that lead to SUD.
- Pediatric care clinicians underestimate the prevalence of adolescent SUD.

The prevalence rates of SUD are also underestimated for older adults. Historically, older adults have not presented in large numbers to substance abuse treatment programs, which perpetuate a misconception that older adults do not misuse substances (Kuerbis, Sacco, Blazer, & Moore, 2014). The aging of the baby boomer generation has created an urgency to effectively identify substance misuse among older adults because aging presents risks for harm when considering even minimal amounts of psychoactive substances. For example, as a person ages, the percentages of lean body mass and total body water decrease, and the ability of the liver to process alcohol is diminished; blood–brain barrier permeability and neuronal receptor sensitivity to alcohol in the brain increase (Kuerbis et al., 2014).

The same biological changes that increase the effect of alcohol among older adults also increase the effect of medications and illicit drugs, causing an increased vulnerability to their effects and interactions. The diagnosis and treatment of comorbid sleep disorders, cognitive impairment, and chronic illnesses are complicated by concurrent use of alcohol, tobacco, and prescription medications.

KEY HISTORY QUESTIONS AND CONSIDERATIONS FOR SUBSTANCE USE DISORDER

APPROACH TO ASSESSMENT OF SUBSTANCE USE: SCREENING, BRIEF INTERVENTION, AND REFERRAL TO TREATMENT

Clinicians have the responsibility for assessing and engaging with individuals who are experiencing mild, moderate, or severe SUD. Their interactions can be complicated by an individual's inability to control or reduce substance use, and continued use despite consequences, which are characteristics consistent with the diagnostic criteria for SUD (American Psychiatric Association [APA], 2014). The criteria to be considered for diagnosing substance use disorder, listed in **Box 23.2**, do not require the clinician to differentiate whether or not an individual is dependent on substances, but do include signs and symptoms that indicate a problematic pattern of use that leads to significant impairment or distress.

Using evidence-based approaches to screening for SUD, and motivational interviewing skills that create engagement and support motivation to change with an unbiased approach, allows clinicians to engage patients and identify motivations, discrepancies, and commitment for sustained behavior change related to the use of substances.

Effective, therapeutic communication is key to establishing patient-centered, evidence-based care. An essential element of therapeutic communication is empathy, the ability to recognize and share the emotions and perceptions of another. Studies suggest that healthcare clinicians have higher levels of empathy when SUD is recognized as a complex disease characterized by use despite consequences, rather than a result of moral failing or personal weakness (van Boekel, Brouwers, van Weeghel, & Garretsen, 2014). Clinicians are also better able to establish therapeutic rapport when they understand that treatment for SUD can be effective, even if an individual has low motivation, denial, or resistance, which are all commonly associated with tobacco, alcohol, or illicit substance misuse (SAMHSA, 2019b).

BOX 23.2
DIAGNOSTIC CRITERIA: SUBSTANCE USE DISORDER

Signs and Symptoms Consistent With Substance Use Disorder:

1. Substance used in larger amounts or over longer periods than intended
2. Unsuccessful efforts to cut down or control substance use, despite the desire to do so
3. Considerable time spent in activities necessary to obtain and use substance or to recover from the effects of substance use
4. Craving or a strong desire to use the substance leading to onset of repeated substance use
5. Tolerance resulting in need for increased amounts of the substance to attain the desired effect, or diminished effect with continued use of the same amount of the substance
6. Withdrawal symptoms experienced, or the substance used to relieve or avoid withdrawal symptoms
7. Recurrent substance use resulting in failure to fulfill major role obligations at work, school, or home
8. Continued substance use despite having persistent or recurrent social or interpersonal problems
9. Social, occupational, or recreational activities discontinued or reduced as a result of substance use
10. Recurrent substance use in hazardous situations or environments
11. Continued substance use despite knowledge of having a persistent or recurrent physical or psychological problem that is likely to have been caused or exacerbated by the substance

Mild SUD is defined by two or three signs/symptoms of 11 listed.
Moderate SUD is defined by four to five signs/symptoms. Severe SUD manifests as six or more.
Source: Adapted from American Psychiatric Association. (2014). *Diagnostic and statistical manual of mental disorders* (5th ed.). Arlington, VA: American Psychiatric Publishing. Retrieved from https://dsm.psychiatryonline.org/doi/book/10.1176/appi.books.9780890425596

Unfortunately, less than 10% of individuals with SUD seek treatment (SAMHSA, 2019a). Barriers to treatment include denial, shame, and self-stigma; individuals fear negative reactions from clinicians; often have difficulty with accepting a diagnosis of SUD, addiction, or alcoholism; and internalize real or perceived clinician bias (Corrigan et al., 2017; van Boekel et al., 2014). The most important first step for any clinician before assessing an individual for SUD is to recognize whether their own views, emotions, or expectations might limit their ability to effectively communicate with the patient. Clinicians who recognize that toxic stress, adverse childhood events, lack of social support, comorbidities, and intergenerational distress can add to an individual's vulnerability for SUD are better able to implement screening, intervention, and referral (Corrigan et al., 2017).

Identifying adults or adolescents who may have SUD and intervening early have been proposed as population-wide health priorities that can be implemented using the clinical model of **SBIRT**, or (S) Screening, (BI) Brief Intervention, and (RT) Referral to Treatment (Harris, Louis-Jacques, & Knight, 2014; Ozechowski, Becker, & Hogue, 2016; Reho, Agley, DeSalle, & Gassman, 2016; SAMHSA, 2019a; U.S. Preventive Services Task Force [USPSTF], 2018; Young et al., 2014). Screening, or assessing the patient using a standardized screening tool, guides patient–clinician interaction. Based on the results of the screening, clinicians engage the patient through brief intervention or meaningful conversation about their substance use. When the screening and brief intervention indicate the need for additional services, referral to treatment is immediately offered. The strength of the SBIRT model is the ease of use and the priority of intervention when needed.

Screening as a Component of the SBIRT Model

The SBIRT model does not require clinicians to use one specific tool to screen for SUD and allows for clinician discretion to choose a tool based on ease of use and appropriateness for patient population. A single-question screen that has been validated in primary care settings to identify illicit substance use is, "How many times in the past year have you used an illegal drug or used a prescription medication for nonmedical reasons?" If clarification of "nonmedical reasons" is needed, the clinician can provide the explanation, "For instance, because of the experience or feeling it caused" (NIDA, 2012; Shapiro, Coffa, & McCance-Katz, 2013). Similarly, screening for alcohol misuse in primary care can begin with the question, "How many times in the past year have you had X or more drinks in a day?" where X is five for men and four for women, and a response of one or more is considered a positive screen (Smith, Schmidt, Allensworth-Davies, & Saitz, 2009, 2010). While a review of the evidence suggests that single-screening questions can be effective, screening for substance misuse includes screening for tobacco, alcohol, *and*

illicit drug use; screening negatively for the misuse of one substance does not negate the need to screen for misuse of other substances (Smith, Cheng, Allensworth-Davies, Winter, & Saitz, 2014). Responses to these single questions serve as the foundation or basis for further dialogue and assessment.

Specifically for adolescents, the AAP recommends screening for tobacco, drugs, and alcohol use with the CRAFFT (**C**ar, **R**elax, **A**lone, **F**orget, **F**riends, **T**rouble) tool. As discussed in Chapter 4, Evidence-Based Assessment of Children and Adolescents, this screening tool takes less than 2 minutes to administer and can help clinicians identify adolescents who may be experiencing the consequence of SUD (USPSTF, 2014).

For adults, including pregnant women, with significant risk factors, signs, symptoms, or concerns related to risky or hazardous drinking or substance use, the screening tools that follow support assessment, brief intervention, and follow-up with referrals to reduce misuse and identify SUDs (Dhalla & Kopec, 2007; Harris et al., 2014; NIDA, 2012; Ozechowski et al., 2016; SAMHSA, 2019a; USPSTF, 2018):

- CAGE: **C**ut down, **A**nnoyed, **G**uilty, **E**ye Opener questionnaire is an internationally used screening to identify alcohol use disorder.
- CAGE-AID: **C**ut down, **A**nnoyed, **G**uilty, **E**ye Opener tool **A**dapted to **I**nclude **D**rug Use expands the CAGE screening to include other substances.
- ASSIST: **A**lcohol, **S**moking, and **S**ubstance **I**nvolvement **S**creening **T**est developed by the World Health Organization. Items are reliable, feasible, and screen for use of tobacco products, alcoholic beverages, cannabis, cocaine, stimulants, inhalants, sedatives, hallucinogens, opioids, and other substances. ASSIST version 3.0 is free and available online in nine languages: https://www.who.int/substance_abuse/activities/assist_test/en.
- AUDIT-C: **A**lcohol **U**se **D**isorders **I**dentification **T**est-Consumption is a three-item screening tool used to identify hazardous or harmful use of alcohol. This tool is also available in the public domain at https://www.integration.samhsa.gov/images/res/tool_auditc.pdf.

Next Steps of the SBIRT Model: Brief Intervention and Referral to Treatment

For the adult or adolescent who screens positively for misuse of alcohol, use of illegal drugs, or use of prescribed medications for nonmedical reasons, the next steps of the SBIRT model of care are brief intervention and referral to treatment (Ozechowski et al., 2016; Reho et al., 2016; SAMHSA, 2019a; USPSTF, 2018; Young et al., 2014).

Brief intervention is a nonconfrontational, patient-centered approach to address unhealthy, hazardous, or ongoing substance use or misuse, using therapeutic communication techniques that include empathy, reflective listening, and statements of support for self-efficacy. Brief interventions are discussions that are intended to raise awareness and motivation to change. Examples of clinician statements that are more effective as components of a brief intervention are included in **Table 23.2**. Authentic feedback offered with respect and empathy by the clinician supports and encourages an individual's self-determination and motivation to change.

Referral to treatment is provided to support cessation of substance use; support and treatment can be provided through referral to specialty care and may include detoxification services, inpatient rehabilitation, outpatient counseling, and recovery support groups. Therapeutic services and interventions can include cognitive-behavioral therapy, complementary therapies, and pharmacological management, with support

---

BOX 23.3
THE 5 A'S: STEPS TO INTERVENTION IN TOBACCO USE DISORDER

1. **Ask:** Identify and document tobacco use status for every patient at every visit.
2. **Advise:** Support the self-efficacy of every person who uses tobacco to quit.
3. **Assess:** Determine each individual's willingness and readiness to quit.
4. **Assist:** Individuals willing to make a quit attempt should be offered options, including counseling and pharmacotherapy, as appropriate.
5. **Arrange:** Schedule follow-up, in person or by phone, within the first week of a quit date.

---

for ongoing recovery. Inherent in this approach is the recognition that an individual can make the choice to change, that the clinician can be a partner in the process, and that individuals have options, no matter what treatment level is needed.

The SBIRT model is aligned with the *5 A's*, which are steps of successful intervention to treat tobacco use disorder (Addo, Maiden, & Ehrenthal, 2011; Kruger, O'Halloran, Rosenthal, Babb, & Fiore, 2016; Patnode et al., 2015). **Box 23.3** lists these steps, which incorporate screening, brief intervention, and referral to treatment for individuals who may have tobacco use disorder.

HISTORY OF PRESENT ILLNESS
Common Presenting Symptoms

For any individual who presents with symptoms or signs suggestive of substance misuse, assessing components of their history as if they were presenting with symptoms of any other chronic illness is appropriate. These include a review of presenting symptoms, past medical history, family and social history, review of systems, and history of primary care preventive practices. Two examples of the history of present illness (HPI) assessments (discussed later in this chapter) can be implemented after the SBIRT framework is initiated, or the SBIRT model may be implemented as a result of the HPI assessment findings.

Example: Individual Who Currently Smokes Cigarettes

For each sign or symptom, targeted HPI questions are required to determine needed physical examination and differential diagnoses. One example is the individual who presents as a current cigarette smoker; OLDCART questions include:

TABLE 23.2 Less Effective and More Effective Clinician Statements Offering Motivational Support

Less Effective	More Effective
"You need to stop smoking because you are damaging your lungs."	"I am wondering: How does it feel to hear that smoking may be damaging your lungs?"
"Now that you are pregnant, you need to think about your baby first, before you drink alcohol."	"Tell me your thoughts and feelings about your alcohol use, now that you are pregnant."
"I am going to refer you to a special program for people who are alcoholics."	"I am interested in hearing what you think about the treatment options that we have discussed."
"You are putting yourself at risk every time that you smoke, and you need to stop."	"What do you think leads you to consider quitting? What do you think leads to your smoking?"
"So you relapsed and started using drugs again. . . . You just have to use your will power and quit."	"So you relapsed and started using again. . . . The fact that you quit for a period of time is a good thing. Are you ready to try again? Let's talk about this."

Source: Adapted from Shapiro, B., Coffa, D., & McCance-Katz, E. F. (2013). A primary care approach to substance misuse. *American Family Physician, 88*(2), 113–121. Retrieved from https://www.aafp.org/afp/2013/0715/p113.html

- Onset: Time of first cigarette in the morning, waking at night to smoke
- Location: Smoking at work, home, in the car, around children
- Duration: Age that smoking began, previous attempts to quit
- Character: Number of cigarettes smoked each day, most recent cigarette; also note if any additional types of nicotine or tobacco are used
- Associated symptoms: Cough, wheezing, or respiratory problems; chest pain; fatigue; and/or symptoms associated with smoking cessation attempts
- Relieving symptoms: Coping skills, pharmacological and/or nonpharmacological methods to quit, previous or current counseling
- Timing or temporal factors: Use related to stress or need to relax, concurrent use of substances, personal beliefs about need or desire to quit (i.e., readiness to change)

Example: Individual Who Is Misusing Alcohol

For the person who may present with a history of alcohol misuse, heavy use, or binge drinking, OLDCART questions can include:

- Onset: Time of first drink, amount of drinks/day
- Location: Drinking alone, socially, before or associated with driving a motor vehicle
- Duration: Occasions of heavy use and binge drinking, average use days/week
- Character: Typical amount of alcohol use, type of alcohol use, history of blackouts, most recent use
- Associated symptoms: Emotions and beliefs related to use, abstinence; consequences of alcohol use (i.e., unable to attend school or work; effect on relationships; legal issues; health issues, including type 2 diabetes, pancreatitis, cancers, heart disease, dementia, hepatitis, and cirrhosis); recent intoxication, disinhibition, or stupor
- Relieving symptoms: Coping skills, support system, pharmacological and/or nonpharmacological methods to quit, previous or current counseling or involvement in recovery groups, previous periods of sobriety, and what worked to achieve this
- Timing or temporal factors: Use related to stress or need to relax, concurrent use of substances, personal beliefs about need or desire to quit (i.e., readiness to change)

PAST MEDICAL HISTORY

- Depression, anxiety, or mental health disorder
- Chronic pain
- Recent or current acute pain
- Constitutional changes

- Physical disabilities or reduced mobility
- Poor health status
- Use of medications/polypharmacy
- Allergies to medications
- Past history of substance misuse
- Motor vehicle accidents
- Past surgical history
- Chronic physical illness/comorbidities
- Recent or past infectious disease
- Current or previous treatment for mental health or SUDs

FAMILY HISTORY

- Substance misuse
- SUDs or addiction
- Mental health disorders
- Trauma—physical or sexual abuse
- Other chronic diseases impacted by smoking, alcohol use, or substances

SOCIAL HISTORY

- Tobacco use/smoking history
- Alcohol intake (current, usual, past)
- Drug use (prescribed, nonprescribed)
- Previous or current SUD
- Stress and coping
- Sleep
- Nutrition
- Social support system/social isolation
- Romantic partner with SUD
- Transitions in care; living situations, homelessness
- Family relationships
- Environmental exposures
- Trauma, including adverse childhood events, bereavement, grief
- Engagement in high-risk sexual behaviors (e.g., multiple partners, unprotected sex)
- Financial problems, employment
- Legal problems, justice involvement, history of driving under the influence (DUI)

REVIEW OF SYSTEMS

- Psychiatric: Sadness, helplessness, hopelessness, worry, insomnia, hypersomnia, fatigue, headaches; changes in memory, concentration, or mood, memory loss, mood swings, mania, risk-taking, anxiety, worry, guilt, shame; suicidal or homicidal ideation, hallucinations, delusions
- Neurologic: Weakness, numbness, loss of consciousness, blackouts, headaches, falls, dizziness, idiopathic seizures, confusion
- Integumentary: Dryness, itching, bruising, rashes, lesions (sores), burns

- Head, Eyes, Ears, Nose, Throat (HEENT): Sensory deficits, congestion, sinus pain, sore throat
- Lymphatic: Bruising, bleeding, lymphadenopathy
- Cardiovascular/respiratory: Chest pain, dyspnea, shortness of breath (SOB), wheezing, cough
- Musculoskeletal: Injury history, pain, stiffness, or swelling
- Gastrointestinal (GI)/genitourinary (GU): Weight and/or appetite changes, constipation, diarrhea, abdominal pain, nausea, vomiting, incontinence, poor nutrition

PREVENTIVE CARE CONSIDERATIONS

- Healthy lifestyle behaviors, including exercise
- Nutrition, including access to fruits and vegetables
- Adequate sleep and rest
- Tobacco cessation
- Alcohol moderation or abstinence
- Family, social, and/or community support, including counseling, recovery groups

DIFFERENTIAL DIAGNOSES

Substance misuse, SUD (mild, moderate, severe)—more specifically alcohol use disorder, opioid use disorder, tobacco use disorder, nicotine dependence, alcoholism, and addiction

PHYSICAL EXAMINATION FOR SUBSTANCE USE DISORDER

Completion of a thorough history leads to the determination of which components of a physical examination are completed and how the findings are interpreted. The likelihood of comorbid mental health and substance disorders is significant and should be considered as the clinician completes the physical examination. Individuals may present with symptoms resulting from ingestion, withdrawal, and/or chronic use of substances, in addition to the symptoms of mental health disorders that are treated or untreated. Substance use can be associated with compromised function in any or every body system related to the substance used, how the substance was ingested, and/or the high-risk behaviors in which an individual engages. **Box 23.4** identifies physical signs that may indicate substance misuse, SUD, or addiction.

While the clinician completes an advanced assessment, that is, history and physical examination, how they communicate with the individual who may have an SUD is a priority. Clinicians should continue to employ the framework of SBIRT and avoid implicit bias when completing the physical examination of an individual using and/or misusing substances in order to avoid triggering shame, guilt, and resistance to treatment. The

---

BOX 23.4
PHYSICAL INDICATORS OF SUBSTANCE USE

Signs may indicate intoxication, withdrawal, or heavy use. Signs may be related to the type of substance used or method of use. Presence or absence of these signs are not the sole assessment of substance use.

- **General Survey:** Thin, altered vital signs; unsteady gait
- **Appearance:** Poor personal hygiene; smell of alcohol, tobacco, or drug use
- **Mental Status:**
  - Combative, aggressive, or bizarre behavior; may appear fatigued, sedated
  - Impaired cognition, confusion, disorientation
  - Slurred speech
- **Integumentary:** Jaundice, diaphoresis, lesions/rashes, burns, scars, abscesses, very dry skin
- **Head, Neck, and Lymphatics:** Bruising, bleeding, lymphadenopathy
- **Eyes:** Eye redness or drainage, pupil dilation or constriction
- **ENT:** Rhinorrhea, deviations or deformities in nasal septum, including perforation, atrophy of the nasal mucosa, epistaxis, pharyngitis
- **Respiratory:** Cough, wheezing, respiratory depression or tachypnea
- **Cardiovascular:** Hypertension, hypotension, tachycardia, edema
- **GI/GU/GYN:** Hepatomegaly, splenomegaly, abdominal distention, signs of sexually transmitted infection
- **Neurologic:** Weakness, numbness, loss of consciousness, jitteriness, seizure activity
- **Musculoskeletal:** Pain with movement; neck pain, stiffness, or swelling

---

use of therapeutic communication strategies, including motivational interviewing (MI), while interacting with the patient is foundational to evidence-based practice and effective patient outcomes.

LABORATORY CONSIDERATIONS FOR SUBSTANCE USE DISORDER

Toxicology tests of blood, urine, hair, saliva, breath, and sweat can provide objective evidence of substance use, but the results do not distinguish between occasional use, chronic use, and impairment (Moeller, Kissack,

Atayee, & Lee, 2017). For this reason, toxicology tests may be more useful for monitoring abstinence repeatedly over time than for one-time assessment.

The basic toxicology screens used in labs across the United States identify primarily five substances: amphetamine, cocaine, cannabis, some opioids, and phencyclidine. Other drugs that may be added to a toxicology screen include barbiturates, methamphetamine, and synthetic opioids. Many substances are not detected by routine drug screening tests, including alcohol (which can be detected by measuring ethyl glucuronide; synthetic cannabinoids; synthetic opioids, such as methadone and fentanyl; and plant-derived substances, such as hallucinogenic mushrooms (Moeller et al., 2017).

Urine drug screens are the most widely used type of toxicology test because they are easy to administer and less invasive than other tests. However, these tests can be misinterpreted and have associated false-positive results; inaccurate results can lead to significant consequences, as urine drug testing is frequently used in clinical, legal, employment, and educational settings. Interpreting the results of urine drug screens requires an understanding of the approximate drug detection time in the urine, acceptable cutoff values for screening versus confirmatory tests, and an ability to evaluate the urine sample for adulteration or dilution (Moeller et al., 2017). Because of the complex nature of result interpretation and test ordering, it is critical that the clinician develops a close working relationship with the laboratory and understands the limitations of any in-office, point-of-care testing (Moeller et al., 2017). Except in emergency situations, consent for conducting a urine drug screen should be obtained from patients because testing for substances without a person's consent may represent a violation of their civil rights. Requirements regarding notification and permission vary by state and jurisdiction.

Legalities and misinterpretation are issues that affect the decision-making about the use of breath analyzers, saliva point-of-care testing, and/or serum tests to evaluate sobriety, acute intoxication, and compliance with abstinence in treatment. Field tests suggest that new methods of saliva testing for alcohol intoxication may have advantages in portability, ease of use, cost, and time efficiency (Bates, Brick, & White, 2015). Clinicians should caution patients, including parents who are keen to "drug test" their adolescent children, that screening tests have limitations.

IMAGING CONSIDERATIONS FOR SUBSTANCE USE DISORDERS

Although much can be revealed about the neuroadaptations of the brain structure and function in response to substance use, brain imaging is not recommended for the assessment or diagnosis of SUD. Brain imaging with magnetic resonance imaging (MRI) and positron emission tomography (PET) scanning, however, have provided key evidence for researchers about the neurobiological effects of substances, including the causes and mechanisms of the brain vulnerability to addiction; the results of imaging studies have yielded important findings about recovery from SUD.

EVIDENCE-BASED PRACTICE CONSIDERATIONS FOR SUBSTANCE USE DISORDERS

The USPSTF (2015, 2016, 2018) has developed recommendations for the screening and prevention of alcohol use disorder and tobacco use; these guidelines support the SBIRT model reviewed earlier in this chapter for adults, pregnant women, and for school-aged children and adolescents in regard to tobacco smoking cessation. The USPSTF recommendations are listed in **Tables 23.3** and **23.4**.

Although the USPSTF has recommended CRAFFT screening be used to assess adolescents who may be

TABLE 23.3 USPSTF Recommendations for Screening and Behavioral Counseling Interventions Related to Unhealthy Alcohol Use

Age/Population	Recommendations
Adults aged 18 years or older, including pregnant women	The USPSTF recommends screening for unhealthy alcohol use in primary care settings and providing persons engaged in risky or hazardous drinking with brief behavioral counseling interventions to reduce unhealthy alcohol use (Grade B).
Adolescents aged 12–17 years	The USPSTF concludes that the current evidence is insufficient to assess the balance of benefits and harms of screening and brief behavioral counseling interventions for alcohol use in primary care settings in adolescents (Grade I).

USPSTF, U.S. Preventive Services Task Force.

Source: From U.S. Preventive Services Task Force. (2018). *Final recommendation statement: Unhealthy alcohol use in adolescents and adults: Screening and behavioral counseling interventions.* Retrieved from https://www.uspreventiveservicestaskforce.org/Page/Document/RecommendationStatementFinal/unhealthy-alcohol-use-in-adolescents-and-adults-screening-and-behavioral-counseling-interventions#consider

TABLE 23.4 USPSTF Recommendations for Tobacco Smoking Cessation	
Age/Population	Recommendations
Adults who are not pregnant	The USPSTF recommends that clinicians ask all adults about tobacco use, advise them to stop using tobacco, and provide behavioral interventions and FDA-approved pharmacotherapy for cessation (Grade A).
Pregnant women	The USPSTF recommends that clinicians ask all pregnant women about tobacco use, advise them to stop using tobacco, and provide behavioral interventions for cessation to pregnant women (Grade A).
School-aged children and adolescents	The USPSTF recommends that primary care clinicians provide interventions, including education or brief counseling, to prevent initiation of tobacco (Grade B).

FDA, U.S. Food and Drug Administration; USPSTF, U.S. Preventive Services Task Force.

Sources: From U.S. Preventive Services Task Force. (2015). *Tobacco smoking cessation in adults, including pregnant Women: Behavioral and pharmacotherapy interventions.* Retrieved from https://www.uspreventiveservicestaskforce.org/Page/Document/UpdateSummary Final/tobacco-use-in-adults-and-pregnant-women-counseling-and-interventions1; U.S. Preventive Services Task Force. (2016). *Tobacco use in children and adolescents: Primary care interventions.* Retrieved from https://www.uspreventiveservicestaskforce.org/Page/Document/ UpdateSummaryFinal/tobacco-use-in-children-and-adolescents-primary-care-interventions

experiencing the consequence of SUD (USPSTF, 2014); their guidelines for the prevention of opioid use disorder, including screening for illicit drug use are currently being developed. Their statement (USPSTF, 2019) is as follows:

"The USPSTF is deeply committed to addressing the opioid epidemic by promoting primary care strategies to prevent opioid misuse and opioid use disorder. After careful consideration of public feedback on this issue, the USPSTF has determined that it can best help address the opioid epidemic by identifying what new research is most needed on primary care strategies for preventing opioid misuse and opioid use disorders." (para. 1)

ABNORMAL/COMMON FINDINGS RELATED TO SUBSTANCE USE DISORDER

SUBSTANCE AND NON-SUBSTANCE ADDICTIVE BEHAVIORS

The diagnoses reviewed in this chapter, with associated signs, symptoms, and diagnostic criteria, include:

- Substance misuse
- SUD
- Tobacco use disorder
- Opioid use disorder
- Alcohol use disorder
- Binge drinking
- Heavy drinking
- Addiction
- Alcoholism

While this chapter focused on substance use, misuse, and addiction, the *Diagnostic and Statistical Manual of Mental Disorders*, Fifth Edition (*DSM-5*) criteria for addiction does allow for behavior to be characterized as non-substance addictive behaviors; for example, Internet gaming addiction and/or gambling addiction (King & Delfabbro, 2014; Potenza, 2014). Clinicians are reminded to assess for behaviors that are causing personal, emotional, social, financial, spiritual, or legal harm to individuals as a component of the well-being assessment. Although controversy exists whether health behaviors such as eating or sex can become addictive, the assessment of a problem in these areas should lead the clinician to recommend support through cognitive-behavioral therapy (Hebebrand et al., 2014; Meule & Gearhardt, 2014).

IMPACT ON FAMILIES

Consequences of substance misuse and SUD are experienced by each member of a family; there are emotional, developmental, social, and/or behavioral effects that can have an impact across time and generations (Lander, Howsare, & Byrne, 2013; Usher, McShane, & Dwyer, 2015). Clinicians should screen for negative outcomes and provide intervention and support to family members experiencing the effects of substance use. Family environments in which a parent or primary caregiver has an SUD are associated with higher rates of abuse and trauma, poor parenting skills, and poor quality parent–child interactions, all of which are risk factors for the development of addiction (SAMHSA, 2019a). Assessment should include screening for comorbid developmental delays, mental and physical health disorders, abuse, neglect, and safety issues; early intervention in families leads to better outcomes for all family members (Lander et al., 2013; SAMHSA, 2019a; Usher et al., 2015).

WITHDRAWAL SYMPTOMS AND NEONATAL ABSTINENCE SYNDROME

Symptoms related to withdrawal from a substance are manifested by either (a) an individual having the characteristic withdrawal symptoms for the substance or (b) an individual using the same or closely related substance to avoid the substance-specific withdrawal symptoms. **Box 23.5** lists withdrawal symptoms for specific substances.

Newborns who are exposed to substances during fetal growth and development can experience short- and long-term sequelae. One example is fetal alcohol syndrome, which is discussed in Chapter 11, Evidence-Based Assessment of the Head and Neck. When an infant is exposed to opiates in utero, the constellation of signs, symptoms, and problems that result is known as *neonatal abstinence syndrome* (NAS). The characteristic symptoms of NAS are highly variable, serious, and include central nervous system (CNS) hyperirritability and autonomic nervous system dysfunction (Stover & Davis, 2015). Pregnancy complications associated with opiate use include intrauterine growth restriction, placental abruption, preterm delivery, oligohydramnios, stillbirth, NAS, and maternal death (Bagley, Wachman, Holland, & Brogly, 2014; Jansson & Patrick, 2019; Stover & Davis, 2015). Opiate use during pregnancy is a major public health crisis, and clinicians are cautioned to carefully assess women of reproductive age, pregnant women, newborns, children, and adolescents regarding use and exposure to substances.

RECOVERY

Although resistance to treatment and relapse are common, individuals with SUD can recover. SAMHSA (2019a) defines recovery as a process of change through which individuals improve their health and wellness, live a self-directed life, and strive to reach their full potential. Being "in recovery" indicates that positive sustained changes have become part of a voluntarily adopted lifestyle. Individuals in recovery have unique and personal stories about their lives before recovery, what happened to motivate their change, and what their lives are like now. Clinicians who want to support continued recovery for individuals with SUD can approach these individuals in a manner similar to any individual with a chronic illness. Assess their health in all dimensions of wellness; ask whether they have a safe and secure place to live; support their involvement in activities of daily living that give them purpose; and assess their connections to others, their relationships, and their social networks. Learning to live 1 day at a time, accepting consequences

BOX 23.5 SUBSTANCE-SPECIFIC WITHDRAWAL SYMPTOMS

Alcohol withdrawal two or more of these symptoms:
- Autonomic hyperactivity
- Increased hand tremor
- Insomnia
- Nausea or vomiting
- Transient visual, tactile, or auditory hallucinations
- Psychomotor agitation
- Generalized tonic–clonic seizures

Cannabis withdrawal three or more of these symptoms:
- Irritability, anger, or depression
- Nervousness or anxiety
- Sleep difficulties (e.g., insomnia or disturbing dreams)
- Decreased appetite or weight loss
- Restlessness
- Depressed mood
- Physical symptom that causes significant discomfort (abdominal pain, shakiness/tremors, sweating, fever, chills, or headache)

Opioid withdrawal three or more of these symptoms:
- Moodiness
- Nausea or vomiting
- Muscle aches
- Lacrimation or rhinorrhea
- Yawning
- Pupillary dilation, piloerection, or sweating
- Diarrhea
- Fever
- Insomnia

Stimulant withdrawal two or more of these symptoms:
- Fatigue
- Vivid, unpleasant dreams
- Insomnia or hypersomnia
- Increased appetite
- Psychomotor retardation or agitation

Tobacco withdrawal four or more of these symptoms:
- Irritability, frustration, or anger
- Anxiety
- Difficulty concentrating
- Increased appetite or weight gain
- Restlessness
- Depressed mood
- Insomnia
- Decreased heart rate

Source: American Psychiatric Association. (2014). Diagnostic and statistical manual of mental disorders. Retrieved from https://dsm.psychiatryonline.org/doi/book/10.1176/appi.books.9780890425596

and responsibility for one's own actions, and developing a sense of health and wellness are not generally accomplished in isolation. Not all individuals in recovery participate in 12-step programs; those who do often find a sense of community and connection that promotes sustained change. Ask about sponsorship and sobriety. Positive clinician feedback can be a significant part of breaking the cycle of shame, guilt, stigma, and secrecy.

CASE STUDY: Illicit Prescription Use

History

A 32-year-old woman presents with concerns of recurrent headaches. She shares that she has used OTC medications without relief. Her headaches are associated with stress, worry, and insomnia. The patient was offered medication not prescribed to her from a friend and admits to using both oxycodone and gabapentin to relieve her headaches and improve sleep. She presents to the clinician because she finds herself unable to stop these medications and is wondering what to do next. She denies ever using prescription medications previously, although she notes that she did binge drink in college. She states that the medications relieved her headaches at first, but now she takes the pills "just to feel normal." If she stops taking the medications, she feels "agitated, nervous, upset, and sad." She's tried to cut back without success.

This individual is married and has one child, age 5 years. She believes that her husband, family, friends, and employer are unaware of her drug use. She does believe that she may be addicted, as she has been using these medications for almost 12 months, but has been afraid to seek treatment for fear of losing her job. She has been purchasing medications from acquaintances and over the Internet. She is worried, wants to cut back, admits to using every day, and notes that she has also started drinking alcohol daily but does not get relief from her alcohol use. She denies drinking or using prior to operating a motor vehicle. She is a nonsmoker. She does not believe that she has a problem with alcohol because she "drank a lot more than this" when she was in college. She is feeling guilt and shame because of her drug use.

Her family history includes alcoholism (her father) and depression (sister). She did experience neglect as a child and previously sought counseling for depression when she was a college student. She was treated for 2 years with bupropion and responded well. She does believe that she may be depressed again, but denies suicidal ideation or plan. She is willing to participate in outpatient treatment if the clinician believes this is necessary.

Differential Diagnoses

Substance use disorder

Additional Assessment, Including Physical Examination

- Blood pressure, heart rate, temperature, and body mass index within normal limits
- Mental status screening within normal limits
- PHQ-9 screening indicates moderate depression
- GAD-7 screening indicates moderate anxiety
- No abnormalities in neurologic examination: Speech is clear and distinct, patient is easily understood, gait is smooth and even, cranial nerves II to XII are intact, upper and lower extremity reflexes are 2+, strength 5/5 all extremities

Laboratory and Imaging

Patient agreed to urine drug testing to be completed during outpatient treatment

Final Diagnosis

Opioid use disorder; substance use disorder

Clinical Pearls

- Assessing and engaging with individuals who are unable to control or reduce their use of substances, and/or whose use continues despite consequences, requires skill in MI techniques, understanding the stages of change, and the ability to recognize and respond effectively to ambivalence.

- Using an unbiased, empathetic, patient-centered approach, clinicians can support substance use treatment and recovery.
- The overall objective for using SBIRT is to engage patients in recognizing their risks related to substance use. Patient–clinician partnerships can positively impact an individual's confidence and commitment for sustained behavior change related to the use of substances.

Key Takeaways

- Substance use can be associated with compromised functioning in virtually every system of the body. Medical conditions may develop as a result of the toxicity of the substance, route of administration, and high-risk behaviors in which the patient engages.
- A family history of SUD has been shown to be a risk factor, with genetic and environmental components, for the development of SUD and/or addiction. Family members require support and guidance.
- Recovery is possible. Screening and interventions can support sustained change, resulting in improved mental and physical wellness. Treatment and recovery are ongoing processes that occur over time.

REFERENCES

Addo, S. F., Maiden, K., & Ehrenthal, D. B. (2011). Awareness of the 5 A's and motivational interviewing among community primary care providers. *Delaware Medical Journal, 83*(1), 17–21.

American Academy of Pediatrics. (2015). *Substance use screening and intervention implementation guide.* Retrieved from https://www.aap.org/en-us/Documents/substance_use_screening_implementation.pdf

American Psychiatric Association. (2014). *Diagnostic and statistical manual of mental disorders* (5th ed.). Arlington, VA: American Psychiatric Publishing. Retrieved from https://dsm.psychiatryonline.org/doi/book/10.1176/appi.books.9780890425596

Anderson, E. M., Penrod, R. D., Barry, S. M., Hughes, B. W., Taniguchi, M., & Cowan, C. W. (2018). It is a complex issue: Emerging connections between epigenetic regulators in drug addiction. *European Journal of Neuroscience, 50*(3), 2477–2491. doi:10.1111/ejn.14170

Bagley, S. M., Wachman, E. M., Holland, E., & Brogly, S. B. (2014). Review of the assessment and management of neonatal abstinence syndrome. *Addiction Science & Clinical Practice, 9*(1), 19. doi:10.1186/1940-0640-9-19

Bates, M. E., Brick, J., & White, H. R. (2015). The correspondence between saliva and breath estimates of blood alcohol concentration: Advantages and limitations of the saliva method. *Journal of Studies on Alcohol, 54*(1), 17–22. doi:10.15288/jsa.1993.54.17

Corrigan, P. W., Schomerus, G., Shuman, V., Kraus, D., Perlick, D., Harnish, A., . . . Smelson, D. (2017). Developing a research agenda for reducing the stigma of addictions, part II: Lessons from the mental health stigma literature. *American Journal on Addictions, 26*(1), 67–74. doi:10.1111/ajad.12436

Dhalla, S., & Kopec, J. A. (2007). The CAGE questionnaire for alcohol misuse: A review of reliability and validity studies. *Clinical and Investigative Medicine, 30*(1), 33–41. doi:10.25011/cim.v30i1.447

Harris, S. K., Louis-Jacques, J., & Knight, J. R. (2014). Screening and brief intervention for alcohol and other abuse. *Adolescent Medicine: State of the Art Reviews, 25*(1), 126–156.

Hebebranda, J., Albayrak, Ö., Adan, R., Antel, J., Dieguez, C., De Jong, J., . . . Dickson, S. L. (2014). "Eating addiction", rather than "food addiction", better captures addictive-like eating behavior. *Neuroscience and Biobehavioral Reviews, 47*, 295–306. doi:10.1016/j.neubiorev.2014.08.016

Jansson, L. M., & Patrick, S. W. (2019). Neonatal abstinence syndrome. *Pediatric Clinics of North America, 66*(2), 353–367. doi:10.1016/j.pcl.2018.12.006

King, D. L., & Delfabbro, P. H. (2014). The cognitive psychology of Internet gaming disorder. *Clinical Psychology Review, 34*(4), 298–308. doi:10.1016/j.cpr.2014.03.006

Kruger, J., O'Halloran, A., Rosenthal, A. C., Babb, S. D., & Fiore, M. C. (2016). Receipt of evidence-based brief cessation interventions by health professionals and use of cessation assisted treatments among current adult cigarette-only smokers: National Adult Tobacco Survey, 2009–2010. *BMC Public Health, 16*, 141. doi:10.1186/s12889-016-2798-2

Kuerbis, A., Sacco, P., Blazer, D. G., & Moore, A. A. (2014). Substance abuse among older adults. *Clinics in Geriatric Medicine, 30*(3), 629–654. doi:10.1016/j.cger.2014.04.008

Lander, L., Howsare, J., & Byrne, M. (2013). The impact of substance use disorders on families and children: From theory to practice. *Social Work in Public Health, 28*(3–4), 194–205. doi:10.1080/19371918.2013.759005

Meule, A., & Gearhardt, A. N. (2014). Food addiction in the light of *DSM-5*. *Nutrients, 6*(9), 3653–3671. doi:10.3390/nu6093653

Moeller, K. E., Kissack, J. C., Atayee, R. S., & Lee, K. C. (2017). Clinical interpretation of urine drug tests: What clinicians need to know about urine drug screens. *Mayo Clinic Proceedings, 92*(5), 774–796. doi:10.1016/j.mayocp.2016.12.007

National Institute on Drug Abuse. (2012). *Screening for drug use in general medical settings: Resource guide.* Bethesda, MD: National Institutes of Health. Retrieved from https://www.drugabuse.gov/sites/default/files/resource_guide.pdf

National Institute on Drug Abuse. (2017). The defining features of drug intoxication and addiction can be traced to disruptions in neuron-to neuron signaling. Retrieved from https://www.drugabuse.gov/news-events/nida-notes/2017/03/impacts-drugs-neurotransmission

National Institute on Drug Abuse. (2018). Drugs and the brain.. Retrieved from https://www.drugabuse.gov/publications/drugs-brains-behavior-science-addiction/drugs-brain

Ozechowski, T. J., Becker, S. J., & Hogue, A. (2016). SBIRT-A: Adapting SBIRT to maximize developmental fit for adolescents in primary care. *Journal of Substance Abuse Treatment, 62*, 28–37. doi:10.1016/j.jsat.2015.10.006

Patnode, C. D., Henderson, J. T., Thompson, J. H., Senger, C. A., Fortmann, S. P., & Whitlock, E. P. (2015). Behavioral counseling and pharmacotherapy interventions for tobacco cessation in adults, including pregnant women: A review of reviews for the U.S. Preventive Services Task Force. *Annals of Internal Medicine, 163*(8), 608–621. doi:10.7326/M15-0171

Potenza, M. N. (2014). Non-substance addictive behaviors in the context of *DSM-5. Addictive Behaviors, 39*(1), 1–2. doi:10.1016/j.addbeh.2013.09.004

Reho, K., Agley, J., DeSalle, M., & Gassman, R. A. (2016). Are we there yet? A review of screening, brief intervention, and referral to treatment (SBIRT) implementation fidelity tools and proficiency checklists. *Journal of Primary Prevention, 37*(4), 377–388. doi:10.1007/s10935-016-0431-x

Shapiro, B., Coffa, D., & McCance-Katz, E. F. (2013). A primary care approach to substance misuse. *American Family Physician, 88*(2), 113–121. Retrieved from https://www.aafp.org/afp/2013/0715/p113.html

Smith, P. C., Cheng, D. M., Allensworth-Davies, D., Winter, M. R., & Saitz, R. (2014). Use of a single alcohol screening question to identify other drug use. *Drug and Alcohol Dependence, 139*, 178–180. doi:10.1016/j.drugalcdep.2014.03.027

Smith, P. C., Schmidt, S. M., Allensworth-Davies, D., & Saitz, R. (2009). Primary care validation of a single-question alcohol screening test. *Journal of General Internal Medicine, 24*(7), 783–788. doi:10.1007/s11606-009-0928-6

Smith, P. C., Schmidt, S. M., Allensworth-Davies, D., & Saitz, R. (2010). A single-question screening test for drug use in primary care. *Archives of Internal Medicine, 170*(13), 1155–1160. doi:10.1001/archinternmed.2010.140

Stover, M. W., & Davis, J. M. (2015). Opioids in pregnancy and neonatal abstinence syndrome. *Seminars in Perinatology, 39*(7), 561–565. doi:10.1053/j.semperi.2015.08.013

Substance Abuse and Mental Health Services Administration. (2019a). *Alcohol, tobacco, and other drugs.* Retrieved from https://www.samhsa.gov/find-help/atod

Substance Abuse and Mental Health Services Administration. (2019b). *Enhancing motivation for change in substance use disorder treatment: Treatment improvement protocol (TIP) series No. 35* [SAMHSA Publication No. PEP19-02-01-003]. Rockville, MD: Author. Retrieved from https://store.samhsa.gov/system/files/pep19-02-01-003_0.pdf

U.S. Department of Health and Human Services. (2016). *Facing addiction in America: The surgeon general's report on alcohol, drugs, and health.* Washington, DC: Author.

U.S. Preventive Services Task Force. (2014). *Drug use, illicit: Primary care interventions for children and adolescents.* Retrieved from https://www.uspreventiveservicestaskforce .org/Page/Document/UpdateSummaryFinal/drug-use -illicit-primary-care-interventions-for-children-and-adoles cents

U.S. Preventive Services Task Force. (2015). *Tobacco smoking cessation in adults, including pregnant women: Behavioral and pharmacotherapy interventions.* Retrieved from https://www.uspreventiveservicestaskforce .org/Page/Document/UpdateSummaryFinal/tobacco -use-in-adults-and-pregnant-women-counseling-and -interventions1

U.S. Preventive Services Task Force. (2016). *Tobacco use in children and adolescents: Primary care interventions.* Retrieved from https://www.uspreventiveservicestask force.org/Page/Document/UpdateSummaryFinal/to bacco-use-in-children-and-adolescents-primary-care-in terventions

U.S. Preventive Services Task Force. (2018). *Final recommendation statement: Unhealthy alcohol use in adolescents and adults: Screening and behavioral counseling interventions.* Retrieved from https://www .uspreventiveservicestaskforce.org/Page/Document /RecommendationStatementFinal/unhealthy-alcohol-use -in-adolescents-and-adults-screening-and-behavioral -counseling-interventions#consider

U.S. Preventive Services Task Force. (2019). *Inactive topic: Prevention of opioid use disorder: Interventions.* Retrieved from https://www.uspreventiveservicestaskforce .org/BrowseRec/InactiveTopic/442

Usher, A. M., McShane, K. E., & Dwyer, C. (2015). A realist review of family-based interventions for children of substance abusing parents. *Systematic Reviews, 4*, 177. doi:10.1186/s13643-015-0158-4

van Boekel, L. C., Brouwers, E. P. M., van Weeghel, J., & Garretsen, H. F. L. (2014). Healthcare professionals' regard towards working with patients with substance use disorders: Comparison of primary care, general psychiatry and specialist addiction services. *Drug and Alcohol Dependence, 134*, 92–98. doi:10.1016/j.drugalcdep.2013.09.012

Young, M. M., Stevens, A., Galipeau, J., Pirie, T., Garritty, C., Singh, K., . . . Moher, D. (2014). Effectiveness of brief interventions as part of the Screening, Brief Intervention and Referral to Treatment (SBIRT) model for reducing the nonmedical use of psychoactive substances: A systematic review. *Systematic Reviews, 3*, 50. doi:10.1186/2046-4053-3-50

24

Evidence-Based Assessment and Screening for Traumatic Experiences: Abuse, Neglect, and Intimate Partner Violence

Gail Hornor, Catherine Davis, Katharine Doughty, Catherine Huber, Rosie Zeno, and Linda Quinlin

> *"We remember the people who show up in our darkest hours."*
>
> —Shauna L. Hoey

LEARNING OBJECTIVES

- Understand the ways in which traumatic experience(s) can vary across individuals.
- Identify the methods of assessment for trauma.
- Recognize the risk factors, history, and physical examination findings that are concerning for child and elder physical and sexual abuse and what workup should subsequently be initiated.
- Understand the role of emotional maltreatment in isolation and its coexistence with other forms of abuse.
- Recognize the risk factors, history, and physical indicators for child and elder neglect and understand the subsequent workup that should be initiated.
- Recognize the significance of the incidence and impact of intimate partner violence.
- Describe evidence-based preventive methods for screening and preventing all forms of abuse and maltreatment.

TRAUMA

Trauma is a word that is now commonly used in every-day language. It is in the news when natural disasters strike. Clinicians and other first responders often use this term. Psychologists, social workers, and other mental health clinicians use this term as well. The actual definition of trauma has been difficult for researchers to agree upon because it is so expansive. The Substance Abuse and Mental Health Services Administration (SAMHSA) defines individual trauma as resulting from "an event, series of events, or set of circumstances that is experienced by an individual as physically or emotionally harmful or [life] threatening and that has lasting adverse effects on the individual's functioning and [mental], physical, social, emotional, or spiritual well-being (SAMHSA, 2012 as cited in SAMHSA, 2014, p. 20). One thing that the experts agree upon is that a trauma is an event that overwhelms a person's capacity to cope. These events can take place in the form of one-time incidents such as natural disasters, crimes, deaths, accidents, or violent events. Trauma can also be caused by chronic conditions or circumstances such as child abuse, neglect, urban violence, combat, and violent relationships (Giller, n.d.). No two individuals will experience trauma in the same way. Subjectively speaking, trauma refers to the unique experience(s) of the

645

individual who has encountered these events. An event that is traumatic for one individual may not be viewed as distressing in the same way for another individual. Defining trauma in this way provides a framework in which to view an event from the perspective of its survivors and in the context of their own lives and experiences rather than defining what is considered traumatic for them (SAMHSA, 2014).

It is best to think of trauma broadly because of the many different forms trauma can have. Traumas can be either natural or man-made. Traumas that occur deliberately, at the hands of another human being, tend to be more difficult for survivors to overcome. Examples include criminal acts that are often violent, such as sexual abuse/assault, domestic violence, child abuse, war, and community violence. Of these examples of man-made traumas, survivors of rape, child sexual abuse, and other forms of sexual violence comprise the largest group of individuals diagnosed with *posttraumatic stress disorder (PTSD)* in this country. Unfortunately, the effects of ongoing trauma are cumulative.

One of the greatest findings in trauma research is the concept of a dose–response relationship, meaning that the greater the dose of trauma, the more damaging the effects are on an individual. The greater the stressor, the greater the likelihood that the victim will develop PTSD. Individuals who have experienced repeated and ongoing trauma throughout their lives tend to be the most difficult to work with, both personally and clinically. Their worldview and attitudes surrounding relationships have been shaped by the expectation that they will ultimately be harmed in some way. Because of the chaotic and unpredictable nature of their experiences, these individuals often develop a deep mistrust of others and a sense that they have no control over what happens next. Resulting emotions include grief, rage, torment, and sorrow (Giller, n.d.).

Despite the fact that the ways in which people experience trauma vary immensely, it is important to remember that there are certain patterns of responses that consistently present across the variety of stressors and the experiences of survivors. The majority of people receiving mental health services have experienced some form of trauma. There is no one diagnosis that encompasses all trauma survivors. Many survivors carry multiple mental health diagnoses. By far, the most commonly diagnosed mental health disorder among trauma survivors is PTSD. This is the only category in the *Diagnostic and Statistical Manual of Mental Disorders* (5th ed.; *DSM-5*; American Psychiatric Association, 2013) that is based on etiology. In order to be diagnosed with PTSD, an individual must have experienced a traumatic event. It is descriptive rather than explanatory and helps to provide the context as to why a set of behaviors or symptoms have developed. The symptoms of PTSD are considered to be adaptive because they

are dysfunctional ways of coping with traumatic stress. PTSD symptoms should be thought of as adaptations that are helping an individual to cope in the best way they can with their overwhelming feelings. Symptoms include hypervigilance, dissociation, numbing in response to the intrusive thoughts, reexperiencing, and depression (Giller, n.d.).

Trauma not only affects a person psychologically and behaviorally, but neurologically as well (**Figure 24.1**). Neurological research has found that a child's development can be interrupted by traumatic experience in significant ways. Bruce Perry has been on the forefront of research, showing that the hard-wiring of the brain is impacted when children live in a constant state of fight-or-flight. The term *family violence* is often used to encompass all forms of intimate violence, including *intimate partner violence* (IPV), child abuse, and *elder abuse* by caregivers (Niolan et al., 2017). When children live in chaotic, unpredictable environments and experience prolonged adversity, cortisol and other hormones are continuously released and this leads to chronic states of anxiety and hyperarousal. Their bodies and brains must learn to always be ready for potential danger, which can lead to behavioral accommodations; symptoms such as aggression, sleeplessness, distrust; and the continuous scanning of their surroundings. This hypervigilance of the autonomic system ultimately results in the hard-wiring of the brain being altered and typical child development being interrupted (Perry, 1994).

The impact of trauma can be devastating and lifelong for many individuals. It is important, however, not to generalize the effect of traumatic experiences. Most individuals who experience trauma are able to recover and function very well in their day-to-day life.

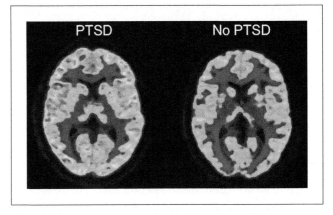

FIGURE 24.1 Changes in brain activity that occur when an individual has experienced PTSD. Numerous studies have found significant structural and functional brain changes, specifically in the hippocampus, amygdala, and prefrontal cortex.

PTSD, posttraumatic stress disorder.

Courtesy of Bill Hathaway (2017). New PTSD study identifies potential path to treatment. Yale University, New Haven, Connecticut.

Just as no two people will experience a traumatic event in the same way, it is also true that not all individuals find themselves permanently impacted in a negative way. Given the sizeable numbers of children who have experienced trauma, fewer than 20% of these children grow up to have serious psychological disturbance as adults. This is because of a number of factors including an individual's degree of resiliency and being met with a supportive and appropriate response from others after the traumatic event has occurred. Clinicians involved in their care play a large role in facilitating an appropriate response in the aftermath of a traumatic experience.

ADVERSE CHILDHOOD EXPERIENCES

Between the years of 1995 and 1997, researchers set out to describe the long-term relationship of childhood adversity to medical and public health issues later in life. This study, known as the **Adverse Childhood Experience (ACE)** study, is considered to be a landmark study that is relevant to professionals across various disciplines. The aims of the study were to determine retrospectively and prospectively the impact that childhood adversity and household dysfunction have on the following outcomes later in life: disease incidence and risk factors, healthcare utilization, quality of life, and mortality. Researchers first described the prevalence and inter-relation among exposures to child abuse and household dysfunctions. Researchers then studied how the number of exposures to childhood adversity may later be related to the incidence of chronic diseases that are the underlying causes of death in adults (Felitti et al., 1998).

The questions included in the ACE questionnaire originated from other published surveys and addressed the following areas: physical and psychological abuse, violence against the respondent's mother, sexual abuse, parental drug use, mental illness, and criminal behavior. All the questions on the survey began with the phrase, "While you were growing up during your first 18 years of life…." The respondents were considered to be exposed to a category if they answered "yes" to one or more of the questions listed in each category (Felitti et al., 1998).

Ten risk factors were then chosen to be examined that are known to contribute to the leading causes of death in the United States. The 10 risk factors that were chosen were severe obesity, depressed mood, alcoholism, suicide attempts, smoking, drug use, parental drug use, physical inactivity, a high number of sexual partners, and having a history of a sexually transmitted infection (STI). Based upon the participant's medical history, researchers then sought to determine if there were any relationships between the number of childhood exposures and disease conditions that are known to be the leading causes of mortality. The disease conditions included were heart disease, emphysema, chronic

bronchitis, cancer, diabetes, stroke, jaundice or hepatitis, and the participant's answer to the question: "Do you consider your physical health to be excellent, very good, good, fair, or poor?" (Felitti et al., 1998).

The results of the study found that substance abuse was the most prevalent of the seven categories of childhood exposure with 25.6% reporting being exposed to substance abuse in the household. Over half of the respondents, 52%, reported being exposed to one or more categories of adverse events and 6.2% reported being exposed to four or more categories of adverse events. These findings also suggest that the greater the number of childhood exposures, the more it increased the prevalence and risk for obesity, smoking, physical inactivity, depressed mood, and suicide attempts. In addition, the rates and risk of using illegal drugs, alcoholism, having more than 50 sexual partners, and having a history of STIs increased as the number of childhood exposures increased.

Another important finding from the ACE study demonstrated a strong relationship between the number of childhood exposures and the number of health risk factors for the leading causes of death. Fifty-six percent of respondents with no childhood exposures had none of the health risk factors, whereas only 14% of those respondents with four or more childhood exposures had no risk factors. The findings from the ACE study clearly suggest a strong dose–response relationship, meaning that the greater amount of exposure to abuse and/or other household dysfunction appears to be closely tied to a higher number of risk factors for several of the leading causes of death in adults (Felitti et al., 1998).

These results led researchers to question how exposure to childhood adversity is linked to health risk behaviors and subsequent diseases later in life. Experiencing childhood adversity can lead to high levels of stress, anxiety, anger, and depression. Many lifestyle behaviors such as smoking, drug abuse, overeating, and sexual behavior have immediate psychological or pharmacological benefit and, because of this, tend to be chronically used as ways to cope. Long-term use of these coping skills can also lead to negative health outcomes. The ACE study findings have made it clear that exposure to childhood adversity not only impacts one's mental health but can also have a devastating impact on an individual's physical health, which may ultimately lead to early death.

Because research has solidly shown the staggering prevalence of childhood adversity, the American Academy of Pediatrics (AAP) released a report and policy statement on childhood toxic stress. The documents contained in the report serve as an ethical guide to address and prevent childhood adversity. These documents also include language that emphasizes the importance of screening for ACEs and trauma (AAP, 2012a,

2012b). The benefits of screening are numerous, no matter the age of the patient. Screening for ACEs early in life can help reduce a child's risk of exposure to ongoing abuse and dysfunction by linking families with appropriate community supports. The vast majority of individuals who have been exposed to ACEs survive into adulthood. Screening for ACEs in the adult population is critical as ACE exposures are often intergenerational (Dube, 2018). Appropriate support and intervention within the adult community can hopefully interrupt the pattern of ongoing abuse and dysfunction commonly seen in families. A 2014 review of 10 studies suggests that screening in primary care clinics leads to reductions in adverse child outcomes such as exposure to domestic violence, child physical abuse, aggression, and delinquent behavior (Flynn et al., 2015).

Finkelhor (2017) has suggested that screening for ACEs should be entered into cautiously owing to the fact that screening is beneficial only when there are effective interventions that are readily available to help mitigate the negative effects from the issue that the screening identifies. Finkelhor raises an interesting argument by pointing out that the range of specific needs stemming from ACE referrals can vary from domestic violence intervention to substance abuse programs to grief and trauma counseling. There are a number of effective interventions available to families experiencing adversity, from parent training courses to individual and family counseling services. It is imperative that clinicians screening for ACEs be familiar with the resources available in their communities and that they feel confident in being able to make appropriate referrals that will target the specific needs of the individual (Finkelhor, 2017). Clinicians must also be cognizant of the fact that as mandated reporters, screening for ACEs will naturally lead to an increase in reporting to child welfare agencies and clinicians must feel comfortable with this process.

ACE measures have only recently begun to be used in clinical practice and there is no consensus among healthcare clinicians on a framework that should be used when evaluating ACE measures. Bethell et al. (2017) evaluated 14 measures, 10 child-focused measures and four adult measures. For a complete list of the measures that were evaluated, see **Box 24.1**.

All but one of the assessments evaluated in the Bethell et al. study (2017) were self-reported measures. The Washington State University School ACEs tool is a teacher-reported instrument. Eight years of age is considered to be the youngest at which a child is capable of self-reporting on their ACE exposure. Out of 14 measures, 12 measures are recommended for use alongside other questionnaires or as part of a larger survey. Other questions that are commonly asked in conjunction with these measures include demographic information, healthcare access, current and past health

---

BOX 24.1
ACE MEASUREMENT METHODS

Child-Focused ACE Measurement Measures

1. 2011/12 NSCH-ACEs
2. National Survey of Child and Adolescent Well-Being (NSCAW)
3. Yale-Vermont Adversity in Childhood Scale (adult, youth, youth self-reported, and clinician-reported versions)
4. Center for Youth Wellness Adverse Childhood Experiences Questionnaire (child, youth, and youth self-reported versions)
5. Marie-Mitchell and O'Connor Child ACEs Algorithm
6. Montefiore Group Attachment–Based Intervention Study Clinical ACEs Measure
7. Philadelphia Childhood Adversity Questionnaire
8. Washington State University (WSU) ACEs Tool for Schools
9. WSU ACEs Tool for Head Start
10. Crittenton Foundation/Aspen Institute ACEs Assessment Tool

Adult ACE Measurement Measures

1. Centers for Disease Control and Prevention (CDC) and Kaiser Permanente Study ACEs Measure
2. The State-Level Behavioral Risk Factor Surveillance Survey (BRFSS) ACEs Module
3. World Health Organization's (WHO) ACEs International Questionnaire
4. Philadelphia Urban ACEs Tool

ACEs, adverse childhood experiences; NSCH, National Survey of Children's Health.

Source: Adapted from Bethell, C. D., Carle, A., Hudziak, J., Gombojav, N., Powers, K., Wade, R., & Braveman, P. (2017). Methods to assess adverse childhood experiences of children and families: Toward approaches to promote child well-being in policy and practice. *Academic Pediatrics, 17*(7 Suppl.), S51–S69. doi:10.1016/j.acap.2017.04.161

---

history, protective factors, and overall well-being (Bethell et al., 2017).

Although there are many examples of formal assessment tools that can be used in a variety of settings to screen for various types of trauma, perhaps the best way to screen for trauma is always approach patients through the lens of **trauma-informed care** (TIC). Finding a universal definition for TIC across literature is difficult; however, Hopper, Bassuk, and Olivet (2010) defined TIC as "a strengths-based framework that is grounded in an understanding of and responsiveness to the impact of trauma, that emphasizes physical, psychological, and emotional safety for both providers and survivors, and that creates opportunities for survivors to rebuild a sense of control and empowerment" (p. 133). How TIC is defined and conceptualized in any given system might vary depending on the needs and uniqueness of each organization. Most organizations implementing TIC focus on work force development (training, awareness, and secondary traumatic stress), trauma-focused services (use of standardized screening measures and evidence-based practices), and organizational environment and practices (collaboration, service coordination, safe physical environment, written policies, and defined leadership; Lang, Campbell, Shanley, Crusto, & Connell, 2016). Lang et al. (2016) also note that the essential rationale for TIC is that addressing trauma earlier and more effectively will result in improved outcomes, less need for more extensive and expensive services, and reduction in long-term costs. Taking appropriate steps to become more trauma-informed will allow clinicians to look for the residue of trauma that will often present in the form of mental health diagnoses, drug and alcohol problems, and behavioral problems in children, among others. Ongoing training in the area of trauma and staying abreast of research within this field will help healthcare clinicians to feel confident, comfortable, and competent in asking patients about their trauma histories. Screening and identifying trauma can be the starting point for patients and families in receiving appropriate intervention and beginning on a path toward healing.

ABUSE AND NEGLECT OF CHILDREN

PHYSICAL AND SEXUAL ABUSE

The Child Abuse Prevention and Treatment Act (CAPTA, 1974) legally defines *child abuse and neglect* as "any recent act or failure to act on the part of a parent or caretaker, which results in death, serious physical or emotional harm, sexual abuse or exploitation . . ., or an act or failure to act, which presents an imminent risk of serious harm." Of the 676,000 children in the United States who were victims of abuse/neglect in 2016, 18.2% were physically abused (U.S. Department of Health and Human Services [USDHHS], 2018). The youngest children are the most vulnerable, with more than a quarter (28.5%) of victims being under the age of 3 years. Males and females had similar rates of victimization overall in 2016. Three races or ethnicities comprised most victims that year—White (44.9%), Hispanic (22.0%), and African American (20.7%); this differs from the overall population distribution for children in the United States—White (51.1%), Hispanic (24.9%), and African American (13.8%; USDHHS, 2018). Child fatality is the most severe result of abuse and neglect; it is estimated

that 1,750 children died because of abuse and neglect in this country in 2016 alone. Almost half of these children were victims of fatal physical abuse (USDHHS, 2018). For all clinicians, this should be considered a major health concern when taking care of young patients.

Although every patient encounter should prompt the clinician to screen for traumatic experiences, there are some risk factors that should heighten one's awareness that a child may need more than standard screening. Having an awareness of the individual patient population being treated as well as the community environment that a patient lives in will assist in this process (Christian, 2015; Flaherty, 2010). Risk factors inherent to the child are considered first. Oftentimes, patients who are abused are considered "difficult" by caregivers, which can mean a number of things. Perhaps the child is medically complicated, requiring frequent appointments, medications, and interventions on a regular basis. They may have developmental delays or disabilities and differ from the typical abilities of their siblings and peers. They could have emotional or behavioral issues that put them at risk for physical abuse. Infants remain at the highest risk for physical maltreatment; children from unwanted or unplanned pregnancies have also been found to be at increased risk. Twins have been shown to be at significantly increased risk of physical abuse in comparison to other sibling dynamics in the family, especially when it comes to sustaining abusive fractures (Lindberg, 2012).

Parents and caregivers have innate risk factors as well. Parents who struggle with self-esteem, impulse control, substance abuse, and mental illness are more at risk for perpetrating maltreatment, as are those who have been previous victims of abuse themselves. Having unrealistic or inappropriate expectations for their children can also put a family at risk. Key times in a young child's life can trigger more frustration and difficulties in parenting, thus increasing the risk for physical abuse. Colic, night crying, separation anxiety, exploratory behavior, negativism, poor appetite, and potty-training all have been shown to trigger physical abuse, despite being parts of normal childhood development (Schmitt, 1987). The community environment can influence the maltreatment of a child. Social isolation, poverty, unemployment, lower educational achievement, and community violence are all factors placing a child at risk for maltreatment. Although many of these factors cannot be alleviated by the clinician when assessing a patient, being aware of these features can influence the clinician in the next steps that may be taken to assess and protect a child.

Child sexual abuse is a problem of epic proportions resulting in significant consequences for victims. According to the USDHHS (2018), more than 57,000 children were documented victims of sexual abuse in 2016. This number grossly underrepresents the actual number of victims. Based upon retrospective studies of adults, approximately only one in 20 cases of sexual abuse is ever reported or investigated (Kellogg, 2005). The prevalence of child sexual abuse is estimated to be one in five girls and one in 20 boys (National Center for Victims of Crime [NCVC], 2012).The ACE study described previously (Felitti et al., 1998) solidified the realization that exposure to sexual abuse impacts the developmental and health outcomes of children in a graded, dose–response fashion (Traub & Boynton-Jarrett, 2017).

The World Health Organization (WHO) established the definition of *child sexual abuse* in 1999 as "the involvement of a child in sexual activity that they cannot fully understand, is unable to give informed consent, for which the child is developmentally unprepared and cannot give consent, or that violates the laws or social taboos of the society." Child sexual abuse involves sexual activity between a child and an adult or another child who by age or development is in a position of responsibility, trust, or power over the child. Sexual abuse includes both touching and nontouching behaviors. Touching behaviors range from fondling of the breasts, genitalia, or buttocks to oral, genital, or anal penetration. Noncontact behaviors include exposure to pornography, voyeurism, or purposeful exposure to adults engaging in sexual activity.

Sexual abuse perpetrators are most often someone the child knows, trusts, and even loves. Although men are much more frequently identified as sexual abuse perpetrators, women also sexually abuse children. Adolescents are perpetrators in 21% of sexual abuse cases (Ryan & Otonichar, 2016). Sexual abuse also includes the exploitive use of a child in prostitution, pornography performance and materials, or other unlawful sexual practices (WHO, 1999). The sex trafficking of minors is a form of child sexual abuse referred to as commercial sexual exploitation of children—crimes of a sexual nature committed against juvenile victims for financial or other economic reasons (Greenbaum, Crawford-Jakubiak, & Committee on Child Abuse and Neglect, 2015).

It is not unusual for sexual abuse to occur in association with other types of maltreatment; in other words, the sexually abused child is at risk for other ACEs. Dong, Dube, Felitti, Giles, and Anda (2003) found that child sexual abuse victimization was frequently associated with emotional and physical abuse, as well as neglect. Sexual abuse is also associated with a home environment, which may be low in family support and high in stress affected by interpersonal violence, substance abuse, mental illness, parental mental retardation, separation or divorce, and criminal activity (Butler, 2013; Murray, Nguyen, & Cohen, 2014). Experiencing child sexual abuse has been linked to a variety of negative consequences for victims, including PTSD, depression, substance abuse, suicidal ideation,

high-risk sexual behaviors, and other behavioral and physical health concerns (Dube et al., 2005; Murray et al., 2014). Child sexual abuse victims are at increased risk for sexual revictimization later in life. Ullman and Vasquez (2015) found child sexual abuse victims to be about twice as likely to experience sexual assault in adolescence or adulthood. Children most at risk for later revictimization are those with multiple familial psychosocial concerns and a parent/caregiver who is not supportive of them or their sexual abuse allegations (Hornor & Fischer, 2016).

Certain characteristics place children at increased risk for sexual abuse, including sex, age, and disability. Females are three to four times more likely to experience sexual abuse than males (NCVC, 2012). However, males may be less likely to disclose abuse when it occurs. The majority of boys who experience sexual abuse are sexually abused by a male; fear of being perceived as homosexual may inhibit a boy from disclosing sexual abuse victimization.

Children between the ages of 7 and 13 years are most vulnerable to sexual abuse (NCVC, 2012). This is not to say that children less than 7 years of age do not experience sexual abuse, but rather that younger children often lack the developmental skills to understand and communicate their experiences to the adults in their lives. The risk of experiencing sexual abuse for girls rises with age, whereas for boys risk peaks around puberty (Finkelhor, 2009). Approximately 60% of girls who suffer sexual abuse by a family member will also experience a rape after age 14 (NCVC, 2012).

Children with disabilities are at increased risk of victimization. Contributing to this increased risk are dependency, need for institutional care, and communication difficulties. Some disabilities, such as cognitive delays, mental illness, and speech disorders, lead to the child being perceived as a noncredible source of information regarding potential sexual abuse, thereby making them a target for sexual abuse (Wissink, van Vugt, Moonen, Stams, & Hendriks, 2015).

EMOTIONAL ABUSE

Abuse is not limited to physical and social maltreatment. *Emotional abuse* is a repeated pattern of damaging interactions between caregivers and a child that becomes typical of the relationship; leaving the child to feel that they are unloved, unwanted, and/or interferes with the child's development and socialization. This can harm the child's emotional, developmental, or psychological well-being. Oftentimes, emotional maltreatment can overlap with other forms of maltreatment, including physical and sexual abuse, emotional neglect, and exposure to IPV. Emotional maltreatment can be overlooked and is often thought to be the most complex, prevalent, and damaging form of child abuse or neglect.

It is often difficult to identify, partly because such maltreatment involves an ongoing relationship between the caregiver and the child rather than a specific or ongoing series of events. Many times, emotional maltreatment will be identified when coexisting with other forms of child abuse and neglect; however, it can exist as the sole form of maltreatment experienced as well (Campbell & Hibbard, 2014; Hibbard, Barlow, & MacMillan, 2012; Kairys, Johnson, & Committee on Child Abuse and Neglect, 2002).

Emotional maltreatment may include a single traumatic event or a repeated pattern of behavior, which can include acts of omission (ignoring a key part of development such as the need for social interaction) or commission (spurning, terrorizing); emotional maltreatment may express itself verbally or in nonverbal forms, actively or passively, and with or without intent to harm. This harm can take on several forms, including spurning; terrorizing; exploiting/corrupting; denying emotional responsiveness; isolating; and mental health, medical, and educational neglect (Campbell & Hibbard, 2014).

A child's brain and nervous system development take on rapid and extensive growth during the first 3 years of life. For this reason, emotional maltreatment can be very impactful to the child in this age group. Brain and nervous system development are greatly influenced by the child's environment to include the relationships, either positive or negative, that the child is exposed to, the way in which a child relates or attaches to their environment and others around them, as well as the way the child is able to process and regulate during periods of growth and stress. Kairys et al. (2002) suggest that the severity of consequences of psychological maltreatment (emotional maltreatment) is influenced by its intensity, extremeness, frequency, and chronicity.

The long-term consequences of this type of maltreatment are extensive and profound. The effects on the child are multifaceted, impacting all aspects of the child's development. These effects can interfere with mental health and emotional well-being, expressing this sequelae as low self-esteem, anxiety, depression, thoughts of self-harm, impulse control problems, anger, emotional instability/lability, and substance abuse disorders. Socially, children can exhibit attachment problems whether they seek out unhealthy relationships or struggle with recognizing and maintaining appropriate boundaries. They may have difficulty expressing empathy toward others and may self-isolate. They may also exhibit learning difficulties leading to low academic achievement as well as compromised physical health expressed as failure to thrive, frequent somatic complaints, poor adult health, and even high mortality (Campbell & Hibbard, 2014; Hibbard et al., 2012; Kairys et al., 2002).

A study by Shin, Lee, Jeon, and Wills (2015) looked at whether emotional maltreatment influenced alcohol use through urgent personality trait. In this study, *urgent personality trait* was defined as the propensity to act on impulses, often under the influence of distress. The study included a sample size of 268 males and females aged 18 to 25 years. They found that emotional maltreatment was related to urgency, which in turn influenced four types of alcohol use: frequency of alcohol use, binge drinking, alcohol-related problems, and alcohol use disorder (AUD). The authors concluded that urgency may play a significant role in linking childhood maltreatment to alcohol use in young adulthood (Potthast, Neuner, & Catani, 2014). Another study by Potthast et al. suggests that emotional maltreatment might have a major role in the etiology of alcohol dependence, more so than other forms of maltreatment and peer-victimization experiences (Perry, 2002). Results of these two studies emphasize the need for one to address child maltreatment experiences when working with adults who have an alcohol disorder.

NEGLECT

Neglect is often an overlooked form of child maltreatment; however, it is the most common and deadliest form of child maltreatment. As previously noted, 676,000 American children were victims of child maltreatment in 2016. Three-quarters (74.8%) of these children experienced neglect compared with physical abuse (18.2%) and sexual abuse (8.5%; U.S. Department of Health and Human Services, 2017). When compared with other forms of child maltreatment, the consequences of neglect are not benign. It is estimated that nearly 2,000 (1,750) American children died in 2016 as a result of child maltreatment (U.S. Department of Health and Human Services, 2017). Of the children who died, 74.6% suffered neglect, 5.7% suffered medical neglect, and 44.2% experienced physical abuse either in isolation or in combination with other forms of child maltreatment.

The WHO (1999) defines *neglect* as the failure to provide for the development of the child in one or more of the following realms: health, education, emotional development, nutrition, shelter, and safe living conditions. The WHO definition also includes abandonment and failure to provide supervision adequate to protect children from harm as facets of neglect. This failure to meet the needs of a child must be measured with an understanding of the resources reasonably available to the parents or caregivers; thus, neglect must be differentiated from circumstances of poverty. Resultant harm or potential for harm to the child's physical, mental, spiritual, moral, or social health must also be considered (Schilling & Christian, 2014).

The consequences of experiencing childhood neglect can be significant and long-term, with children's physical and mental health as well as their psychosocial and cognitive development affected (Dubowitz, 2014). Physical effects of neglect can be relatively immediate, such as complications resulting from a delay/failure to seek healthcare or injuries resulting from lack of supervision (Hornor, 2014). Other consequences are more subtle and can take time to present, such as impaired brain development, inferior academic performance, and emotional or behavioral problems (Dubowitz, 2014). The ACE study, discussed previously, solidified the understanding that even in adulthood the effects of childhood neglect can resurface with liver disease, heart disease, depression, and suicidality (Dong et al., 2003, 2004; Edwards, Holder, Felitti, & Anda, 2003).

There are multiple risk factors that place children at increased risk to experience neglect; many of these risk factors are interrelated and dependent on one another. There are child, familial, and societal factors that contribute to neglect. Similar to the risk factors for physical abuse, children with complex health and/or behavioral problems are at increased risk to experience neglect because of significant needs that can exhaust caregiver resources (Fong & Christian, 2012). Certain caregiver/familial factors limit the caregiver's abilities to adequately meet a child's needs, such as a cognitive/intellectual disability, mental health concerns, IPV, physical illness or disability, substance abuse, and lack of social supports. Societal factors contributing to neglect include poverty, specifically a lack of resources for child care, transportation, and healthy foods; lack of health insurance; unsafe housing conditions; community violence; and cultural or religious beliefs (Fong & Christian, 2012).

Neglect can present in many different forms (Hornor, 2014). **Box 24.2** discusses different types of neglect, with some specific examples of neglectful situations. As previously noted with other forms of child maltreatment, neglect rarely occurs in isolation. Neglected children are at increased risk to also experience physical, sexual, or emotional abuse. Children can also experience multiple types of neglect. Egregious situations of neglect are typically easily identified; however, identification is often dependent on the ongoing observations of healthcare clinicians, teachers, day-care workers, and other professionals who work with the children and who ultimately make a decision about the inadequacy of the overall care of the child within their family context (Appleton, 2012).

INTIMATE PARTNER VIOLENCE

IPV is also a serious public health problem that occurs across the life span and can result in significant morbidity and mortality for the people involved. *IPV* refers

---

BOX 24.2
TYPES OF CHILD NEGLECT

Medical
- Failure/delay in seeking healthcare
- Noncompliance with plan of care

Supervision/Safety
- Ingestions
- Guns/other weapons
- Car seats/seat belts
- Intimate partner violence

Education
- Truancy
- Noncompliance

Dental
- Failure to seek care

Nutrition
- Nonorganic failure to thrive
- Obesity
- Noncompliance with plan of care

Prenatal Drug Exposure

Shelter/Home
- Homelessness
- Safe
- Clean

Hygiene/Clothing

Love/Affection and Nurturance
- Abandonment
- Ignoring/apathetic care

Source: Adapted from Hornor, G. (2014). Child neglect: Assessment and intervention. *Journal of Pediatric Health Care, 28*(2), 186–192. doi:10.1016/j.pedhc.2013.10.002

---

to physical violence, sexual violence, stalking, and psychological aggression by a current or former intimate partner, which may include a spouse, dating partner, domestic partner, or anyone with whom a person has had a close personal relationship; however, the relationship does not require sexual intimacy (Breiding, Basile, Smith, Black, & Mahendra, 2015). See **Table 24.1** for types of IPV behaviors.

IPV is also commonly referred to as *domestic violence* and occurs along a spectrum, ranging from an acute single episode to chronic recurrent episodes. Episodes of IPV may range from minor to severe and may occur in person, electronically, or online.

TABLE 24.1 Types of Intimate Partner Violence Behaviors

Physical violence	A person hurts or tries to hurt a partner by hitting, kicking, or using another type of physical force.
Sexual violence	Forcing or attempting to force a partner to take part in a sex act, sexual touching, or a nonphysical sexual event (e.g., sexting) when the partner does not or cannot consent.
Stalking	A pattern of repeated, unwanted attention and contact by a partner that causes fear for one's own safety or the safety of someone close to the victim.
Psychological aggression	The use of verbal and nonverbal communication with the intent to harm another person mentally or emotionally and/or exert control over another person.

Source: Adapted from Breiding, M. J., Basile, K. C., Smith, S. G., Black, M. C., & Mahendra, R. R. (2015). *Intimate partner violence surveillance: Uniform definitions and recommended data elements, Version 2.0.* Atlanta, GA: National Center for Injury Prevention and Control, Centers for Disease Control and Prevention.

IPV can occur within heterosexual or same-sex relationships and often begins in adolescence and continues throughout the life span. Data from the National Intimate Partner and Sexual Violence Survey (NISVS) show that nearly 8.5 million women and over 5 million men reported experiencing IPV in their lifetime and, importantly, that they first experienced IPV prior to age 18 (S. G. Smith et al., 2017). The National Youth Risk Behavior Surveillance report shows that among students who report dating, 12% of girls and 7% of boys experienced physical dating violence, and 16% of girls and 5% of boys experienced sexual dating violence within the preceding year (Kann et al., 2016). When referring to this particular subset of IPV, it is also commonly termed *teen dating violence.*

The consequences of IPV on a person's health are substantial. Many negative health effects have been linked with IPV, including physical illnesses (gastrointestinal [GI] problems, neurological disorders, chronic pain, hypertension, cancer and cardiovascular diseases), mental illnesses (anxiety, PTSD, and higher risk for developing substance addictions), and reproductive issues (unintended pregnancy and miscarriage; WHO, 2013). Victims of IPV may not only experience physical injuries and chronic health issues, but the violence within a relationship can also result in death. One in six murder victims is killed by an intimate partner and over 40% of female murder victims are killed by an intimate partner according to statistics from U.S. crime reports (Cooper & Smith, 2011).

Families with young children have the highest rates of IPV (Bair-Merritt et al., 2014). One in 15 children are exposed to IPV each year, and 90% of these children are eyewitnesses to this violence (Hamby, Finkelhor, Turner, & Ormrod, 2011). Children exposed to IPV are not only at risk of becoming physically involved in the violence between their caregivers, but they are also at risk for significant psychosocial trauma from experiencing traumatic events. Children may be at risk even before they are born as pregnancy increases a woman's risk for

IPV. It is estimated that up to 19% of pregnant women experience IPV (Sharps, Laughon, & Giangrande, 2007), which can result in poor maternal–infant health outcomes, such as low birth weight, prematurity, and fetal demise. The relationship between IPV and child abuse is well established. Evidence indicates that in up to 60% of families in which IPV or child abuse is occurring, the other form of abuse is also occurring (Edelson, 1999). Millions of children are exposed to IPV each year, and as demonstrated by the ACE study, many suffer serious behavioral, emotional, and physical health consequences across their life span (Felitti et al., 1998).

ELDERLY AND DISABLED ADULT ABUSE

Approximately one out of every 10 individuals over the age of 60 in community settings is estimated to have been affected by some form of elder abuse (Centers for Disease Control and Prevention, 2017; National Center on Elder Abuse, n.d.; WHO, 2018). It is thought that this statistic is likely underestimated because of the fear or inability of many to self-report the abuse. Studies have found that only one in 24 cases of elder abuse is reported (WHO, 2018). The most frequently reported elder abuse in the community setting includes verbal abuse, followed by financial abuse, and lastly physical abuse (National Center on Elder Abuse, n.d.). Rates of elder abuse in institutional settings are just as prevalent as in the community setting. Systematic reviews and meta-analyses of studies on elder abuse identified 64.2% of institutional staff admitting to some form of elder abuse in the past year (WHO, 2018; Yon, Ramiro-Gonzalez, Mikton, Huber, & Sethi, 2019). Elder abuse in institutional settings includes physically restraining residents, loss of dignity (being kept in soiled garments), intentional act of not providing sufficient care (not turning residents resulting in the development of pressure ulcers), and over- or under-medicating residents (WHO, 2018).

Elder abuse is the act of intentionally causing or creating a serious risk of harm to an older adult or failing to act by a caregiver or another person where there is an expectation of trust. Abuse can come in the form of physical, sexual, psychological, emotional, financial, neglect, and abandonment (Centers for Disease Control and Prevention, 2017; National Center on Elder Abuse, n.d.; WHO, 2018). Elder abuse can lead to poor health outcomes such as death and depression. Worldwide, the cases of elder abuse are expected to rise, as the world's aging population increases. By 2050, it is estimated that, globally, the population of individuals over the age of 60 will increase from 900 million in 2015 to approximately 2 billion. The majority of aging individuals will live in low- and middle-income countries (WHO, 2018).

KEY HISTORY QUESTIONS AND CONSIDERATIONS

HISTORY OF PRESENT ILLNESS

Physical Abuse

When there is a concern for physical abuse, the patient encounter should start the same as any other encounter by obtaining a chief concern (Bickley, 2007). Opening the conversation with "What brings you in today?" is a simple way to determine what the caregiver's knowledge is regarding the physical abuse concern or if physical abuse is even a part of the presenting problem. Starting with an open-ended question and letting the patient or caregiver take the lead to provide a narrative gives the best overall summary of information to begin the patient encounter. Once the patient or caregiver has told the story in their own words, the clinician can ask for clarifying details. Other communication techniques can be utilized to build the clinician–patient relationship: active listening, nonverbal communication, empathetic responses, and summarization.

When obtaining the history of present illness, there are some key questions to consider for children when there is a concern for physical abuse. "When was the child last normal?" can be critical in determining if there was a slow onset of symptoms or an abrupt change in the child's health status. Having the caregiver describe the time leading up to the change and what prompted the family to seek medical care can be helpful as well. Historical information that can alert the clinician to be concerned about physical abuse may include a changing history, an unwitnessed event, a lack of detailed information or no history of trauma at all, a delay in seeking medical care, or a history inconsistent with the child's developmental abilities. A 2-month-old infant cannot yet roll over, so the baby should not be able to roll off the adult bed unassisted to cause an injury.

Physical abuse or a traumatic injury may not be the chief concern at a medical appointment and yet this becomes a critical component of the encounter when discovered. When an injury is found on a child during examination, the same questioning regarding the history of present illness should be used to help determine if this finding is concerning for physical abuse. Always ask what happened of the caregiver and child, even if the mark does not appear initially concerning, as this questioning then becomes habit and a routine practice as part of the medical assessment. In older children, caregivers may not know what caused every mark or scrape on their child; this can also be the case if the parent at the medical assessment is the nonoffending caregiver or not the primary caregiver. In these cases, older verbal children are often able to give important historical information regarding their own injuries. Children and caregivers should be asked basic screening questions regarding discipline, the use of corporal punishment, and exposure to IPV (see **Box 24.3**).

BOX 24.3
SCREENING QUESTIONS FOR CORPORAL PUNISHMENT AND INTIMATE PARTNER VIOLENCE

Corporal Punishment Screening
Parent/Caregiver

1. How do you discipline your child?
2. Do you or anyone else ever spank your child with your hand?
   a. Where on the child's body?
   b. How often?
   c. Has it ever left a mark?
3. Do you or anyone else ever hit your child with an object?
   a. What object?
   b. Where on the child's body?
   c. How often?
   d. Has it ever left a mark?
4. Do you ever use other physical means of discipline?
5. Do you ever use nonphysical means of discipline?

Child

1. What happens when you get in trouble?
2. What does Mommy do when you get in trouble?
3. What does Daddy do when you get in trouble?

(continued)

BOX 24.3
SCREENING QUESTIONS FOR CORPORAL PUNISHMENT AND INTIMATE PARTNER VIOLENCE (*continued*)

4. Does anyone ever hit, spank, or whoop you?
   a. What do they hit you with?
   b. Where on your body do they hit?
   c. Who hits you?
   d. How often do you get hit?
   e. Does it ever leave a mark on your body?

Intimate Partner Violence
Parent/Caregiver/Dating Teens

1. Have you ever been hit, kicked, punched, or hurt by a partner/spouse/boyfriend/girlfriend or have they ever threatened to hurt you?
2. Do you feel safe in your current relationship?
3. Do you have a past relationship where you did not feel safe or were afraid?
4. Is there a partner/spouse/boyfriend/girlfriend from a past or current relationship who is making you feel afraid or unsafe?
5. Has a partner/spouse/boyfriend/girlfriend ever made you feel ashamed, embarrassed, or emotionally hurt?
6. Have you ever been forced to have sex?
7. Have weapons ever been used against you?

Child/Adolescent

1. What happens when Mom and Dad fight?
2. Have you ever seen anyone hit/push/hurt Mom?
3. Have you ever seen anyone hit/push/hurt Dad?

Source: Adapted from Hornor, G. (2013). Child maltreatment: Screening and anticipatory guidance. *Journal of Pediatric Health Care, 27*(4), 242–249. doi:10.1016/j.pedhc.2013.02.001

Sexual Abuse

The healthcare presentation of children experiencing sexual abuse is varied. Children may present with a chief concern of sexual abuse; at other times, the abuse is not the stated chief concern and must be identified by the healthcare clinician. Common chief concerns that may raise the concern of possible sexual abuse include pregnancy, anogenital trauma, discharge, bleeding, pain, or lesions. Sometimes the sequelae of sexual abuse manifest themselves before children make a disclosure about their abuse. Knowledge of potential sexual abuse consequences can assist the clinician both in recognizing abuse and understanding children's experience and reaction.

Children experience sexual abuse differently; therefore, the development of physical and mental health consequences from such abuse may vary. Children who are initially asymptomatic may become symptomatic over time. Sexualized behaviors exhibited by children are often part of normal development, such as touching or looking at the genitalia of themselves or peers. Sexual abuse or exposure to sexual behavior (pornography or adults engaging in sexual activity) should be considered when a child exhibits concerning sexual behaviors. Concerning sexualized behaviors exhibited by children include sexual behaviors that are persistent (with the child becoming angry at distraction attempts), coercive, abusive, developmentally abnormal, or involving children who are 4 years or more apart in age. Sexual problems in adolescence and adulthood can also result from experiencing child sexual abuse. Child sexual abuse increases the risk for early initiation of sexual activity and engaging in high-risk sexual behaviors, including multiple sexual partners and having unprotected sex (Abajobir, Kisely, Maravilla, Williams, & Najman, 2017).

Other problematic behaviors and mental health sequelae can develop following child sexual abuse. These problems can extend into adulthood. The most common psychiatric disorder noted in victims of sexual abuse is PTSD. Symptoms of PTSD may develop immediately following the victimization or present months or even years later (Chowdhury, 2011). Sexual abuse victims may exhibit symptoms of attention deficit hyperactivity disorder (ADHD; Fuller-Thomson & Lewis, 2015). They may be misdiagnosed as having ADHD when the symptoms are actually the result of sexual abuse trauma and should more accurately be diagnosed as PTSD or anxiety. Depression, suicidal ideation and behaviors, nonsuicidal self-injury, substance abuse, borderline personality disorder, eating disorders, conduct disorders, and somatization along with other psychiatric disorders can also develop following sexual abuse (Easton & Kong, 2017; Maniglio, 2009).

The optimal healthcare assessment for sexual abuse requires a team approach. The clinician with the most training in sexual abuse assessments should proceed with the evaluation. Depending on the institutional resources available, a pediatric sexual assault nurse examiner may be employed to perform the history and physical examination. A social worker trained in interviewing children may conduct a forensic interview. Triage is the first step in the healthcare assessment for sexual abuse. When talking to a child regarding sexual abuse concerns, questions should be asked in an open-ended, nonleading, and developmentally appropriate manner. Any statements made by the patient regarding their sexual abuse must be clearly documented. This information is necessary for medical assessment and diagnosis; in addition, many courts have allowed

BOX 24.4
SEXUAL ABUSE SCREENING QUESTIONS

Parent/Caregiver

- Do you have any concerns of sexual abuse?
- Is there a history of sexual abuse in your or your partner's family?
- Were you or your partner a victim of child sexual abuse?
- Is your child ever in contact with anyone who has been accused of sexually abusing a child or adolescent?

Child

- Have the child identify body parts.
- Have the child identify their private parts.
- Using the child's words for their private parts, ask if anyone has ever touched, tickled, hurt, or put anything in their private parts.

Adolescent

- Introduce the subject of sex. Clarify the adolescent's meaning of the word.
- Ask the adolescent if they have ever had sex when they wanted to.
- How old were you when you first had sex?
- How many partners have you had?
- How old are the people you have had sex with?
- Has anyone ever forced you to have sex when you did not want to or touch you in a sexual way when you did not want them to?

Source: Adapted from Hornor, G. (2011). Medical evaluation for child sexual abuse: What the PNP needs to know. *Journal of Pediatric Health Care, 25*(4), 250–256. doi:10.1016/j.pedhc.2011.01.004

clinicians to testify regarding specific details of a pediatric patient's statements obtained when gathering a medical history (Kellogg, 2005). It is vital that the clinician understand state laws/sexual abuse protocols defining acute versus nonacute sexual abuse.

Children presenting for care with anogenital symptoms, pregnancy, or the previously discussed behavioral symptoms should be asked a few sexual abuse screening questions (see **Box 24.4**). The anogenital examination, which should be a part of every well-child examination, offers the clinician an opportunity to educate the child about the concept of private parts and to ask a few screening questions (see **Box 24.4**), which may identify a concern for sexual abuse. Children disclosing a concern of sexual abuse to the clinician or presenting with a chief concern of sexual abuse should be asked a few questions on the minimal facts to obtain the information needed to report a concern of suspected sexual abuse to Child Protective Services (CPS) and law enforcement (see **Table 24.2**). A detailed history of the sexual abuse need not be obtained by the clinician, except for those specializing in child sexual abuse, as the clinician understands that the child will need to be interviewed by an individual trained to talk to the child in a forensically sound and child-friendly manner. The clinician should obtain a history from the caregiver and pediatric patient separately.

Children who present with complaints of anogenital symptoms (bleeding, pain, or discharge) or who present acutely (typically within 72 hours of the latest incident of sexual abuse) need to be evaluated as soon as possible that same day. Acutely presenting children may require referral to a child advocacy center or emergency department to facilitate forensic evidence collection. Children presenting nonacutely (typically >72 hours since the latest incident of sexual abuse and/or without complaints of anogenital symptoms) do not require an

TABLE 24.2 Minimal Facts/Information for Reporting Sexual Abuse

	Key Questions	Purpose
WHO	Who sexually abused the child? Does the child live with the alleged perpetrator?	To determine immediate safety of the child.
WHAT	What happened? Brief history of which body part of the perpetrator touched which body part of the child/adolescent victim.	To determine need for sexually transmitted infection testing.
WHEN	When did the sexual abuse last happen or, if child is unable to give the time frame, when did the child last have contact with the alleged perpetrator?	To determine whether the sexual abuse is acute or nonacute.
WHERE	Where does the child live? Where did the sexual abuse occur?	To determine Child Protective Services and law enforcement jurisdiction.

Note: Minimum information that needs to be obtained if child abuse is suspected. Clinicians need to be aware of state laws regarding child abuse reporting.

immediate healthcare assessment. Depending on the institutional protocol and resources, the nonacutely presenting patient may be referred to a child advocacy center or child abuse specialist for evaluation at a later date. For both acutely and nonacutely presenting children, a referral to CPS and local law enforcement should be made immediately to assure the child's safety.

Emotional Abuse

Although many times challenging, assessment of exposure to emotional maltreatment is very important to the child's overall health. It is important for the clinician to be aware of the possibility of this exposure when assessing mental health and behavioral concerns. The AAP recommends that whenever possible, information regarding the specific details related to the mental health or behavioral concern should be gathered from different informants involved in the child's care and well-being, such as teachers, caregiver, and daycare providers. When developmentally appropriate, speaking with the child is an important piece of the assessment as well to obtain details regarding their relationship with the caregiver as well as normative discipline practices. The interview should be completed in a child-friendly, unbiased format. The AAP recommends that the interview be done away from the caregiver as the maltreatment may be perpetrated by the person who brought them to the office (Hibbard et al., 2012).

Although emotional maltreatment can occur in any family, it is most often associated with multiple family stressors (Hibbard et al., 2012). When assessing for emotional maltreatment, it is important to be knowledgeable of the parental risk factors that can carry an association with this form of maltreatment. These risk factors can include poor parenting skills, substance abuse, depression, suicidal ideation, and/or suicide attempts, as well as other mental health concerns such as low self-esteem, inadequate social support including lack of social skills, and added social stress. Emotional maltreatment can also be a sequelae of IPV (Kairys et al., 2002).

Documentation of emotional maltreatment can be difficult. It often requires knowledge of behavioral changes and concerning events that can span a period of time. A clinician will need knowledge of the child's baseline development and behaviors as well. Assessing the child's physical growth is important because often the only physical finding may be weight gain or loss (Kairys et al., 2002). Because of these factors, there is often a delay in diagnosis and reporting to CPS.

Neglect

Neglected children can present to healthcare clinicians in a variety of ways, rarely with neglect being the chief concern. Possible healthcare presentations of child neglect include the following: delay in seeking healthcare, failure to follow through with the prescribed healthcare

---

BOX 24.5

SAFE ENVIRONMENT FOR EVERY KID PARENT QUESTIONNAIRE (SEEK)

- Phone number for poison control
- Need for a smoke detector
- Exposure to tobacco smoke
- Food insecurity
- Child difficult to care for
- Need to hit/spank your child
- Parental depression
- Intimate partner violence
- Parental drugs/alcohol

Source: Dubowitz, H. (2014). The Safe Environment for Every Kid model: Promotion of children's health, development, and safety, and prevention of child neglect. *Pediatric Annals,* *43*(11), e271–e277. doi:10.3928/00904481-20141022-11

---

plan, nutritional concerns (nonorganic failure to thrive or morbid obesity), exposure to environmental hazards (IPV, car accidents, guns, cigarette smoke, unsafe housing), inadequate supervision, injuries, intrauterine drug exposure, childhood drug exposures/ingestions, homelessness, abandonment, or inadequate hygiene or clothing (Dubowitz, Giardino, & Gustavson, 2000). The clinician must be able to recognize the situation as neglectful. There are evidence-based screening tools that can be used to screen for neglect risk factors. One commonly used screening tool is the Safe Environment for Every Kid Parent Questionnaire™ (SEEK-PQ-R). This evidence-based questionnaire (**Box 24.5**) is designed for use in pediatric primary care settings. Its goal is to prevent child maltreatment by identifying risk factors for child maltreatment such as parental depression and substance abuse, domestic violence, harsh punishment, food insecurity, and major stress (www.seek wellbeing.org/background). Identifying these types of psychosocial issues in families and then providing appropriate interventions has been shown to reduce risk for child maltreatment. The SEEK model was developed, in part, to help healthcare clinicians feel more comfortable in addressing family psychosocial issues. Researchers have found that clinicians who implemented the use of SEEK in their clinics improved and sustained levels of confidence and competence in screening for all risk factors (Dubowitz et al., 2011). SEEK training and resources are available via www .seekwellbeing.org.

There are certain factors to consider that can assist the clinician when evaluating for possible child neglect (**Table 24.3**). When considering a healthcare assessment for neglect, the first step involves examining the neglect in terms of extent, severity, frequency, chronicity, and harm/health consequences (Fong & Christian 2012).

TABLE 24.3 Child Neglect Evaluation

Criteria 1	Child's basic needs are not being met, leading to harm or risk of harm.
Criteria 2	Harm is serious or potentially serious.
Criteria 3	Harm is frequent and chronic.
Criteria 4	Assess potential barriers for caregiver in meeting child's needs • Lack of access to resources (e.g., financial, geographic) • Lack of caregiver understanding (e.g., cognitive delay) • Presence of psychosocial risk factors (e.g., caregiver mental health or substance abuse, intimate partner violence) • Previous Child Protective Services involvement
If criteria 1 is met	Neglect evaluation is indicated.
If criteria 2 and/or 3 are met	Report to CPS is indicated • Provide appropriate intervention to address neglect concern • Monitor adherence to plan of care • Reassess after intervention • Communicate to CPS child's needs are now being adequately met • Communicate to CPS continued inadequacy of needs being met
If criteria 4 is met but not 2 or 3	No CPS report indicated at this time • Provide appropriate intervention to address neglect concern • Provide appropriate intervention to address identified barrier • Monitor caregiver's ability to follow care plan • Reassess after intervention • Report to CPS may become necessary if criteria 2 and/or 3 met after reassessment

CPS, Child Protective Services.
Note: Criteria for conducting a thorough, evidence-based assessment when child neglect is suspected.
Source: Boston Medical Center Child Protection Team. (2012). *Evaluation tool for medical neglect.* Boston, MA: Author. Retrieved from http://www.bmc.org/sites/default/files/For_Medical_Professionals/Pediatric_Resources/Pediatrics__Child_Protection_Team__CPT_/Tools_and _Medical_Evaluation_Abuse/field_Attachments/medical-neglect.pdf

Did caregiver action or lack of action result in serious or potentially serious physical, emotional, or developmental harm to the child (Hornor, 2014)? If the answer to that question is "Yes," then the clinician is obligated to report a concern of suspected neglect to CPS. CPS is then responsible for determining a safety plan for the child and deciding if it is safe to discharge the patient home with the caregiver. Best practices dictate that it is crucial to inform the caregiver of the concerns of neglect and discuss the need to report this to CPS. This openness is crucial in ensuring preservation of the professional relationship with the family so that clinician and caregiver can together devise a plan to correct the neglect concern.

An assessment of potential barriers that are present which contribute to the caregiver's ability to provide adequate care to their children will provide vital information to help in the clinician's reporting decision and also to share with CPS, if reported. Gather a thorough psychosocial history assessing for potential barriers. Assess for a repetitive pattern of neglect. Is the neglect concern an isolated issue, or is it one of multiple neglect concerns? Have there been previous reports of suspected physical abuse, sexual abuse, or neglect to CPS? Has the caregiver previously demonstrated an inability to comply with a prescribed plan of care? If the answer is "Yes" to one or more of these questions, then a referral to CPS is most likely indicated. Allen and Fost (2012) describe three criteria for determining the need to report a concern of neglect to CPS: there exists a serious or imminent threat of harm to a child's health or safety, interventions have previously been unsuccessful or unavailable, and there exists a reasonable likelihood that CPS intervention will be effective. The clinician may also seek guidance from a child abuse specialist when available to assist in decision making.

Elder Abuse

When obtaining a health history from an older person, it is important to be familiar with the risk factors for elder abuse. There are particular risk-factor levels that make an older adult more susceptible to abuse. These risk factors can be identified as a combination of individual, relationship, community, and sociocultural levels.

TABLE 24.4 Risk Factors for Elder Abuse: Contributing Risk Factor Levels for Abuse in the Community	
Individual	Poor physical and mental health Functional impairment Level of dependence on a caregiver Dementia and cognitive impairment Gender of the victim (women may be at increased risk of persistent and severe forms of abuse and injury)
Relationship	Shared living arrangements Dysfunctional family relationships Caregiver burden
Community	Social isolation Lack of social support
Sociocultural	Stereotypes of older adults as frail, weak, dependent Loss of family relationships between generations Lack of funds for caregiving
Institutions	Poor standards for healthcare Welfare services Poorly trained staff who are overworked Deteriorating physical environment Policies developed for the institution rather than residents

Source: National Center on Elder Abuse. (n.d.). *Statistics and data.* Retrieved from https://ncea.acl.gov/What-We-Do/Research/Statistics-and-Data.aspx; World Health Organization. (2018, June 8). *Elder abuse.* Retrieved from https://www.who.int/news-room/fact-sheets/detail/elder-abuse

Additionally, both the victim's and the abuser's mental and physical conditions can be risk factors for abuse/likelihood of abusing (Jackson, 2018; National Center on Elder Abuse, n.d.; WHO, 2018). See **Table 24.4** for more information on risk factors that need to be identified when doing a health history in an older adult.

PAST MEDICAL HISTORY

Even when a patient is only a few days old, obtaining a past medical history is an important part of the information gathering process for all medical assessments. Starting from the mother's pregnancy and moving forward to the day of presentation can provide details relevant in a case concerning for abuse. Although a lay person may not classify child birth as traumatic, there are many complicated steps that occur during this process and injuries can occur. Knowing the details of the delivery can help ascertain whether an injury could be caused by a traumatic birth. Information regarding other hospitalizations or emergency department visits, no matter the chief concern, is helpful as well. Whether the child has sustained fractures, burns, needed stitches, or had other significant injuries are all relevant details when assessing a pediatric patient.

Whether the child is routinely treated by a primary care clinician, had surgery, has allergies or routine medication usage, has up-to-date immunizations, and has any chronic medical conditions that are being managed are all important factors to note when assessing past medical history. The developmental abilities of the child at baseline from the caregiver's perspective and from the clinician's assessment will alert the clinician as to if there is or could be a developmental delay, another concern, or some discrepancy between the history given and the abilities of the patient.

When concerns of sexual abuse arise, the following past medical history information will be important to obtain. It is important to know if there have been past concerns of sexual abuse and if they have been reported to and investigated by CPS and law enforcement. Are there current or past complaints of the following: anogenital pain; anogenital bleeding, discharge, or itching; dysuria; pain with bowel movements; constipation; and recent medical treatment of anogenital conditions? Inquire about any history of past surgical interventions to the anogenital region to explain any injuries. Ask about any current or past infection(s) with any sexually transmitted disease(s), including gonorrhea, chlamydia, syphilis, *Trichomonas vaginalis*, HIV, anogenital warts, and anogenital herpes simplex virus type 1 or type 2. This also raises the concern of sexual abuse in a nonconsensually sexually active adolescent.

FAMILY HISTORY

Family medical history should also be noted with all pediatric patient encounters as some rare genetic conditions may initially present with examination findings concerning physical abuse, in particular. It is common to ask what medical conditions run in the family, but eliciting details regarding easy bruising or bleeding, frequent fractures, and metabolic or genetic conditions in extended family members can help guide a medical workup when there is concern for physical abuse.

Caregiver history of experiencing child maltreatment can also affect their ability to parent, and there can be a familial pattern to child maltreatment. Inquire as to a parental/caregiver history of sexual abuse, physical abuse, and/or neglect as a child or involvement with CPS. Parental mental health issues, including depression, and past/current substance use/abuse should be assessed. Although some may consider these social topics "sensitive," families are often forthcoming to medical clinicians when asked in a respectful and open manner. Reassuring parents that these questions are asked of all families in order to best help the patient can alleviate some fears and misgivings that the clinician or family may have. Familial strengths and supports should also be assessed.

SOCIAL HISTORY

Obtaining a social history and being cognizant of the risk factors for the previously discussed maltreatment can help guide medical decision-making. In addition to the previously detailed risk factors, parental age (young), low educational attainment, single parenthood, a large number of dependent children in the home, and low-income households are also associated with perpetration (CDC, 2018). Who lives in the home, who cares for the child, any interactions of the family with CPS and/or law enforcement (LE), and other social stressors (substance abuse, unstable housing, IPV, caregiver mental health concerns, financial concerns) provide information regarding the daily life of the child. Ask about nonbiological, transient caregivers in the home (e.g., mother's male partner) as these individuals can be more likely to be perpetrators (CDC, 2018). Asking about discipline techniques used in the home is informative. Although spanking is common in many households, leaving marks or bruises can qualify this behavior as physical abuse in many states.

It is important to gather a sexual history from adolescents, including past consensual or forced sexual intercourse, timing of past intercourse, number of sexual partners, age of sexual partners, gender of sexual partners, age at initiation of sexual intercourse, and use of birth control and safe sex practices (Hornor, 2011).

REVIEW OF SYSTEMS

Questions included in this section may prompt the caregiver's memory regarding other concerns or details that may be worrisome in relationship to abuse. Especially in young infants, changes in demeanor or behavior (anything from fussiness to lethargy) can be an alert that something abnormal is going on internally. A history of bleeding from the mouth, ears, or nose in a young infant could be a sign of a prior sentinel injury, which should prompt concern. *Sentinel injuries* are described as more minor inflicted injuries in young nonmobile children that sometime precede more severe physical abuse (Sheets, 2013). Vomiting alone or possible seizure activity can signal an intracranial abnormality. Abusive head trauma (AHT), previously known as shaken baby syndrome, has been shown to present in a variety of ways and can be challenging to diagnose (Jenny, 1999); therefore, obtaining a thorough review of systems for any medical changes in a young child is vital.

PREVENTIVE CARE CONSIDERATIONS

Child Abuse

Child maltreatment is preventable. Child maltreatment is the largest preventable causal influence of child mental health disorders in the United States (Constantio, 2016). Healthcare clinicians can play an essential role in the prevention of child maltreatment and other psychosocial traumas. All patients and their caregivers should be screened for exposure to ACEs and linked to appropriate interventions if screenings are positive.

Healthcare clinicians need to consistently encourage parents and caregivers to use positive parenting practices including nonphysical methods of discipline. Educate parents regarding developmentally appropriate behavioral expectations and the power of praising a child for good behavior. Evidence-based child maltreatment programs include Nurse–Family Partnership, Triple P-Positive Parenting Program, Strong Communities for Children, Durham Family Initiative, Stop It Now, and Well Baby Plus (Molnar, Beatriz, & Beardslee, 2016). For example, the Nurse–Family Partnership is a home-visitation program provided by nurses to low-income first-time mothers beginning prenatally and continuing through the child's second birthday. In a study by Eckenrode et al. (2000), they found that families receiving home visitation during pregnancy and infancy had significantly fewer child maltreatment reports involving the mother as perpetrator or the study child as the subject when compared with families not receiving home visitation. Additionally, the study also concluded that the presence of domestic violence may be a limit in the effectiveness of interventions to reduce incidence of child abuse and neglect (Eckenrode et al., 2000). For these reasons, in families where a suspicion of maltreatment or risk factors for maltreatment have been identified, timely referrals to community programs, counseling services, or CPS are vital to prevent further abuse/neglect.

Anticipatory guidance is a valuable tool that the medical clinician can offer in the office during each visit that will help to educate the caregiver on normal growth and development and positive parenting techniques. By understanding normal growth and development, the caregiver will be able to have realistic expectations for their children; this education can also assist the caregiver in providing enriching experiences to support healthy brain development.

Anticipatory guidance specific to the prevention of child sexual abuse includes parental/caregiver understanding of the following concepts: Most children are not sexually abused by strangers but rather by someone they know, trust, and love; never leave your child with someone who has a history of sexually abusing a child as they are at high risk to sexually abuse again; pedophiles present as normal, healthy individuals and parents should pay attention if an adult wants to spend a lot of alone time with the child. Most children who are sexually abused will have no physical signs of abuse even on examination by a healthcare clinician.

Evidence-based familial protective factors include a supportive and stable family environment, support of basic needs including stable housing, nurturing parenting style, exposure to positive role models outside household contacts, household rules, access to healthcare and social services, and parental education and employment. Communities that support parents can also play an important role in child abuse prevention (CDC, 2018).

Intimate Partner Violence

The U.S. Preventive Services Task Force (USPSTF, 2018) recommends that clinicians screen women of childbearing age for IPV and provide (or refer) women who screen positive to intervention services. This recommendation includes women who do not currently exhibit signs of abuse. The American College of Obstetricians and Gynecologists (ACOG), the USDHHS, and the Institute of Medicine (IOM) assert that routine preventive healthcare for women, as well as obstetric care, should include IPV screening at regular intervals (ACOG, 2012). Screening can be performed by the clinician or self-administered via paper form or electronically. The screening tools that have shown the best sensitivity and specificity are shown in **Box 24.6** (USPSTF, 2018).

Although the strongest recommendation is for routine screening of all women of childbearing age, all at-risk populations can be screened. The key to eliciting a disclosure of abuse and gathering an accurate history is establishing a rapport in a private setting. Clinicians should avoid terms that are associated with stigma, such as *battered woman* or *victim of domestic violence*, but rather use terms that focus on *experiencing violence, getting hurt,* or *being fearful.* People who feel judged or shamed are less likely to disclose abuse to the clinician. It is helpful to frame the question first, for example, "Many patients I see have experienced violence in their relationships, so now I talk with everyone about safe relationships." Then, proceed with a

---

BOX 24.6

EVIDENCE-BASED INTIMATE PARTNER VIOLENCE SCREENING TOOLS

- HITS (Hurt, Insult, Threaten, Scream)
- OVAT (Ongoing Violence Assessment Tool)
- STaT (Slapped, Things, and Threaten)
- HARK (Humiliation, Afraid, Rape, Kick)
- CTQ-SF (Modified Childhood Trauma Questionnaire-Short Form)
- WAST (Women Abuse Screen Tool)

Source: U.S. Preventative Services Task Force. (2018, April). *Screening for intimate partner violence, elder abuse, and abuse of vulnerable adults.* Retrieved from https://www.uspreventiveservicestaskforce.org/USPSTF_Admin/Home/GetFileByID/3589

---

nonjudgmental question; for example, "Has your partner ever made you feel afraid?"

Child abuse reporting is mandated in every state, but IPV reporting is controversial and can vary from state to state. It is important for clinicians to understand their state laws regarding mandated reporting and which information can be kept confidential if requested.

Elder Abuse

Whereas the statistics on elder abuse are very troubling, the USPSTF found insufficient evidence that screening for elder abuse reduces harm and the effectiveness of interventions is unclear. The USPSTF notes additional research is needed in regards to how clinicians screen for and address elder abuse. The current USPSTF recommendation for screening older adults is grade I; current evidence is insufficient to assess the balance of benefits and harms of screening (USPSTF, 2018).

Although there is no recommended screening tool, clinicians do have the option of using existing elder abuse screening tools. When using an existing screening tool, clinicians should use the screening as part of a holistic assessment and include their clinical judgment and clinical expertise. They should not rely entirely on the screening tool. Available elder abuse screening tools are noted in the following list. An appropriate time to consider screening would be when abuse is suspected or yearly during preventive health visits.

- Elder Abuse Suspicion Index (EASI)
- Brief Abuse Screen for the Elderly (BASE)
- Hwalek–Sengstock Elder Abuse Screening Test (H-S/EAST)
- Vulnerability to Abuse Screening Scale (VASS)

- Elder Assessment Instrument (EAI)
- Indicators of Abuse (IOA; Jackson, 2018)

PHYSICAL EXAMINATION

PHYSICAL ABUSE

The physical examination begins immediately when the clinician encounters a patient, starting with inspection. The initial visualization can alert the clinician if the child is critically ill and needs emergent intervention, is happy and playful, or is withdrawn and depressed. Vital signs are called such because they can be very informative and of utmost importance. Heart rate, respiratory rate, and blood pressure are routinely obtained for all patients. For pediatric patients, height, weight, and head circumference (if <3 years old) are also performed. Children grow differently, but standard growth charts are used to help the clinician assess if growth is a medical issue. For example, an infant whose head circumference has rapidly grown in a short amount of time may have an intracranial injury, whereas a toddler who is dropping percentiles on the weight curve may have malnutrition secondary to neglect. Although not always possible, being able to compare two or more growth points separated by time can provide more information to the overall trend of the patient's growth than one value on the day of the medical appointment. It is also important to note the child's hygiene and appropriateness of clothing. Oral hygiene and the presence of dental caries/fractures should be assessed. Throughout the examination, the clinician should observe the child's behavior and the interaction between the caregiver and

child. This can give important insight into the family dynamics, the parent–child relationships, and red flags for abuse or neglect.

Once immediate needs have been assessed, the examination continues with complete inspection. This critical examination technique may get overlooked if it is not a conscious decision with every patient. It is very important for a pediatric patient to change their clothing into a gown for a head-to-toe examination as skin injuries are easily concealed by restrictive clothing. The skin is the largest organ in the body and is subject to a variety of injuries. Bruising, although a common accidental injury in a mobile child, is a critical injury in a young infant, as seen in a study by Sugar et al., "Those Who Don't Cruise Rarely Bruise" (1999). Of the children younger than 6 months, only 0.6% had any bruises, and in the children younger than 9 months, only 1.7% had bruises. These numbers only increased slightly to 2.2% in children who were not yet walking with support, or cruising. Bruises became much more common once children were mobile, as 51.9% of walkers had bruises. Typical sites for these injuries in the walker group were the anterior tibia and knee, forehead, and upper leg, whereas bruises to the face and trunk were rare and were not seen at all on the hands and buttocks.

Other studies have demonstrated the common locations for accidental bruises and a clinical decision rule has been developed to help clinicians determine locations that are more concerning than others (Maguire, 2005b; Pierce, 2010; Pierce et al., 2015). Called TEN-4, the clinical decision rule by Pierce et al. (2015) describes the characteristics predictive of abuse as bruising to the torso (**Figure 24.2**), ears (**Figure 24.3**), or neck (TEN; **Figure 24.4**) for any child less than or equal to

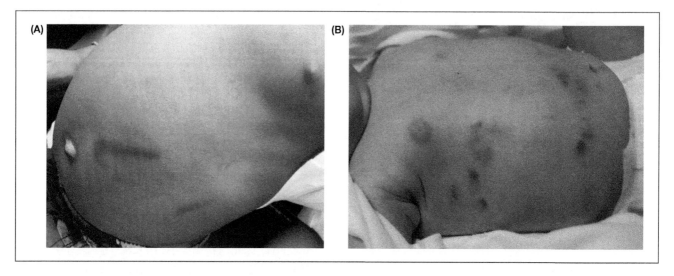

FIGURE 24.2 Torso bruising. (A) Torso ecchymosis in an older child. Note the pattern with the linear and then curved portion. (B) Scattered torso ecchymoses in various stages of healing on an infant.

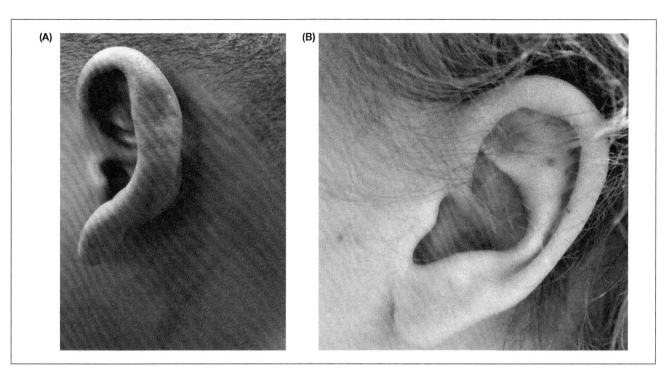

FIGURE 24.3 Ear bruising. (A) Dramatic presentation of ear ecchymosis in a young child. Crescent-shaped ecchymosis found behind the ear (or the Battle sign) can indicate a basilar skull fracture. (B) Scattered pinpoint ecchymoses on the pinna, demonstrating a more subtle presentation of child abuse that could be missed on examination without careful inspection. Ear bruising can be from pinching, twisting, or pulling or a direct blow to the head that compresses the ear between the skull and whatever is hitting the head.

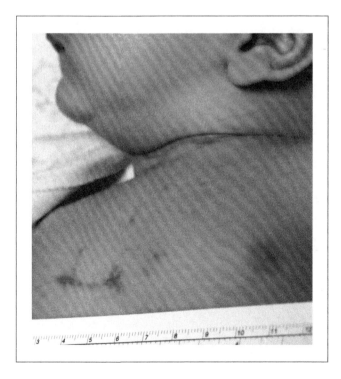

FIGURE 24.4 Neck bruising. Scattered ecchymoses on the neck and upper torso of an infant, aligning with the TEN-4 clinical decision rule.

4 years old and bruising in any location on an infant less than 4 months old. When these injuries are found, it should prompt the clinician to initiate a workup for physical abuse, investigating for other occult injuries. Although bruises to the face (**Figure 24.5**), back, abdomen, arms, buttocks (**Figure 24.6**), ears, and hands are suggestive of physical abuse, any injury can be inflicted and no injury should be interpreted in isolation. Skin injury characteristics that should make a clinician concerned for physical abuse also include different stages of healing, patterns (**Figure 24.7**), bites, burns, and signs of injury to additional body systems. Although a common misconception, Maguire's 2005 systematic review demonstrated that bruises are not able to be accurately dated whether evaluated in person or by photograph and medical clinicians should avoid estimating the age of a bruise when performing their assessment (Maguire, 2005b, 2013).

A discussion of bruising in young children bridges into the concept of sentinel injuries. The most commonly seen sentinel injuries are bruises, intraoral injuries like frenula tears (**Figure 24.8**), and subconjunctival hemorrhages (**Figure 24.9**), especially if associated with facial petechiae. Because these are not life-threatening injuries, they may get dismissed by clinicians and caregivers as unimportant at the time of

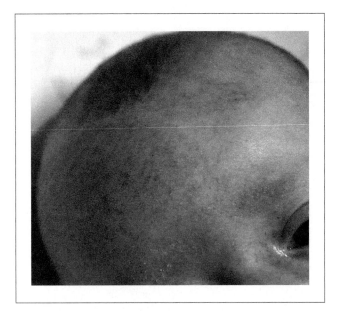

FIGURE 24.5 Facial bruising. Scattered ecchymoses on the forehead and nasal bridge of an infant.

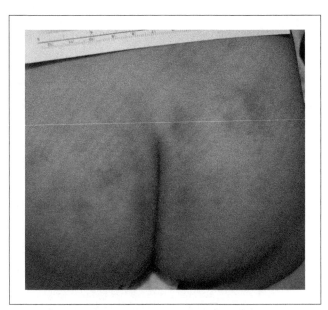

FIGURE 24.6 Buttock bruising. Severe buttock ecchymoses in various stages of healing in a young child.

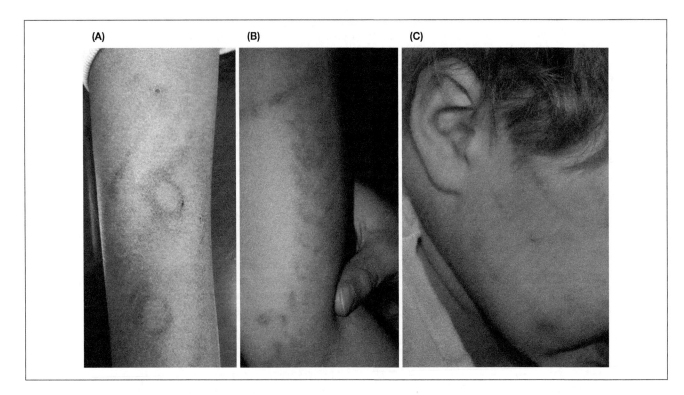

FIGURE 24.7 Pattern bruising. (A and B) These are examples of pattern bruising inflicted by a belt. (C) A common presentation of a healing slap mark on a young child's face.

injury or evaluation. They also may be the first and only injury found. However, studies have shown that the presence of these injuries or historical report of said injuries should heighten concern for physical abuse and the clinician should pursue a medical workup for occult injuries, as this intervention may prevent the abuse from escalating to further harm to the child. Even if the sentinel injury is the only injury found following a thorough workup for physical abuse, this should not diminish the original concern; the child still is in need of protection and is at risk of further harm if there is no intervention.

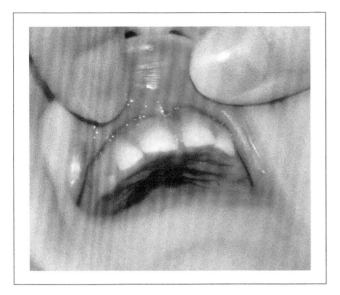

FIGURE 24.8 Upper lip frenulum tear, a common sentinel injury.

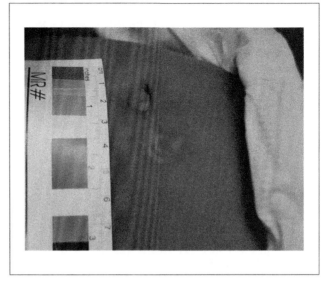

FIGURE 24.10 Lighter burn scar. Abdominal scar on an infant from a lighter burn.

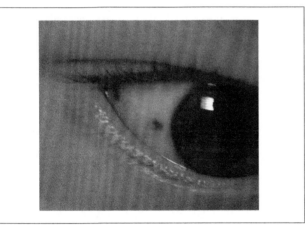

FIGURE 24.9 Small subconjunctival hemorrhages. Increases in intrathoracic pressure, a direct blow to the eye, or covert suffocation can cause rupture of the small blood vessels of the subconjunctiva.

Evaluating the skin for burn injuries is another important aspect of the inspection portion of the examination. Burns are a very common injury in childhood, but up to 20% of cases are secondary to abuse and neglect. When burns are an abusive injury, the child is typically less than 6 years old, is sicker from their injury overall with an increased morbidity, and may have other concerning injuries on their physical examination (Hodgman, 2016; Maguire, 2008). Burns are classified based on the depth of tissue injury. A superficial burn, like a sunburn for example, extends only into the epidermis, the most external layer of skin. If blisters form, the burn is deeper, from superficial to deep partial thickness into the dermis. Finally, a full-thickness burn extends into the subcutaneous tissue and possibly muscle and can damage the nerve endings of the skin (Hettiaratchy, 2004; Krishnamoorthy, 2012).

Thermal burns are the most common type of burn in children overall with scalding by immersion into hot water the most frequently reported abusive burn injury. The location of the burn on the body and the pattern on the skin are the most telling as to whether the history matches the injury. Burn injury to the hands, feet, buttocks, back, or perineum are all extremely concerning for an inflicted burn. Immersion burns typically have a pattern with uniform depth, sparing of the flexor creases of the joints, a sharp line of demarcation between injured and noninjured skin, an absence of splash marks, and areas of sparing if the skin was touching a cool surface, like the bottom of a sink or tub (Maguire, 2008). Contact burns occur secondary to prolonged contact with a solid or smoldering source and produce distinct margins and patterns (**Figure 24.10;** Jinna, 2017). Burns change over time so knowing what the injury looked like when it first occurred in comparison to how it has been healing can help put the pieces together in regards to mechanism of injury. Any cutaneous injuries should be documented and photographed. The presence of rashes or lesions that may be the result of neglect, such as diaper dermatitis, should also be noted.

Palpation is somewhat different in the pediatric patients and has specific aspects to consider. Because of their developmental abilities, young children do not always provide the most reliable examinations. They are not able to clearly verbalize, are often unable to specifically localize their pain, and cannot always follow directions when performing an examination. Because of this, clinicians often should rely on radiological studies when there is concern for physical abuse in a young child and an occult injury is a concern. Palpation may reveal callus formation from a healing fracture or swelling from an acute injury, but these findings would still prompt the clinician to obtain imaging to clarify the diagnosis and are not always readily apparent on examination.

SEXUAL ABUSE

The physical examination for suspected sexual abuse requires a complete head-to-toe physical assessment. It is especially crucial to perform a thorough cutaneous examination as sexual abuse can often be accompanied by other forms of child maltreatment such as physical abuse. Nongenital injuries should be identified and documented in both written and photographic form.

Prepubertal Female Anogenital Examination

The anogenital examination, regardless of age or gender, should begin with a thorough inspection of the external anogenital anatomy for signs of acute or chronic trauma, lesions, or discharge. Sexual maturity should be assessed and documented.

Anatomical differences exist in prepubertal and pubertal female genital anatomy. The clinician must be familiar with normal female prepubertal anogenital anatomy (**Figure 24.11**). Use of a speculum is never indicated in the prepubertal female anogenital examination unless unexplained vaginal bleeding is present; in that situation, the examination is performed under general anesthesia (Adams, Farst, & Kellogg, 2018). The prepubertal hymen is sensitive; touching it should be avoided. An adequate light for visualization is necessary, such as an otoscope. Colposcopy, which provides a source of light and magnification, can assist the clinician with visualization and the ability to photographically document the examination.

Position the pediatric patient in the supine frog-leg position, possibly in the caregiver's lap, or stirrups may be utilized. The prone knee-chest position may facilitate visualization of the hymen and should always be used when there is a suspected abnormal finding noted in the supine position. Crucial for optimal visualization of genital anatomy is utilization of proper traction technique, which involves adequate separation and pulling of the labia majora toward the clinician (**Figure 24.12**).

Normal saline or water can be flushed into the vestibule to facilitate visualization of the hymenal opening

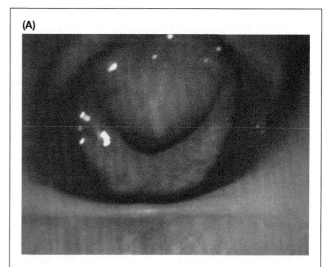
(A)

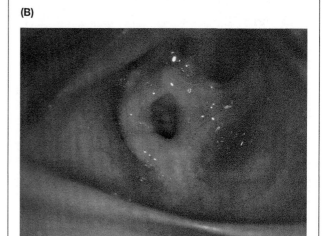
(B)

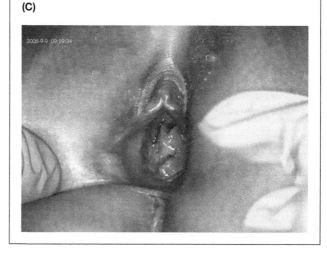
(C)

FIGURE 24.11 Variations in normal female prepubertal anogenital anatomy. Normal prepubertal hymenal configurations are typically crescentic (A), annular (B), or fimbriated (C).

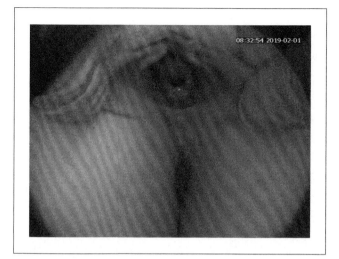

FIGURE 24.12 Traction technique. This clinician is using proper traction technique to examine the anogenital region of a prepubertal child. The labia majora is separated and pulled toward the clinician to ensure adequate visualization of the area.

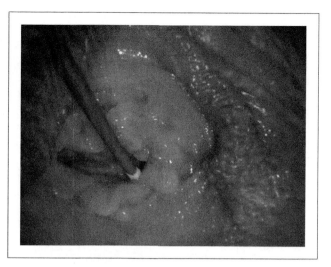

FIGURE 24.13 Normal pubescent female adolescent anogenital anatomy.

and rim. Imagine the hymen as the face of a clock. Attention should be focused on the posterior rim between 3 and 9 o'clock, as this is where abnormalities from sexual abuse generally occur (Adams et al., 2018).

Adolescent Female Anogenital Examination

Note the differences in the estrogenized adolescent genital female anatomy (**Figure 24.13**). Estrogen causes the hymen to hypertrophy and creates redundancy and elasticity in the tissue. The hymenal rim can easily be explored with a swab to check for transections or notches without resulting in discomfort. The inferior portion of the hymen between 3 and 9 o'clock is again where findings consistent with previous injury may be discovered. A speculum can be used and a pelvic examination completed if there is unexplained vaginal bleeding or concerns of pelvic inflammatory disease. Inspection of the hymen should always be conducted prior to speculum insertion as hymenal injury can result with insertion of the speculum.

Male Anogenital Examination

Inspect the penis, scrotum, and anus for signs of acute or chronic trauma, as well as lesions or discharge. If the penis is uncircumcised, retract the foreskin to visualize the urethra. Palpate the scrotum to note the presence of either testes or masses. Note anal folds and the presence of fissures or lacerations. The supine knee-chest and lateral decubitus positions are helpful in accomplishing this examination.

Genital or anal examination findings diagnostic of sexual abuse are rare. Less than 5% of children who

report a history of sexual abuse have a physical finding upon examination (Heger, Ticson, Velasquez, & Bernier, 2002). Explanations for this phenomenon can be explained by a variety of factors, including the nature of the sexual abuse behavior (nontouching, fondling, orogenital contact); elasticity of the hymen and genital structures or anus, allowing for penetration without tearing or injury; healing of anogenital injuries with little to no residual scarring; delayed disclosure of abuse; and sensitivity of the prepubertal hymen to touch (Adams et al., 2018). The ultimate goal of the physical examination for suspected sexual abuse is to ensure positive outcomes for the pediatric patient and family by providing reassurance that despite what has happened, the child's body is normal or will heal.

When children are examined acutely following a sexual abuse incident, physical examination findings are more common. Approximately 20% of children examined acutely following an incident of sexual abuse will have an anogenital finding concerning for sexual abuse (Pilani, 2008). Acute findings include ecchymosis, edema, petechiae, bleeding, abrasions, transections, or tears of the hymen or other anogenital structures (**Figure 24.14**). Nonacute/residual/healed findings are more difficult to detect, but may include healed hymenal transections in the posterior rim extending to the base of the hymen or to the vaginal wall, missing hymenal tissue in the posterior rim, scarring of the posterior fourchette, or perianal scarring (**Figure 24.15**; Adams et al., 2018). Always confirm nonacute anogenital findings in supine and knee-chest position wherever possible.

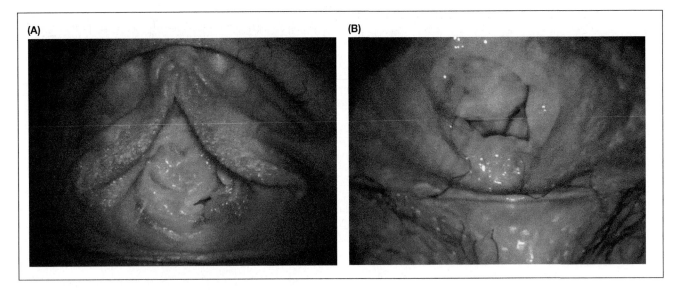

FIGURE 24.14 (A and B) Acute findings of sexual abuse include ecchymosis, edema, petechiae, bleeding, abrasions, transections, or tears of the hymen or other anogenital structures.

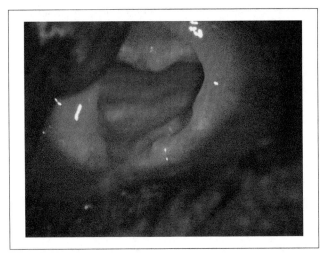

FIGURE 24.15 Nonacute/residual/healed findings of sexual abuse.

Box 24.7 shows findings caused by trauma. Such findings are highly suggestive of sexual abuse even in the absence of a disclosure of sexual abuse by the child (Adams et al., 2018). Traumatic findings can also result from accidental anogenital injury. However, any history given by the child and/or caregiver should be closely examined for timeliness and plausibility. Confirm any history of past surgical interventions given to explain the injuries.

BOX 24.7
INTERPRETATION OF PHYSICAL FINDINGS IN SUSPECTED SEXUAL ABUSE

- Acute injuries to genital/anal tissues
- Acute lacerations or bruising of labia, penis, scrotum, perianal tissues, or perineum
- Acute laceration of the posterior fourchette or vestibule, not involving the hymen
- Bruising, petechiae, or abrasions on the hymen
- Acute laceration (tear) of the hymen, partial or complete
- Vaginal laceration
- Perianal laceration with exposure of tissue below the dermis
- Healing (non-acute/chronic) injuries to genital/anal tissues
- Perianal scar
- Scar of posterior fourchette
- Healed hymenal transection between 4 and 8 o'clock, which extends through to the base of the hymen with no hymenal tissue remaining at the location
- Missing segment of hymen between 4 and 8 o'clock

Source: Adapted from Adams, J., Farst, K., & Kellogg, N. (2018). Interpretation of medical findings in suspected child sexual abuse: An update for 2018. *Journal of Pediatric & Adolescent Gynecology, 31*(3), 225–231. doi:10:1016/j.jpag.2017.12.011

TABLE 24.5 Common Findings in Suspected Elder Abuse	
Physical	Bruises, burns, broken bones
Sexual	Bruises or injury to genital area
Emotional	Withdrawn, anxiety, depression, unusual behavior
Neglect	Malnutrition, medically unexplained weight loss, poor control of medical problems despite access to medications
Financial	Failure to pay bills, uncharacteristic purchases

Sources: Hoover, R., & Polson, M. (2014). Detecting elder abuse and neglect: Assessment and intervention. *American Family Physician,* *89*(6), 453–460. Retrieved from https://www.aafp.org/afp/2014/0315/p453.html; National Center on Elder Abuse. (n.d.). *Statistics and data.* Retrieved from https://ncea.acl.gov/What-We-Do/Research/Statistics-and-Data.aspx

ELDER ABUSE

When examining an elderly patient, the clinician must keep in mind that one sign does not equate abuse. The clinician must keep in mind patterns of injury such as multiple marks, burns, and bruises especially located on the abdomen, neck, posterior extremities, or medial arms. Injuries in these areas do not generally develop for unintentional trauma (Hoover & Polson, 2014). See **Table 24.5**, for common findings in suspected elder abuse.

IMAGING AND LABORATORY CONSIDERATIONS

When generating a differential diagnosis for an injury, physical abuse should always be on the list of considerations. If it is not, this diagnosis is missed every single time. When physical abuse is a concern, specific testing should be performed to both narrow the differential diagnoses as well as look for occult injuries. Fractures, head trauma, and abdominal organ injury may not have physical examination findings that are easily seen by the trained eye; therefore, laboratory and imaging studies are frequently used to further assess the patient for injuries.

Acute fractures are often symptomatic, but the examination findings in young patients with these injuries are variable. The radiologic skeletal survey is a 22-image standard imaging protocol devised by the American College of Radiology and supported by the AAP as the appropriate standard for imaging the bones in children less than 2 years of age when there is a concern for physical abuse (AAP, Section on Radiology, 2009; Flaherty, 2014; **Box 24.8**). There should be a low threshold for obtaining this study in children aged 24 to 36 months when there is a concern for physical abuse as Lindberg's 2014 study identified new fractures

---

BOX 24.8
COMPLETE SKELETAL SURVEY

- Bilateral arms (AP)
- Bilateral forearms (AP)
- Bilateral hands (PA)
- Bilateral thighs (AP)
- Bilateral legs (AP)
- Bilateral feet (AP or PA)
- Thorax (AP and lateral, left and right) to include spine and ribs
- AP abdomen, lumbosacral spine, and bony pelvis
- Lumbar spine (lateral)
- Cervical spine (AP and lateral)
- Skull (frontal and lateral)

AP, anteroposterior; PA posteroanterior.

Source: American Academy of Pediatrics, Section on Radiology. (2009). Diagnostic imaging of child abuse. *Pediatrics, 123,* 1430–1435. doi:10.1542/peds.2009-0558

---

in 10% of these patients (Lindberg, 2014). If a child has significant developmental delays and a thorough musculoskeletal examination is difficult to complete, obtaining a skeletal survey should be considered in older children when evaluating for physical abuse and occult fractures. A follow-up skeletal survey is recommended 2 weeks after the initial study to permit a more accurate determination when abnormal or equivocal findings are noted (Harper, 2013). Injuries can also be more apparent on the follow-up study when the injury shows signs of healing with callus formation. Any fracture in a nonmobile child is concerning and should not be quickly dismissed. Some locations have a high specificity for being abusive fractures in infants and toddlers, such as the ribs, scapula, sternum, spinous processes, and classic metaphyseal lesions. Almost any fracture could be caused by abuse or an accidental mechanism, so putting the entire picture together is critical in these cases. Older children are more often able to verbalize where their pain is located and thus site-specific radiologic imaging would be performed in these children rather than a skeletal survey.

Children with a suspected intracranial injury must undergo a head computed tomography (CT) without contrast at the time the concern for physical abuse arises. For those who are found to have an abnormality, brain magnetic resonance imaging (MRI) should be performed to fully assess the intracranial injury. Early detection is important as head injury is the leading cause of death in young abused children (**Figure 24.16**). Following Rubin's 2003 study in *Pediatrics*, it was recommended that universal screening with head CT or MRI be performed in children less than 6 months of age when there is a concern for physical abuse. If a child older than 6 months has rib fractures, multiple fractures, or facial injury, it is also recommended that they undergo head imaging to assess for further injury (Rubin, 2003). The Pittsburgh Infant Brain Injury Score (PIBIS) is a clinical prediction rule used to identify high-risk infants who should undergo an evaluation with head CT (Berger, 2016). Well-appearing, afebrile infants without a history of trauma who presented for medical care with an apparent-life-threatening event (ALTE), vomiting without diarrhea, seizures, swelling to the scalp, bruising, or other neurologic symptoms were included in this study. "The 5-point PIBIS included abnormality on dermatologic examination (2 points),

age ≥3.0 months (1 point), head circumference >85th percentile (1 point), and serum hemoglobin <11.2 g/dL (1 point)." If the infant had a score of 2, the sensitivity was 93.3% and specificity 53% for having abnormal neuroimaging. This study supports extending the age to 12 months of age for obtaining a head CT to screen for intracranial injury when there is a concern for physical abuse (**Figure 24.17**).

In order to screen for abdominal trauma in children less than 5 years, hepatic transaminase levels (aspartate aminotransferase [AST] and alanine aminotransferase [ALT]) should be obtained. A cutoff level of more than 80 IU/L in either of these would indicate that the patient should undergo imaging with abdominal CT (Lindberg, 2009). If a child is observed to have an injury to the abdomen that is concerning for physical abuse, an abdominal CT with intravenous contrast is recommended, no matter the level of the AST or ALT. Pancreatic enzymes (amylase and lipase) should also be obtained to screen for abdominal trauma.

When a child's bone health is questioned because of a finding of a fracture, initial laboratory testing can be pursued with serum calcium, phosphorus, and alkaline phosphatase levels. At times, vitamin D 25-OH and parathyroid hormone levels are performed; some cases may even need consultation with a metabolic geneticist. When bruising or bleeding injuries are found, an evaluation for possible bleeding disorders should be pursued. This begins with a complete blood count with platelet level, prothrombin time and partial thromboplastin time, factor VIII level, and factor IX level (Anderst, 2013). If the concern is bruising, von Willebrand antigen and activity testing should be done. If the child has an intracranial hemorrhage, d-dimer and fibrinogen levels should be obtained. Further testing and consultation with a pediatric hematologist may be indicated if initial studies are abnormal. If neglect is also a concern, additional laboratory testing may be warranted. See **Table 24.6** for other laboratory testing considerations.

STI testing may be indicated depending on the nature of the sexual abuse disclosure and the presence of any physical findings or complaints (**Box 24.9**). See **Box 24.10**, for interpretation of STI findings and appropriate follow-up. Collection of forensic evidence should be considered for adolescent and pediatric patients who present acutely (as defined by state laws and/or facility protocols) and give a history of orogenital, anogenital, genital-genital, or digital-genital contact; fondling of breasts, genitalia, or buttocks under clothing; or who present with an acute anogenital injury without a consistent history of how the injury occurred (Hornor, 2011). See **Box 24.11** for an example of forensic evidence inclusion and exclusion criteria. A forensic evidence kit should be collected for subsequent forensic analysis by the appropriate local or regional crime laboratory.

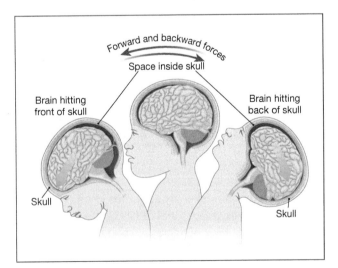

FIGURE 24.16 Mechanism of action during abusive head trauma. Infants are extremely susceptible to injury when they are shaken. Their bone structure, neck muscles, and connecting tissues are underdeveloped and are unable to provide any protection. Their brain gets bruised and can swell, causing tearing of blood vessels, intracranial bleeding, and death.

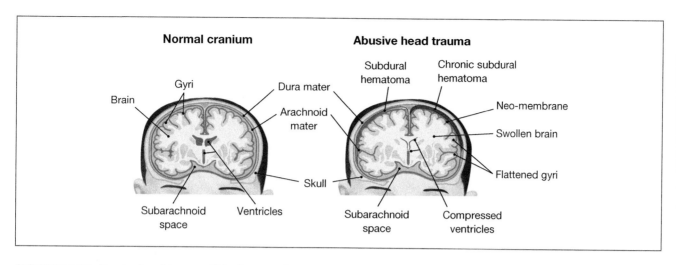

FIGURE 24.17 Abusive head trauma. This diagram shows the differences in brain anatomy in a normal child's brain and the brain of a child who has suffered abusive head trauma. Pathological changes can include subdural hematoma (acute and chronic), compressed ventricles, and flattened gyri.

TABLE 24.6 Examples of Laboratory Testing Indicated Per Neglect Concern

Concern	Laboratory Testing
Intrauterine drug exposure	Maternal drugs of abuse screening (urine/serum) Infant drugs of abuse screening (urine/cord blood)
Ingestion	Child toxicology drug screening (urine/serum) Child drugs of abuse screening (urine/serum)
Obesity	Hemoglobin A1c or fasting blood sugar Fasting lipid profile Liver enzymes
Failure to thrive	Complete blood count, C-reactive protein, and ESR • To screen for anemia, chronic infections, inflammation, and malignancy Urinalysis and culture • To screen for protein or carbohydrates (diabetes mellitus type 1) and indolent renal disease (chronic urinary tract infection or renal tubular acidosis)

ESR, erythrocyte sedimentation rate.

Note: Laboratory tests will vary based on the patient history and presentation. Other additional testing may be indicated.

Sources: Jansson, L. (2019). Neonatal abstinence syndrome. In J. A. Garcia-Prats (Ed.), *UpToDate*. Retrieved from https://www.uptodate.com/contents/neonatal-abstinence-syndrome; Klish, W. (2018). Clinical evaluation of the obese child and adolescent. In K. J. Motil & M. E. Geffner (Eds.), *UpToDate*. Retrieved from https://www.uptodate.com/contents/clinical-evaluation-of-the-obese-child-and-adolescent; Motil, K. & Duryea, T. (2019). Poor weight gain in children younger than two years in research-rich countries: Etiology & evaluation. In J. E. Drutz & C. Jensen (Eds.), *UpToDate*. Retrieved from https://www.uptodate.com/contents/poor-weight-gain-in-children-younger-than-two-years-etiology-and-evaluation

ADDITIONAL CONSIDERATIONS

An essential part of the "workup" when there is a concern for any type of abuse is reporting to CPS and LE. All states have laws that require medical clinicians to report to CPS and/or LE when there is suspected child maltreatment (Child Welfare Information Gateway, 2016). Clinicians can be held legally responsible if they fail to do so. Other professionals who work with children, such as in education, social services, child day care, or foster care, are often considered mandated reporters of suspected child abuse and neglect. The laws vary slightly depending on the state of residence. The Child Welfare Information Gateway website (www.childwelfare.gov) is a helpful resource that clinicians can utilize when there are questions regarding when

BOX 24.9
SEXUALLY TRANSMITTED INFECTION TESTING

Indications for Children and Adolescents

- Signs/symptoms for sexually transmitted infection (STI; anogenital discharge, pain, erythema, bleeding, and/or pruritus; lower abdominal pain)
- Disclosure of genital–genital contact, genital–anal contact, or oral–genital/anal contact
- Anogenital injury without consistent history
- Perpetrator known to have an STI
- Prepubertal child in the home known to have an STI

Laboratory Tests

- Testing of orifices depends on the sexual abuse history given and the presence of any anogenital or oral symptoms.
- Serologies (syphilis, hepatitis B/C, and HIV testing) should be completed with a history of anogenital or genital–genital contact.
  - Gonorrhea: Oral, anal, and/or genital/urine nucleic acid amplification test (NAAT)
  - Chlamydia: Anal and/or genital/urine NAAT
  - Trichomonas: Genital/urine NAAT
- If NAAT testing for chlamydia, gonorrhea, or trichomonas is not available, then oral, anal, or genital culture(s) should be obtained.
- Urine specimen for NAAT testing (chlamydia, gonorrhea, and trichomonas) is the preferred method of testing for genital infection in prepubertal females and males of all ages.
- NAAT genital swab may provide more sensitivity than urine in pubertal females.
- Other testing:
  - Syphilis: Rapid plasma reagin (RPR)
  - Hepatitis B: Hepatitis B surface antigen
  - Hepatitis C: Hepatitis C antibody
  - Human immunodeficiency virus: HIV antibody
  - Vesicular lesions concerning for herpes: Polymerase chain reaction (PCR) assays for HSV DNA
- Serologies collected following an acute sexual abuse/assault should be repeated in 6 weeks, 3 months, and 6 months to ensure continued negativity.

Screening for All Adolescents

- Urine pregnancy test (females)
- Urine NAAT for gonorrhea/chlamydia/trichomonas

Sources: Adapted from Adams, J., Farst, K., & Kellogg, N. (2018). Interpretation of medical findings in suspected child sexual abuse: An update for 2018. *Journal of Pediatric & Adolescent Gynecology, 31*(3), 225–231. doi:10.1016/j.jpag.2017.12.011; Hornor, G. (2017). Sexually transmitted infections and children: What the PNP should know. *Journal of Pediatric Health Care, 31*(2), 222–229. doi:10.1016/j.pedhc.2016.04.016

BOX 24.10
INTERPRETATION OF SEXUALLY TRANSMITTED INFECTION TESTING

Diagnostic Findings (Unless Explained by Consensual Sexual Activity in an Adolescent)

Report to Child Protective Services:

- Positive oral, anal, or genital gonorrhea nucleic acid amplification test (NAAT) or culture
- Positive anal or genital chlamydia nucleic acid amplification test (NAAT) or culture
- Positive genital *Trichomonas vaginalis* NAAT or culture
- Positive RPR or VDRL (syphilis) if perinatal transmission is ruled out
- Positive HIV test if perinatal transmission, contact with contaminated needles, or blood products are ruled out

Indeterminate Findings (Can Be Transmitted Via Sexual and Nonsexual Means)

Report to Child Protective Services unless vertical or horizontal transmission is likely:
- Anogenital warts (*Condyloma accuminata*)
- Anogenital herpes simplex virus type 1 or type 2

HIV, human immunodeficiency virus; RPR, rapid plasma reagin; STI, sexually transmitted infection; VDRL, venereal disease research laboratory.

Source: Adapted from Adams, J., Farst, K., & Kellogg, N. (2018). Interpretation of medical findings in suspected child sexual abuse: An update for 2018. *Journal of Pediatric & Adolescent Gynecology, 31*(3), 225–231. doi:10.1016/j.jpag.2017.12.011

and how to make a report to CPS. Remember, the obligation is to report when there is a suspicion for abuse or neglect; it is not required that the clinician or professional have "proof" or a final diagnosis of abuse to get CPS involved in an investigation. The goal is to protect the child from further harm and the clinician should utilize the resources available in order to do so.

When a report to CPS is made, the clinician initiating the report needs to discuss this decision with the caregivers who are present with the child. The fact that concerns regarding abuse arose should be brought to the attention of the caregivers in an objective and straight-forward manner. The clinician should not be seen as someone who is trying to hide information from the parents. These are often difficult conversations, but families appreciate honesty regarding the health and well-being of their child. The clinician should explain that CPS and LE have investigative roles that the clinician cannot accomplish, like observing the home

BOX 24.11
SAMPLE FORENSIC EVIDENCE INCLUSION/EXCLUSION CRITERIA

Inclusion Criteria

1. Children between the ages of 0 and 15 years who present with a concern of sexual abuse within 72 hours of the latest incident of sexual abuse involving genital–genital, anal–genital, oral–genital, oral–anal, oral–breast, digital–genital, or digital–anal contact, as well as fondling breasts, genitals, or anus under clothes per child history

2. Adolescents aged 16 years and above who present with a concern of sexual abuse within 96 hours of the latest incidence of sexual abuse involving genital–genital, anal–genital, oral–genital, oral–anal, oral–breast, digital–genital, or digital–anal contact, as well as fondling breasts, genitals, or anus under clothes per adolescent history

3. Other high-risk credible concern even if child is not giving history of sexual abuse (e.g., abduction, confession of a perpetrator)

4. All prepubertal children presenting with a positive oral, anal, or genital gonorrhea result; positive anal or genital chlamydia result; or positive genital trichomonas result

5. All children and adolescents presenting with an unexplained acute anal or genital injury

6. Law enforcement requesting evidence collection yet not meeting the previous criteria

Exclusion Criteria

1. Latest incident of sexual abuse is >72 hours for children 0–15 years and 96 hours for adolescents 16 years and above.

2. Child engaging in sexualized behaviors or problematic sexualized behaviors where both children are under the age of 12 years.

conditions and talking to other people who care for the child. Because there is a concern that someone harmed the patient, multiple individuals should be involved to help protect the child going forward. The medical clinician should make clear to families that they will continue in their role as clinician for the patient and family throughout this process as best as they are able.

As with all patient encounters, documentation is an important part of the assessment. The clinician should remain as objective as possible, as well as thorough and accurate in their documentation. When the subjective histories are obtained, the clinician should document specifically who provided what information to them. If one parent provides the history but the other caregiver was the one present for the event, this should be clearly stated in the clinician's documentation. Attention to detail when describing the physical examination findings is critical, as these change over time and the patient may undergo further examinations by other clinicians who could observe different findings. The final diagnosis of "physical abuse" is not always made at the end of a patient encounter, even when there are very strong suspicions for child maltreatment. Documenting all of the findings and concerns that arose regarding the patient will help CPS, LE, and other clinicians going forward with the child.

In the case of neglect, regardless of the need to report to CPS, close follow-up with caregivers will be indicated. The clinician must work with the caregivers to develop a plan to ensure that the child's needs are met, optimally at a higher level than noted currently. It is vital that the plan of care be discussed with caregivers, ensuring that they understand the plan of care, why the plan of care is important, and exactly what they must do to ensure their child receives adequate care (Hornor, 2014). Clinicians must also link the caregiver with community resources to address identified barriers such as financial (e.g., Medicaid, food stamps, food pantries, or public assistance), mental health (e.g., appropriate assessment and treatment), IPV (e.g., local domestic violence shelters, legal assistance, and treatment options), or substance abuse (e.g., an appropriate treatment program). In order to ensure that the child's needs are being adequately addressed, close follow-up is indicated for both adherence to plan of care and linkage with community resources to address identified barriers. Frequent reeducation and reinforcement of the plan of care, including linkage with necessary community resources, is optimal. Close surveillance of care can prevent potential serious harm to the child (Hornor, 2014). A referral to CPS may be necessary if caregiver deviation from the plan of care places the child at risk of harm. Encouragement and positive reinforcement should be given to caregivers for following the plan of care. Gradually decrease surveillance as compliance is demonstrated.

Neglect can result in serious consequences for victims. It is crucial that clinicians recognize child neglect and respond appropriately. Understand that a report to CPS is never a punitive action against a parent or caregiver but rather a positive action to ensure the safety of the child. Working closely with caregivers to address identified neglect concerns often results in positive outcomes for both the child and family.

When reporting elder abuse, one does not have *known* that elder abuse exists, only that there is *suspected* abuse. Anyone can file a voluntary report with the appropriate authority, including LE, Adult Protective Services (APS), or with the long-term care ombudsman. Most states have mandatory elder abuse reporting. States vary on the specific reporting requirements and who is mandated to report, but typically those in positions that will likely detect elder abuse are mandated to report when abuse is suspected. Clinicians are required to report suspected abuse in states that have mandatory reporting. Most states with mandatory reporting are required to report suspected abuse with APS. Some states with mandatory reporting require financial institutions to report suspected financial exploitation of another adult. Information required when filing a report with APS includes victim's age, identity, location of the incident, and the circumstances causing the suspicion (Jackson, 2018).

EVIDENCE-BASED PRACTICE CONSIDERATIONS

Child advocacy centers (CAC) and child abuse specialists are resources for the clinician when performing healthcare assessments for sexual abuse; it is imperative to become familiar with local resources. Consider referral to a CAC or a child abuse specialist for the healthcare assessment for child sexual abuse if it is available in a timely manner. Second-opinion anogenital examinations by a skilled child sexual abuse clinician should be obtained whenever the clinician questions an examination finding or an STI.

STI and pregnancy prophylaxis should be considered for adolescents reporting acute sexual abuse or assault. Prophylactic treatment for STIs (chlamydia, gonorrhea, or trichomonas) in the prepubertal pediatric population is not routinely recommended because of the low risk of ascending infection (Workowski & Berman, 2006). **Box 24.12** identifies indications for STI and pregnancy prophylaxis following acute sexual abuse/assault. The only STI for which postexposure prophylaxis is considered in both the prepubertal and adolescent populations is HIV. HIV prophylaxis (HIV PEP) must be initiated within 72 hours of the latest incident of sexual abuse or assault. HIV PEP must be taken for 28 days and can be toxic to bone marrow and the liver; therefore, baseline laboratory testing must be obtained prior to initiating HIV PEP (see **Box 24.13**). Follow-up with an infectious disease clinician is indicated to monitor patient tolerance of the medication and HIV status. HIV PEP medications, especially those taken by children younger than 12 years, can result in nausea and general malaise; provision of an anti-emetic medication is most often necessary. Note that the risk of contracting HIV from sexual abuse is relatively low. In a study of 9,136 cases of HIV in children, Lindegren et al. (1998) found 26 children to have a confirmed ($n = 17$) or suspected ($n = 9$) exposure to HIV via sexual abuse. Confirmed exposure was defined as HIV-positive children with no other HIV risk factors and a sexual abuse perpetrator

BOX 24.12
ACUTE PRESENTATION: SEXUALLY TRANSMITTED INFECTION AND PREGNANCY PROPHYLAXIS AND TREATMENT OPTIONS

Indications for STI Prophylaxis (Adolescents)
- Perpetrator is known to have an STI.
- Adolescent gives a history of oral–genital, anal–genital, or genital–genital contact.
- Patient is symptomatic: Genital/anal discharge, pain, itching, or bleeding; dysuria; urinary urgency; or lesions.
- Sexual abuse/assault by multiple perpetrators
- Sibling is known to have an STI.
- Unknown perpetrator
- Caregiver or patient request

Indications for Pregnancy Prophylaxis (Adolescent Females)
- Pubertal female with history of genital–genital contact
- Caregiver/patient request

Indications for HIV Prophylaxis (Children and Adolescents)
- Child/adolescent gives history of genital–genital or anal–genital contact.
- Acute genital or anal trauma
- Perpetrator known to be positive or at high risk for HIV (IV drug user; male who has sex with males; prison)
- Unknown perpetrator

STI, sexually transmitted infection.

Sources: Adapted from Kuhar, D., Henderson, D., Struble, K., Heneine, W., Thomas, V., Cheever, L., . . . Panlilio, A. (2015). Updated U.S. Public Health Service guidelines for the management of occupational exposures to human immunodeficiency virus and recommendations for postexposure prophylaxis. Retrieved from https://npin.cdc.gov/publication/updated-us-public-health-service-guidelines-management-occupational-exposures-human; Centers for Disease Control and Prevention. (n.d.). *HIV.* Retrieved from https://www.cdc.gov/hiv/default.html; Smith, D., Grohskopf, L., Black, R., Auerbach, J., Veronese, F., Struble, K., . . . Greenberg, A. (2005). Antiretroviral postexposure prophylaxis after sexual, injection-drug use, or other nonoccupational exposure to HIV in the United States. *MMWR: Recommendations and Reports, 54*(RR02), 1–20. Retrieved from https://www.cdc.gov/mmwr/preview/mmwrhtml/rr5402a1.htm; Workowski, K., & Berman, S. (2006). Sexually transmitted diseases treatment guidelines, 2006. *MMWR: Recommendations and Reports, 55*(RR11), 1–94. Retrieved from https://www.cdc.gov/mmwr/preview/mmwrhtml/rr5511a1.htm

BOX 24.13

BASELINE LABORATORY TESTING PRIOR TO INITIATING HIV PROPHYLAXIS

- HIV antibody
- Hepatitis B virus surface antigen
- Hepatitis C virus antibody
- Complete blood count with differential
- Alanine aminotransferase
- Aspartate aminotransferase
- Alkaline phosphatase
- Blood urea nitrogen
- Creatinine

Follow-up with infectious diseases professional for needed laboratory monitoring.

Source: Adapted from Centers for Disease Control and Prevention. (2016). HIV. Retrieved from https://www.cdc.gov/hiv/default.html

known to be HIV positive. Suspected exposure was defined as HIV-positive children with no other HIV risk factors and a perpetrator of unknown HIV status.

Clinicians are mandated reporters and any suspicion of child abuse or neglect must be reported to CPS and LE. Appropriate mental health treatment is essential in decreasing trauma to child victims and their families. It is essential that the clinician ensure that a referral to a mental health specialist skilled in providing trauma-focused cognitive behavioral therapy for sexual abuse victims and nonoffending family members is made. Providing necessary resources to nonoffending caregivers is crucial as studies suggest that the single most important determinant of resilience for sexually abused children is support from primary caregivers (Kim, Trickett, & Putnam, 2010).

ABNORMAL FINDINGS

ABUSIVE HEAD TRAUMA

The CDC (Parks, Annest, Hill, & Karch, 2012) defines pediatric AHT as "an injury to the skull or intracranial contents of an infant or young child (<5 years of age) due to inflicted blunt impact and/or violent shaking" (p. 10). Still commonly called shaken baby syndrome, the AAP is trying to move away from this definition for reporting purposes and since shaken baby syndrome implies a single mechanism of injury. Children under the age of 1 are at the highest risk for AHT with peak incidence around 2 to 3 months of age. The most common trigger for AHT is thought to be related to episodes of prolonged, inconsolable crying that is developmentally normal in infants of this age. Injuries from AHT can vary with infant mortality occurring in roughly 20% of cases (Parks et al, 2012). Signs and symptoms may be subtle or drastic depending on the severity of the trauma.

Key History and Physical Findings

- Extreme fussiness or irritability
- Facial bruising
- Subconjunctival or retinal hemorrhages
- Difficulty staying awake
- Breathing problems
- Lethargy
- Poor feeding
- Vomiting
- Pale or bluish skin
- Seizures
- Damage to the spinal cord and neck
- Fractures of the ribs and bones
- Cognitive impairments
- Behavioral problems
- Cerebral palsy
- Paralysis
- Coma

CASE STUDY: Well-Child Visit

History

A 2-month-old male presents to the primary care clinician for his first routine well-child visit. He was born at 38 weeks via spontaneous vaginal delivery; the mother had no complications during pregnancy and the patient was discharged home with family after 2 days in the hospital. The mother is exclusively breastfeeding every 3 hours. The infant has been sleeping well between feeds but does get fussier with stooling. Parents have tried gas drops and gripe water but neither seem to help. In the home are the infant's mother, father, 4-year-old brother, and 18-month-old sister.

Physical Examination

The infant is alert and interactive for age. Vitals are within normal limits and his growth parameters (weight, length, and head circumference) are all

(continued)

CASE STUDY: Well-Child Visit (*continued*)

around the 50th percentile. When his clothes are removed, you observe a 1 cm area of blue-purple discoloration over the left rib cage that appears to be a bruise. It blanches when palpated, does not appear tender, and does not have any associated swelling. When you ask the mother about this mark, she states that she gave him a bath yesterday and hadn't noticed it at the time. When asked if she has ever seen other bruises on the baby, she reports that there was a linear mark on his lower leg last week that the father stated was from doing bicycle leg exercises with him. The remainder of the physical examination is normal.

Differential Diagnoses

Trauma (accidental or inflicted), hematological disorder

Laboratory and Imaging

Patient was sent to the local children's hospital emergency department in order to obtain a head CT, skeletal survey, AST/ALT/lipase/amylase, CBC, PT/PTT, Factor VIII and IX levels, and von Willebrand antigen and activity.

Final Diagnosis

Suspected physical abuse. Prior to patient being referred to the emergency department, a report was made to CPS and LE because of unexplained bruising in a nonmobile infant. All laboratory tests were normal, as was the head CT. Patient's skeletal survey demonstrated three left posterior rib fractures as well as a left distal femur classic metaphyseal lesion. These additional injuries greatly increase the likelihood of abuse.

CASE STUDY: Vaginal Discharge and Pain

History

A 4-year-old previously healthy female presents to her primary care clinician accompanied by her mother because of vaginal discharge and pain. Symptoms started 2 to 3 days ago and have become increasingly worse. Her mother has been applying Lotrimin cream to the area because of concerns of a yeast infection. Her mother denies any fevers, genital blisters, or inability to urinate. The child has no significant medical or surgical history, no allergies, and is not currently taking any medications. The child lives with her mother and visits with her father every Friday to Sunday. Living in her mother's home are the mother and child. Her father lives with his girlfriend and her adult brother (Travis). The child was last with her father 5 days ago. The mother denies domestic violence, mental health concerns, drug/alcohol concerns, or previous involvement with Child Protective Services or law enforcement for the father or herself.

Physical Examination

The patient appears well. She is afebrile. Her pulse is 92 and respirations are 20. Her weight is stable

based on her previous well-child visit last month. A focused anogenital examination is completed. Yellow/white discharge is noted in the introitus along with generalized erythema. No acute or chronic anogenital trauma, lesions, or structural abnormalities are noted. No foreign body was visualized. During the anogenital examination, a review of the concept of private parts is completed. The child spontaneously states, "Travis has a big pee pee and it hurts me." No further information can be elicited from the child.

Differential Diagnoses

Sexual abuse, vulvovaginitis, vaginal yeast infection, STI (chlamydia, gonorrhea, or trichomonas), genital strep infection, vaginal foreign body

Laboratory and Imaging

A dirty urine specimen was collected for NAAT testing for chlamydia, gonorrhea, and trichomonas. Genital culture was collected. Vaginal pathogens panel was collected for yeast, gardnerella, and trichomonas.

(continued)

CASE STUDY: Vaginal Discharge and Pain (*continued*)

Final Diagnosis

Suspected sexual abuse:

- Report was made to Child Protective Services and law enforcement because of the child's concerning disclosure during anogenital examination. Report was made prior to the child's discharge from the office. Safety plan was determined by Child Protective Services prior to discharge.

- Referral was made to a local child advocacy center/child abuse program for complete assessment.
- Urine NAAT was positive for gonorrhea.
- The child was treated with ceftriaxone when a positive gonorrhea result was obtained after collection of a confirmatory specimen.
- The child returned in 3 weeks for test of cure.
- Child Protective Services and law enforcement were notified of the positive gonorrhea result, which greatly increased concern for sexual abuse.

Clinical Pearls

- Child maltreatment prevention begins with the first newborn well-child appointment. Consistent encouragement of positive parenting practices, discussing age-appropriate developmental expectations for behavior, and the consistent encouragement of the use of non-physical methods of discipline are all ways to help the caregivers prevent child maltreatment.
- Healthcare clinicians should know their patients' psychosocial histories as well as their medical histories. When psychosocial concerns are identified, it is crucial to link patients/families with appropriate interventions and monitor follow through.
- Prompt recognition and reporting of child and elder abuse by the clinician can prevent further abuse—not only of the patient currently receiving treatment, but also of other potential victims. Educate pediatric and elder patients and caregivers regarding abuse. Be a resource to other clinicians and the community.

- Pregnancy is a high-risk time for interpersonal violence.
- Approximately one out of every 10 individuals over the age of 60 in community settings is estimated to have been affected by some form of elder abuse.
- When generating a differential diagnosis for an injury in a child, elder, or person with disability, physical abuse should always be on the list of considerations. If it is not, this diagnosis is missed every single time.
- Bruising to the torso, ears, or neck for any child less than or equal to 4 years of age and bruising in any location on an infant less than 4 months of age should prompt the clinician to initiate a workup for physical abuse, investigating for other occult injuries.
- A report to CPS is never a punitive action against a parent or caregiver but rather a positive action to ensure the safety of the child.
- Clinicians need to be familiar with the state and federal laws around reporting abuse.

Key Takeaways

- Instead of approaching a patient and thinking "What is wrong with you?" take the approach of "What happened to you?"
- The greater the dose of trauma, the more damaging the effects are on an individual.
- Neglect is often an overlooked form of child maltreatment; however, it is the most common and deadliest form of child maltreatment.

REFERENCES

Abajobir, A., Kisely, S., Maravilla, J., Williams, G., & Najman, J. (2017). Gender differences in the association between childhood sexual abuse and risky sexual behaviors: A systematic review and meta-analysis. *Child Abuse & Neglect, 63*, 249–260. doi:10.1016/j.chiabu.2016.11.023

Adams, J., Farst, K., & Kellogg, N. (2018). Interpretation of medical findings in suspected child sexual abuse: An update for 2018. *Journal of Pediatric & Adolescent Gynecology, 31*(3), 225–231. doi:10:1016/j.jpag.2017.12.011

Allen, D., & Fost, N. (2012). Obesity and neglect: It's about the child. *Journal of Pediatrics, 60,* 898–899. doi:10.1016/j.jpeds.2012.02.035

American Academy of Pediatrics. (2012a). Policy statement: Early childhood adversity, toxic stress, and the role of the pediatrician: Translating developmental science into lifelong health. *Pediatrics, 129*(1), e224–e231. doi:10.1542/peds.2011-2662

American Academy of Pediatrics. (2012b). Technical report: The lifelong effects of early childhood adversity and toxic stress. *Pediatrics, 129*(1), e232–e246. doi:10.1542/peds.2011-2663

American Academy of Pediatrics, Section on Radiology. (2009). Diagnostic imaging of child abuse. *Pediatrics, 123,* 1430–1435. doi:10.1542/peds.2009-0558

American Congress of Obstetricians and Gynecologists. (2012). Intimate partner violence: Committee opinion No. 518. *Obstetrics & Gynecology, 119,* 412–417. doi:10.1097/AOG.0b013e318249ff74

American Psychiatric Association. (2013). *Diagnostic and statistical manual of mental disorders* (5th ed.). Arlington, VA: American Psychiatric Publishing.

Anderst, J. (2013). Evaluation for bleeding disorders in suspected child abuse. *Pediatrics, 131,* 1314–1322. doi:10.1542/peds.2013-0195

Appleton, J. (2012). Perspectives of neglect. *Child Abuse Review, 21,* 77–80. doi:10.1002/car.2208

Bair-Merritt, M. H., Lewis-O'Connor, A., Goel, S., Amato, P., Ismailji, T., Jelley, M., ... Cronholm, P. (2014). Primary care-based interventions for intimate partner violence: A systematic review. *American Journal of Preventive Medicine, 46*(2), 188–194. doi:10.1016/j.amepre.2013.10.001

Berger, R. (2016). Validation of the Pittsburgh infant brain injury score for abusive head trauma. *Pediatrics, 138,* 1–8. doi:10.1542/peds.2015-3756

Bethell, C. D., Carle, A., Hudziak, J., Gombojav, N., Powers, K., Wade, R., & Braveman, P. (2017). Methods to assess adverse childhood experiences of children and families: Toward approaches to promote child well-being in policy and practice. *Academic Pediatrics, 17*(7 Suppl.), S51–S69. doi:10.1016/j.acap.2017.04.161

Bickley, L. (2007). *Bates' guide to physical examination and history taking* (9th ed.). Philadelphia, PA: Lippincott Williams & Wilkins.

Boston Medical Center Child Protection Team. (2012). *Evaluation tool for medical neglect.* Boston, MA: Author. Retrieved from https://www.bmc.org/sites/default/files/For_Medical_Professionals/Pediatric_Resources/Pediatrics__Child_Protection_Team__CPT_/Tools_and_Medical_Evaluation_Abuse/field_Attachments/medical-neglect.pdf

Breiding, M. J., Basile, K. C., Smith, S. G., Black, M. C., & Mahendra, R. R. (2015). *Intimate partner violence surveillance: Uniform definitions and recommended data elements, Version 2.0.* Atlanta, GA: National Center for Injury Prevention and Control, Centers for Disease Control and Prevention.

Butler, A. (2013). Child sexual assault: Risk factors for girls. *Child Abuse & Neglect, 37*(9), 643–652. doi:10/1016/j.chiabu.2013.06.009

Campbell, A. M., & Hibbard, R. (2014). More than words: The emotional maltreatment of children. *Pediatric Clinics of North America, 61,* 959–970. doi:10.1016/j.pcl.2014.06.004

Centers for Disease Control and Prevention. (2016). *HIV.* Retrieved from https://www.cdc.gov/hiv/default.html

Centers for Disease Control and Prevention. (2017, June 5). *Elder abuse prevention.* Retrieved from https://www.cdc.gov/features/elderabuse/index.html

Centers for Disease Control and Prevention. (2018). *Child abuse and neglect: Risk and protective factors.* Retrieved from https://www.cdc.gov/violenceprevention/childabuseandneglect/riskprotectivefactors.html

The Child Abuse Prevention and Treatment Act (CAPTA) P.L. 93-247, 42 U.S.C. §§ 2(b)(6) (1974).

Child Welfare Information Gateway. (2016). *Mandatory reporters of child abuse and neglect.* Washington, DC: U.S. Department of Health and Human Services, Children's Bureau.

Chowdhury, U. (2011). Post-traumatic stress disorder in children and adolescents. *Community Practitioner, 84*(12), 33–35.

Christian, C. (2015). The evaluation of suspected child physical abuse. *Pediatrics, 135*(5), 1337–1354. doi:10.1542/peds.2015-0356

Constantino, J. (2016). Child maltreatment prevention and the scope of child and adolescent psychiatry. *Prevention Psychiatry, 25,* 157–165. doi:10.1016/j.chc.2015.11.003

Cooper, A., & Smith, E. L. (2011). *Homicide trends in the United States, 1980-2008.* Washington, DC: Bureau of Justice Statistics.

Dong, M., Dube, S., Felitti, V., Giles, W., & Anda, R. (2003). Adverse childhood experiences and self-reported liver disease: New insights into a causal pathway. *Archives of Internal Medicine, 163,* 1949–1956. doi:10.1001/archinte.163.16.1949

Dong, M., Giles, W., Felitti, V., Dube, S., Williams, J., Chapman, D., & Anda, R. (2004). Insights into causal pathways for ischemic heart disease: Adverse childhood experiences study. *Circulation, 110,* 1761–1766. doi:10.1161/01.CIR.0000143074.54995.7F

Dube, S. R. (2018). Continuing conversations about adverse childhood experiences (ACEs) screening: A public health perspective. *Child Abuse & Neglect, 85,* 180–184. doi:10.1016/j.chiabu.2018.03.007

Dube, S. R., Anda, R., Whitfield, C., Brown, D., Felitti, V., Dong, M., & Giles, W. (2005). Long-term consequences of childhood sexual abuse by gender of victim. *American Journal of Preventive Medicine, 28*(5), 430–438. doi:10.1016/j.amepre.2005.01.015

Dubowitz, H. (2014). The Safe Environment for Every Kid model: Promotion of children's health, development, and safety, and prevention of child neglect. *Pediatric Annals, 43*(11), e271–e277. doi:10.3928/00904481-20141022-11

Dubowitz, H., Giardino, A., & Gustavson, E. (2000). Child neglect: Guidance for pediatricians. *Pediatric Review, 21,* 111–116. doi:10.1542/pir.21-4-111

Dubowitz, H., Lane, W. G., Semiatin, J. N., Magder, L. S., Venepally, M., & Jans, M. (2011). The Safe Environment for Every Kid Model: Impact on pediatric primary care profes-

sionals. *Pediatrics, 127*(4), e962–e970. doi:10.1542/peds
.2010-1845

Easton, S., & Kong, J. (2017). Mental health indicators fifty
years later: A population-based study of men with histories
of child sexual abuse. *Child Abuse & Neglect, 63,* 272–283.
doi:10.1016/j.chiabu.2016.09.011

Eckenrode, J., Ganzel, B., Henderson, C. R., Smith, E., Olds,
D. L., Powers, J., . . . Sidora, K. (2000). Preventing child
abuse and neglect with a program of nurse home visitation: The limiting effects of domestic violence. *Journal
of the American Medical Association, 284,* 1385–1391.
doi:10.1001/jama.284.11.1385

Edelson, J. (1999). The overlap between child maltreatment
and women battering. *Violence Against Women, 5*(2), 134–
154. doi:10.1177/107780129952003

Edwards, V., Holder, G., Felitti, V., & Anda, R. (2003). Relationship between multiple forms of childhood maltreatment
and adult mental health in community respondents: Results from the adverse childhood experiences study. *American Journal of Psychiatry, 160,* 1453–1460. doi:10.1176/
appi.ajp.160.8.1453

Felitti, V. J., Anda, R. F., Nordenberg, D., Williamson, D. F.,
Spitz, A. M., Edwards, V., & Marks, J. S. (1998). Relationship
of childhood abuse and household dysfunction to many
of the leading causes of death in adults. *American Journal of Preventive Medicine, 14*(4), 245–258. doi:10.1016/
s0749-3797(98)00017-8

Finkelhor, D. (2009). Prevention of childhood sexual abuse.
Future Child, 19(2), 169–194. doi:10.1353/foc.0.0035

Finkelhor, D. (2017). Screening for adverse childhood experiences (ACEs): Cautions and suggestions. *Child Abuse &
Neglect, 85,* 174–179. doi:10.1016/j.chiabu.2017.07.016

Flaherty, E. (2010). Clinical report—The pediatrician's role in
child maltreatment prevention. *Pediatrics, 126*(4), 833–
841. doi:10.1542/peds.2010-2087

Flaherty, E. (2014). Evaluating children with fractures for
child physical abuse. *Pediatrics, 133,* 477–489. doi:10.1542/
peds.2013-3793

Flynn, A. B., Fothergill, K. E., Wilcox, H. C., Coleclough, E.,
Horwitz, R., Ruble, A., . . . Wissow, L. S. (2015). Primary
care interventions to prevent or treat traumatic stress in
childhood: A systematic review. *Academic Pediatrics,
15*(5), 480–492. doi:10.1016/j.acap.2015.06.012

Fong, H., & Christian, C. (2012). Child neglect: A review for
the primary care pediatrician. *Pediatric Annals, 41*(12),
e254–e258. doi:10.3928/00904481-20121126-08

Fuller-Thomson, E., & Lewis, D. (2015). The relationship between early adversities and attention deficit/hyperactivity
disorder. *Child Abuse & Neglect, 47,* 94–101. doi:10.1016/j
.chiabu.2015.03.005

Giller, E. (n.d.). What is psychological trauma? Retrieved from
http://www.theannainstitute.org/What%20Is%20Psycho
logical%20Trauma.pdf?contentID=88

Greenbaum, J., Crawford-Jakubiak, C., & Committee on Child
Abuse and Neglect. (2015). Child sex trafficking & com-
mercial sexual exploitation: Health care needs of victims.
Pediatrics, 135(3), 506–574. doi:10.1542/peds.2014-4138

Hamby, S., Finkelhor, D., Turner, H., & Ormrod, R. (2011).
*Children's exposure to intimate partner violence and
other family violence.* Washington, DC: U.S. Department

of Justice, Office of Juvenile Justice and Delinquency Prevention. Retrieved from https://www.ncjrs.gov/pdffiles1/
ojjdp/232272.pdf

Harper, N. (2013). The utility of follow-up skeletal surveys
in child abuse. *Pediatrics, 131,* 672–678. doi:10.1542/
peds.2012-2608

Heger, A., Ticson, L., Velasquez, O., & Bernier, R. (2002). Children referred for possible sexual abuse: Medical findings
in 2384 children. *Child Abuse & Neglect, 26*(6), 645–659.
doi:10.1016/S0145-2134(02)00339-3

Hettiaratchy, S. (2004). ABC of burns, pathophysiology
and types of burns. *BMJ, 328,* 1427–1429. doi:10.1136/
bmj.328.7453.1427

Hibbard, R., Barlow, J., & MacMillan, H. (2012). Clinical report: Psychological maltreatment. *Pediatrics, 130,* 372–
378. doi:10.1542/peds.2012-1552

Hodgman, E. (2016). The Parkland Burn Center experience
with 297 cases of child abuse from 1974 to 2010. *Burns, 42,*
1121–1127. doi:10.1016/j.burns.2016.02.013

Hoover, R., & Polson, M. (2014). Detecting elder abuse and
neglect: Assessment and intervention. *American Family
Physician, 89*(6), 453–460. Retrieved from https://www
.aafp.org/afp/2014/0315/p453.html

Hopper, E. K., Bassuk, E. L., & Olivet, J. (2010). Shelter from
the storm: Trauma-informed care in homelessness services
settings. *The Open Health Services and Policy Journal,
3*(2), 80–100. Retrieved from http://www.traumacenter
.org/products/pdf_files/shelter_from_storm.pdf

Hornor, G. (2011). Medical evaluation for child sexual abuse:
What the PNP needs to know. *Journal of Pediatric Health
Care, 25*(4), 250–256. doi:10.1016/j.pedhc.2011.01.004

Hornor, G. (2013). Child maltreatment: Screening and anticipatory guidance. *Journal of Pediatric Health Care, 27*(4),
242–249. doi:10.1016/j.pedhc.2013.02.001

Hornor, G. (2014). Child neglect: Assessment and intervention. *Journal of Pediatric Health Care, 28*(2), 186–192.
doi:10.1016/j.pedhc.2013.10.002

Hornor, G. (2017). Sexually transmitted infections and children: What the PNP should know. *Journal of Pediatric
Health Care, 31*(2), 222–229. doi:10.1016/j.pedhc.2016.04
.016

Hornor, G., & Fischer, B. (2016). Child sexual abuse revictimization: Child demographics, familial psychosocial
risk factors, & sexual abuse case characteristics. *Journal of Forensic Nursing, 12*(4), 151–159. doi:10.1097/
JFN.000000000000124

Jackson, S. (2018). *Understanding elder abuse: A clinician's guide.* Washington, DC: American Psychological
Association.

Jansson, L. (2019). Neonatal abstinence syndrome. In J. A.
Garcia-Prats (Ed.), *UpToDate.* Retrieved from https://www
.uptodate.com/contents/neonatal-abstinence-syndrome

Jenny, C. (1999). Analysis of missed cases of abusive head
trauma. *Journal of the American Medical Association,
281*(7), 621–626. doi:10.1001/jama.281.7.621

Jinna, S. (2017). Cutaneous sign of abuse: Kids are not just
little people. *Clinics in Dermatology, 35,* 504–511.
doi:10.1016/j.clindermatol.2017.08.002

Kairys, S. W., Johnson, C. F., & Committee on Child Abuse
and Neglect. (2002). The psychological maltreatment of

children—Technical report. *Pediatrics, 109,* e68–e70. doi:10.1542/peds.109.4.e68

Kann, L., McManus, R., Harris, W. A., Shanklin, S. L., Flint, K. H., Hawkins, J., . . . Zaza, S. (2016). Youth risk behavior surveillance—United States. *MMWR Surveillance Summaries, 65*(6), 1–174. doi:10.15585/mmwr.ss6509a1

Kellogg, N. (2005). The evaluation of sexual abuse in children. *Pediatrics, 116*(2), 992–998. doi:10.1542/peds.2005-1336

Kim, K., Trickett, P., & Putnam, F. (2010). Childhood experiences of sexual abuse and later parenting practices among non-offending mothers of sexually abused and comparison girls. *Child Abuse & Neglect, 34,* 610–622. doi:10.1016/j.chiabu.2010.01.007

Klish, W. (2018). Clinical evaluation of the obese child and adolescent. In K. J. Motil & M. E. Geffner (Eds.), *UpToDate.* Retrieved from https://www.uptodate.com/contents/clinical-evaluation-of-the-obese-child-and-adolescent

Krishnamoorthy, V. (2012). Pediatric burn injuries. *International Journal of Critical Illness and Injury Science, 2*(3), 128–134. doi:10.4103/2229-5151.100889

Kuhar, D., Henderson, D., Struble, K., Heneine, W., Thomas, V., Cheever, L. . . . Panlilio, A. (2015). Updated U.S. public health service guidelines for the management of occupational exposures to human immunodeficiency virus and recommendations for postexposure prophylaxis. Retrieved from https://npin.cdc.gov/publication/updated-us-public-health-service-guidelines-management-occupational-exposures-human

Lang, J. M., Campbell, K., Shanley, P., Crusto, C. A., & Connell, C. M. (2016). Building capacity for trauma-informed care in the child welfare system. *Child Maltreatment, 21*(2), 113–124. doi:10.1177/1077559516635273

Lindberg, D. (2009). Utility of hepatic transaminases to recognize abuse in children. *Pediatrics, 124,* 509–516. doi:10.1542/peds.2008-2348

Lindberg, D. (2012). Prevalence of abusive injuries in siblings and household contacts of physically abused children. *Pediatrics, 130,* 193–201. doi:10.1542/peds.2012-0085

Lindberg, D. (2014). Yield of skeletal survey by age in children referred to abuse specialists. *The Journal of Pediatrics, 164,* 1268–1273. doi:10.1016/j.jpeds.2014.01.068

Lindegren, M., Hanson, I., Hammett, T., Beil, J., Fleming, P., & Ward, J. (1998). Sexual abuse of children: Intersection with HIV epidemic. *Pediatrics, 102*(4), e46. doi:10.1542/peds.102.4.e46

Maguire, S. (2005a). Are there patterns of bruising in childhood which are diagnostic or suggestive of abuse? A systematic review. *Archives of Disease in Childhood, 90,* 182–186. doi:10.1136/adc.2003.044065

Maguire, S. (2005b). Can you age bruises accurately in children? A systematic review. *Archives of Disease in Childhood, 90,* 187–189. doi:10.1136/adc.2003.044073

Maguire, S. (2008). A systematic review of the features that indicate intentional scalds in children. *Burns, 34,* 1072–1081. doi:10.1016/j.burns.2008.02.011

Maguire, S. (2013). Systematic reviews of bruising in relation to child abuse—What have we learnt: An overview of review updates. *Evidence-Based Child Health, 8,* 255–263. doi:10.1002/ebch.1909

Maniglio, R. (2009). The impact of child sexual abuse on health: A systematic review of reviews. *Clinical Psychology Review, 29,* 647–657. doi:10.1016/j.cpr.2009.08.003

Molnar, B., Beatriz, E., & Beardslee, W. (2016). Community-level approaches to child maltreatment prevention. *Trauma, Violence & Abuse, 17*(4), 387–397. doi:10.1177/1524838016658879

Motil, K. & Duryea, T. (2019). Poor weight gain in children younger than 2 years: Etiology & evaluation. In J. E. Drutz & C. Jensen (Eds.), *UpToDate.* Retrieved from https://www.uptodate.com/contents/poor-weight-gain-in-children-younger-than-two-years-etiology-and-evaluation

Murray, L., Nguyen, A., & Cohen, J. (2014). Child sexual abuse. *Child & Adolescent Psychiatric Clinics North America, 23,* 312–337. doi:10.1016/j.chc.2014.01.003

National Center for Victims of Crime. (2012). *Child sexual abuse statistics.* Retrieved from http://victimsofcrime.org/media/reporting-on-child-sexual-abuse/child-sexual-abuse-statistics

National Center on Elder Abuse. (n.d.). *Statistics and data.* Retrieved from https://ncea.acl.gov/What-We-Do/Research/Statistics-and-Data.aspx

Niolon, P. H., Kearns, M., Dills, J., Rambo, K., Irvind, S., Armstead, T., & Gilbert, L. (2017). *Preventing intimate partner violence across the lifespan: A technical package of programs, policies, and practices.* Atlanta, GA: National Center for Injury Prevention and Control, Centers for Disease Control and Prevention.

Parks, S., Annest, J., Hill, H., & Karch, D. (2012). *Pediatric abusive head trauma: Recommended definitions for public health surveillance and research.* Atlanta, GA: Centers for Disease Control and Prevention.

Perry, B. D. (1994). Neurobiological sequelae of childhood trauma: PTSD in children. In M. M. Marburg (Ed.), *Catecholamine function in posttraumatic stress disorder: Emerging concepts* (pp. 253–276). Washington, DC: American Psychiatric Press.

Perry, B. D. (2002). Childhood experience and the expression of genetic potential: What childhood neglect tells us about nature and nurture. *Brain and Mind, 3,* 79–100. doi:10.1023/A:1016557824657

Pierce, M. (2010). Bruising characteristics discriminating physical child abuse from accidental trauma. *Pediatrics, 125,* 67–74. doi:10.1542/peds.2008-3632

Pierce, M., Magana, J. N., Kaczor, K., Lorenz, D. J., Meyers, G., Bennett, B. L., & Kanegaye, J. T. (2015). The prevalence of bruising among infants in pediatric emergency departments. *Annals of Emergency Medicine, 67*(1), 1–8. doi:10.1016/j.annemergmed.2015.06.021

Pilani, M. (2008). Genital findings in prepubertal girls: What can be concluded from an examination? *Journal of Pediatric and Adolescent Gynecology, 21*(4), 177–185. doi:10.1016/j.jpag.2007.08.005

Potthast, N., Neuner, F., & Catani, C. (2014). The contribution of emotional maltreatment to alcohol dependence in a treatment-seeking sample. *Addictive Behaviors, 39,* 949–958. doi:10.1016/j.addbeh.2014.01.015

Rubin, D. (2003). Occult head injury in high-risk abused children. *Pediatrics, 111,* 1382–1386. doi:10.1542/peds.111.6.1382

Ryan, E., & Otonichar, J. (2016). Juvenile sex offenders. *Current Psychiatry Report, 18,* 1–10. doi:10.1007/s11920-016-0706-1

Schilling, S., & Christian, C. (2014). Child physical abuse and neglect. *Child & Adolescent Psychiatric Clinics of North America, 23,* 309–319. doi:10.1016/j.chc.2014.01.001

Schmitt, B. (1987). Seven deadly sins of childhood: Advising parents about difficult developmental phases. *Child Abuse and Neglect, 11,* 421–432. doi:10.1016/0145-2134(87)90015-9

Sharps, P., Laughon, K., & Giangrande, S. (2007). Intimate partner violence and the childbearing year: Maternal and infant health consequences. *Trauma Violence Abuse, 8*(2), 105–116. doi:10.1177/1524838007302594

Sheets, L. (2013). Sentinel injuries in infants evaluated for child physical abuse. *Pediatrics, 131,* 701–707. doi:10.1542/peds.2012-2780

Shin, S. H., Lee, S., Jeon, S. M., & Wills, T. A. (2015). Childhood emotional abuse, negative emotion-driven impulsivity, and alcohol use in young adulthood. *Child Abuse & Neglect, 50,* 94–103. doi:10.1016/j.chiabu.2015.02.010

Smith, D., Grohskopf, L., Black, R., Auerbach, J., Veronese, F., Struble, K., . . . Greenberg, A. (2005). Antiretroviral postexposure prophylaxis after sexual, injection-drug use, or other nonoccupational exposure to HIV in the United States. *MMWR: Recommendations and Reports, 54*(RR02), 1–20

Smith, S. G., Chen, J., Basile, K. C., Gilbert, L. K., Merrick, M. T., Patel, N., . . . Jain, A. (2017). *The National Intimate Partner Violence Survey (NISVS): 2010-2012 state report.* Atlanta, GA: National Center for Injury Prevention and Control, Centers for Disease Control and Prevention.

Substance Abuse and Mental Health Services Administration. (2012). *SAMHSA's working definition of trauma and principles and guidance for a trauma-informed approach* [Draft]. Rockville, MD: Substance Abuse and Mental Health Services Administration.

Substance Abuse and Mental Health Services Administration. (2014). *Trauma-informed care in behavioral health services. Treatment Improvement Protocol (TIP) Series 57* [HHS Publication No. (SMA) 13-4801]. Rockville, MD: Author.

Sugar, N., Taylor, J. A., Feldman, K. W., & Puget Sound Pediatric Research Network (1999). Bruises in infants and toddlers: Those who don't cruise rarely bruise. *Archives of Pediatrics & Adolescent Medicine, 153,* 399–403. doi:10.1001/archpedi.153.4.399

Traub, F., & Boynton-Jarrett, R. (2017). Modifiable resilience factors to childhood adversity of clinical pediatric practice. *Pediatrics, 139*(5), 1–13. doi:10.1542/peds.2016-2569

Ullman, S., & Vasquez, A. (2015). Mediators of sexual revictimization risk in adult sexual assault victims. *Journal of Child Sexual Abuse, 24*(3), 300–314. doi:10.1080/10538712.2015.1006748

U.S. Department of Health and Human Services, Administration for Children and Families, Administration on Children, Youth and Families, Children's Bureau. (2018). *Child maltreatment 2016.* Retrieved from https://www.acf.hhs.gov/sites/default/files/cb/cm2016.pdf

U.S. Preventive Services Task Force. (2018, April). *Screening for intimate partner violence, elder abuse, and abuse of vulnerable adults.* Retrieved from https://www.uspreventiveservicestaskforce.org/USPSTF_Admin/Home/GetFileByID/3589

U.S. Preventive Services Task Force. (2018). Screening for intimate partner violence and abuse of elderly and vulnerable adults: U.S. Preventive Services Task Force Recommendation Statement. *Journal of the American Medical Association, 320*(16), 1678–1687. doi:10.1001/jama.2018.14741

U.S. Preventive Services Task Force. (2018, October). *Final Update Summary: Intimate Partner Violence, Elder Abuse, and Abuse of Vulnerable Adults: Screening.* Retrieved from https://www.uspreventiveservicestaskforce.org/Page/Document/UpdateSummaryFinal/intimate-partner-violence-and-abuse-of-elderly-and-vulnerable-adults-screening1

Wissink, I., van Vugt, E., Moonen, X., Stams, G., & Hendriks, J. (2015). Sexual abuse involving children with intellectual disabilities. *Research Developmental Disabilities, 36,* 20–35. doi:10.1016/j.ridd.2014.09.007

Workowski, K., & Berman, S. (2006, August 4). Sexually transmitted diseases treatment guidelines. *MMWR: Recommendations and Reports, 55*(RR11), 1–94. Retrieved from https://www.cdc.gov/mmwr/preview/mmwrhtml/rr5511a1.htm

World Health Organization. (1999). Report of the consultation on child abuse prevention. Retrieved from https://apps.who.int/iris/handle/10665/65900

World Health Organization. (2013). *Global and regional estimates of violence against women: Prevalence and health effects of intimate partner violence and non-partner sexual violence.* Geneva, Switzerland: WHO Press.

World Health Organization. (2018, June 8). *Elder abuse.* Retrieved from https://apps.who.int/iris/handle/10665/65900

Yon, Y., Ramiro-Gonzalez, M., Mikton, C. R., Huber, M., & Sethi, D. (2019, February). The prevalence of elder abuse in institutional settings: A systematic review and meta-analysis. *European Journal of Public Health, 29*(1), 58–67. doi:10.1093/eurpub/cky093

Evidence-Based Therapeutic Communication and Motivational Interviewing in Health Assessment

Sharon Tucker, Debbie Sheikholeslami, and Haley Roberts

"Most people do not listen with the intent to understand; they listen with the intent to reply."

—STEPHEN R. COVEY

LEARNING OBJECTIVES

- Discuss the importance of communication in the assessment process to create a positive and safe environment for patients to share and express their symptoms, concerns, and health education needs.
- Review key evidence-based communication strategies for conducting health assessments.
- Demonstrate the value and evidence for motivational interviewing for conducting health assessments.

THERAPEUTIC COMMUNICATION IN THE CONTEXT OF HEALTH ASSESSMENT

THERAPEUTIC COMMUNICATION, MOTIVATIONAL INTERVIEWING, AND STAGES OF CHANGE

Therapeutic Communication Skills

Use of **therapeutic communication** is an expected, evidence-based standard of care in clinician–patient encounters, including advanced assessment, with consideration of patient age, developmental level, health literacy level, cultural perspectives, and unique dimensions of health and well-being.

Therapeutic communication involves genuine communication between a clinician and patient or client. Different from social communication, the focus is one sided, that is, all on the patient and meeting the needs and goals of the patient. Clinicians show respect and **empathy** to the individual, aim to understand and encourage expressions, and facilitate problem-solving. The general components of therapeutic communication include the sender (person communicating), receiver (person listening to the information), message (the actual information being communicated), and feedback context (circumstances in which the communication is occurring). The primary goal for the clinician when "sending" a message is to convey clear, useful messages; when "receiving" a message, to accurately interpret what patients are communicating. **Reflection** is a very effective technique to ensure the clinician is accurately interpreting what an individual is communicating.

Clinicians need to consider the context of the communication to best view and understand from the patient's perspective. For example, if a patient conveys that their primary presenting symptom is back pain, the emotion and meaning to the patient may be very different for a woman who works in construction than for a survivor of ovarian cancer. The process of therapeutic communication is dynamic and occurs within the context and dimensions of wellness and illness, which include the physical experience of symptoms, as well as what the individual is experiencing in terms of emotion, thoughts, and meaning. Verbal and nonverbal behaviors intended and perceived are components of the assessment process that clinicians need to be mindful of during interviews and assessments.

Clinicians must attend to a number of factors for their communication to be therapeutic while completing advanced assessment, beginning with consideration of patient characteristics such as age, gender, language, education, attitudes, self-concept, experiences, and cultural and spiritual beliefs. Sensory components such as vision, hearing, smell, taste, and tactile abilities are important to assess. Components of the message must be considered, including denotation, the literal meaning of words being sent; connotation, what the receiver interprets; vocabulary; and pacing. Medical language is important to clarify (or avoid) because many patients do not understand medical terms and definitions. Clinicians regularly use medical language with colleagues, yet patients are often confused by medical terminology and may not choose to ask for clarification, given their vulnerability as patients. Individuals also absorb language at different rates, and knowing when a patient is not keeping up is crucial to effective therapeutic communication. Using pauses and asking the patients to repeat back what they are hearing (also known as **teach-back**) can be useful to avoid losing the patients in the conversation. Setting goals with the patient, being brief, and offering clarity or asking for clarity are also important elements of effective therapeutic communication, which should be completed while maintaining confidentiality, privacy, and a nonjudgmental attitude (verbal and nonverbal).

Motivational Interviewing

A specific evidence-based therapeutic communication approach that has become widespread in use is **motivational interviewing** (MI). Developed by William Miller and Stephen Rollnick, MI is defined as a collaborative, goal-oriented style of communication with particular attention to the language of change. MI is designed to strengthen personal motivation for and commitment to a specific goal by eliciting and exploring the person's own reasons for change within an atmosphere of acceptance and compassion (Miller & Rollnick, 2013). Sharon Tucker, co-author of this chapter, offers the definition as follows: "MI is an evidence-based assessment and coaching process that uses **non-judgmental** listening and other guiding tools to help generate and develop a person's own motivation for changing a behavior that will serve them positively."

MI has its roots in treatment of substance abuse. Psychologists and social workers have long been familiar with MI as an effective behavioral approach in the treatment of substance use disorder. MI has also been successfully applied as an approach in the areas of weight management, self-management of hypertension and diabetes, and medication adherence. There is a growing interest in applying MI to other areas of healthcare, from pain management to fall prevention; the potential applications are endless when behavior change is desired.

MI changes the dynamic of the healthcare clinician's interaction with the patient. Patients do not change their habits/behaviors by being shamed into changing or instructed to change; rather, the patients will consider change if they see it as in their best interest or that it will benefit them more than it will cost them and when they do not feel judged. MI is a **patient-centered** philosophy with a core belief that the answer to commitment to change is within the patient. MI works by activating the patient's own motivation for change and adherence to treatment. MI is nonconfrontational in its approach; however, it is empathetic and involves more of a guiding rather than directing style, listening more than telling. The healthcare clinician works as a partner with patients to overcome ambivalence to change and gently guides them toward their desired goals. This process involves recognizing that individuals vary in their readiness to make a behavior change, even those changes that the clinician thinks are critical to health outcomes. Recognition of an individual's readiness to change as an important factor in changing health behaviors developed as a behavioral approach concurrent to MI; both MI techniques and the assessment of readiness to change can be used successfully to affect sustained change in healthy lifestyle behaviors.

Stages of Change

In the 1970s, James Prochaska and Carlo DiClemente developed the Transtheoretical Model of Change (TTM), which defined six stages of change a person goes through for successful behavior change (Prochaska, DiClemente, & Norcross, 1992).

- Stage 1 – Precontemplation: The individual is not yet considering change or is unwilling or unable to change.
- Stage 2 – Contemplation: The individual recognizes the possibility of change, but is ambivalent and uncertain.
- Stage 3 – Determination: The individual is committed to changing, but is still considering what to do.
- Stage 4 – Action: The individual is taking steps toward change, but the change is not yet stabilized.
- Stage 5 – Maintenance: The individual's goals have been achieved, and efforts are focused on maintaining the change.

- Stage 6 – Recurrence: The individual experiences a recurrence or relapse of the old behaviors and is deciding what to do next.

The model in **Figure 25.1** represents the stages of change a person goes through for successful behavior change. The stages are not linear; movement back and forward occurs depending on many factors. If or when relapse happens, an individual can go back one stage or more, or all the way back to precontemplation. For example, a patient made the decision to quit smoking (Contemplation), devised a plan (Determination), stopped smoking for 6 months (Action), but returned to smoking because of a stressful life event and is not sure if they will be able to quit again (Contemplation). In this example, the individual did not enter the maintenance stage but took several steps back. This example is not uncommon, as stages of change are not linear; as such, the work for this example patient will be about addressing their ambivalence.

KEY SKILLS AND CONSIDERATIONS WHEN ELICITING PATIENT HISTORY

THERAPEUTIC SKILLS TO ELICIT CHIEF CONCERN AND REASON FOR VISIT

Before a healthcare team member first meets a patient, whether inpatient or outpatient, the clinician is likely to have reviewed the individual's medical record, including vital signs, medications, and diagnosis list, and may have received a handoff report or reviewed a health summary; this information often leads the clinician to consider their own goals/initiatives to accomplish during the patient encounter. To be most therapeutic, one must set these expectations aside and first talk with the patient about their health and wellness concerns, allow the individual to clarify the reason for seeking care and verbalize their own goals for the visit (or for their health), and determine the patient's stage of readiness for change (**Figure 25.2**).

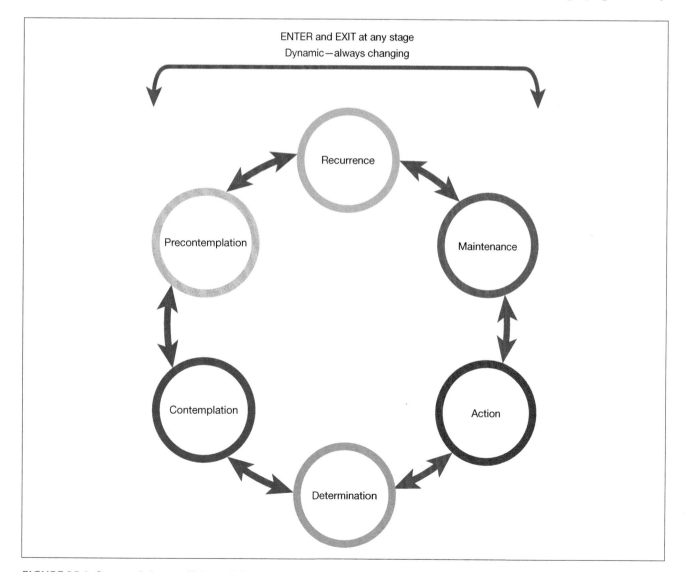

FIGURE 25.1 Stages of change. This model represents the stages of change that lead to successful, sustained behavior change.

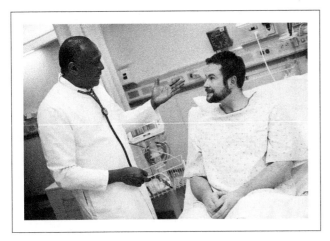

FIGURE 25.2 Clinician speaking with patient.
Source: National Institutes of Health Clinical Center.

TABLE 25.1 Core Motivational Interviewing Skills	
Core Skills	**Description**
Open-ended questions	Used to establish acceptance and trust between the clinician interviewer and the patient or client. The client should be doing the majority of the talking, while the interviewer listens and encourages
Affirmations	This can be done in the manner of a compliment, highlighting an individual's strengths and efforts of behavioral change
Reflection: Simple	Repeat: Adds little to no meaning or emphasis to what the patient or client has said Rephrase: Slightly altering what a patient or client has said
Reflections: Complex	A clinician interviewer's reflection that adds additional or different meaning beyond what the patient has just said; a guess as to what the individual may have meant
Continuing the paragraph	A method of reflective listening in which the clinician offers what may be next (as yet unspoken) by the patient or client's paragraph
Amplified	Reflects back on what an individual has said in an amplified or exaggerated form—to state in an even more extreme manner than the client or patient has done
Reflection of feeling	Emphasizing the emotional content of what the individual has said; guess about emotion(s) patient may be experiencing
Paraphrase	Speculation about what a patient or client means
Double sided	Reflects both sides of an individual's ambivalence
Metaphor	Painting a picture that can clarify the patient or client's position

Note: Core skills of motivational interviewing described are patient-centered, strength-based, authentic strategies that lead to patient activation and motivation to change.

The spirit of MI conveys that both the individual seeking care and clinician are equal, collaborative partners in the relationship. From the introduction through the health assessment, motivation to change is noted and elicited from the individual. The patient or client is the best expert on self. People are almost always ambivalent about change—this is normal. They are more likely to change when they hear their own discussion about their ambivalence. This discussion is called **change talk**.

There are **four processes of MI** that are relevant to advanced assessment: Engaging, Focusing, Evoking, and Planning. There is a hierarchy to these four processes; each builds off the previous level. **Engaging** skills are essential to the spirit of MI and are used throughout assessments, including when resistance is encountered. **Focusing** is the next phase and includes attention to a patient problem or concern and goal. This may take one or more sessions. The next phase involves **Evoking,** which integrates the MI spirit and a process of evoking change talk from patients. The use of open-ended questions assists in evoking what is important to the patient and what is working and not working. Individual strengths and past successes are assessed and recognized to facilitate self-efficacy and motivation for change. Finally, the **Planning** stage involves guiding the individual to form a concrete plan of action. The patient or client must be ready for this stage, bringing back the importance of assessing stages of change and the need to re-engage and maybe refocus and evoke more change talk.

Important components of MI include empathizing and empowering the individuals to take steps toward change and affirming their strengths. Being genuine is important, along with the MI spirit, empathy, open-ended questions, validation and affirmation, and use of **reflective listening**. The core skills of MI are listed in **Table 25.1**. Assess for (a) signs of change talk, such as "I've been struggling with headaches every morning and I would like to get rid of them," (b) increased confidence or self-efficacy, such as "I truly believe I can do this," and (c) self-monitoring, such as "I have been keeping track of my physical activity levels and seeing a gradual increase daily."

ELICITING THE PAST MEDICAL HISTORY

This chapter highlights the importance of eliciting an accurate patient history; the process is influenced heavily by the communication process and style that a clinician employs. The communication process will be most effective when therapeutic communication principles and skills are used to develop rapport. Again, this means conveying reflective listening, nonjudgment, empathy, and sensitivity to the context of the patient's particular situation. Respect for the individual is essential, as are privacy, confidentiality, and sufficient time to ensure the collection of accurate information.

Verbal and nonverbal behaviors by clinicians are validated in the literature as influential in promoting the best assessment. Examples of verbal behaviors described earlier are language, pace, intonation, pitch, and volume. Examples of nonverbal behaviors include eye contact, interested posture, nodding of head, hand gestures, clothing, and facial gestures. Patients need to feel they are in a safe, trusting environment with a clinician who respects and values them and their situations to be able to share all history experiences without fear of shame, judgment, and less quality care. Conditions that are behavior related, such as obesity, will invoke shame when the complexity is not appreciated, and possibly lead to the withholding of information vital to the assessment and diagnosis.

FAMILY HEALTH HISTORY

As noted throughout this chapter, family history of illness is one of the key risk factors for common, chronic disease, and is an important genomic tool for disease prevention and population health. Use of therapeutic communication and MI skills are strategies that can help a patient understand the link(s) between their illness, or risk of illness, and family history. Examples of therapeutic statements while assessing family history include the following: "Tell me about your family and what struggles with illness you recall family members experiencing" or "May I ask you about your family's health history as this can assist me in understanding your risks for illness as well as what treatment options might be best for you?"

SOCIAL HISTORY

Use of therapeutic communication and MI can also improve a clinician's ability to complete a social history. Wu (2013) proposes that a patient-centered approach to the health assessment interview is to begin with the social history because this allows the clinician to convey interest in the individuals beyond their medical illness/condition and fosters the clinician–patient relationship. Assessment of social history, including current living arrangements, social support system including spiritual support, educational background, occupation, marital status, birth history, functional status, gender identity, and sexual health history; assessment of healthy lifestyle behaviors including diet/nutrition, sleep and rest, tobacco use, and alcohol intake; and assessments related to substance use and coping allow the clinician to appreciate the individual's dimensions of health and wellness. As noted in Chapter 3, Approach to Implementing and Documenting Patient-Centered, Culturally Sensitive Evidence-Based Assessment, asking about the environments in which an individual resides, works, learns, plays, worships, and connects socially offers insight into the impact of community in their lives. Each chapter in this text has offered culturally sensitive, patient-centered history questions related to social history to improve the clinician's ability to ask social history questions. Review these within the context of the practice of therapeutic communication to avoid implied judgment or implicit bias. To begin an assessment with a therapeutic approach to social history with a broad, open-ended question such as, "What is a typical day like for you—in terms of your daily routine for work, school, meals, and bedtime?" stands in contrast to a closed-ended, negative question such as "You don't smoke, do you?" which can make the patient to feel defensive.

An essential communication tool to use during the assessment of social history is to remember to respond to the patient's response. As previously noted, reflection is an excellent tool that allows the assessment to move forward and provides clarity. Often, novice clinicians uncover information during the history taking that is difficult for them (as the healthcare clinician) to assimilate; if/when this happens, the novice clinician can use reflection and respond by stating, "Thank you for sharing. May I have your permission to revisit this information after completing your exam?" This type of statement acknowledges the information that was shared and allows the clinician time to assimilate the meaning of the information within the context of the patient's health and wellness.

PREVENTIVE CARE CONSIDERATIONS

Life-Span Considerations for History

Patient age and level of development must be considered in the therapeutic communication process. Clearly, infants will largely communicate through behavioral cues such as crying and smiling, and clinicians will offer gentle touches and positive facial expressions (**Figure 25.3**). Younger children (toddlers and preschoolers) will have a limited receptive and expressive vocabulary and understanding, and clinicians need to use language accordingly and/or speak with their parents. Messages that are angry, reflect dissatisfaction, or invoke fear will be important to avoid with young children. Working with parents to get a good history,

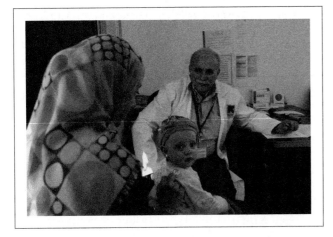

FIGURE 25.3 Clinician talking with parent and child.

Source: DFID-UK Department for International Development.

without judging, to understand the situation and make sense of observations using the same approach as if they were the patients will be important. The clinician will also want to be mindful of parents' interpretations of their child's presenting concerns and what role they play as parents, and be supportive and encourage the parents along with the child. Building confidence among parents will also be important. Adolescents can be treated as young adults with adjustments for their self-image issues, sensitivity to specific issues, and physical examination. Clinicians will want to support their self-efficacy, utilizing empathy, open-ended questions to understand their perceptions, nonjudgment, affirmation, and good listening with reflective statements.

Unique Population Consideration for History

Use of therapeutic communication and MI are appropriate skills to assess and promote preventive care, whether encouraging routine immunizations, regular physical examinations, completing appropriate screenings such as mammography or colon cancer screening, or self-care behaviors such as meeting recommendations for daily physical activity, meeting dietary guideline recommendations, or monitoring stress levels or use of alcohol. Good holistic listening, nonjudgment, empathy, and sensitivity to the context of the patient's particular situation are important. Respect for the patient is essential; this includes privacy, confidentiality, and sufficient time to ensure the collection of accurate information. Verbal and nonverbal behaviors by clinicians are validated in the literature as influential in promoting the best assessment. MI skills of open-ended questions, validation and affirmation, and use of reflective listening can be most effective for promoting the behaviors desired and working in partnership with individuals to meet their personal goals that are consistent with their values.

PHYSICAL EXAMINATION

During every step of the physical assessment, therapeutic, respectful communication should be used. If the clinician has concerns about an individual's ability to communicate or understand communication, special considerations for adjusting communication strategies are required. These include situations where cognition may be impaired.

SPECIAL CONSIDERATIONS FOR COMMUNICATING DURING THE PHYSICAL EXAM

If there are indications for impaired cognition, clinicians can use a standardized assessment tool to assess cognition, such as The Mini-Mental State Examination (MMSE). The MMSE is an 11-question standardized assessment that measures five areas of cognitive impairment: orientation, registration, attention and calculation, recall, and language. The maximum score of the assessment is 30, whereas a score of 23 or lower is indicative of cognitive impairment. The MMSE takes approximately 5 to 10 minutes to administer and is, therefore, feasible to use repeatedly and routinely. A recent meta-analysis conducted by Mitchell (2013) on the reliability and validity of the MMSE indicates reliability to be moderate and test–retest good. There are concerns about using it to discriminate dementia, mild cognitive impairment, and delirium; however, it performs adequately as a screening instrument. Thus, it can be used in routine assessments to rule out general concerns about cognitive challenges. Any identified concerns must be further assessed with additional diagnostic tools.

Clinicians will need to adjust their communication style somewhat with cognitive impairment. Listening remains highly relevant, along with being nonjudgmental, empathetic, sensitive, and respectful. Use of reflective statements, types of questions, and goal setting may need to be modified depending on the patient's level of understanding and ability to speak.

For patients with altered cognition due to psychosis, communication style will also need to be adjusted. For example, McCabe et al. (2016) examined a specific training program for psychiatrists focusing on understanding the patient with psychotic experiences, communication techniques for working with the symptoms, empowering the patient using agenda setting (an MI technique), explaining normalizing psychosis, and involving the patient in decision-making about medications. In a randomized controlled trial, they found the training can improve relationships in treating psychosis. Although expertise in such skills is beyond the expectations for general health clinicians, the study demonstrates the importance of understanding the patient's experience and empowering patients in decision-making, which are skills consistent with general therapeutic communication and MI. Similarly, working with other mental health conditions such as depression and anxiety will require unique attention to listening, observing the patient's nonverbal cues, using silence, understanding transference, maintaining empathy and compassion, seeking clarification, and dealing with suicidal ideations (Martin & Chanda, 2016). Additional training and supervision may be needed by clinicians to develop skills in working with patients with mental illness.

For individuals with speech disorders or conditions, the same therapeutic general skills are important, but the degree of patient participation through interview methods may need to be modified. Finally, the same considerations will be needed with cultural and language barriers. Individuals who speak through an interpreter will need the same general skills; however, the extent of what the individual is able to convey may differ. The interpretation might also change meanings; clinicians can talk with interpreters and family members as appropriate, as well as other clinicians, to best meet the patient's goals and concerns.

EVIDENCE-BASED PRACTICE CONSIDERATIONS

Substantial evidence exists to support therapeutic communication approaches and strategies related to health assessment and treatment. Three particular approaches related to health assessment and prevention coaching are highlighted here. These are the 5 A's, MI, and trauma-informed care (TIC).

THE 5 A'S APPROACH

The U.S. Preventive Services Task Force recognizes a number of behavioral counseling interventions that are evidence based. They endorsed a paper originally published by Whitlock, Orleans, Pender, and Allan (2002) that reviews the evidence supporting behavioral counseling strategies. The authors report there is no simple model that captures the range of behaviors perceived as posing health risks and in need of change; however, they identified a 4 A's framework that offers a workable model that can be used in multiple settings and with a range of behaviors.

The 4 A's are ask, advise, assist, and arrange. Originally developed by the National Cancer Institute for guiding smoking cessation, others have recommended the 4 A's for use in general clinical practice and for a variety of behaviors. The Canadian Task Force on Preventive Health Care added a fifth A, "agree," and changed the word "ask" to "assess"; this model was recommended as a general approach for behavioral counseling. The U.S. Preventive Services Task Force endorses the 5 A's for

TABLE 25.2 The 5 A's to Support Behavioral Change

Term	Definition
Assess	Beliefs, behavior, and knowledge
Advise	Provide clear and specific health benefits and risks
Agree	Collaboratively set goals for patient's interest and their confidence to change the behavior
Assist	Using a behavior change approach, identify personal barriers, strategies, and problem-solving techniques
Arrange	Specify a plan for follow-up (in person or through phone) to provide consistent assistance/support; adjust the treatment plan as needed

Note: As an evidence-based model, the 4 A's can be used as an approach to behavior change. The fifth A (agree) reflects the importance of setting goals collaboratively.

clinicians; these can be applied when performing health assessments and prevention coaching. See **Table 25.2** for definitions of the terms included in the model.

MOTIVATIONAL INTERVIEWING

As highlighted considerably in this chapter, MI is an approach recommended for both behavioral counseling and as an approach to health assessment. A number of systematic reviews have been published on MI (Burke, Arkowitz, & Menchola, 2003; Dunn, Deroo, & Rivara, 2001; McKenzie, Pierce, & Gunn, 2015; Purath, Keck, & Fitzgerald, 2014; Rubak, Sandbaek, Lauritzen, & Christensen, 2005). Knight, McGowan, Dickens, and Bundy (2006) examined MI effectiveness in physical healthcare settings and found most studies identified positive outcomes from MI; however, most studies faced methodological issues. In a 2010 review, MI was examined for general healthcare professionals (Söderlund, Madson, Rubak, & Nilsen, 2011). Findings were generally favorable for MI to improve communication and counseling lifestyle-related issues; however, similar to the 2006 review, studies were again evaluated as limited by methodological quality.

Lundahl and colleagues (2013) reviewed 48 studies (9,618 participants) in their systematic review and meta-analysis of MI efficacy in medical care settings. Their findings indicated a modest advantage for MI across a number of health behaviors, delivery settings, and patient characteristics. Likewise, VanBuskirk and Wetherell (2014) found MI to be useful in primary care populations with as few as one session to enhance readiness to change and promote health behaviors to reach patient goals.

In a systematic review by Copeland, McNamara, Kelson, and Simpson (2015), motivation and MI spirit were identified as the most promising mechanisms of MI. They found that MI spirit was linked to patient change talk and that patient health behaviors were associated with positive health outcomes. More high-quality research is needed; however, various factors support the general approach in working with patients, including listening to them, establishing a true partnership in identifying behavior change needs, supporting the patients' ideas, and promoting patients' decisions about change and behavior.

Apodaca et al. (2016) aimed to identify individual therapist behaviors that elicit patient change talk or sustain talk in MI via a single session for alcohol intervention among college students. A therapist behavior that significantly increased student change talk and reduced sustain talk (reasons to not change) was the use of affirm. Affirm is described as statements made by the therapist/clinician that convey something positive or complimentary to the patient. It may be in the form of expressed appreciation, confidence, or reinforcement.

This technique can be used when interviewing patients during health assessments and is likely to create a positive encounter and candidness from the patient about concerns and needs.

Motivational Interviewing for Fall-Risk Assessment

The authors of this chapter conducted a study to examine if nurses working within the hospital setting could utilize MI skills for brief encounters and assessments with hospitalized patients. They evaluated the effects of training nurses in MI to specifically incorporate into their existing falls assessment and prevention program on an oncology inpatient unit. The project built on an earlier project which revealed that among oncology patients who were interviewed about their fall history (Tucker et al., 2019), 70% who had a history of falls did not see themselves as at risk for falling. As falls are a major safety concern, this study serves as exemplar of how MI can be an approach for both behavioral counseling and as advanced assessment of health and well-being. See **Box 25.1** for an exemplar on utilizing MI for fall-risk assessment.

BOX 25.1
MOTIVATIONAL INTERVIEWING FOR FALL-RISK ASSESSMENT: AN EXEMPLAR

As falls are a major safety concern for hospitalized patients and their caregivers, staff members wondered if the use of MI could actively engage hospitalized patients in accurately assessing their risks for falling and identifying a plan for reducing these risks. The first step was to examine if nurses could be trained in the techniques and the spirit of MI, specifically related to engaging patients in discussing fall-risk assessment and prevention planning.

A convenience sample of 14 staff nurses volunteered to participate in the 8-week project, which included a 3-hour MI training program and pre- and post-training evaluations. These nurses worked on a designated inpatient oncology unit. The training included didactic content on MI principles and strategies, viewing videos of MI scenarios with discussion, and small group role-playing exercises.

Participants learned to facilitate a fall-risk conversation with patients. At time of admission, the nurse may have begun with, "We have a falls prevention program on our unit to help prevent patients from falling while in the hospital. Would it be OK for us to talk about this program?" Then, the nurse would say, "Before I tell you about the program, would you share with me what you know about your risks of falling while in the hospital?" The nurse would listen to the patient and use reflective statements to ensure they heard and interpreted what the patient intended. The nurse may have validated what the patient knew and then asked permission to share a bit more about the facts. The nurse then asked the patient what they thought about these facts. After validating the patient's understanding, the participants using MI might ask the patient, "Would you be willing to establish a plan that would work for you to reduce your risks?" A goal would be established with action strategies that worked for the patient and a confidence rating was assessed to determine the patient's readiness to stick to the plan. The plan was shared in the hospital room and medical record, assessed routinely, and modified as indicated.

After the initial training session was completed for all members of the project, the nurse participants were instructed to use the skills and knowledge learned in training in their patient care specific to fall prevention for the next 6 weeks. A single 3-hour training session was not expected to lead to nurse experts in MI; however, nurses' knowledge about MI increased after the training and practice period. Fifty-seven percent of the nurses showed improvement in their knowledge scores with the post-test. The observation data (Video Assessment of Simulated Encounters–Revised [VASE-R]) findings were consistent with data reported by Rosengren, Hartzler, Baer, Wells, and Dunn (2008) in their report of reliability and validity of the VASE-R. This study's baseline scores compared favorably to VASE-R study scores for individuals not trained

(continued)

in MI, MI-trained individuals, and experts in MI. Significant improvements were noted for the full-scale scores, with reflective listening and eliciting change talk driving the overall change. This was very consistent with expectations for newly trained MI clinicians and reflects that the nurse participants were developing awareness and achieving the spirit of MI. See **Table 25.3** for nurse participants' pre- and post-training MI scores.

Although not expected given the short intervention period, fall rates on the unit were also evaluated. Interestingly, fall rates decreased during and for a short time after the study to 0. See **Figure 25.4** for fall-rate data on the study unit. In the 1½ years before the study, the fall rates never reached 0. Moreover, no other fall initiatives were started during the study period. Although the sustainability of the fall rates is unlikely with no permanent program in place, this project demonstrated that engaging patients through MI strategies in assessing their risks of falling while hospitalized and in a prevention plan may indeed be an appropriate approach for hospitalized patients at risk for hospital-acquired conditions. Feedback from the nurses in the project included seeing value in developing MI skills for patient care, appreciating role-playing in the training as a useful training method, desiring more training with good reminders of the skills and how-to guidance, and expanding MI to other behaviors.

TABLE 25.3 Fall-Risk Assessment: Nurse Participant Pre- and Post-Training Motivational Interviewing Scores

Study Data Compared to VASE-R Author Reported Data*

	Pre-Training		Study's Pre-Training		Post-Training		Study's Post-Training	
	M	SD	*M*	SD	*M*	SD	*M*	SD
Full VASE-R score	18.21	7.41	19.93	5.28	24.13	6.74	24.13**	4.19
Reflective listening	4.88	2.26	5.43	1.99	6.13	2.04	6.14*	1.61
Responding to resistance	5.72	2.56	5.07	3.15	7.41	2.49	6.07	2.07
Summarizing	1.53	1.67	2.93	1.92	2.83	1.59	3.71	1.14
Eliciting change talk	2.79	1.69	1.93	2.23	3.66	1.76	3.64*	1.39
Developing discrepancy	3.29	1.86	4.57	1.34	4.10	1.61	4.57	1.60

*$p < 0.05$; **$p < 0.01$.

M, mean; SD, standard deviation; VASE-R, Video Assessment of Simulated Encounters–Revised.

Note: Study scores for pre- and post-MI training were (a) similar to the VASE-R reported data and (b) indicated significant improvement with eliciting change talk to drive overall change.

Motivational Interviewing for Special Populations

Children and Adolescents

MI has been found increasingly effective in incorporated weight-loss programs in obese children and adolescents. Pakpour, Gellert, Dombrowski, and Fridlund (2015) completed a study of 357 Iranian adolescents aged 14 to 18 years. The adolescents were selected randomly to receive MI intervention, MI intervention + parent, or assessments only (passive control). Data including anthropometric, biochemical, psychosocial, and behavioral measures were collected at baseline and 12 months later. Results demonstrated significant effects on most of the outcome parameters for MI + parent involvement (e.g., mean ± standard deviation

[SD] body mass index [BMI] z score: 2.58 ± 0.61) in comparison to the passive control group (2.76 ± 0.70; post hoc test, $p = 0.02$), also including an additional dominance of MI + parental involvement compared with MI only (2.81 ± 0.76; post hoc test, $p = 0.05$). This pattern was shown for most of the measures listed. To conclude, MI in addition to parental involvement is an effective strategy in changing obesity-related outcomes and has additional effects-surpassing benefits of MI with adolescents solely.

Individuals With Substance Use Disorder

As noted in Chapter 23, Evidence-Based Assessment of Substance Use Disorder, "[t]here are 76.3 million people

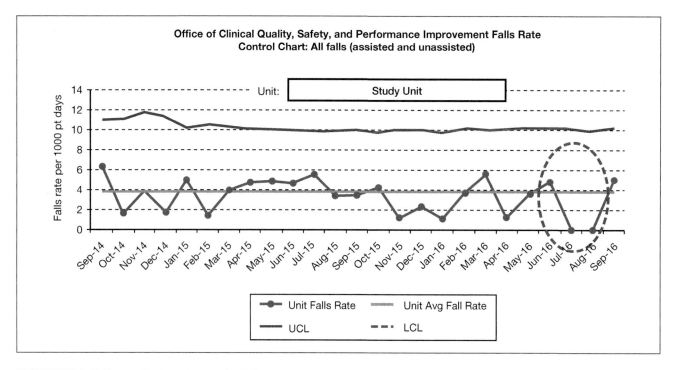

FIGURE 25.4 Fall rates for inpatient study. Fall rates dropped significantly after engaging patients through motivational interviewing strategies in assessing their risks of falling and in creating a plan to prevent falls while hospitalized. LCL, lower control limit; UCL, upper control limit.

with alcohol use disorders worldwide and 15.3 million with drug use disorders" (Smedslund et al, 2011, "Background"). A systematic review and meta-analysis published by Smedslund et al. (2011) investigated the effectiveness of MI for substance abuse or drug use, retention in treatment, readiness for change, and number of repeat convictions. The study included 59 randomized controlled trials with persons dependent on or abusing substances, with a total of 13,342 participants. Compared to no treatment control, MI participants showed a significant effect on substance use, which was the strongest at postintervention with a standard mean difference (SMD) 0.79 (95% confidence interval [CI] 0.48–1.09) and weaker at short follow-up, SMD 0.17 (95% CI 0.09–0.26) and the medium follow-up, SMD 0.15 (95% CI 0.04–0.25). For long-term follow-up, the effect was not significant SMD 0.06 (95% CI 0.16–0.28). There were no significant differences between MI and treatment for follow-up postintervention, and short and medium follow-up.

Adults Who Have Experienced Stroke

Strokes are not only life-threatening, but they can also create psychological issues that can cause those who have experienced a stroke to lose motivation in day-to-day activities. MI offers a specific way to promote intrinsic motivation. Cheng, Qu, Xiao, and Wang (2015) completed a systematic review of studies comparing MI with no intervention. Only one study of 411 adult stroke patients met inclusion criteria. Patients

received either MI or usual care between 5 and 28 days following stroke; the follow-up period was 12 months. Those who received MI had one session per week for four individual sessions, with each of the sessions lasting about 30 to 60 minutes. With only one study, the evidence was insufficient to support the use of MI for improving activities of daily living after stroke. However, participants receiving MI were more likely to have a normal mood than those who received usual care.

TRAUMA-INFORMED CARE

As outlined in Chapter 24, Evidence-Based Assessment and Screening for Traumatic Experiences: Abuse, Neglect, and Intimate Partner Violence, individuals who have experienced trauma have specific assessment needs. TIC is an evidence-based approach that emerged in the 1990s in recognition of the high prevalence of trauma exposure and significant impact of trauma on well-being and health states. In a Treatment Improvement Protocol published by the Substance Abuse and Mental Health Services Administration (SAMHSA), TIC is defined as "an intervention and organizational approach that focuses on how trauma may affect an individual's life and there response to behavioral health services from prevention through treatment" (SAMHSA, 2014, p. 32). Three elements are identified in TIC: recognition of the prevalence; recognizing impact of trauma on people, settings, and organizations, including one's workforce; and importance of using this knowledge in practice.

In a systematic review of evidence, the effects of organizational trainings related to TIC were evaluated (Purtle, 2018). Improved staff knowledge, attitudes, and behaviors and significant improvement in patient outcomes were positively correlated with clinician trainings in TIC.

CASE STUDY: Therapeutic Communication

Introduction

Clinicians can complete accurate, thorough, evidence-based assessment of health and well-being using therapeutic communication, specifically employing principles and techniques from MI, the 5 A's, and TIC. How these strategies are utilized for best practice depends on the patient and context, including case scenario, setting, and the patient's unique characteristics, including (but not limited to) age, gender, race, ethnicity, developmental status, culture and language, and presenting-disease comorbidities.

Therapeutic Communication in Assessing a Patient With Dizziness

A patient presenting with dizziness would first be welcomed to the clinical setting with a greeting from the clinician. Orienting the patient to the assessment process, including setting an agenda of what to expect during the interview and assessment, is a first step in MI. The clinician then asks the patient to describe what brings them to the office, perhaps starting with social history questions to convey interest in the patient as a whole and not just as a condition to be quickly assessed and treated. An opening statement might be, "Tell me a little about yourself and then we will move to what brings you here today."

Active listening is the most important skill of therapeutic communication with use of reflective statements, a great technique to ensure accurate interpretation of the patient's story and primary concerns. Use of open-ended questions (rather than closed-ended questions that require one-word answers) helps the clinician learn more about the story and allows the patient to direct what they shares. Expressing empathy as to the story and suffering, as well as avoiding judgments of the patient and building the patient's confidence in finding solutions are key strategies. Once the patient shares how dizziness affected them and caused fears, the clinician asks permission to focus the interview a bit more to assess the common types of dizziness symptoms (e.g., vertigo, near-faint, lightheaded/woozy, out of body/floating, motion sickness, gait unsteadiness). Again, open-ended questions are used by the clinician, with affirmation of the story components. This will include focusing on what triggers bring the dizziness on, when it began, how long an episode lasts if not constant, what makes it worse, what improves it, and what solutions the patient has tried. Additionally, it is important to assess the patient's goal regarding the dizziness. Giving the patient affirmation for their strengths and solution-finding will help build trust and confidence in the clinician.

Once the problem is shared, the focused interview is completed, and the patient is validated and affirmed about the characteristics of the dizziness, the clinician can seek permission from the patient to perform a physical examination and order indicated laboratory tests and imaging studies. General therapeutic techniques should be used throughout the examination, including maintaining privacy, showing patience and respect, observing nonverbal cues, asking permission and informing the patient along the way of each examination procedure, individualizing language, using reflective statements, showing empathy, and maintaining confidentiality.

Following completion of the physical examination and any immediate testing or studies, the clinician can review the results with the patient; overall, the clinician reviews and discusses the possibilities for the dizziness, possible solutions, patient resources to manage the solutions, patient confidence in being able to implement solutions, and action strategies to initiate first. This might include the need for laboratory and imaging tests first before a diagnosis can be made, which requires the clinician to be mindful of the different meaning for each patient of the experience of dizziness, of having this disorder, and for whether the requirement to wait for answers is anxiety producing. Using sensitive communication, affirming any anxiety, and asking the patient what will help them most during the waiting period demonstrates powerful therapeutic communication.

Once the problem is identified, the clinician needs to partner with the patient to develop strategies to meet the patient's goals and manage the medical problem. Creating a SMART goal or goals is key; SMART goals are those that are specific, measurable, action-oriented, realistic, and time-sensitive. Factors to consider and integrate into the goals are

(continued)

CASE STUDY: Therapeutic Communication (*continued*)

patient age, gender, language, education, attitudes, self-concept, previous and current health experiences, sensory limitations, abilities/disabilities, and cultural and spiritual beliefs. If concerns about cognitive impairment surface, use of the MMSE can provide screening data to decide if further assessment for cognitive decline is needed.

If behavior change is indicated for the dizziness, such as a need for reduction of stress, nonpharmacological interventions, or self-care strategies, readiness for change using stages of change is recommended. Asking open-ended questions about change readiness will help guide the SMART goal and action strategies. Scaling readiness on a scale ranging from 1 to 10 can be helpful, with the patient rating used to discuss what strategies might be first and most useful. If determined to be in precontemplation for change, the clinician might ask permission to review facts with the patient for consideration. If contemplating behavior change such as adding physical activity or changing

diet, exploring pros and cons of strategies will be important. As greater readiness stages are identified, selecting action strategies with confidence ratings that the patient can accomplish will be important.

Remaining empathic, offering validation and affirming the patients for the sharing, reviewing their strengths and past successes, and evoking change talk regarding behaviors that will help them resolve ambivalence and move in a positive health behavior direction are all important as part of the health assessment process; when conducted with therapeutic communication and particularly MI, it can lead into the treatment process and health behavior recommendations. Following up as agreed upon is essential for patient trust and building the relationship that will facilitate further testing, treatment follow-through, and behavioral change strategies. These are all strategies consistent with MI, the 5 A's, and TIC as a basis for doing all health and wellness assessments with patients.

Clinical Pearls

- Understanding patient values and goals in the assessment process offers tremendous insight into patient circumstances and presenting symptoms.
- To support behavioral change, remember 5 A's: **A**ssess beliefs and behaviors, **A**dvise about benefits and risks related to behavior change, **A**gree to goal setting collaboratively, **A**ssist with identifying strategies to reach goals, and **A**rrange a plan for follow-up.

Key Takeaways

- Listening to patients using simple and complex reflections and open-ended questions can promote communication vital to assessment.
- Practicing nonjudgmental and empathic listening is crucial in the assessment process.
- Therapeutic rapport is promoted through listening compassionately and opens the door for patient trust, transparency, and reduced resistance.

REFERENCES

Apodaca, T. R., Jackson, K. M., Borsari, B., Magill, M., Longabaugh, R., Mastroleo, N. R., . . . Barnett, N. P. (2016). Which individual therapist behaviors elicit client change talk and sustain talk in motivational interviewing? *Journal of Substance Abuse Treatment, 61,* 60–65. doi:10.1016/j.jsat.2015.09.001

Burke, B. L., Arkowitz, H., & Menchola, M. (2003). The efficacy of motivational interviewing: A meta-analysis of controlled clinical trials. *Journal of Consulting and Clinical Psychology, 5,* 843–861. doi:10.1037/0022-006X.71.5.843

Cheng, D., Qu, Z., Xiao, Y., & Wang, J. (2015). Motivational interviewing for improving recovery after stroke. *Cochrane Database of Systematic Reviews,* (6), CD011398. doi:10.1002/14651858.CD011398.pub2

Copeland, L., McNamara, R., Kelson, M., & Simpson, S. (2015). Mechanisms of change within motivational interviewing in relation to health behaviors outcomes: A systematic review. *Patient Education and Counseling, 98*(4), 401–411. doi:10.1016/j.pec.2014.11.022

Dunn, C., Deroo, L., & Rivara, F. P. (2001). The use of brief interventions adapted from motivational interviewing across behavioral domain: A systematic review. *Addiction, 96,* 1725–1742. doi:10.1046/j.1360-0443.2001.961217253.x

Knight, K. M., McGowan, L., Dickens, C., & Bundy, C. (2006). A systematic review of motivational interviewing in physical health care settings. *British Journal of Health Psychology, 11,* 319–332. doi:10.1348/135910705X52516

Lundahl, B., Moleni, T., Burke, B. L., Butters, R., Tollefson, D., Butler, C., & Rollnick, S. (2013). Motivational interviewing in medical care settings: A systematic review and meta-analysis of randomized controlled trials. *Patient Education and Counseling, 93*(2), 157–168. doi:10.1016/j.pec.2013.07.012

Martin, C. T., & Chanda, N. (2016). Mental health clinical simulation: Therapeutic communication. *Clinical Simulation in Nursing, 12*(6), 209–214. doi:10.1016/j.ecns.2016.02.007

McCabe, R., John, P., Dooley, J., Healey, P., Cushing, A., Kingdon, D., . . . Priebe, S. (2016). Training to enhance psychiatrist communication with patients with psychosis (TEMPO): Cluster randomised controlled trial. *The British Journal of Psychiatry, 209*, 517–524. doi:10.1192/bjp.bp.115.179499

McKenzie, K. J., Pierce, D., & Gunn, J. M. (2015). A systematic review of motivational interviewing in healthcare: The potential of motivational interviewing to address the lifestyle factors relevant to multimorbidity. *Journal of Comorbidity, 5*, 162–174. doi:10.15256/joc.2015.5.55

Miller, W. R., & Rollnick, S. (2013). *Motivational interviewing: Helping people change* (3rd ed.). New York, NY: Guilford Press.

Mitchell, A. J. (2013). The Mini-Mental State Examination (MMSE): An update on its diagnostic validity for cognitive disorder. In A. Larner (Ed.), *Cognitive screening instruments* (pp. 15–46). London, UK: Springer.

Pakpour, A. H., Gellert, P., Dombrowski, S. U., & Fridlund, B. (2015). Motivational interviewing with parents for obesity: An RCT. *Pediatrics, 135*(3), e6440652. doi:10.1542/peds.2014-1987

Prochaska, J. O., DiClemente, C. C., & Norcross, J. C. (1992). In search of how people change: Applications to addictive behaviors. *American Psychologist, 47*(9), 1102–1114. doi:10.1037/0003-066X.47.9.1102

Purath, J., Keck, A., & Fitzgerald, C. (2014). Motivational interviewing for older adults in primary care: A systematic review. *Geriatric Nursing, 35*, 219–224. doi:10.1016/j.gerinurse.2014.02.002

Purtle, J. (2018). Systematic review of evaluations of trauma-informed organizational interventions that include staff trainings. *Trauma, Violence, & Abuse*, 1–16. doi:10.1177/1524838018791304

Rosengren, D. B., Hartzler, B., Baer, J., Wells, E. A., & Dunn, C. W. (2008). The Video Assessment of Simulated Encounters–Revised (VASE-R): Reliability and validity of a revised measure of motivational interviewing skills. *Drug and Alcohol Dependence, 97*(1/2), 130–138. doi:10.1016/j.drugalcdep.2008.03.018

Rubak, S., Sandbaek, A., Lauritzen, T., & Christensen, B. (2005, April). Motivational interviewing: A systematic review and meta-analysis. *British Journal of General Practice, 55*(513), 305–312. Retrieved from https://www.ncbi.nlm.nih.gov/pmc/articles/PMC1463134

Smedslund, G., Berg, R. C., Hammerstrom, K. T., Steiro, A., Leiknes, K. A., . . . Karlsen, K. (2011). Motivational interviewing for substance abuse. *Cochrane Database of Systematic Review*, (5), CD008063. doi:10.1002/14651858.CD008063.pub2

Söderlund, L. L., Madson, M. B., Rubak, S., & Nilsen, P. (2011). A systematic review of motivational interviewing training for general health care practitioners. *Patient Education and Counseling, 84*(1), 16–26. doi:10.1016/j.pec.2010.06.025

Substance Abuse and Mental Health Services Administration. (2014). *A Treatment Improvement Protocol (TIP) Series 57: Trauma-informed care in behavioral health services* (HHS Publication No. [SMA] 13-4801). Rockville, MD: Author.

Tucker, S., Sheikholeslami, D., Farrington, M., Picone, D., Johnson, J., Matthews, G., . . . & Cullen, L (2019). Patient, nurse, and organizational factors that influence evidence-based fall prevention for hospitalized oncology patients: An exploratory study. *Worldviews on Evidence-Based Nursing, 16*(2), 111–120. doi:10.1111/wvn.12353

VanBuskirk, K. A., & Wetherell, J. L. (2014). Motivational interviewing with primary care populations: A systematic review and meta-analysis. *Journal of Behavioral Medicine, 37*(4), 768–780. doi:10.1007/s10865-013-9527-4

Whitlock, E. P., Orleans, C. T., Pender, N., & Allan, J. (2002). Evaluating primary care behavioral counseling interventions: An evidence-based approach. *American Journal of Preventive Medicine, 22*(4), 267–284. doi:10.1016/S0749-3797(02)00415-4

Wu, B. (2013). History taking in reverse: Beginning with the social history. *Consultant 360, 53*(1), 34–36. Retrieved from https://www.consultant360.com/article/history-taking-reverse-beginning-social-history

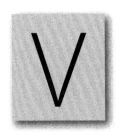

SPECIAL TOPICS IN EVIDENCE-BASED ASSESSMENT

26

Evidence-Based History and Physical Examinations for Sports Participation Evaluation

Marjorie A. Vogt

"Do or do not—there is no try!"

—YODA (STAR WARS)

 VIDEO

- Well Exam: Sports Physical

LEARNING OBJECTIVES

- Define the purpose of the pre-participation sports physical.
- Describe key essential components of the pre-participation sports physical in the adolescent.
- Distinguish between expected findings and common variations or abnormal findings on the pre-participation sports physical.
- Identify commonly used diagnostic testing for clearance prior to participation in sports.

ANATOMY AND PHYSIOLOGY OF THE ADOLESCENT

Adolescents are undergoing rapid physiological changes beginning with the onset of puberty. A surge

Visit https://connect.springerpub.com/content/book/978-0-8261 -6454-4/chapter/ch00 to access the videos.

in growth hormone results in typical body changes of increasing muscle mass or mesomorphic somatotypes in males and increasing subcutaneous adipose tissue or endomorphic somatotypes in women. In addition, there is an increase in gender-specific hormones, causing secondary sexual characteristics. These bodily changes can impact the adolescent's functional and athletic abilities.

In addition to increased mesomorphic somatotypes and the rapid growth in muscles seen particularly in the **adolescent athlete**, there may be increased joint flexibility and lack of coordination. Bones also become denser and slightly more brittle. The increase in androgen production can result in maturation of the skeletal systems and closure of the epiphyseal plates.

Cardiovascular and respiratory function may also change in the adolescent period, usually resulting in an increase in size and capacity of both the heart and lungs. Certain somatotypes, such as endomorphic types, can be associated with increased cardiovascular risk such as hypertension. This may appear during adolescence. Specific athletic training can result in respiratory physiological changes such as increased forced vital capacity in swimmers.

Brain development is also undergoing rapid changes during this period with a later-onset of maturity in the frontal lobes of the brain, which is responsible for decision-making, judgment, and planning. This lack of decision-making ability may result in increased risk-taking, lack of impulse control, and inconsistent

699

self-confidence at times. With the increase in release of serotonin and dopamine, there can be increases in mood swings and emotional behavior in this population.

Because of the rapid physiological and anatomical changes that are occurring in the adolescent body, and the rapid changes in brain and cognitive development, a **pre-participation screening examination** can help direct the adolescent to appropriate exercise and sports activities. The pre-participation examination can also identify potential risk(s) or safety factors that may influence sports performance and help develop a strategic plan of action to avoid sports-related injuries. Ideally, the pre-participation examination should occur at least 6 weeks before the onset of the planned sport (Evidence Category C; Mick & Dimeff, 2004).

KEY HISTORY QUESTIONS AND CONSIDERATIONS

The history is a key component for the **pre-participation physical examination**. Although the history may be limited in determining all sports-related risk factors, it is an important component of the pre-participation process. Guidelines for standardization of pre-participation sports examinations are available from national organizations such as the American College of Sports Medicine (ACSM), the American Academy of Family Physicians (AAFP), the American Academy of Pediatrics (AAP), the American Medical Society for Sports Medicine (AMSSM), the American Orthopaedic Society for Sports Medicine (AOSSM), and the American Osteopathic Academy of Sports Medicine (AOASM). Standardization of the history and physical examination forms can be found at various websites and may be individualized in each state. The majority of the history and physical examination for the pre-participation examination will be dictated by state requirements, and clinicians will need to adhere to these specific forms when providing medical clearance. In addition, requirements for athletes with special needs are also available and will often need specific forms completed prior to their participation in a particular sport (**Table 26.1**).

The history should focus on the type of sport that the athlete has chosen and the risks associated with that specific sport. For example, athletes participating in golf may have very different risks than athletes participating in football or hockey. Assessing the athlete's knowledge related to the individualized sport risks can help in focusing appropriate health counseling related to safety, risk reduction, training, and sports participation.

HISTORY OF PRESENT ILLNESS

The majority of adolescents who present for a pre-participation physical assessment do not have a presenting illness or concern. The pre-participation

TABLE 26.1 Specialty Organization Recommended Sports Participation Forms

Organization	Link
American College of Sports Medicine	www.acsm.org
American Academy of Family Physicians	www.aafp.org
American Academy of Pediatrics	www.aap.org
American Medical Society for Sports Medicine	www.amssm.org
American Orthopaedic Society for Sports Medicine	www.sportsmed.org
American Osteopathic Academy of Sports Medicine	www.aoasm.org
American Sports Medicine Institute	www.asmi.org
International Federation of Sports Medicine	www.fims.org

assessment is similar to a well examination and often includes anticipatory guidance and preventive healthcare considerations. Occasionally an athlete may present for clearance to return to sports participation after an injury or illness. In this situation, the assessment related to the history of the presenting illness should focus on the injury or situation that may have caused the athlete to avoid active sports participation (Arden et al., 2016).

PAST MEDICAL HISTORY

The past medical history can be a significant determinant for future risks related to sports participation. Assessment related to previous acute injury and associated rehabilitation is critically important, especially if related to hospitalization or surgical interventions required for management of injuries.

The past medical history can also be significant if the athlete currently has a chronic disease, such as cardiovascular disease, asthma, diabetes, obesity, or sickle cell trait. Management of the chronic disease, including number of exacerbations in the past year, influence of the chosen sport on the chronic disease management if sports participation has occurred previously, and complications related to the chronic disease should be assessed. Any type of intervention associated with management of the chronic disease and its impact on sports, such as the use of a bronchodilator inhaler prior to sports participation, should be assessed. Previous restrictions on sports activities because of chronic disease exacerbation or rehabilitation need to be explored in detail prior to clearance for sports. See **Table 26.2**, for sample questions on past medical history.

TABLE 26.2 Past Medical History: Sample Questions	
Body System	**Sample Questions**
Chronic illnesses	Any chronic illnesses currently receiving treatment? Any missing organs, such as a kidney?
HEENT	Any sustained visual or hearing impairments? Use of hearing or visual aids? Glasses or contact lens? Any environmental allergies?
Lymphatic	Any history of mononucleosis? Any history of spleen injury or abnormality?
Cardiovascular	History of congenital or acquired heart disease, including murmurs? Any heart-related illnesses? Previous high or low blood pressure? Any history of elevated cholesterol? Any history of anemia? Any history of sickle cell disease or other blood disorders?
Respiratory	History of asthma?
Neurological	Previous history and consequences of concussion? Previous head injury?
Musculoskeletal	Previous musculoskeletal injuries, treatment, rehabilitation? Previous x-rays or MRI, CT scan, injections, and results?

HEENT, head, eyes, ears, nose, throat.

A priority history should be completed on the athlete using the guidelines set forth by the American Heart Association (Maron et al., 2014). The American Heart Association Cardiovascular Screening Checklist has 14 key indicators that can identify the possible risk factors related to cardiovascular disease such as cardiomyopathy or congenital abnormalities. The key indicators assessed during the health history are listed in **Table 26.3**. Certain eye conditions that may be associated with Marfan syndrome should also be screened for, including any history of lens dislocation, lens abnormality, myopia, and ectopia lentis.

Medication history is critical in the older school-aged or adolescent age groups. A history of routine prescription and/or over-the-counter (OTC) use of medications should be assessed. Athletes who are routinely utilizing energy supplements such as creatinine or other herbals need to be educated and understand the possible side effects or adverse reactions associated with these supplements.

TABLE 26.3 American Heart Association Cardiovascular Screening Checklist

Personal History

Yes	No	Criteria
		Chest pain/discomfort/tightness/pressure related to exertion
		Unexplained syncope/near-syncope; judged not to be of neurocardiogenic (vasovagal) origin; of particular concern when occurring during or after physical exertion
		Excessive exertional and unexplained dyspnea/fatigue or palpitations, associated with exercise
		Prior recognition of a heart murmur
		Elevated systemic blood pressure
		Prior restriction from participation in sports
		Prior testing for the heart, ordered by a clinician

Family History

Yes	No	
		Premature death (sudden and unexpected, or otherwise) before age 50 attributable to heart disease in one or more relative
		Disability from heart disease in close relative <50 years of age
		Hypertrophic or dilated cardiomyopathy, long-QT syndrome, or other ion channelopathies, Marfan syndrome, or clinical significant arrhythmias; specific knowledge of certain cardiac conditions in family members

Physical Examination

Yes	No	Criteria
		Heart murmur (likely to be organic and unlikely to be innocent); auscultation should be performed with the patient in both the supine and standing position (or with Valsalva maneuver); specifically to identify murmur of dynamic left ventricular outflow tract obstruction
		Femoral pulses to exclude aortic coarctation
		Physical stigmata of Marfan syndrome
		Brachial artery blood pressure in sitting position (both arms)

Note: Clinicians should use the American Heart Association's evidence-based checklist when evaluating healthy, young individuals aged 12 to 25 years for congenital and genetic heart disease. This 14-item checklist should be used in lieu of doing initial screenings using electrocardiograms.

Source: Adapted from Maron, B. J., Friedman, R. A., Kligfield, P., Levine, B. D., Viskin, S., Chaitman, B. R., . . . Thompson, P. D. (2014). Assessment of the 12-lead ECG as a screening test for detection of cardiovascular disease in healthy general populations of young people (12–25 years of age). *Circulation, 130,* 1303–1334. doi:10.1161/CIR.0000000000000025. © 2014 American Heart Association, Inc.

In addition to a comprehensive medication history, it is important to solicit a history related to allergies, both medication and environmental. Assessment of allergies should include identification of the allergen, prior allergy testing, type of allergic reaction that may occur, and management of the allergy. Exacerbation of the allergy, frequency of occurrence, duration, and complications should also be determined.

The past medical history should also include information related to previous hospitalizations or surgeries, particularly if they have occurred as a result of a sports injury. Athletes who have previously suffered a concussion, loss of consciousness, or traumatic brain injury may need additional history questions related to long-term consequences and cognitive concerns (McCrory et al., 2017).

Changes in mood, emotions, cognitive functioning, behavioral changes, and sleep disturbances should all be explored thoroughly in the athlete who has sustained a concussion. Any unexpected or long-term consequences of the hospitalization or surgical intervention should be explored in detail as related to sports participation. The athlete should also be screened for a history of any sensory deficits such as vision or hearing loss.

FAMILY HISTORY

A comprehensive family history may help to identify potential risks associated with the athlete's health and chosen sport. A thorough three-generation genogram identifying familial tendencies for chronic illness will help to identify risk factors in the athlete. Familial risk factors associated with cardiovascular, respiratory, and musculoskeletal disorders should be the priority. Specific questions should include any family history of the following conditions: premature death or disability because of heart disease in a relative younger than 50 years, hypertrophic or dilated cardiomyopathy, long-QT syndrome, Marfan syndrome, or any cardiac arrhythmias.

SOCIAL HISTORY

The social history may not only identify the risk factors associated with sports participation, but may also identify other risk factors associated with the age-related population. Risk factors such as the use of cigarettes or illicit substances, such as marijuana or steroids, and the use of medications other than those prescribed for the athlete may be identified. Additional social history questions related to behaviors such as seat belt use, school extracurricular activities, stress and coping, use of personal protective sports equipment, employment, sexual activity, and peer relationships can help identify factors that may influence sports participation. In some instances, the pre-participation sports examination may be the only opportunity the healthcare clinician has to interact with this adolescent athlete, as there is often less routinely scheduled well-examinations in the late school-aged and adolescent populations. Therefore, the risk factors identified in the social history may allow the clinician to offer anticipatory guidance and provide additional support resources as needed.

An important component of the social history is a nutritional history to identify eating disorders that may be associated with the individualized sports. Desired weight loss or gain may be required to meet weight parameters in sports such as wrestling, gymnastics, ballet, or football. Increase in caloric consumption related to increased activity may need to be discussed based on the nutritional history and/or significant weight loss.

REVIEW OF SYSTEMS

The review of systems helps to identify areas of concern that may impact sports participation (**Table 26.4**). Although it may primarily focus on areas identified in the past medical history, review of all systems will help to detect other disorders that may be present. The review of systems is typically conducted as part of the history and may be expanded from the past medical history.

PREVENTIVE CARE CONSIDERATIONS

In addition to anticipatory guidance related to social history, the pre-participation sports physical allows the clinician to determine any additional preventive healthcare needs, such as immunizations. This is also an opportunity to discuss important issues such as diet, strength and flexibility training/activities, coping and stress, familial or peer relationships, dental care, substance abuse avoidance, and risk-taking behaviors.

PHYSICAL EXAMINATION

VITAL SIGNS

Vital signs are an important assessment finding that may indicate risk factors associated with sports participation. Height and weight can be important indicators related to issues such as eating disorders, certain genetic abnormalities such as Marfan syndrome, and overweight or obesity concerns. Irregularities in the pulse related to rate and rhythm may indicate need for further evaluation for disorders such as cardiomyopathy, prolonged QT syndrome, pathological arrhythmias, or congenital malformations. Respiratory rate and effort should be evaluated when assessing vital signs. A rapid respiratory rate, with increased respiratory effort while at rest, may indicate further evaluation is needed.

TABLE 26.4 Review of Systems: Sample Questions	
Body System	**Sample Questions**
Current illnesses	Any fevers, night sweats, extreme fatigue, weight loss, or weight gain?
HEENT	Any vision problems? Any ongoing rhinorrhea or nasal congestion?
Lymphatic	Any lymph gland swelling or tenderness?
Skin	Any rashes or skin concerns? Any skin infections or erythema?
Cardiovascular	Any syncope or lightheadedness? Any shortness of breath (with or without exertion)? Any chest pain or tightness (with or without exertion)? Any palpitations ("missed beats"; with or without exertion)? Any sensation of "heart racing"? Any swelling of feet or hands? Increased bleeding or bruising? Unexpected or excess fatigue after exercise?
Respiratory	Any shortness of breath (with or without exertion)? Any wheezing or difficulty "catching breath" (with or without exertion)? Excess coughing with exertion?
Abdominal	Any abdominal pain (with or without exertion)? Changes in bowel or bladder habits with exercise? Any masses or "lumps"?
Neurological	Changes in mood/behavior or cognition? Headaches? Seizures or tremors? Dizziness or lightheadedness? Sleep disturbances?
Musculoskeletal	Pain in joints or muscles? Weakness in joints or muscles? Tingling or numbness in extremities? Current use of braces or wraps?
Endocrine	Increased thirst or urination? Increased sensation of hot or cold body temperature?
Reproductive	Changes in menses? Any testicular or groin pain?

HEENT, head, eyes, ears, nose, throat.

Blood pressure in the young athlete should be evaluated using appropriate technique and cuff size. The athlete should have it completed in both the sitting and standing positions and in both arms several minutes apart. Hypertension is the most common condition affecting athletes. If the blood pressure is elevated at the time of the visit, the clinician should ask about the common causes of acute blood pressure elevation (tobacco, caffeinated beverages, stimulants, supplements, etc.) to help determine whether the elevation could be transient. If an elevated blood pressure is found at the initial examination, the athlete is permitted to participate in the sport until their follow-up visit. Elevated blood pressures need to be repeated in several days to ensure there is a sustained elevation (Berger, Isern, & Berge, 2015; McCambridge et al., 2010).

Per the AAFP, the AAP, the ACSM, the AMSSM, the AOSSM, and the AOASM, pre-participation examination guidelines (2010), the athlete with stage I or stage II hypertension *without* signs of target organ damage should have no restrictions on sports participation. If the athlete has stage I or stage II hypertension *with* signs of target organ damage, sports participation should be restricted until the athlete's blood pressure is controlled (as evidenced by two blood pressure readings under 130/80 at least 2 weeks apart) and any symptoms of target organ damage have resolved.

INSPECTION

The general examination should begin as the athlete enters the examination area through inspection. Overall appearance, facial features, mood, skin, respiratory effort, posture, gait, symmetry and length of limbs, and somatotype can all be identified within the first few minutes of the examination. Inspection should occur in a systematic fashion as described previously, using a head-to-toe approach or a systems approach.

Skin should be inspected for rashes, lesions, moles, hydration status, and injuries. Some types of skin lesions may limit sports participation such as tinea corporis or herpes simplex in the athlete wrestler.

The head, eyes, ears, nose, throat (HEENT) inspection should initially focus on symmetry of facial features, ear and eye alignments, and unusual movements such as tics or spasms. The ophthalmoscopic and otoscopic examinations should inspect the internal structures of the eye, ear, and oral cavity for any unexpected findings. Visual acuity should be assessed and documented with Snellen and Rosenbaum eye charts. Hearing should be assessed through the use of the whisper test. A cranial nerve assessment may be included as part of the HEENT inspection. The neck and thyroid should be inspected for masses or asymmetry.

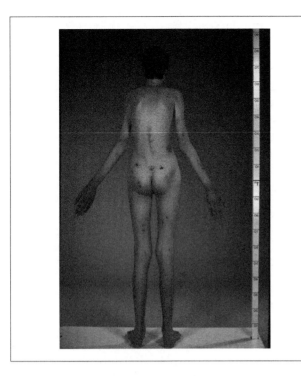

FIGURE 26.1 Individual with Marfan syndrome.
Source: Medical Images RM/Bob Tapper/DIOMEDIA.

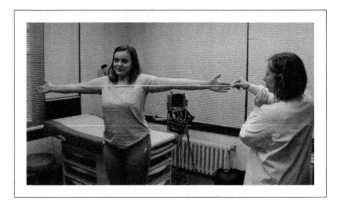

FIGURE 26.2 Measurement of arm span.

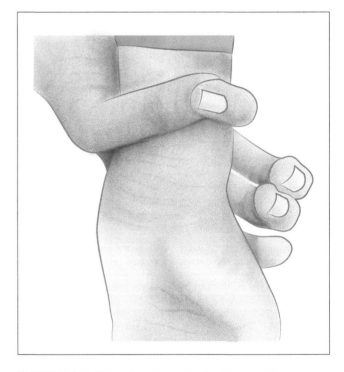

FIGURE 26.3 Wrist–thumb sign. Index finger and thumb overlap when grasping the opposite wrist.

Inspection of the anterior and posterior thorax can provide valuable clues related to the health of the cardiac and respiratory system. Abnormal findings such as asymmetrical chest expansion with respiration or a prominent cardiac pulsation at the point of maximal impulse requires further evaluation. Certain body characteristics, such as an elongated skeleton, hyperflexibility of the small joints of the hands and wrists, and pectus carinatum deformity, may indicate the presence of Marfan syndrome (**Figure 26.1**), which is often accompanied by cardiac risk factors such as a dilated aorta. These athletes need further comprehensive cardiac examinations and should be referred to a cardiologist for further evaluation (Braverman, Harris, Kovacs, & Maron, 2015).

Inspection of the musculoskeletal system is a priority assessment for the student athlete. Range of motion of all joints should be inspected looking for symmetry and/or limitations in both the anterior and posterior planes. Flexion, extension, abduction, adduction, pronation, and supination should be evaluated as appropriate for each joint. Arm span should be measured and arm span/height should be calculated (**Figure 26.2**). If the arm span exceeds the individual's height (ratio >1.05), Marfan syndrome should be considered. Various techniques that can be employed to assess range of motion include having the patient duck-walk, squat, hop, and heel-to-toe gait walk. Feet should be inspected for hindfoot deformity or misalignment that may contribute to ankle instability and increased risk of injury. The hands should be inspected

for the wrist–thumb sign (**Figure 26.3**), where the index finger and thumb overlap when grasping the opposite wrist (Temples, Rogers, Willoughby, & Holaday, 2017). The U.S. Preventive Services Task Force (2015) currently recommends against the routine screening of asymptomatic adolescents for scoliosis.

In some instances, student athletes with a missing limb may choose to participate in school sports versus sports activities such as Special Olympics and Paralympics. During the pre-participation physical examination, it would be important to discuss barriers, challenges, or facilitators for the athlete and the chosen sport activity. Referral to a rehabilitation team for additional sports clearance may be indicated at times (Ahmed et al., 2017). Special Olympics and Paralympics have specific medical forms that must be completed prior to the athletic participation. Clinicians should refer to these forms to determine medical clearance and consider individualized risks and circumstances.

The neurological system includes inspection of the face for cranial nerve abnormalities, as well as inspection of muscle symmetry, gait, posture, balance, and coordination. Visual acuity and reaction time should be undertaken with an athlete who has sustained a sports-related concussion or traumatic brain injury (McCrory et al., 2017). In some instances, the athlete may need to return for serial examinations of the neurological systems, especially if the concussion was recent.

PALPATION

Palpation should occur in a head-to-toe fashion as typically seen in a comprehensive well examination. Specific focus should be in areas where previous injury has occurred, or evidence of discomfort with palpation. Palpation of each major system should occur using a similar systematic approach. Skin turgor, warmth, and moisture should be assessed through palpation of the skin and is best assessed in the inferior clavicular area.

Palpation of the lymph nodes in the head and neck area, the axillae, and inguinal areas should be completed as part of the comprehensive examination. The clinician, if palpating an unexpected enlarged lymph node, should be cognizant of the lymph node drainage pattern and may need to conduct additional examination of the area. The thyroid should also be palpated for assessment of symmetry or masses.

Palpation of the anterior and posterior chest wall should reveal smooth, symmetrical unrestricted respiratory effort and an apical pulse at the point of maximal impulse. Pulses at the carotid, brachial, radial, femoral, popliteal, and pedal should be assessed. Symmetrical femoral and radial pulses should be assessed for coarctation of the cardiac vessels with any unusual or unexpected findings receiving additional examination.

The abdomen should be palpated in order to assess any tenderness, organ enlargement, hernias, unusual palpitations, or masses. The male athlete, in particular, should be examined for testicular symmetry and descent as well as inguinal hernias.

In addition to inspecting each joint in the musculoskeletal system for range of motion and symmetry, it is important to palpate each joint for abnormal findings such as clicks, grating, or crepitus. Assessing muscle strength and symmetry through active resistance can help determine any abnormalities in the musculoskeletal or neurological system. Particular attention should be noted of the cervical spine if there is a previous history of concussion, spinal cord stenosis/compression, or injury. Any of these abnormal findings indicate additional examination and possible referral needs to be completed (McCriskin, Cameron, Orr, & Waterman, 2015).

AUSCULTATION

Auscultation is a priority assessment in the pre-participation physical. The presence or absence of normal versus adventitious sounds need to be evaluated comprehensively.

The lungs should be auscultated carefully, identifying normal and any adventitious sounds such as wheezing. Any abnormal finding will require additional evaluation.

A thorough cardiac examination may help to identify potential risk factors or problems that may lead to sudden cardiac arrest or underlying cardiac abnormalities. The past medical history, particularly related to exertional chest pain or family medical history of early cardiac events, can help guide the cardiovascular examination; however, the history and physical examination can be limited in identifying athletes at risk for sudden cardiac arrest (Drezner et al., 2017).

The cardiac examination should include listening to the heart at all five points previously described. Rate, rhythm, and usual heart sounds should be evaluated. Abnormal sounds, such as a click, murmur, rub, gallop, or additional sounds should be described in detail related to the location, relationship to systole or diastole, audibility, and any changes in rate and/or rhythm with position changes. Sinus arrhythmia, an increase in heart rate with inspiration, is a common variation in the student athlete and does not need further evaluation.

The heart should be assessed with the student athlete in several positions, including standing, sitting, supine, and left lateral. The heart should also be auscultated when the student athlete is in a squatting position or doing the Valsalva maneuver (**Figure 26.4**). A harsh, crescendo–decrescendo systolic murmur auscultated at the left lower sternal border and/or apex could indicate hypertrophic cardiomyopathy.

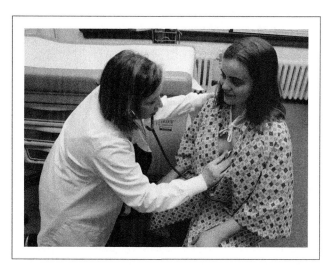

FIGURE 26.4 Valsalva maneuver. Listening to heart while patient is squatting.

This murmur classically increases with any maneuver that decreases venous return like the Valsalva maneuver. Similarly, this murmur diminishes when preload is increased. Any unusual or unexpected finding requires further evaluation.

According to the AHA 14-Element Cardiovascular Screening Checklist, key indicators found on the physical examination that indicate the need for further evaluation include criteria in **Table 26.3** (Maron et al., 2014).

CONTRAINDICATIONS AND RESTRICTIONS FOR SPORTS PARTICIPATION

Although it is not optimal, there may be instances where a student athlete may require further evaluation for an examination finding, and thus may need to be restricted from sports participation. In addition, there may be sports that are inappropriate for a student athlete related to their medical history or physical examination findings. Sports are classified by physical intensity, with sports such as triathlon events being classified as high intensity and sports such as bowling may be of lower intensity (Levine et al., 2015). Some sports have increased risk of contact or collision, such as football or hockey, and other sports have increased risk of elevation of blood pressure or cardiac output, such as weight lifting.

Disqualification from sports may also be indicated if the student athlete has a chronic disease that is less than optimally controlled. For example, a student with an uncontrolled seizure disorder would not be qualified to do scuba diving or weight lifting. Students with certain types of symptomatic congenital heart disease may be restricted from all but the lowest intensity sports (Van Hare et al., 2015).

In general, restriction from sports participation should be considered in student athletes with:

- Uncontrolled chronic illnesses, including seizures, diabetes mellitus, bleeding disorders, hypertension, symptomatic cardiac disease, asthma, vision or hearing deficits, and sickle cell disease
- Concussion, and subsequent persistent symptoms
- Cardiac disorders, such as cardiomyopathy, arrhythmias, and cardiac infections
- Enlarged liver or spleen
- Missing limb or organ
- Unresolved previous injury with persistent sequelae

However, restriction or disqualification from sports participation should be individualized based on the student's health status, physical examination findings, type and intensity of desired sports activity, and conditioning. Restriction or disqualification should be used if there is a concern about safety or risk to the student athlete if participation occurs (Clifton, Grooms, Hertel, & Onate, 2016).

Students with chronic illnesses that are well controlled may be able to participate in select sports activities.

LABORATORY CONSIDERATIONS

In the past decade, there has been much debate about the use of screening laboratory testing in the asymptomatic athlete. Urine tests were frequently screened for glucose and protein; however, recently, those screenings have fallen out of favor because of inadequate evidence to support their inclusion. Proteinuria in the athlete can be a result of intense exercise and is usually transient in nature, resolving within 24 to 48 hours (Goldberg, Saraniti, Witman, Gavin, & Nicholas, 1980; Saeed, Devaki, Mahendrakar, & Holley, 2012). Because of the transient nature of proteinuria in the exercising athlete, there is a recommendation of B (inconsistent or limited quality patient-oriented evidence) specifically related to repeat testing after a random urinalysis detects proteinuria, particularly in an exercising athlete (Conley et al., 2014).

Laboratory diagnostic testing may be considered in female athletes with a history of irregular or absent menses, especially if there is also a history of anemia or increased fatigue. A pregnancy test, follicle-stimulating hormone, thyroid-stimulating hormone, prolactin level, a complete blood count, ferritin, electrolyte panel (including calcium, magnesium, and phosphorus) glucose testing, urinalysis, and electrocardiogram should be considered (Evidence Category C; American College of Obstetricians and Gynecologists, 2017; Conley et al., 2014).

Athletes with chronic illnesses such as diabetes, sickle cell/trait, and/or asthma may need individualized laboratory screening to evaluate compliance, management, and stability of their medication and disease. Modifications to the usual and customary management routine may be required with the addition of sports activity, and restriction from sports participation should be considered during exacerbations of chronic conditions. Spirometry should also be considered in athletes with a history of exercise-induced bronchospasm to exclude undiagnosed asthma, but overall athletes with asthma who do not have symptoms at rest or activity may be permitted to play (Evidence Category C; Hong, & Mahamitra 2005; Mirabelli, Devine, Singh, & Mendoza, 2015).

IMAGING CONSIDERATIONS

When the history or examination presents a concern for further evaluation, especially in the area of unusual cardiac findings, it may be necessary to complete further diagnostic testing. However, routine testing of all athletes using electrocardiograms or echocardiograms has not been widely accepted in the United States (Class III, no evidence of benefit: level of Evidence C), although routine testing using imaging on all athletes does occur in other countries (Maron et al., 2014; Roberts et al., 2014). Although there are some calls for the use of the electrocardiogram because of a greater sensitivity than just the history (20% vs. 94%) and physical examination (9% vs. 94%), at this point, it has not been universally accepted as a usual component of the pre-participation evaluation (Harmon, Zigman, & Drezner, 2015). Part of the controversy related to the use of routine cardiac testing is the sensitivity of the tests, the availability and access to the diagnostic testing and cardiology specialty follow-up, the education and training of the healthcare clinician in the use and interpretation of the test findings, the heightened athlete and parental anxiety related to the testing, and the cost–benefit ratio (Drezner et al., 2017; Maron et al., 2014). Early detection, however, can benefit the individual athlete and possibly the family, if cardiovascular disease was previously undetected.

Diagnostic testing for athletes who have suffered a concussion is rarely indicated. The AMSSM (2014) recommends against ordering brain computed tomography (CT) or magnetic resonance imaging (MRI) to evaluate acute concussions unless there are progressive neurological symptoms, focal neurological findings on examination, or there is concern for a skull fracture.

When an athlete is diagnosed with mononucleosis, sport participation should be restricted because of splenic enlargement and potential for splenic rupture with impact or contact sports. Routine abdominal ultrasound to determine splenic enlargement is discouraged and not seen as a valid method to assess splenic enlargement because of significant variations in the population (AMSSM, 2014).

EVIDENCE-BASED PRACTICE CONSIDERATIONS

It should be noted that the overall effectiveness of the pre-participation examination is controversial as it has not been shown to be effective at decreasing rates of sudden cardiac death during sports in young athletes (Drezner et al., 2017; Winkelmann & Crossway, 2017). The majority of athletes (80%) who have sudden cardiac death have no reported warning symptoms at the time of the pre-participation examination (Alapati, Strobel, Hashmi, Bricker, & Gupta-Malhotra, 2013; Sealy, Pekarek, Russ, Sealy, & Goforth, 2010). Other factors that contribute to low effectiveness include reliability of the patient to report symptoms, development of symptoms after the examination, unknown familial history, inconsistencies and lack of uniformity in approach by clinicians when conducting the examinations, clinicians' ability to differentiate physiologic murmurs from pathologic murmurs, and the clinicians'

ability to identify the physical stigmata and characteristics of Marfan syndrome (Drezner et al., 2017; O'Connor, Johnson, Chapin, Oriscello, & Taylor, 2005).

A number of the recommendations previously discussed are based on evidence-based guidelines proposed by national clearinghouses, medical boards such as the AAP or the AAFP, and specialty organizations such as the AMSSM, or the National Athletic Trainers' Association. Recommendations and resources can be located at specific clearing houses such as Choosing Wisely®, an initiative of the American Board of Internal Medicine. Resources related to recommendations are available to clinicians and patients to stimulate discussion and promote appropriate patient care management (Arden et al., 2016; Huggins et al., 2017).

ABNORMAL FINDINGS

HYPERTROPHIC CARDIOMYOPATHY

Hypertrophic cardiomyopathy is an enlargement of the left ventricle of the heart (**Figure 26.5**). The ventricle size may remain normal but the walls of the left ventricle or septum thicken and stiffen. This makes the inside of the ventricle smaller so it holds less blood. If blood flow is blocked or restricted out of the left ventricle, it is called obstructive hypertrophic cardiomyopathy. If blood flow is not restricted, it is called nonobstructive hypertrophic cardiomyopathy. Hypertrophic cardiomyopathy can be either pathological or physiological in nature (Levis, 2013). It may occur in athletes who have undergone increased conditioning resulting in increased cardiac workload and mild left

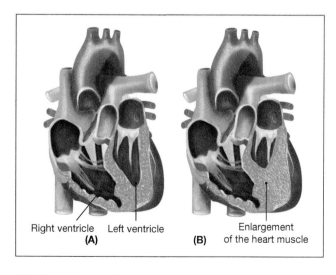

FIGURE 26.5 (A) Normal heart. (B) Heart with hypertrophic cardiomyopathy. The heart muscle cells enlarge and cause the walls of the ventricles (typically the left ventricle and/or septum) to thicken. This enlargement causes many pathological changes in the body.

ventricular enlargement. Pathologic hypertrophic cardiomyopathy, however, is one of the most common causes of sudden cardiac death in athletes, particularly in the adolescent population, and can result in electrical abnormalities and diastolic dysfunction. Hypertrophic cardiomyopathy is an autosomal-dominant disorder, so there is a 50% chance that the children of a parent with hypertrophic cardiomyopathy will inherit the genetic mutation for the disease (Beutler & Deweber, 2009).

Key History and Physical Findings

- Often asymptomatic
- Shortness of breath with exercise
- Palpitations
- Chest pain
- Lightheadedness
- Syncope especially during exercise or exertion
- High blood pressure
- Mid-systolic murmur at the apex radiating to the axilla or a mid-systolic, crescendo–decrescendo murmur, often heard loudest at the left lower sternal border, and increases intensity with the Valsalva maneuver or a squat to stand (Houston & Stevens, 2015)
- Presence of S4
- Arrhythmias
- Mitral valve regurgitation
- Abnormal electrocardiogram (i.e., S wave in lead V1 plus R wave in lead V5 or V6 >35 mm, QRS complex in V1 and V2, deep symmetric T-wave inversion and/or ST-segment depression in leads I, aVL, V5, and V6; pseudo-delta waves; Houston & Stevens, 2015)
- Left ventricle or septal hypertrophy on MRI or transthoracic echocardiogram

For athletes presenting with these symptoms on a pre-participation sports examination, additional diagnostic testing and/or referral to pediatric cardiology are indicated. Although some changes may be evident on an electrocardiogram, the most effective tool for diagnosing pathological hypertrophic cardiomyopathy remains the cardiac MRI (Maron et al., 2007; Maron, Zipes, & Kovacs, 2015; **Figure 26.6**). If detected, athletes may be able to participate in less strenuous athletic activities, depending on the severity of the hypertrophic cardiomyopathy (Fletcher et al., 2013).

MARFAN SYNDROME

Marfan syndrome is an autosomal-dominant disease that can affect many areas of the body but typically presents with skeletal, ocular, and cardiovascular manifestations (see **Figure 26.1**). It is caused by mutation of the *FBN1* gene on chromosome 15, which causes a multisystem disorder of the body's connective tissues (Graffunder, Sties, Gonzales, & Carvalho, 2017; Summers et al., 2012). The greatest concern for athletes with Marfan syndrome

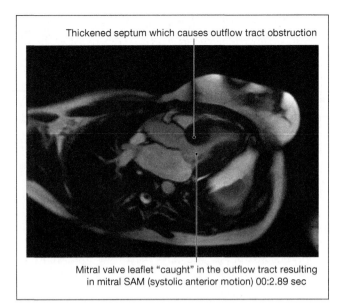

Thickened septum which causes outflow tract obstruction

Mitral valve leaflet "caught" in the outflow tract resulting in mitral SAM (systolic anterior motion) 00:2.89 sec

FIGURE 26.6   MRI of hypertrophic cardiomyopathy.

is aortic aneurysm and potential rupture, especially with strenuous or contact sport activities. The Revised Ghent Criteria (**Box 26.1**) provide standardized criteria to assist in the diagnosis of Marfan syndrome. It differentiates between symptoms associated with a family history and those not associated with a family history. A comprehensive family history related to early-onset cardiac disease or events should be evaluated (Braverman et al., 2015; von Kodolitsch et al., 2015). Adolescent athletes exhibiting symptoms of Marfan syndrome should be referred to pediatric cardiology for further evaluation, including echocardiogram to evaluate the size of the aortic root and detection of potential aneurysm(s) (Classification of Evidence: C; Braverman et al., 2015). Even if Marfan syndrome is diagnosed, athletes may be able to participate in less strenuous athlete activities or noncontact sports.

Key History and Physical Findings

- Family history of Marfan syndrome
- *FBN1* mutation
- Aortic root aneurysm or dissection
- Mitral valve prolapse
- Joint hyperflexibility
- Increased limb length
- Pectus deformities (pectus carinatum)
- Hindfoot deformities
- Connective tissue disorders
- Scoliosis
- Visual abnormalities such as ectopia lentis and myopia
- Facial characteristics including dolichocephaly, downward slanting palpebral fissures, enophthalmos, retrognathia, and malar hypoplasia
- Striae in uncommon location such as the mid-back, lumbar region, the upper arm, and axillary region

---

BOX 26.1
REVISED GHENT CRITERIA FOR DIAGNOSIS OF MARFAN SYNDROME

In the Absence of Family History:
1. Ao (Z ≥2) AND EL = MFS
2. Ao (Z ≥2) AND FBN1 = MFS
3. Ao (Z ≥2) AND Syst (≥7 pts) = MFS
4. EL AND FBN1 with known Ao = MFS

EL with or without Syst AND with an FBN1 not known with Ao or no FBN1 = ELS Ao (Z <2) AND Syst (≥5 with at least one skeletal feature) without EL = MASS MVP AND Ao (Z <2) Syst (<5) without EL = MVPS

In the Presence of Family History:
5. EL AND FH of MFS (as defined above) = MFS
6. Syst (≥7 pts) AND FH of MFS (as defined above) = MFS
7. Ao (Z ≥2 above 20 years old, ≥3 below 20 years) + FH of MFS = MFS

Ao, aortic diameter at the sinuses of Valsalva above indicated z-score or aortic root dissection; EL, ectopia lentis syndrome; FBN1, fibrillin-1 mutation, FH, family history; MASS, mitral valve prolapse, borderline (Z <2) aortic root dilatation; MFS, Marfan syndrome; MVPS, mitral valve prolapse syndrome; Striae, skeletal findings phenotype; Syst, systemic score; Z, Z-score.

Source: Loeys, B. L., Dietz, H. C., Braverman, A. C., Callewaert, B. L., De Backer, J., Devereux, R. B., . . . De Paepe, A. M. (2010). The revised Ghent nosology for the Marfan syndrome. *Journal of Medical Genetics*, *47*(7), 476–485. doi:10.1136/jmg.2009.072785. Reprinted with permission from BMJ Publishing Group Limited

FEMALE ATHLETE TRIAD

The **female athlete triad** is characterized by menstrual, energy, and bone density abnormalities. Often there is a history of amenorrhea or irregular menstrual patterns. Low energy may be impacted by eating disorders, such as bulimia or anorexia, especially in female athletes for whom weight is important, such as gymnasts, dancers, figure skaters, runners, or cheerleaders. In females who participate in these types of sports that focus on aesthetic appearance or being thin, the prevalence of secondary amenorrhea can be as high as 69% compared with 2% to 5% in the general population (Nazem & Ackerman, 2012). Related to the hormonal abnormalities and disordered eating, the female athlete can exhibit decreased bone mineral density and increased fatigue. Athletes with low bone mineral density are at risk for increased stress fractures and even early-onset osteopenia or osteoporosis. The history and physical examination may lead the clinician to this diagnosis, although there are other disorders that can have similar symptoms such as thyroid disorders. Often a multidisciplinary team approach is needed to help normalize menstrual patterns, one of the primary objectives. The female athlete may also need nutritional and psychological counseling with a focus on the possible eating disorders.

Key History and Physical Findings
- Participation in sports that emphasize aesthetic appearance and leanness
- Harmful dieting or disordered eating patterns
- Depression
- Fear of weight gain
- Low self esteem
- Poor body image
- Anxiety disorders
- Low energy availability
- Diminished athletic performance
- Fatigue
- Low body mass index
- Low bone density for age (including diagnosis of osteopenia or osteoporosis)
- Primary or secondary amenorrhea
- Stress fractures
- Weakened immune system
- Susceptible to injuries

CASE STUDY: Pre-Participation Sports Evaluation

History

Chris, age 16 years, presents without a parent to the retail health clinic for a pre-participation sports examination. After reviewing the standardized health history form, the clinician seeks additional information. Chris is planning on wrestling in the fall, playing basketball in the spring, and playing softball in the summer. Although he has wrestled the past two seasons, he has not previously played basketball or softball.

(continued)

CASE STUDY: Pre-Participation Sports Evaluation (*continued*)

On his standardized health history form, a line has been drawn through all questions, indicating there are no health concerns. However, when questioned, Chris indicates that he is in the habit of using a ketogenic diet to maintain his weight limit for wrestling, that he has not started any conditioning for basketball or softball, and is unable to keep up with the other athletes when they run laps for training. He states he occasionally gets "out of breath" with running and has chest tightness which resolves when he sits and rests.

He was hospitalized twice before the age of 8 years for asthma exacerbations, but states he is "cured" of asthma and no longer uses any inhalers or medications. He has never had surgery, or sustained any sports injuries. Chris is on no medications, and states he has "hay-fever allergies only" that are untreated. He believes his immunizations are all up-to-date, but can't recall when or what his last immunization was. He has never been immunized for influenza.

His family history is significant in that his father has hypertension, controlled through diet, and his mother has type 2 diabetes. He has no siblings, and his grandparents' medical histories are unknown.

He denies risk-taking behaviors, consistently uses his seatbelt, and denies sexual activity. He occasionally drinks a beer at a party, but denies use of illicit medications or medications that are not prescribed for him. He does use protein shakes daily to supplement his diet and uses an occasional herbal caffeine supplement for energy.

Physical Examination

On examination, Chris appears well nourished, appropriate in conversation, and in no acute distress. He is 72 inches tall, weighs 206 (BMI 28). Vital signs are:

- T: 98.2°F
- Pulse: 90/min
- Respirations: 16/min
- BP: 142/92

HEENT examination is unremarkable and his visual acuity is 20/20 od and 20/70 os.

Lung sounds reveal an occasional expiratory wheeze bilaterally in lower lobes. Cardiac examination reveals S1, S2 with soft systolic murmur that increases with intensity with the Valsalva maneuver, at the right sternal border. Pulses are symmetrical in extremities, and no bruits are noted at carotids or abdomen. Inguinal and radial pulses are consistent bilaterally. Abdomen is obese with few striae noted, but no tenderness, organomegaly, hernias, or masses noted on palpation. He has bilateral descended testicles. He is a Tanner stage 5.

His musculoskeletal examination reveals slight limitation in spinal flexion (he is unable to touch his toes), but full range of motion in all other major joints. His gait is smooth and symmetrical, and he is able to heel–toe walk, and hop without limitation. He has difficulty squatting to duck-walk.

Final Diagnoses

Myopia, obesity and possible eating disorder, elevated blood pressure, systolic murmur of unknown origin

Management

Although Chris protests, he is unable to be cleared for sports participation at this time. The clinician discusses further evaluation that is needed related to visual acuity, blood pressure, and cardiac murmur. Chris was referred to his primary care clinician for further evaluation.

Clinical Pearls

- Although athletes and parents may protest if clearance for sports participation is denied, it is important to emphasize the need for sports safety and risk reduction.
- Recommend that when beginning an exercise program, patients use the "10% rule": limit to no more than 10% per week any increase of intensity of exercise (e.g., pace and distance for running or repetitions and resistance for weight training).

- If something is causing an athlete pain, this should not be ignored. This can cause worsening of the condition, more severe injury, and longer rehabilitation than if it were addressed at the onset.
- Restricting or denying sport participation can be very upsetting for adolescents and parents. It is important to discuss your reasoning for denial as it relates to the health and safety of the athlete.

Key Takeaways

- Pre-participation examination requirements may vary state-to-state. Utilize the AHA's evidence-based cardiovascular screening checklist in addition to the state required form to ensure all essential aspects of the history and examination are covered.
- A thorough cardiovascular family history should be explored during the pre-participation examination.
- The pre-participation examination may be the only encounter an adolescent has with a healthcare clinician during the year. The clinician should take the opportunity to assess and educate the adolescent about risky behaviors and health maintenance needs.
- Any patient with a mid-systolic murmur that increases in intensity with the Valsalva maneuver or a squat to stand needs a referral to cardiology to rule out cardiac pathology.
- Chronic illnesses do not exclude sports participation but need to be monitored. The intensity and vigor of the sport need to be considered and weighed against the nature of the illness.

REFERENCES

Ahmed, B., Lamy, M., Cameron, D., Artero, L., Ramdial, S., Leineweber, M., & Andrysek, J. (2017). Factors impacting participation in sports for children with limb absence: A qualitative study. *Disability Rehabilitation, 12*, 1–8. doi: 10.1080/09638288.2017.1297496

Alapati, S., Strobel, N., Hashmi, S., Bricker, J. T., & Gupta-Malhotra, M. (2013). Sudden unexplained cardiac arrest in apparently healthy children: A single-center experience. *Pediatric Cardiology, 34*(3), 639–645. doi:10.1007/s00246-012-0516-0

American Academy of Family Physicians, American Academy of Pediatrics, American College of Sports Medicine, American Medical Society for Sports Medicine, American Orthopaedic Society for Sports Medicine & American Osteopathic Academy of Sports Medicine. (2010). *Pre-participation physical evaluation* (4th ed.). Itasca, IL: American Academy of Pediatrics.

American College of Obstetricians and Gynecologists, Committee Opinion No. 702. (2017). Female athlete triad. *Obstetrics & Gynecology, 129*(6), e160–e167. doi:10.1097/AOG.0000000000002113

American Medical Society for Sports Medicine. (2014). *Five things physicians and patients should question.* Retrieved from http://www.choosingwisely.org/societies/american-medical-society-for-sports-medicine

Arden, C., Glasgow, P., Schneiders, A., Witvrouw, E., Clarsen, B., Cools, A., . . . Bizzini, M. (2016). Consensus statement

of return to sport from the First World Congress in Sports Physical Therapy, Bern. *British Journal of Sports Medicine, 50*, 853–864. doi:10.1136/bjsports-2016-096278

Berger, H., Isern, C., & Berge, E. (2015). Blood pressure and hypertension in athletes: A systematic review. *British Journal of Sports Medicine, 49*(11), 716–723. doi:10.1136/bjsports-2014-093976

Beutler, A., & Deweber, K. (2009). Hypertrophic cardiomyopathy: Ask athletes these nine questions. *Journal of Family Practice, 58*(11), 576–584. Retrieved from https://www.mdedge.com/familymedicine/article/63755/cardiology/hypertrophic-cardiomyopathy-ask-athletes-these-9-questions

Braverman, A., Harris, K., Kovacs, R., & Maron, B. (2015). Eligibility and disqualification recommendations for competitive athletes with cardiovascular abnormalities: Task Force 7: Aortic diseases, including Maran syndrome. *Journal of the American College of Cardiology, 66*(21), 2398–2405. doi:10.1016/j.jacc.2015.09.039

Clifton, D., Grooms, D., Hertel, J., & Onate, J. (2016). Predicting injury: Challenges in prospective injury risk factor identification. *Journal of Athletic Training, 51*(8), 658–661. doi:10.4085/1062-6050-51.11.03

Conley, K., Bolin, D., Carek, P., Konin, J., Neal, T., & Violette, D. (2014). National Athletic Trainer's Association Position Statement: Pre-participation physical examinations and disqualifying conditions. *Journal of Athletic Training, 49*(1), 102–120. doi:10.4085/1062-6050-48.6.05

Drezner, J., O'Connor, F., Harmon, K., Fields, K., Asplund, C., Asif, I., . . . Roberts, W. (2017). AMSSM position statement of cardiovascular pre-participation screening in athletes: Current evidence, knowledge gaps, recommendations and future directions. *British Journal of Sports Medicine, 51*, 153–167. doi:10.1136/bjsports-2016-096781

Fletcher, G. F., Ades, P. A., Kligfield, P., Arena, R., Balady, G. J., Bittner, V. A., . . . Williams, M. A. (2013). Exercise standards for testing and training: A statement from the American Heart Association. *Circulation, 128*, 873–934. doi:10.1161/CIR.0b013e31829b5b44

Goldberg, B., Saraniti, A., Witman, P., Gavin, M., & Nicholas, J. (1980). Pre-participation sports assessment—An objective evaluation. *Pediatrics, 66*(5), 736–745. doi: 10.1097/01241398-198110000-00046

Graffunder, F., Sties, S., Gonzales, A., & Carvalho, T. (2017). Differential diagnosis of Marfan syndrome in a teenage volleyball athlete. *International Journal of Cardiovascular Sciences, 30*(2), 182–185. doi:10.5935/2359-4802.20170036

Harmon, K., Zigman, M., & Drezner, J. (2015). The effectiveness of screening history, physical exam and ECG to detect potentially lethal cardiac disorders in athletes: A systematic review/meta-analysis. *Journal of Electrocardiology, 48*, 329–338. doi:10.1016/j.jelectrocard.2015.02.001

Hong, G., & Mahamitra, N. (2005). Medical screening of the athlete: How does asthma fit in? *Clinical Review of Allergy and Immunology, 29*(2), 97–111. doi:10.1385/CRIAI:29:2:097

Houston, B. A., & Stevens, G. R. (2015). Hypertrophic cardiomyopathy: A review. *Clinical Medicine Insights Cardiology, 8*(Suppl. 1), 53–65. doi:10.4137/CMC.S15717

Huggins, R., Scarneo, S., Casa, D., Belval, L., Carr, K., Chiampas, G., . . . Weston, T. (2017). The inter-association task force document on emergency health and safety:

Best-practice recommendations for youth sports leagues. *Journal of Athletic Training*, *52*(4), 384–400. doi: 10.4085/1062-6050-52.2.02

Levine, B., Baggish, A., Kovacs, R., Link, M., Maron, M., & Mitchell, J. (2015). Eligibility and disqualification recommendations for competitive athletes with cardiovascular abnormalities: Task force 1: Classification of sports: Dynamic, static and impact. *Circulation, 132*(22), e262–e266. doi:10.1161/CIR.0000000000000237

Levis, J. T. (2013). ECG diagnosis: Apical hypertrophic cardiomyopathy. *The Permanente Journal, 17*(2), 84. doi: 10.7812/TPP/12-089

Loeys, B. L., Dietz, H. C., Braverman, A. C., Callewaert, B. L., De Backer, J., Devereux, R. B., . . . De Paepe, A. M. (2010). The revised Ghent nosology for the Marfan syndrome. *Journal of Medical Genetics, 47*(7), 476–485. doi:10.1136/jmg.2009.072785

Maron, B. J., Friedman, R. A., Kligfield, P., Levine, B. D., Viskin, S., Chaitman, B. R., . . . Thompson, P. D. (2014). Assessment of the 12-lead electrocardiogram as a screening test for detection of cardiovascular disease in healthy general populations of young people (12–25 years of age). *Journal of the American College of Cardiology, 64*(14), 1479–1514. doi:10.1016/j.jacc.2014.05.006

Maron, B., Thompson, P., Ackerman, M., Balady, G., Berger, S., Cohen, D., . . . Puffer, J. (2007). Recommendations and considerations related to pre-participation screening for cardiovascular abnormalities in competitive athletes: 2007 update. *Circulation, 115*(12), 1643–1655. doi:10.1161/CIRCULATIONAHA.107.181423

Maron, B. J., Zipes, D. P., & Kovacs, R. J. (2015). Eligibility and disqualification recommendations for competitive athletes with cardiovascular abnormalities: Preamble, principles, and general considerations. *Journal of the American College of Cardiology, 132*(22), e256–e261. doi:10.1161/CIR.0000000000000236

McCambridge, T., Benjamin, H., Brenner, J., Cappetta, C. T., Demorest, R. A., Gregory, A. J., . . . Rice, S. G. (2010). Council on Sports Medicine and Fitness. Athletic participation by children and adolescents who have systemic hypertension. *Pediatrics, 125*(6), 1287–1294. doi:10.1542/peds.2010-0658

McCriskin, B. J., Cameron, K. L., Orr, J. D., & Waterman, B. R. (2015). Management and prevention of acute and chronic lateral ankle instability in athletic patient populations. *World Journal of Orthopedics, 6*(2), 161–171. doi:10.5312/wjo.v6.i2.161

McCrory, P., Meeuwisse, W., Dvorak, J., Aubry, M., Bailes, J., Broglio, S., . . . Vos, P. (2017). Consensus statement on concussion in sport—The 5th International Conference on Concussion in Sport held in Berlin, October 2016. *British Journal of Sports Medicine, 51*, 838–847. doi:10.1136/bjsports-2017-097699

Mick, T., & Dimeff, R. (2004). What kind of physical examination does a young athlete need before participating in sports. *Cleveland Clinical Journal of Medicine, 71*(7), 587–597. doi:10.3949/ccjm.71.7.587

Mirabelli, M., Devine, M., Singh, J., & Mendoza, M. (2015). The pre-participation sports evaluation. *American Family Physician, 92*(5), 371–376. Retrieved from https://www.aafp.org/afp/2015/0901/p371.html

Nazern, T., & Ackerman, K. (2012). The female athlete triad. *Sports Health, 4*(4), 302–311. doi:10.1177/1941738112439685

O'Connor, F. G., Johnson, J. D., Chapin, M., Oriscello, R. G., & Taylor, D. C. (2005). A pilot study of clinical agreement in cardiovascular pre-participation examinations: How good is the standard of care? *Clinical Journal of Sport Medicine, 15*, 177–179. doi:10.1097/01.jsm.0000156150.09811.63f

Roberts, W., Lollgen, H., Matheson, G., Royalty, A., Meeuwisse, W., Levine, B., . . . Pigozzi, F. (2014). Advancing the pre-participation physical evaluation: An ACSM and FIMS joint consensus statement. *Clinical Journal of Sports Medicine, 24*(6), 442–447. doi:10.1097/JSM.0000000000000168

Saeed, F., Devaki, P., Mahendrakar, L., & Holley, J. (2012). Exercise-induced proteinuria? *Journal of Family Practice, 61*(1), 23–26. Retrieved from https://www.mdedge.com/familymedicine/article/64604/nephrology/exercise-induced-proteinuria

Sealy, D. P., Pekarek, L., Russ, D., Sealy, C., & Goforth, G. (2010). Vital signs and demographics in the pre-participation sports exam: Do they help us find the elusive athlete at risk for sudden cardiac death? *Current Sports Medicine Reports, 9*, 338–341. doi:10.1249/JSR.0b013e3182014ed6

Summers, K. M., West, J. A., Hattam, A., Stark, D., McGill, J. J., & West, M. J. (2012). Recent developments in the diagnosis of Marfan syndrome and related disorders. *Medical Journal of Australia, 197*(9), 494–497. doi:10.5694/mja12.10560

Temples, H., Rogers, C., Willoughby, D., & Holaday, B. (2017). Marfan syndrome (MFS): Visual diagnosis and early identification. *Journal of Pediatric Health Care, 31*(5), 609–617. doi:10.1016/j.pedhc.2017.05.002

U.S. Preventive Services Task Force. (2015, July). *Final update summary: Idiopathic scoliosis in adolescents: Screening.* Retrieved from https://www.uspreventiveservicestaskforce.org/Page/Document/UpdateSummaryFinal/idiopathic-scoliosis-in-adolescents-screening

Van Hare, G. F., Ackerman, M. J., Evangelista, J. K., Kovacs, R. J., Myerburg, R. J., Shafer, K. M., . . . Washington, R. L. (2015). Eligibility and disqualification recommendations for competitive athletes with cardiovascular abnormalities: Task Force 4: Congenital heart disease: A scientific statement from the American Heart Association and American College of Cardiology. *Journal of the American College of Cardiology, 66*(21), 2372–2384. doi:10.1016/j.jacc.2015.09.036

von Kodolitsch, Y., De Backer, J., Schüler, H., Bannas, P., Behzadi, C., Bernhardt, A. M., . . . Robinson, P. N. (2015). Perspectives on the revised Ghent criteria for the diagnosis of Marfan syndrome. *The Application of Clinical Genetics, 8*, 137–155. doi:10.2147/TACG.S60472

Winkelmann, Z., & Crossway, A. (2017). Optimal screening methods to detect cardiac disorders in athletes: An evidence-based review. *Journal of Athletic Training, 52*(12), 1168–1170. doi:10.4085/1062-6050-52.11.24

27

Using Health Technology in Evidence-Based Assessment

Lisa K. Militello and Janna D. Stephens

> *"Every once in a while, a new technology, an old problem, and a big idea turn into an innovation."*
>
> —DEAN KAMEN

 VIDEO

- Patient Case: Telehealth Visit for Woman With Dysuria

LEARNING OBJECTIVES

- Identify evidence-based tools to assess the quality of digital health technology.
- Identify health technology strategies beneficial in the clinical decision-making process.
- Review how health technology can be incorporated into evidence-based assessments and clinical decision support.

HEALTH TECHNOLOGY IN EVIDENCE-BASED PRACTICE

Technology is transforming healthcare and providing clinicians with an unprecedented ability to monitor health status, capture data, and intervene as needed to save lives, manage illness, and support wellness. The rapid and continuous evolution of technology creates challenges for clinicians who recognize the importance

Visit https://connect.springerpub.com/content/book/978-0-8261 -6454-4/chapter/ch00 to access the videos.

of providing accurate and timely information to individuals who may be able to access technologies to prioritize their health and who will want to know the value relative to the quality and complexity of technological innovations. Technology has paved new paths to extend assessment and clinical care beyond hospitals and clinics, and into the everyday lives of patients. This chapter provides an overview of how innovative technologies to support health and well-being may be assessed for quality and incorporated into evidence-based assessments and clinical decision support.

TERMINOLOGY ACROSS DISCIPLINES

The World Health Organization (WHO) defines **health technology** broadly as the application of evidence-based knowledge and/or skills that result in a device, intervention, procedure, or system that solves a health problem and/or improves lives (WHO, 2019a). Fields of study historically separate from one another, rapidly evolving fields, and disciplines infrequently associated with the health professions are remarkably consistent in how they describe and define health technology. These fields of study, including computer science, engineering, nursing, social work, statistics, applied mathematics, design, and human–computer interaction, also have distinct differences. **Table 27.1** lists terminology related to health technology that is representative of multiple disciplines; relevant resources are noted for clarity.

When health technology interventions utilize digital devices such as mobile phones, tablets, computers, sensors, activity trackers, or other applications to support behavior change related to health and wellness, these

713

TABLE 27.1 Terminology Related to Health Technology and Digital Health Interventions	
Health Technology	
Term	*Definition*
Health Information Technology	Secure exchange of health information across an electronic environment (U.S. Department of Health and Human Services, n.d.)
Health Technology	Devices, medicines, vaccines, procedures, and systems intended to improve quality of life and/or solve a health problem (World Health Organization [WHO], 2019a)
Health Technology Assessment	Direct and indirect systematic evaluation of health technologies and interventions' effects and/or impacts on health (WHO, 2019a)
Mobile health (mHealth)	Application of mobile technologies (e.g., wireless devices and sensors) for monitoring health status or improving health outcomes (Kumar, Nilsen, Pavel, & Srivastava, 2013)
eHealth	Broad concept to represent an emerging transdisciplinary field that uses the Internet and related technologies to deliver or enhance health services and information (Eysenbach, 2001)
Telehealth	Broad term for remote healthcare services across services, including, but not limited to, patient and professional health-related education, public health and health administration, and nonclinical services (e.g., clinician training, administrative meetings; The Office of the National Coordinator for Health Information Technology [ONC], n.d.)
Telemedicine	Specific term indicating remote clinical services, such as two-way, real-time interactive communication between the patient and the clinician from a distant site. Telehealth is a broader, more inclusive term than telemedicine. (Centers for Medicare & Medicaid Services, n.d.; ONC, n.d.)
Multidisciplinary	General use term, when multiple disciplines are involved, but specific nature of involvement is unspecified; drawing upon knowledge from different disciplines, yet bounded by a discipline (Choi & Pak, 2006)
Interdisciplinary	Linking disciplines to yield coordinated and coherent whole (Choi & Pak, 2006)
Transdisciplinary	Transcends traditional boundaries of a discipline to integrate natural, social, and health sciences in a humanities context (Choi & Pak, 2006)
Digital Health Interventions	
Behavioral Intervention Technologies	Behavioral and psychological interventions that use information and communication technology features to support behavior change related to health, mental health, and wellness outcomes (Mohr et al., 2015)
Digital Behavior Change Interventions	Programs that are delivered via technology or use technology to promote or support behavior change (Michie, Yardley, West, Patrick, & Greaves, 2017; Murray et al., 2016)

interventions are referred to as **digital health interventions** (DHIs). See Table 27.1 for definitions and terminology related to DHIs. This chapter includes a review of how and where to search the literature for DHIs and how to assess for DHI quality, as the design, development, and implementation of technology into healthcare is reshaping traditional ways of thinking about the analysis and interpretation of health assessment.

ETHICAL AND LEGAL CONSIDERATIONS

Drawing from the multiple disciplines that contribute to health technology, it is important to acknowledge that what might be implicitly obvious in one discipline may not hold true across disciplines. For example, more technical fields such as engineering may be more willing to "fail fast, fail often," which is in sharp contrast to that of healthcare professionals trained to "do no harm" (Michie, Yardley, West, Patrick, & Greaves, 2017). Prior to adopting technology in clinical practice, current regulations and ethical considerations should be reviewed.

Food and Drug Administration

The U.S. Food and Drug Administration (FDA, 2018) is examining the use of real-world evidence from real-world data (RWD) to make critical decisions about the regulation of medical devices. Data are often collected during assessment of a patient and are usually not considered as a step in the rigorous generation of evidence. However, with the use of new health technologies (e.g., mobile devices and applications) and the expanding capabilities of older technology (e.g., electronic health records), the FDA recommends to use data from these devices to generate evidence to inform their regulatory processes (FDA, 2018). In order for RWD to be suitable for the FDA to use for regulatory decisions, several criteria must be met:

- The data collected from the device contain enough detail to answer questions about a specific population.
- When appropriate analytical methods are used, the data collected from the device are capable of addressing the specified question.
- The data and evidence provided from the device can inform clinical and scientific judgment.

It is important for the clinician who is recommending and implementing technology-driven devices in clinical practice to consider using the data collected to help generate evidence for the regulation of the specific type of device. In situations where electronic devices are used for collection of assessment data, clinicians may gather a multitude of data that can be compiled to examine specific health questions related to specific populations. Quality improvement measures are being implemented within inpatient and outpatient electronic health record systems to compile the data that inform evidence-based practice.

Health Insurance Portability and Accountability Act

The use of digital technologies, both in assessment and across the care continuum, brings important questions related to the safety and confidentiality of patient records. The **Health Insurance Portability and Accountability Act (HIPAA)**, passed by the Congress in 1996, mandates industry-wide standards for handling healthcare information and requires the protection and confidentiality of protected health information. With the ever-changing world of digital technologies, the HIPAA has now been adapted to handle an electronic environment similar to that of the paper-based environment.

Individuals have a right to access their health information (U.S. Department of Health and Human Services [USDHHS] & Office for Civil Rights [OCR], 2013). The use of electronic devices to assess and document health findings can allow individuals to have more convenient access to their own personal, protected health information; patients can access electronic copies of visit summaries, lab work results, and referral notes through the use of secure online websites, or **patient portals**. The HIPAA grants access to an individual or

a personal representative to obtain their healthcare records electronically or in person. In a digital world, however, it may be more difficult to verify the identity of a personal representative. The HIPAA states that covered entities must develop and implement "reasonable policies" for the verification of the identity or a personal representative before granting access to protected health information (HIPAA Journal Team, n.d.; USDHHS & OCR, 2013).

Specific technologies frequently used for assessment of patients, or communication about/with patients, may lead to compliance concerns in regard to the HIPAA. For example, clinicians may use SMS (short message service), Skype, or email to share information regarding a patient or may take assessment notes on such devices (USDHHS & OCR, 2013). To be compliant with the HIPAA, one must follow the Security Rule, which states that all protected health information must be encrypted and accessed with a unique identifier, and the technology must have an automatic log off (HIPAA Journal Team, n.d.). These important regulations must be kept in mind when utilizing technology for patient assessment.

Children's Online Privacy Protection Rule

The Children's Online Privacy Protection Act (COPPA, 1998) imposes certain requirements on operators of websites or online services directed to children under 13 years of age, as well as on operators of other websites or online services that have actual knowledge that they are collecting personal information online from a child under 13 years of age. This rule was designed to keep parents in control of the information being collected on their children via online services or websites. The rule states that consent must be obtained, must display a privacy policy that complies with COPPA, and must give parents the right to review information collected on their children. This rule applies to a multitude of technology that is used in healthcare. For example, if a child's clinician wanted the child to use an application designed to increase physical activity or wanted them to play an Internet-enabled game focused on nutrition, the COPPA rule would apply.

Practice Requirements

Clinicians considering providing care using telecommunications should review federal and state laws regarding the provision of care. Although the use of telehealth is steadily increasing, states vary in the type of assessments and care that can be legally implemented from a distance. A clinician's ability to assess and/or manage patient care may be limited by where they are physically located and/or where the individual is located during a telehealth visit; licensing and regulations vary from state to state, especially regarding the provision of care across state lines. Reimbursement for care offered by

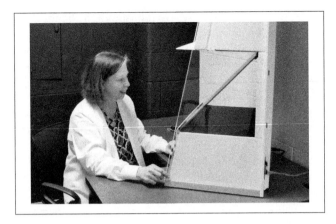

FIGURE 27.1 Telehealth kiosk. A telehealth kiosk is a type of digital health intervention that allows for patient check-in, assessments, video conferencing, and/or access to electronic health records.

telecommunications is expanding because telehealth is correlated with patient satisfaction, positive health outcomes, decreased readmission rates, improved clinician–patient communication, and increased access to care (Kruse et al., 2017). Establishing clinical practice using telehealth, as depicted in **Figure 27.1**, requires the implementation of health technology that allows for patient confidentiality, high-quality assessments, recognition of state policy regarding practice, and an understanding of reimbursement policies.

EVALUATION OF EVIDENCE TO SUPPORT USE OF HEALTH TECHNOLOGY

VARIATIONS IN APPROACH TO EVIDENCE

Prior to incorporating health technology into clinical practice, it is imperative to determine the quality of the technology itself. Across disciplines and relevant to the priorities of each discipline, best practices to disseminate evidence vary. For example, researchers and clinicians from health professions may favor the process of disseminating scholarly work via a peer-reviewed journal publication. Although thorough, the peer-review process and resulting revisions for journal publication can be lengthy, requiring evaluation over a specified length of time (Nature Publishing Group, 2017). To keep pace with rapid changes occurring in technology, it is not uncommon for researchers in technical fields (e.g., engineering, computer science) to expedite the process of scholarly dissemination and publish in conference proceedings. Conference proceedings, technical reports, and policy institute reports are among the notable types of grey literature. Grey literature is scholarly or substantive information not formally published in journals or books (Cornell University Library, 2017;

Higgins & Green, 2011). Historically, grey literature has been considered less prestigious, reliable, and "official" than publication in a peer-reviewed journal, yet these works are fully legitimate avenues of publication (Cornell University Library, 2017) and important to consider when evaluating health technology.

LOCATING HEALTH TECHNOLOGY EVIDENCE

It is beneficial to employ an interdisciplinary or transdisciplinary approach when searching for relevant literature. Health professionals searching for Level-1 Evidence, the highest level of evidence to inform evidence-based clinical practice, are likely to use search engines or databases such as the Cochrane Library (www.cochranelibrary.com); PubMed, which is maintained by the U.S. National Library of Medicine (www.ncbi.nlm.nih.gov/pubmed); or Web of Science (https://webofknowledge.com). While colleagues from technical sciences are also likely to utilize these resources, additional resources such as the Institute of Electrical and Electronics Engineers (IEEE) *Xplore* digital library (https://ieeexplore.ieee.org/Xplore/home.jsp) or the Association for Computing Machinery (ACM) Digital Library (https://dl.acm.org) may be more apropos to locate significant technical publications. Similarly, supplementing searches (especially when narrowed down by year) with support from web-based academic search engines such as Google Scholar (https://scholar.google.com) is not uncommon.

As health technology continues to evolve, inclusion of grey literature (but not standalone) is essential to understand emerging approaches in health and can serve as powerful additions to traditional search methods (Cooper, 2009; Haddaway, Collins, Coughlin, & Kirk, 2015; Higgins & Green, 2011). However, debate regarding best strategies to search for and identify grey literature still exists, which can limit efforts to search for relevant evidence (Cornell University Library, 2017). Searching the grey literature can be structured using databases that specialize in grey literature like OpenGrey (www.opengrey.eu), identifying professional organizations that might have researchers presenting work relevant to their field, and identifying government and international nongovernmental organizations that might publish relevant reports (Cornell University Library, 2017).

KEEPING PACE WITH EVOLVING HEALTH TECHNOLOGY

The landscape of technology is likely to continue to evolve and change. Broadly speaking, clinically relevant DHIs, including telecommunications, should be capable of protecting and securing data, showing evidence of usability, demonstrating cost-effectiveness, and providing support to benefit health and well-being. However, DHIs are complex, frequently encompassing multiple intervention components comprised of cognitive, behavioral, delivery, or implementation factors that may have individual or combined effects on outcomes (Chakraborty, Collins, Strecher, & Murphy, 2009; Collins, Chakraborty, Murphy, & Strecher, 2009; Collins, Dziak, & Li, 2009). Deviating from traditional methodology where interventions are fixed, testing a "fixed" intervention that uses technology has little public health value because the shelf life of the fixed intervention is short or unknown. DHIs capable of providing rich data streams are better suited for randomized controlled trials when they are deemed to be "relatively stable" over the medium term (opposed to the long term; Murray et al., 2016). This determination is made at the discretion of the researchers, guided by causal models and optimization data, keeping in mind how changes in technology will influence generalizability of the findings (Mohr et al., 2015; Murray et al., 2016). To move digital health science forward and yield clinically meaningful benefits, rather than focus on evaluating a fixed DHI, researchers in digital health advocate for evaluating whether the DHI acted as intended on guiding principles/strategies (Collins, Dziak,

& Li, 2009; Klasnja, Consolvo, & Pratt, 2011; Michie et al., 2017; Mohr et al., 2015; Murray et al., 2016; Torous, Chan, Yellowlees, & Boland, 2016). Guiding principles may include theory and behavior change techniques (e.g., self-monitoring, self-belief), user experience, and privacy/ethical considerations.

Strategies to increase knowledge and awareness of various technologies available to both clinicians and patients requires an ongoing process. Guidelines published by the WHO (2019b) recommend an ongoing, critical evaluation of the evidence on emerging DHIs that are contributing to health systems improvements. The critical appraisal process is subject to logistical challenges owing to broad users, challenges with system integration, proprietary considerations, resource requirements, and equity considerations. When attempting to integrate DHIs into clinical practice, clinicians are often challenged with these questions: "Where do I look?" or "How do I know if this provides high-quality, accurate information?" To help answer these questions, **Box 27.1** provides links to repositories, clearinghouses, assessment tools, and applications that are evidence-based, high-quality, and/or have proven stability.

BOX 27.1
DIGITAL HEALTH INTERVENTIONS: TOOLS, REPOSITORIES, AND CLEARINGHOUSES

Assessment Tools: How to Assess Quality

- Mobile Application Rating Scale (MARS; Stoyanov et al., 2015): Reliable tool for classifying and assessing the quality of mobile health apps, specifically assessing engagement, functionality, aesthetics, and information/content quality
- System Usability Scale (SUS; Bangor, Kortum, & Miller, 2008; Brooke, 1996; Peres, Pham, & Phillips, 2013): Scale provides global view of subjective usability; provides an overall usability and user satisfaction index
- User Burden Scale (UBS; Suh, Shahriaree, Hekler, & Kientz, 2016): Assesses difficulty of use, physical, time and social, mental and emotional, privacy, and financial burdens to determine the negative impact of computing systems on users

Repositories + Quality Assessment: Evidence in Action

- Common Sense Media: Independent, nonprofit organization dedicated to providing developmentally appropriate, unbiased information on pediatric media. https://www.commonsensemedia.org
  Quality Assessment: Rates technology and media based on age appropriateness and learning potential. Fifteen-point rubric evaluating three key essential qualities—engagement, pedagogy, and support—with consideration to how engrossing the tool is to use, whether it promotes conceptual understanding and creativity, and how it adapts to individual needs and supports knowledge transfer.
- PsyberGuide: Clearinghouse of mental health apps; established in 2013 in response to a growing need for guidelines to help people navigate the mental health app marketplace. The aim is to help people make responsible and informed decisions about apps and other digital tools for mental health by providing unbiased reviews. Funded by OneMind, a nonprofit organization in brain health research. https://psyberguide.org
  Quality Assessment: Evaluates credibility (i.e., research evidence, funding, clinical expertise, updates and maintenance, specificity), user experience (i.e., MARS), and transparency (i.e., data privacy and handling policies; Torous & Shore, 2018).

(continued)

BOX 27.1
DIGITAL HEALTH INTERVENTIONS: TOOLS, REPOSITORIES, AND CLEARINGHOUSES (*continued*)

- National Health Services (NHS) Digital NHS Digital (United Kingdom): National information and technology partner to the health and social care system; specific app library focused on patient-facing apps to support social care, maternity, mental health, or chronic conditions. https://apps.beta.nhs.uk
  Quality Assessment: Digital assessment questionnaire to assess patient-facing technology across areas of clinical safety, data protection, security, usability, interoperability, technical stability, and benefits to health and well-being.

Repositories and Clearinghouses: Where to Look

- American Academy of Pediatrics: Provides parents and healthcare clinicians with mobile apps for "fast, convenient answers and information." https://www.aap.org/en-us/Pages/Get-the-AAP-Mobile-App.aspx
- iMedicalApps: Independent online medical publication for medical professionals, patients, and analysts interested in mobile medical technology; led by a team of physicians, allied health professionals, and mHealth analysts. http://www.imedicalapps.com

CASE STUDY: How Technology Can Support Evidence-Based Assessment

Introduction

In the examples that follow, health technology is being used to expand the clinician–patient relationship, include patient-centered assessments in care, integrate DHI information within the patient's electronic health record (EHR), and better utilize the EHR in a manner that allows the information within it to be accessible and relevant. Although EHRs have been around for years, best practices for using the data within the EHR to improve the lives of patients are still being developed.

Integrating Patient Self-Assessment and Mobile Health Data Into the Electronic Health Record

The U.S. Department of Veterans Affairs (VA) is currently working to develop a mobile health application that will support mental health symptom monitoring. Assessing mental health in an ongoing and meaningful manner is a complex process, often not completed as frequently as needed, and often not indicative of how an individual is functioning at home or in the community (The National Academies of Sciences, Engineering, Medicine, 2018; Torous et al., 2016). This application allows a veteran to monitor their symptoms using a mobile device. The monitoring of the mobile health application will automatically sync to the individual's EHR at the VA, which will allow for a more accurate and ongoing assessment of mental health symptoms from the patient's perspective. This mobile health application is being developed with respect for the autonomy of the individual veteran in monitoring their own symptoms, supports patient self-efficacy related to mental health disorders, and allows for improved clinician–patient communication concerning mental health assessment.

CASE STUDY: How Technology Can Support Evidence-Based Practice

Improved Use of Current Technology in Patient Assessments

Caring for individuals with multiple health conditions can be challenging. Utilizing technology in ways that can identify risks, concerns, screenings, and health interventions related to comorbidities, as well as alert the clinician to changes in patient status, are key to achieving the best outcomes for their care. A study completed at Cincinnati Children's Medical Center examined the use of the EHR for population identification and stratification for care support in children with medical complexities (Lail, Fields, & Schoettker, 2017). As part of the assessment phase, the clinicians assigned a risk stratification based on the Pediatric Medical Complexity Algorithm, which

then was embedded into the EHR. This allowed for the availability of on-demand reports. Although there were additional interventions as part of this study, the overall goal was to improve the outcomes and experiences of children in the complex care unit. The team at Cincinnati Children's Medical Center saw improvement in the percent of active patients who attended a well-child visit in the previous 13 months (47.8% at baseline to 91.3%). While at baseline only 28% of these children received all of the recommended vaccines; within 10 months of the intervention, the value exceeded 90%. This initiative demonstrates how a project that is focused on integration of new algorithms or other technology into an already established system can improve outcomes.

CONCLUSION

As the landscape of healthcare continues to evolve, so does the role and prominence of technology utilization within the healthcare system. Fully appreciating all aspects of technology utilization in healthcare would require reviewing and condensing vast amounts of information, and this is beyond the capability of any one clinician. Information provided within this chapter is intended to reflect underlying principles congruent with the most current evidence in order to provide a holistic approach to assessing and evaluating health technologies that is attainable.

Health technologies adopted for use in patient diagnosis and treatment, chronic disease management, and primary prevention are "still mainly in the age of promise rather than delivery" (Michie et al., 2017). As even the most innovative technologies can become obsolete, clinicians are best served by asking themselves, "How can I determine if a technology is of high quality?" Given the potential for health technology to revolutionize healthcare delivery and to promote health

and wellness, prioritizing health technology research is necessary to inform evidence-based practice and will require ongoing investigations to represent a rapidly changing healthcare landscape.

Key Takeaways

- When using technology to support health and wellness, rely on the science and leverage the technology to support the science.
- Employ a multidisciplinary approach.
- Ensure compliance with ethical and regulatory standards.
- Search relevant academic and grey literature to ensure accurate and timely evidence.
- Seek out and search reputable repositories and clearinghouses for health technology.
- Look for transparency and quality assessments based on empirically supported tools.

REFERENCES

Bangor, A., Kortum, P. T., & Miller, J. T. (2008). An empirical evaluation of the system usability scale. *International Journal of Human–Computer Interaction, 24*(6), 574–594. doi:10.1080/10447310802205776

Brooke, J. (1996). SUS: A "quick and dirty" usability scale. In P. W. Jordan, B. Thomas, B. A. Weerdmeester, & I. L. McClelland (Eds.), *Usability evaluation in industry* (pp. 189–194). London, UK: Taylor & Francis.

Centers for Medicare & Medicaid Services. (n.d.). *Telemedicine.* Retrieved from https://www.medicaid.gov/medicaid/benefits/telemed/index.html

Chakraborty, B., Collins, L. M., Strecher, V. J., & Murphy, S. A. (2009). Developing multicomponent interventions using fractional factorial designs. *Statistics in Medicine, 28*(21), 2687–2708. doi:10.1002/sim.3643

Children's Online Privacy Protection Act, 15 U.S.C. §§ 6501–6506 (1998).

Choi, B. C. K., & Pak, A. W. P. (2006). Multidisciplinarity, interdisciplinarity and transdisciplinarity in health research, services, education and policy: 1. Definitions, objectives, and evidence of effectiveness. *Clinical and Investigative Medicine, 29*(6), 351–364.

Collins, L. M., Chakraborty, B., Murphy, S. A., & Strecher, V. (2009). Comparison of a phased experimental approach and a single randomized clinical trial for developing multicomponent behavioral interventions. *Clinical Trials (London, England), 6*(1), 5–15. doi:10.1177/1740774508100973

Collins, L. M., Dziak, J. J., & Li, R. (2009). Design of experiments with multiple independent variables: A resource management perspective on complete and reduced factorial designs. *Psychological Methods, 14*(3), 202–224. doi:10.1037/a0015826

Cooper, H. M. (2009). *Research synthesis and meta-analysis: A step-by-step approach* (4th ed.). Los Angeles, CA: SAGE Publications.

Cornell University Library. (2017, February 6). *Gray literature: Gray literature.* Retrieved from http://guides.library.cornell.edu/c.php?g=293667&p=1955919

Eysenbach, G. (2001). What is e-health? *Journal of Medical Internet Research, 3*(2), e20. doi:10.2196/jmir.3.2.e20

Haddaway, N. R., Collins, A. M., Coughlin, D., & Kirk, S. (2015). The role of Google Scholar in evidence reviews and its applicability to grey literature searching. *PLoS One, 10*(9), e0138237. doi:10.1371/journal.pone.0138237

Health Insurance Portability and Accountability Act (HIPAA), P.L. No. 104-191, 110 Stat. 1938 (1996).

Higgins, J., & Green, S. (Eds.). (2011). *Cochrane handbook for systematic reviews of interventions Version 5.1.0* [updated March 2011]. West Sussex, England: Wiley-Blackwell. Retrieved from http://training.cochrane.org/handbook

HIPAA Journal Team. (n.d.). The use of technology and HIPAA compliance. Retrieved from https://www.hipaajournal.com/the-use-of-technology-and-hipaa-compliance

Klasnja, P., Consolvo, S., & Pratt, W. (2011). *Proceedings of the SIGCHI conference on human factors in computing systems* (pp. 3063–3072). New York, NY: Association for Computing Machinery. Retrieved from http://dl.acm.org/citation.cfm?id=1979396

Kruse, C. S., Krowski, N., Rodriguez, B., Tran, L., Vela, J., & Brooks, M. (2017). Telehealth and patient satisfaction: A systematic review and narrative analysis. *BMJ Open, 7*(8), e016242. doi:10.1136/bmjopen-2017-016242

Kumar, S., Nilsen, W., Pavel, M., & Srivastava, M. (2013). Mobile health: Revolutionizing healthcare through transdisciplinary research. *Computer, 46*(1), 28–35. doi:10.1109/MC.2012.392

Lail, J., Fields, E., & Schoettker, P. J. (2017). Quality improvement strategies for population management of children with medical complexity. *Pediatrics, 140*(3), e20170484. doi:10.1542/peds.2017-0484

Michie, S., Yardley, L., West, R., Patrick, K., & Greaves, F. (2017). Developing and evaluating digital interventions to promote behavior change in health and health care: Recommendations resulting from an international workshop. *Journal of Medical Internet Research, 19*(6), e232. doi:10.2196/jmir.7126

Mohr, D. C., Schueller, S. M., Riley, W. T., Brown, C. H., Cuijpers, P., Duan, N., . . . Cheung, K. (2015). Trials of intervention principles: Evaluation methods for evolving behavioral intervention technologies. *Journal of Medical Internet Research, 17*(7), e166. doi:10.2196/jmir.4391

Murray, E., Hekler, E. B., Andersson, G., Collins, L. M., Doherty, A., Hollis, C., . . . Wyatt, J. C. (2016). Evaluating digital health interventions: Key questions and approaches. *American Journal of Preventive Medicine, 51*(5), 843–851. doi:10.1016/j.amepre.2016.06.008

The National Academies of Sciences, Engineering, Medicine. (2018). *Evaluation of the Department of Veterans Affairs Mental Health Services* (pp. 253–264). Washington, DC: National Academies Press. Retrieved from https://www.nap.edu/read/24915/chapter/14

Nature Publishing Group. (2017). Preprints under peer review. *Nature Communications, 8.* doi:10.1038/s41467-017-00950-5

The Office of the National Coordinator for Health Information Technology. (n.d.). What is telehealth? How is telehealth different from telemedicine? Retrieved from https://www.healthit.gov/faq/what-telehealth-how-telehealth-different-telemedicine

Peres, S. C., Pham, T., & Phillips, R. (2013). Validation of the system usability scale (SUS), SUS in the Wild. *Proceedings of the Human Factors and Ergonomics Society Annual Meeting, 57*(1), 192–196. doi:10.1177/1541931213571043

Stoyanov, S. R., Hides, L., Kavanagh, D. J., Zelenko, O., Tjondronegoro, D., & Mani, M. (2015). Mobile app rating scale: A new tool for assessing the quality of health mobile apps. *JMIR MHealth and UHealth, 3*(1), e27. doi:10.2196/mhealth.3422

Suh, H., Shahriaree, N., Hekler, E. B., & Kientz, J. (2016). Developing and validating the user burden scale: A tool for assessing user burden in computing systems. Retrieved from https://www.hcde.washington.edu/files/news/Suh-UserBurdenScale-CHI2016.pdf

Torous, J., & Shore, J. (2018, September). Mental Health Mobile Apps and Videoconferencing-based Telemental Health. Presented as SAMHSA Behavioral Health IT Webinar. Retrieved from https://www.youtube.com/watch?v=GA9FvOtZdwQ&t=47s

Torous, J. B., Chan, S. R., Yellowlees, P. M., & Boland, R. (2016). To use or not? Evaluating ASPECTS of smartphone apps and mobile technology for clinical care in psychiatry. *The Journal of Clinical Psychiatry, 77*(6), e734–e738. doi:10.4088/JCP.15com10619

U.S. Department of Health and Human Services. (n.d.). Health information technology. Retrieved from https://www.hhs.gov/hipaa/for-professionals/special-topics/health-information-technology/index.html

U.S. Department of Health and Human Services & Office for Civil Rights. (2013, July 26). Health information technology; right to access and HIT. Retrieved from https://www.hhs.gov/civil-rights/for-individuals/fact-sheets.html

U.S. Food & Drug Administration. (2018). Framework for FDA's Real-World Evidence Program. Retrieved from https://www.fda.gov/media/120060/download

World Health Organization. (2019a). What is a health technology? Retrieved from https://www.who.int/health-technology-assessment/about/healthtechnology/en

World Health Organization. (2019b). *WHO guideline: Recommendations on digital interventions for health system strengthening.* Retrieved from https://apps.who.int/iris/bitstream/handle/10665/311980/WHO-RHR-19.10-eng.pdf?ua=1

28

Evidence-Based Assessment of Personal Health and Well-Being for Clinicians: Key Strategies to Achieve Optimal Wellness

Bernadette Mazurek Melnyk, Kate Gawlik, and Alice M. Teall

"If you don't take time to prioritize your own health and well-being today, you will have to take time for illness later. Take action NOW!"

—Bern Melnyk

LEARNING OBJECTIVES

- Discuss the prevalence of clinician burnout and its adverse consequences.
- Describe the National Academy of Medicine's Action Collaborative on Clinician Well-Being and Resilience.
- Conduct a self-assessment of one's own health and well-being.
- Evaluate one's own personal health and well-being (strengths and needs) related to the nine dimensions of wellness.
- Identify key strategies for improving one's well-being in each of the nine wellness dimensions.

THE IMPORTANCE OF CLINICIAN HEALTH AND WELL-BEING

The prevalence of depression, burnout, suicidal ideation, and chronic health conditions (e.g., hypertension, diabetes) tends to be higher in healthcare clinicians than that in the general population (Melnyk, Orsolini, et al., 2018). **Burnout** consists of emotional exhaustion; no longer finding work meaningful; feeling ineffective; and a tendency to view patients, students, and colleagues as objects rather than as human beings (Fred & Scheid, 2018). Conditions associated with burnout include headaches, tension, insomnia, fatigue, anger, impaired memory, decreased attention, thoughts of quitting work, drug and alcohol use, and suicide. Burnout not only has adverse effects on clinician population health and healthcare quality and **healthcare safety**, but it also contributes to high turnover and substantial financial losses (Willard-Grace et al., 2019). For every physician who leaves a practice, it is estimated that $500,000 to $1,000,000 in revenue is lost (Fred & Scheid, 2018). For every newly licensed registered nurse (NLRN) who is lost in the first year of practice, it costs the organization up to three times the nurse's annual salary when taking into consideration the cost of recruitment, training, and orientation (Unruh & Zhang, 2014). Burnout currently affects more than 50% of health professionals (Shanafelt et al., 2015) and impacts the quality and safety of healthcare. Depression and burnout in clinicians are related to reductions in healthcare quality, increased medical errors, patient dissatisfaction, reduced productivity, and very costly staff turnover (Hall, Johnson, Watt, Tsipa, & O'Connor, 2016; Melnyk, Orsolini, et al., 2018). Because burnout can lead to adverse consequences for both clinicians and patients, urgent attention must be given to this public health epidemic. Preventable medical errors are the third leading cause of death in America (Makary, 2016). In a national study of nearly 1,900 nurses from 19 healthcare systems throughout the United States, more than 50% of them reported poor physical and mental health. Approximately one-third of the nurses reported depression, which was the leading cause of medical errors (Melnyk, Orsolini, et al., 2018).

Clinicians typically do a wonderful job of caring for their patients and family members, but they often do not prioritize their own self-care. Coupled with healthcare system challenges, including documentation requirements of electronic health records that results in clinicians spending less time with patients, maintenance of certification, loss of autonomy, unhealthy workplace cultures, and heavy workloads, these issues are a prescription for an unhealthy population and unsafe provision of care.

THE NATIONAL ACADEMY OF MEDICINE'S ACTION COLLABORATIVE ON CLINICIAN WELL-BEING AND RESILIENCE

Because of the high prevalence of clinician burnout, depression, and suicide, the National Academy of Medicine (NAM) launched an *Action Collaborative on Clinician Well-Being and Resilience* in 2017 in order to enhance visibility on this issue and to develop evidence-based solutions to tackle this public health epidemic and improve **clinician health and well-being** (Dzau, Kirch, & Nasca, 2018). The NAM collaborative identified both external and individual factors that affect clinician well-being and resistance (**Figure 28.1**).

The NAM also emphasized the urgent need for healthcare systems to implement system interventions to combat this problem, including prioritizing the hiring of Chief Wellness Officers (CWOs) whose responsibility is to lead a culture of well-being and implement strategies to create a healthier workforce (Kishore et al., 2018). CWOs should have a role within the executive suite to elevate the importance of the position and be equipped with the needed resources to effectively build cultures of well-being and implement evidence-based interventions to enhance well-being in clinicians. A knowledge hub with best practices has been developed by the NAM collaborative, and this can

be accessed at https://nam.edu/clinicianwellbeing. This hub provides several resources and solutions to combat clinician burnout, compassion fatigue, depression, and anxiety symptoms at both the individual and organizational levels.

HEALTHCARE SYSTEM INTERVENTIONS

Healthcare organizations should implement a comprehensive, multicomponent wellness strategy that targets evidence-based interventions to individual clinicians, the family and social network, the workplace culture and environment, and organizational policies that are built on a clear vision and mission (Melnyk, Gascon, Amaya, & Mehta, 2018). Central to this strategy must include the building of a wellness culture that makes healthy choices—the easy choices for clinicians to make (Melnyk, Szalacha, & Amaya, 2018). Leaders as well as supervisors and managers must role model and provide support for wellness; if not, it is unlikely that their clinicians will engage in healthy lifestyle behaviors (Melnyk, 2019).

It should be made clear to all clinicians that their **well-being** is a high priority for the organization and that they should be made aware of wellness resources within the institution that are available to them. It is critical to have a "menu of options" for wellness because not all clinicians will benefit from the same interventions (Melnyk, 2019). Grassroots tactics, such as wellness champions, are an effective and low-cost strategy in creating a wellness culture throughout the organization (Amaya, Melnyk, Buffington, & Battista, 2017).

Efforts must be made to decrease mental health stigma within organizations because it is still a barrier for clinicians seeking care. Clinicians should be screened annually for burnout, depression, and anxiety. The Healer Education Assessment and Interactive Screening Program by the American Foundation for Suicide Prevention offers useful system that provides anonymous, encrypted risk screening at low cost. Counseling with cognitive-behavioral therapy (CBT) should be made available for those clinicians who are affected, as it is the gold-standard, evidence-based treatment for depression (Melnyk, Orsolini, et al., 2018). Findings from a recent study using a CBT-based program entitled MINDBODYSTRONG with new nurse residents showed decreases in depressive symptoms, anxiety, and stress as well as increases in healthy lifestyle behaviors and job satisfaction in the nurses who received MINDBODYSTRONG versus those who received an attention control program (Sampson, Melnyk, & Hoying, 2019).

EXTERNAL FACTORS

SOCIETY & CULTURE

- Alignment of societal expectations and clinician's role
- Culture of safety and transparency
- Discrimination and overt and unconscious bias
- Media portrayal
- Patient behaviors and expectations
- Political and economic climates
- Social determinants of health
- Stigmatization of mental illness

LEARNING/PRACTICE ENVIRONMENT

- Autonomy
- Collaborative vs. competitive environment
- Curriculum
- Health IT interoperability and usability/electronic health records
- Learning and practice setting
- Mentorship program
- Physical learning and practice conditions
- Professional relationships
- Student affairs policies
- Student- and patient-centered focus
- Team structures and functionality
- Workplace safety and violence

RULES & REGULATIONS

- Accreditation, high-stakes assessments, and publicized quality ratings
- Documentation and reporting requirements
- Human resources policies and compensation issues
- Initial licensure and certification
- Insurance company policies
- Litigation risk
- Maintenance of licensure and certification
- National and state policies and practices
- Reimbursement structure
- Shifting systems of care and administrative requirements

HEALTHCARE RESPONSIBILITIES

- Administrative responsibilities
- Alignment of responsibility and authority
- Clinical responsibilities
- Learning/career stage
- Patient population
- Specialty-related issues
- Student/trainee responsibilities
- Teaching and research responsibilities

ORGANIZATIONAL FACTORS

- Bureaucracy
- Congruent organizational mission and values
- Culture, leadership, and staff engagement
- Data collection requirements
- Diversity and inclusion
- Harassment and discrimination
- Level of support for all healthcare team members
- Power dynamics
- Professional development opportunities
- Scope of practice
- Workload, performance, compensation, and value attributed to work elements

INDIVIDUAL FACTORS

PERSONAL FACTORS

- Access to a personal mentor
- Inclusion and connectivity
- Family dynamics
- Financial stressors/economic vitality
- Flexibility and ability to respond to change
- Level of engagement/connection to meaning and purpose in work
- Personality traits
- Personal values, ethics, and morals
- Physical, mental, and spiritual well-being
- Relationships and social support
- Sense of meaning
- Work-life integration

SKILLS & ABILITIES

- Clinical competency level/experience
- Communication skills
- Coping skills
- Delegation
- Empathy
- Management and leadership
- Mastering new technologies or proficient use of technology
- Optimizing work flow
- Organizational skills
- Resilience skills/practices
- Teamwork skills

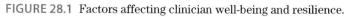

FIGURE 28.1 Factors affecting clinician well-being and resilience.

Source: Adapted from National Academies of Sciences. (2018). *Factors affecting clinician well-being and resilience.* Retrieved from https://nam.edu/clinicianwellbeing/wp-content/uploads/2019/07/Factors-Affecting-Clinician-Well-Being-and-Resilience-July-2019.pdf. Copyright 2018 National Academy of Sciences.

Healthcare systems also must address staffing where patient-to-clinician ratios are high, and 12-hour shifts should be eliminated (Melnyk, 2019). In addition, changes to the electronic health record also are necessary so that clinicians can spend more time with their patients. Systems should also consider using scribes because they can decrease the data entry workload of healthcare clinicians.

Findings from cost analyses indicate that, for every dollar invested in wellness, there is a $3 to $6 return on investment (Baicker, Cutler & Song, 2010). At The Ohio State University, the first university in the United States to appoint a CWO, investment in wellness has resulted in a negative faculty and staff healthcare trend for the third year in a row.

KEY QUESTIONS FOR SELF-ASSESSMENT OF CLINICIAN HEALTH AND WELL-BEING

In reflecting upon your own health and well-being, it is important to answer the following questions:

1. Have you had a wellness examination in the past year? If not, is one scheduled?
2. Do you follow the U.S. Preventive Services Task Force (USPSTF) recommendations for **your own** preventive health screenings that apply to your age, sex, and smoking status? The USPSTF has an online calculator that can be used to determine applicable and individualized screenings and preventive measures. To access it and determine what screenings apply to you, please visit https://epss.ahrq.gov/ePSS/search.jsp.
3. How high is your current level of stress according to the 10-item Perceived Stress Scale (PSS-10)? Please answer the 10-question PSS-10 (**Exhibit 28.1**) and total your score.
4. Are you currently experiencing depressive symptoms according to the 9-item Patient Health Questionnaire (PHQ-9)? Please answer the nine-question PHQ-9 (**Exhibit 28.2**) and total your score.
5. Are you currently experiencing anxiety symptoms according to the 7-item Generalized Anxiety Disorder Questionnaire (GAD-7)? Please answer the GAD-7 scale (**Exhibit 28.3**) and total your score.
6. Are you currently experiencing burnout according to the scale in **Exhibit 28.4**?

If you are currently experiencing elevated symptoms of stress, depressive symptoms, anxiety, or burnout according to your scores on the previously mentioned scales, are they interfering with your ability to concentrate or function? If yes, it is time to seek assistance. Do not let stigma interfere with you seeking help for your symptoms. Everyone has difficulty coping or functioning at certain times in their lives. For the sake of your own health and the people who love you as well as for the patients for whom you care, *seek help now!*

> *If you ever have thoughts of suicide, immediately seek help or call the national suicide prevention hotline at 1-800-273-8255.*

The Suicide Lifeline provides 24/7, free, and confidential support for people in distress. It also provides prevention and crisis resources for you or your loved ones, in addition to best-practice resources for clinicians.

KEY STRATEGIES FOR OPTIMIZING PERSONAL HEALTH AND WELL-BEING IN THE NINE DIMENSIONS OF WELL-BEING

When we board an airplane and hear safety messaging, we are told by a flight attendant to place the oxygen mask on ourselves first before placing it on your child or loved one. Remember, you cannot take good care of your family and/or your patients unless you practice good **self-care**. As briefly discussed in Chapter 1, Approach to Evidence-Based Assessment of Health and Well-Being, good self-care should encompass the **nine dimensions of wellness**. These dimensions of wellness are physical, emotional, financial, social, intellectual, career, creative, environmental, and spiritual. Each of these are discussed in the subsequent sections.

PHYSICAL WELLNESS

Chronic disease affects one in two Americans, yet approximately 80% of chronic disease can be prevented with just a few healthy lifestyle behaviors. Although cardiovascular disease remains the number one killer of Americans, if all causes of death and disease are taken into consideration, it is really our behaviors that are the

EXHIBIT 28.1 Perceived Stress Scale (PSS-10)

	Never	Almost Never	Sometimes	Fairly Often	Very Often
1. In the past month, how often have you been upset because of something that happened unexpectedly?	0	1	2	3	4
2. In the past month, how often have you felt that you were unable to control the important things in your life?	0	1	2	3	4
3. In the past month, how often have you felt nervous and stressed?	0	1	2	3	4
4. In the past month, how often have you felt confident about your ability to handle your personal problems?	4	3	2	1	0
5. In the past month, how often have you felt that things were going your way?	4	3	2	1	0
6. In the past month, how often have you found that you could not cope with all the things that you had to do?	0	1	2	3	4
7. In the past month, how often have you been able to control irritations in your life?	4	3	2	1	0
8. In the past month, how often have you felt that you were on top of things?	4	3	2	1	0
9. In the past month, how often have you been angered because of things that happened that were out of your control?	0	1	2	3	4
10. In the past month, how often have you felt difficulties were piling up so high that you could not overcome them?	0	1	2	3	4
Column totals					
Sum of columns (total score)					

Interpretation of Score for the Perceived Stress Scale (PSS-10)

Total Score	Perceived Stress Severity
0–13	Low perceived stress
14–26	Moderate perceived stress
27–40	High perceived stress

Source: Adapted from Cohen, S., Kamarch, T., & Mermelstein, R. (1983). A global measure of perceived stress. *Journal of Health and Social Behavior, 24,* 385–396. doi:10.2307/2136404

EXHIBIT 28.2 Patient Health Questionnaire (PHQ-9)

Over the past 2 weeks, how often have you been bothered by any of the following problems?

	Not at All	Several Days	More Than 7 Days	Nearly Every Day
1. Little interest or pleasure in doing things	0	1	2	3
2. Feeling down, depressed, or hopeless	0	1	2	3
3. Trouble falling or staying asleep, or sleeping too much	0	1	2	3
4. Feeling tired or having little energy	0	1	2	3
5. Poor appetite or overeating	0	1	2	3
6. Feeling bad about yourself or that you are a failure or have let yourself or your family down	0	1	2	3
7. Trouble concentrating on things, such as reading the newspaper or watching television	0	1	2	3
8. Moving or speaking so slowly that other people have noticed. Or the opposite—being so fidgety or restless that you have been moving around a lot more than usual	0	1	2	3
9. Thoughts that you would be better off dead or of hurting yourself	0	1	2	3
Column totals				
Sum of columns (total score)				

Interpretation of Score for the Patient Health Questionnaire (PHQ-9)

Total Score	Depression Severity
1–4	Minimal depression
5–9	Mild depression
10–14	Moderate depression
15–19	Moderately severe depression
20–27	Severe depression

Note: Developed by Drs. Robert L. Spitzer, Janet B.W. Williams, Kurt Kroenke, and colleagues, with an educational grant from Pfizer, Inc.
Source: Adapted from Kroenke, K., Spitzer, R. L., & Williams, J. B. (2001). The PHQ-9: Validity of a brief depression severity measure. *Journal of General Internal Medicine, 16*(9), 606–613. doi:10.1046/j.1525-1497.2001.016009606.x

EXHIBIT 28.3 Generalized Anxiety Disorder Screener (GAD-7)

Over the past 2 weeks, how often have you been bothered by the following problems?

	Not at All	Several Days	More Than 7 Days	Nearly Every Day
1. Feeling nervous, anxious, or on edge	0	1	2	3
2. Not being able to stop or control worrying	0	1	2	3
3. Worrying too much about different things	0	1	2	3
4. Trouble relaxing	0	1	2	3
5. Being so restless that it is hard to sit still	0	1	2	3
6. Becoming easily annoyed or irritated	0	1	2	3
7. Feeling afraid as if something awful might happen	0	1	2	3
Column totals				
Sum of columns (total score)				

Interpretation of Score for the Generalized Anxiety Disorder Questionnaire (GAD-7)	
Total Score	Provisional Diagnosis
0–7	None
8+	Probable anxiety disorder

Note: Developed by Drs. Robert L. Spitzer, Janet B.W. Williams, Kurt Kroenke, and colleagues, with an educational grant from Pfizer, Inc.
Source: Adapted from Spitzer, R. L., Kroenke, K., Williams, J. B., & Lowe, B. (2006). A brief measure for assessing generalized anxiety disorder: The GAD-7. *Archives of Internal Medicine, 166*(10), 1092–1097. doi:10.1001/archinte.166.10.1092

EXHIBIT 28.4 Assessment of Burnout

Overall, how would you rate your level of burnout?

Response	Score
I enjoy my work. I have no symptoms of burnout.	1
Occasionally, I am under stress, and I do not always have as much energy as I once did, but I do not feel burned out.	2
I am definitely burning out and have one or more symptoms of burnout, such as physical and emotional exhaustion.	3
The symptoms of burnout that I am experiencing will not go away. I think about frustration at work a lot.	4
I feel completely burned out and often wonder if I can go on. I am at the point where I may need some changes or may need to seek some sort of help.	5

Interpretation of Score for the Assessment of Burnout	
Total Score	Interpretation
≤2	No symptoms of burnout
≥3	Symptoms of burnout

Source: Adapted from Dolan, E. D., Mohr, D., Lempa, M., Joos, S., Fihn, S. D., Nelson, K. M., & Helfrichm, C. D. (2014). Using a single item to measure burnout in primary care staff: A psychometric evaluation. *Journal of General Internal Medicine, 30*(5), 582–587. doi:10.1007/s11606-014-3112-6

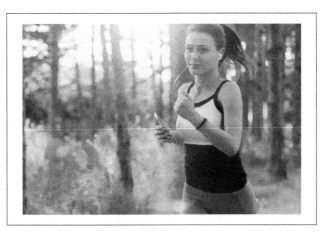

FIGURE 28.2 Engage in some physical activity each day; even small amounts can increase your energy and decrease fatigue.

number one killer, including lack of physical activity, unhealthy eating, drug abuse, and smoking. In order to substantially reduce your risk of chronic disease, make a commitment to achieve the following, including:

- Thirty minutes of moderate-intensity physical activity 5 days/week (**Figure 28.2**)
- Five servings of fruits and vegetables per day
- Do not smoke
- If you drink alcohol, limit it to no more than one drink a day if you are a woman and two a day if you are a man (Ford, Zhao, Tsai, & Li, 2011).

Aim for at least 7 hours of sleep per night, sit less, and practice regular stress reduction for even more preventive benefits (Melnyk & Neale, 2018). For a person who is inactive, even small increases in moderate-intensity physical activity (e.g., 11 minutes a day) has health benefits (Physical Activity Guidelines Advisory Committee, 2018). There is no threshold that has to be exceeded before benefits occur. For more energy, it is also important to sit less and stand more. Several chronic diseases and conditions result from prolonged sitting. One recent study found that prolonged sitting (i.e., 6 or more hours/day vs. <3 hours/day) was related to a higher risk of mortality from all causes, including cardiovascular disease, cancer, diabetes, kidney disease, suicide, chronic obstructive pulmonary disease, pneumonitis due to solids and liquids, liver disease, peptic ulcer and other digestive diseases, Parkinson's disease, Alzheimer's disease, nervous disorders, and musculoskeletal disorders (Patel, Maliniak, Rees-Punja, Matthews, & Gapstur, 2018). Try having standing meetings instead of sitting meetings. In addition to being good for your cardiovascular health, you will get through your meetings more quickly! Instead of waiting until January 1 to set a new healthy lifestyle behavior goal, consider today your January 1. Remember, it takes 30 to 60 days to make or break a new health habit. It is important to write down your new healthy lifestyle behavior goal and place that goal where you can see it every day (e.g., by where you brush your teeth or at your computer). If you do fall off track, just start again the following day. Habits take consistent practice to make or break.

In addition, know your own numbers, including total cholesterol, low-density lipoproteins, high-density lipoproteins, body mass index, hemoglobin A1C, and waist circumference. The 2017 American College of Cardiology (ACC)/American Heart Association (AHA) guideline defines normal blood pressure (BP) as less than 120/80 mmHg and recommends BP checks at every healthcare clinician visit, or at least once every 2 years if your BP is normal (Whelton et al., 2017).

It is also important to engage in strength training at least twice a week because it provides several benefits, including increased muscle mass, increased bone strength, better stability, and lower BP. Resistance bands are an ideal and convenient way to build strength, as you can keep them at your desk and place one in your suitcase when you travel. Many websites contain resistance band workouts (e.g., https://greatist .com/fitness/resistance-band-exercises).

It is also important to limit your sodium intake to less than 1,500 mg/day and drink plenty of water because even mild dehydration can make you feel fatigued. The recommended amount is approximately 15.5 cups for men and 11.5 cups a day for women.

EMOTIONAL WELLNESS

Emotional wellness is the ability to identify, express, and manage the full range of your feelings. It includes practicing techniques to deal with stress, depression, and anxiety and seeking help when your feelings become overwhelming or interfere with everyday functioning.

There is a wise saying: Change your thinking; change your life! CBT or cognitive-behavioral skills building is the gold-standard, first-line treatment for mild-to-moderate depression and anxiety; however, only a few people having these symptoms receive it because of a lack of mental health professionals throughout the United States. In CBT, people are taught that how they think is related to how they feel and how they behave. The ABCs are taught in CBT. The letter "A" stands for an activating event that triggers a negative belief or thought. The consequence of the negative belief is feeling stressed, anxious, or depressed or acting in unhealthy ways. In CBT, individuals are taught how to monitor for activating events and stop negative beliefs when they occur. The consequence is feeling emotionally better and behaving in healthier ways. The next time when you feel stressed, anxious, angry, or depressed, ask yourself, "What was I just thinking?" Chances are it was a negative thought. Monitoring for these activating events and turning negative thought patterns around is key to experiencing less negative moods. A recent randomized controlled trial testing a CBT-based program entitled MINDBODYSTRONG, originally created by Bernadette Melnyk and also known in several studies as COPE, with new nurse residents in a large academic medical center in the Midwest revealed that those who received the MINDBODYSTRONG program versus those who received an attention control program had less stress, anxiety, and depression as well as healthier behaviors and job satisfaction (Sampson et al., 2019). For more information on this MINDBODYSTRONG program, please contact mindstrong@osu.edu.

Try monitoring your thoughts for the next 30 days or keeping a journal of negative thought patterns and the emotions that come with them. Write down how you will respond to the stressor the next time. With time and practice, you can actually change your thinking in response to the stressors in your life and that will change how you feel (Melnyk & Neal, 2018). Other tactics that can enhance your emotional well-being include:

- Engage in some physical activity each day; even small amounts can increase your energy and decrease fatigue.
- Keep a journal of what causes your stress and strategies that help to reduce it.
- Get at least 7 hours of sleep a night to avoid excess cortisol from being released.
- Practice mindfulness—the ability to stay in the present moment. Mindfulness decreases worry about the future and guilt about the past, which are two wasted emotions.
- Manage your energy by taking short recovery breaks throughout the day (even 5 minutes of activity every hour can increase your level of energy).
- Read 5 minutes in a positive-thinking book of your choice every morning to elevate your mood and protect yourself from negativity that can arise each day.
- When stressed, take just five slow deep breaths in and out—a deep breathing decreases stress and lowers BP. As you breathe in, say "I am calm." As you breathe out, say "I am blowing out all of my stress."
- Help others and be kind; compassion for others helps you feel good.
- Talk to someone you trust about how you feel.
- Resolve to keep your workplace positive.
- Practice a daily attitude of gratitude. Naming or writing down three people or things you are grateful for every morning and evening can boost your mood.

If symptoms of anxiety, stress, or depression persist for more than 2 weeks and interfere with your daily functioning, do not wait; seek help from a qualified therapist or your healthcare clinician. Emotional wellness includes seeking help when needed (Melnyk & Neale, 2018).

FINANCIAL WELLNESS

Financial well-being includes being fully aware of your financial state and budget and managing your finances to achieve your goals. Detailed analysis and planning is important so that you can make decisions regarding how you will spend and save your income. According to a study conducted by the American Psychological Association (APA, 2015), approximately three in four Americans experience financial stress, which typically affects physical and emotional well-being. According to the APA, high levels of financial stress are associated with an increased risk for ulcers, migraines, heart attacks, depression, anxiety, and sleep disturbance and may lead to unhealthy coping mechanisms, such as binge drinking, smoking, and overeating. By analyzing, planning, and managing your spending, you can improve your financial well-being. The following are helpful strategies:

- **Evaluate your finances.** Analyze your monthly income and how you are currently spending it. Three months' worth of credit card and bank statements will give you a clear picture of your income and expenses. Identify your fixed expenses, such as mortgage, car payments, student loans, and utility bills, and your variable expenses, such as money spent on food, clothing, vacations, emergencies, and health.
- **Prioritize.** Decide what you want to spend your income on every month and draw up a realistic budget. Online resources such as Quicken, YNAB, and Moneydance can help you.
- **Save rather than borrow.** Paying cash for things is best. If you use a credit card to obtain airline miles or other benefits, be sure to pay it off at the end of the month. It is much better to save to pay for something rather than borrow it. If you are thinking about a big purchase, sit on it overnight and see if you feel the same sense of urgency to buy it as you did when you saw it.
- **Protect yourself from unexpected expenses.** Reduce worry about financial emergencies by saving at least 6 months of pay.
- **Seek help.** A certified financial planner (CFP) can help you evaluate your current situation and show you ways to pay off debt and invest in your future. Look for fee-based CFPs, who charge a one-time fee rather than taking a percentage of your investments' earnings.
- **Find healthy outlets for your stress that are free.** Physical activity and stress reduction practices can reduce your overall stress, which will help you think more clearly and get a better handle on your finances (Melnyk & Neale, 2018).

SOCIAL WELLNESS

Social wellness can be defined as our ability to effectively interact with people around us and to create a support system that includes family and friends (Melnyk & Neale, 2018). Findings from studies indicate that social connections help people deal with stress and keep us healthy. It is important to build positive relationships at home and work and to learn to have crucial conversations. It is fine to disagree with coworkers or loved ones as long as the disagreements are handled respectfully. Disconnecting from emails and technology to connect with the important people in your life on a regular basis will improve your mood. If you are feeling frustrated with how little time you have to connect with the people in your life who are important, consider saying "no" more to opportunities that create work overload in your life. Studies on the impact of loneliness on physical and mental health are alarming. Loneliness has been found to cause inflammation and raise stress hormone levels, which can increase the risk of heart disease, arthritis, type 2 diabetes, depression, pain, fatigue, and dementia (Jaremka et al., 2014). Jaremka and colleagues (2013) also found that people who are lonely may have suppressed immune systems, brought on by stress. Bottom line: Prioritize taking time to connect to people and activities that bring you joy (**Figure 28.3**).

INTELLECTUAL WELLNESS

When a person is intellectually healthy, they appreciate lifelong learning, foster critical thinking, develop moral reasoning, expand worldviews, and engage in education for the pursuit of knowledge. Any time that you learn a new skill or concept and attempt to understand a different viewpoint or exercise your mind with puzzles and games, you are building intellectual well-being. Studies show that intellectual exercise may improve the physical structure of your brain to help prevent cognitive decline (Melnyk & Neale, 2018). Research reported that physical and mental

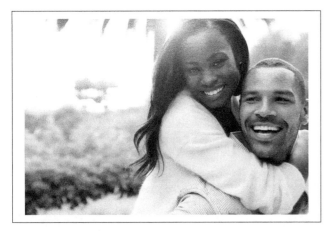

FIGURE 28.3 Take time to connect to people and activities that bring you joy.

exercise supports the growth of new neurons, whereas stress and depression can hinder it (Barry, 2011). Challenging your brain also helps existing neurons to form new connections. Combining intellectual growth with mindfulness can enhance your brain's health and prevent the cognitive decline that often occurs with aging.

Strategies that can help with intellectual well-being include reading 5 to 10 minutes in a positive-thinking book every day, which can also elevate your mood; giving your brain a rest with at least a few minutes of quiet time every few hours; not multitasking as it is the enemy of full engagement; disrupting your typical routines; and engaging in lifelong learning.

CAREER WELLNESS

If you are engaged in work that you are truly passionate about throughout your career, you will never feel like you work a day in your life. It is important to answer the following question:

*What will you do in the next 5 to 10 years if
you know that you cannot fail?*

Then, write the answer down, put a date on it, and place it where you can see it every day. So many people get immersed in day-to-day living and "to do's" or grinding chores or work that they lose their ability to dream. "Nothing happens without first a dream" is a famous quote by Carl Sandburg. When your work is aligned with your dreams and passions, you will wake up every day with energy and enthusiasm. If you are experiencing chronic stress, dissatisfaction, and burnout at work, it should prompt you to do an evaluation of your career wellness. People who are the happiest in their careers are those who have purpose, passion, and pride (Buettner, 2017).

Even if you cannot change where you work right now, you can change your approach to the stressors and challenges you face at work. Several strategies can help you reevaluate your career, cope with change and stress, and reenergize your work life.

- Practice mindfulness at select times during the day at work. Research supports that mindfulness can increase on-the-job resiliency and improve effectiveness and safety.
- Cultivate a positive mind-set. By staying positive, you will feel emotionally better and be more productive.
- Do not multitask. Multitasking can drain your energy.
- Evaluate your work hours, including time you spend commuting. If you cannot cut your commuting time, try making use of drive time to listen to audiobooks or positive music. Use your vacation hours to disconnect and get away at regular intervals.

CREATIVE WELLNESS

Creativity has long been a part of well-being. A review of more than 100 studies of the benefits of the arts (such as music, visual arts, dance, and writing) found that creative expression has a powerful impact on health and well-being among various populations. Findings from studies indicate that participating in the arts decreases depressive symptoms, increases positive emotions, reduces stress, and, in some cases, improves immune-system functioning. Creative wellness means valuing and participating in a diverse range of arts and cultural experiences to understand and appreciate your surrounding world (Melnyk & Neale, 2018; **Figure 28.4**). If you do not consider yourself creative, attempt doodling in a blank journal to relieve stress, or try a free doodling app like Doodle Buddy and You Doodle. Freewriting, journaling, and writing poetry and stories can be stress reducing and healing. Creativity can include cooking, gardening, redecorating your home or office, and more. Research shows that creative pursuits also boost intellectual wellness and may delay cognitive decline in older people.

ENVIRONMENTAL WELLNESS

Environmental wellness means recognizing the responsibility to preserve, protect, and improve the environment and to appreciate your connection to nature (Melnyk & Neale, 2018). Environmental wellness intersects with social wellness when you work to conserve the environment for future generations and improve conditions for others around the world. Studies have shown that green space, such as parks, forests, and river corridors, are good for our physical and mental health (World Health Organization, 2016). Your environment includes everything that surrounds you—your home, your car, your workplace, the food you eat, and the people with whom you interact.

Paying attention to environment is especially important at work, where our surroundings can have a profound effect on how we feel and function. We tend to thrive better when we are surrounded by people who support our goals and provide support to help us to succeed. We cannot usually choose the people with whom we work, but we can support an environment of workplace civility and choose to spend more time with those who support and uplift us. Also, we can contribute to making our physical surroundings healthier, from recycling to creating a culture of respect and gratitude (Melnyk & Neale, 2018).

You can improve your environment by taking steps to be conscious about how you use natural resources, such as recycling; turning off water or electric appliances and lights when not in use; saving gas by walking, biking, or taking public transportation instead of driving; and supporting your colleagues' efforts to recycle at the office. When you show respect for the natural environment, you show respect for others and for future generations.

SPIRITUAL WELLNESS

Spiritual wellness is largely about your purpose, not religion. Dossey (2015) contends that our spirituality involves a sense of connection outside ourselves and includes our values, meaning, and purpose. Your spiritual well-being is about what inspires you, what gives you hope, and what you feel strongly about (Melnyk & Neale, 2018). Your spirit is the seat of your deepest values and character.

Although religion and spirituality can be connected, they are different. A faith community can give you an outlet for your spirituality, but religion is not spirituality's only expression. Hope, purpose, job, love, meaning, connection, appreciation of beauty, and caring and compassion for others are associated with spiritual well-being.

Our purpose is at the foundation of our spiritual nature. If you are feeling disconnected from your values and purpose, try the following strategies:

- Set aside some quiet time to think about your purpose and whether you are fulfilling it. Identify what you need to do to adjust. Ask yourself what you would do in the next 5 to 10 years if you knew you could not fail.
- Retain a positive outlook. Actively seek ways to increase positivity, such as keeping a gratitude journal, celebrating your strengths, and recognizing and practicing small acts of kindness daily.

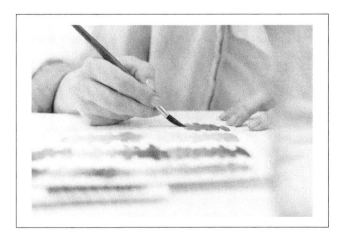

FIGURE 28.4 Participating in the arts decreases depressive symptoms, increases positive emotions, reduces stress, and, in some cases, improves immune-system functioning.

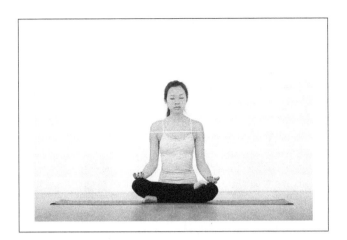

FIGURE 28.5 Adopt a meditative practice to reflect on what inspires you, gives you hope, and what you feel strongly about.

- Adopt a meditative practice (**Figure 28.5**). Traditional forms of meditation can include prayer or sitting in stillness with a quiet mind. Some people prefer physical action that incorporates meditation, such as yoga, tai chi, or walking. Find out what you like best and do what works for you.

TAKE ACTION TO IMPROVE YOUR HEALTH AND WELL-BEING NOW: BERN'S STORY

Do not procrastinate taking good self-care. Your life and others' lives depend on it.

Now that you have nearly completed this chapter and reviewed evidence-based strategies that can assist you in achieving optimal health and well-being, evaluate your strengths and needs in each of the nine dimensions of well-being. Choose one dimension that you will focus on in the next 30 to 60 days. If you are finding it difficult to prioritize your own self-care, think about all of the people who love you and want you to be around for a long time. The first author of this chapter (Bernadette [Bern] Melnyk) lost her mom suddenly at the age of 15. After a wonderful breakfast interchange when they were home alone, Bern's mom sneezed, suffered a stroke, and died. The sad part of this story is that Bern's mother had a history of headaches for over a year. She finally visited her physician for an evaluation a week before she died, was diagnosed with high BP, and given a prescription for a BP medication. However, she never filled the prescription; Bern's father found it in her mom's purse after she died. Owing to this traumatic event, Bern had posttraumatic stress disorder for a few years. Unfortunately, there was no help or counseling for her in

the small town of Republic, Pennsylvania, where she grew up. In the next 4 years, Bern also lost a cousin after a motor vehicle accident, the only grandparent she ever knew and loved, and her father had a major heart attack. However, what does not break us only makes us stronger. As a result of these adversities, Bern developed a passion and purpose to become a nurse, a pediatric nurse practitioner and psychiatric nurse practitioner, and obtain a PhD so that she could develop and test evidence-based programs to improve mental health outcomes in children, teens, college students, and parents. These programs are now bringing her evidence-based Creating Opportunities for Personal Empowerment (COPE) cognitive-behavioral skills-building intervention programs to thousands of children and youth with depression and anxiety across the United States and five other countries. We tell this story to encourage you because we often do not understand why we are experiencing life's challenges when they are happening, but as a result of these types of experiences, we grow stronger and pursue our purpose to make a positive impact in the world.

If it is difficult for you to prioritize your own self-care, think about doing it for the people who love you—who want you to be around for a very long time. Bern lost her mom suddenly when she was 15 years old due to a stroke that may have been able to be prevented if she had filled her prescription and started taking the medication. She did not have a mother to see her graduate from high school, become a nurse, and go on to have her three beautiful daughters. When she lacks the energy to exercise or the motivation to make healthy food choices, Bern thinks about her husband, three daughters, and two small grandsons who provide the motivation for her to continue to make healthy lifestyle choices. Who is the person/people in your life that will serve as the motivator(s) for you to make healthy choices and take better self-care?

ACT NOW: Take one step today and commit to improving one wellness dimension that can lead you on a better path to optimal health and well-being. If you do not take the time for good self-care today, you will need to take the time to deal with chronic illness in the future. We believe in you; you can do it!

ACKNOWLEDGMENTS

Special thanks to the *American Nurse Today* "Nine Dimensions of Wellness" by Bernadette Melnyk and Susan Neale with Brenda C. Buffington, EdD, NBC-HWC, EP-C; David Hrabe, PhD, RN, NC-BC; and Laura Newpoff. Excerpts from this series were adapted for this chapter.

REFERENCES

Amaya, M., Melnyk, B. M., Buffington, B., & Battista, L. (2017) Workplace wellness champions: Lessons learned and implications for future programming. *Building Healthy Academic Communities Journal, 1*(1), 59–67. doi:10.18061/bhac.v1i1.5744

American Psychological Association. (2015). *Paying with our health.* Retrieved from https://www.apa.org/news/press/releases/stress/2014/stress-report.pdf

Baicker, K., Cutler, D., & Song, Z. (2010). Workplace wellness programs can generate savings. *Health Affairs, 29*(2), 304–311. doi:10.1377/hlthaff.2009.0626

Barry, S. R. (2011). How to grow new neurons in your brain. *Psychology Today.* Retrieved from https://www.psychologytoday.com/intl/blog/eyes-the-brain/201101/how-grow-new-neurons-in-your-brain

Buettner, D. (2017). *The blue zones of happiness: Lessons from the world's happiest people.* Washington, DC: National Geographic Partners.

Cohen, S., Kamarch, T., & Mermelstein, R. (1983). A global measure of perceived stress. *Journal of Health and Social Behavior, 24*, 385–396. doi:10.2307/2136404

Dolan, E. D., Mohr, D., Lempa, M., Joos, S., Fihn, S. D., Nelson, K. M., & Helfrichm, C. D. (2014). Using a single item to measure burnout in primary care staff: A psychometric evaluation. *Journal of General Internal Medicine, 30*(5), 582–587. doi:10.1007/s11606-014-3112-6

Dossey, B. M. (2015). Integrative health and wellness assessment. In B. M. Dossey, S. Luck, & B. S. Schaub (Eds.), *Nurse coaching: Integrative approaches for health and well-being* (pp. 109–121). North Miami, FL: International Nurse Coach Association.

Dzau, V. J., Kirch, D. G., & Nasca, T. J. (2018). To care is human—Collectively confronting the clinician-burnout crisis. *New England Journal of Medicine, 378*(4), 312–314. doi:10.1056/NEJMp1715127

Ford, E. S., Zhao, G., Tsai, J., & Li, C. (2011). Low-risk lifestyle behaviors and all-cause mortality: Findings from the national health and nutrition examination survey III mortality study. *American Journal of Public Health, 101*, 1922–1929. doi:10.2105/AJPH.2011.300167

Fred H. L., Scheid M. S. (2018). Physician burnout: Causes, consequences and (?) cures. *Texas Heart Institute Journal, 45*(4), 198–202. doi:10.14503/THIJ-18-6842

Hall, L. H., Johnson, J., Watt, I., Tsipa, A., & O'Connor, D. B. (2016). Healthcare staff wellbeing, burnout, and patient safety: A systematic review. *PLoS One, 11*(7), e0159015. doi:10.1371/journal.pone.0159015

Jaremka, L. M., Andridge, R. R., Fagundes, C. P., Alfano, C. M., Povoski, S. P., Lipari, A. M., . . . Kiecolt-Glaser, J. K. (2014). Pain, depression, and fatigue: Loneliness as a longitudinal risk factor. *Health Psychology, 33*(9), 948–957. doi:10.1037/a0034012

Jaremka, L. M., Fagundes, C. P., Peng, J., Bennett, J. M., Glaser, R., Malarkey, W. B., & Kiecolt-Glaser, J. K. (2013). Loneliness promotes inflammation during acute stress. *Psychological Science, 24*(7), 1089–1097. doi:10.1177/0956797612464059

Kishore, S., Ripp, J., Shanafelt, T., Melnyk, B. M., Rogers, D., Brigham, T., . . . Dzau, V. (2018, October 26). Making the case for the chief wellness officer in America's health systems: A call to action [Blog post]. *Health Affairs.* Retrieved from https://www.healthaffairs.org/do/10.1377/hblog20181025.308059/full

Kroenke, K., Spitzer, R. L., & Williams, J. B. (2001). The PHQ-9: Validity of a brief depression severity measure. *Journal of General Internal Medicine, 16*(9), 606–613. doi:10.1046/j.1525-1497.2001.016009606.x

Makary, M. A. (2016). Medical error—the third leading cause of death in the US. *BMJ, 353*, i2139. doi:10.1136/bmj.i2139

Melnyk, B. M. (2019). Making an evidence-based case for urgent action to address clinician burnout. *American Journal of Accountable Care, 7*(2), 12–14. Retrieved from https://www.ajmc.com/journals/ajac/2019/2019-vol7-n2/making-an-evidencebased-case-for-urgent-action-to-address-clinician-burnout

Melnyk, B. M., Gascon, G. M., Amaya, M., & Mehta, L. S. (2018). A comprehensive approach to university wellness emphasizing Million Hearts demonstrates improvement in population cardiovascular risk. *Building Healthy Academic Communities Journal, 2*(2), 6–11. doi:10.18061/bhac.v2i2.6555

Melnyk, B. M., & Neale, S. (2018). *9 Dimensions of wellness. Evidence-based tactics for optimizing your health and wellbeing.* Columbus: The Ohio State University.

Melnyk, B. M., Szalacha, L. A., & Amaya, M. (2018). Psychometric properties of the perceived wellness culture and environment scale. *American Journal of Health Promotion, 32*(4), 1021–1027. doi:10.1177/0890117117737676

Melnyk, B. M., Orsolini, L., Tan, A., Arslanian-Engoren, C., Melkus, G. D., Dunbar-Jacob, J., . . . Lewis, L. M. (2018). A national study links nurses' physical and mental health to medical errors and perceived worksite wellness. *Journal of Occupational and Environmental Medicine, 60*(2), 126–131. doi:10.1097/JOM.0000000000001198

National Academies of Sciences. (2018). *Factors affecting clinician well-being and resilience.* Retrieved from https://nam.edu/clinicianwellbeing/wp-content/uploads/2019/07/Factors-Affecting-Clinician-Well-Being-and-Resilience-July-2019.pdf

Patel, A. V., Maliniak, M. L., Rees-Punia, E., Matthews, C. E., & Gapstur, S. M. (2018). Prolonged leisure time spent sitting in relation to cause-specific mortality in a large US cohort. *American Journal of Epidemiology, 187*(10), 2151–2158. doi:10.1093/aje/kwy125

Physical Activity Guidelines Advisory Committee. (2018). *2018 Physical Activity Guidelines Advisory Committee.* Washington, DC: U.S. Department of Health and Human Services.

Sampson, M., Melnyk, B. M., & Hoying, J. (2019). Intervention effects of the MINDBODYSTRONG cognitive behavioral skills building program on newly licensed registered nurses' mental health, healthy lifestyle behaviors, and job satisfaction. *Journal of Nursing Administration, 49*(10), 487–495. doi:10.1097/NNA.0000000000000792

Shanafelt, T. D., Hasan, O., Dyrbye, L. N., Sinsky, C., Satele, D., Sloan, J., & West, C. P. (2015). Changes in burnout and satisfaction with work-life balance in physicians and the general US working population between 2011 and 2014. *Mayo Clinic Proceeding, 90*, 1600–1613. doi:10.1016/j.mayocp.2015.08.023

Spitzer, R. L., Kroenke, K., Williams, J. B., & Lowe, B. (2006). A brief measure for assessing generalized anxiety disorder: The GAD-7. *Archives of Internal Medicine, 166*(10), 1092–1097. doi:10.1001/archinte.166.10.1092

Unruh, L. Y., & Zhang, N. J. (2014). Newly licensed registered nurse job turnover and turnover intent. *Journal of Nurses in Professional Development, 30*(5), 220–230. doi:10.1097/NND.0000000000000079

Whelton, P. K., Carey, R. M., Aronow, W. S., Casey, D. E., Jr., Collins, K. J., Dennison Himmelfarb, C., . . . Wright, J. T., Jr. (2017). 2017 ACC/AHA/AAPA/ABC/ACPM/AGS/APhA/ASH/ASPC/NMA/PCNA guideline for the prevention, detection, evaluation, and management of high blood pressure in adults: A report of the American College of Cardiology/American Heart Association Task Force on Clinical Practice Guidelines. *Hypertension, 71,* e13–e115. doi:10.1161/HYP.0000000000000065

Willard-Grace, R., Knox, M., Huang, B., Hammer, H., Kivlahan, C., & Grumbach, K. (2019). Burnout and health care workforce turnover. *Annals of Family Medicine, 17*(1), 36–41. doi:10.1370/afm.2338

World Health Organization. (2016). *Urban green spaces and health: A review of evidence.* Retrieved from http://www.euro.who.int/__data/assets/pdf_file/0005/321971/Urban-green-spaces-and-health-review-evidence.pdf?ua=1

29

Evidence-Based Health and Well-Being Assessment: Putting It All Together

Alice M. Teall and Kate Gawlik

"The only place success comes before work is in the dictionary."

—VINCE LOMBARDI

LEARNING OBJECTIVES

- Review the components of the comprehensive health history.
- Review the components that may be included in a comprehensive physical examination.

INTRODUCTION

This chapter provides a summary listing of the components of a comprehensive health history and physical examination. Clinicians are advised to adapt the summary lists to meet the needs of the individual who may be presenting with acute, episodic, chronic, or preventive healthcare needs. Best practice for how to adapt the history and/or physical exam is based on the clinician's expertise and use of evidence to guide a patient-centered approach to advanced assessment. For the novice clinician or student, the lists in this chapter can be used as guides to practice the techniques of assessment.

The reader of this chapter will note that physical assessment of the breasts, inguinal lymph nodes, and male/female genitalia and examination of the anus/rectum are not in the summary lists, as these elements are not routinely included when practicing physical exam skills. Please note, however, that the authors recommend review and practice of these assessments in appropriate lab and clinical settings. In addition, much of the neurologic examination is incorporated within the head-to-toe

examination. These lists are intended to help the novice clinician to complete the history in a concise and comprehensive manner and to complete the physical examination in a manner that avoids excessive repositioning.

COMPONENTS OF ADVANCED ASSESSMENT

EPISODIC/ACUTE VISIT: REVIEW OF HISTORY OF PRESENT ILLNESS

- Onset
- Location
- Duration
- Character/characteristics
- Aggravating factors/associated symptoms
- Relieving factors
- Timing
- Severity

CHRONIC CARE MANAGEMENT VISIT: SUPPORT SELF-MANAGEMENT

- Functional and psychosocial assessment, with disease-specific concerns
- Assessment of wellness, dimensions of wellness, and healthy lifestyle behaviors
- Individual health goals; motivation and readiness, confidence, and self-efficacy
- Problem list, treatment goals, expected outcomes, and collaborative management
- Self-management support; options for coaching, team-based care, and group visits

HEALTH HISTORY

- Past medical conditions, chronic diseases, including physical, mental, and behavioral
- History of hospitalizations and surgeries; emergency department or urgent care visits
- Recent illness, accidents, injuries, and environmental or occupational exposures
- History of trauma, victim of violence, and adverse childhood events
- Medications including prescribed, over-the-counter (OTC), vitamins, supplements, herbs, and essential oils
- Allergies to medication, food, and environment including reaction
- Immunization status, record of vaccines
- Gender identity and sexual orientation with age-appropriate considerations
  ○ Women's health history: Menstrual, gynecological, sexual health, obstetric
  ○ Men's health history: Sexual and reproductive health
  ○ Pediatric health history: Birth history, growth and development

FAMILY HISTORY

- Chronic disease: Hypertension, heart disease, obesity, diabetes, cancer, epilepsy, and asthma
- Intellectual disabilities, learning disorders, genetic disorders, and developmental delays
- Mental health disorders: Anxiety, depression, and bipolar disorder

SOCIAL HISTORY

- Use of tobacco, smoking history
- Substance use, including alcohol; use of prescription drugs not prescribed
- Family dynamics, relationships, including marital status; living arrangements
- Friends and social support system
- Safety of home, work, and/or school environments
- Social determinants of health; socioeconomic factors impacting health
- Behaviors involving risk-taking; risk of falls; participation in sports and physical activities
- Strengths, including spiritual, religious, and ethnic/cultural support systems

REVIEW OF SYSTEMS: FOCUSED, EXTENDED, OR COMPLETE

- Constitution: Recent illness? Weight gain or loss? Fatigue? Fever? Irritability?
- Integumentary: Lesions or rashes? Changes in skin or moles? Itching? Bruising?
- Head, neck, lymph: Headache? Neck pain? Dizziness? Swollen or tender lymph nodes?
- Ears, Eyes, Nose, Throat (EENT): Eye drainage or redness? Vision changes? Itchy eyes/ears/nose? Ear pain? Hearing loss? Rhinorrhea or congestion? Pharyngitis?
- Cardiovascular: Chest pain? Palpitations? Exercise intolerance? Orthopnea? Edema?
- Respiratory: Cough? Dyspnea? Wheezing? Hemoptysis?
- Breast: Tenderness? Palpable lumps or masses? Skin changes or discharge?
- Gastrointestinal: Pain? Change in bowel habits? Blood in the stool? Nausea? Vomiting?
- Genitourinary: Urinary frequency? Dysuria? Nocturia? Hematuria? Vaginal/penile discharge? Pelvic or groin pain?
- Musculoskeletal: Back pain? Muscle aches? Joint swelling? Limitations of function?
- Neurologic/endocrine: Numbness or tingling? Increased thirst? Heat or cold intolerance?
- Psychiatric: Worry? Sadness, helplessness, hopelessness? Insomnia? Change in mood? Difficulty coping with stress? Trouble concentrating?

PREVENTIVE CARE CONSIDERATIONS

- Healthy lifestyle behaviors, including diet/nutrition, physical activity/exercise, and sleep
- Management of stress, coping with stressors
- Concerns or worries about health/wellness
- Recent/needed health screenings, (e.g., blood pressure, anxiety, depression, mammogram, colonoscopy, cholesterol, lead, sexually transmitted infections [STIs], and vision/hearing)

PHYSICAL EXAMINATION COMPONENTS

GENERAL SURVEY

- Assess for distress using ABCDE (**a**irway, **b**reathing, **c**irculation, **d**isability, and **e**xposure)
- Vital signs (e.g., temperature, pulse rate, respiratory rate, blood pressure)

MENTAL STATUS

- Appearance: Affect (facial expression), posture, hygiene, and grooming; body habitus (height, weight, waist circumference)
- Behavior: Verbal or nonverbal expressions of pain, anxiety, or illness; body movements and mobility, coordination
- Cognition: Orientation to time, person, and place; attention and concentration, pattern and pace of speech, judgment, memory, and mood
- Additional screenings if needed for anxiety, depression, and substance use disorder

HEAD AND NECK (INCLUDING LYMPHATICS)

- Inspect the position of the head and the quality and condition of the hair and scalp.
- Inspect the face and facial expressions for symmetry (cranial nerve [CN] VII).
- Inspect alignment of the eyebrows, eyes, ears, nose, and mouth.
- Palpate the head for areas of edema and tenderness.
- Test sensation of light touch on the forehead, cheeks, and chin (CN V).
- Palpate while the patient clenches jaw (CN V).
- Palpate the temporomandibular joint (TMJ), with opening and closing the mouth.
- Palpate the thyroid gland.
- Palpate the submental, submandibular, retropharyngeal, tonsillar, preauricular, postauricular, and anterior and posterior cervical lymph nodes.
- Palpate for supraclavicular lymph nodes and infraclavicular lymph nodes.
- Palpate axillary and epitrochlear lymph nodes.

EYES

- Inspect the eyelids, eyelashes, conjunctivae, sclera, corneas, and irises.
- Assess the corneal light reflex or cover test (depending on age).
- Assess that the pupils are symmetrical (i.e., equal and round).
- Assess that the pupils accommodate for both near and far vision.
- Assess direct and consensual pupillary light reflex (CN II).
- Test visual fields by confrontation (CN II).
- Test extraocular muscles using cardinal fields of gaze (CN III, CN IV, CN VI).
- Use the ophthalmoscope to assess red reflex and complete the fundal examination.
- Assess visual acuity (CN II).

EARS

- Inspect the outer ears for erythema, edema, tissue deformity, lesions, or masses.
- Palpate the tragus, pinna, and mastoid process for tenderness (each ear).
- Use an otoscope to complete the internal examination of the ears.
- Assess auditory acuity; use whisper, finger rub, or tuning-fork test (CN VIII).

NOSE

- Inspect the nose for deformity, lesions, asymmetry, and deviation.
- Assess the patency of the nares.

- Palpate the sinuses to evaluate for tenderness.
- Use an otoscope to complete the internal examination of the nose.

MOUTH AND THROAT

- Inspect the lips for symmetry, color, lesions, and closure.
- Inspect the gingiva, teeth, buccal mucosa, tongue, and subglossal areas.
- Assess the tongue for fasciculation, symmetry, function, and movement (CN XII).
- Assess for movement of uvula with phonation and the ability to swallow (CN IX, CN X).
- Inspect posterior pharynx, tonsillar pillars, retromolar trigone, soft palate, and uvula.
- Inspect tonsils for symmetry, size, crypts, exudates, tonsilliths, and/or masses.
- Palpate the mouth, jaw, and tongue.

ANTERIOR, POSTERIOR, AND LATERAL CHEST

- Observe the rate, rhythm, and depth of respirations.
- Inspect the anterior and posterior chest wall for skin lesions, masses, or discolorations; note shape and symmetry; note the ratio of the anteroposterior (AP) and lateral diameter.
- Palpate for crepitus and tactile fremitus.
- Palpate for symmetric expansion.
- Percuss anterior, posterior, and lateral chest.
- Auscultate anterior, posterior, and lateral chest.
- Auscultate for bronchophony, egophony, or whispered pectoriloquy.

CARDIOVASCULAR AND PERIPHERAL VASCULAR

- Auscultate precordium at all sites with diaphragm—with person seated.
- Auscultate precordium at all sites with bell—with person seated.
- Auscultate base of heart for murmurs—ask person to lean forward, use diaphragm.
- Inspect precordium for heaves and lifts—with person supine.
- Palpate the precordium for thrill—with person supine.
- Auscultate precordium at all sites with diaphragm—with person supine.
- Auscultate precordium at all sites with bell—with person supine.
- Auscultate apex for murmurs—ask person to turn on the left side and assess with bell.
- Auscultate precordium at all sites—with patient standing and while patient squats.
- Assess for jugular venous distention (JVD).
- Auscultate for carotid bruits.
- Inspect the upper and lower extremities for lesions, hair distribution, and varicosities.

- Evaluate nail angle and nail beds for color and capillary refill.
- Assess the extremities for edema.
- Palpate radial and brachial pulses bilaterally.
- Palpate popliteal, posterior tibial, and dorsalis pedis pulses bilaterally.

ABDOMEN

- Inspect skin and note contour, scars, pulsations, bruises, discoloration, and lesions.
- Auscultate for vascular sounds over aorta and iliac and renal arteries.
- Percuss lightly across all quadrants of the abdomen.
- Percuss the liver span (may use optional scratch test).
- Percuss for splenic dullness.
- Palpate the abdomen lightly and then deeply in all the quadrants.
- Palpate for the liver, spleen, and kidneys.
- Palpate for aorta.
- With person seated or standing, percuss for left and right costovertebral angle (CVA) tenderness.

MUSCULOSKELETAL AND NEUROLOGIC

- Test the range of motion of cervical spine.
- Assess head turn and shoulder shrug against resistance (CN XI).
- Test the ability to sense light touch in the upper and lower extremities.
- Test reflexes of biceps, triceps, and brachioradialis.
- Test patellar and Achilles' reflexes.
- Test rapidly alternating movements, finger-to-nose testing, and heel-to-shin testing.
- Test position sense of great toe and plantar reflex.
- Assess Romberg's test for vestibular function and balance.
- Assess for pronator drift.
- Assess for symmetry of the trunk, shoulders, and extremities, with person standing.
- Assess the range of motion of shoulders; include internal and external rotation.

- Assess the range of motion of elbows, wrists, and hands.
- Assess strength against resistance of the shoulders, elbows, wrists, and hands.
- Inspect and palpate spine as person bends at the waist, and assess spinal curvature.
- Test the range of motion of the pelvis as person hyperextends, rotates, and laterally bends.
- Assess gait and tandem walking.
- Ask person to walk a few steps on toes and a few steps on heels.
- Ask the person to either duck walk or perform a shallow knee bend.
- Assess strength against resistance for knees, ankles, and feet.

Clinical Pearls

- The clinician begins the history and physical examination by introducing themselves, clarifying the reason for seeking care, and washing their hands.
- The clinician completes the history and physical examination by reviewing the assessment findings with the individual and clarifying any concerns or questions.

Key Takeaways

- Advanced assessment includes the priority skills of observation and listening.
- Assessment includes a review of the dimensions of wellness and self-care.
- Evidence-based assessment guides the clinician to determine the important components of the history and physical examination and evaluate the findings within the context of health and well-being.

Index